Radiology Illustrated: Uroradiology

Seung Hyup Kim, M.D.

Department of Radiology

Seoul National University Hospital

Seoul, Korea

SAUNDERS

An Imprint of Elsevier Science

SAUNDERS
An Imprint of Elsevier Science

The Curtis Center
Independence Square West
Philadelphia, PA 19106

RADIOLOGY ILLUSTRATED: URORADIOLOGY ISBN 0–7216–3920–8

Copyright © 2003, Elsevier Science (USA). All rights reserved.

Notice

Radiology is an ever-changing field. Standard safety precautions must be followed, but as new research and clinical experience broaden our knowledge, changes in treatment and drug therapy may become necessary or appropriate. Readers are advised to check the most current product information provided by the manufacturer of each drug to be administered to verify the recommended dose, the method and duration of administration, and contraindications. It is the responsibility of the treating physician, relying on experience and knowledge of the patient, to determine dosages and the best treatment for each individual patient. Neither the Publisher nor the author assumes any liability for any injury and/or damage to persons or property arising from this publication.

The Publisher

Library of Congress Cataloging in Publication Data

Radiology illustrated. Uroradiology / [edited by] Seung Hyup Kim.
  p. ; cm.
    ISBN 0–7216–3920–8
  1. Urinary organs—Radiography. I. Title: Uroradiology. II. Kim, Seung Hyup.
    [DNLM: 1. Urologic Diseases—radiography. WJ 141 R1275 2003]
    RC901 .R26 2003
616.6'07572—dc21

2002070830

Editor-in-Chief: Richard Lampert
Acquisitions Editor: Allan Ross
Developmental Editor: Josh Hawkins
Project Manager: Linda Van Pelt
Book Designer: Gene Harris

EH/MVY

Printed in the United States of America

Last digit is the print number: 9 8 7 6 5 4 3 2 1

To my patients, teachers, and families

Seung Hyup Kim

Preface

In the daily practice of imaging diagnosis, radiologists expect a variety of imaging findings for each disease entity, and in turn many different disease entities have similar imaging findings. Usually, a certain diagnosis is made based on one's memory of having seen other cases with similar imaging features. This practical guide provides approximately 3000 selected and categorized illustrations along with short, key text passages that will help the reader easily recall the correct images and work through to a differential diagnosis.

I owe so much to my colleagues—radiologists, urologists, nephrologists, and pathologists—for collecting the materials in this illustrative book, which comprehensively covers topics in uroradiology. The biggest debt I have in publishing this book is to my patients. I imagine that the more beautiful the images in this book, the more severe the patients' suffering, and I hope that the readers who are helped by the images in this book can appreciate the pain that the patients might have experienced.

This task could not have been completed without the guidance of Dr. Man Chung Han, Professor Emeritus of Radiology, Seoul National University College of Medicine. From the beginning of my career, he showed me how to be a radiologist as well as a physician, a researcher, and a teacher. When I was discussing this book project with him, I was very surprised that the style of the book and the title, *Radiology Illustrated*, were exactly the same as he had imagined.

The year I spent in Philadelphia with Dr. Howard Pollack was a turning point in my career as a uroradiologist. At that time, Pollack's *Clinical Urography* had just been published. I learned how the materials in his book had been collected, categorized, and retrieved. His collaborative style in working with his clinical counterparts as a uroradiologist strongly influenced mine. I am very fortunate to have the generous dedication of my co-editors on this book, Dr. William Bush and Dr. Lee Talner. I am also lucky to have worked with the finest publisher, Elsevier Science, and I appreciate the perfect job that its staff did. Above all, the strongest support to finish this book was the love, encouragement, and patience given to me by my dearest wife Byung Hee and my son Jin Woong.

Seung Hyup Kim

Contributing Authors

William H. Bush Jr., M.D.
Department of Radiology
University of Washington
Seattle, Washington

Jeong Yeon Cho, M.D.
Department of Diagnostic Radiology
Samsung Cheil Hospital
Sungkyunkwan University School of Medicine
Seoul, Korea

Jin Wook Chung, M.D.
Department of Radiology
Seoul National University Hospital
Seoul, Korea

Bohyun Kim, M.D.
Department of Radiology
Samsung Medical Center
Seoul, Korea

In-One Kim, M.D.
Department of Radiology
Seoul National University Hospital
Seoul, Korea

Woo Sun Kim, M.D.
Department of Radiology
Seoul National University Hospital
Seoul, Korea

Hak Jong Lee, M.D.
Department of Diagnostic Radiology
Samsung Cheil Hospital Center & Women's Healthcare
  Center
Seoul, Korea

Chang Kyu Seong, M.D.
Department of Diagnostic Radiology
Kyungpook National University School of Medicine
Daegu, Korea

Jung Suk Sim, M.D.
Department of Radiology
National Cancer Center
Koyang, Korea

Lee B. Talner, M.D.
Department of Radiology
University of Washington
Seattle, Washington

Radiology Illustrated:
Uroradiology

Contents

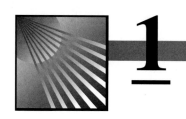

1

Normal Findings and Variations of the Urinary Tract

JEONG YEON CHO

NORMAL RADIOLOGIC FINDINGS

On plain radiograph of the abdomen, the kidneys, liver, spleen, and urinary bladder are usually identified by surrounding radiolucent fat. The kidneys are parallel to the outer border of the psoas muscle. The left kidney is usually slightly higher than the right. The length of the kidney is approximately 3.7 times the height of the L2 vertebral body. The psoas muscle is usually outlined by the fat, and disappearance of this outline may represent accumulation of fluid or mass adjacent to the psoas muscle. The outline of the quadratus lumborum muscle is parallel and about 1 cm lateral to the outline of the psoas muscle. The "flank fat stripe" is the continuation of the posterior pararenal space and is located between the transversalis fascia and the parietal peritoneum. The top of the bladder is outlined by perivesical fat.

In the early nephrogram phase, an intravenous urogram (IVU) shows the renal outline. The densities of both renal nephrogram should be similar and even. The normal kidney is sharply marginated and smooth in contour. On the 5-minute image, both collecting systems should be opacified. The difference in renal excretion of two kidneys or delayed excretion of both kidneys can be estimated on this image. The normal kidney has 10 to 15 calyces. The calyces should be sharply defined and deeply curved. The renal calyx can be divided into a simple calyx and a compound calyx. In simple calyces, each minor calyx drains one papilla, while multiple papillae enter into a compound calyx. Compound calyces are common in polar regions of the kidney. The infundibula should be straight without distortion. The renal pelvis is variable in appearance. The usual funnel-shaped pelvis lacks clear demarcation of the ureteropelvic junction, whereas the box-shaped pelvis has clear demarcation of the ureteropelvic junction. There are normal constrictions of the ureter: at the ureteropelvic junction, crossing over the psoas muscle, crossing over the iliac vessels, and at the ureterovesical junction. The size and contour of the bladder are variable depending on the degree of filling. The normal bladder is round and smooth in contour.

On ultrasonography (US), the echogenicity of the normal renal cortex is slightly lower than that of liver and slightly higher than that of renal medulla. The central echo complex of the renal sinus is usually bright. The cortex and medulla can be differentiated in about half of normal adults. The low echo of medulla may be confused with cyst or diverticulum. The upper-polar area is usually hypoechoic due to compound papilla, which may be confused with a mass. Arcuate arteries at the cor-

ticomedullary junction may be demonstrated with high echo. Normal minor calyces are usually not identifiable on US, but major calyces and pelvis appear anechoic with a thin wall. The ureter is usually not identified unless dilated. The fluid-filled urinary bladder is symmetrical with a thin wall.

On color Doppler US, renal vessels, including interlobar and arcuate vessels, are well visualized. Power Doppler US can demonstrate slow blood flow and renal parenchymal perfusion. Spectral Doppler US is usually performed at an interlobar artery to estimate the peripheral renal vascular resistance. The normal resistive index of interlobar artery is less than 0.7.

Computed tomography (CT) can demonstrate detailed anatomy of the urinary tract and surrounding structures. The kidney and adrenal gland are located in the perirenal space bound by the anterior and posterior renal fasciae. The anterior pararenal space lies between the posterior parietal peritoneum and anterior renal fascia. The lateral border of the anterior pararenal space is lateroconal fascia. The renal hilum, containing renal pelvocalyces and vessels, opens toward the anteromedial direction. The attenuation of the renal cortex and medulla is similar and cannot be distinguished without contrast enhancement. Corticomedullary demarcation can be obtained in the early phase of contrast-enhanced CT, and cortex and medulla reach equilibrium on the delayed image. The renal pelvis and continuing ureter can usually be traced on CT. The ureter turns downward in front of the psoas muscle, crosses over the iliac vessels, and opens into the base of the urinary bladder. The urinary bladder and surrounding structures are well demonstrated on CT. The bladder lies in the perivesical space. Thickness of bladder wall is even and depends on the degree of bladder filling.

T1-weighted spin-echo magnetic resonance (MR) image demonstrates distinct corticomedullary contrast of the kidney by higher intensity of the renal cortex and lower intensity of the medulla. On T2-weighted MR image, the signal intensities of both renal cortex and medulla are increased and they cannot be differentiated. The signal intensity of sinus fat is high on both T1- and T2-weighted images. The signal intensity of urine-containing renal pelvis is low on T1-weighted image and high on T2-weighted image. The signal intensities of the renal vessels are low on both T1- and T2-weighted images except for the high signal intensity of slow venous flow on T2-weighted image. When the ureter is obstructed and invisible on IVU, MR urography is useful to delineate the ureter and the cause of obstruction. The urinary bladder and surrounding structures are

well demonstrated on MR images. The sagittal and coronal images are helpful to evaluate the lesion in the dome or base of the bladder.

On renal arteriography, branches of the renal artery are well demonstrated. The main renal artery divides into ventral and dorsal rami that further divide into segmental arteries. Interlobar arteries divided from the segmental arteries penetrate renal parenchyma and divide into arcuate arteries that run between the renal cortex and medulla.

NORMAL VARIATIONS AND PSEUDOLESIONS

A variety of normal variations and pseudolesions may produce variable unusual appearances on the radiologic images of the urinary tract. Pseudotumor of the renal parenchyma is the most common pseudolesion in the urinary tract. It refers to normal renal tissue that mimics an abnormal mass. The causes of pseudotumor are variable, including prominent column of Bertin, dromedary hump, fetal lobulation, and localized compensatory hypertrophy.

Prominent column of Bertin

The column of Bertin, originally described by Bertin as a septum, is a thickened aggregate of the cortical tissue instead of the usual thin cortical septum that separates two pyramids. It is the most common cause of renal pseudotumors on IVU and cross-sectional images. The junction of the upper and middle thirds of the kidney is the most common site of prominent column. It causes deformity of adjacent calyces and infundibula and focal dense nephrogram on IVU or angiography. It can also mimic low or isoechogenic renal mass on the US and isoattenuated mass on CT. However, it usually does not cause any bulge on the outer cortex. Color or power Doppler US may demonstrate blood vessels passing through the lesion, unlike the true parenchymal tumor, in which the vessels are usually stretched and displaced in the periphery of the mass.

Dromedary hump

A prominent bulge on the lateral border of the kidney is sometimes appreciated on imaging studies such as IVU or CT. This hump may be present on either kidney but is more often on the left side. It is caused by thick parenchyma and does not cause any deformity on the pelvocalyceal system. This is called *dromedary hump* and represents molding by the spleen and liver.

Fetal lobulation

At the 4th month of gestation, there are classically 14 renal lobules separated by longitudinal fibrous grooves. Following the 28th week of gestation, assimilation of the boundary between these lobules occurs. Persistence of these grooves into adulthood results in the lobulation on the renal contour known as *persistent fetal lobulation*. We can differentiate fetal lobulation from pathologic scarring of chronic pyelonephritis by smooth renal contour, regular spacing, and the absence of calyceal blunting or deformity in fetal lobulation.

Localized compensatory hypertrophy of renal parenchyma

The kidneys affected by severe focal disease such as reflux nephropathy frequently have islands of unaffected parenchyma adjacent to the lesion. These islands are usually hypertrophied to compensate for the impaired renal function of the adjacent scarred parenchyma. They can mimic a mass lesion by producing displacement or impression on the neighboring calyces.

Junctional parenchymal defect

A triangular echogenic area is identified most often in the upper pole of the right kidney. Similar echogenic defect also can be seen in the lower pole of the left kidney. These defects in the parenchyma result from extension of the renal sinus fat due to incomplete fusion of two embryogenic parenchymatous masses. This normal variation can be differentiated from pathologic conditions such as parenchymal scarring or angiomyolipoma by its characteristic location and continuity with the renal sinus.

Sinus lipomatosis and abnormal echo of sinus fat

A variable amount of fat and fibrous tissue is present in the renal sinus extending around the calyceal infundibuli. When the fat and fibrous tissue increase in amount, the renal pelvis is compressed and the infundibuli are elongated and stretched. At times increased sinus fat and fibrous tissue may have an echogenicity lower than that of the normal sinus fat tissue and can mimic urothelial tumor of the renal pelvis on US.

Obesity is the most common cause of sinus lipomatosis. Aging is also a common cause of increased amount of sinus fat, which replaces the atrophied renal parenchyma. Chronic infection, particularly associated with calculi, tends to produce asymmetrical increase of sinus fat tissue. CT is helpful to differentiate the sinus lipomatosis from multiple parapelvic cysts and urothelial tumor of the renal pelvis.

Unidentified bright objects on the US

On US, tiny echogenic foci are occasionally seen in the renal parenchyma. They are called *unidentified bright objects* (UBOs). These echogenic foci frequently accompany reverberation artifact, but posterior sonic shadowing is absent. The possible causes of these UBOs in the kidney are tiny stones, tiny cysts, small calyceal diverticulum with wall calcification or milk of calcium, calcified arteries, and tiny angiomyolipoma. CT may be helpful to differentiate among the causes of the renal UBOs.

Nephroptosis

Normal kidneys may displace downward within the distance of two lumbar vertebral bodies when the patients change their positions from supine to standing. Displacement of a greater degree is referred to as *nephroptosis*. In contrast to ectopic kidneys, ptotic kidneys have a normal-length ureter with tortuous appearance on IVU taken in standing position. Most ptotic kidneys are asymptomatic but may cause intermittent obstruction, which is called *Dietl's crisis*.

Pseudohydronephrosis

Variable conditions can mimic hydronephrosis on the radiologic images. Prominent renal vessels may be confused with dilated pelvocalyces on gray-scale US. We can easily differentiate these vessels from the dilated pelvocalyces using color Doppler US. On contrast-enhanced CT in early phase, the renal pelvis and ureter that are not opacified with contrast material may mimic hydronephrosis. Multiple parapelvic cysts also can mimic dilated pelvocalyces on gray-scale US, which can be differentiated from hydronephrosis by demonstrating the absence of communication between the cystic lesions. IVU demonstrates the normal pelvocalyceal system with subtle compression or displacement. Contrast-enhanced CT easily distinguishes the pelvocalyces filled with contrast material and cystic lesions creeping between the calyceal infundibuli. Extrarenal pelvis usually mimics renal pelvis dilation. It appears as a box-shaped pelvis on urography and as a dilated pelvis on CT. However, the excretion of the contrast media is not delayed without an obstructing lesion.

Variations in calyces and papillae

Compound calyces are a common variation produced by fusion of minor calyces. These are commonly seen in the polar areas, particularly in the upper pole. Multiple minor calyces are drained into one major calyx, with the resultant appearance of one major calyx possessing multiple papillae. The intrarenal reflux occurs most easily in compound calyces, because their orifices are more patulous than those of simple calyces. This explains the tendency for reflux nephropathy to be most frequent and most severe in the polar areas of the kidney.

When the calyceal infundibula arise from the pelvis outside of the kidney and penetrate the renal parenchyma individually, they are called *extrarenal calyces*. They are usually asymptomatic.

Rarely, a renal papilla is ectopic or aberrant and protrudes into a calyx in an unusual position. It is not symptomatic, but it may be confused with a lesion since it appears as a round, well-circumscribed filling defect in the pelvis on urography. Polyps, neoplasms, and blood clots can produce similar appearances.

The normal human kidney has 10 to 14 minor calyces. Polycalycosis is an anomaly in which an excessive number of calyces are present. Polycalycosis is usually associated with congenital megacalycosis. Rarely, a unipapillary kidney can be found, which is usually associated with renal hypoplasia.

Vascular impressions on pelvocalyces

On IVU, intrarenal vascular impressions are commonly seen on the upper infundibulum and renal pelvis. Renal artery as well as renal vein can produce impressions. The crossing veins produce large filling defects, whereas the arteries produce sharply defined small defects on IVU. Hematuria may be associated with vascular impressions. Occasionally, vascular impressions may cause pain, especially when the patient takes in a large amount of fluid. Fraley described such a sequence in the upper infundibulum; therefore, it is called *Fraley's syndrome*. Extrarenal vascular impressions are common in the presence of multiple renal arteries. The aberrant lower-pole arteries may cause impressions near the ureteropelvic junction.

Papillary blush and renal backflow

Papillary blush is produced by the contrast material concentrated in the normal collecting ducts. It appears as a fan-shaped density in the renal papilla. This finding is seen more often when non-ionic contrast material is used instead of ionic and is more evident when IVU is performed with compression of the ureter. It should not be confused with the finding of the papillary blush that represents the collection of contrast material in abnormal dilated collecting ducts in medullary sponge kidney.

Several types of backflow are described: pyelosinus, pyelotubular, pyelovenous, and pyelolymphatic. Pyelosinus or pyelointerstitial backflow is the most common type, which results from rupture of the fornix. It occasionally occurs during IVU when an acute obstruction is present in the urinary tract.

Medial position of ureters

Medial displacement of the ureter may be a normal variation or a manifestation of an abnormal lesion. Mild and abrupt medial deviations usually appear on the margin of the normal psoas muscle or in the area where the ureter crosses common iliac vessels. Obstruction and progression are absent in these normal variations. Hypertrophy of the psoas muscle may cause anterolateral deviation of the upper ureter and medial deviation of the mid-lower ureter. The lower portion of ureters may appear straight and medially displaced after pelvic surgery such as radical hysterectomy.

Miscellaneous variations of the urinary tract

Fetal valve of ureter

In the infant and young child, mucosal redundancy is common, with the appearance of folds or webs in the ureter. They usually appear in the upper ureter and are multiple. Usually they do not cause obstruction, and most disappear with aging.

Ureteral jet

The spurt or jet of urine emerging from the ureteral orifice may be observed on various imaging studies, including IVU, color or power Doppler US, and contrast-enhanced CT or MR imaging. It is not only a normal finding but also a good sign that vesicoureteral reflux or obstruction is not present.

Bladder ear

In young infants, inferomedial protrusions of the bladder lumen may be present, which are called *bladder ears*. They are probably due to the close relationship of the bladder and persistent large inguinal canal in infants. The protrusions are usually transitory and most often seen when the bladder is partially filled. Bladder ears usually disappear when the bladder is filled and when the infant grows up.

Vicarious excretion

On IVU or contrast-enhanced CT, most contrast material is excreted by the kidney, but a small amount is excreted by the liver, intestine, lacrimal gland, and salivary gland. In case of renal insufficiency these extrarenal excretory pathways become important. In such cases, contrast material within the

gallbladder or intestine is well visualized on the plain radiograph or CT obtained 12 to 24 hours after intravascular administration of the contrast material. This process is known as *vicarious excretion*.

References

1. Friedenberg RM, Harris RD: Excretory urography. In Pollack HM, McClennan BL (eds): Clinical Urography, 2nd ed, vol 1. Philadelphia, WB Saunders, 2000, pp 147–281.
2. Lee GH, Kim SH, Cho JY, et al: Pseudohydronephrosis in two-phase spiral CT of the abdomen. Korean J Radiol Soc 1997; 37:889–892.
3. Dunnick NR, Sandler CM, Amis ES, Newhouse JH: Congenital anomalies. In Textbook of Uroradiology, 2nd ed. Baltimore, Lippincott Williams & Wilkins, 1997, pp 15–43.
4. Saxton HM: Opacification of collecting ducts at urography. Radiology 1989; 170:16–17.
5. Lafortune M, Constantine A, Greton G, et al: Sonography of the hypertrophied column of Bertin. AJR Am J Roentgenol 1986; 146:53–56.
6. Carter AR, Horgan JG, Jennings TA, et al: The junctional parenchymal defect: A sonographic variant of renal anatomy. Radiology 1985; 154:499–502.
7. Subramanyam BR, Bosniak MA, Horii SC, et al: Replacement lipomatosis of the kidney: Diagnosis by computed tomography and sonography. Radiology 1983; 148:791–792.
8. Amis ES Jr, Cronan JJ, Pfister RC: Pseudohydronephrosis on noncontrast computed tomography. J Comput Assist Tomogr 1982; 6:511–513.
9. Kuhns LR, Hernandez R, Koff S, et al: Absence of vesicoureteral reflux in children with ureteral jet. Radiology 1977; 124:185–187.

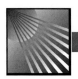

Illustrations • Normal Findings and Variations of the Urinary Tract

1 • Normal findings: plain radiograph and IVU

2 • Normal findings: US of the kidney

3 • Normal findings: CT of the kidney

4 • Normal findings: MR imaging of the kidney

5 • Variations of renal position

6 • Various appearances of the renal pelvis and calyx

7 • Vascular indentations on the urinary tract

8 • Renal backflows

9 • Renal pseudotumors

10 • Fetal lobulation

11 • Junctional parenchymal defect

12 • Renal unidentified bright objects (UBOs) on US

13 • Sinus lipomatosis and prominent perirenal fat

14 • Pseudohydronephrosis

15 • Ureter: normal findings and variations

16 • Urinary bladder: normal findings and variations

1. Normal Findings: Plain Radiograph and IVU

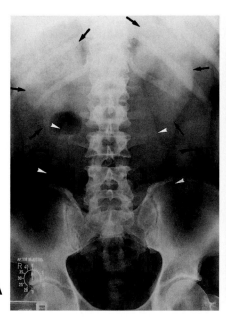

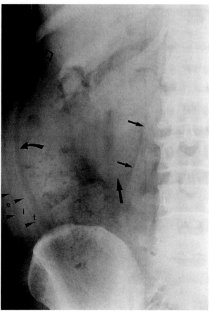

A

B

Fig. 1. Normal plain radiograph.
A. Normal plain radiograph (KUB) obtained as a scout image of an IVU well delineates the outlines of the kidneys *(arrows)* and psoas muscles *(arrowheads)*. Note well-demonstrated properitoneal fat layers or flank stripes *(curved arrows)*. **B.** Magnified image of a plain radiograph shows the lower margin of the right kidney *(large arrow)*, liver edge *(open arrow)*, and outlines of the psoas muscles *(small arrows)*. Also note the right properitoneal fat layer *(curved arrow)* and the fat layers *(arrowheads)* between the muscles of the abdominal wall. e, external oblique muscle; i, internal oblique muscle; t, transversalis abdominis muscle.

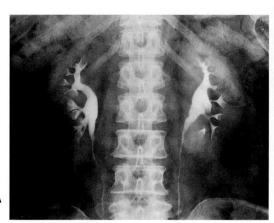

A

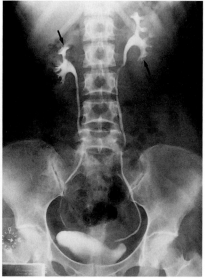

B

Fig. 2 *See legend on opposite page*

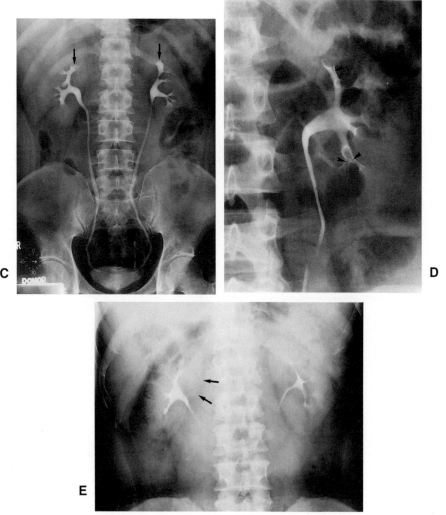

Fig. 2. Normal IVU.
A. IVU obtained 5 minutes after injection of contrast material shows various shapes of calyces. Note the sharp margin of the calyceal fornices. **B.** A 15-minute IVU in another patient shows well-opacified urinary tracts. Note compound calyces *(arrows)* in the upper pole of the right kidney and the lower pole of the left kidney. Also note that the position of the right kidney is lower than that of the left kidney. **C.** A 15-minute IVU in a donor for renal transplantation shows well-opacified urinary tracts. Compound calyces are noted in the upper poles of both kidneys *(arrows)*. **D.** A 5-minute IVU in another patient shows linear radiolucencies *(arrowheads)* connecting two adjacent papillae. **E.** A 15-minute IVU shows focal bulging of renal contour in suprahilar portion of the right kidney *(arrows)*. This is a normal finding and is called a *suprahilar lip*.

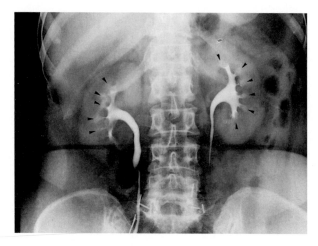

Fig. 3. Normal papillary blush in a 57-year-old woman. An IVU taken 15 minutes after an injection of non-ionic contrast material shows homogeneous staining of the renal papillae *(arrowheads)* due to collection of contrast material in normal collecting ducts.

2. Normal Findings: US of the Kidney

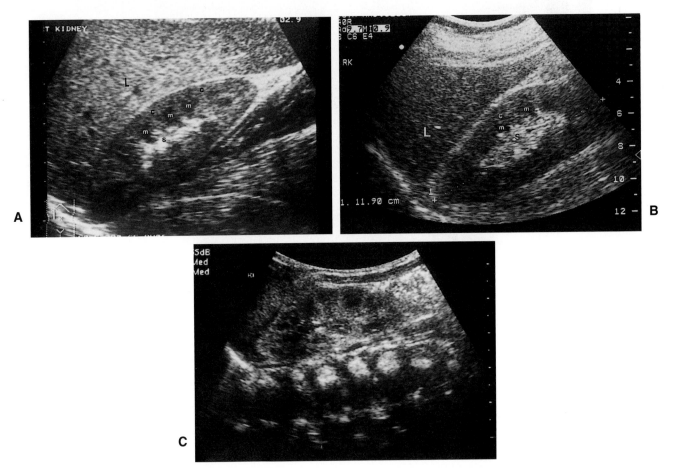

Fig. 1. Normal gray-scale US of the kidney.
A. Longitudinal US of the right kidney in a 50-year-old woman shows normal echogenicity of the renal parenchyma. Note that the echogenicity of the renal cortex (c) is lower than that of the liver (L) and is higher than that of the renal medulla (m). s, renal sinus. **B.** Longitudinal US of the right kidney in a 40-year-old man shows that renal cortical echogenicity (c) is similar to that of the liver (L). Note that the renal medulla (m) is less well differentiated from renal cortex than in **A.** s, renal sinus. **C.** Longitudinal US of the right kidney in a 16-day-old female infant shows a slightly hyperechoic cortex and prominent hypoechoic medulla. Note that renal sinus echo is less well defined.

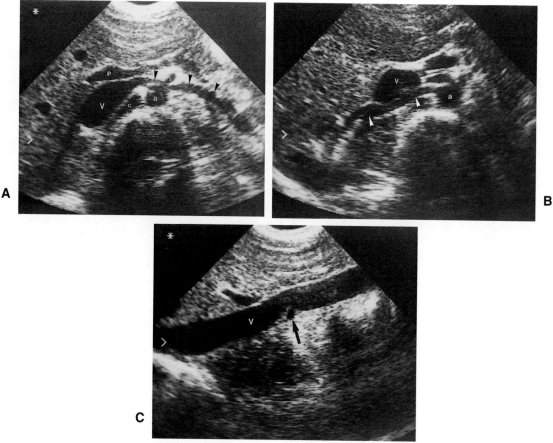

Fig. 2. Gray-scale US findings of the renal vessels: normal findings.
A. Transverse US shows left renal vein *(arrowheads)* coursing between the aorta (a) and superior mesenteric artery (s) to the inferior vena cava (v). c, crus of the diaphragm; p, portal vein. **B.** US in oblique plane shows the right renal artery *(arrowheads)* arising from the aorta (a), coursing behind the inferior vena cava (v) to the right kidney. **C.** Longitudinal US along the inferior vena cava (v) shows the right renal artery *(arrow)* coursing behind the inferior vena cava.

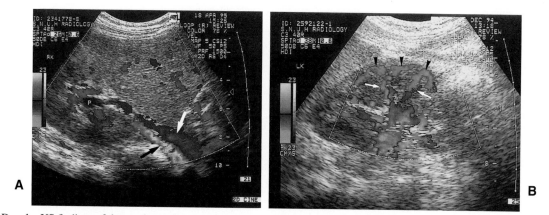

Fig. 3. Color Doppler US findings of the renal vessels: normal findings. (**A, B,** See also Color Section.)
A. Color Doppler US along the right renal vessels shows the right renal artery *(black arrow)* and the right renal vein *(white arrow)*. Anechoic structure without flow signal indicates the renal pelvis (p). **B.** Color Doppler US of the left kidney well demonstrates intrarenal vessels, including interlobar *(arrows)* and arcuate vessels *(arrowheads)*.

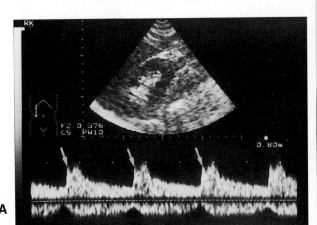

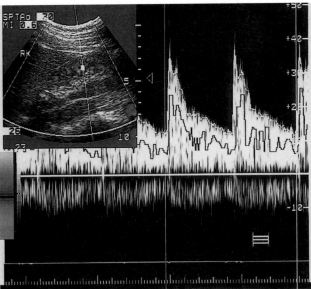

A

B

Fig. 4. Spectral Doppler US findings of the intrarenal arteries: normal findings.
A. Spectral Doppler US of the right kidney performed at the level of the interlobar artery in a 49-year-old man shows a normal spectral pattern with early systolic compliance peak *(arrows)*. The resistive index is 0.67 in this case. **B.** Spectral Doppler US of the right kidney in another 25-year-old man shows a normal Doppler spectral pattern with a resistive index of 0.65. In this patient, early systolic compliance peak is not seen. (**B**, See also Color Section.)

3. Normal Findings: CT of the Kidney

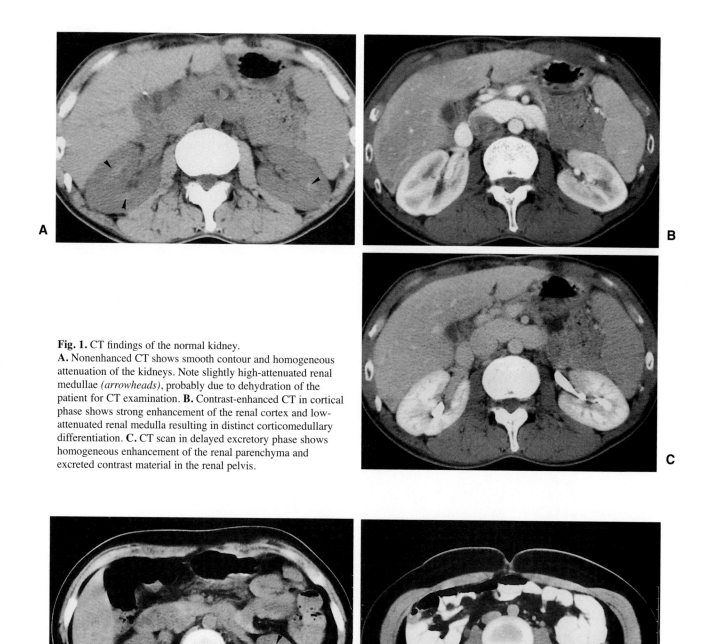

Fig. 1. CT findings of the normal kidney.
A. Nonenhanced CT shows smooth contour and homogeneous attenuation of the kidneys. Note slightly high-attenuated renal medullae *(arrowheads)*, probably due to dehydration of the patient for CT examination. **B.** Contrast-enhanced CT in cortical phase shows strong enhancement of the renal cortex and low-attenuated renal medulla resulting in distinct corticomedullary differentiation. **C.** CT scan in delayed excretory phase shows homogeneous enhancement of the renal parenchyma and excreted contrast material in the renal pelvis.

Fig. 2. Renal excretion of gastrointestinal contrast material.
A. Nonenhanced CT at the level of the kidneys shows excretion of contrast material in the right pelvocalyceal system *(arrow)*. Also note faintly enhanced renal medullae *(arrowheads)*. **B.** Nonenhanced CT at lower level shows small bowel filled with iodinated contrast material, which is diluted but basically the same iodinated agent as that used as intravenous contrast material. This phenomenon does not occur when microbarium is used as a gastrointestinal contrast material.

4. Normal Findings: MR Imaging of the Kidney

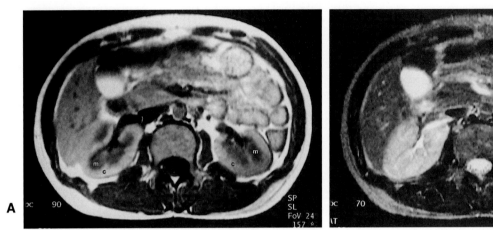

Fig. 1. Normal spin-echo MR images of the kidney in a 22-year-old woman.
A. T1-weighted spin-echo MR image (TR/TE = 500/15 msec) shows distinct corticomedullary contrast demonstrated by high intensity of the renal cortex (c) and low intensity of the renal medulla (m). **B.** On T2-weighted spin-echo MR image (TR/TE = 2700/80 msec), the signal intensities of the renal cortex and medulla are increased, and they are not more differentiated.

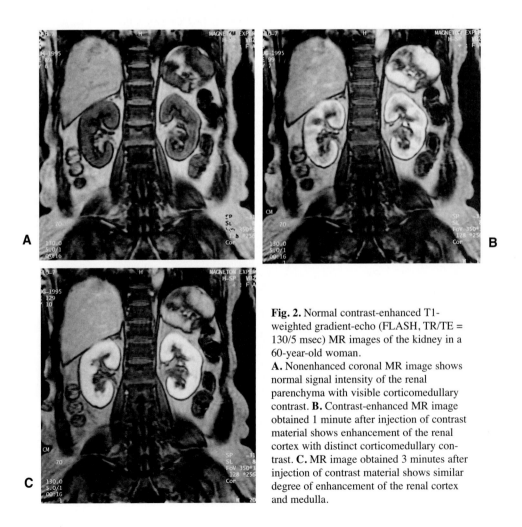

Fig. 2. Normal contrast-enhanced T1-weighted gradient-echo (FLASH, TR/TE = 130/5 msec) MR images of the kidney in a 60-year-old woman.
A. Nonenhanced coronal MR image shows normal signal intensity of the renal parenchyma with visible corticomedullary contrast. **B.** Contrast-enhanced MR image obtained 1 minute after injection of contrast material shows enhancement of the renal cortex with distinct corticomedullary contrast. **C.** MR image obtained 3 minutes after injection of contrast material shows similar degree of enhancement of the renal cortex and medulla.

5. Variations of Renal Position

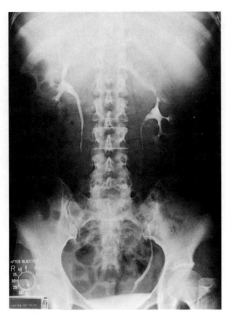

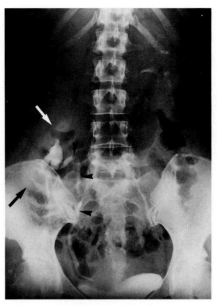

Fig. 1. The right kidney is higher than the left kidney in a 53-year-old woman with liver cirrhosis and splenomegaly. A 15-minute IVU shows higher right kidney and lower left kidney because of a shrunken liver and splenomegaly due to liver cirrhosis.

Fig. 2. Nephroptosis in a 50-year-old woman. IVU in erect position shows the low position of the right kidney *(arrows)*. The right ureter has normal length and so is tortuous *(arrowheads)*.

6. Various Appearances of the Renal Pelvis and Calyx

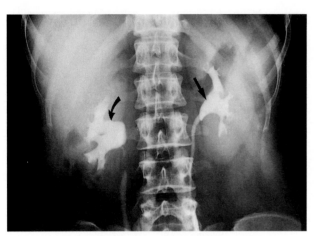

Fig. 1. Various shapes of the renal pelvis on IVU. IVU shows two typical shapes of normal renal pelvis: a funnel-shaped pelvis on the left kidney *(arrow)* and a box-shaped pelvis on the right kidney *(curved arrow)*.

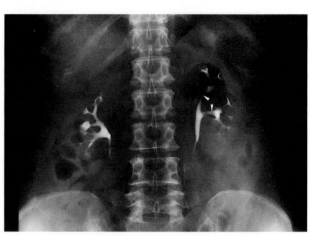

Fig. 2. Bifid pelvis in a 60-year-old woman. A 15-minute IVU shows a bifid pelvis *(arrowheads)* separated by invagination of the renal parenchyma. This is the mildest form of duplication anomaly of the renal pelvis and ureter.

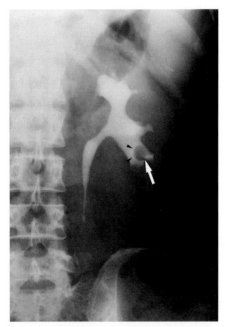

Fig. 3. Prominent end-on papilla mimicking a calyceal filling defect in a 42-year-old woman. A 15-minute IVU shows a round radiolucency *(arrow)* in the lower polar calyx of the left kidney due to a prominent end-on papilla. This radiolucency may mimic a urothelial tumor or blood clot. Note that the radiolucency is surrounded by a thin, ringlike radiopacity *(arrowheads)*, which represents contrast material in the calyceal fornix.

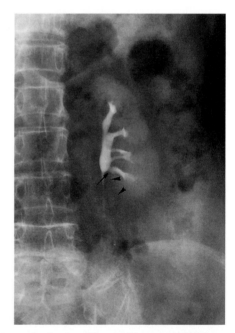

Fig. 4. Extrarenal calyx in a 67-year-old woman. IVU shows an elongated left renal pelvis, which is mainly extrarenal in location. Note that the infundibulum of the lower polar calyx *(arrow)* is located outside of the lower medial margin of the left kidney *(arrowheads)*.

7. Vascular Indentations on the Urinary Tract

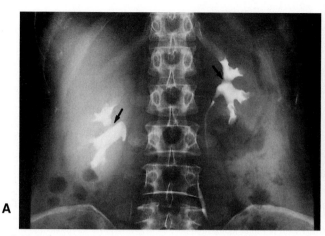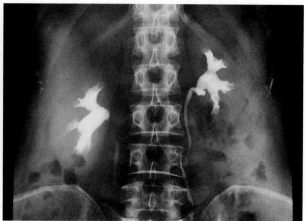

Fig. 1. Vascular indentations on the calyceal infundibulum in a 52-year-old woman with intermittent flank pain.
A. IVU obtained 25 minutes after injection of contrast material shows well-defined linear impressions *(arrows)* on the upper calyceal infundibula of both kidneys. **B.** The vascular impressions were less well demonstrated on a 15-minute IVU.

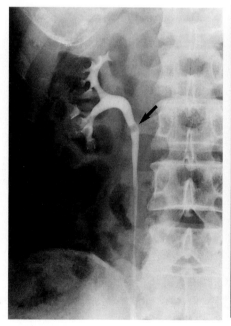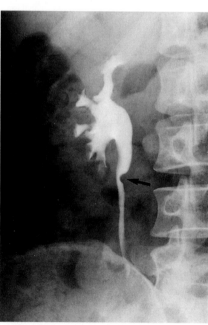

Fig. 2. Arterial indentation on the proximal ureter.
A. IVU in a 64-year-old man shows a well-defined arterial impression on the right proximal ureter *(arrow)* mimicking a true filling defect. **B.** IVU in another 38-year-old woman shows a sharp indentation on the right proximal ureter *(arrow)*.

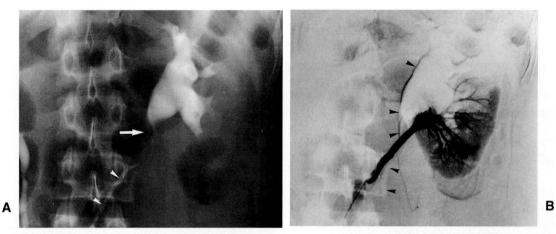

Fig. 3. Impression on the right ureteropelvic junction by an accessory renal artery to the lower pole of the left kidney in a 50-year-old woman.
A. IVU obtained before arteriography shows slight dilation of the left renal pelvis and narrowing of the ureteropelvic junction *(arrow)*. Note a catheter in the accessory lower-polar artery *(arrowheads)*. **B.** Selective arteriography of the accessory lower-polar artery demonstrates the relation of the artery and the urinary tract. Note that the renal pelvis and proximal ureter that are filled with contrast material appear as bright shadow *(arrowheads)* on this digital subtraction arteriogram.

8. Renal Backflows

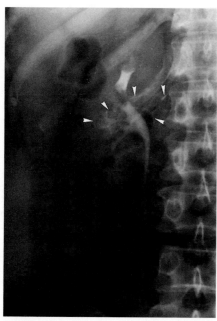

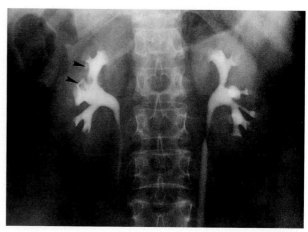

Fig. 2. Calyceal rupture due to ureteral compression during IVU. A 15-minute IVU shows leak of contrast material *(arrowheads)* from the calyceal fornix in the upper pole area of the right kidney. This patient does not have ureteral obstruction, and this leak of contrast material is probably due to rupture of calyceal fornix caused by ureteral compression applied during IVU.

Fig. 1. Pyelosinus backflow demonstrated on IVU in a 45-year-old woman with uterine cervical carcinoma. IVU shows leakage of contrast material from the interpolar calyces to the renal sinus *(arrowheads)*, probably due to forniceal rupture.

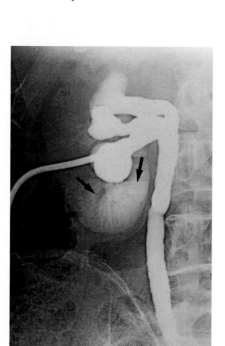

Fig. 3. Pyelotubular backflow in an 84-year-old man with stomach cancer who underwent percutaneous nephrostomy for ureteral obstruction by periureteral metastasis. A nephrostomy tubogram shows reflux of contrast material into the collecting ducts in the lower polar area *(arrows)*.

9. Renal Pseudotumors

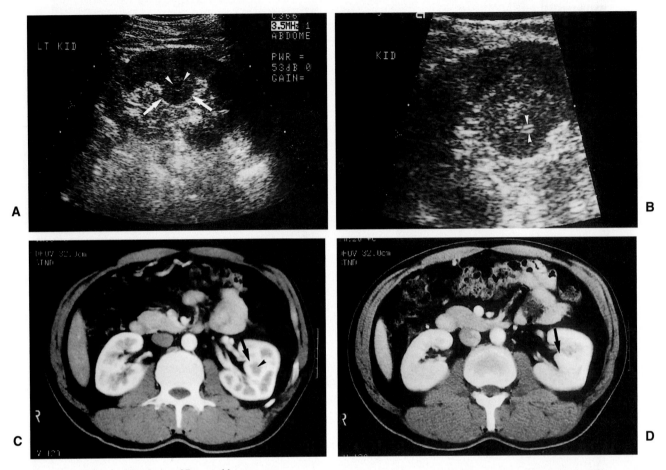

Fig. 1. Prominent column of Bertin in a 37-year-old man.
A. US shows a prominent column of renal parenchyma *(arrows)* projecting into the renal sinus. The column contains a focal hypoechoic area *(arrowheads)* that probably represents a medulla surrounded by septal cortical tissues. **B.** Magnified image of US, obtained in a slightly different angle from **A,** shows a small tubular structure with echogenic walls *(arrowheads)* that probably represents an arcuate artery in the column. **C.** Contrast-enhanced CT in cortical phase shows a prominent column *(arrow)* projecting into the renal sinus. Note that the column contains a medulla *(arrowhead)* that is not enhanced yet. **D.** Contrast-enhanced CT scan in nephrographic phase shows that the attenuation of the column *(arrow)* is identical to that of the renal parenchyma in other parts of the kidney.

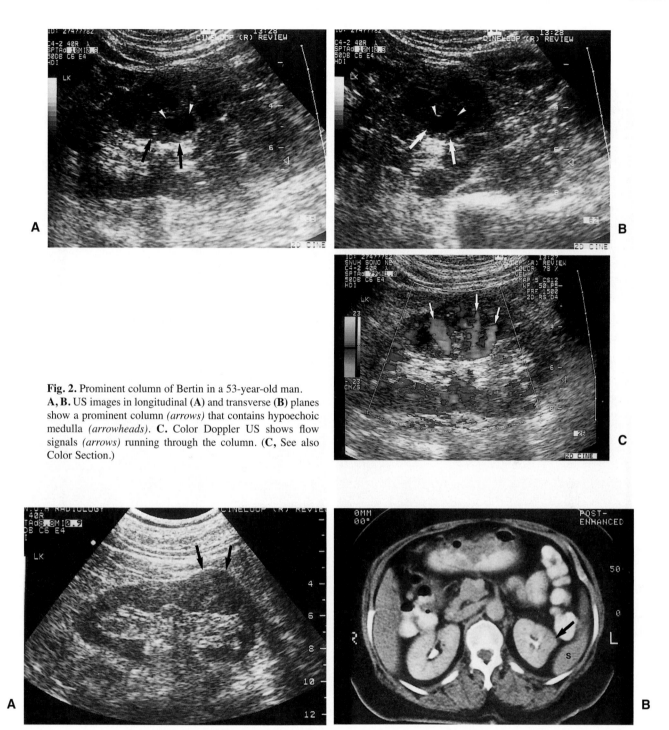

Fig. 2. Prominent column of Bertin in a 53-year-old man.
A, B. US images in longitudinal (**A**) and transverse (**B**) planes show a prominent column *(arrows)* that contains hypoechoic medulla *(arrowheads)*. **C.** Color Doppler US shows flow signals *(arrows)* running through the column. (**C,** See also Color Section.)

Fig. 3. Dromedary hump demonstrated on US and CT in a 56-year-old man.
A. Longitudinal US shows a localized bulge on the lower lateral border of the left kidney *(arrows)*. **B.** Contrast-enhanced CT shows a parenchymal bulge *(arrow)* on the lateral border of the left kidney. S, spleen.

10. Fetal Lobulation

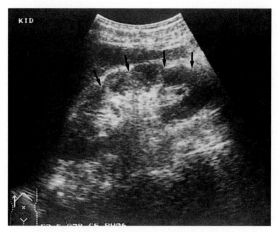

Fig. 1. US findings of fetal lobulation in a 80-year-old man. Longitudinal US of the right kidney shows lobulation of the renal parenchyma with regular indentations *(arrows)* on the outer margin of the kidney.

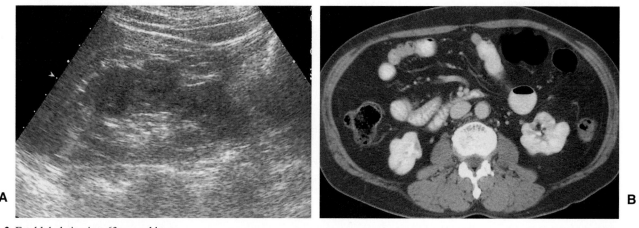

A   B

Fig. 2. Fetal lobulation in a 63-year-old man.
A. Longitudinal US of the right kidney shows lobulated renal outline. **B.** Contrast-enhanced CT scan shows severe fetal lobulation in both kidneys.

11. Junctional Parenchymal Defect

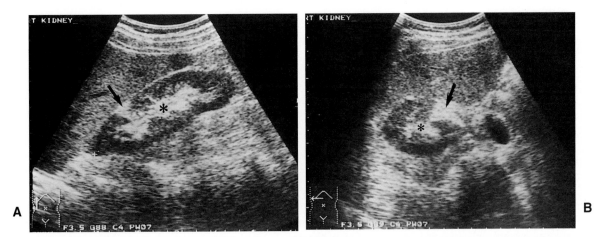

Fig. 1. Junctional parenchymal defect demonstrated on US in a 61-year-old man.
A, B. US images of the right kidney in longitudinal (**A**) and transverse (**B**) planes show a wedge-shaped, hyperechoic lesion *(arrow)* in the anteromedial aspect of the upper pole of the right kidney. The lesion is continuous with renal sinus fat *(asterisk)* and shows similar echogenicity.

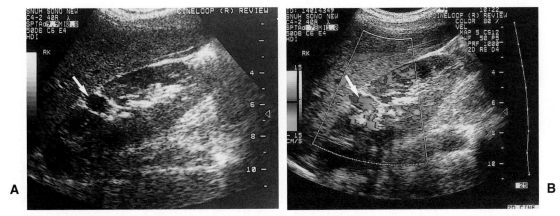

Fig. 2. Renal vein in a junctional parenchymal defect that mimics a cyst in a 41-year-old man.
A. Longitudinal US of the right kidney shows an anechoic structure *(arrow)* in the junctional parenchymal defect. **B.** Color Doppler US reveals that the anechoic structure seen on gray-scale US is a renal vessel *(arrow).* (**B**, See also Color Section.)

12. Renal Unidentified Bright Objects (UBOs) on US

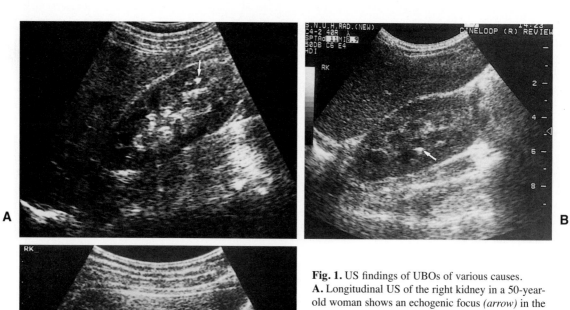

Fig. 1. US findings of UBOs of various causes.
A. Longitudinal US of the right kidney in a 50-year-old woman shows an echogenic focus *(arrow)* in the lower pole, which probably represents a specular reflective echo from an arcuate artery. **B.** Longitudinal US of the right kidney in a 67-year-old man shows an echogenic lesion *(arrow)* in the interpolar area, probably caused by a tiny calcification in the papilla. **C.** Transverse US in a 54-year-old man shows echogenic foci *(arrows)* in the anterior aspect of the right kidney. Also note a small anechoic lesion *(arrowheads)* anterior to the echogenic foci, suggesting that these echogenic foci probably represent the strong sonic reflection at the posterior wall of a tiny cyst.

13. Sinus Lipomatosis and Prominent Perirenal Fat

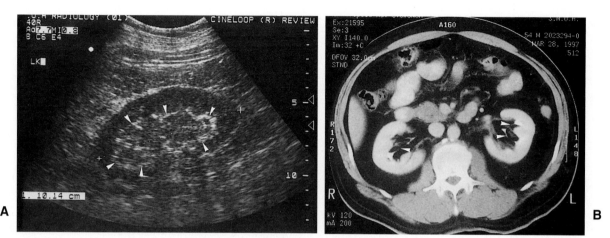

Fig. 1. Sinus lipomatosis in a 54-year-old man, which mimics a renal pelvis tumor on US.
A. Longitudinal US of the left kidney shows unusual hypoechogenicity of the renal sinus echo mimicking a mass filling the pelvocalyceal system. Note that the hypoechoic sinus is marginated by an echogenic rim *(arrowheads)*. **B.** Contrast-enhanced CT shows prominent renal sinus fat in both kidneys stretching the calyceal infundibula (arrowheads).

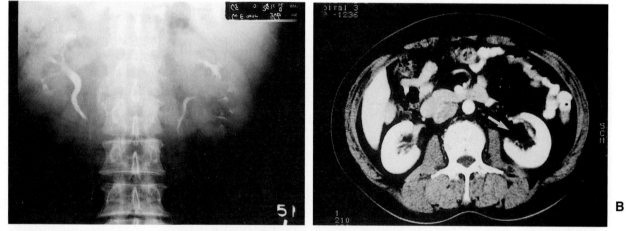

Fig. 2. Prominent renal sinus fat in a 57-year-old man with liver cirrhosis.
A. IVU shows lower position of the left kidney due to splenomegaly and indistinct calyceal infundibula in the left kidney. **B.** Contrast-enhanced CT reveals prominent sinus fat in the left kidney *(arrow)*, which is the cause of compression effect on calyceal infundibula.

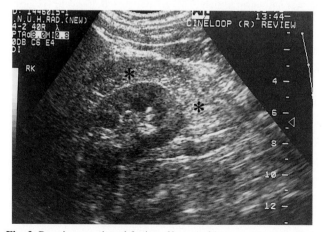

Fig. 3. Prominent perirenal fat in a 60-year-old woman. Longitudinal US shows the right kidney and prominent, hyperechoic, perirenal fat *(asterisks)*.

14. Pseudohydronephrosis

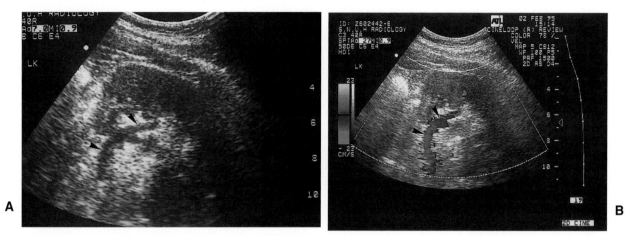

Fig. 1. US findings of pseudohydronephrosis by prominent renal vessels in a 27-year-old man.
A. US of the left kidney in transverse plane shows a tubular anechoic structure *(arrowheads)* in the renal hilar region mimicking dilated pelvocalyceal system. **B.** Color Doppler US reveals flow signal in the tubular structure *(arrowheads)* confirming that the structure is a blood vessel and is not dilated pelvocalyces. (**B**, See also Color Section.)

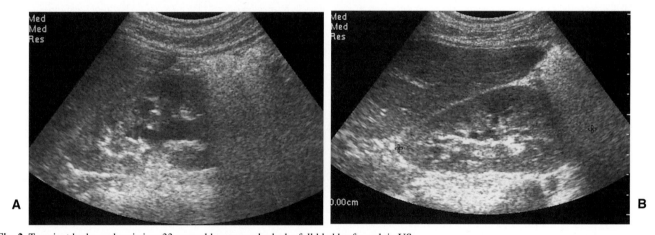

Fig. 2. Transient hydronephrosis in a 33-year-old woman who had a full bladder for pelvic US.
A. US of the right kidney when the bladder was full shows dilation of the pelvocalyces. **B.** Repeated US after voiding shows disappeared pelvocalyceal dilation.

15. Ureter: Normal Findings and Variations

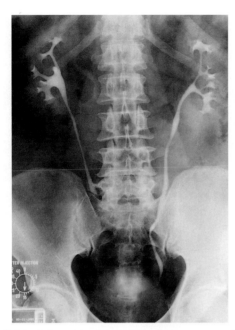

Fig. 1. Medial deviation of the ureters due to large psoas muscle in a 53-year-old man. IVU shows medial deviation of bilateral distal ureters probably due to prominent psoas muscles.

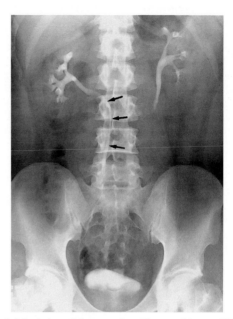

Fig. 2. Medial deviation of the ureter in a 33-year-old man. IVU shows medial deviation of the right proximal ureter *(arrows)* without any abnormality.

16. Urinary Bladder: Normal Findings and Variations

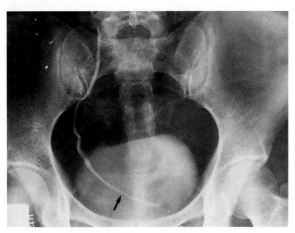

Fig. 1. Ureteral jet on IVU in a 55-year-old woman. IVU shows a jet of urine from the ureteral orifice *(arrow)* into the bladder.

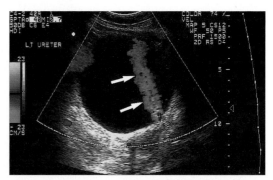

Fig. 2. Ureteral jet on color Doppler US in a 20-year-old woman. Color Doppler US of the bladder shows jetting of urine *(arrows)* from the left ureteral orifice. This finding of ureteral jet virtually excludes the possibility of significant obstruction of the urinary tract. (See also Color Section.)

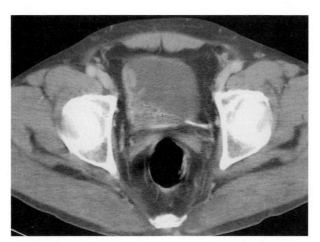

Fig. 3. Ureteral jet on CT, which may mimic an enhancing bladder tumor in a 32-year-old man. Contrast-enhanced CT shows jetting of opacified urine from the left ureteral orifice to the right wall of the bladder. This contrast material in the bladder may mimic an enhancing tumor of the bladder.

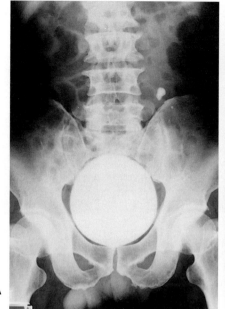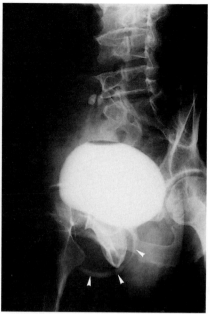

Fig. 4. Normal bladder on VCU in a 53-year-old man.
A, B. VCU images in rest (**A**) and voiding (**B**) states show smooth contour of the bladder and absence of vesicoureteral reflux. Also note normal urethra on **B** *(arrowheads)*.

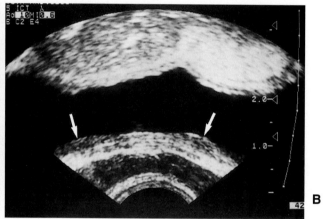

Fig. 5. Normal bladder on US in a 73-year-old man.
A. US of the bladder in parasagittal plane shows localized bulging of the bladder mucosa at the ureteropelvic junction *(arrow).* **B.** US of the bladder in transverse plane shows prominent bladder mucosa at the ureterovesical junctions on both sides *(arrows).*

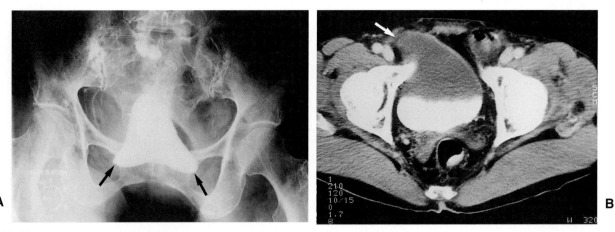

Fig. 6. Bladder ears.
A. A 75-year-old woman who underwent radical hysterectomy and radiation therapy for uterine cervical carcinoma. IVU shows protrusion of the bladder into both inguinal rings *(arrows)*. **B.** Unilateral bladder ear in a 60-year-old man. Contrast-enhanced CT demonstrates protrusion of the right inferolateral aspect of the bladder into the inguinal ring *(arrow)*.

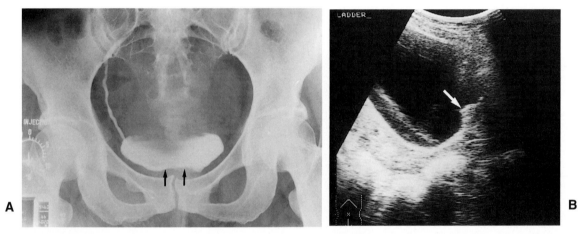

Fig. 7. Female prostate in a 41-year-old woman.
A. IVU shows smooth elevation of the bladder neck *(arrows)*. This IVU finding is called female prostate because it closely mimics a finding of prostatic enlargement in the male. **B.** Longitudinal US of the bladder shows elevation of the bladder neck *(arrow)* due to prominent soft tissue of the proximal urethra.

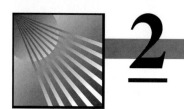

2

Congenital Anomalies of the Upper Urinary Tract

JEONG YEON CHO

CONGENITAL ANOMALIES OF THE KIDNEY
Renal agenesis and hypoplasia
Unilateral renal agenesis

Unilateral renal agenesis occurs in about 1 in 1000 births. Agenesis of ipsilateral ureter, ureteral orifice, and trigone is usually associated. In most cases the contralateral kidney is large due to compensatory hypertrophy. Ipsilateral genital abnormalities are common. In men, seminal vesicle cyst, absence of the vas deferens, hypoplasia or agenesis of the testicle, and hypospadias may occur. In women, varying fusion anomalies of uterus and absence or hypoplasia of the uterus and vagina may occur. Often one of the duplicated uterovaginal systems is obstructed, causing hematocolpometra.

Bilateral renal agenesis

Bilateral renal agenesis is rare. It occurs more often in males than females. About 40% of involved fetuses die during fetal life and the remainder die immediately after the birth. The major cause of death is pulmonary hypoplasia due to severe oligohydramnios. On prenatal ultrasound (US), there is severe oligohydramnios, and the fetal kidneys and bladder are persistently invisible.

Renal hypoplasia

Renal hypoplasia is an incomplete development of the kidney. The kidney is small and has few calyces and papillae. The hypoplastic kidney is usually unilateral and functionally normal for its size. The hypoplastic kidney may appear as a miniature of the normal kidney, but more often it is combined with a varying degree of renal dysplasia. Therefore, differential diagnosis from chronic pyelonephritis, ischemia, and long-standing obstruction may be difficult.

Renal ectopy and anomalies of fusion
Renal ectopy

Renal ectopy occurs as a result of failure of renal migration from the pelvic cavity to the normal renal fossa. The most common type is the pelvic kidney. Most ectopic kidneys are also malrotated. Their ureters are usually short compared with the normal. This finding helps differentiate from nephroptosis, in which the ureter has normal length and therefore is tortuous. Most are asymptomatic and detected occasionally on the imaging studies performed for other reasons. Rarely intratho-racic kidney occurs when the kidney ascends to a position that is a higher than normal location. Ectopic kidney may be confused with renal agenesis or a mass.

Crossed renal ectopy

Crossed renal ectopia is defined as a kidney located on the opposite side from its ureter. The crossed kidney usually lies below the normally situated kidney. Most are associated with malrotation and fusion anomalies. The ureteral insertion and the trigone of the bladder are usually normal. Most cases are asymptomatic. This anomaly can be readily detected on intravenous urography (IVU) but may be misdiagnosed as unilateral renal agenesis on US.

Horseshoe kidney

Horseshoe kidney is a common congenital anomaly, occurring in approximately 1 in 400 births. Two kidneys are fused usually at the lower poles. The connecting isthmus is composed of normal renal parenchyma or connective tissue. Varying degrees of ureteropelvic junction obstruction with resultant infection and stones often accompany horseshoe kidney. Horseshoe kidneys are prone to injury, and reportedly the prevalence of Wilms' tumor and renal carcinoid tumor is increased. On IVU, the renal axis is vertical or reversed, with the lower poles being medial to the upper poles. The lower-pole calyces are often medial to the pelvis and ureter. The renal pelvis is often large and extrarenal. On computed tomography (CT) and US, the isthmus is readily detected.

Anomalies of rotation

Malrotation of the kidney most commonly occurs as a result of incomplete inward rotation about its longitudinal axis. This results in abnormal anterior facing of the renal pelvis. The renal pelvis and proximal ureter appear to be located in the more lateral position of the calyces on IVU. Rarely over-rotation occurs and results in posterior facing of the renal hilum.

Anomalies of the renal calyces
Calyceal diverticulum

Calyceal diverticulum is an intraparenchymal cavity lined by transitional epithelium. It usually communicates with the fornix by a narrow neck. Most cases are unilateral and single in the upper pole of the kidney. The size of diverticulum is usually

small, less than 1 cm. Most diverticula are asymptomatic, but infection or obstruction may occur. Stone formation, especially milk of calcium, is a frequent complication. On IVU, calyceal diverticulum is readily detected as a round lesion filled with contrast material through the channel communicating with the fornix. On US and CT, differentiation from a renal cyst may be difficult.

Congenital hydrocalycosis

Congenital obstruction of the calyceal infundibulum refers to a hydrocalycosis. Dilated calyx has a fornix and a papilla, which is different from a calyceal diverticulum. However, the differentiation from a large calyceal diverticulum may be difficult.

Congenital megacalycosis

Congenital megacalycosis is defined as symmetrical enlargement of calyces without obstruction or reflux. This anomaly is usually unilateral, and the involved kidney is normal in size or mildly enlarged. Most cases are asymptomatic and functionally normal. On IVU, opacification of calyces may be slightly delayed due to large calyceal spaces, and differentiation from postobstructive change of calyces may be difficult. Congenital megaureter often accompanies.

CONGENITAL ANOMALIES OF THE RENAL PELVIS AND URETER

Congenital ureteropelvic junction obstruction

Congenital ureteropelvic junction (UPJ) obstruction is the most common cause of abdominal mass in a neonate. Most cases are functional obstruction by abnormal alignment of the smooth muscle fibers in the UPJ area. Anatomic obstruction rarely presents by adhesion, kinking, valves, or aberrant vessels. Many UPJ obstructions are diagnosed in the antenatal period because of routine use of antenatal US, but significant numbers of unilateral UPJ obstructions are detected in later adulthood because most of those cases are clinically silent. On IVU, calyces and pelvis are dilated and the opacification is delayed or invisible. In some cases, the pelvis is markedly dilated to form a huge cyst occupying the entire abdomen. In these circumstances, it is difficult to determine the exact site of UPJ. Surgical pyeloplasty has been considered the treatment of choice, but it can also be treated with percutaneous pyeloplasty or endoscopic pyelotomy.

Congenital megaureter

Congenital megaureter is functional obstruction of the distal ureter. The ureter proximal to the aperistaltic segment just above the ureteral orifice is variably dilated. Dilation usually involves the distal one third of the ureter, and the calyces are usually not dilated or blunted. Congenital megaureter may occur in association with congenital megacalycosis. Most cases are asymptomatic, but urinary tract infection, abdominal pain, hematuria, and urolithiasis may be complications.

Circumcaval ureter

Circumcaval ureter is a rare congenital anomaly in which the ureter passes posterior to and around the inferior vena cava.

The anomaly occurs when the infrarenal vena cava segment is formed from the right subcardinal vein instead of right supracardinal vein. On IVU, the proximal right ureter is tortuous and dilated with associated hydronephrosis. The course of the proximal ureter has a reverse-J configuration before it crosses behind the vena cava, and then it descends medial to the ipsilateral pedicle of the lumbar vertebra. CT may also demonstrate the ureter passing posterior and medial to the vena cava.

Duplication of collecting system

Duplication of the collecting system is the most common congenital urinary tract anomaly. Partial duplication results from the branching of the ureteral bud before it connects with the metanephric blastema. Complete duplication occurs when two separate ureteric buds arise from the mesonephric duct. When the junction of duplicated ureters is extravesical or intravesical, it is called *Y-duplication* or *V-duplication*, respectively. The mildest form of incomplete duplication is a bifid pelvis, in which only renal pelvis is duplicated and joins at the UPJ. In complete type, although the lower-moiety ureter usually inserts into the trigone, the upper-moiety ureter usually inserts into the inferior and medial portion of the urinary bladder. Ectopic insertion of the upper-moiety ureter causes stenosis of orifice and ureterocele. Lower-moiety ureter may be complicated by vesicoureteral reflux or UPJ obstruction.

Most of the partial duplications and uncomplicated complete duplication are incidentally detected on IVU. In case of complete duplication with severe obstruction of the upper-moiety ureter, the dilated upper pole may compress the lower pole to make a "drooping lily" configuration on IVU. Vesicoureteral reflux to the lower-moiety ureter may cause severe scarring of the lower pole, producing a so-called nubbin sign on IVU. In case of partial duplication with distal obstruction, the peristalsis down in one ureter may force urine via reflux up the other, which is called the "yo-yo" phenomenon.

On US, sinus echo complex and pelvis are separated by intervening renal parenchymal tissue. In case of complete duplication with upper-moiety obstruction, US typically shows an anechoic cystic area in the upper medial part of the kidney. Duplication artifact of the left kidney, which is caused by US beam refraction between the spleen and adjacent fat, may be confused with a duplicated system.

Ureterocele

Ureterocele is defined as dilation of the intramural segment of the distal ureter either congenitally or by acquired stenosis at the distal ureteral orifice. Although simple ureterocele occurs in a normal single collecting system, rare ectopic ureterocele occurs in the upper-moiety ureter of the duplicated system. Most simple ureteroceles are small and asymptomatic. Calculi within the ureterocele are common.

On IVU, the ureterocele typically appears as a smooth, round or ovoid lesion in the bladder base with a "cobra-head" appearance. Usually the ureter is not dilated in case of small ureterocele, but marked dilation may occur. On US, the ureterocele appears as a well-defined cystic lesion in the bladder base.

Pseudoureterocele is defined as a lesion causing similar lucent filling defect at the ureterovesical junction on IVU. Edema caused by impaction of a small stone or bladder tumor appears as a lucent filling defect. Pseudoureteroceles show ill-defined margin and irregular thick wall, in contrast to the smooth and thin wall of true ureteroceles.

Ectopic ureteral insertion

Extravesical ureteral insertion is most commonly associated with complete duplication. Unduplicated ectopic ureteral insertion is more common than previously recognized. Ectopic ureteral insertion occurs more frequently in females than in males. In cases of complete duplication, the upper-moiety ureter usually inserts into the lower medial portion of the bladder. In some instances, the ureter inserts not into the bladder but into the posterior urethra, vagina, uterus, broad ligament, vas deferens, or seminal vesicle. The ectopic orifice may be obstructed or associated with incontinence of urine. The kidneys associated with unduplicated ectopic ureters are usually dysplastic. The more ectopic the position of the ureteral orifice, the more dysplastic the kidney.

References

1. Friedland GW: Developmental and congenital disorders. In Pollack HM, McClennan BL (eds): Clinical Urography, 2nd ed, vol 2. Philadelphia, WB Saunders, 2000, pp 661–912.
2. Talner LB, O'Reilly PH, Wasserman NF: Specific causes of obstruction. In Pollack HM, McClennan BL (eds): Clinical Urography, 2nd ed, vol 2. Philadelphia, WB Saunders, 2000, pp 1967–1978.
3. Dunnick NR, Sandler CM, Amis ES, Newhouse JH: Congenital anomalies. In Textbook of Uroradiology, 2nd ed. Baltimore, Lippincott Williams & Wilkins, 1997, pp 15–43.
4. Middleton WD, Melson GL: Renal duplication artifact in US imaging. Radiology 1989; 173:427–429.
5. Cope JR, Trickey SE: Congenital absence of the kidney: Problems in diagnosis and management. J Urol 1982; 227:10–12.
6. Scott JE: The single ectopic ureter and dysplastic kidney. Br J Urol 1981; 53:300–305.
7. Curtis JA, Pollack HM: Renal duplication with a diminutive lower pole: The nubbin sign. Radiology 1979; 131:327–331.
8. Siegel MJ, McAlister WH: Calyceal diverticula in children: Unusual features and complications. Radiology 1979; 131:79–82.
9. Prewitt LH Jr, Lebowitz RL: The single ectopic ureter. AJR Am J Roentgenol 1976; 127:941–948.

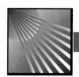

Illustrations • Congenital Anomalies of the Upper Urinary Tract

1 • Renal agenesis

2 • Renal hypoplasia

3 • Ectopic kidney

4 • Crossed renal ectopy

5 • Fusion anomaly

6 • Rotation anomaly

7 • Calyceal diverticulum

8 • Hydrocalycosis

9 • Congenital ureteropelvic junction obstruction

10 • Congenital ureteral obstruction

11 • Congenital megaureter

12 • Circumcaval ureter

13 • Duplication of the collecting system

14 • Ureterocele

15 • Ectopic ureteral insertion

1. Renal Agenesis

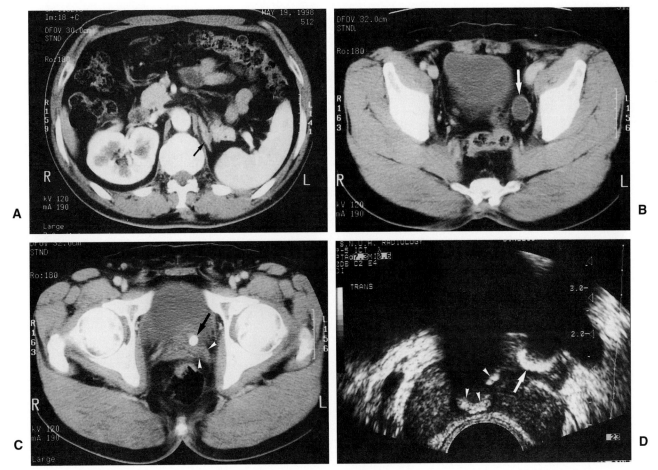

Fig. 1. Left renal agenesis with remnant distal ureter communicating with left seminal vesicle in a 58-year-old man with history of recurrent epididymitis on the left side.
A. Contrast-enhanced CT shows absent left kidney and prominent left adrenal gland *(arrow)* in a location lower than usual. **B.** CT scan of the pelvic cavity shows a dilated remnant in the distal part of the left ureter *(arrow)*. **C.** CT scan of the lower pelvic cavity shows a round stone *(arrow)* in the left distal ureter joining the left seminal vesicle *(arrowheads)*. **D.** Transrectal US in transverse plane shows a stone *(arrow)* with posterior sonic shadowing in the left seminal vesicle. Also note calcifications in the prostate *(arrowheads)*.

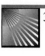

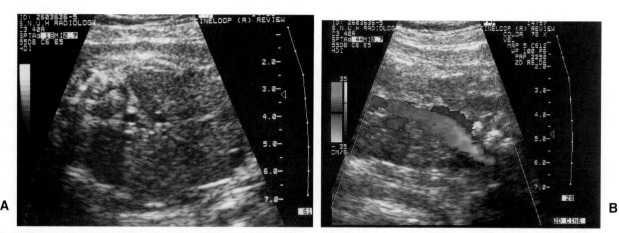

Fig. 2. Bilateral renal agenesis detected on prenatal US of a 28-week fetus.
A. US of the fetal abdomen in axial plane shows severe oligohydramnios and no demonstrable fetal kidneys. **B.** Color Doppler US of the fetal abdomen in coronal plane well demonstrates the abdominal aorta, but renal arteries are not demonstrable. (**B**, See also Color Section.)

2. Renal Hypoplasia

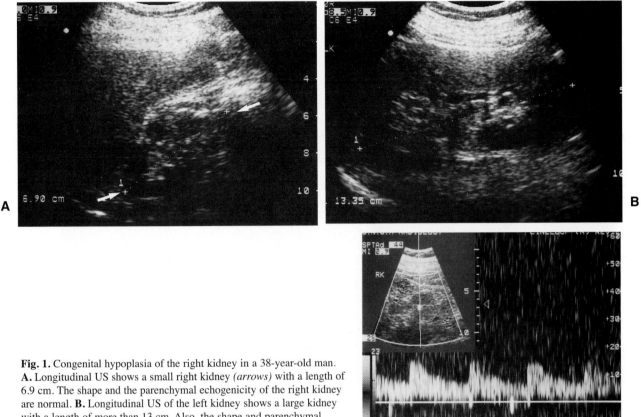

Fig. 1. Congenital hypoplasia of the right kidney in a 38-year-old man. **A.** Longitudinal US shows a small right kidney *(arrows)* with a length of 6.9 cm. The shape and the parenchymal echogenicity of the right kidney are normal. **B.** Longitudinal US of the left kidney shows a large kidney with a length of more than 13 cm. Also, the shape and parenchymal echogenicity of the left kidney are normal. **C.** Doppler US of the right kidney shows normal spectral pattern.

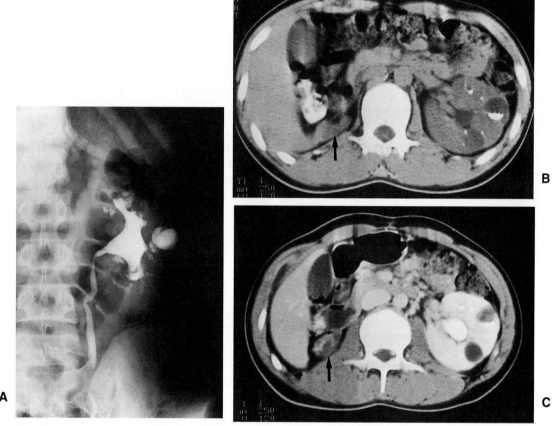

Fig. 2. Congenital renal hypoplasia associated with contralateral cystic medullary sponge kidney in an 18-year-old male patient.
A. IVU shows collection of contrast material in the dilated collecting ducts with tubular and cystic appearances in the left kidney. **B.** Nonenhanced CT shows a small right kidney *(arrow)*. The left kidney is large and has cystic lesions containing calcifications in the dependent portions. **C.** Contrast-enhanced CT shows small cysts in the hypoplastic right kidney *(arrow)* and large cystic lesions in the left kidney.

3. Ectopic Kidney

Fig. 1. Pelvic kidney in a 23-year-old man.
A, B. Plain radiograph (**A**) and 15-minute IVU (**B**) show nonopacification of the left kidney in the usual location. Instead there is a kidney *(arrows)* in the left pelvic cavity with opacification of the pelvocalyces and ureter *(arrowheads)*.

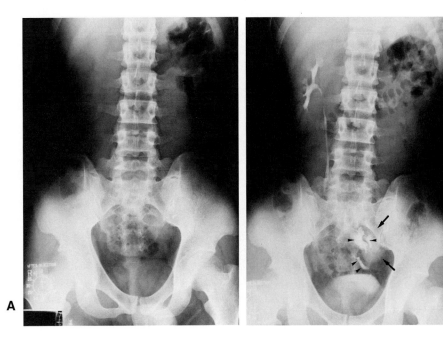

4. Crossed Renal Ectopy

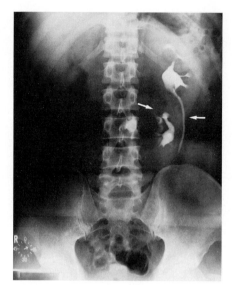

Fig. 1. Crossed fused ectopic kidney in a 30-year-old man. IVU shows two kidneys in the left abdomen. The upper pole of the right kidney is fused to the lower pole of the left kidney *(arrows)*.

5. Fusion Anomaly

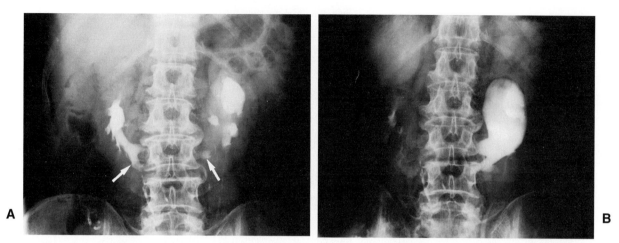

Fig. 1. Horseshoe kidney in a 67-year-old man.
A, B. IVU images show vertical orientation of the kidneys and fusion of the lower poles. Note that the isthmus consists of renal parenchyma and has calyces in it *(arrows)*. Also note that the left renal pelvis is dilated due to associated ureteropelvic junction obstruction.

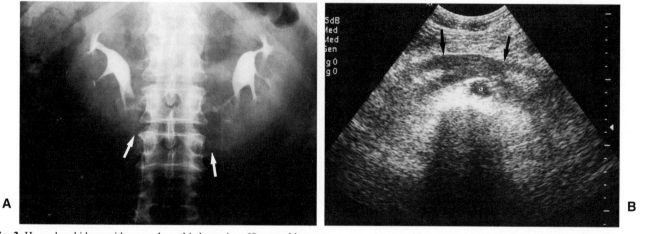

Fig. 2. Horseshoe kidney with parenchymal isthmus in a 60-year-old woman.
A. IVU shows vertical renal axes and fused lower poles *(arrows)*. **B.** US of the abdomen in transverse plane well demonstrates parenchymal isthmus *(arrows)* anterior to the abdominal aorta (a).

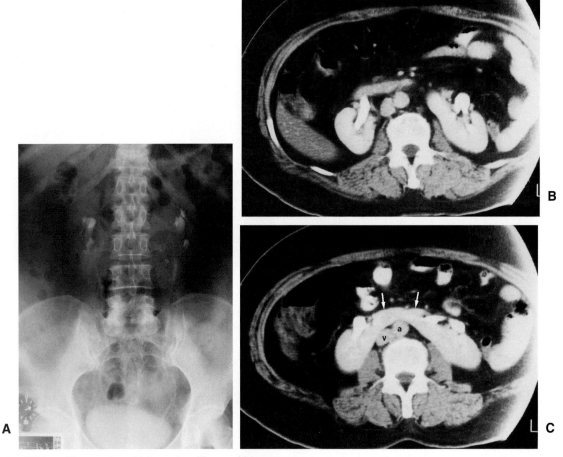

Fig. 3. Horseshoe kidney with parenchymal isthmus in a 57-year-old woman.
A. A 10-minute IVU shows vertical orientation of the kidneys suggesting a horseshoe kidney. **B, C.** Contrast-enhanced CT scans demonstrate the horseshoe kidney with the isthmus composed of enhancing renal parenchyma *(arrows)* anterior to the abdominal aorta (a) and inferior vena cava (v).

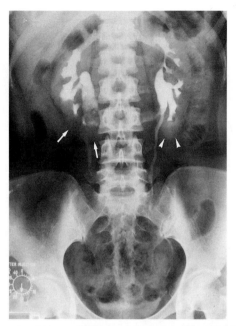

Fig. 4. Horseshoe kidney with fibrous isthmus in a 39-year-old woman. IVU shows vertical orientation of both kidneys indicating horseshoe kidney. Note that the right kidney has contour abnormality with calyceal deformity in the lower polar region *(arrows)*, but the lower pole of the left kidney is well demarcated *(arrowheads)*. This finding suggests that the isthmus of the horseshoe kidney is thin and composed of fibrous tissue. On US, no parenchymal isthmus was demonstrated (not shown).

Fig. 5. Left renal ectopia with fusion in a 29-year-old man. (**A**, **B**, Courtesy of Hae Jeong Jeon, MD.)
A. IVU shows ectopic left kidney *(arrows)* that is fused with lower pole of the right kidney. **B.** Three-dimensional reconstruction image of spiral CT well demonstrates both urinary tracts and fusion of both kidneys.

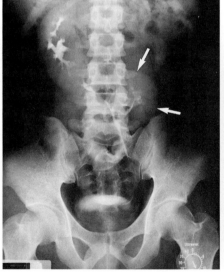

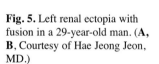

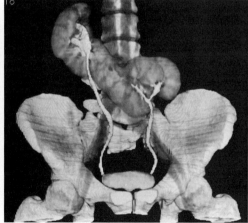

6. Rotation Anomaly

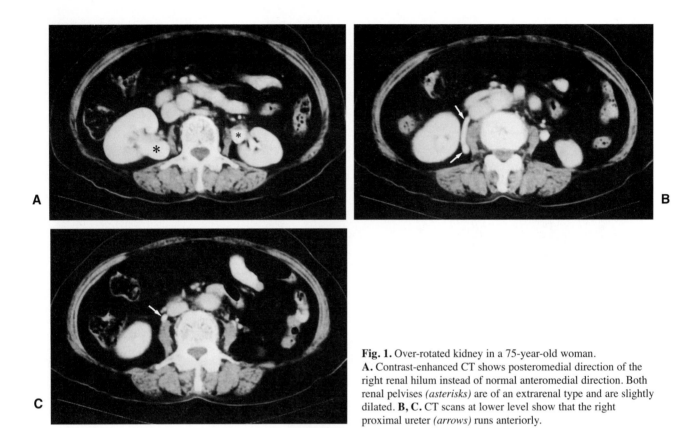

Fig. 1. Over-rotated kidney in a 75-year-old woman.
A. Contrast-enhanced CT shows posteromedial direction of the right renal hilum instead of normal anteromedial direction. Both renal pelvises *(asterisks)* are of an extrarenal type and are slightly dilated. **B, C.** CT scans at lower level show that the right proximal ureter *(arrows)* runs anteriorly.

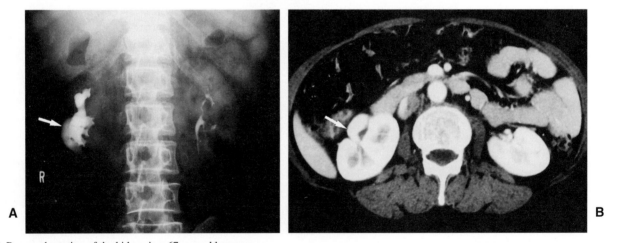

Fig. 2. Reversed rotation of the kidney in a 67-year-old woman.
A. IVU shows malrotation of the right kidney. Note that the renal pelvis is directed laterally *(arrow)*. **B.** Contrast-enhanced CT scan of the kidney demonstrates anterolateral direction of the renal pelvis *(arrow)*.

7. Calyceal Diverticulum

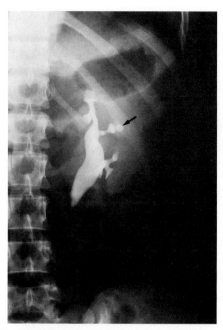

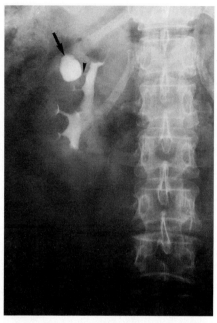

Fig. 1. Small calyceal diverticulum in a 34-year-old woman. A 25-minute IVU shows a small diverticulum *(arrow)* in the interpolar calyx of the left kidney. Note that the left kidney is malrotated.

Fig. 2. Calyceal diverticulum in a 68-year-old woman. A 5-minute IVU shows a round calyceal diverticulum *(arrow)* connected to the fornix of the upper polar calyx *(arrowhead)* of the right kidney.

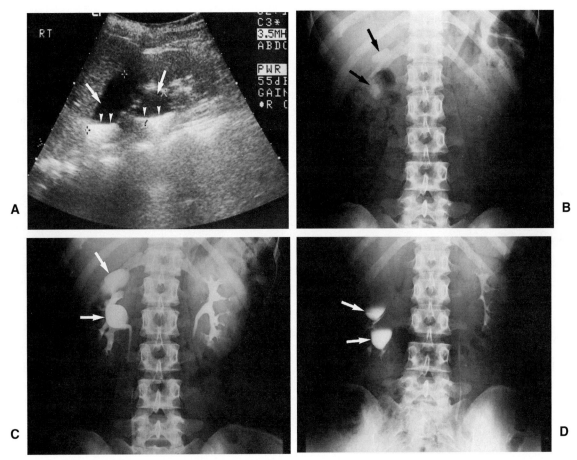

Fig. 3. Calyceal diverticulum with milk of calcium urine in a 26-year-old woman.
A. Longitudinal US of the right kidney shows two cystic lesions *(arrows)* that contain echogenic materials layered in the dependent portion *(arrowheads)*. **B.** Plain radiograph shows homogeneous radiopacities *(arrows)* in the right kidney. **C, D.** IVU images obtained with the patient in supine **(C)** and upright **(D)** positions show two large calyceal diverticula *(arrows)*.

8. Hydrocalycosis

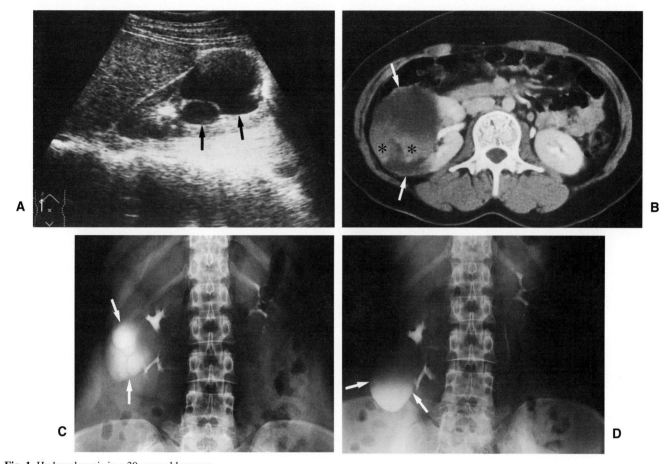

Fig. 1. Hydrocalycosis in a 30-year-old woman.
A. Longitudinal US of the right kidney shows a large, lobulated cystic lesion *(arrows)* in the lower polar area. **B.** Contrast-enhanced CT shows a large cystic lesion *(arrows)* in the right kidney containing excreted contrast material *(asterisks)*. **C, D.** IVU images obtained with the patient in supine **(C)** and erect **(D)** positions show a large, lobulated, cystic lesion *(arrows)* containing excreted contrast material in the right kidney.

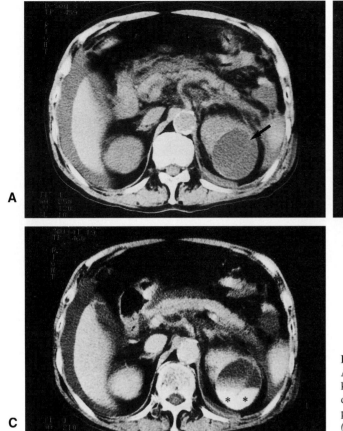

A

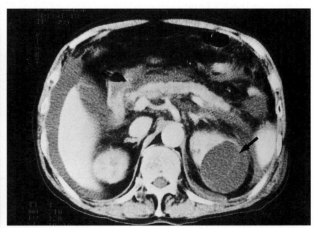

B

C

Fig. 2. Hydrocalycosis in a 73-year-old woman.
A. Nonenhanced CT shows a round cystic mass *(arrow)* in the left kidney. **B.** Contrast-enhanced CT in cortical phase well demonstrates the cystic lesion *(arrow)*. **C.** CT scan in excretory phase demonstrates layering of excreted contrast material *(asterisks)* in the dependent portion of the cystic lesion. Note ascites in the abdomen.

9. Congenital Ureteropelvic Junction Obstruction

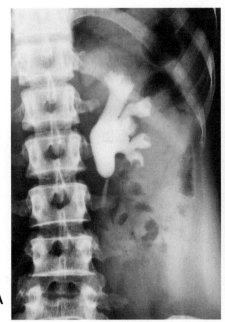

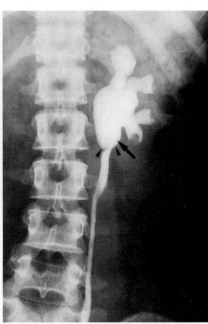

Fig. 1. Congenital ureteropelvic junction obstruction in a 33-year-old woman. **A.** A 1-hour IVU shows dilated left pelvocalyces due to an obstruction at the ureteropelvic junction. The exact site of the ureteropelvic junction is not clear on this IVU image. **B.** RGP shows that the narrowed ureteropelvic junction *(arrow)* is higher than the bottom of the dilated renal pelvis *(arrowheads)*.

A

B

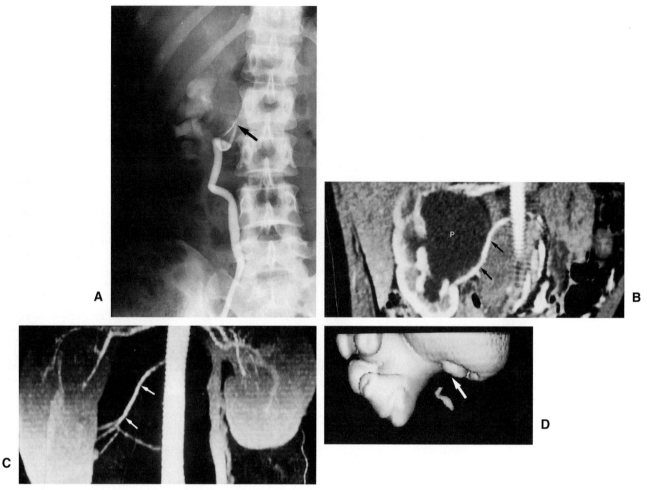

Fig. 2. Congenital ureteropelvic junction obstruction due to aberrant vessel in a 35-year-old woman.
A. RGP shows narrowing of the ureteropelvic junction *(arrow)* and dilated pelvocalyces. **B.** Coronal reformation image of the contrast-enhanced spiral CT shows dilated, urine-filled renal pelvis (P) and an aberrant lower polar artery *(arrows)* crossing the ureteropelvic junction. **C.** Maximal intensity projection image of spiral CT shows the aberrant vessel *(arrows)*. **D.** Shaded surface display image of spiral CT shows dilated renal pelvis and obstructed ureteropelvic junction *(arrow)*.

Fig. 3. Congenital ureteropelvic junction obstruction with massive dilation of the renal pelvis occupying the whole abdomen in a 30-year-old woman. **A.** A 10-minute IVU shows nonopacification of the left urinary tract. **B.** US of the abdomen in the transverse plane shows a huge mass with a lobulating contour occupying the whole abdomen. a, aorta. **C.** RGP obtained with the catheter in the left ureteral orifice shows the left ureter deviated to the right side and narrowed ureteropelvic junction *(arrow)*. Injected contrast material fills markedly dilated pelvocalyces of the left kidney *(arrowheads)*. **D.** Nonenhanced CT scan obtained following RGP shows markedly dilated renal pelvis *(asterisks)* and calyces (C) of the left kidney, which are opacified with contrast material due to previous RGP.

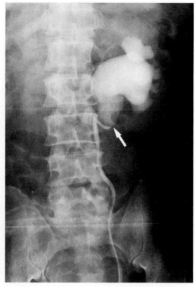

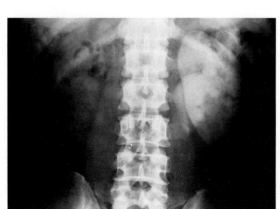

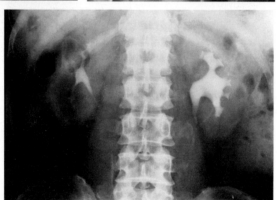

A

B

C

Fig. 4. Congenital ureteropelvic junction obstruction improved after surgical pyeloplasty in a 55-year-old man.
A. A 24-hour delayed IVU shows persistent dense nephrogram and dilated pelvocalyces of the left kidney. The right kidney already excreted contrast material. **B.** RGP well demonstrates obstruction of the ureteropelvic junction *(arrow)* with proximal dilation. **C.** A 30-minute IVU obtained 5 months after surgical pyeloplasy shows relieved obstruction at the left ureteropelvic junction.

10. Congenital Ureteral Obstruction

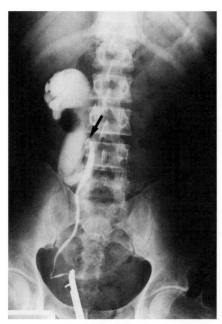

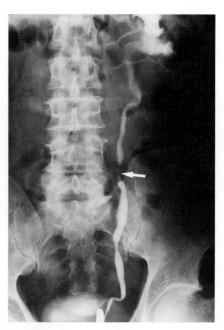

Fig. 1. Congenital obstruction of the proximal ureter in a 35-year-old man due to an aberrant vessel supplying the lower pole of the kidney. RGP shows an S-shaped configuration with obstruction *(arrow)* in the right ureter with dilation of the pelvocalyces and proximal ureter. Note that the S-shaped loop of the ureter is narrow and does not run medial to the vertebral pedicle. At surgery, there was an aberrant vessel supplying the lower pole of the right kidney crossing the narrowed portion of the ureter.

Fig. 2. Congenital obstruction of the left mid-ureter in a 39-year-old man. RGP shows a short-segment stricture in the left mid-ureter *(arrow)* with mild dilation of the proximal urinary tract. The lesion was confirmed to be a congenital stenosis at surgery and pathologic examination.

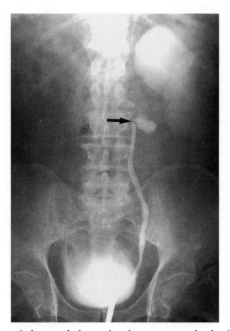

Fig. 3. Congenital ureteral obstruction due to a ureteral valve in a 66-year-old man. RGP shows obstruction of the left proximal ureter by a valve *(arrow)* with severe hydronephrosis.

11. Congenital Megaureter

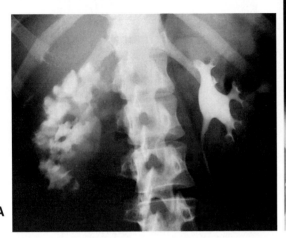

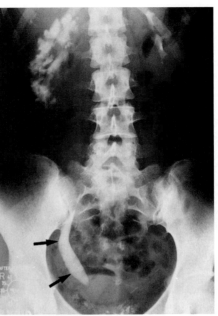

A

B

Fig. 1. Congenital megaureter and megapolycalycosis in a 30-year-old woman. **A.** A 5-minute IVU shows large number of calyces with slight dilation in the right kidney. Note that the right renal pelvis is not dilated. **B.** A 30-minute IVU shows fusiform dilation of the right distal ureter *(arrows)* without significant obstruction.

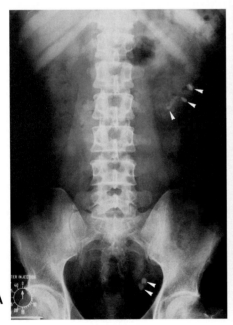

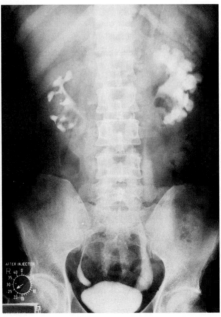

A

B

Fig. 2. Congenital megaureter and megacalycosis with multiple stones in a 30-year-old woman. **A.** Plain radiograph shows multiple stones *(arrowheads)* in the left kidney and left distal ureter. **B.** A 25-minute IVU shows dilated calyces and distal ureter on the left side. Note that the left renal pelvis and proximal ureter are not dilated. Also note similar changes in the right urinary tract.

12. Circumcaval Ureter

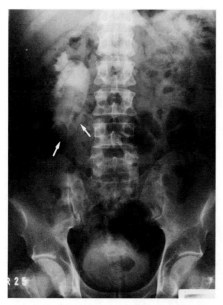

Fig. 1. Circumcaval ureter in a 60-year-old woman. The proximal right ureter is dilated, with reversed-J configuration *(arrows)*.

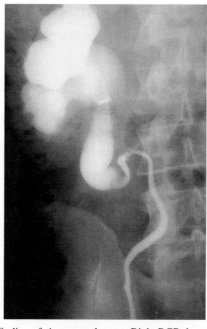

Fig. 2. RGP finding of circumcaval ureter. Right RGP shows a medial swing of the proximal ureter due to circumcaval ureter. (Courtesy of Cheol Min Park, MD.)

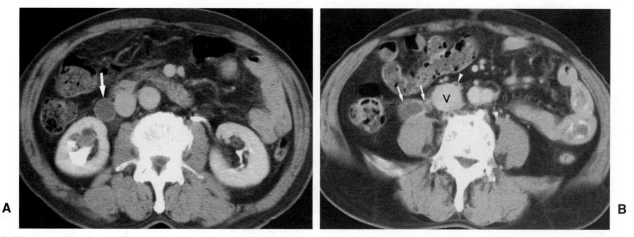

Fig. 3. Circumcaval ureter in a 72-year-old man.
A. Contrast-enhanced CT shows dilation of pelvocalyces and proximal ureter *(arrow)* on the right side. **B.** CT scan at slightly lower level shows dilated proximal ureter *(arrows)* going behind the inferior vena cava (V). Also note the nondilated portion of the right ureter *(arrowhead)* after turning around the inferior vena cava.

13. Duplication of the Collecting System

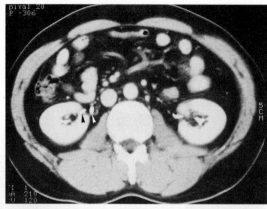

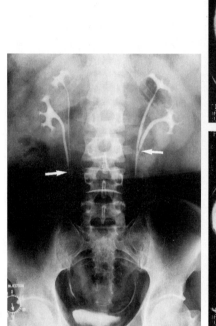

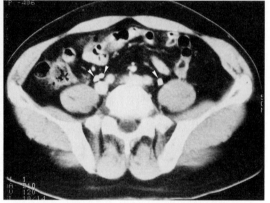

Fig. 1. Bilateral incomplete duplication in a 41-year-old man. **A.** A 15-minute IVU shows incomplete Y-duplications in both urinary tracts. Duplicated ureters join each other at mid-ureter *(arrows)*. **B, C.** Contrast-enhanced CT scans well demonstrate duplicated and joined ureters *(arrowheads)*.

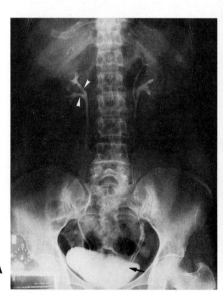

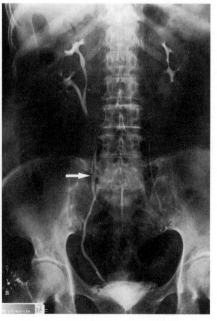

Fig. 2. Duplication of the collecting systems.
A. IVU of a 62-year-old woman shows duplication of collecting systems in both kidneys. The left ureter is duplicated down to the ureterovesical junction *(arrow)*, the so-called V-duplication. Note that the right renal pelvis is bifid *(arrowheads)*. **B.** IVU of a 69-year-old woman shows incomplete duplication of the right collecting system joining at the mid-ureter *(arrow)*, the so-called Y-duplication.

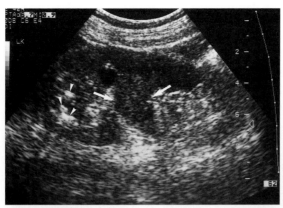

A

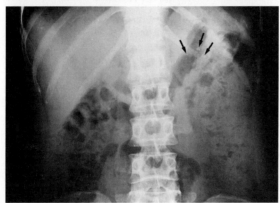

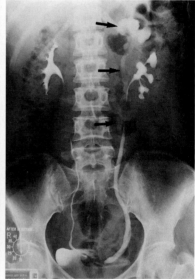

Fig. 3. Y-duplication with stones in the upper moiety calyx in a 40-year-old woman.
A. US shows a duplicated left collecting system. The central echo complex is separated by renal parenchyma *(arrows)*. The upper pole calyces are dilated and have small stones *(arrowheads)*.
B. Plain radiograph shows multiple small calcifications *(arrows)* in the upper pole area of the left kidney. **C.** IVU shows duplicated collecting system on the left side with dilation and faint opacification of the upper-moiety system *(arrows)*.

B

C

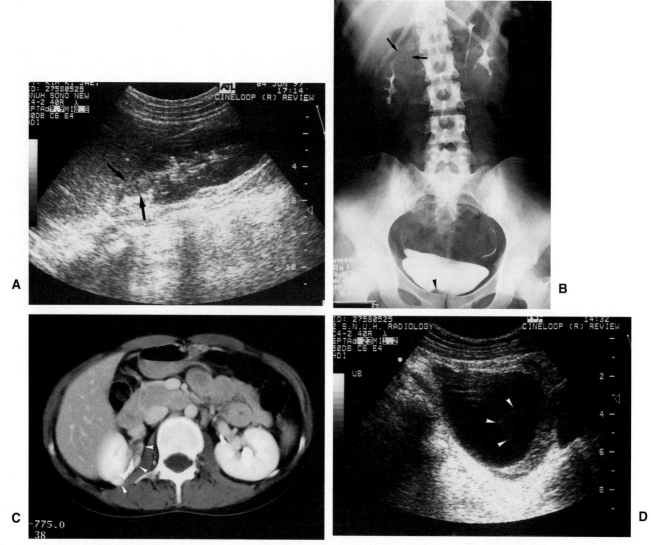

Fig. 4. Complete duplication of the collecting system with upper-moiety contraction and ureterocele in a 23-year-old woman.
A. Longitudinal US of the right kidney shows contracted upper-polar region with markedly increased echogenicity *(arrows)*. **B.** IVU shows faint opacification of the upper-moiety calyces in the right kidney *(arrows)* and an indentation on the right base of the urinary bladder suggesting a ureterocele *(arrowhead)*. Note that the left collecting system is also duplicated. **C.** Contrast-enhanced CT shows contracted posteromedial aspect of the upper pole of the right kidney *(arrowheads)*. **D.** US of the urinary bladder in right parasagittal plane shows a thin-walled ureterocele in the bladder base suggesting an ectopic ureterocele *(arrowheads)*.

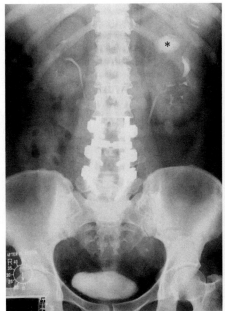 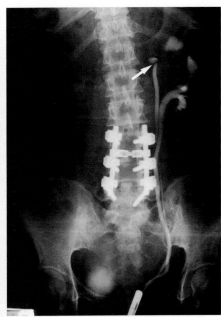

Fig. 5. Complete duplication of the collecting system with ureteropelvic junction obstruction in the upper moiety in a 45-year-old woman.
A. IVU shows dilated calyx in the upper moiety of the left kidney with collection of contrast material in the dependent portion of a calyx *(asterisk)*. Note that the lower-moiety calyces are displaced by the dilated calyces in the upper part of the kidney. **B.** At cystoscopy there were two ureteral orifices. A catheter was inserted into each ureteral orifice and RGP was taken. RGP shows severe stenosis at the ureteropelvic junction of the upper moiety *(arrow)*.

A

B

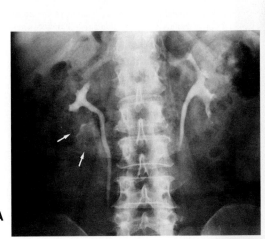 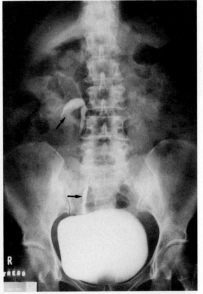

A

B

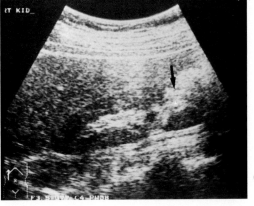

Fig. 6. Complete duplication with vesicoureteral reflux into the lower-moiety ureter causing parenchymal scar, producing a nubbin sign.
A. IVU shows contracted lower pole of the right kidney with faint calyceal opacification *(arrows)*. **B.** VCU shows vesicoureteral reflux into the lower moiety urinary tract *(arrows)*. **C.** US of the right kidney shows atrophic lower pole with echogenic scar *(arrow)*.

C

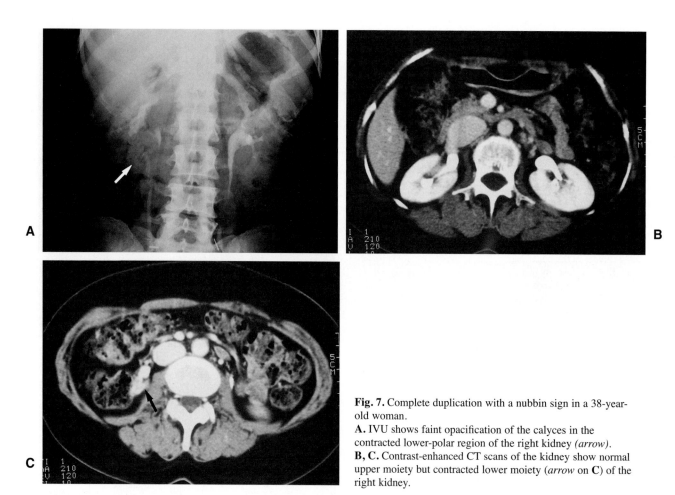

Fig. 7. Complete duplication with a nubbin sign in a 38-year-old woman.
A. IVU shows faint opacification of the calyces in the contracted lower-polar region of the right kidney *(arrow).*
B, C. Contrast-enhanced CT scans of the kidney show normal upper moiety but contracted lower moiety *(arrow on* **C***)* of the right kidney.

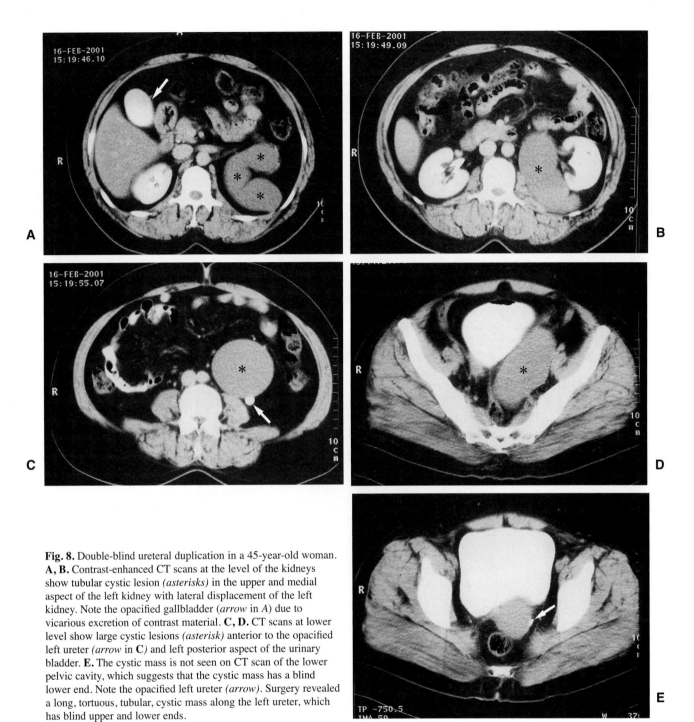

Fig. 8. Double-blind ureteral duplication in a 45-year-old woman. **A, B.** Contrast-enhanced CT scans at the level of the kidneys show tubular cystic lesion *(asterisks)* in the upper and medial aspect of the left kidney with lateral displacement of the left kidney. Note the opacified gallbladder *(arrow in A)* due to vicarious excretion of contrast material. **C, D.** CT scans at lower level show large cystic lesions *(asterisk)* anterior to the opacified left ureter *(arrow in C)* and left posterior aspect of the urinary bladder. **E.** The cystic mass is not seen on CT scan of the lower pelvic cavity, which suggests that the cystic mass has a blind lower end. Note the opacified left ureter *(arrow)*. Surgery revealed a long, tortuous, tubular, cystic mass along the left ureter, which has blind upper and lower ends.

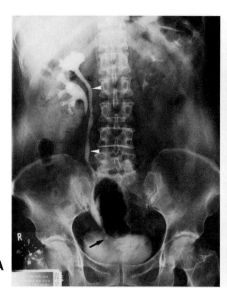

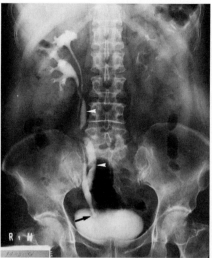

Fig. 9. Duplication with obstruction of the ureterovesical junction due to a stone producing a "yo-yo" phenomenon in a 51-year-old woman.
A. IVU shows incomplete duplication of the right collecting system. There is an obstructing stone in the ureterovesical junction *(arrow)*. While the lower-moiety ureter is contracted by forward peristalsis, the upper-moiety ureter is dilated by backward reflux *(arrowheads)*. **B.** Delayed image shows the contracted upper-moiety ureter and dilated lower-moiety ureter *(arrowheads)*. Note a stone in the ureterovesical junction with surrounding edema *(arrow)*.

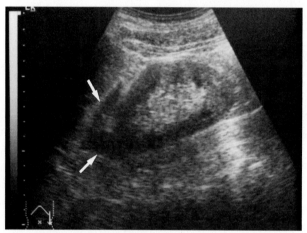

Fig. 10. Renal duplication artifact on US. Longitudinal US of the left kidney shows renal duplication artifact *(arrows)* caused by refraction of US beam traveling through the spleen. This artifact may be confused as a duplication anomaly or a suprarenal mass.

14. Ureterocele

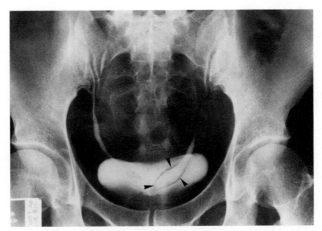

Fig. 1. Simple ureterocele in a 50-year-old woman. IVU shows fusiform dilation of intramural portion of the left ureter with sharply defined lucent wall *(arrowheads)*, which has a typical "cobra-head" appearance.

Fig. 2. Simple ureterocele in a 49-year-old man.
A, B. IVU images show a round ureterocele in the terminal portion of the left ureter with a thin radiolucent rim *(arrowheads)*.

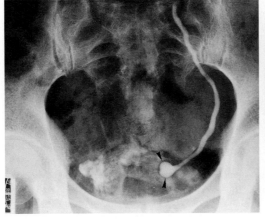

A

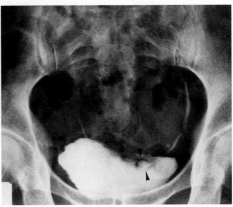

B

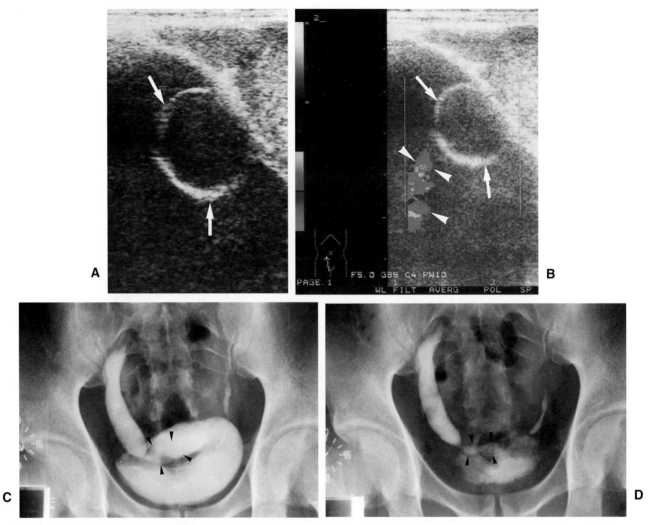

Fig. 3. Simple ureterocele in a 29-year-old man.
A. Transrectal US in right parasagittal plane shows a round cystic lesion *(arrows)* in the posterior wall of the urinary bladder. **B.** Color Doppler US in the same plane demonstrates urine flow *(arrowheads)* jetting from the top of the ureterocele *(arrows)*. (**B**, See also Color Section.) **C, D.** IVU images show changing size of the right ureterocele *(arrowheads)* and dilated right distal ureter.

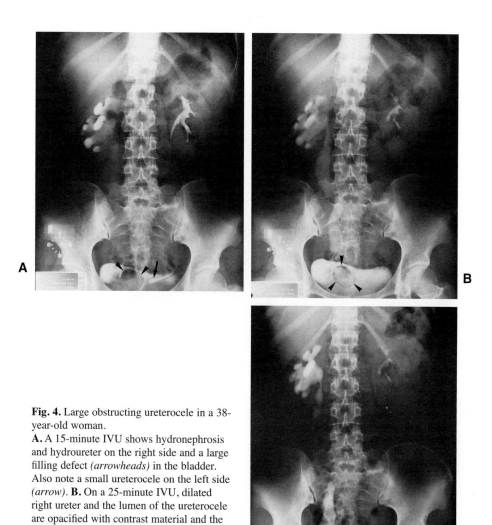

Fig. 4. Large obstructing ureterocele in a 38-year-old woman.
A. A 15-minute IVU shows hydronephrosis and hydroureter on the right side and a large filling defect *(arrowheads)* in the bladder. Also note a small ureterocele on the left side *(arrow)*. **B.** On a 25-minute IVU, dilated right ureter and the lumen of the ureterocele are opacified with contrast material and the radiolucent wall of the ureterocele is well defined *(arrowheads)*. **C.** Postvoiding image shows densely opacified ureterocele *(arrowheads)*.

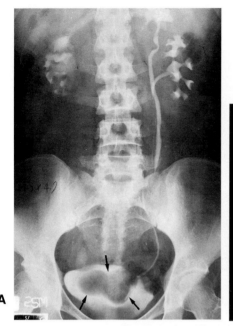

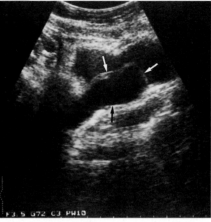

Fig. 5. A large ureterocele in a 36-year-old woman.
A. A 25-minute IVU shows shrunken right kidney with faint opacification. The right ureter is not opacified, and there is a large filling defect *(arrows)* in the urinary bladder. **B.** Longitudinal US of the bladder in the right parasagittal plane shows a dilated right distal ureter and a large ureterocele *(arrows)* bulging into the urinary bladder.

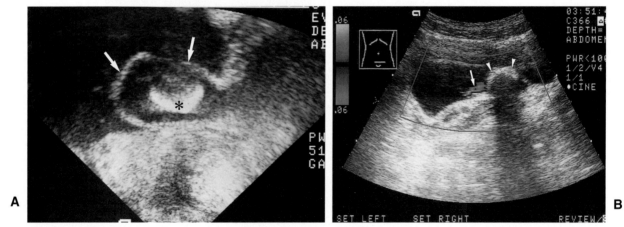

Fig. 6. US findings of ureterocele with a stone in a 34-year-old woman.
A. Transrectal US shows a round cystic lesion *(arrows)* in the left posterior aspect of the urinary bladder. Note a large stone *(asterisk)* in the ureterocele. **B.** Color Doppler US shows color signal of urine flow *(arrow)* jetting from the ureterocele containing a stone *(arrowheads)*. (**B,** See also Color Section.)

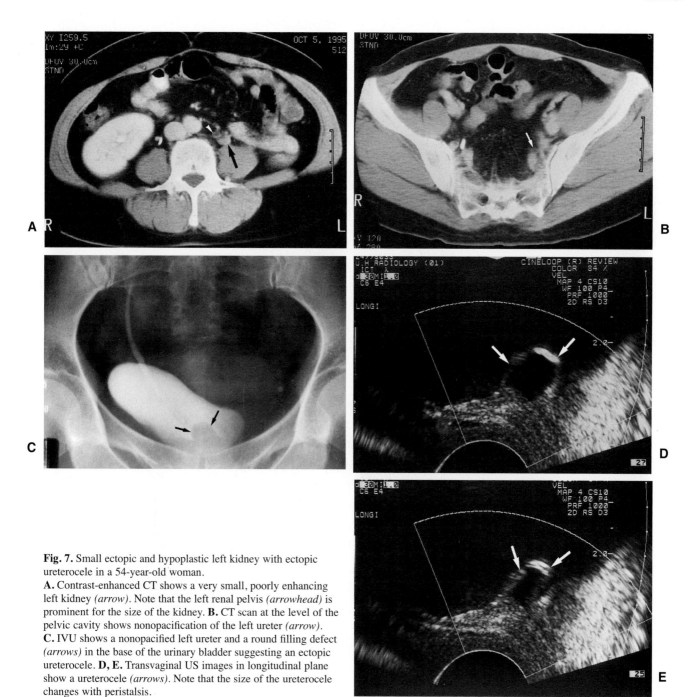

Fig. 7. Small ectopic and hypoplastic left kidney with ectopic
ureterocele in a 54-year-old woman.
A. Contrast-enhanced CT shows a very small, poorly enhancing
left kidney *(arrow)*. Note that the left renal pelvis *(arrowhead)* is
prominent for the size of the kidney. **B.** CT scan at the level of the
pelvic cavity shows nonopacification of the left ureter *(arrow)*.
C. IVU shows a nonopacified left ureter and a round filling defect
(arrows) in the base of the urinary bladder suggesting an ectopic
ureterocele. **D, E.** Transvaginal US images in longitudinal plane
show a ureterocele *(arrows)*. Note that the size of the ureterocele
changes with peristalsis.

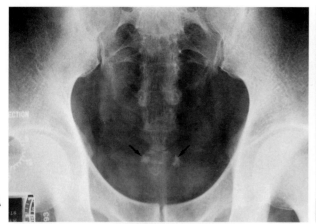

A

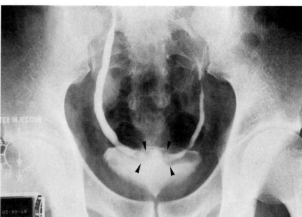

B

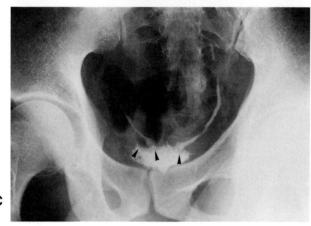

C

Fig. 8. Bilateral pseudoureteroceles due to stones in the ureterovesical junctions in a 26-year-old man. This condition should be differentiated from congenital ureterocele containing stones.

A. Plain radiograph shows two calcified stones *(arrows)* in the pelvic cavity. **B, C.** IVU images of the urinary bladder show dilated distal ureters and irregular, thick radiolucencies representing edema *(arrowheads)*.

15. Ectopic Ureteral Insertion

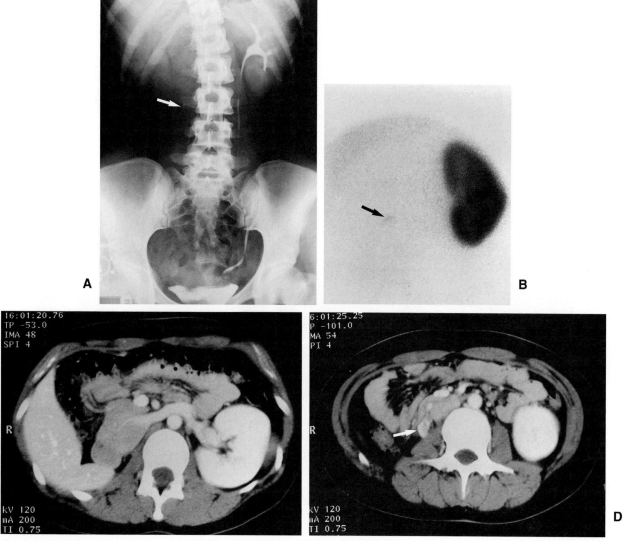

Fig. 1. Severe hypoplasia with ectopic ureteral orifice in a 19-year-old woman with incontinence.
A. A 15-minute IVU shows nonopacification of the right urinary tract, but there is a suspicious linear opacification in the right paravertebral region *(arrow)*. The left kidney is large due to compensatory hypertrophy. **B.** Dimercaptosuccinic acid (DMSA) radioisotope scan shows a large left kidney and a faint radioactivity in the right abdomen *(arrow)*. **C, D.** Contrast-enhanced CT scans show an absent right kidney in the normal location but a small enhancing kidney in the right paravertebral region *(arrow in* **D***)*. This hypoplastic right kidney was removed and the patient's incontinence disappeared.

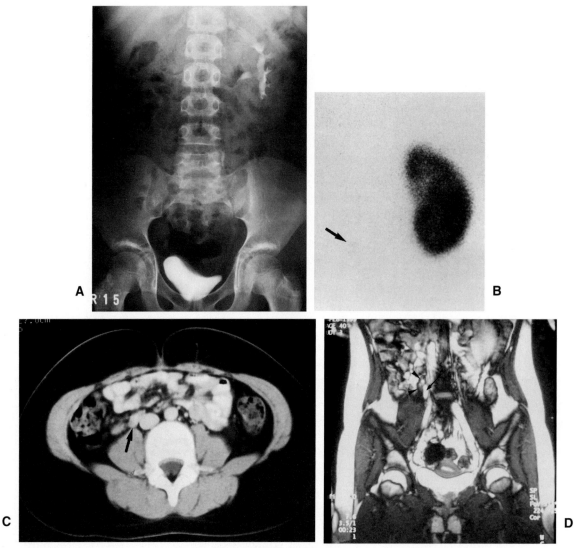

Fig. 2. Severe hypoplasia with ectopic ureteral orifice in a 10-year-old girl with incontinence.
A. A 15-minute IVU shows nonopacification of the right urinary tract. The left kidney is large due to compensatory hypertrophy. **B.** Dimercaptosuccinic acid (DMSA) scan shows large left kidney and a faint radioactivity in the right abdomen *(arrow)*. **C.** Contrast-enhanced CT shows a small enhancing kidney in the right paravertebral region *(arrow)*. **D.** T2-weighted coronal MR image well demonstrates the hypoplastic right kidney *(arrowheads)* and its renal pelvis *(arrow)*. This hypoplastic right kidney was removed and the patient's incontinence disappeared.

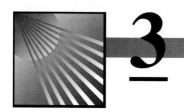

3

Benign Renal Tumors

JUNG SUK SIM AND WILLIAM H. BUSH, JR.

Benign renal tumors, excluding renal cysts, include angiomyolipoma, adenoma, oncocytoma, multilocular cystic nephroma, hemangioma, lymphangioma, and juxtaglomerular tumor. Many benign renal tumors are surgically removed because they cannot be differentiated from renal cell carcinoma.

ANGIOMYOLIPOMA

Angiomyolipoma is a hamartoma of the kidney and is composed of a varying proportion of blood vessels, smooth muscle, and fat. However, it may contain only one or two tissue elements, thus being a lipoma, leiomyoma, angiolipoma, angiomyoma, or myolipoma. About 10% of patients with angiomyolipoma have tuberous sclerosis, and 80% of patients with tuberous sclerosis have renal angiomyolipomas. Angiomyolipomas associated with tuberous sclerosis tend to be multiple and bilateral, whereas those not associated with tuberous sclerosis tend to be unilateral, solitary, large, and symptomatic.

Angiomyolipoma is a nonencapsulated, slow-growing, and expansile mass. Since angiomyolipoma has various components of tissues, its overall appearance is heterogeneous by both computed tomography (CT) and ultrasonography (US). It has abundant acoustic interfaces, so its echogenicity on US is usually very high. Although some small renal cell carcinomas have echogenicity higher than that of normal renal cortex, angiomyolipomas, especially small ones, are usually much more echogenic than renal cell carcinoma. Small echogenic renal cell carcinomas often have a peritumoral hypoechoic halo or intratumoral cysts, but these findings are not found with angiomyolipoma. Frequently the echogenicity of angiomyolipoma is similar to or even higher than that of the renal sinus. A quantitative method for representing the echogenicity of renal masses has been proposed. The gray-scale value of the renal sinus is designated as 100% and the renal cortex as 0%, and the echogenicity of the renal mass is a percentage value. Most of the renal cell carcinomas have a relative gray-scale value less than 80%, whereas nearly all of the angiomyolipomas have values higher than 80%. However, confirmation by nonenhanced CT is advised.

With CT, a renal tumor with fatty attenuation is almost always an angiomyolipoma. Therefore, detection of fatty attenuation in a mass is virtually diagnostic for angiomyolipoma. CT scanning should be done without intravenous contrast material, and thin-section collimation is needed since angiomyolipomas may have only small amounts of fat. The contrast-enhancing angiomyoma-

tous tissue may obscure the low Hounsfield values of fat. Of the few reported renal cell carcinomas containing fat, large tumors had engulfed perirenal or sinus fat, or the smaller tumors contained fat plus calcifications or heterogeneous ossification.

ADENOMA

It had been reported that renal cortical glandular tumors less than 3 cm in diameter rarely metastasize, so the tumors less than 3 cm should be considered benign. There had been a long controversy over the presence of benign renal tubular neoplasm until 1997, when the Union Internationale Contre le Cancer (UICC) and the American Joint Committee on Cancer (AJCC) Classification of Renal Cell Carcinoma workgroup classified the benign adenoma as a separate category of renal tumors. There are three kinds of renal adenoma on the basis of histology: papillary adenoma, metanephric adenoma, and oncocytoma. Papillary adenoma can have the appearance of solid, mixed solid and cystic, or cystic according to the amount of papillary elements. Imaging findings of metanephric adenoma are not well known.

ONCOCYTOMA

The oncocyte is a proximal tubular epithelial cell that has abundant acidophilic granules. Oncocytoma is a benign renal parenchymal tumor of proximal tubular epithelium and therefore is a renal tubular adenoma. The gross appearance of oncocytoma is of a well-encapsulated mass that sometimes has a central fibrous scar.

Radiologic findings of an oncocytoma are nonspecific, usually a well-marginated enhancing mass. When a cartwheel-like central scar is found, the diagnosis of oncocytoma is highly suggestive; however, the central scar appearance is not pathognomonic because a renal cell carcinoma can have central necrosis that resembles a scar.

MULTILOCULAR CYSTIC NEPHROMA

Multilocular cystic nephroma is a rare benign tumor consisting of multiple small cysts with intervening fibrous septa within a single large capsule. No communications exist between small cysts. Usually the tumor is large and calcification is often present on septa or capsule. There is no renal parenchymal tissue within septa, except dysplastic tissues that can be found

occasionally. Some fibrous tissues can enhance, and differentiation from cystic renal cell carcinoma can be difficult at times. Multilocular cystic nephroma does not change into renal cell carcinoma.

MISCELLANEOUS BENIGN RENAL TUMORS

Tumors of the juxtaglomerular cells, or reninoma, produce renin. It is a rare but a curable cause of hypertension. Usually the mass is small and solid.

Renal hemangiomas often occur in the renal pelvis and others occur in the renal parenchyma. They are usually small but can reach a size over 10 cm.

References

1. D'Angelo PC, Gash JR, Horn AW, et al: Fat in renal cell carcinoma that lacks associated calcifications. AJR Am J Roentgenol 2002; 178: 931–932.
2. Kim KW, Seo JB, Lee HJ, et al: Renal and pulmonary lymphangioleiomyomatosis: A case report. Eur J Radiol 2000; 36:126–129.
3. Lee CS, Lee SJ, Kang JH, et al: A case of renal oncocytomatosis with chronic renal failure. Korean J Nephrol 2000; 19:1173–1177.
4. Sim JS, Seo CS, Kim SH, et al: Differentiation of small hyperechoic renal cell carcinoma from angiomyolipoma: Computer-aided tissue echo quantification. J Ultrasound Med 1999; 18:261–264.
5. Lee W, Kim TS, Chung JW, et al: Renal angiomyolipoma: Embolotherapy with a mixture of alcohol and iodized oil. J Vasc Interv Radiol 1998; 9:255–261.
6. Storkel S, Eble JN, Adlakha K, et al: Classification of renal cell carcinoma: Workgroup No. 1. Union Internationale Contre le Cancer (UICC) and the American Joint Committee on Cancer (AJCC). Cancer 1997; 80:987–989.
7. Tongaonkar HB, Sampat MB, Dalal AV, et al: Bilateral renal angiomyolipoma. J Surg Oncol 1994; 57:65–70.
8. Davidson AJ, Hayes WS, Hartman DS, et al: Renal oncocytoma and carcinoma: Failure of differentiation with CT. Radiology 1993; 186:693–696.
9. Helenon O, Chretien Y, Paraf F, et al: Renal cell carcinoma containing fat: Demonstration with CT. Radiology 1993; 188:429–430.
10. Kurosaki Y, Tanaka Y, Kuramoto K, et al: Improved CT fat detection in small kidney angiomyolipomas using thin sections and single voxel measurements. J Comput Assist Tomogr 1993; 17:745–748.
11. Strotzer M, Lehner KB, Becker K: Detection of fat in a renal cell carcinoma mimicking angiomyolipoma. Radiology 1993; 188:427–428.
12. Takahashi K, Honda M, Okubo RS, et al: CT pixel mapping in the diagnosis of small angiomyolipomas of the kidneys. J Comput Assist Tomogr 1993; 17:98–101.
13. Radin DR, Chandrasoma P: CT demonstration of fat density in renal cell carcinoma. Acta Radiol 1992; 33:365–367.
14. Kim SH, Choi BI, Han MC, et al: Multilocular cystic nephroma: MR findings. AJR Am J Roentgenol 1989; 153:1317.
15. Banner MP, Pollack HM, Chatten J, et al: Multilocular renal cysts: Radiologic-pathologic correlation. AJR Am J Roentgenol 1981; 136:239–247.
16. Klein MJ, Valensi QJ: Proximal tubular adenomas of kidney with so-called oncocytic features: A clinicopathologic study of 13 cases of a rarely reported neoplasm. Cancer 1976; 38:906–914.

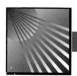

Illustrations • Benign Renal Tumors

1. Angiomyolipoma: Typical Findings

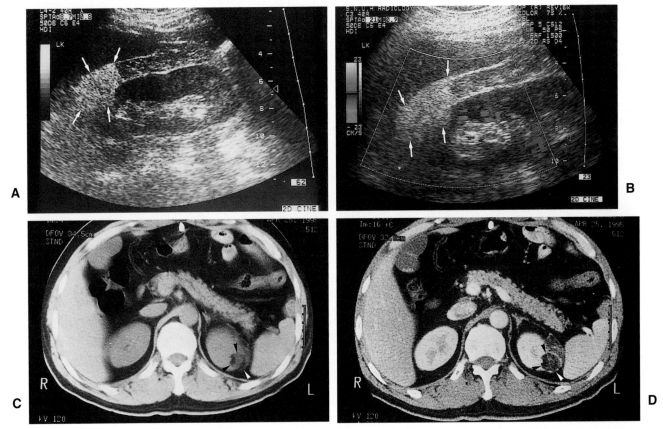

Fig. 1. Exophytic angiomyolipoma in a 45-year-old man.
A. Longitudinal US of the left kidney shows an exophytically growing echogenic mass *(arrows)* in the upper pole of the left kidney. Note that the echogenicity of the mass is similar to that of the renal sinus, and the posterior margin of the mass is ill-defined. **B.** Color Doppler US shows absence of flow signals within the mass *(arrows)*. (**B**, See also Color Section.) **C.** Nonenhanced CT shows a mass of fat attenuation *(arrowheads)* in the upper pole of the left kidney. **D.** Contrast-enhanced CT shows mottled enhancement in the mass *(arrowheads)*.

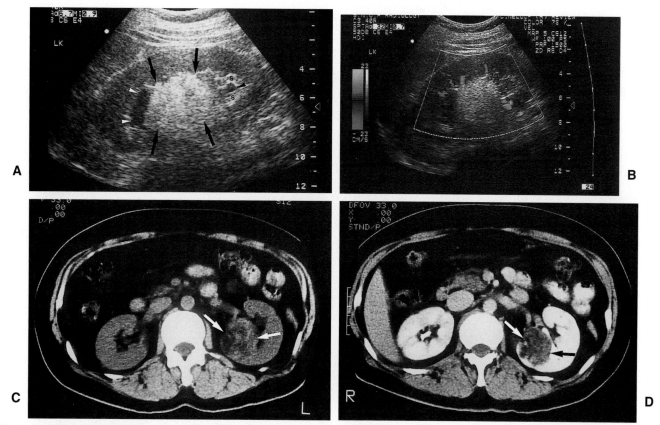

Fig. 2. Endophytic angiomyolipoma in a 46-year-old man.
A. Longitudinal US of the left kidney shows a large echogenic mass *(arrows)* with ill-defined posterior margin in the left kidney. Note that the echogenicity of the mass is higher than that of the renal sinus (s), and calyces are slightly dilated in the upper and lower poles *(arrowheads)*. **B.** No flow signals are demonstrated in the tumor on color Doppler US. (**B**, See also Color Section.) **C.** Nonenhanced CT shows an ill-defined mass *(arrows)* of mixed attenuation. **D.** Contrast-enhanced CT demonstrates the low-attenuated mass *(arrows)* in the left kidney.

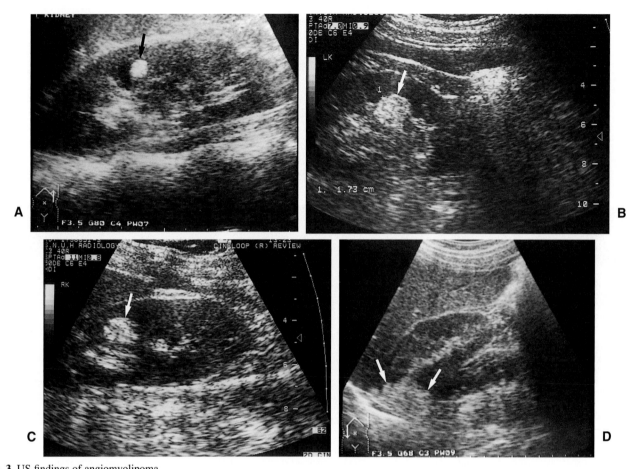

Fig. 3. US findings of angiomyolipoma.
A–D. US images of four different cases of angiomyolipoma show round echogenic masses *(arrows)*. Note that the echogenicity of the masses is the same or higher than that of the renal sinus. The masses do not show peritumoral halo or intratumoral cysts, which are characteristic US findings of small echogenic renal cell carcinomas.

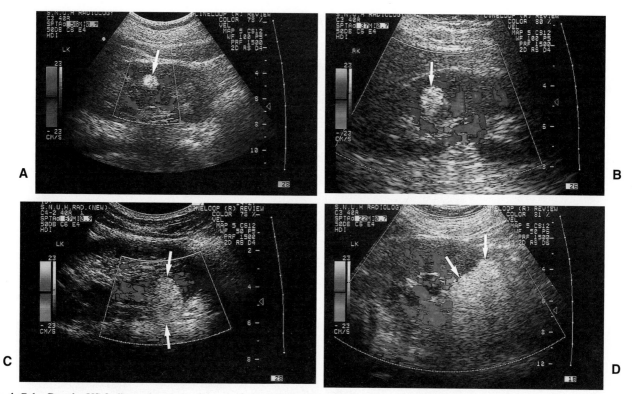

Fig. 4. Color Doppler US findings of angiomyolipoma. (**A–D**, See also Color Section.)
A–D. Color Doppler US images of four different cases of angiomyolipoma show no demonstrable flow signals in the mass *(arrows)* due to slow intratumoral blood flow even though most angiomyolipomas have vascular components by contrast-enhanced CT or angiography.

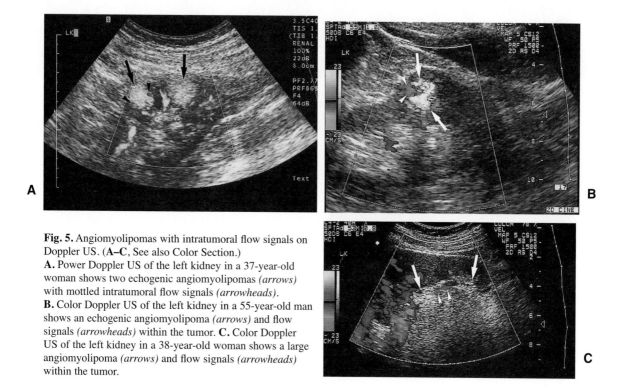

Fig. 5. Angiomyolipomas with intratumoral flow signals on Doppler US. (**A–C**, See also Color Section.)
A. Power Doppler US of the left kidney in a 37-year-old woman shows two echogenic angiomyolipomas *(arrows)* with mottled intratumoral flow signals *(arrowheads)*.
B. Color Doppler US of the left kidney in a 55-year-old man shows an echogenic angiomyolipoma *(arrows)* and flow signals *(arrowheads)* within the tumor. **C.** Color Doppler US of the left kidney in a 38-year-old woman shows a large angiomyolipoma *(arrows)* and flow signals *(arrowheads)* within the tumor.

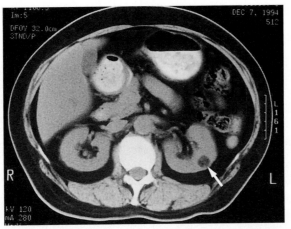

Fig. 6. Small angiomyolipoma in a 40-year-old woman. Nonenhanced CT shows a small, round mass of fatty attenuation *(arrow)* in the left kidney.

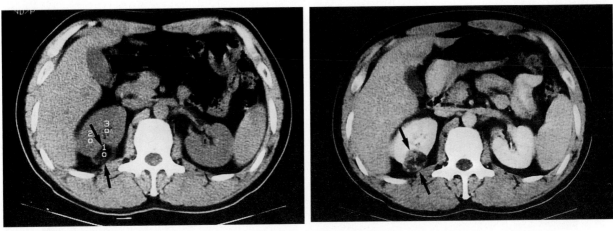

Fig. 7. Angiomyolipoma in a 39-year-old man.
A. Nonenhanced CT demonstrates only fatty component of the tumor *(arrows)*. **B.** Contrast-enhanced CT demonstrates the fatty and nonfatty components of the tumor *(arrows)*.

2. Angiomyolipoma: Atypical Findings

Pat. Name:
Pat. ID: 2661180-6
Report #4

Exam: 13917
Series: 3
Image: 10

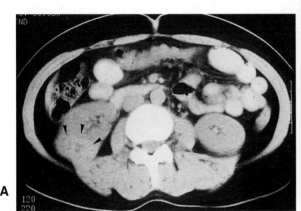

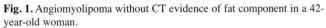

	120	121	122	123	124	125	126	127	128	129	130
321	27	34	34	24	13	8	13	13	15	24	23
322	38	34	20	9	10	15	19	25	33	40	37
323	38	35	23	13	11	15	22	36	45	46	43
324	30	25	18	21	23	25	27	35	38	33	33
325	31	33	29	30	35	36	39	43	39	27	23
326	13	21	30	31	20	18	27	36	36	26	23
327	6	4	19	25	12	10	27	40	43	42	37
328	1	4	18	28	21	23	40	41	40	50	59
329	10	10	22	29	22	20	35	36	28	39	51
330	16	8	21	35	29	25	37	43	46	51	48
331	20	13	25	34	29	27	35	43	48	54	54

A

B

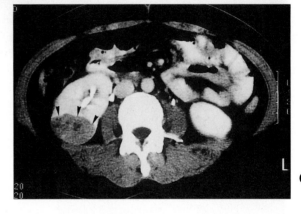

Fig. 1. Angiomyolipoma without CT evidence of fat component in a 42-year-old woman.
A. Nonenhanced CT shows a right renal mass *(arrowheads)* that has an attenuation slightly higher than that of the renal parenchyma. **B.** CT number mapping does not reveal any evidence of fat in the tumor. **C.** Contrast-enhanced CT shows a heterogeneous, low-attenuated mass *(arrowheads)* in the right kidney. This mass would need to be treated as if it were a renal cell carcinoma since the CT images do not permit a confident diagnosis of angiomyolipoma or suggest oncocytoma.

C

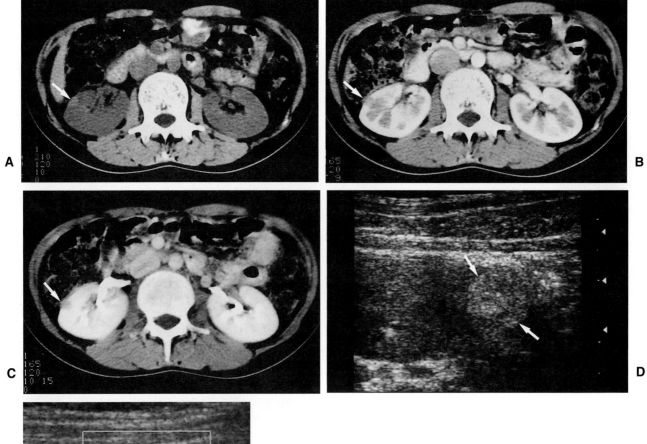

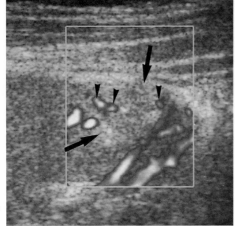

Fig. 2. Small angiomyolipoma appearing as a high-attenuated nodule on nonenhanced CT in a 37-year-old woman.
A. Nonenhanced CT shows a small, round, high-attenuated mass *(arrow)* in the right kidney. **B, C.** Contrast-enhanced CT scans in cortical (**B**) and excretory (**C**) phases show slight but prolonged enhancement of the mass *(arrow)*. **D.** Magnified US image shows heterogeneous hyperechogenicity of the mass without hypoechoic halo or intratumoral cysts *(arrows)*. **E.** Power Doppler US of the kidney shows subtle flow signals *(arrowheads)* within the mass *(arrows)*. Therefore, imaging does not provide a specific diagnosis of angiomyolipoma. (**E**, See also Color Section.)

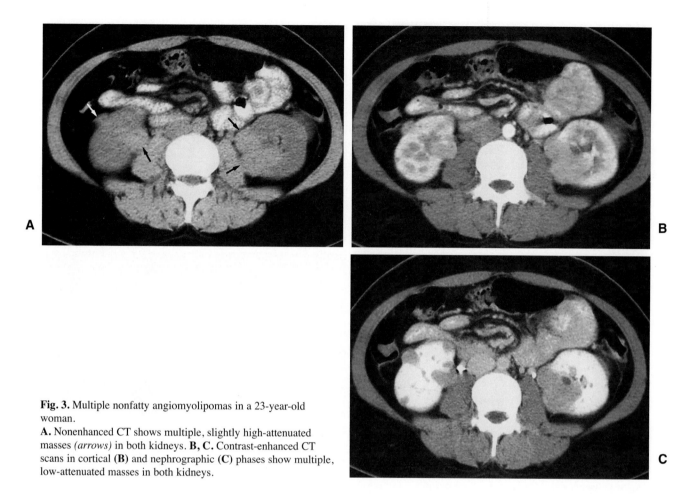

Fig. 3. Multiple nonfatty angiomyolipomas in a 23-year-old woman.
A. Nonenhanced CT shows multiple, slightly high-attenuated masses *(arrows)* in both kidneys. **B, C.** Contrast-enhanced CT scans in cortical **(B)** and nephrographic **(C)** phases show multiple, low-attenuated masses in both kidneys.

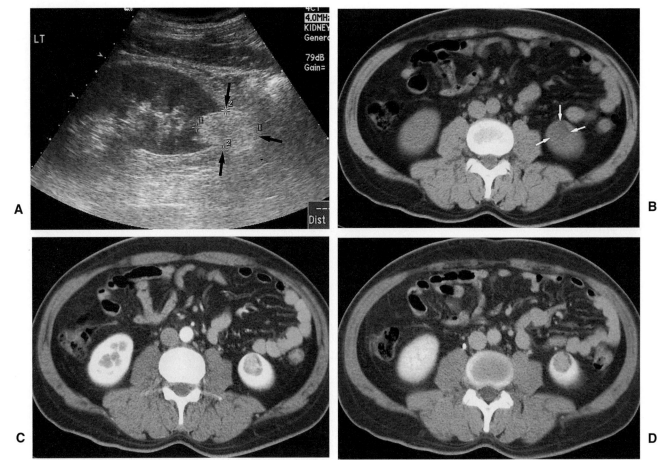

Fig. 4. Angiomyolipoma without definite fatty component in a 44-year-old man.
A. Longitudinal US of the left kidney shows an exophytic, echogenic mass *(arrows)* in the lower polar region. **B.** Nonenhanced CT shows suspicious mass in the lower pole of the left kidney with subtle, low-attenuated component in the periphery of the mass *(arrows)*. However, measurement of CT numbers in this region did not reveal fat. **C, D.** Contrast-enhanced CT scans in cortical **(C)** and nephrographic **(D)** phases show slightly heterogeneous and persistent contrast enhancement.

3. Angiomyolipoma in Tuberous Sclerosis

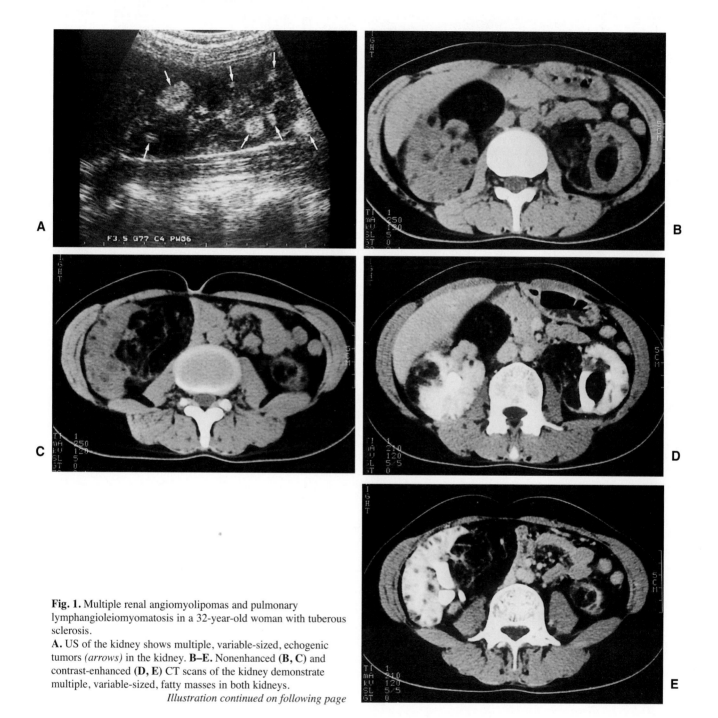

Fig. 1. Multiple renal angiomyolipomas and pulmonary lymphangioleiomyomatosis in a 32-year-old woman with tuberous sclerosis.
A. US of the kidney shows multiple, variable-sized, echogenic tumors *(arrows)* in the kidney. **B–E.** Nonenhanced **(B, C)** and contrast-enhanced **(D, E)** CT scans of the kidney demonstrate multiple, variable-sized, fatty masses in both kidneys.

Illustration continued on following page

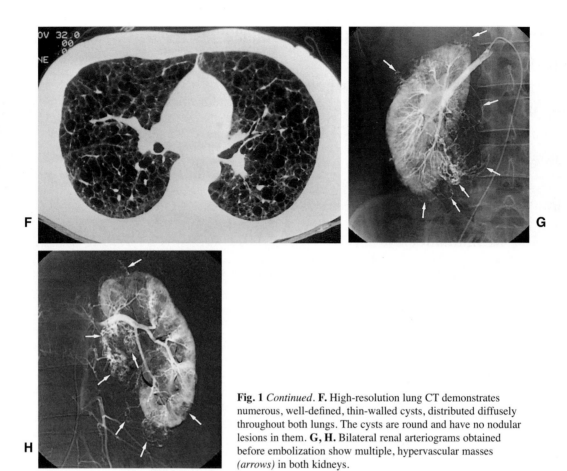

Fig. 1 *Continued*. **F.** High-resolution lung CT demonstrates numerous, well-defined, thin-walled cysts, distributed diffusely throughout both lungs. The cysts are round and have no nodular lesions in them. **G, H.** Bilateral renal arteriograms obtained before embolization show multiple, hypervascular masses *(arrows)* in both kidneys.

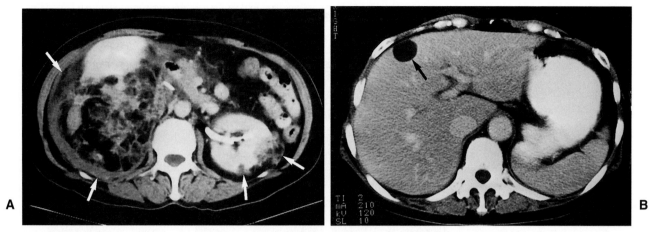

Fig. 2. Renal angiomyolipomas and a hepatic lipoma in a 59-year-old woman with tuberous sclerosis.
A. Contrast-enhanced CT scan shows large angiomyolipomas *(arrows)* in both kidneys. **B.** CT scan of the liver shows a round fatty mass *(arrow)* in the liver.

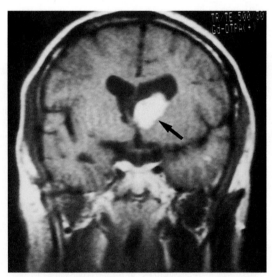

Fig. 3. Giant cell astrocytoma in a 22-year-old man with tuberous sclerosis and multiple renal angiomyolipomas. T1-weighted contrast-enhanced brain MR image in coronal plane shows a strongly enhancing mass *(arrow)* in the floor of the left lateral ventricle.

4. Angiomyolipoma with Retroperitoneal Hemorrhage

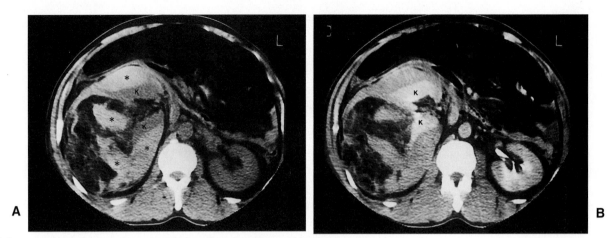

Fig. 1. Large angiomyolipoma with perirenal hemorrhage in a 44-year-old man.
A, B. Nonenhanced (**A**) and contrast-enhanced (**B**) CT scans show a large fatty mass in the right kidney associated with large amount of perirenal hematoma *(asterisks in* **A***)*. Right nephrectomy was done in this patient. K, remnant renal parenchyma.

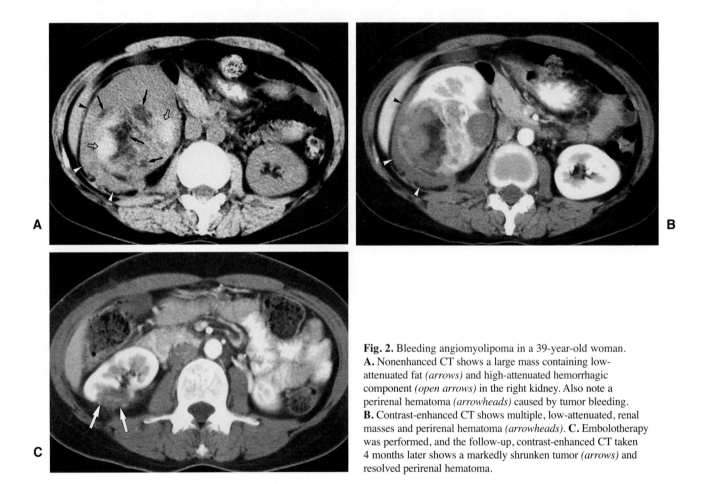

Fig. 2. Bleeding angiomyolipoma in a 39-year-old woman.
A. Nonenhanced CT shows a large mass containing low-attenuated fat *(arrows)* and high-attenuated hemorrhagic component *(open arrows)* in the right kidney. Also note a perirenal hematoma *(arrowheads)* caused by tumor bleeding.
B. Contrast-enhanced CT shows multiple, low-attenuated, renal masses and perirenal hematoma *(arrowheads)*. **C.** Embolotherapy was performed, and the follow-up, contrast-enhanced CT taken 4 months later shows a markedly shrunken tumor *(arrows)* and resolved perirenal hematoma.

5. Angiomyolipoma: Postembolization Changes

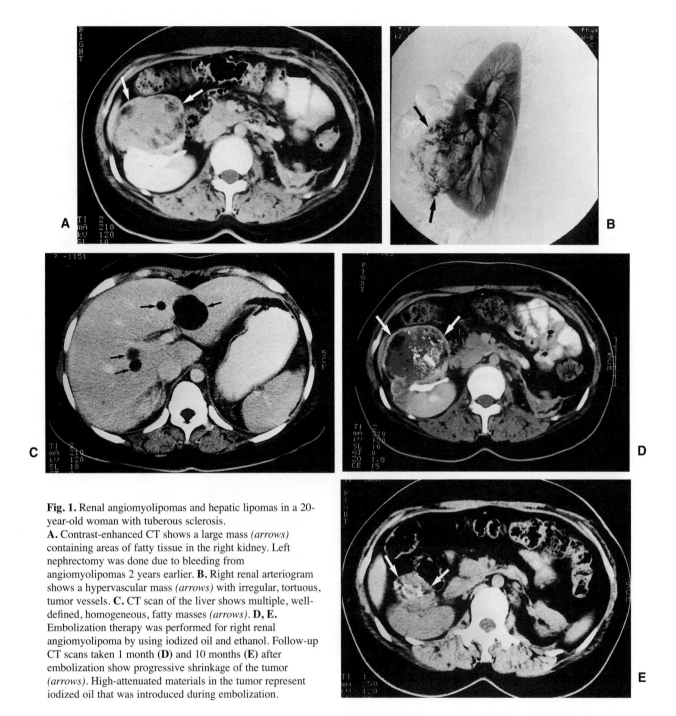

Fig. 1. Renal angiomyolipomas and hepatic lipomas in a 20-year-old woman with tuberous sclerosis.
A. Contrast-enhanced CT shows a large mass *(arrows)* containing areas of fatty tissue in the right kidney. Left nephrectomy was done due to bleeding from angiomyolipomas 2 years earlier. **B.** Right renal arteriogram shows a hypervascular mass *(arrows)* with irregular, tortuous, tumor vessels. **C.** CT scan of the liver shows multiple, well-defined, homogeneous, fatty masses *(arrows)*. **D, E.** Embolization therapy was performed for right renal angiomyolipoma by using iodized oil and ethanol. Follow-up CT scans taken 1 month **(D)** and 10 months **(E)** after embolization show progressive shrinkage of the tumor *(arrows)*. High-attenuated materials in the tumor represent iodized oil that was introduced during embolization.

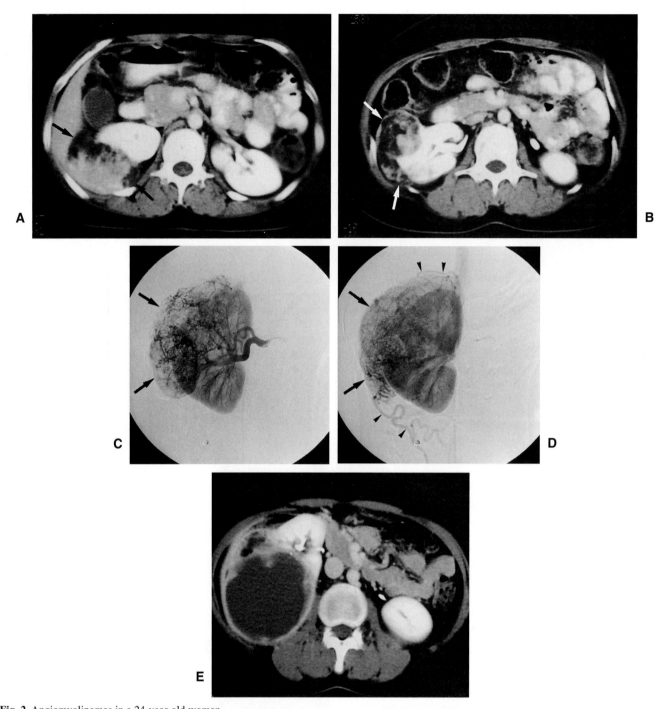

Fig. 2. Angiomyolipomas in a 24-year-old woman.
A, B. Contrast-enhanced CT scans show renal masses *(arrows)* that contain fatty and nonfatty components. **C.** Right renal arteriograms in arterial phase shows large hypervascular masses *(arrows)* in the peripheral portion of the right kidney. **D.** The tumor vessels are still opacified in a venous-phase angiogram, suggesting slow blood flow in the tumor *(arrows)*. Note the prominent veins *(arrowheads)* draining the tumors. **E.** Embolization was performed with iodized oil and ethanol. Follow-up CT scan taken 8 months later shows a markedly enlarged right kidney due to cystic changes of the tumor.

6. Renal Adenoma

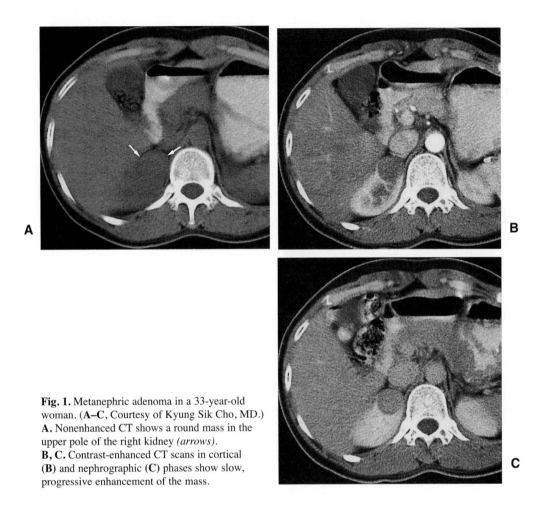

Fig. 1. Metanephric adenoma in a 33-year-old woman. (**A–C**, Courtesy of Kyung Sik Cho, MD.)
A. Nonenhanced CT shows a round mass in the upper pole of the right kidney *(arrows)*.
B, C. Contrast-enhanced CT scans in cortical (**B**) and nephrographic (**C**) phases show slow, progressive enhancement of the mass.

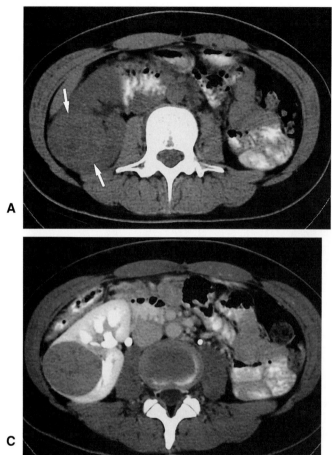

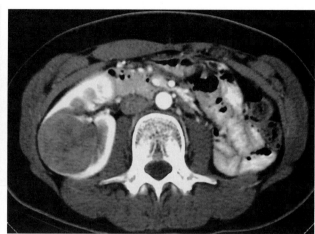

Fig. 2. Metanephric adenoma in a 25-year-old woman (**A–C**, Courtesy of Bohyun Kim, MD.)
A. Nonenhanced CT shows a large, well-defined, round mass *(arrows)* in the right kidney. The attenuation of the mass is slightly higher than that of the renal parenchyma. **B, C.** Contrast-enhanced CT scans in cortical (**B**) and pyelographic (**C**) phases show persistent, homogeneous enhancement of the mass.

7. Renal Oncocytoma

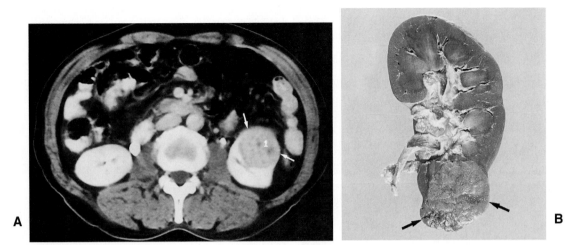

Fig. 1. Renal oncocytoma in a 56-year-old man.
A. Contrast-enhanced CT shows a round mass *(arrows)* in the left kidney. The mass shows strong, homogeneous enhancement in this excretory-phase CT. **B.** Photograph of the removed kidney shows a well-defined mass *(arrows)* with fibrous scar and focal hemorrhage in the lower pole of the left kidney. (**B**, See also Color Section.)

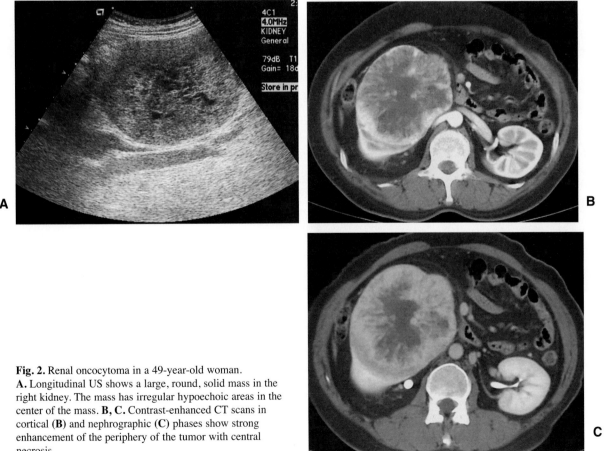

Fig. 2. Renal oncocytoma in a 49-year-old woman.
A. Longitudinal US shows a large, round, solid mass in the right kidney. The mass has irregular hypoechoic areas in the center of the mass. **B, C.** Contrast-enhanced CT scans in cortical (**B**) and nephrographic (**C**) phases show strong enhancement of the periphery of the tumor with central necrosis.

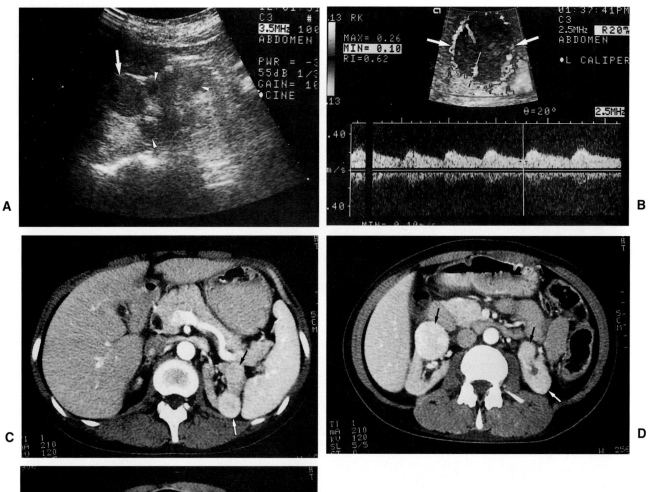

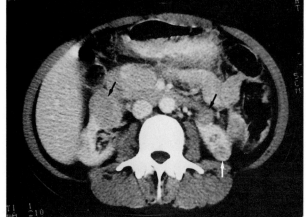

Fig. 3. Renal oncocytomatosis in a 30-year-old woman with chronic renal failure.
A. US of the right kidney shows a round, hypoechoic mass *(arrow)* in the left kidney. Also note suspicious, multiple, small, hypoechoic masses *(arrowheads)* in the same kidney. **B.** Doppler US performed on one of the right renal masses shows spoke wheel–pattern vessels *(arrows)* in the tumor. Spectral Doppler US demonstrates low-resistance arterial flow pattern.
C, D. Contrast-enhanced CT scans in early arterial phase show contracted kidneys and multiple, round, enhancing masses *(arrows)* in both kidneys. **E.** CT scan in delayed phase shows that the attenuation of the masses *(arrows)* is lower than that of the renal parenchyma. (**E,** From Lee CS, Lee SJ, Kang JH, et al: A case of renal oncocytomatosis with chronic renal failure. Korean J Nephrol 2000; 19:1173–1177.)

8. Multilocular Cystic Nephroma

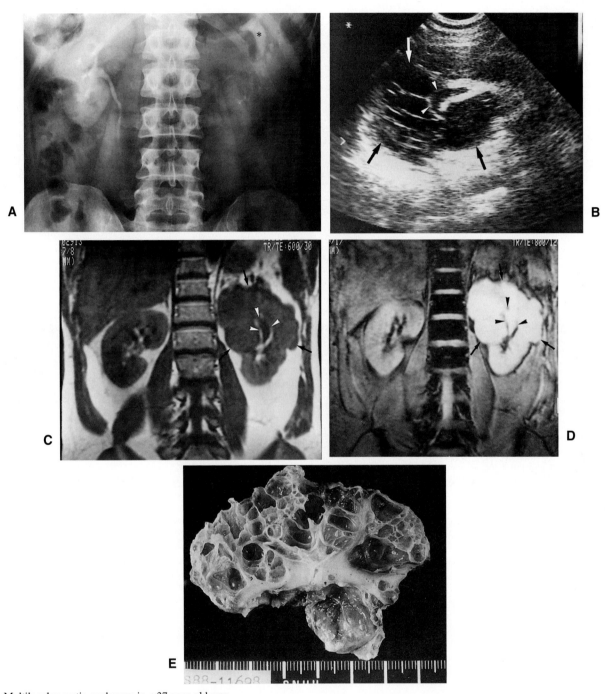

Fig. 1. Multilocular cystic nephroma in a 37-year-old man.
A. IVU shows compression effect on the pelvocalyces of the left kidney with dilation of the upper pole calyx *(asterisk)*. **B.** Longitudinal US of the left kidney demonstrates a multiloculated cystic mass *(arrows)* in the upper pole and a dilated upper polar calyx *(arrowheads)*. **C, D.** T1-weighted spin-echo **(C)** and T2-weighted gradient-echo **(D)** MR images in coronal plane show a large, multiloculated, cystic mass *(arrows)* in the upper pole of the left kidney. Note the dilated upper-pole calyx *(arrowheads)*. (**C,** From Kim SH, Choi BI, Han MC, et al: Multilocular cystic nephroma: MR findings. AJR Am J Roentgenol 1989; 153:1317.) **E.** Photograph of the removed mass shows multiloculated appearance.

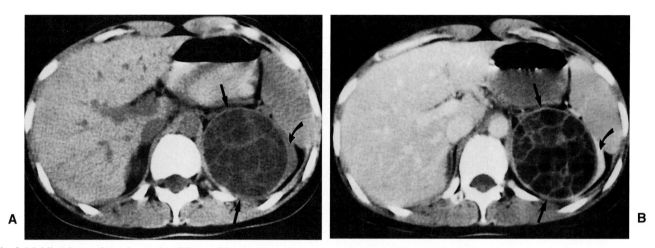

Fig. 2. Multilocular cystic nephroma in a 26-year-old woman.
A, B. Nonenhanced (**A**) and contrast-enhanced (**B**) CT scans show a large, round, multiloculated cystic mass surrounded by a thick capsule *(arrows)* in the upper pole of the left kidney. Note abundant internal septa and compressed renal parenchyma *(curved arrow)* lateral to the mass.

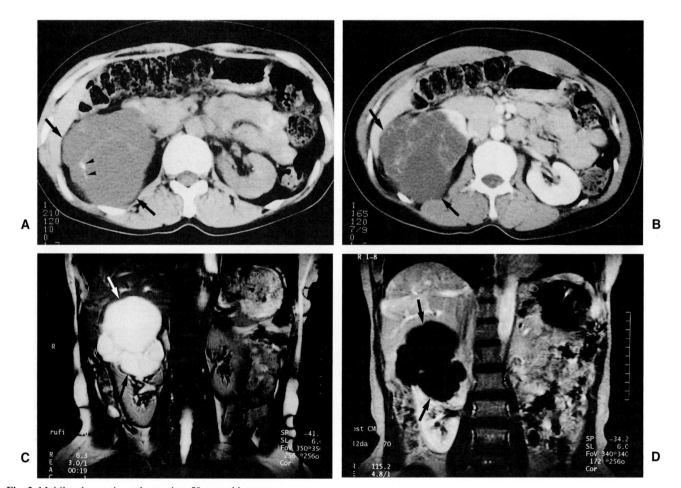

Fig. 3. Multilocular cystic nephroma in a 50-year-old woman.
A, B. Nonenhanced (**A**) and contrast-enhanced (**B**) CT scans show a large, multiloculated cystic mass *(arrows)* in the right kidney. Note calcifications *(arrowheads* in **A**) in the septa. **C, D.** T2-weighted (**C**) and contrast-enhanced T1-weighted gradient-echo (**D**) MR images in coronal plane demonstrate the multiloculated cystic mass *(arrows)* in the upper pole of the right kidney.

9. Miscellaneous Benign Renal Parenchymal Tumors

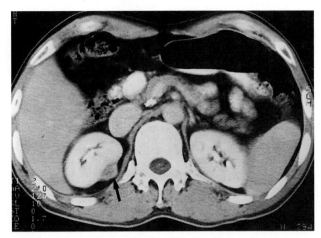

Fig. 1. Renal capsular leiomyoma in a 45-year-old man. Contrast-enhanced CT shows a small, lentiform, low-attenuated mass *(arrow)* in the right kidney. Note that the mass is slightly heterogeneous in attenuation.

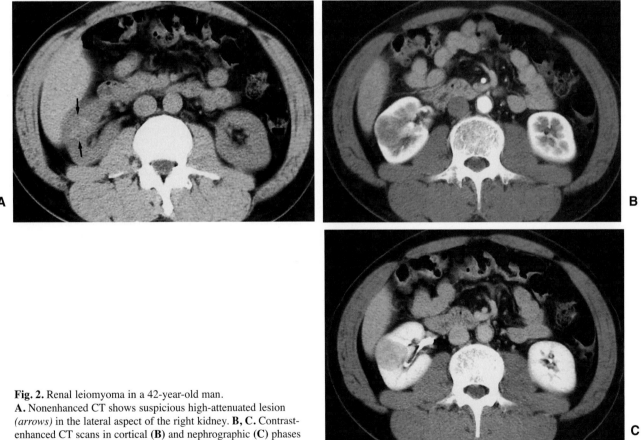

A

B

C

Fig. 2. Renal leiomyoma in a 42-year-old man.
A. Nonenhanced CT shows suspicious high-attenuated lesion *(arrows)* in the lateral aspect of the right kidney. **B, C.** Contrast-enhanced CT scans in cortical **(B)** and nephrographic **(C)** phases show a round mass in the right kidney.

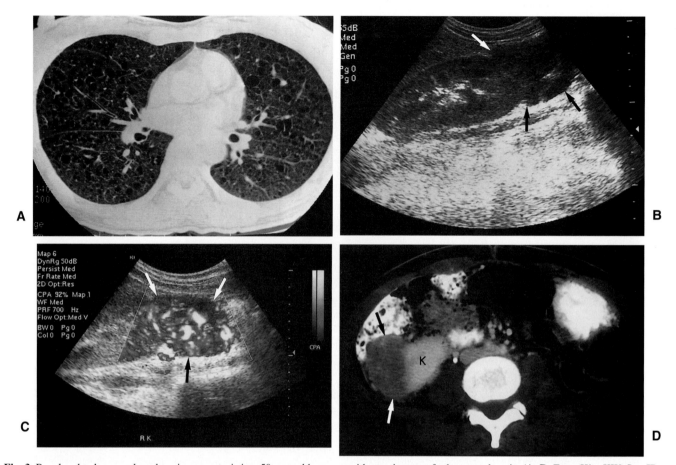

Fig. 3. Renal and pulmonary lymphangiomyomatosis in a 50-year-old woman without stigmata of tuberous sclerosis. (**A, D**, From Kim KW, Seo JB, Lee HJ, et al: Renal and pulmonary lymphangioleiomyomatosis: A case report. Eur J Radiol 2000; 36:126–129.)
A. High-resolution lung CT shows numerous, well-defined, thin-walled cysts, distributed diffusely throughout both lungs. **B.** Longitudinal US shows a large hypoechoic mass *(arrows)* in the lower pole of the right kidney. **C.** Power Doppler US shows hypervascularity of the mass *(arrows)*. (**C,** See also Color Section.) **D.** Contrast-enhanced CT shows a low-attenuated mass *(arrows)* in the lower pole of the right kidney (K).

9. Miscellaneous Benign Renal Parenchymal Tumors

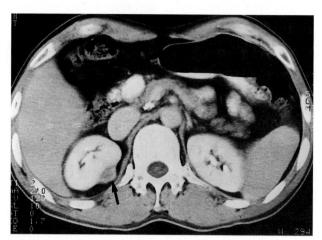

Fig. 1. Renal capsular leiomyoma in a 45-year-old man. Contrast-enhanced CT shows a small, lentiform, low-attenuated mass *(arrow)* in the right kidney. Note that the mass is slightly heterogeneous in attenuation.

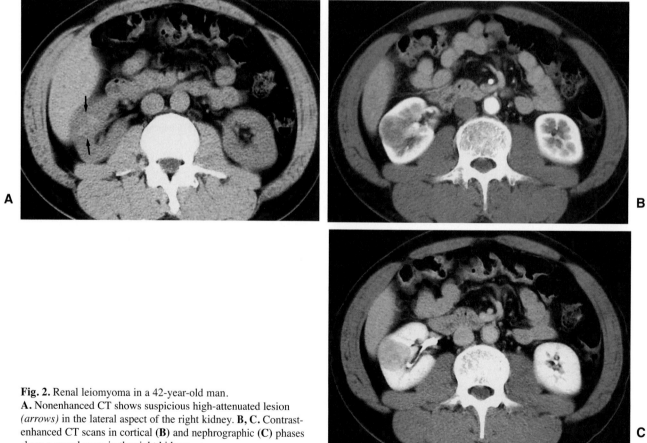

Fig. 2. Renal leiomyoma in a 42-year-old man.
A. Nonenhanced CT shows suspicious high-attenuated lesion *(arrows)* in the lateral aspect of the right kidney. **B, C.** Contrast-enhanced CT scans in cortical **(B)** and nephrographic **(C)** phases show a round mass in the right kidney.

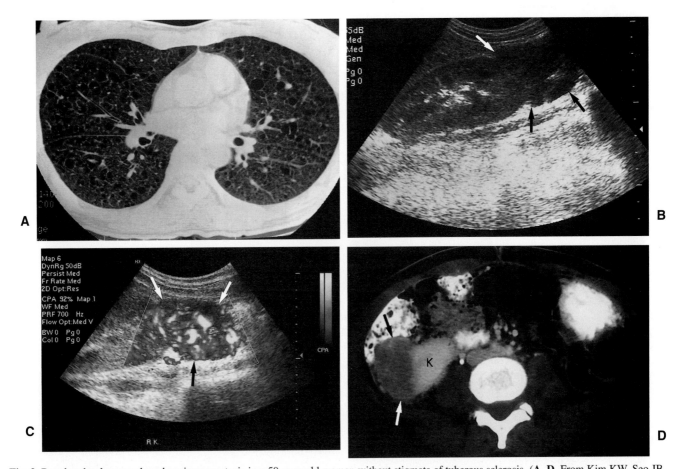

Fig. 3. Renal and pulmonary lymphangiomyomatosis in a 50-year-old woman without stigmata of tuberous sclerosis. (**A, D,** From Kim KW, Seo JB, Lee HJ, et al: Renal and pulmonary lymphangioleiomyomatosis: A case report. Eur J Radiol 2000; 36:126–129.)
A. High-resolution lung CT shows numerous, well-defined, thin-walled cysts, distributed diffusely throughout both lungs. **B.** Longitudinal US shows a large hypoechoic mass *(arrows)* in the lower pole of the right kidney. **C.** Power Doppler US shows hypervascularity of the mass *(arrows)*. (**C,** See also Color Section.) **D.** Contrast-enhanced CT shows a low-attenuated mass *(arrows)* in the lower pole of the right kidney (K).

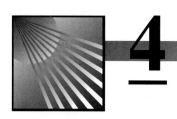

4

Malignant Renal Parenchymal Tumors

JUNG SUK SIM

Because renal cell carcinoma is the most common solid renal neoplasm, diagnosis of a renal mass is virtually a differentiation of renal cell carcinoma from other tumors. A solid mass in the kidneys can be considered renal cell carcinoma unless strong evidence that suggests another diagnosis is found. Cystic renal cell carcinomas comprise a smaller portion of all cystic renal masses, but differentiation of cystic renal cell carcinoma from the benign renal cysts is critical in the management of renal tumors. Lymphomas, metastases, and various sarcomas are other solid tumors of the kidney. Because lymphomas and metastases have unique clinical settings, most cases can be diagnosed easily. Sarcomas are unusually large and have grotesque appearance.

RENAL CELL CARCINOMA

Renal cell carcinomas originate from renal tubular epithelium, usually in the cortex. Peak incidence is between the 4th and 6th decades of life with a male predominance. Gross appearance of renal cell carcinoma is spherical and often shows areas of necrosis and hemorrhage. Growing larger, renal cell carcinoma involves perirenal space, renal vein, renal pelvis, and sinus.

A new histologic classification proposed by the Union Internationale Contre le Cancer (UICC) and the American Joint Committee on Cancer (AJCC) in 1997 is widely accepted. It is based on morphology and genetics and correlates well with prognosis. This is divided into clear cell type (70%), papillary type (10% to 15%), chromophobe type (5%), collecting duct carcinoma (1%), and unclassified type (4% to 5%). Sarcomatoid variant, previously known as sarcomatoid type, is not considered a type of its own since it arises from all other types of carcinomas and there is no evidence of de novo development of sarcomatoid carcinoma. Clear cell–type renal cell carcinomas have a tendency toward stronger enhancement than other subtypes. Chromophobe type shows a solid and silent appearance, whereas others are mixed solid and cystic and infiltrative.

Staging of renal cell carcinoma designed by Robson is widely used. The stages are the following:

I: tumor within the renal capsule
II: tumor spread to the perirenal fat and/or adrenal gland
IIIA: venous tumor invasion
IIIB: regional lymph node metastasis
IIIC: venous invasion and regional node metastasis

IVA: direct invasion beyond Gerota's fascia
IVB: distant metastasis

Classic findings of renal cell carcinoma on intravenous urography (IVU) consist of mass effect, notching of the renal pelvis and ureter due to collateral venous engorgement, obstruction or invasion of the collecting system, and calcification.

With wide use of abdominal ultrasonography (US), renal cell carcinomas are first detected more and more at the time a US is performed. Larger tumors are usually hypoechoic or isoechoic to renal parenchyma, whereas more than half of small renal cell carcinomas are hyperechoic. Typically small renal cell carcinomas show hyperechogenicity, intratumoral cyst, and thin hypoechoic rim. Major differential diagnosis of small renal cell carcinoma is a small angiomyolipoma that shows higher echogenicity with strong sonic attenuation. As renal cell carcinomas grow, they often show heterogeneous echogenicity due to internal necrosis and hemorrhage. US is useful to demonstrate the extent of venous thrombosis but is not adequate to detect lymph node metastasis.

Computed tomography (CT) is the modality of choice in staging renal cell carcinoma. On nonenhanced CT, renal cell carcinoma usually has an attenuation similar to the surrounding parenchyma but may show high attenuation if hemorrhage is present in the tumor. After injection of contrast material, it usually shows heterogeneous enhancement, but its enhancement seldom exceeds that of the surrounding normal parenchyma. Most larger tumors and some small tumors show areas of necrosis or hemorrhage. CT scan well demonstrates calcification in the tumor.

Differentiation between stages I and II, such as absence or presence of perirenal fat involvement, is not so important since stage I and II disease are treated the same, that is, with radical nephrectomy. Radiologic findings suggesting perirenal fat invasion consist of stranding, collateral vessels, fat obliteration, discrete soft tissue mass, and fascial thickening. Among them, a mass larger than 1 cm is the only strong evidence of perirenal invasion and thus would be considered stage II. Other findings are neither sensitive nor specific, with both sensitivity and specificity around 50%. Findings of renal vein invasion include filling defect in the renal vein, enlargement of the renal vein, and development of collateral vessels.

Magnetic resonance (MR) imaging is not commonly used to diagnose a renal cell carcinoma. However, it is regarded as the most accurate method to evaluate the extent of venous thrombosis.

CYSTIC RENAL CELL CARCINOMA

Most renal cell carcinomas contain some cystic portions, but the lesion is called *cystic renal cell carcinoma* when the cystic component predominates. About 15% of renal cell carcinomas are radiologically cystic. Cystic renal cell carcinomas can be divided into three different patterns: unilocular, multilocular, and discrete. Among them, unilocular cystic renal cell carcinoma is most common. Pathogenesis of cystic renal cell carcinoma is suggested variously according to the necrotic and solid component, intrinsic cystic growth (cystadenocarcinoma), or origin from the wall of benign cyst.

Unilocular cystic renal cell carcinoma contains a large area of cystic component. The wall of the cyst is usually thick and irregular, and the internal content usually looks dirty or has debris. Variable-sized, noncommunicating cysts separated by irregular, thick, fibrous septa characterize multilocular cystic renal cell carcinoma. Dystrophic calcification in the capsule or septa may be present. Differentiation between complicated cyst and cystic renal cell carcinoma is often problematic.

Bosniak proposed a classification system for cystic renal masses. Category I lesions are simple benign cysts. Category II lesions are minimally complicated cysts that may have thin septa, minimal calcification, and high internal density. Category III lesions are more complicated cysts that exhibit features of malignancy. Category IV lesions are definitively malignant ones. However, differentiation of class II lesion from class III is still problematic. Class II lesions are exophytic (more than a quarter of the lesion) and show a smooth outer margin, homogeneous internal content, and no enhancement. When a lesion fulfills all these criteria, then it can be classified into category II. When a lesion does not neatly fall into category II but does not need surgical exploration, we categorize that lesion into IIF and do a 6-month follow-up to detect any change.

RENAL LYMPHOMA

Because the kidney has no intrinsic lymphoid tissue, primary renal lymphoma is rare. However, the kidney is one of the most common extranodal sites of metastatic lymphoma. Lymphoma is the third most common metastatic cancer to the kidney, following breast and lung cancers. Non-Hodgkin's lymphoma is more common than Hodgkin's disease, but its appearance is not different.

Radiologic findings of renal lymphoma depend on the mechanism of renal involvement. The most common finding is direct invasion of retroperitoneal mass into the renal sinus, closely followed by multiple nodules in the kidney. Other manifestations of renal lymphoma include solitary mass, gross enlargement of the kidneys due to diffuse infiltration, and perirenal mass. On CT and US, lymphoma mass is characteristically homogeneous. On CT the mass enhances little, and on US the mass appears hypoechoic without posterior enhancement. Sometimes the echogenicity of the mass is very low and therefore the lesion may be mistaken for a cystic lesion.

RENAL SARCOMAS

Various sarcomas can occur in the kidney, and they include leiomyosarcoma, hemangiopericytoma, liposarcoma, rhab-domyosarcoma, and malignant fibrous histiocytoma. Renal sarcomas are usually very large, center at the periphery of kidney, and grow exophytically. Leiomyosarcoma is the most frequent, accounting for more than half of all sarcomas of the kidney. It often arises from the renal capsule, but there is no specific finding for leiomyosarcoma and it is often indistinguishable from renal cell carcinoma. Radiologic findings are not specific for a specific sarcoma.

METASTATIC TUMORS

Metastatic tumors are not difficult to diagnose because they are usually multiple and bilateral and have a known site of the origin. However, a large solitary renal mass in a patient with controlled malignancy is problematic. Metastatic renal tumors tend to have a multiple, small, ill-marginated, and less exophytic nature on CT and homogeneous, isoechoic appearance on US. The incidence of metastasis of solitary renal nodule in a known cancer patient is higher than that of the primary renal cell carcinoma. When the differentiation between primary and metastatic tumor is uncertain, biopsy confirmation is needed to make a therapeutic plan. The most common original site is lung, followed by breast, contralateral kidney, and colon.

WILMS' TUMORS IN ADULTS

Wilms' tumor is a disease of childhood and is rare in the adult population. There is no distinguishing feature from renal cell carcinoma, and preoperatively Wilms' tumor is frequently mistaken for renal cell carcinoma.

References

1. Moch H, Gasser T, Amin MB, et al: Prognostic utility of the recently recommended histologic classification and revised TNM staging system of renal cell carcinoma: A Swiss experience with 588 tumors. Cancer 2000; 89:604–614.
2. Sheafor DH, Hertzberg BS, Freed KS, et al: Nonenhanced helical CT and US in the emergency evaluation of patients with renal colic: Prospective comparison. Radiology 2000; 17:792–797.
3. Sim JS, Seo CS, Kim SH, et al: Differentiation of small hyperechoic renal cell carcinoma from angiomyolipoma: Computer-aided tissue echo quantification. J Ultrasound Med 1999; 18:261–264.
4. Jose MD, Bannister KM, Clarkson AR, et al: Diffuse kidney infiltration with T-cell lymphoblastic lymphoma. Nephrol Dial Transplant 1998; 13:1877–1878.
5. Storkel S, Eble JN, Adlakha K, et al: Classification of renal cell carcinoma: Workgroup No. 1. Union Internationale Contre le Cancer (UICC) and the American Joint Committee on Cancer (AJCC). Cancer 1997; 80:987–989.
6. Jamis-Dow CA, Choyke PL, Jennings SB, et al: Small (±3 cm) renal masses: Detection with CT versus US and pathologic correlation. Radiology 1996; 198:785–788.
7. Siegel CL, Middleton WD, Teefey SA, et al: Angiomyolipoma and renal cell carcinoma: US differentiation. Radiology 1996; 198:789–793.
8. Kim SH: CT and US findings of the renal metastases. J Korean Radiol Soc 1995; 32:307–313.
9. Tomaszewski JE: The pathology of renal tumors. Semin Roentgenol 1995; 30:116–127.
10. Bosniak MA: Problems in the radiologic diagnosis of renal parenchymal tumors. Urol Clin North Am 1993; 20:217–230.
11. O'Toole KM, Brown M, Hoffmann P: Pathology of benign and malignant kidney tumors. Urol Clin North Am 1993; 20:193–205.
12. Yamashita Y, Ueno S, Makita O, et al: Hyperechoic renal tumors: Anechoic rim and intratumoral cysts in US differentiation of renal cell carcinoma from angiomyolipoma. Radiology 1993; 188:179–182.
13. Dinney CP, Awad SA, Gajewski JB, et al: Analysis of imaging modalities, staging systems, and prognostic indicators for renal cell carcinoma. Urology 1992; 39:122–129.

14. Yamashita Y, Takahashi M, Watanabe O, et al: Small renal cell carcinoma: Pathologic and radiologic correlation. Radiology 1992; 184:493–498.

15. Warshauer DM, McCarthy SM, Street L, et al: Detection of renal masses: Sensitivities and specificities of excretory urography/linear tomography, US, and CT. Radiology 1988; 169:363–365.

16. Zeman RK, Cronan JJ, Rosenfield AT, et al: Renal cell carcinoma: Dynamic thin-section CT assessment of vascular invasion and tumor vascularity. Radiology 1988; 167:393–396.

17. Johnson CD, Dunnick NR, Cohan RH, et al: Renal adenocarcinoma: CT staging of 100 tumors. AJR Am J Roentgenol 1987; 148:59–63.

18. Parienty RA, Pradel J, Parienty I: Cystic renal cancers: CT characteristics. Radiology 1985; 157:741–744.

19. Heiken JP, Gold RP, Schnur MJ, et al: Computed tomography of renal lymphoma with ultrasound correlation. J Comput Assist Tomogr 1983; 7:245–250.

Illustrations • Malignant Renal Parenchymal Tumors

1 • Exophytic hypervascular renal cell carcinoma: most common manifestation

2 • Renal cell carcinoma: endophytic growth

3 • Renal cell carcinoma: papillary type

4 • Renal cell carcinoma: chromophobe type

5 • Renal cell carcinoma: collecting duct carcinoma

6 • Small renal cell carcinoma

7 • Cystic renal cell carcinoma

8 • Calcified renal cell carcinoma

9 • Renal cell carcinoma: Doppler US

10 • Multiple renal cell carcinomas

11 • Renal cell carcinoma: various appearances

12 • Renal cell carcinoma: venous invasion

13 • Renal cell carcinoma: lymph node metastasis

14 • Renal cell carcinoma: direct invasion of surrounding organs

15 • Renal cell carcinoma: distant metastasis

16 • Renal cell carcinoma: changes and recurrence after treatment

17 • Wilms' tumor

18 • Renal lymphoma

19 • Metastatic tumors of the kidney

20 • Sarcomas and other malignant tumors of renal parenchyma

1. Exophytic Hypervascular Renal Cell Carcinoma: Most Common Manifestation

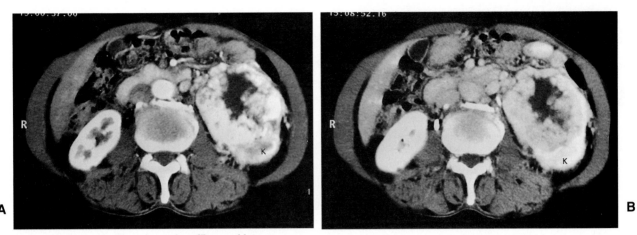

Fig. 1. Hypervascular renal cell carcinoma in a 67-year-old man.
A, B. Contrast-enhanced CT scans in cortical (**A**) and excretory (**B**) phases show a large hypervascular mass with central necrosis in the left kidney. Note that the attenuation of the mass is higher than that of the remainder of the left kidney (K) on cortical phase CT but lower than that of the kidney (K) on excretory phase CT.

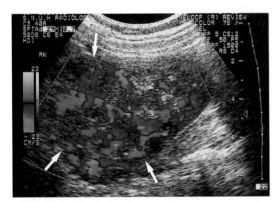

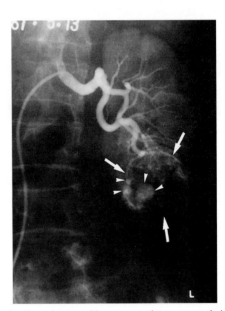

Fig. 2. Hypervascular renal cell carcinoma in a 47-year-old woman. Color Doppler US shows a large mass (*arrows*) in the upper pole of the right kidney. Note that the vascularity of the mass is higher than that of the remainder of the kidney. (See also Color Section.)

Fig. 3. Renal cell carcinoma with aneurysmal tumor vessels in a 66-year-old woman. Left renal arteriogram shows a round hypervascular mass (*arrows*) in the lower pole of the left kidney. Note aneurysmal vessels (*arrowheads*) in the tumor.

2. Renal Cell Carcinoma: Endophytic Growth

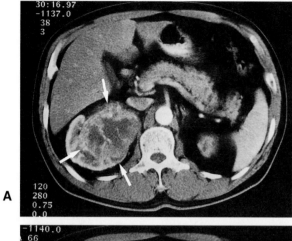

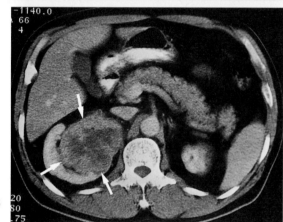

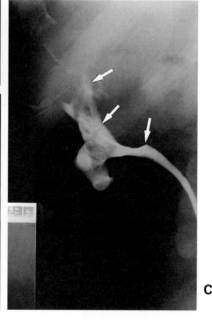

Fig. 1. Renal cell carcinoma growing into the renal sinus in a 60-year-old man.
A, B. Contrast-enhanced CT scans in cortical (**A**) and nephrographic (**B**) phases show a mass *(arrows)* growing into the renal sinus. Note that the tumor vessels are seen on the cortical-phase image, but the tumor has central necrosis and is low attenuated on the nephrographic-phase image. **C.** RGP shows compression and deviation of the calyces *(arrows)* without invasion by the mass.

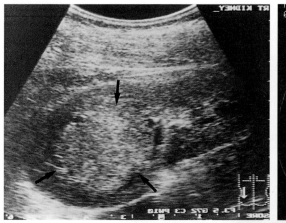

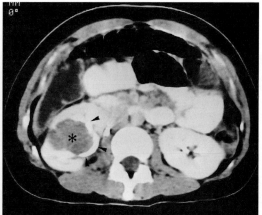

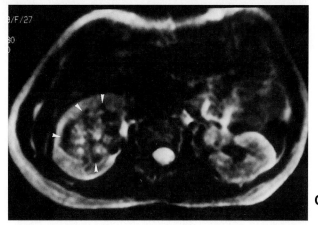

Fig. 2. An echogenic and endophytically growing renal cell carcinoma in a 27-year-old woman.
A. Longitudinal US of the right kidney shows a large echogenic mass *(arrows)* growing in the renal sinus in the upper pole of the right kidney. **B.** Contrast-enhanced CT scan in excretory phase shows a low-attenuated mass *(asterisk)* with compression on the pelvocalyces *(arrowheads)*. **C.** T2-weighted MR imaging shows heterogeneous signal intensity of the mass. Note that the mass is surrounded by a low-intensity rim *(arrowheads)* that represents a pseudocapsule formed by the compressed renal parenchyma.

3. Renal Cell Carcinoma: Papillary Type

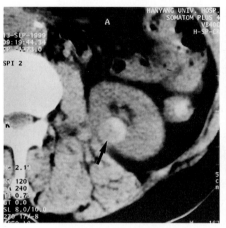
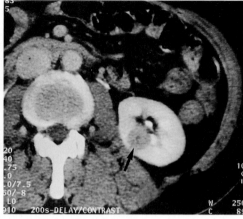

Fig. 1. Papillary renal cell carcinoma in a 47-year-old woman.
A. Nonenhanced CT shows a small, round, high-attenuated mass *(arrow)* in the left kidney. **B.** Contrast-enhanced CT shows a homogeneous low attenuation of the mass *(arrow)*.

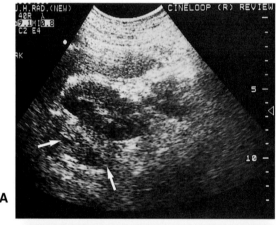
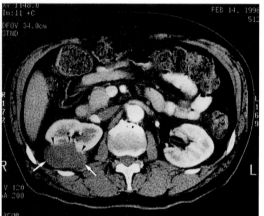

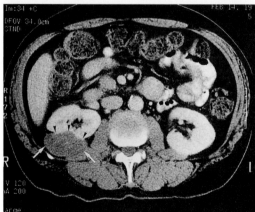

Fig. 2. Papillary renal cell carcinoma in a 71-year-old man.
A. US of the right kidney in transverse plane shows a mass *(arrows)* growing exophytically from the posterior surface of the right kidney. Note that the echogenicity of the mass is higher than that of the renal parenchyma. **B, C.** Contrast-enhanced CT scans in cortical **(B)** and nephrographic **(C)** phases show a mass *(arrows)* growing exophytically in the posterior aspect of the right kidney *(arrowheads)*. Note that the mass does not enhance well.

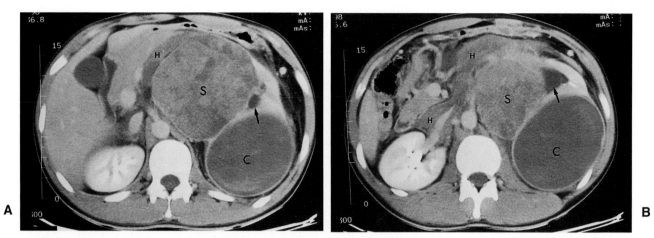

Fig. 3. Papillary renal cell carcinoma in a 23-year-old man who had experienced blunt abdominal trauma 1 week earlier.
A, B. Contrast-enhanced CT scans show a large dumbbell-shaped mass in the left kidney. The anterior part of the mass is an enhancing solid mass (S) and the posterior part is a nonenhancing, thick-walled, cystic one (C). Note the dilated adjacent calyces *(arrow)* and perirenal hematoma (H) anterior to the mass.

4. Renal Cell Carcinoma: Chromophobe Type

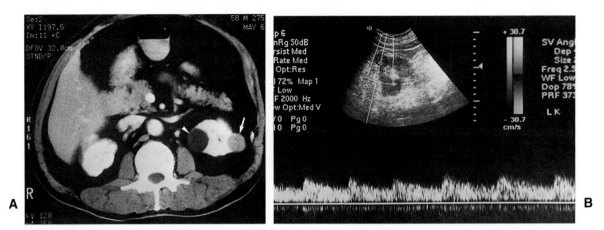

Fig. 1. Renal cyst and a small renal cell carcinoma of chromophobe type in a 58-year-old man with colon cancer.
A. Contrast-enhanced CT shows a simple cyst *(arrowhead)* and a small solid mass *(arrow)* in the left kidney. The solid mass has homogeneous attenuation. **B.** Spectral Doppler US performed at the solid mass shows arterial flow of low-resistance pattern.

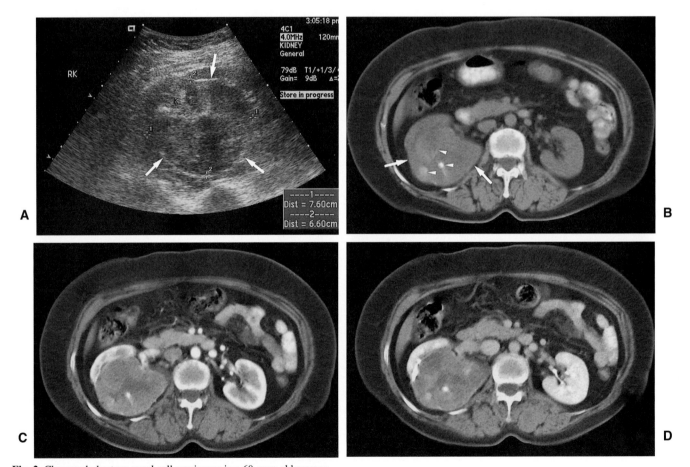

Fig. 2. Chromophobe-type renal cell carcinoma in a 60-year-old woman.
A. US of the right kidney in transverse plane shows a large mass of heterogeneous echogenicity *(arrows)* in the right kidney (K). **B.** Nonenhanced CT shows a large mass *(arrows)* with calcifications *(arrowheads)* in the posterior aspect of the right kidney. **C, D.** Contrast-enhanced CT scans in cortical (**C**) and excretory (**D**) phases show poor enhancement of the mass.

5. Renal Cell Carcinoma: Collecting Duct Carcinoma

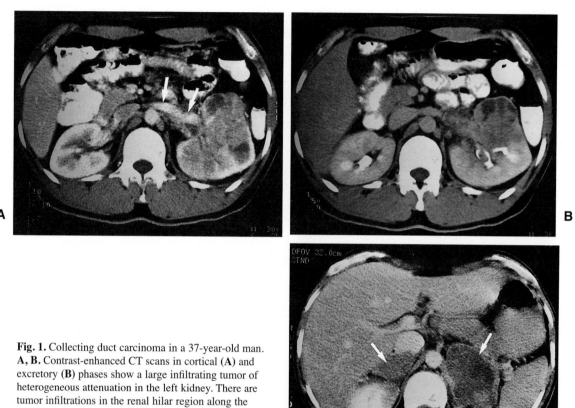

Fig. 1. Collecting duct carcinoma in a 37-year-old man.
A, B. Contrast-enhanced CT scans in cortical (**A**) and excretory (**B**) phases show a large infiltrating tumor of heterogeneous attenuation in the left kidney. There are tumor infiltrations in the renal hilar region along the renal vein, but the renal vein itself is intact *(arrows)*.
C. Follow-up CT obtained 10 months after radical nephrectomy reveals large metastatic masses in both adrenal glands *(arrows)*.

6. Small Renal Cell Carcinoma

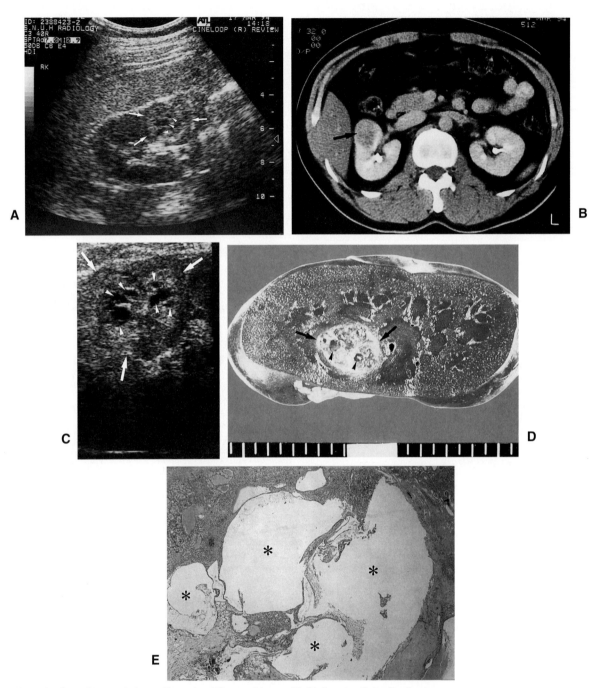

Fig. 1. Small renal cell carcinoma of clear cell type in a 39-year-old man. (**D, E,** See also Color Section.)
A. US of the right kidney shows a round echogenic mass. The mass has a thin hypoechoic halo *(arrows)* and small intratumoral cysts *(arrowheads)*.
B. Contrast-enhanced CT shows a round, low-attenuated mass *(arrow)* in the anterior aspect of the right kidney. **C.** Intraoperative US well demonstrates the mass *(arrows)* and intratumoral cysts *(arrowheads)*. **D.** Color photograph of the removed kidney shows the tumor *(arrows)* that contains small cysts *(arrowheads)*. **E.** Color photomicrograph of the tumor shows intratumoral cysts *(asterisks)*.

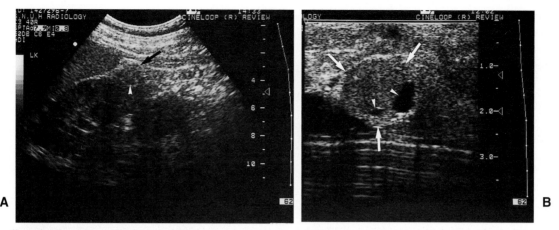

Fig. 2. Small renal cell carcinoma in a 50-year-old man.
A. US of the left kidney shows a small, exophytic mass *(arrow)* of slight hyperechogenicity in the anterior aspect of the left kidney. A peritumoral halo is not seen, but there is a suspicious intratumoral cyst *(arrowhead)*. **B.** Intraoperative US well demonstrates the tumor *(arrows)* and intratumoral cysts *(arrowheads)*.

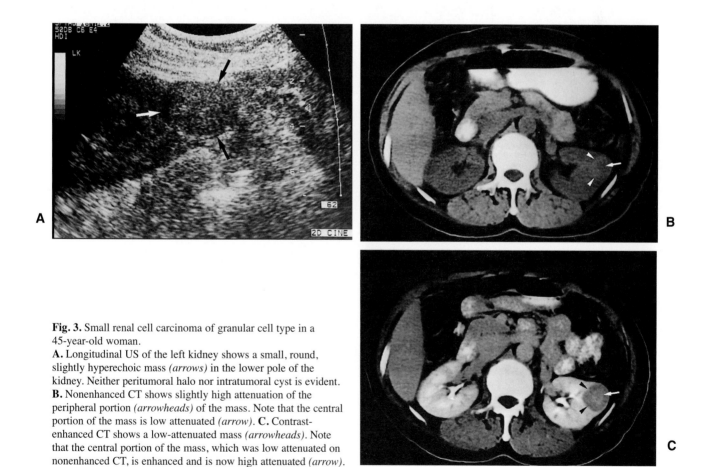

Fig. 3. Small renal cell carcinoma of granular cell type in a 45-year-old woman.
A. Longitudinal US of the left kidney shows a small, round, slightly hyperechoic mass *(arrows)* in the lower pole of the kidney. Neither peritumoral halo nor intratumoral cyst is evident. **B.** Nonenhanced CT shows slightly high attenuation of the peripheral portion *(arrowheads)* of the mass. Note that the central portion of the mass is low attenuated *(arrow)*. **C.** Contrast-enhanced CT shows a low-attenuated mass *(arrowheads)*. Note that the central portion of the mass, which was low attenuated on nonenhanced CT, is enhanced and is now high attenuated *(arrow)*.

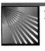

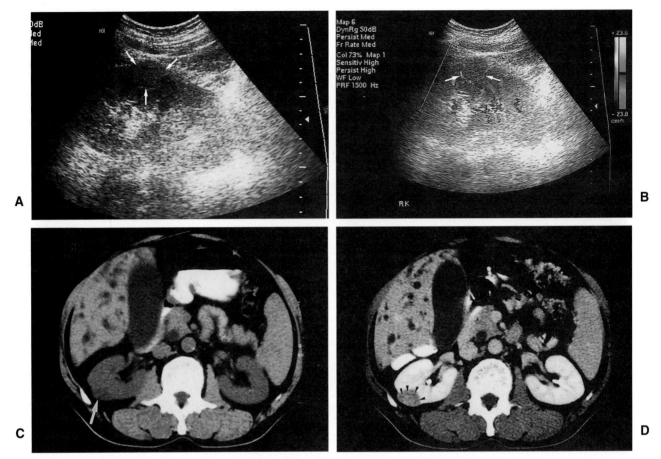

Fig. 4. Small renal cell carcinoma of clear cell type in a 65-year-old man with carcinoma of the common bile duct.
A. Longitudinal US of the right kidney shows a round, hyperechoic mass *(arrows)* in the interpolar region. **B.** Color Doppler US shows vessels draping the tumor *(arrows)*. (**B,** See also Color Section.) **C.** Nonenhanced CT shows a low-attenuated mass *(arrow)* in the right kidney. **D.** Contrast-enhanced CT shows enhancement of the mass and small intratumoral cysts *(arrowheads)*. Note the dilated intrahepatic biliary trees due to carcinoma of the common bile duct.

7. Cystic Renal Cell Carcinoma

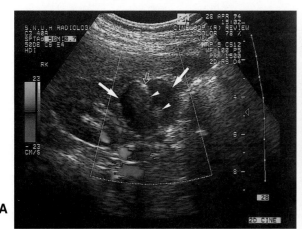

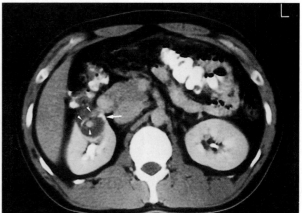

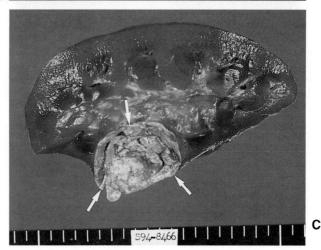

Fig. 1. Cystic renal cell carcinoma in a 36-year-old man. (**A, C**, See also Color Section.)
A. Color Doppler US of the right kidney shows a round cystic mass *(arrows)* that contains echogenic solid nodules *(arrowheads)*, but there is no demonstrable flow signal in the solid part of the mass. A small echogenic dot *(open arrow)* in the mass is probably a calcification. **B.** Contrast-enhanced CT shows the cystic mass and well-enhancing nodules *(arrowheads)* in the mass. Note a small calcification *(arrow)* in the mass. **C.** Partial nephrectomy was performed, and a color photograph of the resected specimen shows the cystic mass with solid lesions *(arrows)*.

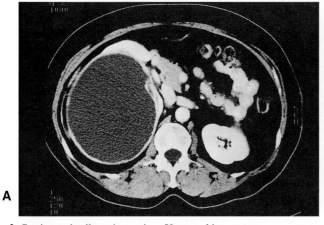

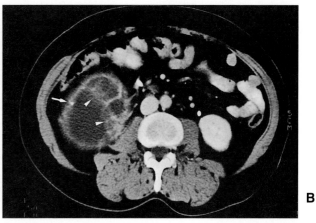

Fig. 2. Cystic renal cell carcinoma in a 59-year-old woman.
A, B. Contrast-enhanced CT scans show a large, thick-walled, cystic mass in the right kidney. Note that there are thick, irregular septa *(arrowheads)* and calcification *(arrow)* in the lower part of the mass.

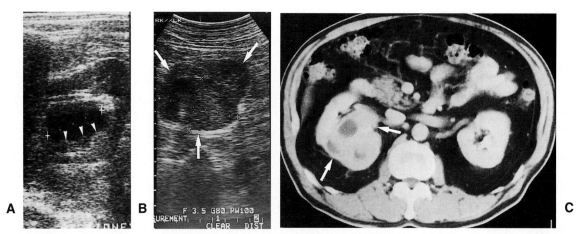

Fig. 3. Cystic renal cell carcinoma misdiagnosed as a simple cyst in a 62-year-old man.
A. Longitudinal US of the right kidney shows a cystic lesion in the lower polar area. At that time, the lesion was interpreted as a simple cyst, but note that the posterior wall of the cyst is irregular *(arrowheads)*. **B.** Follow-up US obtained 2 years later shows that the cystic lesion is filled with solid mass *(arrows)*. **C.** Contrast-enhanced CT shows a large solid mass *(arrows)* with low-attenuated areas of degeneration.

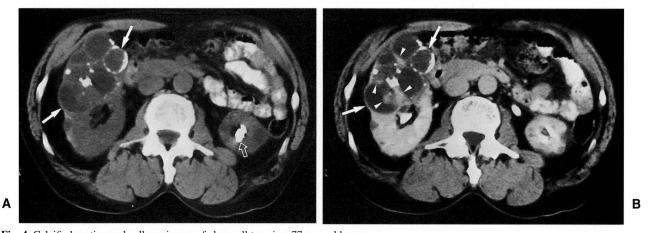

Fig. 4. Calcified cystic renal cell carcinoma of clear cell type in a 77-year-old man.
A, B. Nonenhanced (**A**) and contrast-enhanced (**B**) CT scans show a large, multiloculated, cystic mass *(arrows)* in the anterior aspect of the right kidney. The mass has dense calcifications and exhibits areas of enhancement *(arrowheads in **B**)* after injection of contrast material. Also note that the left kidney has a large stone *(open arrow in **A**)* and there are small cysts in both kidneys. Percutaneous nephrostolithotomy was performed for a left renal stone, and 1 week later a right radical nephrectomy was done for renal cell carcinoma.

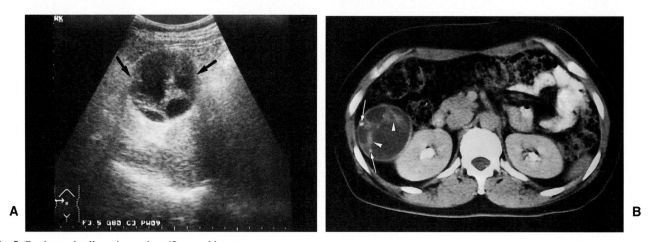

Fig. 5. Cystic renal cell carcinoma in a 43-year-old woman.
A. US of the right kidney shows a round cystic mass *(arrows)* with irregular thick septa. **B.** Contrast-enhanced CT shows a thick-walled cystic mass with irregular enhancing septa *(arrowheads)*. Note small calcifications *(arrows)* in the mass.

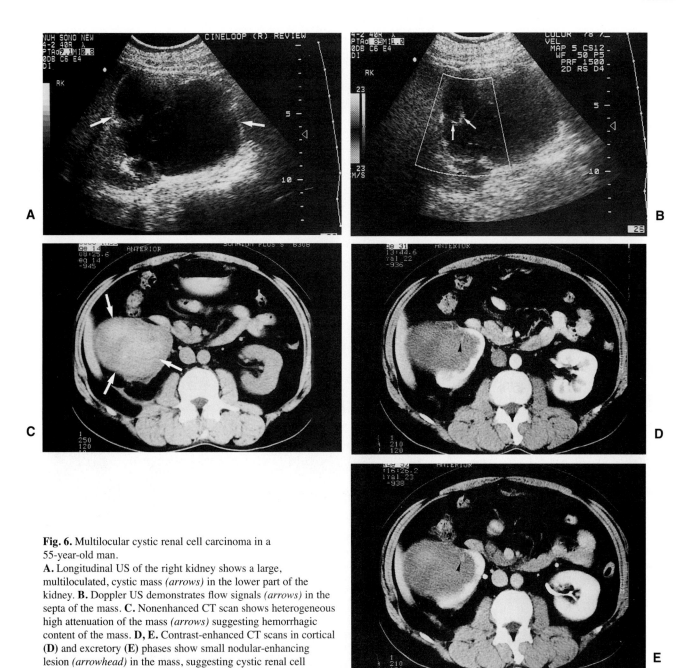

Fig. 6. Multilocular cystic renal cell carcinoma in a 55-year-old man.
A. Longitudinal US of the right kidney shows a large, multiloculated, cystic mass *(arrows)* in the lower part of the kidney. **B.** Doppler US demonstrates flow signals *(arrows)* in the septa of the mass. **C.** Nonenhanced CT scan shows heterogeneous high attenuation of the mass *(arrows)* suggesting hemorrhagic content of the mass. **D, E.** Contrast-enhanced CT scans in cortical (**D**) and excretory (**E**) phases show small nodular-enhancing lesion *(arrowhead)* in the mass, suggesting cystic renal cell carcinoma.

8. Calcified Renal Cell Carcinoma

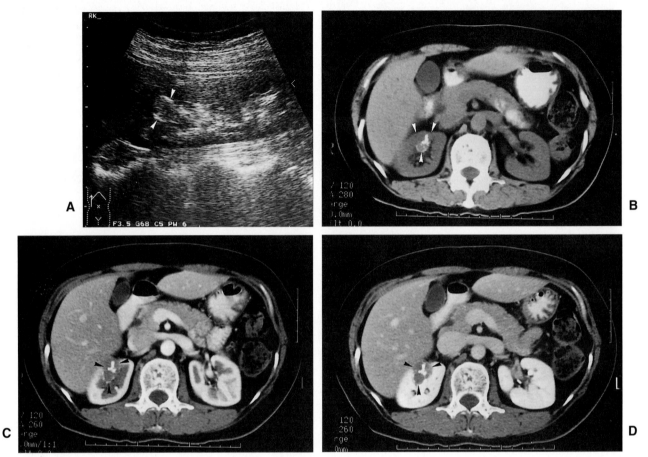

Fig. 1. Small calcified renal cell carcinoma of clear cell type in a 50-year-old woman.
A. Longitudinal US of the right kidney shows a small echogenic mass surrounded by a highly echogenic rim *(arrowheads)* in the upper polar region.
B. Nonenhanced CT shows that the mass *(arrowheads)* has dense central and peripheral calcifications. **C, D.** Contrast-enhanced CT scans in cortical
(C) and nephrographic **(D)** phases well demonstrate the mass *(arrowheads)*, but the enhancement of the mass is not evident.

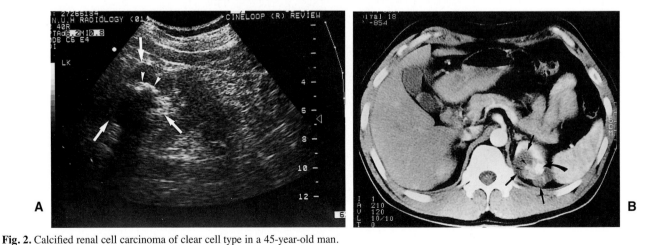

Fig. 2. Calcified renal cell carcinoma of clear cell type in a 45-year-old man.
A. Longitudinal US of the left kidney shows a mass *(arrows)* of heterogeneous echogenicity in the upper pole of the kidney. There is a calcification
(arrowheads) with posterior sonic shadowing in the mass. **B.** Contrast-enhanced CT shows the mass *(arrows)* with enhancing nodule *(arrowheads)* in
the left kidney. Also note a calcification *(curved arrow)* in the mass.

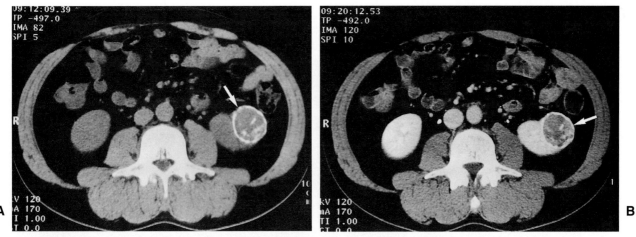

Fig. 3. Calcified renal cell carcinoma of mixed papillary and clear cell type in a 41-year-old man.
A. Nonenhanced CT shows a round, calcified mass *(arrow)* in the lower pole of the left kidney. The mass has peripheral, rimlike calcifications and mottled, central calcifications. **B.** Contrast-enhanced CT shows subtle enhancement in the lateral aspect of the mass *(arrow)*.

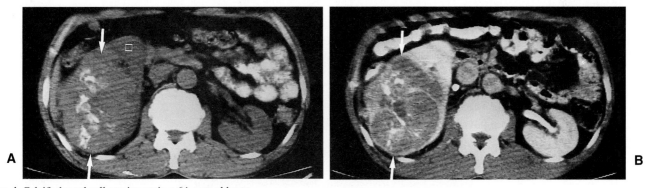

Fig. 4. Calcified renal cell carcinoma in a 64-year-old man.
A, B. Nonenhanced **(A)** and contrast-enhanced **(B)** CT scans show a large solid mass *(arrows)* that contains amorphous calcifications. The mass shows heterogeneous enhancement and has central necrosis.

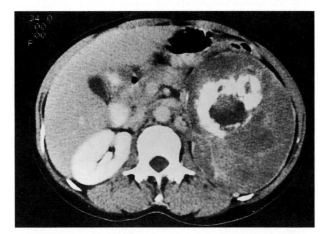

Fig. 5. Calcified renal cell carcinoma in a 47-year-old woman. Contrast-enhanced CT shows a large renal mass with dense calcifications.

9. Renal Cell Carcinoma: Doppler US

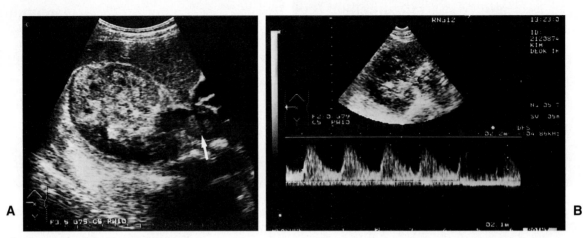

Fig. 1. Renal cell carcinoma in a 63-year-old woman.
A. US of the right kidney in transverse plane shows a large renal mass and echogenic thrombus *(arrow)* in the right renal vein. **B.** Spectral Doppler US performed in the mass demonstrates peak systolic frequency shift of 4.86 KHz at an insonation frequency of 2.2 MHz.

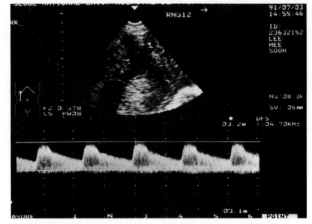

Fig. 2. Renal cell carcinoma in a 54-year-old woman. Spectral Doppler US shows 4.7-KHz frequency shift in peak systole at an insonation frequency of 2.2 MHz.

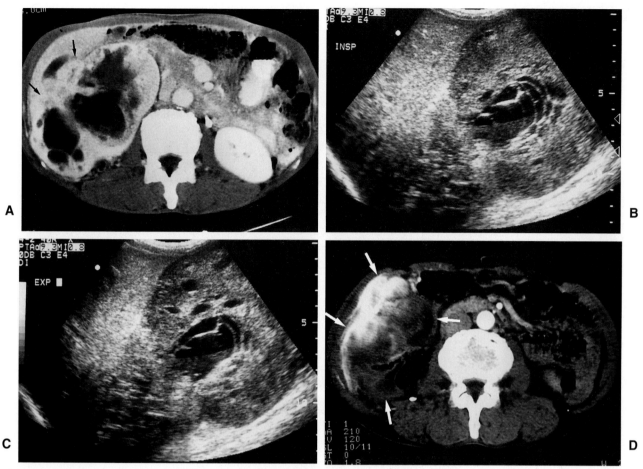

Fig. 3. Renal cell carcinoma of sarcomatoid type in a 53-year-old man.
A. Contrast-enhanced CT shows a large mass with necrosis in the right kidney. Note that the interface between the mass and liver is not clear *(arrows)*. **B, C.** Longitudinal US images of the right renal mass in deep inspiration (**B**) and expiration (**C**) show that the renal mass and liver do not slide at their interface but move together, indicating that there is invasion or at least adhesion to the liver. At surgery there was severe adhesion to the liver, and focal resection was done on the liver together with radical nephrectomy. **D.** Follow-up CT scan obtained 5 months after the surgery shows recurrent tumors *(arrows)* of heterogeneous attenuation with invasion of the bowels.

10. Multiple Renal Cell Carcinomas

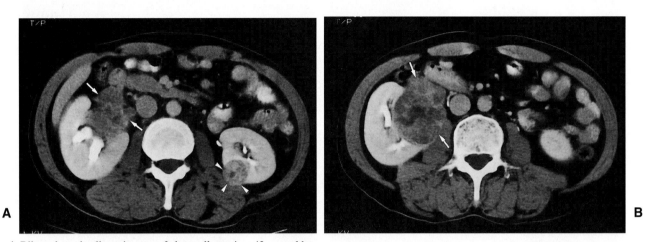

Fig. 1. Bilateral renal cell carcinomas of clear cell type in a 43-year-old man.
A, B. Contrast-enhanced CT scans show a large mass in the right kidney *(arrows)* and a small mass in the left kidney *(arrowheads* in **A**). Both masses are solid with focal necroses. After tumorectomy of the left renal mass, right radical nephrectomy was performed.

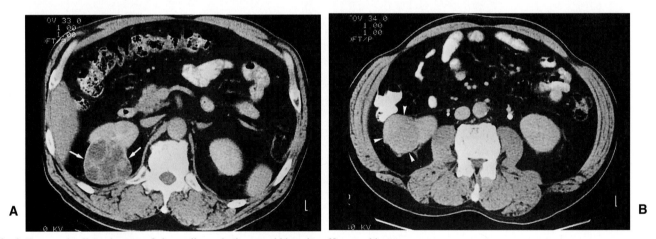

Fig. 2. Two renal cell carcinomas of clear cell type in the same kidney in a 68-year-old man.
A. Contrast-enhanced CT scan shows a mass *(arrows)* with multifocal, low-attenuated lesions growing exophytically from the posterior aspect of the right kidney. **B.** A lower-level CT scan shows another mass *(arrowheads)*. This mass has homogeneous attenuation and shows only subtle enhancement.

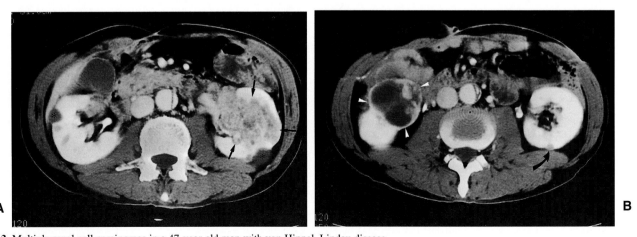

Fig. 3. Multiple renal cell carcinomas in a 47-year-old man with von Hippel–Lindau disease.
A, B. Contrast-enhanced CT scans show a cystic tumor with internal solid nodules in the right kidney *(arrowheads* in **B**) and an ill-demarcated solid tumor in the left kidney *(arrows* in **A**). Also note a small solid tumor in the posterior aspect of the left kidney *(curved arrow)* and multiple cysts *(asterisks* in **A**) in both kidneys.

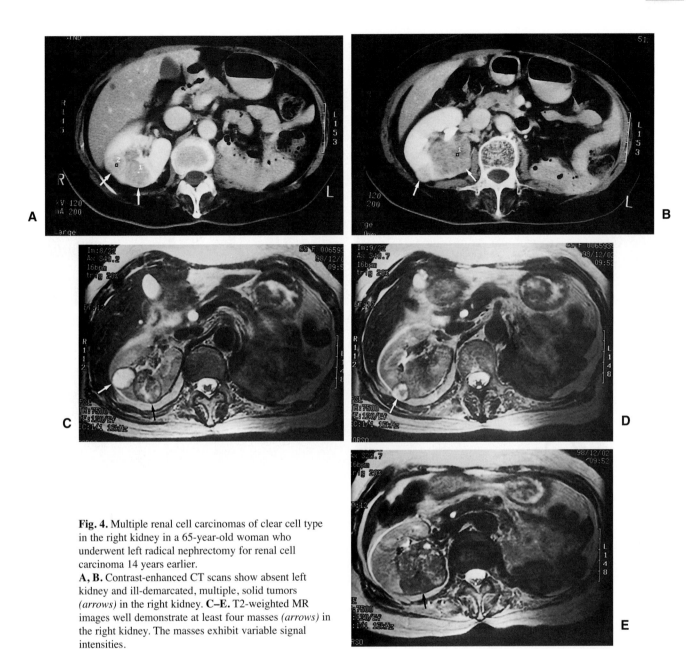

Fig. 4. Multiple renal cell carcinomas of clear cell type in the right kidney in a 65-year-old woman who underwent left radical nephrectomy for renal cell carcinoma 14 years earlier.
A, B. Contrast-enhanced CT scans show absent left kidney and ill-demarcated, multiple, solid tumors *(arrows)* in the right kidney. **C–E.** T2-weighted MR images well demonstrate at least four masses *(arrows)* in the right kidney. The masses exhibit variable signal intensities.

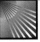

11. Renal Cell Carcinoma: Various Appearances

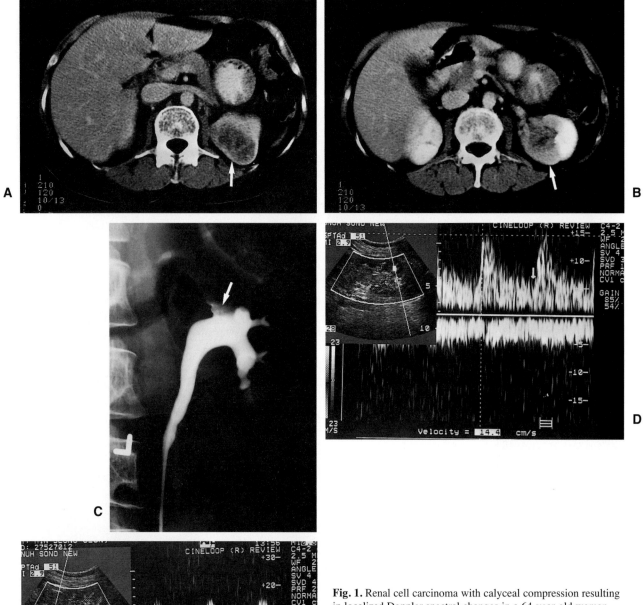

Fig. 1. Renal cell carcinoma with calyceal compression resulting in localized Doppler spectral changes in a 64-year-old woman. **A, B.** Contrast-enhanced CT scans show low-attenuated tumor *(arrow)* in the upper pole of the left kidney. **C.** RGP shows compressed upper pole calyx *(arrow)* of the left kidney without marginal irregularity. **D.** Spectral Doppler US performed at the lower pole of the left kidney shows a normal spectral pattern. **E.** Spectral Doppler US performed at remnant renal parenchyma in the upper pole of the left kidney shows a high-resistance pattern with resistive index of 1.0. This localized Doppler spectral change is probably caused by the calyceal compression by the tumor, which in turn results in difficulty in excreting urine from the upper pole parenchyma.

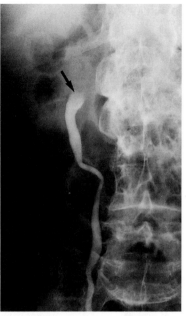

Fig. 2. Renal cell carcinoma mimicking a renal pelvis tumor in a 69-year-old woman. **A.** Contrast-enhanced CT shows an ill-defined, dumbbell-shaped mass *(asterisks)* in the right kidney with preserved form of the kidney. **B.** RGP shows obstruction of ureteropelvic junction *(arrow)* by the tumor. Note smooth margin of obstruction. At surgery, a right renal parenchymal mass was bulging into the renal pelvis.

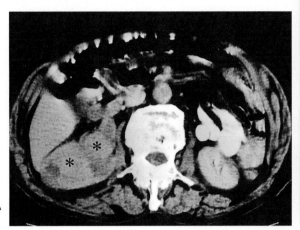

Fig. 3. Renal cell carcinoma of clear cell type mimicking a renal artery aneurysm in a 67-year-old man.
A. Nonenhanced CT shows a round mass in the hilar portion of the left kidney *(arrow)*. The mass has slightly higher attenuation than the renal parenchyma. **B.** Contrast-enhanced CT scan in cortical phase shows strong enhancement of the mass *(arrow)*. The attenuation of the mass is similar to that of the aorta (A). **C.** CT scan in excretory phase shows homogeneous washout of contrast material from the mass *(arrow)*. **D.** Doppler US was performed to evaluate the vascularity of the lesion, and it shows tumor vessels *(arrowheads)* within a solid mass *(arrows)*.

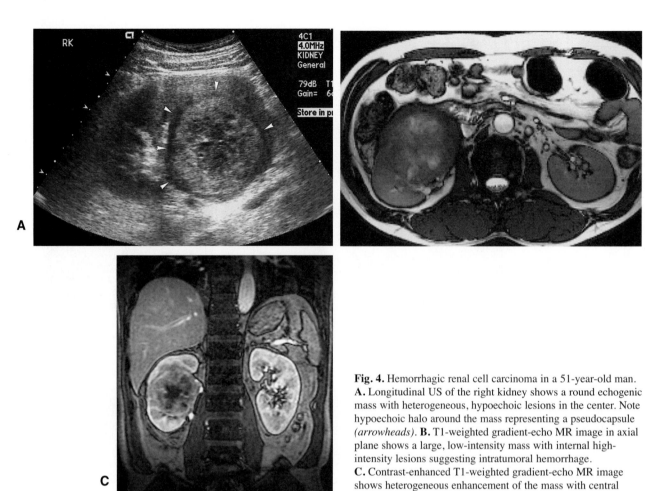

Fig. 4. Hemorrhagic renal cell carcinoma in a 51-year-old man. **A.** Longitudinal US of the right kidney shows a round echogenic mass with heterogeneous, hypoechoic lesions in the center. Note hypoechoic halo around the mass representing a pseudocapsule *(arrowheads)*. **B.** T1-weighted gradient-echo MR image in axial plane shows a large, low-intensity mass with internal high-intensity lesions suggesting intratumoral hemorrhage. **C.** Contrast-enhanced T1-weighted gradient-echo MR image shows heterogeneous enhancement of the mass with central necrosis.

12. Renal Cell Carcinoma: Venous Invasion

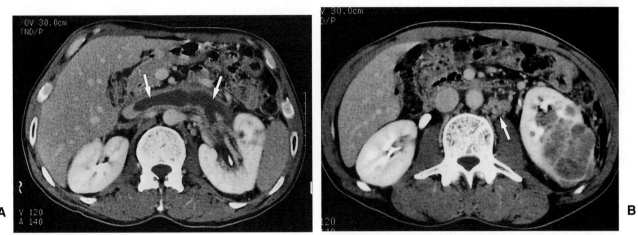

Fig. 1. Renal cell carcinoma with venous invasion and metastasis to the brain in a 51-year-old man.
A. Contrast-enhanced CT shows dilated left renal vein filled with low-attenuated thrombi *(arrows)*. **B.** CT scan at lower level shows a large, low-attenuated tumor in the lower pole of the left kidney. Note multiple enlarged para-aortic lymph nodes *(arrow)*.

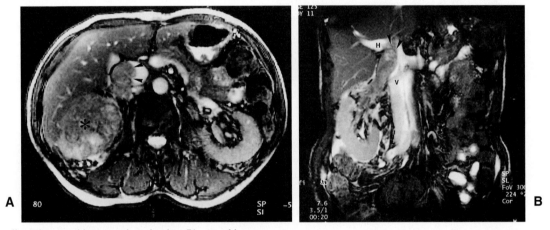

Fig. 2. Renal cell carcinoma with venous invasion in a 71-year-old man.
A. T2-weighted MR image in axial plane shows a large mass in the right kidney *(asterisk)* and thrombi *(arrowheads)* in the inferior vena cava.
B. T2-weighted coronal MR image well demonstrates the extent of the thrombi. Note that the cranial end of the thrombi *(arrowheads)* is at the level of confluence of the hepatic vein (H) with inferior vena cava (V).

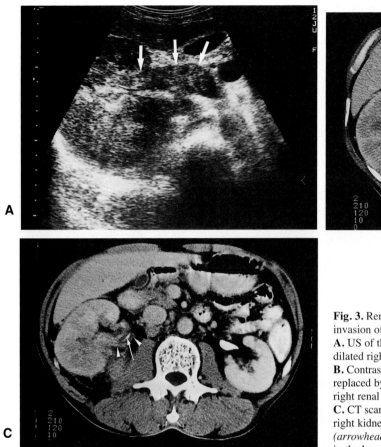

Fig. 3. Renal cell carcinoma with venous thrombosis and invasion of renal pelvis in a 41-year-old man.
A. US of the right kidney shows enlarged right kidney and dilated right renal vein filled with echogenic thrombi *(arrows)*.
B. Contrast-enhanced CT shows enlarged right kidney replaced by low-attenuated infiltrating tumor. Note the dilated right renal vein filled with low-attenuated thrombi *(arrows)*.
C. CT scan at lower level shows low-attenuated tumor in the right kidney and thickened wall of the renal pelvis *(arrowheads)* surrounding excreted contrast material *(arrow)* in the lumen of the renal pelvis.

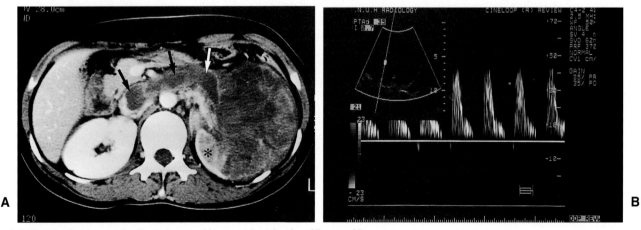

Fig. 4. Diffuse infiltrating renal cell carcinoma with venous invasion in a 27-year-old woman.
A. Contrast-enhanced CT scan shows a large, low-attenuated tumor of infiltrating nature in the left kidney with thrombosis *(arrows)* of the left renal vein and inferior vena cava. Note that only a small area of the left kidney *(asterisk)* is not involved by the tumor. **B.** Spectral Doppler US obtained at the tumor shows a markedly elevated resistive index of 1.0.

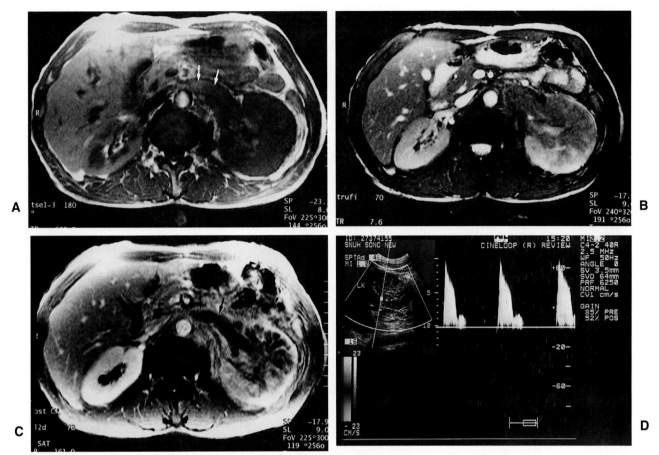

Fig. 5. Diffuse infiltrating renal cell carcinoma in a 60-year-old man with renal vein thrombosis.
A. T1-weighted MR image shows enlarged left kidney with decreased signal intensity and loss of normal corticomedullary contrast. Note that the left renal vein is dilated and is filled with high-intensity thrombi *(arrows)*. **B.** T2-weighted MR image shows marked low signal intensity of the left renal tumor. Renal vein thrombosis is not well demonstrated on this image. **C.** Contrast-enhanced T1-weighted MR image well demonstrates the low-intensity tumor and thrombi in the left renal vein *(arrows)*. **D.** Spectral Doppler US of the left kidney shows markedly elevated resistive index of 1.0.

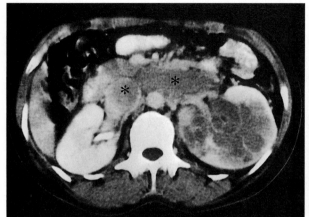

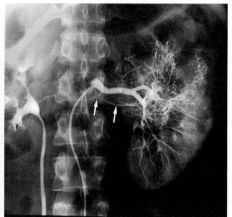

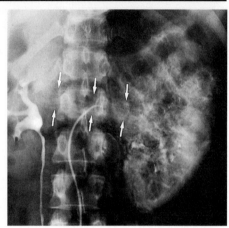

Fig. 6. Papillary renal cell carcinoma with thrombosis of the renal vein and inferior vena cava in a 38-year-old woman.
A. Contrast-enhanced CT shows a large, ill-demarcated, low-attenuated tumor in the left kidney and dilated left renal vein and inferior vena cava filled with low-attenuated thrombi *(asterisks)*. **B, C.** Selective left renal arteriograms in arterial **(B)** and nephrographic **(C)** phases show a large hypervascular tumor in the upper part of the left kidney and linear tumor vessels in the left renal vein producing so-called thread-and-streak sign *(arrows)*.

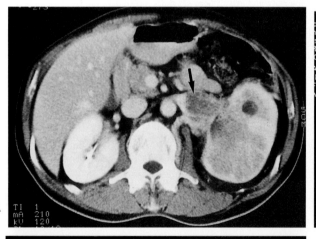

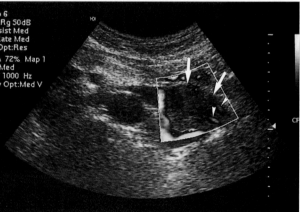

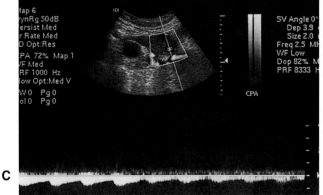

Fig. 7. Renal cell carcinoma with venous thrombosis in a 47-year-old woman.
A. Contrast-enhanced CT scan shows diffusely infiltrating tumor in the left kidney with large thrombi in the dilated left renal vein *(arrow)*. **B.** Doppler US of the left renal vein well demonstrates the thrombi *(arrows)* and tumor vessels *(arrowheads)* within them. **C.** Spectral Doppler US obtained in the thrombi shows arterial, low-resistance flow pattern confirming the presence of tumor vessels in the thrombi.

13. Renal Cell Carcinoma: Lymph Node Metastasis

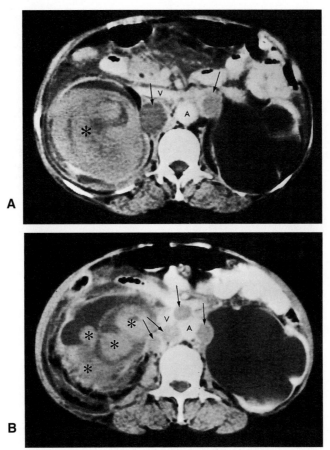

Fig. 1. Renal cell carcinoma with retroperitoneal lymph node metastases in a 61-year-old woman with bilateral ureteropelvic junction obstruction. Lymph node biopsy revealed metastatic renal cell carcinoma.
A, B. Contrast-enhanced CT scans show bilateral ureteropelvic junction obstruction and a large solid mass *(asterisks)* bulging into the dilated renal pelvocalyces in the right kidney. Note multiple, low-attenuated, metastatic lymph nodes *(arrows)* in the retroperitoneum. A, aorta; V, vena cava.

14. Renal Cell Carcinoma: Direct Invasion of Surrounding Organs

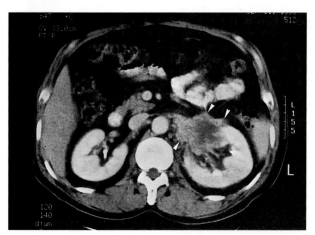

Fig. 1. Renal cell carcinoma with perirenal invasion in a 58-year-old man. Contrast-enhanced CT shows a low-attenuated mass in the anteromedial aspect of the left kidney with direct invasion into the perirenal space *(arrowheads)*.

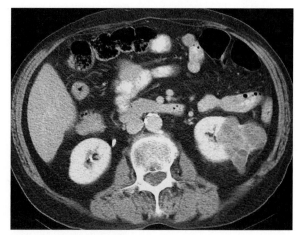

Fig. 2. Renal cell carcinoma with perirenal invasion in a 68-year-old man. Contrast-enhanced CT shows a large, low-attenuated mass in the left kidney. The mass has lobulated contour with extension into the perirenal space.

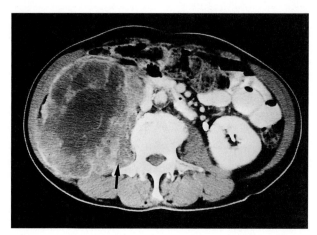

Fig. 3. Renal cell carcinoma with direct invasion into the psoas muscle in a 72-year-old man. Contrast-enhanced CT shows a large mass of heterogeneous attenuation in the right kidney with direct invasion into the right psoas muscle *(arrow)*.

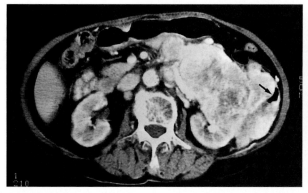
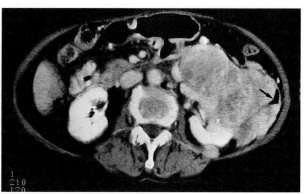

Fig. 4. Renal cell carcinoma with direct invasion into the descending colon in a 79-year-old woman.
A, B. Contrast-enhanced CT scans in cortical (**A**) and excretory (**B**) phases show a large mass in the left kidney with invasion of the surrounding structures through the renal fascia. Note that the descending colon *(arrow)* is encased by the tumor.

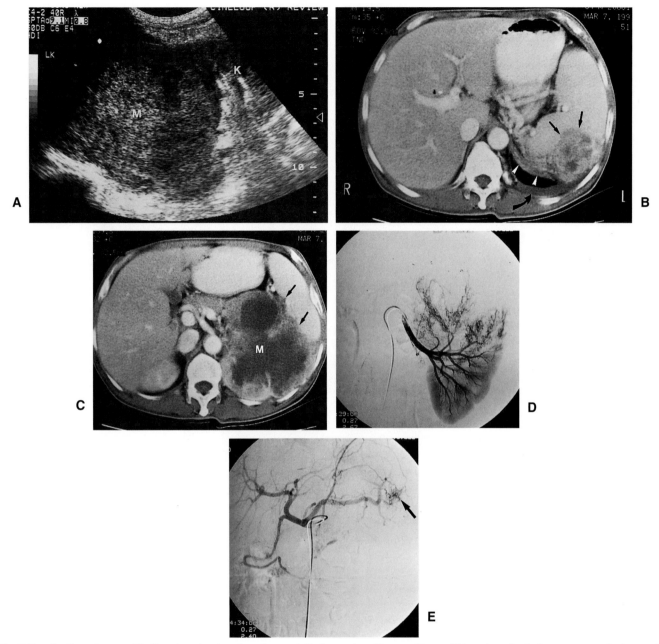

Fig. 5. Renal cell carcinoma with direct invasion into the spleen and diaphragm in a 53-year-old man. This patient also had metastases to the lung and brain.
A. Longitudinal US of the left kidney shows a large mass (M) in the upper pole of the left kidney. K, remnant lower pole of the left kidney.
B, C. Contrast-enhanced CT scans show a large necrotic mass (M) in the left kidney with invasion into the spleen *(arrows)*. Also note thickening of the left diaphragm *(arrowheads* in **B**) suggesting invasion. Pleural effusion is seen in the left thorax *(curved arrow* in **B**). **D.** Left renal arteriogram shows a hypervascular mass in the upper pole. **E.** Celiac angiogram shows hypervascularity in the spleen *(arrow)*.

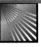
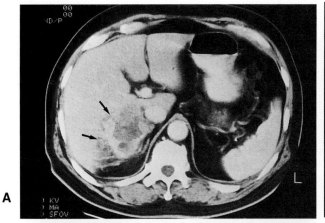

A

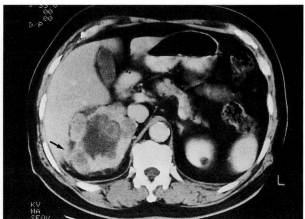

B

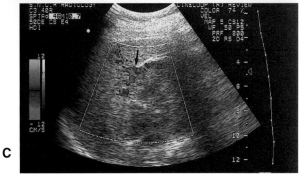

C

Fig. 6. Renal cell carcinoma of the right kidney with invasion of the liver in a 74-year-old man.
A, B. Contrast-enhanced CT scans show a large mass in the upper pole of the right kidney with ill-defined interface with the liver *(arrows)*. Note a small cyst in the upper pole of the left kidney.
C. On US, the mass and the liver did not slide on their interface and color Doppler US shows prominent vessels *(arrow)* crossing the interface between the mass and the liver. (**C,** See also Color Section.)

15. Renal Cell Carcinoma: Distant Metastasis

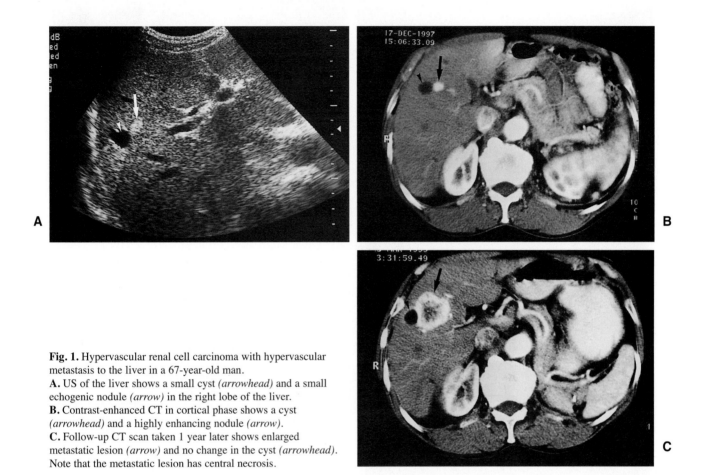

Fig. 1. Hypervascular renal cell carcinoma with hypervascular metastasis to the liver in a 67-year-old man.
A. US of the liver shows a small cyst *(arrowhead)* and a small echogenic nodule *(arrow)* in the right lobe of the liver.
B. Contrast-enhanced CT in cortical phase shows a cyst *(arrowhead)* and a highly enhancing nodule *(arrow)*.
C. Follow-up CT scan taken 1 year later shows enlarged metastatic lesion *(arrow)* and no change in the cyst *(arrowhead)*. Note that the metastatic lesion has central necrosis.

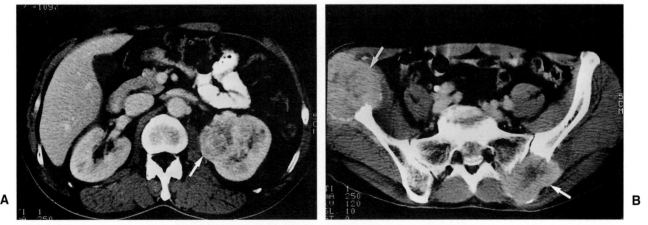

Fig. 2. Renal cell carcinoma with metastases to the pelvic bones in a 53-year-old man.
A. Contrast-enhanced CT shows a tumor *(arrow)* in the left kidney. **B.** CT scan at lower level shows large metastatic lesions in the iliac and sacral bones *(arrows)*.

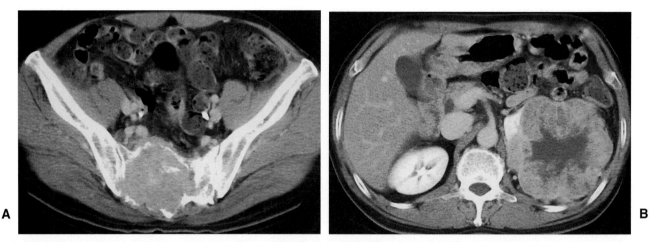

Fig. 3. Solitary bony metastasis in the sacrum that was discovered earlier than renal cell carcinoma in a 63-year-old man.
A. Contrast-enhanced CT shows a large expansile mass in the sacrum with severe bony destruction. **B.** Contrast-enhanced CT at upper level shows a large mass with central necrosis in the left kidney.

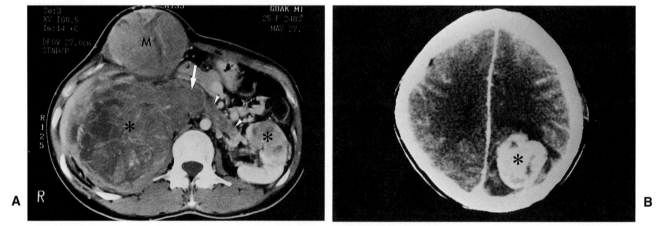

Fig. 4. Bilateral renal cell carcinomas with metastases to the brain and abdominal wall in a 25-year-old woman.
A. Contrast-enhanced CT shows renal tumors in both kidneys *(asterisks)* with thromboses of the inferior vena cava *(arrow)* and left renal vein *(arrowheads)*. Note a large metastatic mass (M) in the anterior abdominal wall. **B.** Contrast-enhanced CT of the brain shows a large, hypervascular, metastatic mass in the left parietal lobe *(asterisk)*.

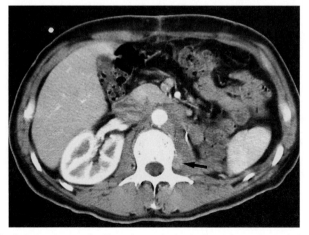

Fig. 5. Recurrent renal cell carcinoma in the ipsilateral psoas muscle in a 38-year-old man who underwent radical nephrectomy 4 months earlier. Contrast-enhanced CT in the cortical phase shows a small enhancing mass in the left psoas muscle *(arrow)*.

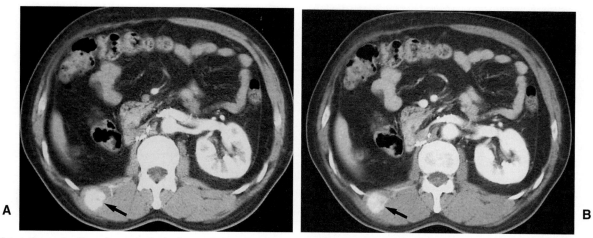

Fig. 6. Metastatic renal cell carcinoma in the back muscle in a 60-year-old man who underwent radical nephrectomy 8 years earlier.
A, B. Contrast-enhanced CT scans in cortical (**A**) and nephrographic (**B**) phases show a mass in the right back muscle *(arrow)*. The mass shows early strong enhancement and prominent washout on nephrographic-phase CT.

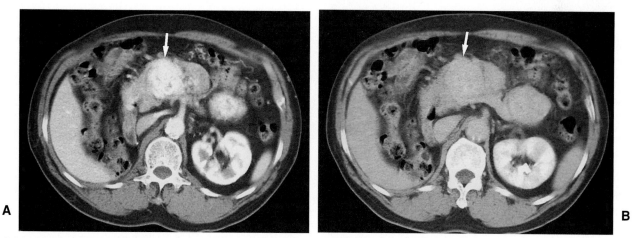

Fig. 7. Metastatic renal cell carcinoma in the pancreas in a 73-year-old man who underwent radical nephrectomy 6 years earlier.
A. Contrast-enhanced CT in cortical phase shows a mass in the pancreas with strong enhancement *(arrow)*. **B.** On nephrographic CT, the mass *(arrow)* is not well demonstrated due to early washout of contrast material.

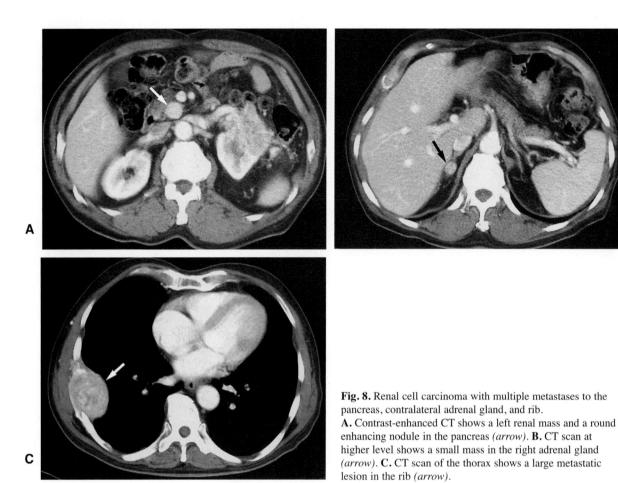

Fig. 8. Renal cell carcinoma with multiple metastases to the pancreas, contralateral adrenal gland, and rib.
A. Contrast-enhanced CT shows a left renal mass and a round enhancing nodule in the pancreas *(arrow)*. **B.** CT scan at higher level shows a small mass in the right adrenal gland *(arrow)*. **C.** CT scan of the thorax shows a large metastatic lesion in the rib *(arrow)*.

16. Renal Cell Carcinoma: Changes and Recurrence after Treatment

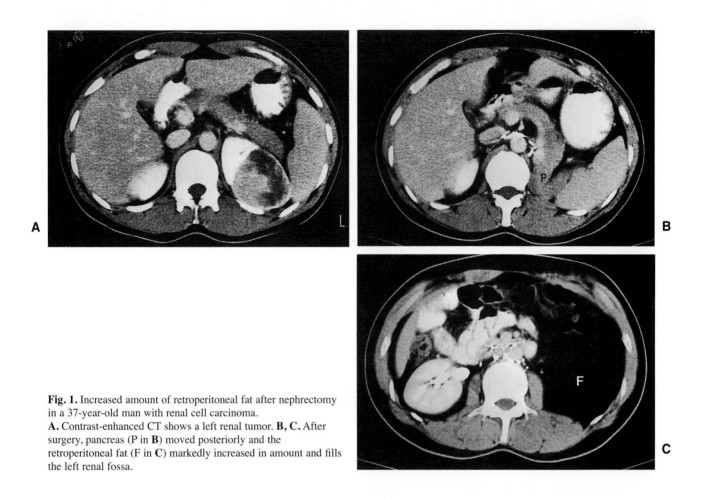

Fig. 1. Increased amount of retroperitoneal fat after nephrectomy in a 37-year-old man with renal cell carcinoma.
A. Contrast-enhanced CT shows a left renal tumor. **B, C.** After surgery, pancreas (P in **B**) moved posteriorly and the retroperitoneal fat (F in **C**) markedly increased in amount and fills the left renal fossa.

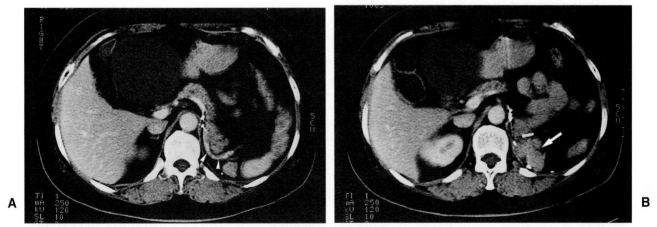

Fig. 2. Postoperative CT in a 57-year-old man, in which the tail of the pancreas may mimic a recurrent tumor.
A, B. Contrast-enhanced CT scans taken 1 year after radical nephrectomy show posteriorly moved pancreas. The tail of the pancreas (*arrow* in **B**) rotates over the splenic vein (*arrowheads* in **A**) and may be misinterpreted as a locally recurrent tumor, but note that it shows homogeneous attenuation.

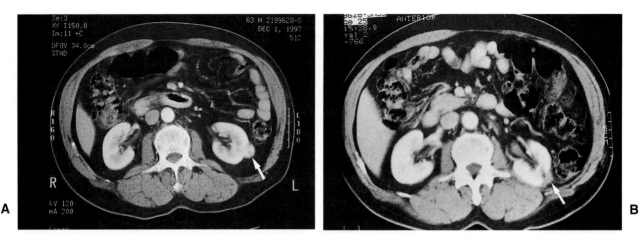

Fig. 3. The changes after tumorectomy in a 63-year-old woman with a small renal cell carcinoma.
A. Contrast-enhanced CT shows a small tumor *(arrow)* in the left kidney. **B.** Follow-up CT scan taken 1 year later shows ill-defined soft tissue lesion in the surgical defect *(arrow)*, but biopsy of the lesion revealed only fibrotic scar.

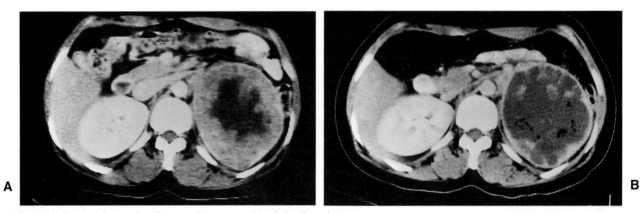

Fig. 4. Postembolization changes in a 33-year-old woman with renal cell carcinoma.
A. Contrast-enhanced CT shows a large tumor in the left kidney. **B.** Because the patient had metastatic lesions, renal artery embolization was performed with ethanol, and follow-up CT scan obtained 2 weeks after embolization shows necrosis and mottled gas in the tumor.

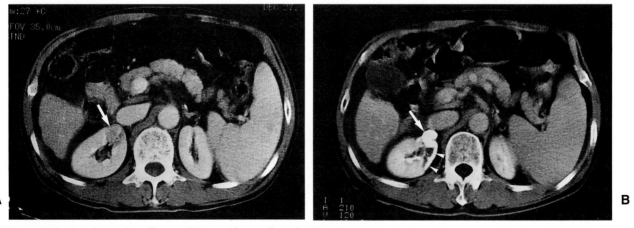

Fig. 5. Postembolization changes in a 63-year-old man with a small renal cell carcinoma.
A. Contrast-enhanced CT shows a small tumor *(arrow)* in the right kidney. Because this patient had severe liver cirrhosis, embolization was done instead of surgery using ethanol and iodized oil. **B.** Follow-up CT taken 5 months later shows a shrunken tumor with retention of iodized oil *(arrow)*. Also note the retention of iodized oil in the adjacent renal parenchyma *(arrowheads)*.

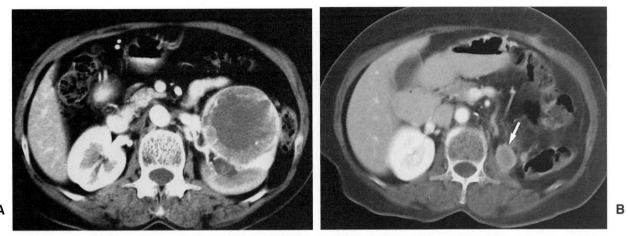

Fig. 6. Local recurrence of renal cell carcinoma of alpha-fetoprotein–producing clear cell type in a 63-year-old woman.
A. Contrast-enhanced CT scan in cortical phase shows a large mass in the left kidney. The mass has extensive central necrosis with subtle enhancement in the periphery. **B.** Follow-up CT scan obtained 4 months after radical nephrectomy shows a locally recurrent tumor *(arrow)* with central necrosis adjacent to the psoas muscle.

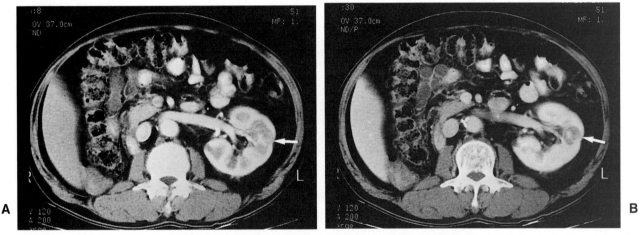

Fig. 7. Recurrent renal cell carcinoma in the opposite kidney in a 65-year-old man who underwent radical nephrectomy for renal cell carcinoma 6 years earlier.
A, B. Contrast-enhanced CT scans in cortical (**A**) and nephrographic (**B**) phases well demonstrate a round mass of heterogeneous attenuation *(arrow)*.

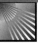

17. Wilms' Tumor

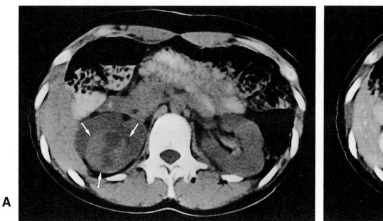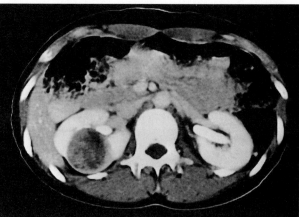

Fig. 1. Wilms' tumor in a 16-year-old girl.
A. Nonenhanced CT shows a round mass *(arrows)* in the right kidney, which has heterogeneous high attenuation. **B.** Contrast-enhanced CT shows heterogeneous enhancement of the lesion. The tumor does not exhibit any specific findings.

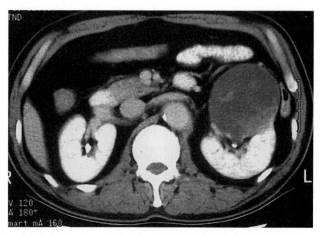

Fig. 2. Wilms' tumor in a 52-year-old man with history of left flank pain and microscopic hematuria. Contrast-enhanced CT shows a well-defined, exophytic, cystic mass with enhancing solid components in the left kidney. (Courtesy of Seung Eun Jung, MD.)

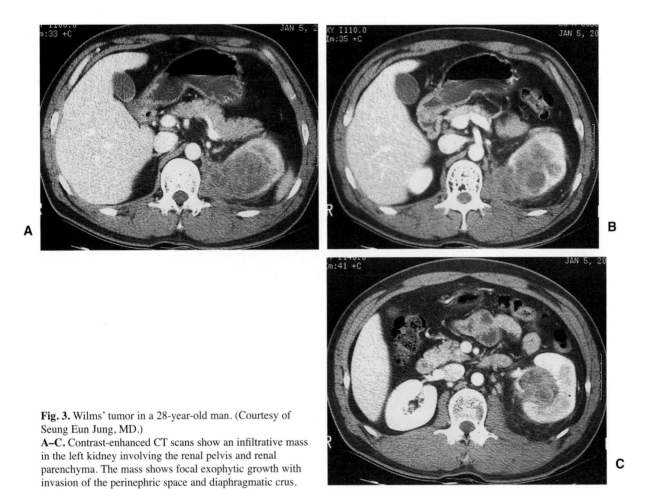

Fig. 3. Wilms' tumor in a 28-year-old man. (Courtesy of Seung Eun Jung, MD.)
A–C. Contrast-enhanced CT scans show an infiltrative mass in the left kidney involving the renal pelvis and renal parenchyma. The mass shows focal exophytic growth with invasion of the perinephric space and diaphragmatic crus.

18. Renal Lymphoma

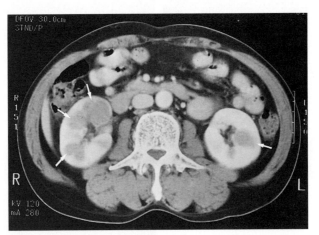

Fig. 1. Renal lymphoma in a 60-year-old man. Contrast-enhanced CT shows multiple, ill-defined, homogeneous, low-attenuated lesions *(arrows)* in both kidneys. Note that the renal contour is preserved.

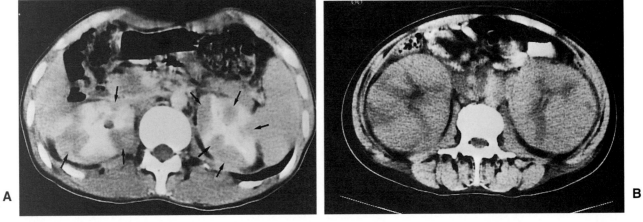

Fig. 2. Renal lymphoma in a 24-year-old man.
A. Contrast-enhanced CT shows multiple, round or wedge-shaped, homogeneous, low-attenuated lesions *(arrows)* in both kidneys. **B.** Follow-up nonenhanced CT scan shows markedly enlarged kidneys replaced by high-attenuated masses. The patient was in a state of acute renal failure and improved after radiation therapy to both kidneys.

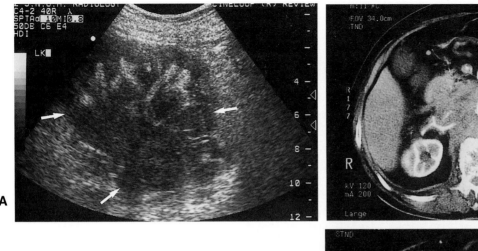

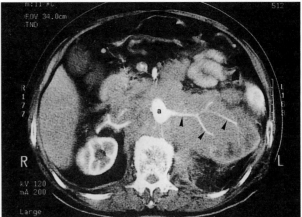

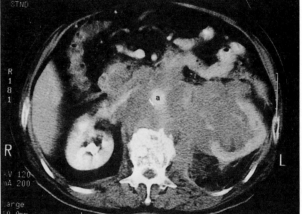

Fig. 3. Retroperitoneal lymphoma involving the kidney in a 76-year-old man.
A. Longitudinal US of the left kidney shows a large, ill-defined, hypoechoic mass *(arrows)* in the renal sinus region.
B, C. Contrast-enhanced CT scans in cortical (**B**) and excretory (**C**) phases show a large, homogeneous, retroperitoneal mass infiltrating into the left renal sinus. Note that the abdominal aorta (a) and renal vessels *(arrowheads in **B**)* are encased by the mass.

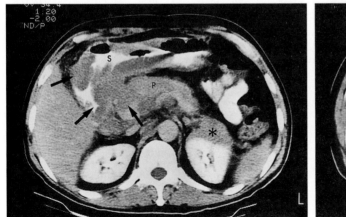

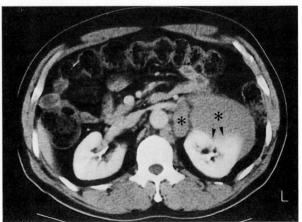

Fig. 4. Lymphoma involving perirenal space and the kidney in a 50-year-old man.
A, B. Contrast-enhanced CT scans show homogeneous, soft tissue masses in the perirenal space *(asterisks)*. Note involvement of the kidney *(arrowheads in **B**)* by the perirenal mass. Also note tumor involvement *(arrows in **A**)* of the stomach (S) and pancreas (P).

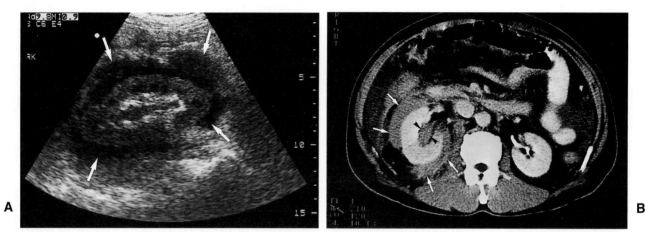

Fig. 5. Lymphoma involving perirenal space and renal sinus in a 65-year-old man.
A. Longitudinal US of the right kidney shows a perirenal mass *(arrows)* encircling the right kidney. Note that the echogenicity of the mass is very low so that it may be mistaken for perirenal fluid collection. **B.** Contrast-enhanced CT shows homogeneous soft tissue masses in the right perirenal spaces *(arrows)* and the renal sinus *(arrowheads).*

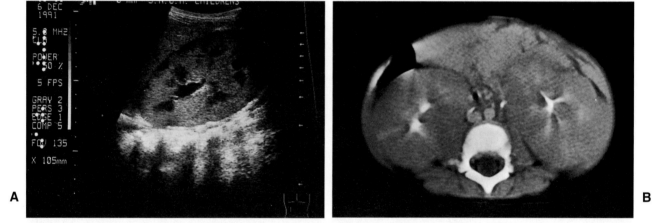

Fig. 6. Diffuse involvement of both kidneys in a 2-year-old boy who has lymphoma with leukemic transformation.
A. US of the right kidney shows globular enlargement with diffusely increased cortical echogenicity. Note that the renal medullae appear prominent.
B. Contrast-enhanced CT shows severe enlargement of both kidneys without focal lesions.

19. Metastatic Tumors of the Kidney

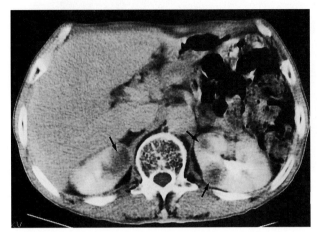

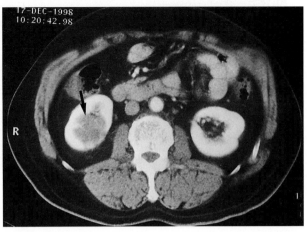

Fig. 1. Renal metastases from lung cancer in a 77-year-old man. Contrast-enhanced CT shows multiple renal masses *(arrows)*. Note most of the masses are ill-defined and are located within the renal contour. (From Kim SH: CT and US findings of the renal metastases. J Korean Radiol Soc 1995; 32:307–313.)

Fig. 2. Solitary renal metastasis from lung cancer in a 57-year-old man. Contrast-enhanced CT scan shows an ill-defined mass in the right kidney *(arrow)*. The mass has homogeneous attenuation and is within the renal contour.

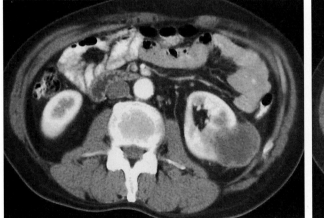

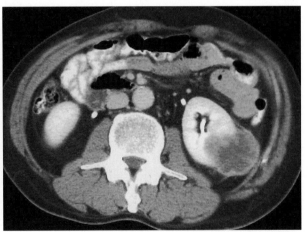

A

B

Fig. 3. Solitary exophytic renal metastasis from lung cancer in a 51-year-old man.
A, B. Contrast-enhanced CT scans in cortical **(A)** and nephrographic **(B)** phases show an exophytic mass in the left kidney. The mass is homogeneous and low attenuated and accompanies perirenal changes.

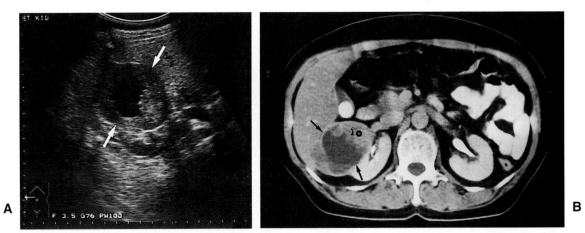

Fig. 4. A 58-year-old woman with solitary renal metastasis from adenoid cystic carcinoma of the parotid gland that was removed 7 years earlier. **A.** US of the right kidney in transverse plane shows a large renal mass *(arrows)* with central necrosis. **B.** Contrast-enhanced CT shows a large mass *(arrows)* in the right kidney, which grows exophytically and has heterogeneous attenuation. This CT finding is indistinguishable from the findings of renal cell carcinoma.

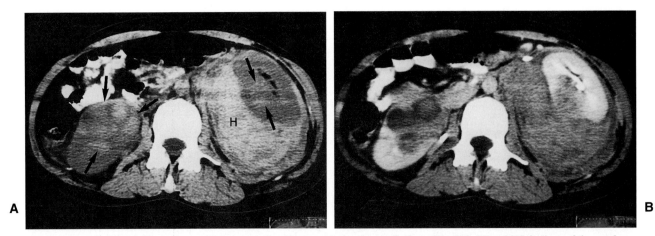

Fig. 5. Renal metastasis from choriocarcinoma of the uterus in a 33-year-old woman. (**A, B,** From Kim SH: CT and US findings of the renal metastases. J Korean Radiol Soc 1995; 32:307–313.) **A.** Nonenhanced CT shows large, high-attenuated, perirenal hematoma on the left side (H) and ill-defined, high-attenuated masses *(arrows)* in both kidneys. **B.** Contrast-enhanced CT demonstrates low-attenuated masses in both kidneys and left perirenal hematoma.

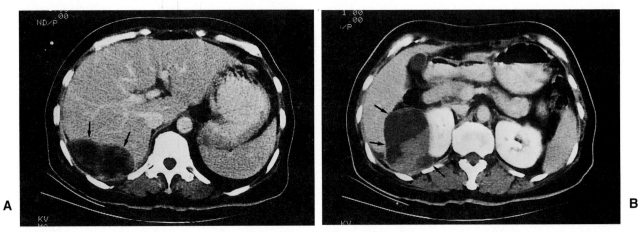

Fig. 6. Perirenal and retrohepatic metastases from endometrial carcinoma in a 57-year-old woman. **A.** Contrast-enhanced CT shows a low-attenuated mass *(arrows)* in the bare area of the liver. **B.** CT scan at a lower level shows a similar low-attenuated mass *(arrows)* in the right perirenal space with compression of the right kidney.

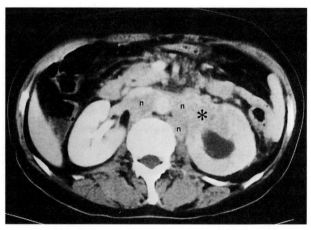

Fig. 7. Uterine cervical carcinoma with metastases to the retroperitoneal lymph nodes and kidney in a 62-year-old woman. Contrast-enhanced CT shows multiple, conglomerated, retroperitoneal lymphadenopathy (n) infiltrating into the left renal sinus *(asterisk)*, causing hydronephrosis.

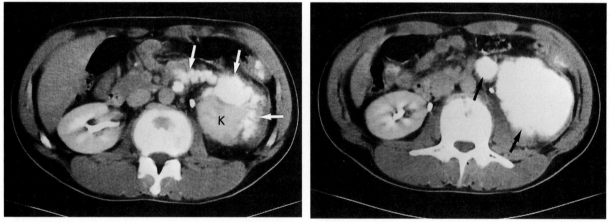

A   B

Fig. 8. Renal metastasis with dense ossification in a 19-year-old man with osteogenic sarcoma.
A, B. Contrast-enhanced CT scans show densely ossified masses in the left perirenal space *(arrows)*. K, lower pole of the left kidney.

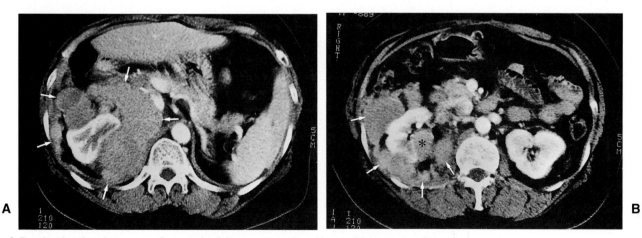

A   B

Fig. 9. Renal and perirenal metastases from uterine leiomyosarcoma in a 44-year-old woman.
A, B. Contrast-enhanced CT scans show multiple masses in the right perirenal space *(arrows)* and a mass *(asterisk in B)* in the right kidney.

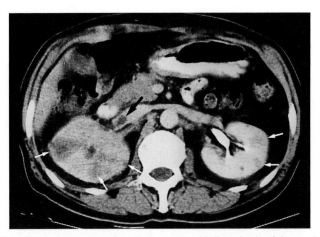

Fig. 10. Renal metastases from lung cancer with thrombosis of the renal vein in a 65-year-old man. Contrast-enhanced CT shows multiple, ill-defined, low-attenuated masses *(white arrows)* in both kidneys. Note a low-attenuated thrombus *(black arrow)* in the right renal vein.

20. Sarcomas and Other Malignant Tumors of Renal Parenchyma

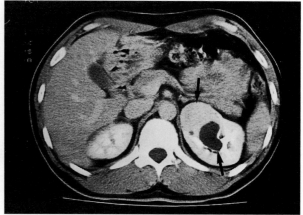
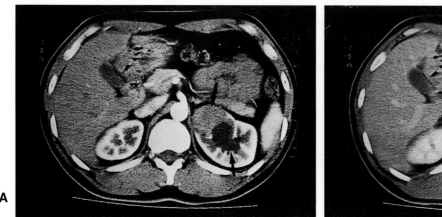

A

B

Fig. 1. Renal capsular leiomyosarcoma in a 34-year-old man.
A, B. Contrast-enhanced CT scans in cortical **(A)** and excretory **(B)** phases show a mass *(arrows)* composed of solid and cystic components in the anterior aspect of the left kidney.

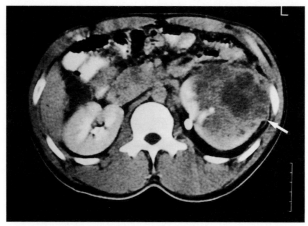

Fig. 2. Malignant fibrous histiocytoma of the kidney in a 36-year-old man. Contrast-enhanced CT shows a large low-attenuated mass in the left kidney. Note that the mass is ill-demarcated and extends into the perirenal space *(arrow)* with thickening of the renal fascia.

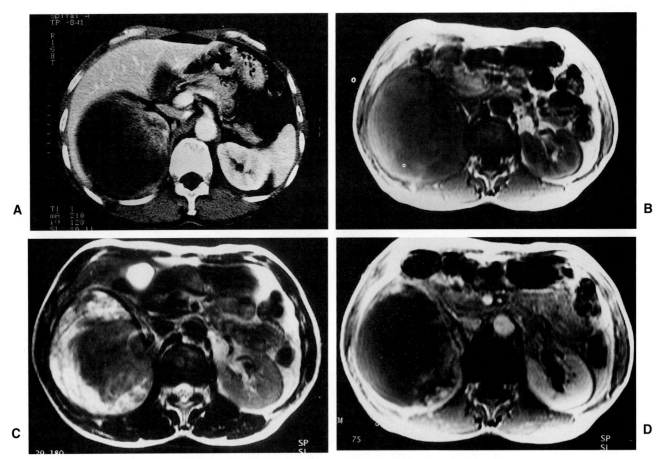

Fig. 3. Carcinosarcoma of the kidney in a 40-year-old man who underwent left pneumonectomy for squamous cell carcinoma of the lung 2 years earlier.
A. Contrast-enhanced CT shows a large, nonenhancing mass in the right kidney. **B.** T1-weighted MR image shows diffuse low signal intensity of the mass. **C.** T2-weighted MR image shows peripheral high intensity and central low intensity of the right renal mass. **D.** Contrast-enhanced T1-weighted image shows poor enhancement of the mass.

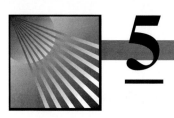

5

Urothelial Tumors of the Pelvocalyces and Ureter

JUNG SUK SIM

Urinary collecting systems, including calyces, pelvis, and ureters, originate in the ureteric bud and consist of urothelium and mesodermal tissues. Transitional cell epithelium covering the urinary tract has a potential for metaplasia to glandular or squamous epithelium. Therefore, any benign or malignant tumors from transitional, glandular, or squamous epithelium can occur in urothelium. The most common tumor from urothelium is transitional cell carcinoma (85%), followed by squamous cell carcinoma. Mesodermal tumors arise from smooth muscles or neural, vascular, fibrous, or lymphoid tissues. The most common mesodermal tumor is fibroepithelial polyp.

TRANSITIONAL CELL CARCINOMA

Transitional cell carcinoma is a cancer of transitional epithelium. It is believed that exposure to industrial carcinogens such as dyes, rubber, cable, and plastics, cigarette smoking, and abuse of analgesics are important risk factors for developing transitional cell carcinoma. Because elderly men are usually exposed to them longer and more intensively, the incidence of transitional cell carcinoma is highest in the age group of 50 to 70 years and occurs more frequently in men than in women. Transitional cell carcinoma occurs more frequently in the bladder than in the pelvis and ureter by 30 to 50 times, since urine that contains carcinogen stays longer in the bladder.

Multiplicity of transitional cell carcinoma is relatively common. Bilateral transitional cell carcinomas occur in the renal pelvis and ureter in 1% and 5% of cases, respectively. Patients with bladder carcinoma may have upper tract carcinoma in 3%, whereas about 30% to 40% of patients with upper tract transitional cell carcinoma have bladder cancer.

Transitional cell carcinoma has two growth patterns: papillary and nonpapillary, or invasive. About half of papillary tumors have a base on mucosa and grow into lumen, whereas nonpapillary tumors usually grow invasively deep into the wall. Calcification of transitional cell carcinoma is rare, found in less than 3% of cases. When it is found, it shows a diffuse, punctate pattern, although in rare instances it is very dense and looks like a stone.

The staging system proposed by the International Union Against Cancer and the American Joint Committee on Cancer is practical to use. In this system, the following criteria apply:

T1: tumor invades subepithelial connective tissue
T2: tumor invades muscularis

T3: renal pelvis tumor invades beyond muscularis into peripelvic fat or renal parenchyma, or ureter tumor invades beyond muscularis into periureteral fat
T4: tumor invades adjacent organs or through the kidney into perirenal fat

Transitional cell carcinoma of the pelvocalyces

Transitional cell carcinoma comprises less than 10% of intrarenal tumors, but it is two or three times more common than transitional cell carcinoma of the ureter.

Intravenous urography (IVU) findings of papillary transitional cell carcinomas are basically filling defects, whereas nonpapillary tumors, which cause wall thickening, may show smooth surfaces. Tumors that obstruct pelvocalyces cause dilation of calyces or pelvis. Tumors that fill a calyx can cause disappearance of a calyx, which is referred to as the "phantom calyx" or "amputated calyx."

Computed tomography (CT) is a useful tool for detection and staging of transitional cell carcinoma of the pelvocalyceal system. On nonenhanced CT, transitional cell carcinoma may be seen as a mass in the pelvocalyceal system that has attenuation higher than urine. On contrast-enhanced CT, transitional cell carcinoma is enhanced, but much less than the renal parenchyma. On delayed CT scan, the tumors appear as filling defects in the pelvocalyces.

The findings that suggest renal parenchymal invasion of pelvocalyceal tumor are focal areas of decreased enhancement in the renal parenchyma, vague interface between the mass and the renal parenchyma, and focal dilation of calyces. Renal parenchymal involvement is an important prognostic factor in pelvocalyceal transitional cell carcinoma.

If a transitional cell carcinoma grows larger, differentiation from renal cell carcinoma may be problematic. In this instance, the findings that favor transitional cell carcinoma are central location of the mass, centrifugal growth pattern, maintenance of reniform contour, relatively homogeneous attenuation, and weak enhancement.

Ultrasonography (US) and magnetic resonance (MR) imaging play only a small role in diagnosis and staging of pelvocalyceal transitional cell carcinomas. The most common US appearance of transitional cell carcinoma is a homogeneous hypoechoic mass, but it may show heterogeneous echogenicity when the tumor is larger. On T1- and T2-weighted MR images, pelvocalyceal transitional cell carcinoma shows similar signal intensity as renal parenchyma.

The most important factor indicating poor prognosis of pelvocalyceal transitional cell carcinoma is infiltration beyond the pelvic wall. If one can find excreted contrast material or sinus fat between the mass and renal parenchyma, that tumor can be assigned as stage T2 or less.

Transitional cell carcinoma of the ureter

Ureteral transitional cell carcinoma is unique because of its infiltrative and well-metastasizing nature. It is believed to be due to a thin ureteral wall and abundant lymphatics around the ureters.

Urography is useful in detecting transitional cell carcinomas of the ureter. If transitional cell carcinoma of any site is detected, IVU should be performed thoroughly to find additional transitional cell carcinomas in the urinary tract. IVU findings of ureteral transitional cell carcinoma are most commonly nonfunctioning kidney or hydronephrosis. IVU may demonstrate ureteral filling defects or circumferential or eccentric masses in the ureteral wall. Goblet sign or Bergman's sign is useful in differentiating a ureteral tumor from a ureteral stone. A typical feature of an intraluminal tumor is dilation of the adjacent proximal ureter as well as the distal ureter. Distal ureteral dilation in ureteral tumor is believed to be due to mechanical expansion by tumor and repeated intussusceptions of tumor into the distal segment of the ureter. On the other hand, acute obstruction due to a ureteral stone does not cause distal ureteral dilation. Instead, the distal segment of the ureter is narrowed in acute obstruction due to spasm and decreased urine flow.

CT is on the second line in the diagnosis of ureteral transitional cell carcinoma. CT may demonstrate hydronephrosis and mass or wall thickening of the ureter. CT is superior in differentiating ureteral tumor from stone or hematoma and in demonstrating the changes in adjacent structures such as periureteral infiltration or regional lymph node enlargement.

SQUAMOUS CELL CARCINOMA

Squamous cell carcinoma is the second most common tumor of the urinary tract. It comprises 15% of all renal pelvis tumors. Longstanding irritation to the urothelium, typically by stone, indwelling catheter, or schistosomiasis, causes metaplasia of the transitional epithelium to squamous epithelium. Hypertrophy of metaplastic squamous epithelium results in leukoplakia, and then leukoplakia changes into a squamous cell carcinoma if it is continuously exposed to concentrated carcinogen in urine.

It is difficult to differentiate squamous cell carcinoma from transitional cell carcinoma radiologically. Squamous cell carcinoma is usually larger than transitional cell carcinoma at the time of diagnosis and frequently has stones or signs of chronic irritation.

ADENOCARCINOMA AND CARCINOSARCOMA

Adenocarcinoma

Adenocarcinoma of the urinary tract is much rarer than transitional cell carcinoma and squamous cell carcinoma. Like squamous cell carcinoma, adenocarcinoma is caused by malignant transformation of metaplastic mucosa. It is commonly associated with stone disease or chronic inflammatory disease. Like adenocarcinoma of other organs, dystrophic calcification is rather common, especially in mucin-producing adenocarcinoma.

Carcinosarcoma

Sometimes, carcinoma and sarcoma are found together. Sarcomatoid transformation of carcinoma or collision of two tumors is possible. The carcinomatous component is transitional cell or squamous cell, whereas the sarcomatous component is various types. The prognosis of carcinosarcoma is poor.

PAPILLOMA AND INVERTED PAPILLOMA

Papilloma is a benign tumor of transitional epithelium. Inverted papilloma is also a benign tumor of transitional epithelium, but the direction of growth is different. Papilloma grows toward the luminal direction, whereas an inverted papilloma grows into submucosa. Histologic features of the two tumors are the same, but whether they are the same tumors is still being debated. They may be premalignant lesions. A usual radiologic finding is a round, mucosa-based filling defect that is quite similar to low-grade transitional cell carcinoma.

References

1. Yoo SY, Kim SH, Lee KH, et al: Intraureteral recurrence of renal cell carcinoma following nephrectomy: A case report. J Korean Radiol Soc 2000; 43:607–609.
2. Wong-You-Cheong JJ, Wagner BJ, Davis CJ Jr: Transitional cell carcinoma of the urinary tract: Radiologic-pathologic correlation. Radiographics 1998; 18:123–142.
3. Weeks SM, Brown ED, Brown JJ, et al: Transitional cell carcinoma of the upper urinary tract: Staging by MRI. Abdom Imaging 1995; 20:365–367.
4. Ramchandani P, Pollack HM: Tumors of the urothelium. Semin Roentgenol 1995; 30:149–167.
5. Badalament RA, Bennett WF, Bova JG, et al: Computed tomography of primary transitional cell carcinoma of upper urinary tracts. Urology 1992; 40:71–75.
6. Nyman U, Oldbring J, Aspelin P: CT of carcinoma of the renal pelvis. Acta Radiol 1992; 33:31–38.
7. Leder RA, Dunnick NR: Transitional cell carcinoma of the pelvicalices and ureter. AJR Am J Roentgenol 1990; 155:713–722.
8. Milestone B, Friedman AC, Seidmon EJ, et al: Staging of ureteral transitional cell carcinoma by CT and MRI. Urology 1990; 36:346–349.
9. Anderstrom C, Johansson SL, Pettersson S, et al: Carcinoma of the ureter: A clinicopathologic study of 49 cases. J Urol 1989; 142:280–283.
10. Narumi Y, Sato T, Hori S, et al: Squamous cell carcinoma of the uroepithelium: CT evaluation. Radiology 1989; 173:853–856.
11. Kim YI, Yoon DH, Lee SW, et al: Multicentric papillary adenocarcinoma of the renal pelvis and ureter: Report of a case with ultrastructural study. Cancer 1988; 62:2402–2407.
12. Goldman SM, Bohlman ME, Gatewood OM: Neoplasms of the renal collecting system. Semin Roentgenol 1987; 22:284–291.
13. Ostrovsky PD, Carr L, Goodman J: Ultrasound of transitional cell carcinoma. J Clin Ultrasound 1985; 13:35–36.
14. Mirone V, Prezioso D, Palombini S, et al: Mucinous adenocarcinoma of the renal pelvis. Eur Urol 1984; 10:284–285.
15. Chen KT, Workman RD, Flam MS, et al: Carcinosarcoma of renal pelvis. Urology 1983; 22:429–431.

16. Markovic B, Antic N, Stanojevic V, et al: Epidermoid carcinoma of the renal pelvis with a large renal stone. Br J Urol 1983; 55:577–578.
17. McClennan BL, Balfe DM: Oncologic imaging: Kidney and ureter. Int J Radiat Oncol Biol Phys 1983; 9:1683–1704.
18. Watters G, Grant A, Wiley S, et al: Inverted papilloma of the upper urinary tract. Br J Urol 1983; 55:176–179.
19. Gatewood OM, Goldman SM, Marshall FF, et al: Computerized tomography in the diagnosis of transitional cell carcinoma of the kidney. J Urol 1982; 127:876–887.
20. Nocks BN, Heney NM, Daly JJ, et al: Transitional cell carcinoma of renal pelvis. Urology 1982; 19:472–477.
21. Banner MP, Pollack HM: Fibrous ureteral polyps. Radiology 1979; 130:73–76

Illustrations • Urothelial Tumors of the Pelvocalyces and Ureter

1 • Transitional cell carcinoma of the renal pelvocalyces

2 • Transitional cell carcinoma with renal parenchymal invasion

3 • Transitional cell carcinoma with renal vein thrombosis

4 • Transitional cell carcinoma in congenital ureteropelvic junction obstruction

5 • Transitional cell carcinoma of the ureter

6 • Multiple transitional cell carcinomas in the urinary tract

7 • Calcified transitional cell carcinoma

8 • Transitional cell carcinoma with other histologic differentiation

9 • Adenocarcinoma of the urinary tract

10 • Squamous cell carcinoma of the urinary tract

11 • Metastatic tumors of the urinary tract

12 • Brush biopsy for urothelial tumor

1. Transitional Cell Carcinoma of the Renal Pelvocalyces

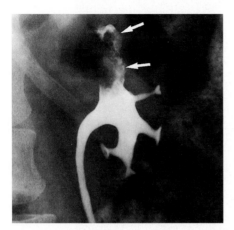

Fig. 1. Papillary transitional cell carcinoma of the calyx in a 45-year-old man. RGP shows papillary tumor involving upper-pole calyx of the left kidney *(arrows)*. Note a mottled and streaky collection of contrast material in the surface of the tumor, suggesting the papillary nature of the tumor.

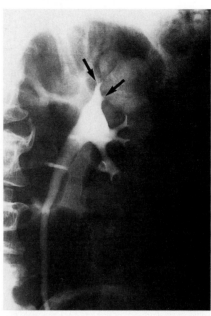

Fig. 2. Transitional cell carcinoma with calyceal amputation in a 66-year-old man. IVU shows amputation of calyceal infundibula *(arrows)* in the upper pole of the left kidney. Note irregularities in the margin of the amputated calyces.

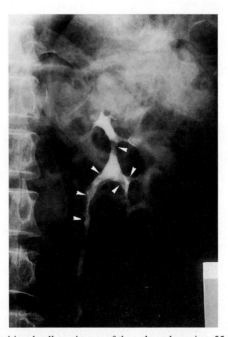

Fig. 3. Transitional cell carcinoma of the pelvocalyces in a 55-year-old man who had transitional cell carcinoma of the bladder that was treated by repeated transurethral resection for 10 years. IVU shows fine nodularities and irregularities in the left pelvocalyces and proximal ureter *(arrowheads)*.

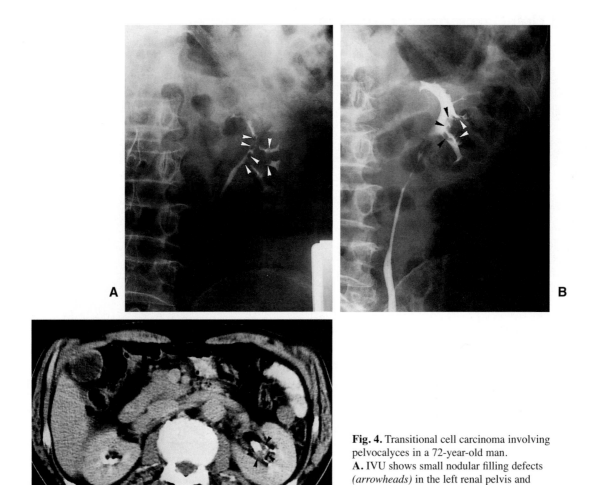

Fig. 4. Transitional cell carcinoma involving pelvocalyces in a 72-year-old man.
A. IVU shows small nodular filling defects *(arrowheads)* in the left renal pelvis and calyces. **B.** RGP well demonstrates filling defects with irregular margin *(arrowheads)*. **C.** Contrast-enhanced CT shows filling defects *(arrowheads)* in the renal pelvis.

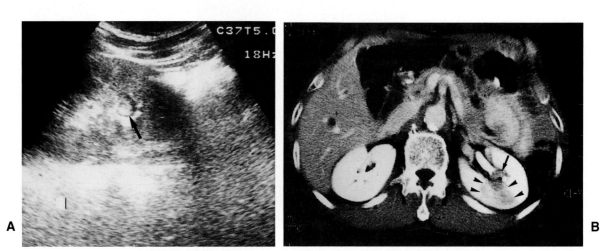

Fig. 5. Small transitional cell carcinoma in a 67-year-old man.
A. Longitudinal US of the left kidney shows a small echogenic mass *(arrow)* in the lower pole area within the renal sinus. **B.** Contrast-enhanced CT shows a small mass *(arrow)* in the tip of the calyx in the left kidney. Note focal area of diminished parenchymal perfusion *(arrowheads)* in the posterior aspect of the left kidney adjacent to the calyceal mass.

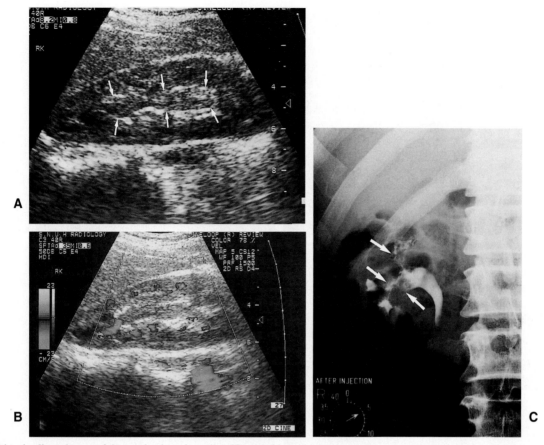

Fig. 6. Transitional cell carcinoma of the renal pelvocalyces in a 47-year-old man.
A. US of the right kidney shows separation of renal sinus echoes by the lesion of intermediate echogenicity *(arrows)*. **B.** Color Doppler US shows hypovascular nature of the lesion. (**B,** See also Color Section.) **C.** IVU shows irregular filling defects in the pelvocalyces of the right kidney *(arrows)*. Note that the surface of the lesions has mottled and streaky contrast material, suggesting the papillary nature of the lesion (the stipple sign).

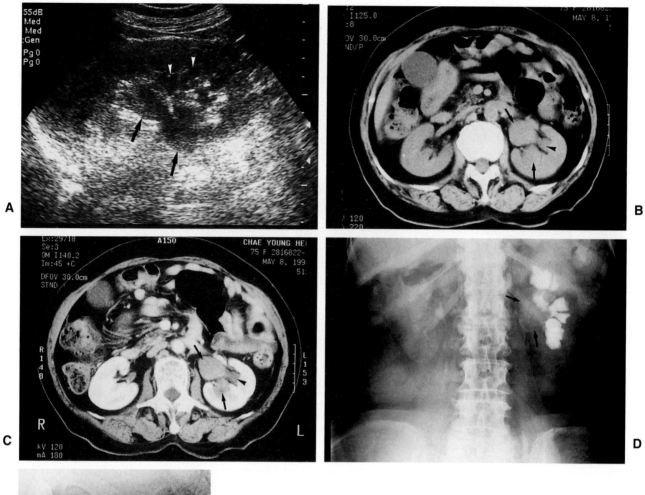

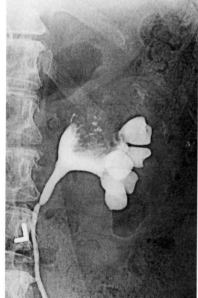

Fig. 7. Papillary transitional cell carcinoma of the pelvocalyces in a 75-year-old woman. **A.** Longitudinal US of the left kidney shows masses *(arrows)* in the dilated renal pelvis and upper-polar calyx. Also note caliectasis in the interpolar and lower-polar regions *(arrowheads)*. **B, C.** Nonenhanced **(B)** and contrast-enhanced **(C)** CT scans at the level of the renal hilum show the masses *(arrows)* in the renal pelvis and posterior calyx with dilation of the anterior calyx *(arrowhead)*. **D.** IVU shows filling defects *(arrows)* in the renal pelvis and upper-polar calyx in the left kidney. **E.** RGP well demonstrates the papillary nature of the tumors.

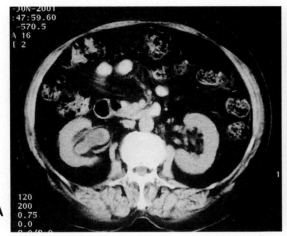

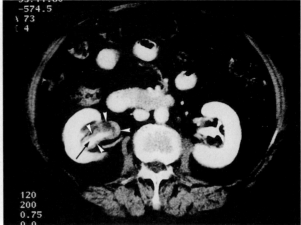

A

B

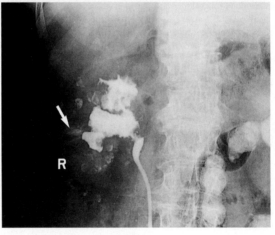

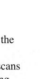

R

C

Fig. 8. Diffuse infiltrative transitional cell carcinoma of the pelvocalyces in a 75-year-old woman.
A, B. Nonenhanced (**A**) and contrast-enhanced (**B**) CT scans show dilated right renal pelvis and diffuse wall thickening (*arrowheads* in **B**). Note that the lumen of the right renal pelvis (*arrow* in **B**) is filled with excreted contrast material. **C.** RGP shows diffuse nodularities and irregularities in the right pelvocalyces. Note pyelotubular backflow *(arrow)* from the lower-pole calyx.

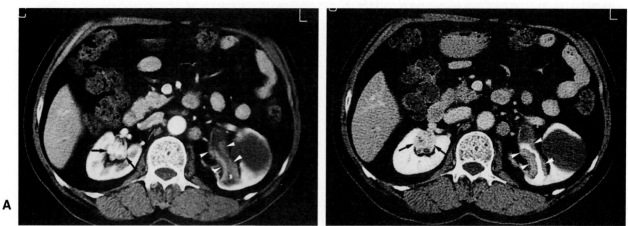

Fig. 9. Simultaneous transitional cell carcinoma and renal cell carcinoma in a 62-year-old man.
A. Contrast-enhanced CT scan in cortical phase shows lesions in both kidneys. The right kidney has a well-enhancing, spherical mass *(arrows)* in the sinus region. Note that the attenuation of the right renal mass is similar to that of the renal cortex. In the left kidney, the wall of the renal pelvis enhances and is thickened and irregular *(arrowheads)*. Also note a simple cyst in the left kidney. **B.** CT scan in excretory phase shows the right renal mass *(arrows)* and thickened pelvic wall *(arrowheads)* in the left kidney more clearly. The right renal mass was a renal cell carcinoma, and transitional cell carcinoma was found in the left renal pelvis.

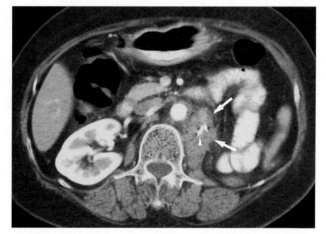

Fig. 10. Postoperative recurrence of transitional cell carcinoma of the renal pelvis in a 70-year-old woman. Contrast-enhanced CT obtained 18 months after left nephroureterectomy shows a soft tissue mass in the left paravertebral region *(arrows)* that engulfs a surgical clip *(arrowhead)*.

2. Transitional Cell Carcinoma with Renal Parenchymal Invasion

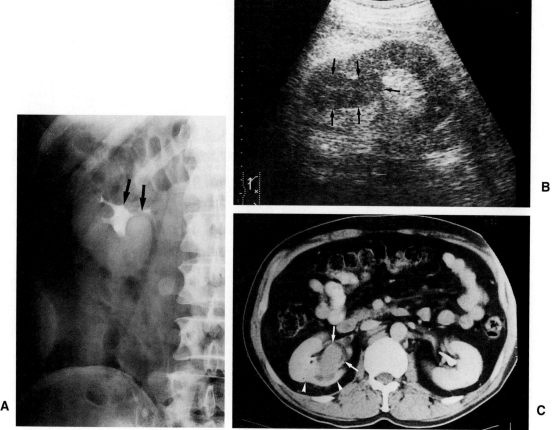

Fig 1. Transitional cell carcinoma causing calyceal amputation in a 52-year-old man.
A. IVU shows nonopacification of the upper-pole calyx and irregularity in the upper margin of the renal pelvis *(arrows)* in the right kidney.
B. Longitudinal US of the right kidney shows an ill-defined, hypoechoic lesion *(arrows)*. **C.** Contrast-enhanced CT shows a homogeneous mass in the right renal pelvis *(arrows)* infiltrating into the posterior renal parenchyma *(arrowheads)*. At pathologic examination, papillary transitional cell carcinoma was found in the renal pelvis and upper-pole calyx with infiltration into the renal parenchyma in the upper-polar region.

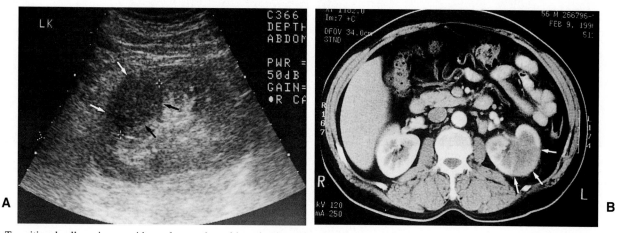

Fig 2. Transitional cell carcinoma with renal parenchymal invasion in a 56-year-old man.
A. Longitudinal US of the left kidney shows an ill-defined, hypoechoic mass *(arrows)* in the upper-polar region. **B.** Contrast-enhanced CT scan in cortical phase shows an ill-defined, low-attenuated lesion in the left kidney *(arrows)*. Note that the renal sinus fat is obliterated but the renal contour is preserved.

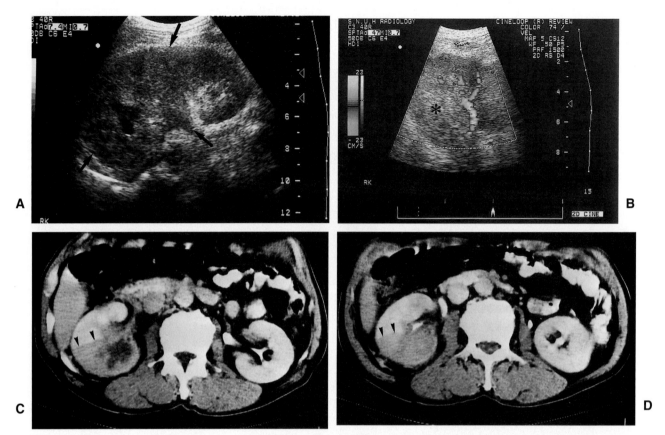

Fig 3. Transitional cell carcinoma with segmental arterial invasion in a 63-year-old man with a history of colon cancer.
A. Longitudinal US of the right kidney shows a diffusely enlarged upper pole *(arrows)* with heterogeneous echogenicity. **B.** Color Doppler US of the right kidney in transverse plane with the patient in lateral decubitus position shows that the posterior aspect of the right kidney is poorly perfused *(asterisk)*. (**B,** See also Color Section.) **C, D.** Contrast-enhanced CT scans show sharp and straight margin of the lesion *(arrowheads)* suggesting involvement of the segmental renal artery by the tumor. Note that the lesion has an area of necrosis and the renal sinus fat is obliterated.

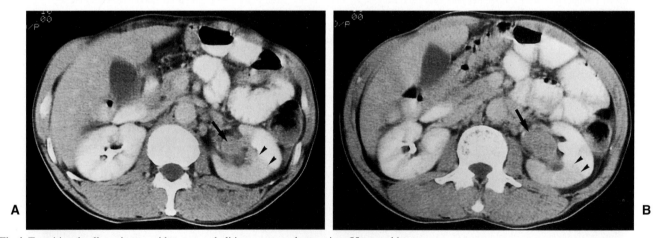

Fig 4. Transitional cell carcinoma with tumor emboli in a segmental artery in a 55-year-old man.
A, B. Contrast-enhanced CT shows a homogeneous, low-attenuated mass in the renal pelvis *(arrow)*. Note poor enhancement of the posterior part of the renal parenchyma with sharp and linear border *(arrowheads)* suggesting involvement of the arterial branch supplying that portion of the kidney.

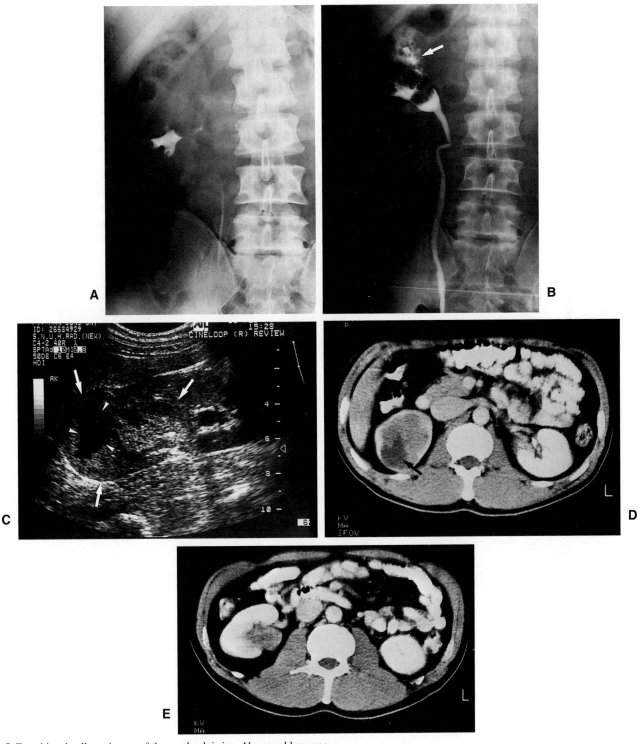

Fig. 5. Transitional cell carcinoma of the renal pelvis in a 41-year-old woman.
A. IVU shows a large filling defect in the renal pelvis and amputated calyces. Only the lower-pole calyx is opacified and is slightly dilated. **B.** RGP well demonstrates a filling defect with an irregular margin in the pelvocalyces of the right kidney. Note the filling of contrast material in the upper-polar region probably in the necrotic cavity of the tumor *(arrow)*. **C.** Longitudinal US of the right kidney demonstrates a large tumor *(arrows)* in the renal pelvis extending into the renal parenchyma in the upper-pole area. Note an irregular cavity *(arrowheads)* in the tumor, which was opacified on RGP. Also note that the lower-pole calyx is slightly dilated. **D, E.** Contrast-enhanced CT scans show the dilated right renal pelvis filled with tumor and the upper-polar region replaced by the low-attenuated tumor. Note the low-attenuated necrotic area *(arrow in **D**)* within the tumor.

3. Transitional Cell Carcinoma with Renal Vein Thrombosis

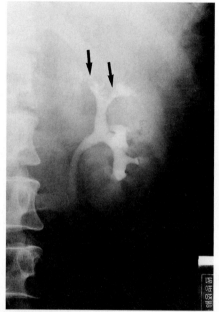

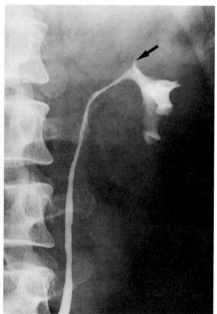

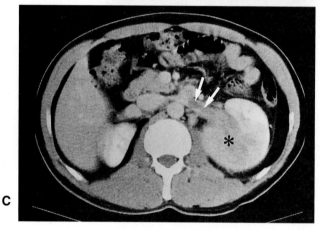

Fig. 1. Renal vein invasion in a 46-year-old man with transitional cell carcinoma mixed with squamous cell carcinoma of the renal pelvocalyces.
A. IVU shows papillary tumors *(arrows)* in the tip of the upper-pole calyx of the left kidney. **B.** RGP taken 2 months later shows marked progression of the disease with amputation of the upper calyceal infundibulum *(arrow)*. **C.** Contrast-enhanced CT shows extensive parenchymal invasion by the tumor *(asterisk)* and invasion of the left renal vein with thrombosis *(arrows)*.

4. Transitional Cell Carcinoma in Congenital Ureteropelvic Junction Obstruction

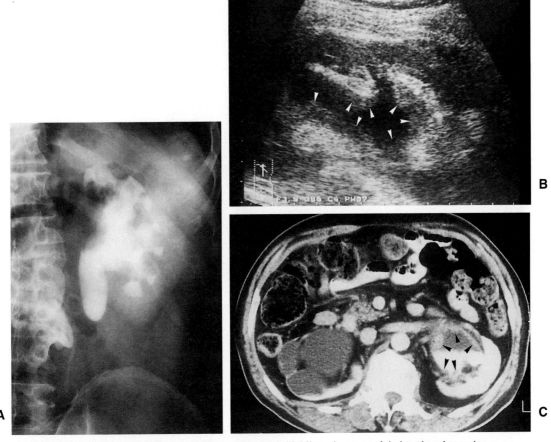

Fig. 1. Transitional cell carcinoma of the pelvocalyces in a 55-year-old man with bilateral ureteropelvic junction obstruction.
A. IVU shows multiple masses arising in the wall of the dilated pelvocalyces of the left kidney. **B.** Longitudinal US of the left kidney shows nodular masses *(arrowheads)* in the wall of the dilated pelvocalyces. **C.** Contrast-enhanced CT shows dilated pelvocalyces of both kidneys. Note thickening and nodular masses *(arrowheads)* in the left pelvocalyces.

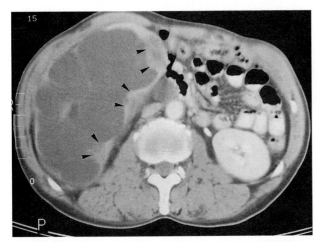

Fig. 2. Transitional cell carcinoma of the renal pelvis in a 62-year-old man with ureteropelvic junction obstruction. Contrast-enhanced CT shows markedly dilated pelvocalyces of the right kidney and thickening with nodular masses *(arrowheads)* in the wall of the dilated pelvis.

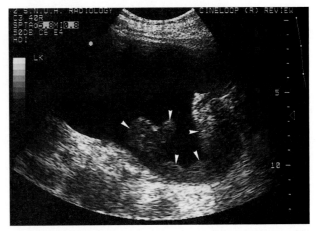

Fig. 3. Transitional cell carcinoma of the renal pelvis in a 68-year-old man with ureteropelvic junction obstruction. US of the left kidney shows markedly dilated renal pelvis and fungating masses *(arrowheads)*.

5. Transitional Cell Carcinoma of the Ureter

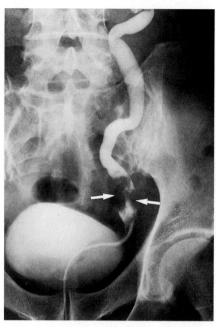

Fig. 1. Transitional cell carcinoma of the ureter in a 64-year-old woman. RGP shows a dilated left ureter and filling defects with papillary surface *(arrows)*.

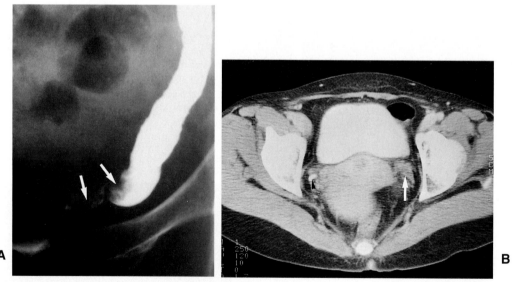

A   B

Fig. 2. Transitional cell carcinoma of the distal ureter in a 52-year-old woman.
A. AGP shows a dilated left ureter due to distal ureteral obstruction. The lesion has an irregular papillary surface *(arrows)*.
B. Contrast-enhanced CT shows a soft tissue tumor in the left distal ureter *(arrow)* with periureteral infiltration. The right distal ureter is well opacified *(arrowhead)*.

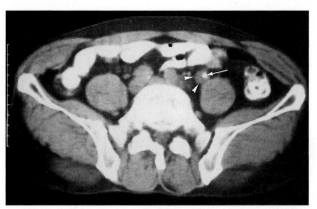

Fig. 3. Transitional cell carcinoma of the ureter in a 55-year-old man. Nonenhanced CT shows a lesion in the left ureter appearing as eccentric thickening *(arrowheads)* of the ureteral wall around the ureteral stent *(arrow)*.

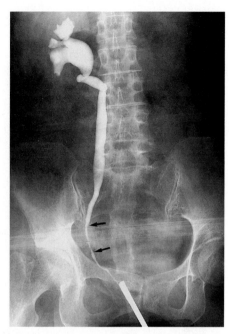

Fig. 4. Transitional cell carcinoma manifesting as a long-segment stenosis of the ureter in a 69-year-old woman. RGP shows a long-segment stenosis of the right distal ureter *(arrows)* with relatively smooth margin.

6. Multiple Transitional Cell Carcinomas in the Urinary Tract

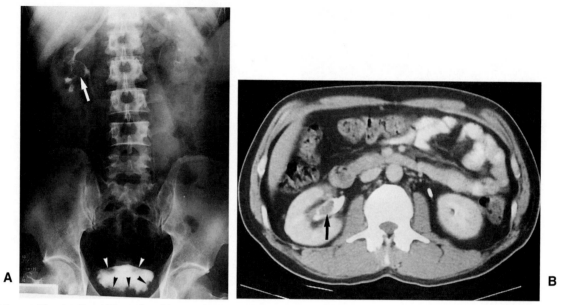

Fig 1. Multiple transitional cell carcinomas in a 56-year-old man.
A. IVU shows multiple papillary tumors in the right renal pelvis *(arrow)* and urinary bladder *(arrowheads)*. **B.** Contrast-enhanced CT of the kidney demonstrates the tumor in the right renal pelvis *(arrow)*.

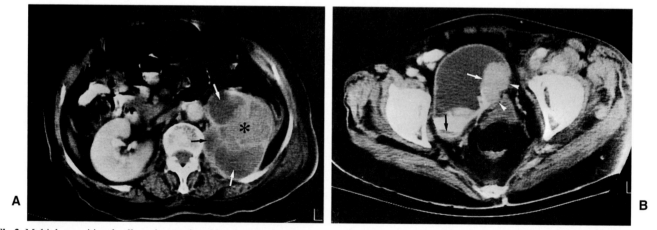

Fig 2. Multiple transitional cell carcinomas in a 80-year-old woman.
A. Contrast-enhanced CT shows a large soft tissue tumor *(asterisk)* and adjacent caliectasis *(arrows)* in the left kidney. **B.** CT scan of the urinary bladder shows multiple masses *(arrows)* in the bladder. Note the deformed contour of the bladder with an irregular outline in the left posterolateral aspect of the bladder *(arrowheads)* suggesting perivesical tumor infiltration.

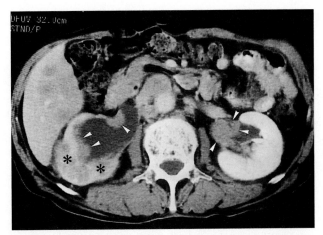

Fig 3. Recurrent bilateral pelvocalyceal transitional cell carcinomas in a 68-year-old man with history of bladder cancer. Contrast-enhanced CT shows multiple masses *(arrowheads)* in the pelvocalyces of both kidneys. Note that there is renal parenchymal invasion *(asterisks)* in the right kidney. This patient also had metastatic lesions in the liver.

7. Calcified Transitional Cell Carcinoma

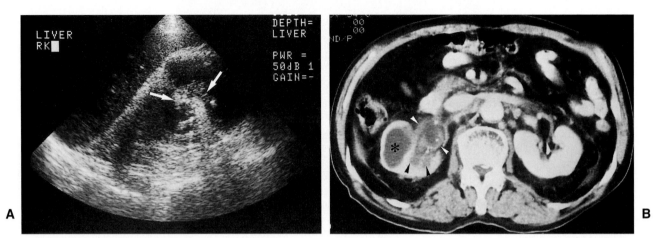

Fig. 1. Calcified transitional cell carcinoma in a 77-year-old man.
A. Longitudinal US of the right kidney shows an irregular-marginated, echogenic mass *(arrows)* in the renal sinus with peripheral caliectases.
B. Contrast-enhanced CT demonstrates the tumor *(arrowheads)* with mottled calcification in the pelvocalyces of the right kidney. Note a dilated calyx *(asterisk)* due to obstruction by the tumor.

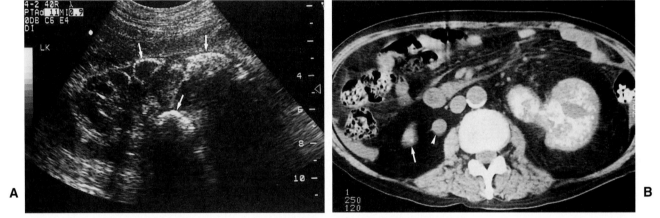

Fig. 2. Calcified transitional cell carcinoma in a 77-year-old man with end-stage renal disease and history of bladder cancer.
A. Longitudinal US of the left kidney shows dilated pelvocalyces filled with echogenic masses *(arrows)* accompanying posterior sonic shadowing.
B. Nonenhanced CT shows an enlarged left kidney replaced by the calcified masses in the dilated pelvocalyces. Note the lower pole of the contracted right kidney *(arrow)* and right renal pelvis *(arrowhead)*.

8. Transitional Cell Carcinoma with Other Histologic Differentiation

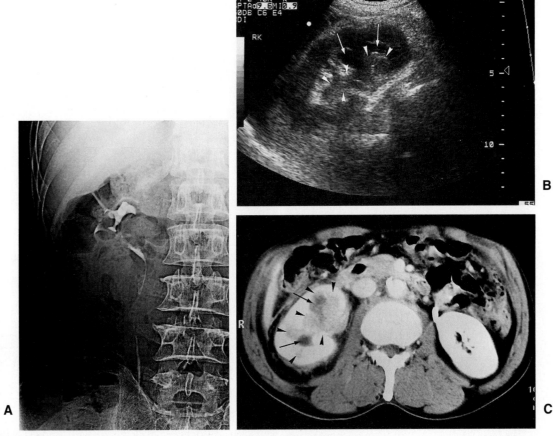

Fig. 1. Transitional cell carcinoma with squamous and glandular differentiation in a 56-year-old man.
A. IVU shows amputated lower-pole calyx and nodular lesions in the renal pelvis and proximal ureter. **B.** Longitudinal US of the right kidney shows soft tissue masses *(arrowheads)* in the pelvocalyces with peripheral caliectasis *(arrows)*. **C.** Contrast-enhanced CT shows ill-defined, low-attenuated mass *(arrowheads)* and dilated calyces *(arrows)*.

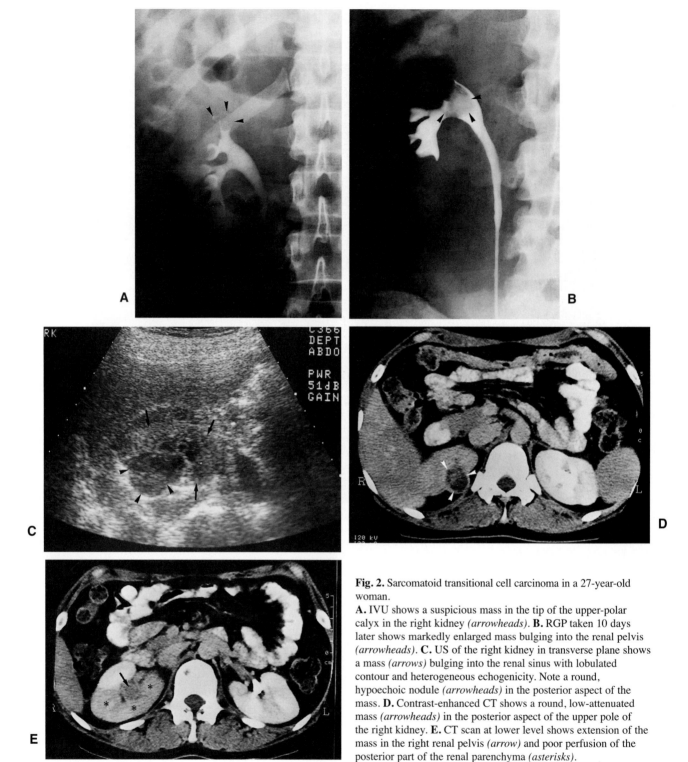

Fig. 2. Sarcomatoid transitional cell carcinoma in a 27-year-old woman.
A. IVU shows a suspicious mass in the tip of the upper-polar calyx in the right kidney *(arrowheads)*. **B.** RGP taken 10 days later shows markedly enlarged mass bulging into the renal pelvis *(arrowheads)*. **C.** US of the right kidney in transverse plane shows a mass *(arrows)* bulging into the renal sinus with lobulated contour and heterogeneous echogenicity. Note a round, hypoechoic nodule *(arrowheads)* in the posterior aspect of the mass. **D.** Contrast-enhanced CT shows a round, low-attenuated mass *(arrowheads)* in the posterior aspect of the upper pole of the right kidney. **E.** CT scan at lower level shows extension of the mass in the right renal pelvis *(arrow)* and poor perfusion of the posterior part of the renal parenchyma *(asterisks)*.

9. Adenocarcinoma of the Urinary Tract

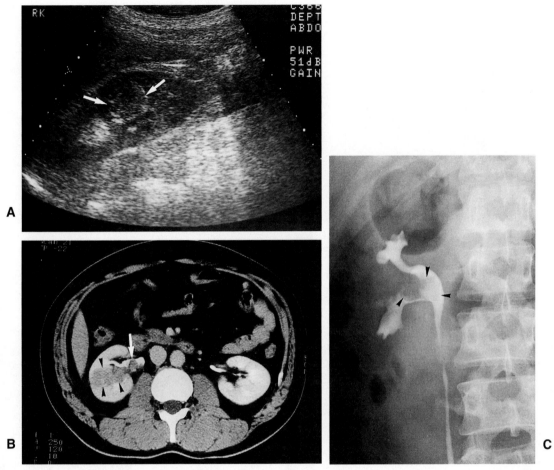

Fig. 1. Papillary adenocarcinoma of the renal pelvis in a 36-year-old man.
A. Longitudinal US of the right kidney shows a round, echogenic mass *(arrows)* in the interpolar region. **B.** Contrast-enhanced CT shows an ill-defined, low-attenuated lesion in the interpolar region of the right kidney *(arrowheads)* that bulges into the renal pelvis (arrow). **C.** RGP well demonstrates the mass bulging into the renal pelvis *(arrowheads)*.

10. Squamous Cell Carcinoma of the Urinary Tract

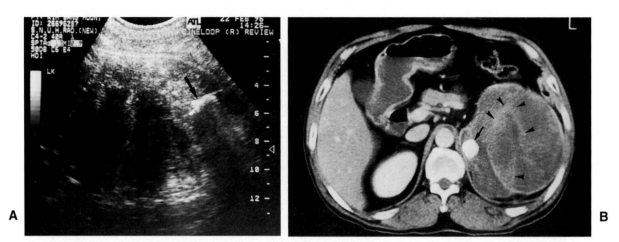

Fig. 1. Squamous cell carcinoma of the pelvocalyces with urolithiasis in a 59-year-old man.
A. Longitudinal US of the left kidney shows an enlarged kidney with heterogeneous echogenicity. Note a large stone *(arrow)* with posterior sonic shadowing in the left kidney. **B.** Contrast-enhanced CT shows a markedly enlarged left kidney containing a large stone *(arrow)*. The left renal enlargement is probably due to dilated pelvocalyces that have the areas of heterogeneous enhancement *(arrowheads)* suggesting a tumorous condition.

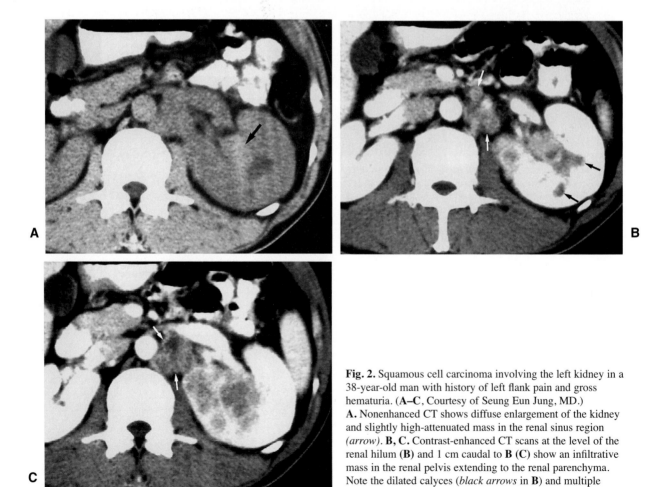

Fig. 2. Squamous cell carcinoma involving the left kidney in a 38-year-old man with history of left flank pain and gross hematuria. (**A–C**, Courtesy of Seung Eun Jung, MD.)
A. Nonenhanced CT shows diffuse enlargement of the kidney and slightly high-attenuated mass in the renal sinus region *(arrow)*. **B, C.** Contrast-enhanced CT scans at the level of the renal hilum (**B**) and 1 cm caudal to **B** (**C**) show an infiltrative mass in the renal pelvis extending to the renal parenchyma. Note the dilated calyces *(black arrows* in **B**) and multiple metastatic lymph nodes in the para-aortic area *(white arrows)*.

11. Metastatic Tumors of the Urinary Tract

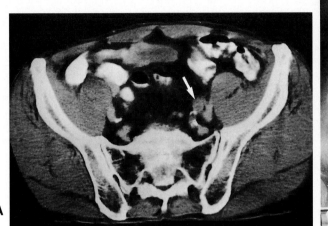

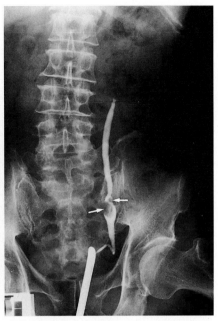

Fig. 1. Recurrent renal cell carcinoma in the remnant ureter in a 75-year-old man who underwent left radical nephrectomy 5 years earlier. (**A, B,** From Yoo SY, Kim SH, Lee KH, et al: Intraureteral recurrence of renal cell carcinoma following nephrectomy: A case report. J Korean Radiol Soc 2000; 43:607–609.)

A. Contrast-enhanced CT shows a dilated left ureter filled with a homogeneous soft tissue mass *(arrow)*. **B.** RGP shows filling defects *(arrows)* in the distal portion of the remnant left ureter.

12. Brush Biopsy for Urothelial Tumor

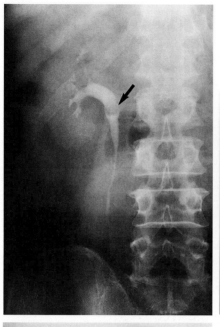

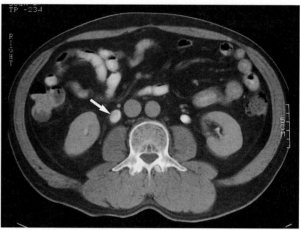

Fig. 1. Papillary transitional cell carcinoma of the ureteropelvic junction that was diagnosed with brush biopsy in a 64-year-old man.
A. IVU shows a round mass in the right ureteropelvic junction *(arrow)* without obstruction. **B.** Contrast-enhanced CT shows a nodular filling defect *(arrow)* in the ureteropelvic junction of the right kidney. **C.** Urine cytology did not reveal tumor cells and therefore brush biopsy of the mass was performed under fluoroscopic guidance, revealing transitional cell carcinoma. Note a biopsy brush *(arrows)* within the mass *(arrowheads)*.

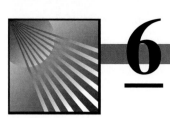

6

Renal Cysts and Cystic Diseases

BOHYUN KIM

Renal cystic disease refers to a heterogeneous entity of various causes, including simple or complicated cysts, hereditary polycystic diseases, developmental cystic diseases such as multicystic dysplastic kidney, acquired cystic disease, and cystic lesions associated with von Hippel-Lindau disease or tuberous sclerosis. Although the diagnosis can be made on the basis of the history of the patient and imaging findings, it is often difficult to differentiate benign from malignant cystic lesions.

SIMPLE CYST

Simple cyst is the most common cystic lesion in the kidney. Renal cysts commonly arise in the cortex but may be located in the medulla. They are more common in older age groups and thus are believed to be acquired lesions. Although the pathogenesis is not well known, ductal or tubular obstruction and vascular compromise are considered to be causative factors.

Simple cysts contain clear fluid and are lined by a thin layer of cuboidal epithelium. With imaging study, the diagnosis of renal cysts can be made by demonstrating a well-demarcated cystic lesion having clear fluid and a very thin wall. On plain radiographs, renal cyst is seen as a bulging mass if located in the periphery. Intravenous urography (IVU) may demonstrate a radiolucent mass that splays or displaces renal pelvocalyceal systems. When a renal cyst is located peripherally, surrounding normal parenchyma may demonstrate a typical crescentic margin, designated as "beak sign" or "claw sign."

On ultrasonography (US), a simple cyst is seen as a round, well-circumscribed, anechoic mass with a sharp interface with normal parenchyma and posterior sonic enhancement. On computed tomography (CT), a renal cyst is seen as a round, thin-walled, low-attenuated lesion with no significant enhancement following administration of intravenous contrast material. Renal parenchyma around the cyst may mimic a thick wall in cross section, which is called "pseudo-thick wall sign." This is most commonly seen in the polar areas but can also be seen near the renal sinus. A low-attenuated lesion of less than 15 HU on nonenhanced scan and less than 10 HU increase on contrast-enhanced scan suggests a benign renal cyst on CT. However, simple renal cysts may demonstrate an artifactual increase in CT attenuation following administration

of intravenous contrast material, so-called pseudoenhancement. This phenomenon, resulting from multiple factors including beam-hardening effect and partial-volume averaging, is more common with small renal cysts than larger cysts.

On magnetic resonance (MR) imaging, simple cyst appears as a thin-walled cystic lesion of low signal intensity on T1-weighted images and homogeneous high signal intensity on T2-weighted images.

COMPLICATED CYST

A simple cyst may be complicated most often by hemorrhage or infection. Complicated renal cyst may have septations, calcifications, thick walls, or high-attenuated content on nonenhanced CT.

The septa can be well seen on US, often better than on CT. Thin, smooth septa suggest benign cyst, whereas thick, irregular septa with or without a solid nodule suggest malignancy.

Calcification is seen on plain radiograph in about 1% to 3% of benign renal cysts. The calcification is usually dystrophic in nature and is often curvilinear in shape at the periphery of the cyst. Evaluation with US is often limited due to posterior sonic shadowing. CT is most suitable for detecting calcifications in renal cysts. Sometimes a calcified cyst is difficult to differentiate from a cystic renal cell carcinoma. Evidence of contrast enhancement, along with the presence of mural nodules or heavy calcifications, may suggest malignancy.

A *hyperdense* cyst refers to a cyst that demonstrates high attenuation on nonenhanced CT. Hemorrhagic cyst is the most common cause, but renal cell carcinoma may demonstrate similar findings. Because internal structures within a hyperdense cyst cannot be well evaluated by CT, the presence or absence of contrast enhancement in the cystic lesion is an important criterion for the differentiation between benign and malignant renal lesions. In such cases, US or MR imaging can be helpful for the differentiation.

Milk of calcium cyst is a renal cyst containing calcific debris in cystic fluid. It is most commonly seen in calyceal diverticula but may be seen in simple cysts as well. The calcific debris is mainly composed of calcium carbonate. CT often demonstrates fluid-calcium levels in the dependent portion of the cyst.

BOSNIAK CLASSIFICATION OF CYSTIC RENAL MASSES

To categorize characteristics of renal cystic lesions, Morton A. Bosniak has proposed a four-category classification system, as follows:

Class I lesions are simple cysts satisfying imaging criteria of an uncomplicated cyst: a well-defined, round, homogeneous, low-attenuated lesion with a very thin wall and without enhancement on contrast-enhanced CT scan.

Class II lesions are minimally complicated benign cysts with thin septa or minimal wall calcifications. The septa are usually less than 1 mm, smooth, and non-nodular, and the lesion does not show areas of soft tissue density or contrast enhancement. Some hyperdense cysts or slightly more complicated cysts such as those with more calcifications in the wall, for which follow-up studies are needed, are classified as class IIF.

Class III lesions are complicated cysts with more numerous or thickened septa or thick, irregular calcifications.

Class IV lesions are obviously malignant lesions with solid enhancing components and irregular wall thickening.

Surgery is not needed for the category I and II cysts, whereas surgical exploration or removal is usually required for the category III and IV cysts.

AUTOSOMAL DOMINANT POLYCYSTIC KIDNEY DISEASE

Autosomal dominant polycystic kidney disease (ADPKD) is a common genetic disorder characterized by innumerable bilateral renal cysts involving both the renal cortex and medulla. It is a common cause of renal failure and accounts for approximately 10% to 12% of patients receiving hemodialysis. ADPKD is inherited as autosomal dominant trait. At least three genes are involved in ADPKD, and the severity of the disease varies from patient to patient. A family history of ADPKD can be obtained in only about 60% of cases due to spontaneous mutation and variable expressivity. ADPKD is often accompanied by cysts in the liver, pancreas, and spleen. Other organs that may contain cysts include the uterus, ovary, epididymis, and thyroid. Seminal vesicles also may have cysts or may be dilated in patients with ADPKD. ADPKD may be associated with intracranial aneurysm, cardiac valvular disease, and colonic diverticulosis.

The disease process is believed to begin in utero but often presents between the third and sixth decades of life. Usually after 30 years of age, renal cysts grow and compress renal parenchyma, which may eventually lead to chronic renal failure. Most common clinical presentations include abdominal pain, hematuria, and hypertension. Hypertension occurs in 50% to 75% of the patients. In affected patients, renal stones and infection are more common than in the normal population, but the risk of renal cell carcinoma is not increased. Most patients with advanced disease are associated with renal failure. Renal involvement is usually symmetrical and bilateral but may be unilateral or partial. However, the supposedly normal kidneys in these cases often contain microscopic cysts. Renal cyst may rupture into the perirenal space.

IVU may demonstrate enlarged kidneys with diminished enhancement and splayed renal collecting system. Cyst wall calcifications and nephrocalcinosis are often seen. On US and CT, numerous cysts of variable size are seen. The presence of calcification or hemorrhage can be depicted on nonenhanced CT.

To relieve the symptoms related to the abdominal distention, cyst volume should be reduced. However, there is no effective medical treatment. Simple aspiration of the cyst is ineffective because the fluid reaccumulates in the cyst. Sclerotherapy of the renal cysts using various sclerosing agents has been reported to be moderately successful.

UNILATERAL CYSTIC DISEASE OF THE KIDNEY

Unilateral renal cystic disease is a multicystic renal disease characterized by multiple variable-sized cysts confined within one kidney. Although the gross and histologic findings are identical to those of ADPKD, unilateral renal cystic disease does not show genetic inheritance or progress to chronic renal failure. Because ADPKD may manifest as unilateral renal cystic disease particularly in children and initial unilateral disease can evolve into an asymmetrical bilateral disease, the possibility of ADPKD should be excluded in patients with presumed unilateral renal cystic disease by phenotype screening of family members or by a long-term follow-up. Although anecdotal cases of coexisting renal cell carcinoma have been reported in the literature, the association of unilateral renal cystic disease with higher rate of renal tumor is unclear.

The differential diagnoses include ADPKD, multilocular cystic nephroma, cystic dysplasia, and multiple simple cysts. US, CT, and radionuclide scans may be helpful for this differentiation. Multilocular cystic nephromas are usually seen as discrete, encapsulated masses and do not contain the islands of enhancing parenchyma on CT, whereas unilateral renal cystic disease has intervening normal parenchyma among the cysts. Although multiple renal cysts may be difficult to differentiate from unilateral renal cystic disease, the number of cysts is smaller and the kidney commonly retains normal parenchymal architecture.

LOCALIZED CYSTIC DISEASE OF THE KIDNEY

Localized cystic disease refers to numerous small cystic lesions localized in one portion of the kidney. It is not a genetically transmitted disease and is not associated with renal tumors. Histologically the lesion consists of a nonencapsulated cluster of simple cysts. The differentiation from a multilocular cystic nephroma is often difficult. The absence of a capsule surrounding the cystic lesions and the presence of cysts outside the cluster can help make a correct diagnosis of this entity.

AUTOSOMAL RECESSIVE POLYCYSTIC KIDNEY DISEASE

Autosomal recessive polycystic kidney disease (ARPKD) is a hereditary disease transmitted by autosomal recessive inheritance. It is characterized by dilation of the renal collecting tubules and varying degree of hepatic fibrosis. The affected infants frequently present with renal insufficiency at birth and often die within the first few days of life. In older children, the

hepatic disease is more dominant than renal disease and the patients commonly present with portal hypertension and varices.

ARPKD may be diagnosed prenatally by US. Prenatal US often demonstrates enlarged echogenic kidneys, although milder diseases are difficult to detect. Similar findings can be seen on postnatal US. Parenchymal echogenicity is increased due to multiple acoustic interfaces between multiple cysts and cystic walls. Enlarged kidneys usually maintain a reniform shape. With a high-resolution scanner, the kidneys may demonstrate tiny cysts within echogenic areas in the cortex and medulla and a peripheral sonolucent rim, which may represent compressed normal parenchyma or increased cystic changes in the outer cortex. In older children, the liver may show increased echogenicity or bile duct dilation.

IVU is not commonly used, but the findings include bilateral enlarged kidneys with faint nephrogram and radiating streaks extending from the medulla to the cortex, which is a characteristic finding. CT may demonstrate enlarged kidneys of water attenuation on nonenhanced scan and poor opacification with striated nephrogram on contrast-enhanced scan. On MR imaging, the enlarged kidneys may demonstrate high signal intensity on T2-weighted images.

MEDULLARY CYSTIC DISEASE OF THE KIDNEY

Medullary cystic disease is a renal disease characterized by renal tubular atrophy and medullary cystic lesions. It can be divided into two entities: juvenile and adult forms. The juvenile form is more common, being transmitted by an autosomal recessive trait and often associated with ophthalmologic and neurologic abnormalities, skeletal dysplasia, and hepatic fibrosis. The adult form is inherited as an autosomal dominant trait and is not associated with extrarenal abnormalities.

The kidneys are normal to slightly small and have a smooth contour. Histologically the disease is characterized by small cysts within the medulla or at the corticomedullary junction, interstitial fibrosis, and glomerular sclerosis. Affected patients often present with polyuria, polydipsia, anemia, and end-stage renal failure.

Plain radiography or IVU may demonstrate smoothly contoured normal-sized to small kidneys. US or CT may show a characteristic finding of small echogenic kidneys with multiple small cysts in the medulla.

MULTICYSTIC DYSPLASTIC KIDNEY

Multicystic dysplastic kidney is a nonhereditary, developmental abnormality characterized by the presence of multiple renal cysts and the absence of functioning renal parenchyma in the affected kidney. Complete obstruction of the ureters during nephrogenesis is thought to be the major cause of multicystic dysplastic kidney.

Multicystic dysplastic kidney is mostly unilateral but may be bilateral or segmental. In the classic type, multiple cysts do not communicate with each other. However, in the hydronephrotic type, in which an incomplete obstruction of the urinary tract occurs during nephrogenesis, the cysts communicate with other cysts or renal pelvis. Clinically, multicystic dysplastic kidney often presents as an abdominal mass in infancy. The contralateral diseases such as multicystic dysplastic kidney, vesicoureteral reflux, and ureteropelvic junction

obstruction have been reported to occur in about 50% of the patients.

Prenatal diagnosis of multicystic dysplastic kidney can be made as early as 20 weeks of gestation. Characteristic US findings include multiple, small, noncommunicating cysts and increased parenchymal echogenicity of the kidneys. On follow-up examinations, the cysts may increase in number and size.

On plain radiographs, the affected kidney is seen as a lobulated soft tissue mass with or without cyst wall calcifications. IVU may demonstrate no contrast enhancement in the kidney. On CT, multiple noncommunicating cysts can be clearly identified. There is no parenchymal enhancement on contrast-enhanced CT.

ACQUIRED CYSTIC DISEASE OF THE KIDNEY

Acquired cystic renal disease is a nonhereditary renal cystic disease occurring in patients with chronic renal insufficiency. Most commonly it occurs in patients treated with dialysis but may occur in patients with chronic renal insufficiency who do not receive dialysis. Although the pathogenesis of acquired cystic renal disease is not fully understood, the duration of renal dialysis is strongly related to its occurrence. The prevalence of acquired cystic renal disease is 10% to 20% after 1 to 3 years after dialysis, 40% to 60% after 3 to 5 years, and more than 90% after 5 to 10 years. The prevalence is similar between the patients treated with hemodialysis and those with peritoneal dialysis.

Acquired cystic renal disease is associated with increased incidence of renal cell carcinoma. These tumors commonly occur in patients with dialysis, and they are found in younger patients than is renal cell carcinoma in the general population.

Evaluation with US is often limited, because small and echogenic kidneys cannot be differentiated from echogenic perinephric fat. Hemorrhage and calcification are frequently seen. Any solid mass should be suspected to be renal cell carcinoma unless proven otherwise.

On CT, multiple small cysts with or without hemorrhage or calcifications are seen in small kidneys. Renal cell carcinoma can be suspected when a low-attenuated lesion shows contrast enhancement.

RENAL CYSTS IN VON HIPPEL-LINDAU DISEASE

Von Hippel-Lindau disease is a hereditary disease transmitted by autosomal dominant trait. It is characterized by retinal angioma, cerebellar or spinal cord hemangioma, renal cell carcinoma, islet cell tumor, pheochromocytoma, and papillary cystadenoma of the epididymis. Renal cysts occur in 59% to 63% of patients, and renal cell carcinoma occurs in 24% to 45%. However, many of the renal lesions that are thought to be cysts on US or CT may represent microscopic foci of renal cell carcinoma. Renal tumors are usually multiple and bilateral.

Although US may differentiate renal cell carcinoma from cysts, contrast-enhanced CT is best suitable for the diagnosis of renal lesions in von Hippel-Lindau disease. MR imaging can be used for patients in whom CT is contraindicated.

RENAL CYSTS IN TUBEROUS SCLEROSIS

Tuberous sclerosis is a hereditary phakomatosis, transmitted by autosomal dominant trait. It is characterized by angiofibroma on the face and hamartomas in multiple organs, including the

brain, skin, and kidneys. In the kidneys, angiomyolipomas occur in about 80% of affected patients, and multiple small renal cysts are frequently seen. Angiomyolipomas often bleed spontaneously, resulting in subcapsular or retroperitoneal hematoma.

US easily differentiates echogenic angiomyolipomas from renal cysts, but it is often difficult to differentiate angiomyolipomas from echogenic small renal cell carcinomas with US. On CT, the presence of fat confirms the diagnosis of angiomyolipoma. However, fat-deficient angiomyolipoma may show findings similar to renal cell carcinoma and thus cannot be differentiated from it.

PARAPELVIC CYST

Parapelvic cyst refers to renal cysts that arise from the lymphatic tissues in the renal sinus. It is also called *renal sinus cyst, peripelvic cyst,* or *parapelvic lymphangiectasia.* They are often multiple and bilateral.

On IVU, renal pelvis and calyces are compressed, and calyceal infundibula are bowed and displaced. US demonstrates multiple cysts within the renal sinus. Sometimes, cysts appear to communicate with each other and thus may mimic hydronephrosis. In this circumstance, IVU or contrast-enhanced CT in delayed phase can differentiate multiple cysts from a dilated pelvocalyceal system.

References

1. Bae KT, Heiken JP, Siegel CL, et al: Renal cysts: Is attenuation artifactually increased on contrast-enhanced CT images? Radiology 2000; 216:792–796.
2. Coulam CH, Sheafor DH, Leder RA, et al: Evaluation of pseudoenhancement of renal cysts during contrast-enhanced CT. AJR Am J Roentgenol 2000; 174:493–498.
3. Kawashima A, Goldman SM: The simple renal cyst. In Pollack HM, McClennan BL (eds): Clinical Urography, 2nd ed, vol 2. Philadelphia, WB Saunders, 2000, pp 1251–1289.
4. Levine E: Autosomal dominant polycystic kidney disease. In Pollack HM, McClennan BL (eds): Clinical Urography, 2nd ed, vol 2. Philadelphia, WB Saunders, 2000, pp 1290–1315.
5. Hwang DY, Ahn C, Lee JG, et al: Unilateral renal cystic disease in adults. Nephrol Dial Transplant 1999; 14:1999–2003.
6. Maki DD, Birnbaum BA, Chakraborty DP, et al: Renal cyst pseudoenhancement: Beam-hardening effects on CT numbers. Radiology 1999; 213:468–472.
7. Elzouki AY, Al-Suhaibani H, Mirza K, et al: Thin-section computed tomography scans detect medullary cysts in patients believed to have juvenile nephronophthisis. Am J Kidney Dis 1996; 27:216–219.
8. Wilson TE, Doelle EA, Cohan RH, et al: Cystic renal masses: A reevaluation of the usefulness of the Bosniak classification system. Acad Radiol 1996; 3:564–570.
9. Choyke PL, Glenn GM, Walther MM, et al: von Hippel-Lindau disease: Genetic, clinical, and imaging features. Radiology 1995; 194:629–642.
10. Keith DS, Torres VE, King BF, et al: Renal cell carcinoma in autosomal dominant polycystic kidney disease. J Am Soc Nephrol 1994; 4:1661–1669.
11. Gabow PA: Autosomal dominant polycystic kidney disease. N Engl J Med 1993; 329:332–342.
12. Atiyeh B, Husmann D, Baum M: Contralateral renal abnormalities in multicystic-dysplastic kidney disease. J Pediatr 1992; 121:65–67.
13. Aronson S, Frazier HA, Baluch JD, et al: Cystic renal masses: Usefulness of the Bosniak classification. Urol Radiol 1991; 13:83–90.
14. Bosniak MA: Difficulties in classifying cystic lesions of the kidney. Urol Radiol 1991; 13:91–93.
15. Sigmund G, Stover B, Zimmerhackl LB, et al: RARE-MR-urography in the diagnosis of upper urinary tract abnormalities in children. Pediatr Radiol 1991; 21:416–420.
16. Choi BI, Yeon KM, Kim SH, et al: Caroli disease: Central dot sign in CT. Radiology 1990; 174:161–163.
17. Matson MA, Cohen EP: Acquired cystic kidney disease: Occurrence, prevalence, and renal cancers. Medicine 1990; 69:217–226.
18. Bosniak MA: The current radiological approach to renal cysts. Radiology 1986; 158:1–10.
19. Kleiner B, Filly RA, Mack L, et al: Multicystic dysplastic kidney: Observations of contralateral disease in the fetal population. Radiology 1986; 161:27–29.
20. Levine E, Cook LT, Grantham JJ: Liver cysts in autosomal dominant polycystic kidney disease: Clinical and computed tomography study. AJR Am J Roentgenol 1985; 145:229–233.
21. Rego JD Jr, Laing FC, Jeffrey RB: Ultrasonic diagnosis of medullary cystic disease. J Ultrasound Med 1983; 2:433–436.
22. Curry NS, Brock G, Metcalf JS, et al: Hyperdense renal mass: Unusual CT appearance of a benign renal cyst. Urol Radiol 1982; 4:33–35.
23. Segal AJ, Spitzer RM: Pseudo-thick-walled renal cyst by CT. AJR Am J Roentgenol 1979; 132:827–828.

Illustrations • Renal Cysts and Cystic Diseases

1 • Simple cysts

2 • Simple cysts with pseudo-thick wall

3 • Septated cysts

4 • Calcified cysts

5 • Hemorrhagic cysts

6 • Infected cysts

7 • Autosomal dominant polycystic kidney disease

8 • Autosomal dominant polycystic kidney disease with hemorrhage

9 • Autosomal dominant polycystic kidney disease with infection

10 • Autosomal dominant polycystic kidney disease: associated lesions

11 • Unilateral cystic disease

12 • Localized cystic disease

13 • Autosomal recessive polycystic kidney disease

14 • Medullary cystic disease

15 • Multicystic dysplastic kidney

16 • Acquired cystic disease

17 • Parapelvic cysts

1. Simple Cysts

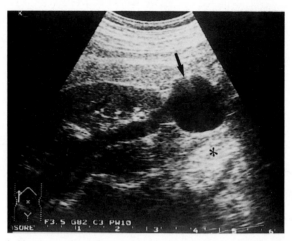

Fig. 1. Simple cyst in a 47-year-old man. Longitudinal US of the right kidney shows a simple, uncomplicated renal cyst *(arrow)*. The cyst is well circumscribed and has a thin, smooth wall. Note posterior sonic enhancement *(asterisk)* and the absence of internal echoes.

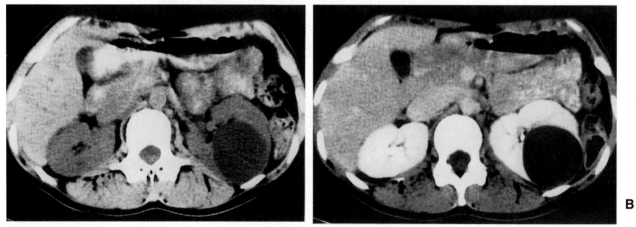

Fig. 2. Simple cyst in a 38-year-old woman.
A. Nonenhanced CT shows a round, well-demarcated, low-attenuated lesion in the left kidney. **B.** Contrast-enhanced CT demonstrates a clear margin, very thin wall, and no enhancement.

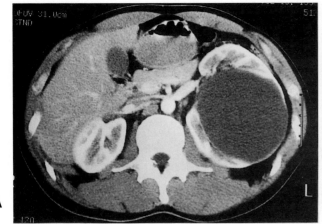 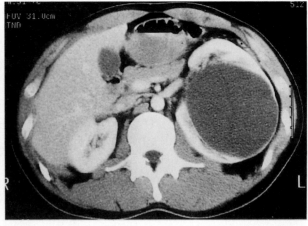

Fig. 3. Large simple cyst in a 28-year-old man.
A, B. Contrast-enhanced CT scans in cortical (**A**) and nephrographic (**B**) phases show a large cyst in the left kidney with a thin wall and homogeneous nonenhancing content.

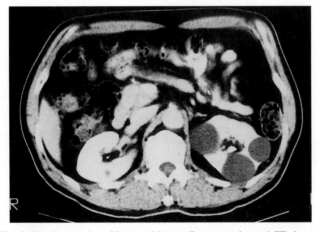

Fig. 4. Simple cysts in a 50-year-old man. Contrast-enhanced CT shows three low-attenuated lesions of water attenuation in the left kidney. Note that the cyst wall is very thin and almost imperceptible.

Fig. 5. Small simple cyst in a 60-year-old woman.
A, B. T2-weighted (**A**) and contrast-enhanced T1-weighted (**B**) MR images in coronal plane show a small cyst (*arrow*) in the left kidney that reveals homogeneous high intensity on T2-weighted image and no enhancement on contrast-enhanced T1-weighted image.

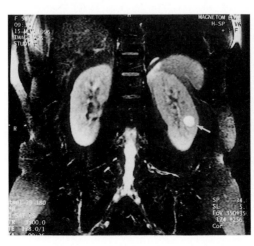 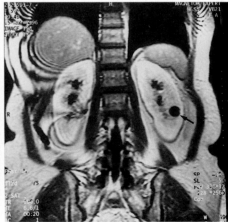

2. Simple Cysts with Pseudo-thick Wall

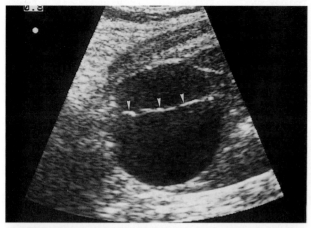

A

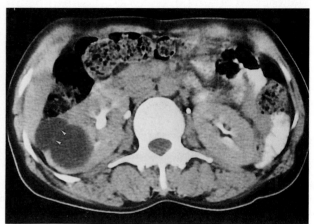

B

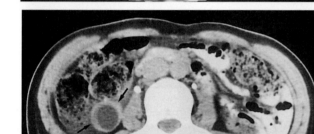

C

Fig. 1. Benign septated cyst with a pseudo-thick wall in a 47-year-old woman.
A. US of the right kidney in transverse plane shows a thin-walled cystic lesion in the lower pole of the right kidney. Note a thin, linear septum *(arrowheads)* in the cystic lesion.
B. Contrast-enhanced CT shows a thin-walled, septated cystic lesion in the right kidney. Note that the septum *(arrowheads)* on CT is less well defined than on US. **C.** CT scan at a lower level shows an apparently thick, enhancing wall at the periphery of cyst *(arrows)*. This pseudo-thick wall is due to partial volume averaging by normal renal parenchyma surrounding the cyst in cross section.

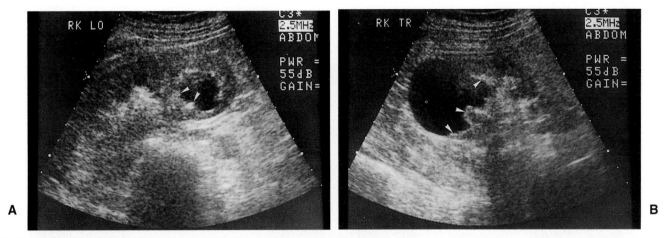

Fig. 2. Benign cyst with an irregular, thick wall abutting the renal sinus in a 61-year-old woman.
A, B. US images of the right kidney in longitudinal (**A**) and transverse (**B**) planes show a cyst in the lower pole area. Note irregular nodularity of the cyst wall *(arrowheads)* abutting the renal sinus fat.

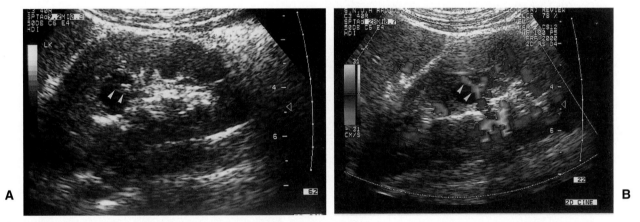

Fig. 3. Benign cyst with a pseudo-thick wall abutting renal sinus in a 40-year-old man.
A. Longitudinal US of the left kidney shows a cyst with suspicious irregular wall *(arrowheads)* abutting the renal sinus. **B.** Color Doppler US well demonstrates that the apparent irregularity of the cyst wall on gray-scale US was due to the vessels *(arrowheads)* in the renal sinus. (**B,** See also Color Section.)

3. Septated Cysts

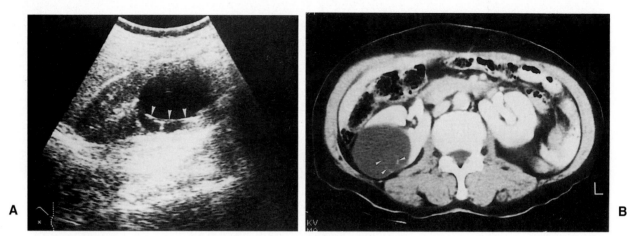

Fig. 1. Benign septated renal cyst in a 69-year-old woman with horseshoe kidney.
A. Longitudinal US of the right kidney shows a large renal cyst containing relatively thin septa *(arrowheads)*. **B.** On contrast-enhanced CT, the septa *(arrowheads)* are faintly visualized. Renal axes of both kidneys are rotated anteriorly due to horseshoe kidney.

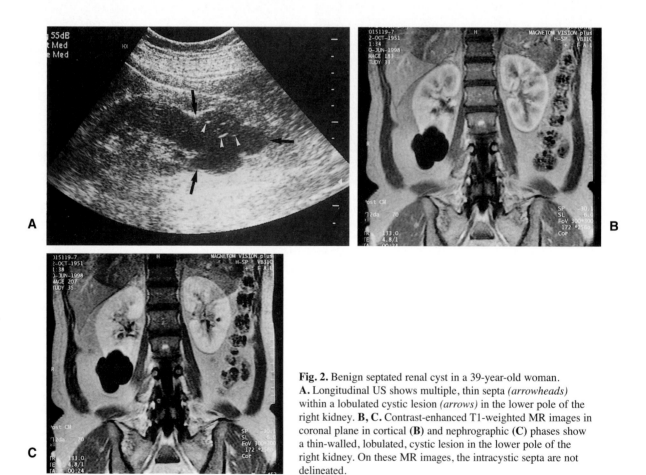

Fig. 2. Benign septated renal cyst in a 39-year-old woman.
A. Longitudinal US shows multiple, thin septa *(arrowheads)* within a lobulated cystic lesion *(arrows)* in the lower pole of the right kidney. **B, C.** Contrast-enhanced T1-weighted MR images in coronal plane in cortical **(B)** and nephrographic **(C)** phases show a thin-walled, lobulated, cystic lesion in the lower pole of the right kidney. On these MR images, the intracystic septa are not delineated.

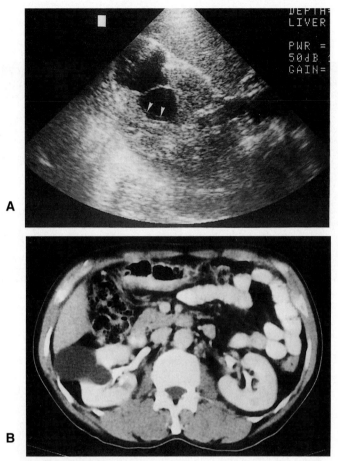

Fig. 3. Simple cysts in a 60-year-old man.
A. Transverse US of the right kidney shows two simple cysts. Note a thin septum *(arrowheads)* in an inner cyst. **B.** Contrast-enhanced CT demonstrates the cysts, and there is no enhancement within the cysts.

4. Calcified Cysts

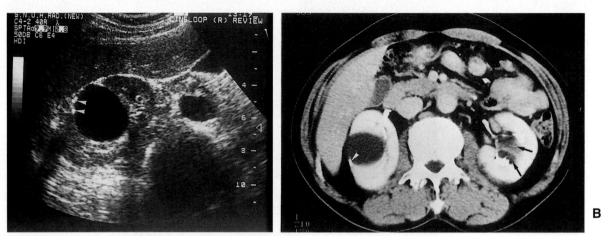

Fig. 1. Simple renal cyst with calcification in the wall in a 52-year-old man.
A. Transverse US of the right kidney reveals a cystic mass in the right kidney. Note a small, echogenic focus *(arrowheads)* with posterior sonic shadowing due to calcification in the wall of the cyst. **B.** Contrast-enhanced CT scan shows a small calcification *(arrowhead)* in the cyst wall. Also note multiloculated parapelvic cysts in the left renal sinus *(arrows)*.

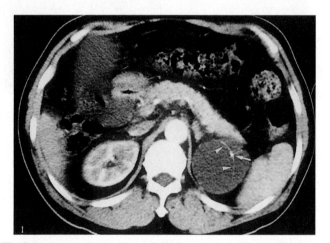

Fig. 2. Benign renal cyst with a calcified septum in a 53-year-old woman. Contrast-enhanced CT scan in cortical phase shows a cyst in the upper pole of the left kidney with a thin septum *(arrowheads)*. Note a small calcification *(arrow)* in the septum.

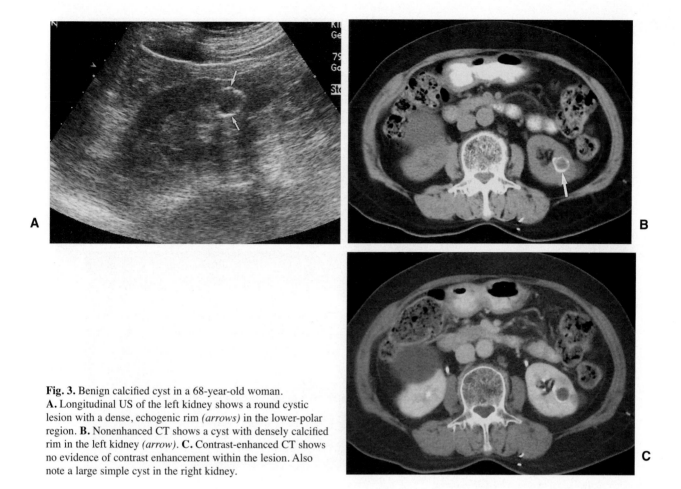

Fig. 3. Benign calcified cyst in a 68-year-old woman.
A. Longitudinal US of the left kidney shows a round cystic
lesion with a dense, echogenic rim *(arrows)* in the lower-polar
region. **B.** Nonenhanced CT shows a cyst with densely calcified
rim in the left kidney *(arrow)*. **C.** Contrast-enhanced CT shows
no evidence of contrast enhancement within the lesion. Also
note a large simple cyst in the right kidney.

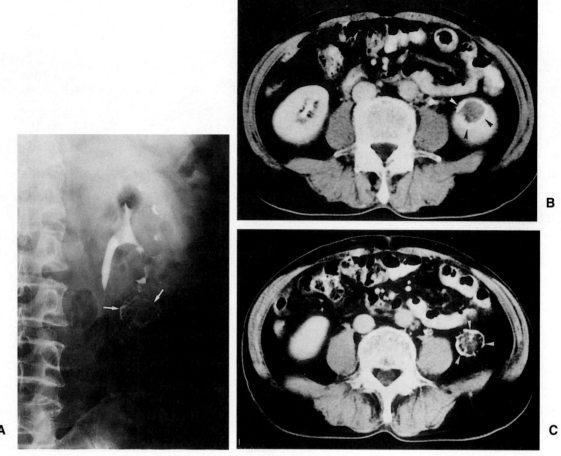

Fig. 4. Benign calcified renal cyst in a 74-year-old man.
A. IVU shows amorphous and rimlike calcifications in lower pole of the left kidney *(arrows)*. **B.** Contrast-enhanced CT demonstrates a low-attenuated lesion with thick calcifications along the wall *(arrowheads)* in the lower pole of the left kidney. **C.** A consecutive scan at a lower level shows heavy calcifications both at the periphery and inside of the low-attenuated lesion *(arrowheads)*.

5. Hemorrhagic Cysts

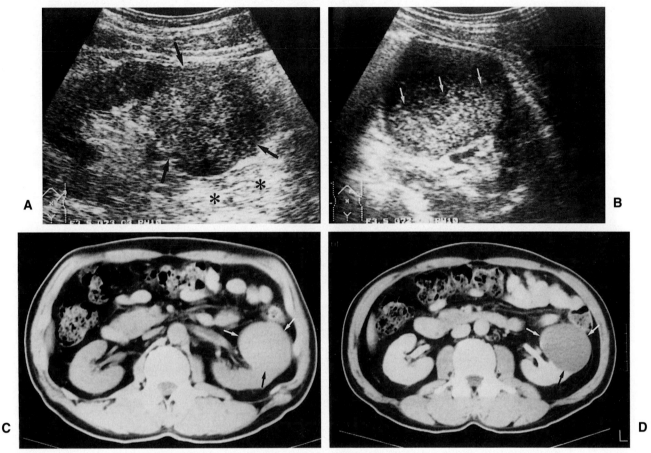

Fig. 1. Hemorrhagic cyst of the left kidney in a 49-year-old man.
A. Longitudinal US shows a cystic mass containing low-level internal echoes *(arrows)*. Although posterior sonic enhancement *(asterisks)* is evident in this case, it is often difficult to differentiate a complicated cyst from a solid mass. **B.** After a change in the patient's position, the cyst shows layering of the internal debris. Note the fluid-debris level within the cyst *(arrows)*. **C.** Nonenhanced CT shows a round, homogeneous, hyperdense mass *(arrows)* in the left kidney. **D.** On contrast-enhanced CT, the mass *(arrows)* appears low attenuated as compared to the adjacent renal parenchyma. There was no significant increase in the CT attenuation of the lesion as compared with the nonenhanced CT.

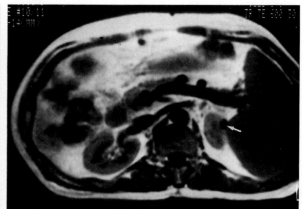

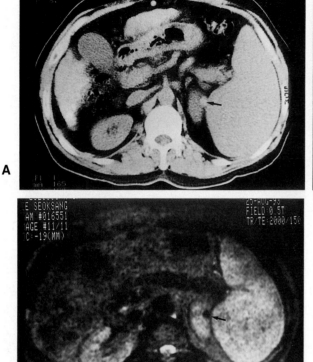

Fig. 2. Small hemorrhagic renal cyst in a 62-year-old man.
A. Nonenhanced CT shows a high-attenuated mass *(arrow)* in the upper pole of the left kidney. **B, C.** T1-weighted **(B)** and T2-weighted **(C)** MR images in the transverse plane show low signal intensity of the lesion *(arrow)* at both pulse sequences. These signal intensities suggest subacute hemorrhage within the cyst.

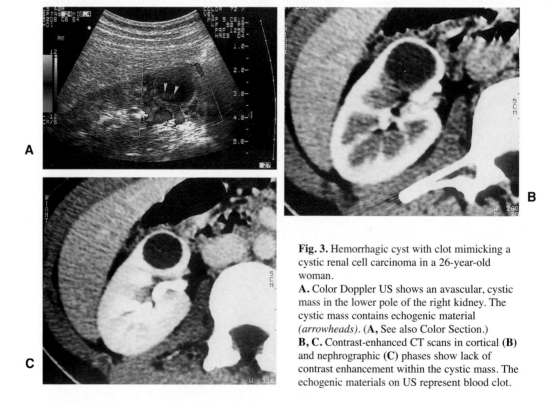

Fig. 3. Hemorrhagic cyst with clot mimicking a cystic renal cell carcinoma in a 26-year-old woman.
A. Color Doppler US shows an avascular, cystic mass in the lower pole of the right kidney. The cystic mass contains echogenic material *(arrowheads)*. (**A,** See also Color Section.)
B, C. Contrast-enhanced CT scans in cortical **(B)** and nephrographic **(C)** phases show lack of contrast enhancement within the cystic mass. The echogenic materials on US represent blood clot.

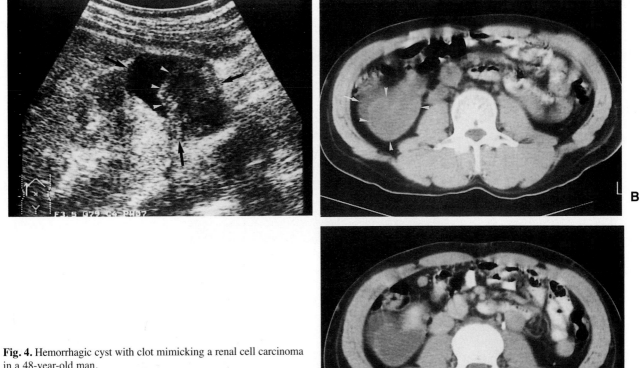

Fig. 4. Hemorrhagic cyst with clot mimicking a renal cell carcinoma in a 48-year-old man.
A. Longitudinal US shows a cystic mass *(arrows)* with solid component *(arrowheads)* in the lower pole of the right kidney.
B. On nonenhanced CT, the solid part *(arrowheads)* of the mass demonstrates high attenuation. Note a crescentic cystic area *(arrow)* surrounding the solid portion. **C.** Contrast-enhanced CT shows no significant enhancement of the mass.

6. Infected Cysts

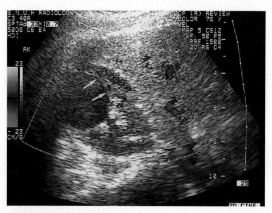

Fig. 1. Infected renal cyst in a 20-year-old woman. Color Doppler US shows a round cystic mass with a slightly thickened wall and low-level internal echoes. Note increased blood flow in the thickened wall *(arrows)*. (See also Color Section.)

7. Autosomal Dominant Polycystic Kidney Disease

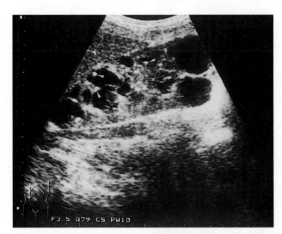

Fig. 1. Autosomal dominant polycystic kidney disease in a 46-year-old man. Longitudinal US of the left kidney shows a large kidney containing innumerable, variable-sized cysts replacing nearly the entire renal parenchyma.

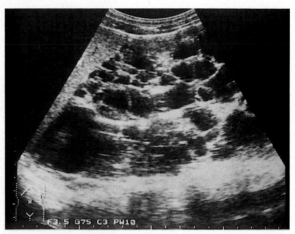

Fig. 2. Autosomal dominant polycystic kidney disease with cyst wall calcifications in a 35-year-old woman. Longitudinal US demonstrates multiple, variable-sized cysts in the right kidney. Note echogenic dots projecting into the cyst lumen, which represent small calcifications in the cyst wall.

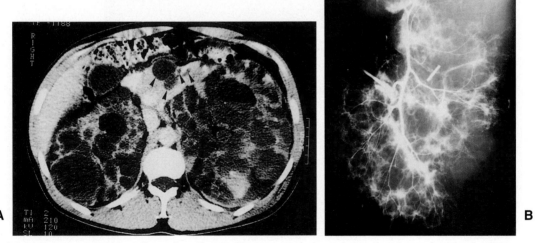

Fig. 3. Autosomal dominant polycystic kidney disease in a 40-year-old man.
A. Contrast-enhanced CT shows marked enlargement of both kidneys with variable-sized cysts occupying the entire kidneys. Note the lack of normal-functioning renal parenchyma. Several cysts are also seen in the pancreas *(arrowheads)*. **B.** Bilateral nephrectomy was performed before renal transplantation. Arteriogram of the removed kidney demonstrates splaying of the intrarenal arteries.

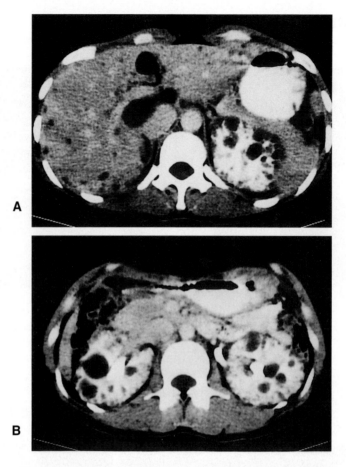

Fig. 4. Autosomal dominant polycystic kidney disease in early stage in a 37-year-old woman.
A, B. Contrast-enhanced CT scans show multiple small cysts in both kidneys and liver. Note that renal enlargement is mild and normally enhancing renal parenchyma is partly spared.

8. Autosomal Dominant Polycystic Kidney Disease with Hemorrhage

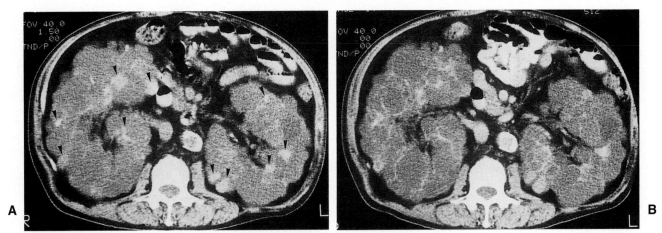

Fig. 1. Autosomal dominant polycystic kidney disease with intracystic hemorrhage in a 59-year-old man.
A. Nonenhanced CT shows marked enlargement of both kidneys with innumerable, variable-sized cysts. Note multiple high-attenuated cysts, which represent hemorrhagic cysts *(arrowheads)*. **B.** Contrast-enhanced CT reveals thin, enhancing, intervening renal parenchyma.

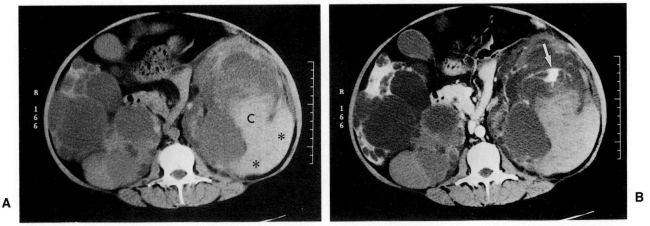

Fig. 2. Autosomal dominant polycystic kidney disease with active bleeding in a 40-year-old woman.
A. Nonenhanced CT reveals enlargement of both kidneys with multiple cysts. Note a hemorrhagic cyst (C) in the left kidney, which has been ruptured, causing perirenal hematoma *(asterisks)*. **B.** On contrast-enhanced CT, there is a leak of contrast material *(arrow)* in the left kidney suggesting active bleeding.

9. Autosomal Dominant Polycystic Kidney Disease with Infection

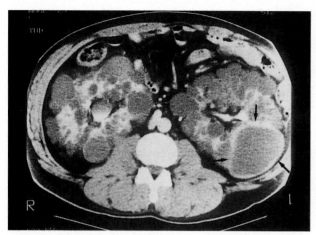

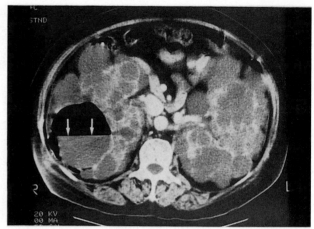

Fig. 1. Autosomal dominant polycystic kidney disease with cyst infection in a 49-year-old man. Contrast-enhanced CT reveals multiple, variable-sized cysts in both enlarged kidneys. Note a thick-walled, high-attenuated cyst *(arrows)* in the left kidney, which was confirmed as an infected cyst at aspiration.

Fig. 2. Autosomal dominant polycystic kidney disease with gas-forming infection of a cyst in a 65-year-old woman. Contrast-enhanced CT shows typical findings of autosomal dominant polycystic kidney disease. Note a large, gas-containing cyst in the mid portion of the right kidney with gas-fluid level *(arrows)*.

10. Autosomal Dominant Polycystic Kidney Disease: Associated Lesions

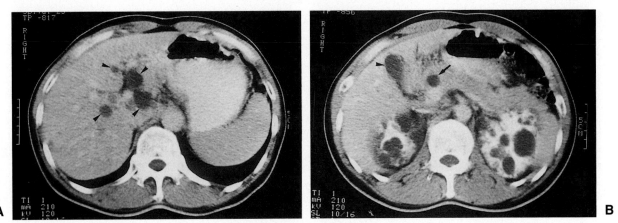

Fig. 1. Multiple hepatic and pancreatic cysts associated with autosomal dominant polycystic kidney disease in a 47-year-old man.
A, B. Contrast-enhanced CT scans show multiple cysts in both kidneys, liver *(arrowheads)*, and pancreas *(arrow in **B**)*.

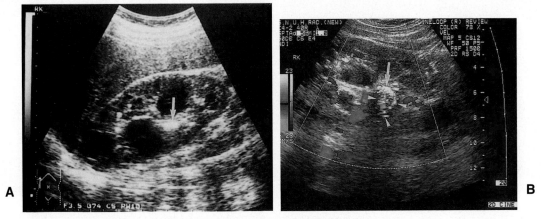

Fig. 2. Autosomal dominant polycystic kidney disease with a renal stone in a 42-year-old man.
A. Longitudinal US of the right kidney shows a large kidney with multiple cysts. Note an echogenic lesion *(arrow)* with faint posterior sonic shadowing suggesting a stone in the renal sinus. **B.** Color Doppler US shows color twinkling artifacts *(arrowheads)* behind the echogenic lesion *(arrow)*, suggesting that the lesion is a stone. (**B,** See also Color Section.)

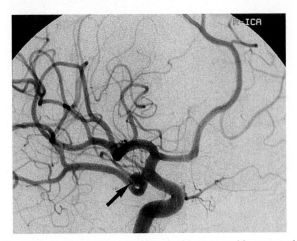

Fig. 3. Cerebral aneurysm in a 58-year-old woman with autosomal dominant polycystic kidney disease. Cerebral arteriogram shows a saccular aneurysm *(arrow)* in the posterior communicating artery.

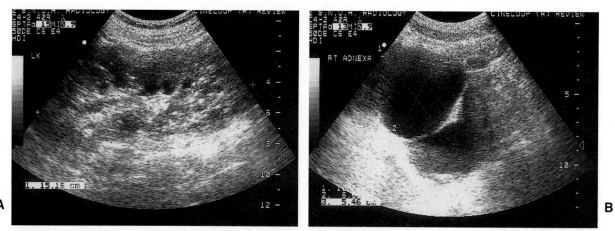

Fig. 4. Ovarian cysts associated with autosomal dominant polycystic kidney disease in a 37-year-old woman.
A. Longitudinal US of the left kidney shows an enlarged kidney and multiple, variable-sized cysts, typical of autosomal dominant polycystic kidney disease. **B.** Transverse US of the pelvis shows large cysts in the right ovary.

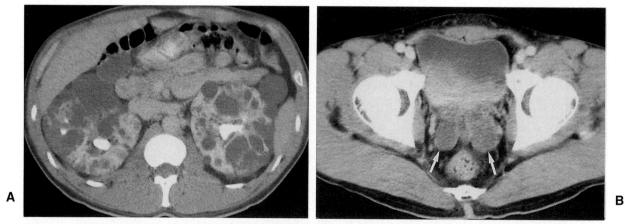

Fig. 5. Dilation of seminal vesicles in a 32-year-old man with autosomal dominant polycystic kidney disease.
A. Contrast-enhanced CT shows large kidneys occupied by innumerable cysts. **B.** CT scan of the pelvic cavity shows dilated seminal vesicles *(arrows)*.

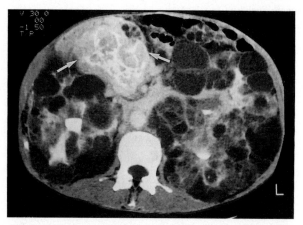

Fig. 6. Renal cell carcinoma occurring in a 35-year-old woman with autosomal dominant polycystic kidney disease. Contrast-enhanced CT reveals multiple, variable-sized cysts in both enlarged kidneys. A large, well-enhancing tumor with irregular calcifications is seen in the anterior aspect of the right kidney *(arrows)*. US-guided biopsy revealed renal cell carcinoma of clear cell type.

11. Unilateral Cystic Disease

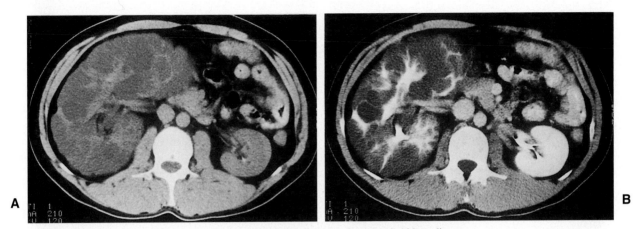

Fig. 1. Unilateral cystic disease in a 30-year-old woman without family history of polycystic kidney disease.
A, B. Nonenhanced (**A**) and contrast-enhanced (**B**) CT scans demonstrate a large right kidney with variable-sized cysts. This finding is indistinguishable from the findings of autosomal dominant polycystic kidney disease. Note the normal-sized left kidney without evidence of cystic disease.

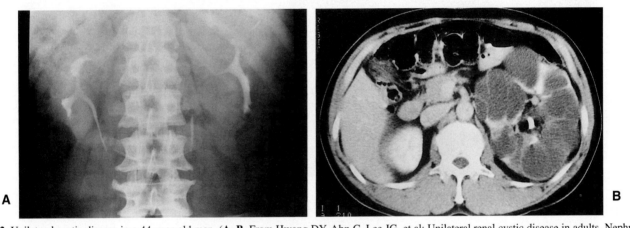

Fig. 2. Unilateral cystic disease in a 44-year-old man. (**A, B,** From Hwang DY, Ahn C, Lee JG, et al: Unilateral renal cystic disease in adults. Nephrol Dial Transplant 1999; 14:1999–2003.)
A. IVU shows enlarged left kidney with stretched pelvocalyces. **B.** Contrast-enhanced CT shows large left kidney with multiple, variable-sized cysts and thinned renal parenchyma.

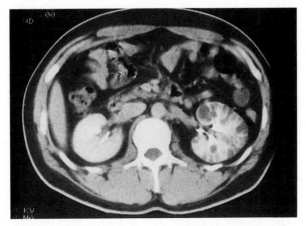

Fig. 3. Unilateral cystic disease in a 26-year-old man. Contrast-enhanced CT shows slightly large left kidney with innumerable small cysts.

12. Localized Cystic Disease

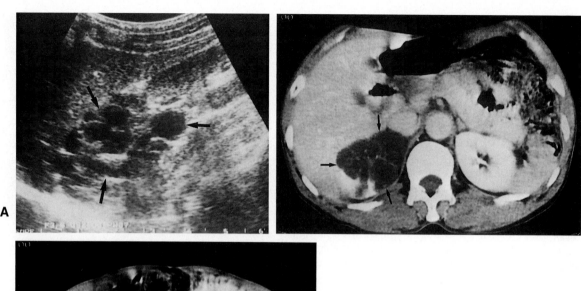

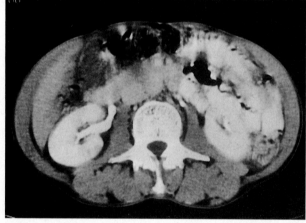

Fig. 1. Localized cystic disease in a 65-year-old woman.
A. Longitudinal US shows a cluster of renal cysts in the upper pole of the right kidney *(arrows)*.
B. Contrast-enhanced CT well demonstrates the cluster of renal cysts in the upper pole of the right kidney *(arrows)*. **C.** CT scan at lower level demonstrates normal renal parenchyma without evidence of renal cysts in the lower pole of the right kidney.

11. Unilateral Cystic Disease

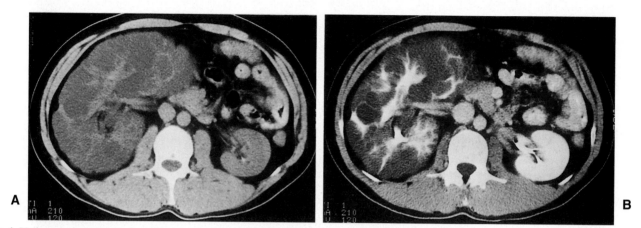

Fig. 1. Unilateral cystic disease in a 30-year-old woman without family history of polycystic kidney disease.
A, B. Nonenhanced (**A**) and contrast-enhanced (**B**) CT scans demonstrate a large right kidney with variable-sized cysts. This finding is indistinguishable from the findings of autosomal dominant polycystic kidney disease. Note the normal-sized left kidney without evidence of cystic disease.

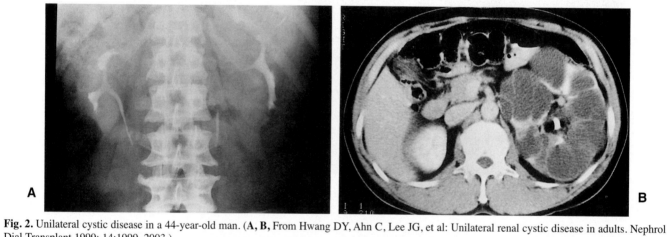

Fig. 2. Unilateral cystic disease in a 44-year-old man. (**A, B,** From Hwang DY, Ahn C, Lee JG, et al: Unilateral renal cystic disease in adults. Nephrol Dial Transplant 1999; 14:1999–2003.)
A. IVU shows enlarged left kidney with stretched pelvocalyces. **B.** Contrast-enhanced CT shows large left kidney with multiple, variable-sized cysts and thinned renal parenchyma.

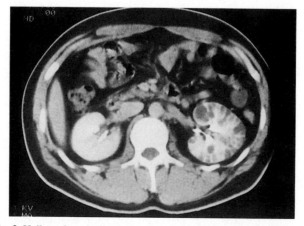

Fig. 3. Unilateral cystic disease in a 26-year-old man. Contrast-enhanced CT shows slightly large left kidney with innumerable small cysts.

12. Localized Cystic Disease

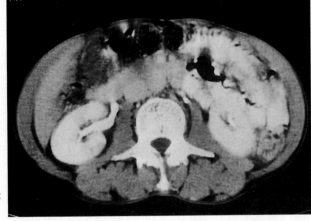

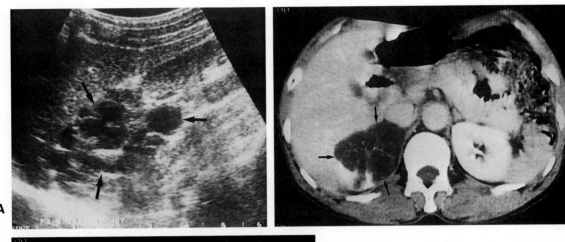

Fig. 1. Localized cystic disease in a 65-year-old woman. **A.** Longitudinal US shows a cluster of renal cysts in the upper pole of the right kidney *(arrows)*. **B.** Contrast-enhanced CT well demonstrates the cluster of renal cysts in the upper pole of the right kidney *(arrows)*. **C.** CT scan at lower level demonstrates normal renal parenchyma without evidence of renal cysts in the lower pole of the right kidney.

13. Autosomal Recessive Polycystic Kidney Disease

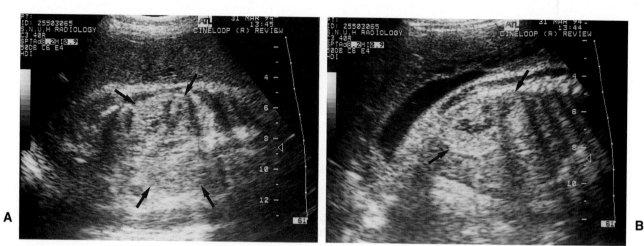

Fig. 1. Autosomal recessive polycystic kidney disease detected at prenatal US in a 35-week fetus.
A. Longitudinal US of the fetal abdomen in coronal plane shows oligohydramnios and both kidneys enlarged *(arrows)* with diffusely increased echogenicity. **B.** US of the fetal right kidney in sagittal plane well demonstrates diffusely increased renal echogenicity *(arrows)*.

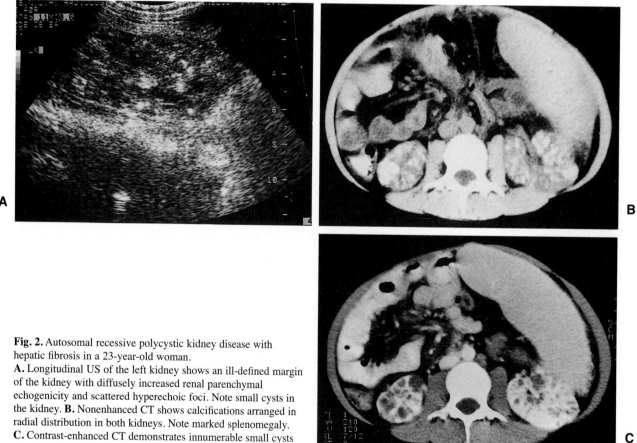

Fig. 2. Autosomal recessive polycystic kidney disease with hepatic fibrosis in a 23-year-old woman.
A. Longitudinal US of the left kidney shows an ill-defined margin of the kidney with diffusely increased renal parenchymal echogenicity and scattered hyperechoic foci. Note small cysts in the kidney. **B.** Nonenhanced CT shows calcifications arranged in radial distribution in both kidneys. Note marked splenomegaly. **C.** Contrast-enhanced CT demonstrates innumerable small cysts in both kidneys.

14. Medullary Cystic Disease

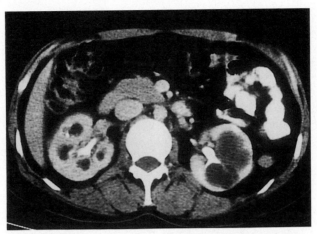

Fig. 1. Medullary cystic disease in a 47-year-old woman. Contrast-enhanced CT shows several cysts in the medullary regions of both kidneys. This patient had proteinuria and polydipsia for 20 years.

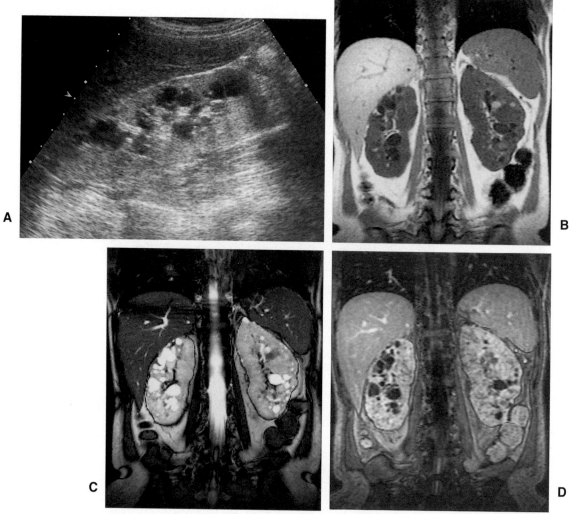

Fig. 2. Medullary cystic disease in a 29-year-old woman with progressive azotemia.
A. US of the right kidney shows innumerable small cysts in the renal parenchyma, predominantly in the medullary region. Some cysts are round and others are tubular. Note the diffusely increased renal parenchymal echogenicity. **B, C.** T1-weighted (**B**) and T2-weighted (**C**) coronal MR images show both kidneys enlarged with innumerable cysts. Some cysts show high signal intensity on T1-weighted image, suggesting intracystic hemorrhage.
D. Contrast-enhanced T1-weighted MR image well demonstrates nonenhancing cysts. US-guided biopsy of the kidney revealed the findings of medullary cystic disease.

15. Multicystic Dysplastic Kidney

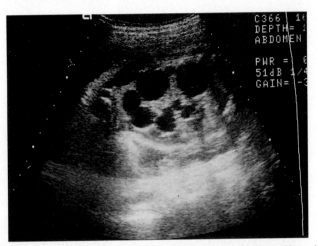

Fig. 1. Multicystic dysplastic kidney detected at prenatal US in a 32-week fetus. US shows large fetal right kidney that contains multiple, variable-sized, noncommunicating cysts. The contralateral kidney was normal at US.

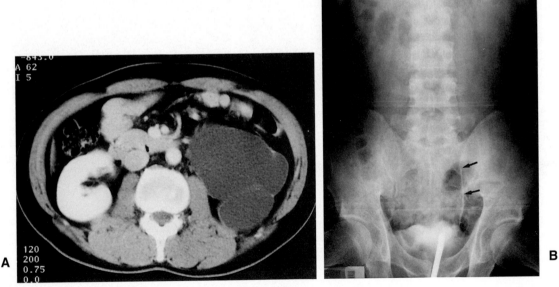

Fig. 2. Multicystic dysplastic kidney of hydronephrotic type in a 46-year-old man.
A. Contrast-enhanced CT shows markedly dilated pelvocalyces of the left kidney without identifiable remnant renal parenchyma. **B.** RGP demonstrates narrow rudimentary ureter at distal portion *(arrows)*.

16. Acquired Cystic Disease

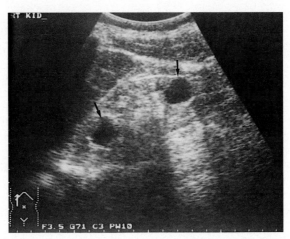

Fig. 1. Acquired cystic disease in a 54-year-old woman with chronic renal failure. Longitudinal US shows a small right kidney with increased parenchymal echogenicity. Note two cysts in the polar areas *(arrows)*.

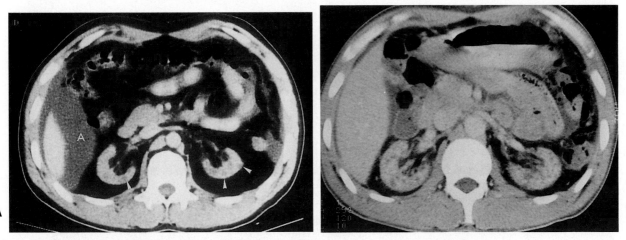

Fig. 2. Acquired cystic disease in a 60-year-old man with chronic renal failure.
A. Contrast-enhanced CT shows both kidneys shrunken and a few small cysts *(arrowheads)*. Note the presence of ascites (A). **B.** On follow-up contrast-enhanced CT taken 18 months later, the kidneys are enlarged as compared with previous CT and the number of the cysts is increased.

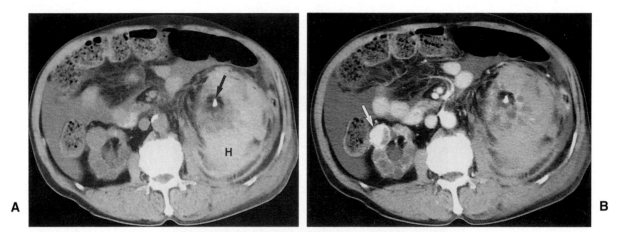

Fig. 3. Acquired cystic disease complicated by perirenal hemorrhage and renal cell carcinoma in a 65-year-old man.
A. Nonenhanced CT shows large amount of perirenal hemorrhage (H) on the left side. Also note a stone in the left kidney *(arrow)*. **B.** Contrast-enhanced CT in cortical phase shows both kidneys poorly enhancing with innumerable cysts. Note a highly enhancing mass *(arrow)* arising in one of the cysts in the right kidney.

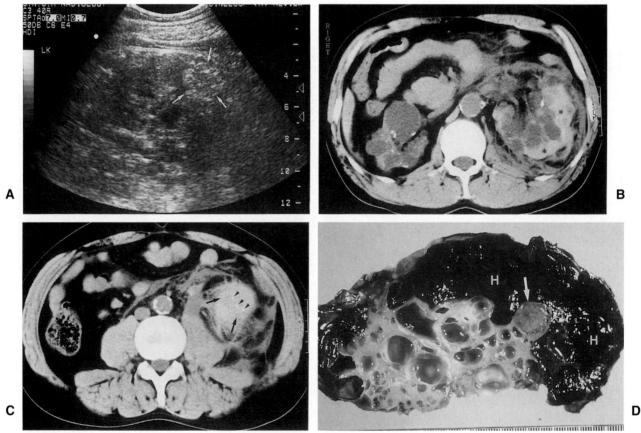

Fig. 4. Oncocytoma and perirenal hematoma associated with acquired cystic renal disease in a 48-year-old man.
A. Longitudinal US shows large left kidney with ill-defined outline. The renal parenchymal echogenicity is increased and there is a round, echogenic mass *(arrows)* in the lower pole of the left kidney. **B.** Contrast-enhanced CT scan at the level of the kidneys shows multiple cysts in both kidneys with mural calcifications. Note high-attenuated, perirenal hematoma on the left side *(asterisks)*. **C.** CT scan at a lower level reveals a homogeneously enhancing mass *(arrows)* with mottled calcifications *(arrowheads)*. Also note the perirenal hematoma with thickened renal fasciae. At surgery the mass was confirmed as an oncocytoma. **D.** Gross specimen of the removed left kidney shows multiple cysts and perirenal hematoma (H). Note a small solid mass *(arrow)* in the lower pole of the kidney, which was confirmed as an oncocytoma. (**D,** See also Color Section.)

17. Parapelvic Cysts

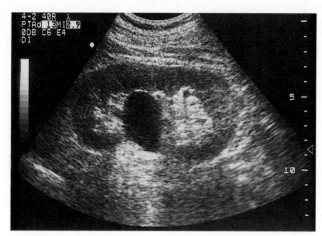

Fig. 1. A parapelvic cyst in a 52-year-old man. Longitudinal US shows a round, unilocular cyst within the renal sinus.

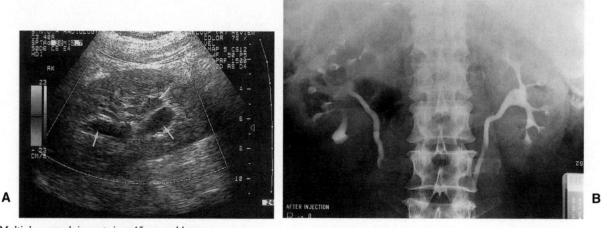

A   **B**

Fig. 2. Multiple parapelvic cysts in a 45-year-old man.
A. Color Doppler US of the right kidney shows several ovoid, anechoic lesions *(arrows)* within the renal sinus, which may mimic dilated renal collecting system. Note that the cysts do not communicate with each other. (**A,** See also Color Section.) **B.** IVU reveals splaying of the renal calyces with elongation of the infundibula in the right kidney.

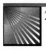
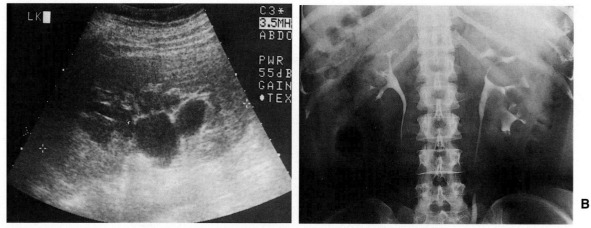

Fig. 3. Parapelvic cysts in a 41-year-old woman.
A. Longitudinal US of the left kidney shows multiple fusiform cystic structures in the renal sinus area, some of which seem to communicate with each other. These findings closely mimic hydronephrosis. **B.** IVU reveals splaying of the collecting systems without evidence of hydronephrosis, confirming that the lesions seen on US are parapelvic cysts.

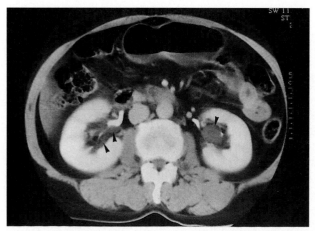

Fig. 4. Bilateral parapelvic cysts in a 50-year-old man. Contrast-enhanced CT shows multiple, homogeneous, low-attenuated lesions (*arrowheads*) in the renal sinuses. Note that the pelvocalyces are well opacified.

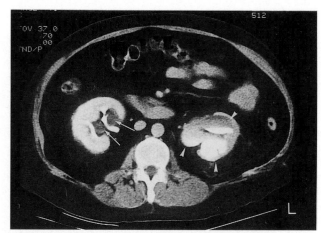

Fig. 5. Parapelvic cyst in one kidney and hydronephrosis in the other kidney in a 60-year-old woman. Contrast-enhanced CT shows low-attenuated, parapelvic cysts in the right kidney (*arrows*) and hydronephrosis with layering of excreted contrast material in the left kidney (*arrowheads*).

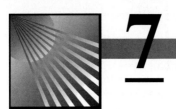

7

Pediatric Renal Masses

WOO SUN KIM

Renal masses are the most common abdominal masses encountered in childhood. Conditions that present as pediatric renal masses include developmental anomalies, cystic renal diseases, and primary renal neoplasms.

The most common renal mass detected in the neonatal period is hydronephrosis, although multicystic dysplastic kidney is the most common in the first day of life. Many neonatal renal masses are now found antenatally by ultrasonography (US).

Wilms' tumor is by far the most common renal neoplasm in children. Other less common tumors include clear cell sarcoma, rhabdoid tumor, multilocular cystic renal tumor, mesoblastic nephroma, renal cell carcinoma, and lymphoma. Mesoblastic nephroma is the most common renal neoplasm in the first year of life.

Because hydronephrosis and cystic renal diseases are the major causes of pediatric abdominal or renal masses, US is the most appropriate and cost-effective initial radiologic study. In most patients with cystic renal masses such as multicystic dysplastic kidney or polycystic kidney disease, no further studies are needed after US diagnosis. Computed tomography (CT) plays an important role in further characterization, staging, and follow-up of children with solid renal masses.

HYDRONEPHROSIS

Hydronephrosis can result from urinary tract obstruction or vesicoureteral reflux. In the evaluation of hydronephrosis, intravenous urography (IVU) with delayed imaging has been replaced by US in most cases. With US, we can easily determine whether a renal mass is a hydronephrotic kidney or a solid mass and can be informed further of the degree and extent of urinary tract dilation. For the evaluation of patients with renal duplication, IVU is still sometimes useful.

Once hydronephrosis is detected by US, renal scintigraphy by using diethylene triamine pentaacetic acid (DTPA) with wash-out phase scan after administration of diuretics is performed to identify obstruction, to confirm the degree and level of obstruction, and to determine remaining renal function. Voiding cystourethrography (VCU) is also performed to exclude vesicoureteral reflux and bladder outlet obstruction such as are seen with the posterior urethral valve.

The most common cause of obstructive hydronephrosis in children is ureteropelvic junction obstruction of variable degree

that may be due to intrinsic abnormality of the wall of the ureteropelvic junction or to extrinsic compression by a crossing blood vessel. Anomalies of the contralateral kidney are present in up to 30% of these patients, including bilateral ureteropelvic junction obstruction in 18% of cases. Other causes of hydronephrosis that can present as renal masses include ureterovesical junction obstruction, massive vesicoureteral reflux, ectopic ureterocele of upper moiety ureter in duplex system, posterior urethral valve, and prune belly syndrome. In these diseases, the ureter is also dilated.

MULTICYSTIC DYSPLASTIC KIDNEY

Multicystic dysplastic kidney is the most common abdominal mass in the neonatal period and is type 2 cystic disease of the kidney according to Potter's classification. It is believed to be secondary to severe obstruction of the upper urinary tract occurring during the early stage of intrauterine development. Pelvoinfundibular atresia or atresia of the ureter is a common cause of the obstruction.

Histologically the multicystic dysplastic kidney consists of multiple noncommunicating cysts of variable size and an intervening primitive dysplastic element. Less commonly, multicystic dysplastic kidney of hydronephrotic type can also be found. The involved kidney typically has no renal function and the contralateral kidney shows compensatory hypertrophy. Unilateral involvement is usual and bilaterality results in increased fetal death or severe oligohydramnios, causing lethal pulmonary hypoplasia. Segmental involvement of the kidney can be detected less frequently. It is more common in boys, and the involvement of the left kidney is more common. Abnormalities of the contralateral kidney are frequently found, with quite different incidence rates reported. Vesicoureteral reflux of the contralateral kidney also occurs more frequently than in the general population.

US findings are mostly diagnostic. A typical case shows a large kidney composed of cysts of varying size that are distributed randomly with an intervening echogenic portion of a dysplastic element. In many patients, however, the involved kidney is not enlarged and rather atrophic. US follow-up of patients shows that cysts of the affected kidney usually regress but can be stable or enlarged. In some patients, involved kidneys cannot be demonstrated on follow-up US.

AUTOSOMAL RECESSIVE POLYCYSTIC KIDNEY DISEASE

Autosomal recessive polycystic kidney disease, also known as *infantile polycystic kidney disease* (Potter's type 1), is the most common heritable disease among all of the cystic renal diseases manifesting in infancy and childhood. It affects the kidney and liver, and the severity of abnormalities of each organ is inversely proportional: patients with severe renal disease have milder hepatic involvement and those with severe liver disease usually have milder renal involvement. Although renal disease is a major problem in infancy, congenital hepatic fibrosis and associated portal hypertension and variceal bleeding are major problems in the juvenile period. Patients who present immediately after birth with markedly enlarged kidneys often have a poor prognosis due to renal failure or respiratory distress secondary to bilateral pulmonary hypoplasia resulting from oligohydramnios in fetal life. Pathologically, the renal lesion is characterized by varying degrees of nonobstructive dilation of the collecting tubules. The liver lesion consists of periportal fibrosis accompanying the malformed and dilated bile ducts. Less commonly, Caroli's disease (nonobstructive dilation of the intrahepatic bile ducts) or choledochal cyst can be associated.

At US, both kidneys are large and of increased echogenicity with no or poor corticomedullary differentiation. Increased echogenicity is thought to be due to the numerous acoustic interfaces between the dilated tubules in the cortex and medulla. With a high-frequency transducer, some of the dilated collecting tubules of radiating pattern can be demonstrated. Small cysts that tend to become larger and more numerous over time can also be found in many patients. In some patients, a thin hypoechoic rim at the periphery is seen on US. There are controversies with regard to the pathologic basis of this US finding. It is generally thought that this finding is due to residual compressed renal parenchyma. In patients with mild renal involvement, the kidneys are not enlarged and increased renal echogenicity is usually confined to the medulla.

Delayed nephrogram or poor opacification of the kidneys is seen on IVU and contrast-enhanced CT. Although IVU is not recommended anymore, CT is performed in some patients mainly for further characterization of liver disease and for evaluation of variceal veins and spleen size. On both studies, contrast pooling in ectatic tubules produces a radially arrayed, striated nephrogram that usually persists for hours or even days. Fine calcifications that are best seen on nonenhanced CT are commonly found in older children, and they show a radiating pattern in some cases.

WILMS' TUMOR

Epidemiology

Wilms' tumor is the most common pediatric abdominal malignancy, although it is less common than neuroblastoma in infants. It is the most common renal malignancy of childhood, accounting for 87% of all renal neoplasms in children. Its peak incidence is at 3 to 4 years of age, and approximately 80% of patients present before 5 years of age. It is rare in neonates and young infants. Approximately 15% of cases have an associated syndrome or renal anomalies. There is an increased incidence of Wilms' tumor in children with nephroblastomatosis, hemihypertrophy, sporadic aniridia, Beckwith-Wiedemann syndrome, Drash syndrome

(male pseudohermaphroditism, progressive glomerulonephritis, and Wilms' tumor), WAGR syndrome (Wilms' tumor, aniridia, genitourinary anomalies, and mental retardation), chromosome abnormalities, and genitourinary anomalies such as cryptorchidism, hypospadias, and horseshoe kidney.

Wilms' tumor is bilateral in 4% to 13% of cases. Although most bilateral tumors occur synchronously, metachronous tumors do occur. Bilateral tumors are correlated with a higher incidence of nephroblastomatosis, a higher incidence of associated congenital anomalies or syndromes, and an earlier presentation than seen in unilateral Wilms' tumor.

Histopathology

Wilms' tumor, also known as *nephroblastoma*, is a malignant embryonal tumor of renal origin. Wilms' tumor usually arises from primitive metanephric blastema within the renal cortex. Rare extrarenal variants may occur from extrarenal metanephric rests and most commonly present in the retroperitoneum. A classic Wilms' tumor has a triphasic histology: it contains variable amounts of blastemal, stromal, and epithelial cell lines. Fat, which can be found in Wilms' tumor, can be differentiated from the stromal elements. The term *teratoid Wilms' tumor* may be applied if there is differentiation along tissue lines not normally found in the kidney, such as bone, cartilage, and muscle. The prognosis and response to chemotherapy of Wilms' tumor are dependent on the presence of anaplasia. According to the presence of anaplastic component, Wilms' tumors are classified into favorable and unfavorable histology. Approximately 90% of Wilms' tumors demonstrate favorable histopathologic findings. Anaplastic Wilms' tumor tends to occur in older age groups and is associated with an increased prevalence of lymph node metastases at the time of diagnosis.

Wilms' tumor manifests as a solid intrarenal mass with a pseudocapsule. The renal parenchyma and collecting system are distorted by the tumor. Hemorrhage and necrosis are common and contribute to cystic degeneration. The tumor spreads in various ways. Wilms' tumor may extend into contiguous vascular structures. Extension into the ipsilateral renal vein is frequent. Propagation of tumor thrombus into the inferior vena cava has been reported in about 4% of Wilms' tumor. Tumor thrombus extends into the right atrium in about 20% of patients with caval involvement. Direct extension into the adjacent organs can occur following capsular invasion. Rarely the tumor may extend into the collecting system in a botryoid fashion. Metastases are most commonly found in the lungs and regional lymph nodes. More than 10% of patients have lung metastases at the time of diagnosis. Pleural or liver metastases occur, but less frequently. Bone metastases are rare.

Clinical features

Children with Wilms' tumor most often present with a palpable abdominal mass. Some patients present with tumor bleeding after minor trauma. Less than 30% have abdominal pain. Hematuria or hypertension is not uncommon. Hypertension may be due to renin production by the tumor or vascular compressions. The prognosis of Wilms' tumor is generally good. Cure rates are based on histologic features and tumor stage at the time of diagnosis. Recently, the rates have improved to 90% or higher.

Imaging

US evaluation of Wilms' tumor demonstrates a large, well-demarcated mass with heterogeneous echogenicity. The tumor-kidney interface is usually sharply defined presumably by pseudocapsule or compressed renal parenchyma. Hypoechoic or cystic lesion may be tumor necrosis, deposit of mucin, or trapped calyces. Fat or calcification may contribute to the hyperechoic areas within the mass. The renal vein and inferior vena cava should be examined to exclude tumor extension, because their presence may change the therapeutic approach. The contralateral kidney must be observed carefully for synchronous tumor or accompanying congenital anomalies. US is considered not sufficient for detection of a small synchronous tumor or nephrogenic rests in the ipsilateral or contralateral kidney. For screening of Wilms' tumor in children at high risk for developing Wilms' tumor, initial CT followed by serial US may be appropriate. Screening protocols vary from institution to institution.

CT has been the most important imaging study for the diagnosis and follow-up of patients with Wilms' tumor. Wilms' tumor is seen as a large, well-defined mass of heterogeneous attenuation on CT. The tumor is usually well circumscribed, and a beak or claw of renal tissue may extend partly around the mass, helping confirm its renal origin. Areas of low attenuation coincide with tumor necrosis or fat deposition. Calcifications may be identified on nonenhanced CT in approximately 15% of cases. When the tumor is predominantly cystic (so-called cystic Wilms' tumor), it may be difficult to differentiate it from multilocular cystic renal tumor. Intravenous administration of contrast material is mandatory to detect tumor extension into the renal vein or inferior vena cava, contralateral and ipsilateral synchronous tumor and/or associated nephrogenic rests, tumor extension into the adjacent perirenal fat, and retroperitoneal lymph node or hepatic metastases. Wilms' tumor does not encase the aorta, whereas the encasement is characteristic in neuroblastoma. With continuation of CT scan up to the chest, lung metastases from the tumor that frequently are invisible on chest radiography can be identified. CT is also the imaging modality of choice for evaluation of patients with postoperative Wilms' tumor. Because most relapses occur within the abdomen and chest, follow-up CT of the abdomen and chest is performed.

Magnetic resonance (MR) imaging is usually performed in selected cases. MR imaging can be useful in assessment of caval patency and multifocal diseases, in which multiplanar imaging is more helpful. With MR imaging, lung metastases cannot be evaluated.

NEPHROBLASTOMATOSIS

Nephroblastomatosis is defined as the presence of multifocal or diffuse nephrogenic rests in the renal cortex. Nephrogenic rests are foci of metanephric blastema that persist beyond 36 weeks of gestation and have the potential for malignant transformation into Wilms' tumor. They are found incidentally in 1% of infants. They have been identified in approximately 30% to 40% of Wilms' tumors, and they are found in up to 99% of bilateral Wilms' tumors. Nephrogenic rests can be classified into perilobar and intralobar types on the basis of location of lesions within the kidneys and the associated syndromes. Although the two types are different in incidence and rate of association with Wilms' tumor development, they cannot be differentiated by imaging studies.

Imaging studies can detect only macroscopic nephrogenic rests. Contrast-enhanced CT scan demonstrates poorly enhancing cortical nodules in cases of multifocal nephroblastomatosis. In diffuse (infantile) nephroblastomatosis, both kidneys are usually enlarged, with distortion of the calyces by a thick, peripheral rind of abnormal tissue. At MR imaging, the nodules of multifocal nephroblastomatosis have low signal intensity on both T1-weighted and T2-weighted images, although hyperplastic nephrogenic rests can be isotense or slightly hyperintense on T2-weighted images. Nephroblastomatosis is far better delineated on contrast-enhanced T1-weighted MR images than on nonenhanced images. At US, diffuse nephroblastomatosis is seen as enlarged kidneys with diffusely decreased echogenicity. US can demonstrate hypoechoic nodules but lacks the sensitivity of CT and MR imaging, especially in cases with lesions smaller than 1 cm. It is difficult to differentiate macroscopic nephrogenic rests from small Wilms' tumor by imaging studies. Although nodules of nephroblastomatosis are small (usually <2 cm), the size of the lesions is not a reliable criterion in the differentiation. Nephrogenic rests are seen as homogeneous nodules at US, CT, or MR imaging, whereas Wilms' tumors are generally heterogeneous.

CLEAR CELL SARCOMA

Clear cell sarcoma, which was considered a highly aggressive variant of Wilms' tumor, is now recognized as a distinct entity. It has also been termed *bone-metastasizing renal tumor of childhood*. It constitutes 4% of all childhood renal neoplasms and has a male predilection. It has a worse prognosis than Wilms' tumor, and its peak incidence is in a similar or slightly younger age group than that of Wilms' tumor. This entity has not been reported in association with nephroblastomatosis or somatic abnormalities such as sporadic aniridia or hemihypertrophy, which has strong associations with Wilms' tumor.

Clear cell sarcoma has no specific imaging features that can reliably distinguish it from Wilms' tumor. It is usually seen as a solid mass with varying areas of cystic necrosis. Calcification within the mass can be found in 25% of cases. Vascular invasion is not common. Because the incidence of skeletal metastases is high, periodic skeletal surveys and bone scan are recommended. Involvement of skull is the most common. The bone metastases usually occur after initial presentation. It can also metastasize to the lungs, lymph nodes, brain, liver, and soft tissue such as periorbital fat or skeletal muscle.

RHABDOID TUMOR

Rhabdoid tumor of the kidney, which is the most aggressive renal neoplasm in children, accounts for 2% to 3% of all renal neoplasms. It commonly presents in infancy (~60%) and may be detected prenatally. It carries a poor prognosis, and many patients have metastases at presentation. Rhabdoid tumor is unique among other renal tumors in children in its significant association with the synchronous or metachronous development of primary brain tumors of mostly posterior fossa origin, including medulloblastoma, ependymoma, glioma, and primitive neuroectodermal tumor. It also commonly metastasizes to the brain.

By imaging studies, it cannot be reliably differentiated from Wilms' tumor in most cases. However, subcapsular fluid collection or hematoma, lobulated surface of the tumor, and

calcifications outlining tumor lobules can be seen in typical instances. The masses are usually large at presentation and frequently central in location, involving the renal hilum. Invasion into the renal vein is common. It frequently metastasizes to the retroperitoneal lymph nodes, lung, liver, brain, and bone.

CONGENITAL MESOBLASTIC NEPHROMA

Congenital mesoblastic nephroma is the most common solid renal tumor in the neonatal period or early infancy. A mean age at presentation is approximately 3 months. It is the most common fetal renal neoplasm, which is usually associated with maternal polyhydramnios. It is a hamartomatous tumor due to proliferation of early nephrogenic mesenchyma and has also been called *fetal renal mesenchymal hamartoma*. Although it is generally considered a benign lesion, it has some malignant potential. Metastatic diseases to the lungs or brain and local recurrence after nephrectomy have been reported rarely.

Pathologically the tumor is solid and unencapsulated. Spindle cells and connective tissue tend to infiltrate between the intact nephrons and entrap them. Histology varies from a benign to a more hypercellular, aggressive variant. Tumor necrosis is uncommon except with the aggressive variant. It may invade the perinephric space but does not infiltrate the vascular pedicle.

The imaging features of mesoblastic nephroma are indistinguishable from those of Wilms' tumor in most instances. On US examination of a typical case, the lesion is a large, solid renal mass. The mass shows variable echoes or may be hypoechoic. Alternating concentric hypoechoic and hyperechoic rings (ring sign) are described in some cases. On CT, some contrast material may occasionally be seen within the tumor due to functioning nephrons or urine, which is interspersed with neoplastic tissue or entrapped within the mass. In larger lesions, areas of low attenuation representing necrosis or hemorrhage can be seen, and they may indicate more aggressive potential. Calcifications within the tumor are rarely seen.

RENAL CELL CARCINOMA

Renal cell carcinoma is rare in children, and it represents a small percentage (2.3% to 6.6%) of all renal neoplasms in childhood. The average age at presentation of 9 to 11 years is considerably older than with Wilms' tumor. The association of renal cell carcinoma with von Hippel-Lindau disease, tuberous sclerosis, and Beckwith-Wiedemann syndrome has been reported in children. Compared with Wilms' tumor, this tumor is more likely to metastasize to bone.

By imaging studies, renal cell carcinoma in children cannot be distinguished from Wilms' tumor. It tends to be smaller than Wilms' tumor at presentation. Calcifications are seen within the tumors in 25% of patients, and they tend to be denser than those in Wilms' tumor. Intravascular extension is as frequent as in adult patients.

MULTILOCULAR CYSTIC RENAL TUMOR

The term *multilocular cystic renal tumor* refers to two types of generally benign cystic tumors: cystic nephroma and cystic partially differentiated nephroblastoma. These are well-encapsulated lesions consisting of multiple, noncommunicating cysts and septa. Two types of multilocular cystic renal tumor are indistinguishable on gross examination. The difference between two entities is that septa of cystic partially differentiated nephroblastoma contain foci of blastemic cells, whereas those of cystic nephroma do not. These two types can be differentiated from cystic Wilms' tumor by the absence of expansile solid portions of nephroblastomatous tissue within the tumor. Although these tumors follow a generally benign course, local recurrences can occur rarely. The relationship between these two entities and Wilms' tumor has been controversial.

Multilocular cystic renal tumor usually presents as an asymptomatic mass. It tends to manifest at two age incidence peaks: in children aged 3 months to 4 years with a male predilection and in adults with a female predilection.

Two entities are indistinguishable on the basis of imaging features. Imaging studies demonstrate a well-circumscribed mass consisting of multiple cysts from several millimeters to a few centimeters in diameter. Septa can be enhanced variably on CT or MR imaging after contrast enhancement. In some cases, the cystic spaces may be quite small, resulting in the appearance of a solid mass, which is usually expected as an imaging finding of cystic Wilms' tumor. Variable signal intensity of cyst contents can be seen on T1-weighted MR images. Because cystic partially differentiated nephroblastoma may demonstrate behavior with a potential for recurrence following resection and it is not always reliably differentiated from Wilms' tumor by imaging studies, the treatment of multilocular cystic renal tumor is complete surgical resection.

LYMPHOMA AND LEUKEMIA

Lymphoma commonly involves the kidneys secondarily from hematogenous metastases or direct retroperitoneal extension. However, lymphoma confined to the kidneys has been reported rarely, although the kidneys contain no lymphoid tissue. In children, non-Hodgkin's lymphoma, especially Burkitt lymphoma, involves the kidneys more commonly than does Hodgkin's lymphoma. Renal lymphoma is usually silent until late in the disease. The most common imaging finding is multiple, bilateral, parenchymal nodules. US usually shows hypoechoic nodules with increased "through" transmission. Nodules are usually low attenuated on CT scans both before and after contrast enhancement. In cases of diffuse infiltration, the kidneys are diffusely enlarged and excretion of contrast material is diminished. Renal failure may be induced on initiation of chemotherapy due to uric acid nephropathy. Direct invasion from contiguous retroperitoneal mass can also occur. The presence of associated findings such as lymph node enlargement and/or hepatosplenomegaly can be helpful for imaging diagnosis.

Although leukemia is the most common malignancy in childhood, gross renal involvement is uncommonly encountered. Leukemic involvement of the kidneys is more common with lymphocytic types than with granulocytic types. The kidneys are symmetrically enlarged and calyceal architecture is distorted. At US, corticomedullary differentiation is lost or decreased. Rarely, renal involvement presents as a focal mass or multiple nodules.

References

1. Han TI, Kim MJ, Yoon HK, et al: Rhabdoid tumour of the kidney: Imaging findings. Pediatr Radiol 2001; 31:233–237.
2. Lonergan GJ, Rice RR, Suarez ES: Autosomal recessive polycystic kidney disease: Radiologic-pathologic correlation. Radiographics 2000; 20:837–855.
3. Lowe LH, Isuani BH, Heller RM, et al: Pediatric renal masses: Wilms' tumor and beyond. Radiographics 2000; 20:1585–1603.
4. Beckwith JB: Children at increased risk for Wilms' tumor: Monitoring issues. J Pediatr 1998; 132:377–379.
5. Lonergan GJ, Martinez-Leon MI, Agrons GA, et al: Nephrogenic rests, nephroblastomatosis, and associated lesions of the kidney. Radiographics 1998; 18:947–968.
6. Rohrschneider WK, Weirich A, Rieden K, et al: US, CT, and MR imaging characteristics of nephroblastomatosis. Pediatr Radiol 1998; 28:435–443.
7. Strouse PJ: Pediatric renal neoplasm. Radiol Clin North Am 1996; 34:1081–1100.
8. Geller E, Smergel EM, Lowry PA: Renal neoplasms of childhood. Radiol Clin North Am 1997; 35:1391–1413.
9. Agrons GA, Kingsman KD, Wagner BJ, et al: Rhabdoid tumor of the kidney in children: A comparative study of 21 cases. AJR Am J Roentgenol 1997; 168:447–451.
10. Broecker B: Renal cell carcinoma in children. Urology 1991; 38:54–56.
11. Freedman AL, Vates TS, Stewart T, et al: Renal cell carcinoma in children: The Detroit experience. J Urol 1996; 155:1708–1710.
12. Fernbach SK, Feinstein KA: Renal tumors in children. Semin Roentgenol 1995; 30:200–217.
13. Navoy JE, Royal SA, Vaid YN, et al: Wilms' tumor: Unusual manifestations. Pediatr Radiol 1995; 25:76–86.
14. Agrons GA, Wagner BJ, Davidson AJ, et al: Multilocular cystic renal tumor in children: Radiologic-pathologic correlation. Radiographics 1995; 15:653–669.
15. Chung CJ, Lorenzo R, Rayder S, et al: Rhabdoid tumors of the kidney in children: CT findings. AJR Am J Roentgenol 1995; 164:697–700.
16. Wootton SL: The child with an abdominal mass. In Hilton SW, Edwards DK (eds): Practical Pediatric Radiology. Philadelphia, WB Saunders, 1994, pp 57–388.
17. Lucaya J, Enriquez G, Nieto J, et al: Renal calcifications in patients with autosomal recessive polycystic kidney disease: Prevalence and cause. AJR Am J Roentgenol 1993; 160:359–362.
18. Strife JL, Souza AS, Kirks DR, et al: Multicystic dysplastic kidney in children: US follow-up. Radiology 1993; 186:785–788.
19. Green DM, Breslow NE, Beckwith JB, et al: Screening of children with hemihypertrophy, aniridia, and Beckwith-Wiedemann syndrome in patients with Wilms' tumor: A report from the National Wilms' Tumor Study. Med Pediatr Oncol 1993; 21:188–192.
20. Gylys-Morin V, Hoffer FA, Kozakewich H, et al: Wilms' tumor and nephroblastomatosis: Imaging characteristics at gadolinium-enhanced MR imaging. Radiology 1993; 188:517–521.
21. Andrews PE, Kelalis PP, Haase GM: Extrarenal Wilms' tumor: Results of the National Wilms' Tumor Study. J Pediatr Surg 1992; 27:1181–1184.
22. Kissane JM, Dehner LP: Renal tumors and tumor-like lesions in pediatric patients. Pediatr Nephrol 1992; 6:365–382.
23. White KS, Kirks DR, Bove KE: Imaging of nephroblastomatosis: An overview. Radiology 1992; 182:1–5.
24. White KS, Grossman H: Wilms' and associated renal tumors of childhood. Pediatr Radiol 1991; 21:81–88.
25. Glass RBJ, Davidson AJ, Fernbach SK: Clear cell sarcoma of the kidney: CT, sonographic, and pathologic correlation. Radiology 1991; 180:715–717.
26. Jafri SZ, Freeman JL, Rosenberg BF, et al: Clinical and imaging features of rhabdoid tumor of the kidney. Urol Radiol 1991; 13:94–97.
27. Beckwith JB, Kiviat NB, Bonadio JF: Nephrogenic rests, nephroblastomatosis, and the pathogenesis of Wilms' tumor. Pediatr Pathol 1990; 10:1–36.
28. Weeks DA, Beckwith JB, Mierau GW, et al: Rhabdoid tumor of kidney: A report of 111 cases from the National Wilms' Tumor Study Pathology Center. Am J Surg Pathol 1989; 13:439–458.
29. Kirks DR, Kaufman RA: Function within mesoblastic nephroma: Imaging-pathologic correlation. Pediatr Radiol 1989; 19:136–139.
30. Joshi VV, Beckwith JB: Multilocular cyst of the kidney (cystic nephroma) and cystic partially differentiated nephroblastoma. Cancer 1989; 64:466–479.
31. Currarino G, Stannard MW, Rutledge JC: The sonolucent cortical rim in infantile polycystic kidneys: Histologic correlation. J Ultrasound Med 1989; 8:571–574.
32. Ritchey ML, Kelalis PP, Breslow N, et al: Intracaval and atrial involvement with nephroblastoma: Review of National Wilms' Tumor Study III. J Urol 1988; 140:1113–1118.
33. Sisler CL, Siegel MJ: Malignant rhabdoid tumor of the kidney: Radiologic features. Radiology 1988; 172:211–212.
34. Chan HS, Cheng MY, Mancer K, et al: Congenital mesoblastic nephroma: A clinicoradiologic study of 17 cases representing the pathologic spectrum of the disease. J Pediatr 1987; 111:64–70.
35. Hayden CK, Swischuk LE, Smith TH, et al: Renal cystic disease in childhood. Radiographics 1986; 6:97–116.
36. Hartman DS, Lesar MSL, Madewell JE, et al: Mesoblastic nephroma: Radiologic-pathologic correlation of 20 cases. AJR Am J Roentgenol 1981; 136:69–74.

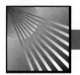

Illustrations • Pediatric Renal Masses

1 • Ureteropelvic junction obstruction

2 • Hydronephrosis associated with duplication of the collecting system

3 • Ureterovesical junction obstruction

4 • Hydronephrosis due to vesicoureteral reflux

5 • Multicystic dysplastic kidney

6 • Autosomal recessive polycystic kidney disease

7 • Wilms' tumor

8 • Nephroblastomatosis

9 • Clear cell sarcoma

10 • Rhabdoid tumor

11 • Congenital mesoblastic nephroma

12 • Renal cell carcinoma in children

13 • Multilocular cystic renal tumor

14 • Lymphoma and leukemia

1. Ureteropelvic Junction Obstruction

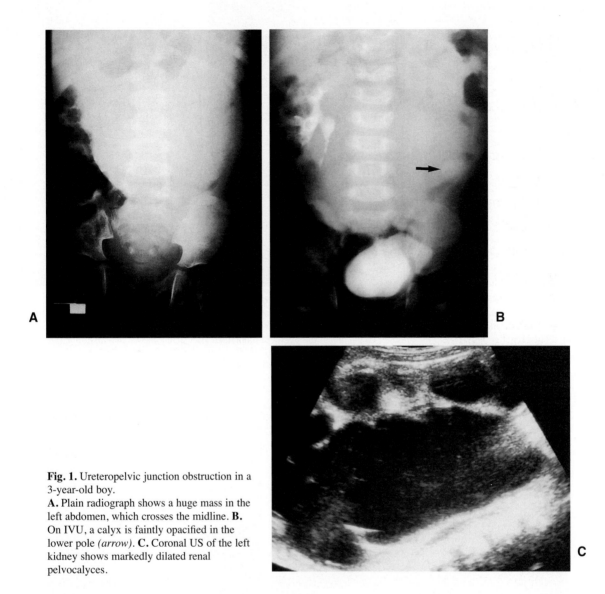

Fig. 1. Ureteropelvic junction obstruction in a 3-year-old boy.
A. Plain radiograph shows a huge mass in the left abdomen, which crosses the midline. **B.** On IVU, a calyx is faintly opacified in the lower pole *(arrow)*. **C.** Coronal US of the left kidney shows markedly dilated renal pelvocalyces.

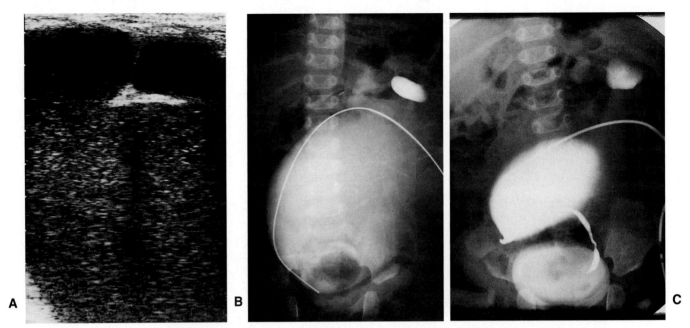

Fig. 2. Ureteropelvic junction obstruction in a 5-month-old boy with urinary tract infection.
A. Longitudinal US of the left kidney shows markedly distended renal pelvocalyces and paper-thin renal parenchyma. Echogenic debris is seen in the urine. **B.** A radiograph taken during percutaneous nephrostomy. A guide wire is located within the renal pelvis, which is opacified by contrast material. Note the markedly dilated renal pelvis crossing the midline. **C.** On antegrade pyelogram obtained after percutaneous nephrostomy, the left ureter is opacified by contrast material that has passed through the ureteropelvic junction.

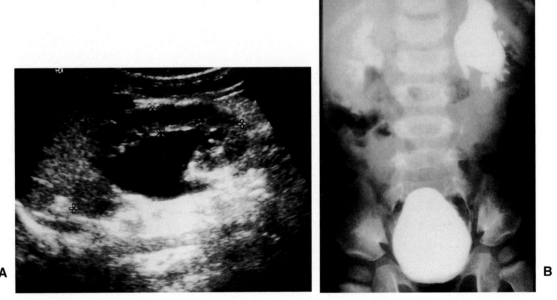

Fig. 3. Mild ureteropelvic junction obstruction.
A. Coronal US of the left kidney shows mild hydronephrosis. **B.** IVU shows mildly dilated pelvocalyces of the left kidney. The left ureter is also visualized.

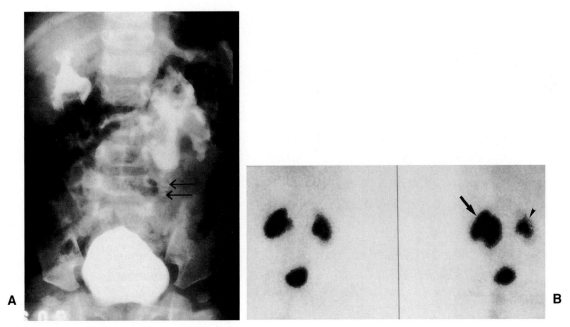

Fig. 4. Ureteropelvic junction obstruction in a 1-year-old boy.
A. IVU taken 1 hour after contrast medium injection shows dilated renal pelvocalyces in the left kidney and slightly prominent renal pelvis of the right kidney as well. Note the left proximal ureter *(arrows)*, which is kinked but not dilated. **B.** A posterior view of DTPA renal scintigraphy before *(left)* and after *(right)* furosemide injection. Diuretic renogram shows more accumulation of isotope in the left renal pelvis *(arrow)*, whereas there is a decrease of isotope in the right renal pelvis *(arrowhead)*. It suggests that there is a ureteropelvic junction obstruction in the left kidney, whereas the right kidney has a prominent extrarenal pelvis without obstruction.

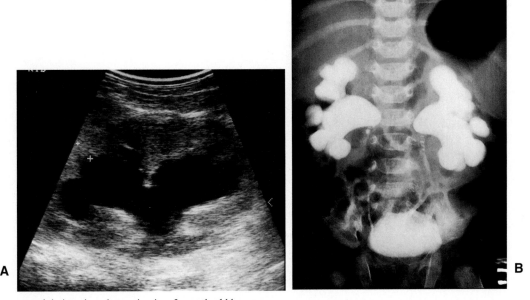

Fig. 5. Bilateral ureteropelvic junction obstruction in a 3-month-old boy.
A. Longitudinal US of the left kidney shows dilated pelvocalyces. **B.** A 30-minute IVU shows dilated renal pelvocalyces in both kidneys. Both ureters are demonstrated and are not dilated.

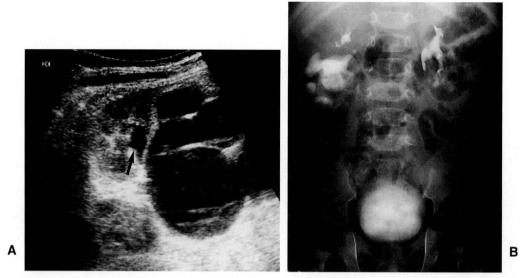

Fig. 6. Ureteropelvic junction obstruction in the lower moiety of the duplicated system in a 3-month-old boy.
A. Longitudinal US of the right kidney shows hydronephrosis confined to the lower moiety. The pelvis of the upper moiety *(arrow)* is compressed by the dilated lower moiety pelvis. **B.** IVU performed 2 months after dismembered pyeloplasty shows improved hydronephrosis in the lower moiety of the right kidney.

2. Hydronephrosis Associated with Duplication of the Collecting System

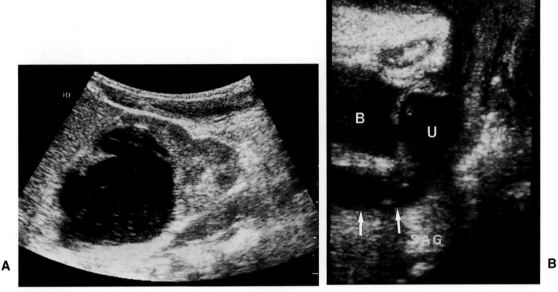

Fig. 1. Duplicated renal system with ectopic ureterocele in a 1-month-old girl.
A. Coronal US of the right kidney shows hydronephrosis in the upper moiety. The right ureter was also dilated (not shown). **B.** Transperineal US in sagittal plane shows a large ureterocele (U) in the inferior aspect of the urinary bladder base. The distal ureter of the upper moiety is dilated *(arrows)*. Ectopic insertion of the ureterocele was confirmed at cystoscopy. B, urinary bladder.

Fig. 2. Bilateral duplicated renal system in a 1-month-old girl with voiding difficulties.
A, B. Three-minute (**A**) and 30-minute (**B**) IVU images show duplicated system in both kidneys. The large filling defect obstructing the bladder outlet is the ureterocele *(arrows)* draining the upper moiety of the left kidney. Note the distended urinary bladder (B). The lower moiety of the left kidney is displaced downward and laterally by nonfunctioning hydronephrotic upper moiety *(asterisk)*, resulting in a "drooping lily sign."

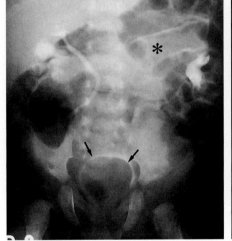

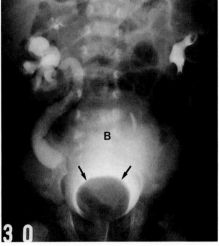

3. Ureterovesical Junction Obstruction

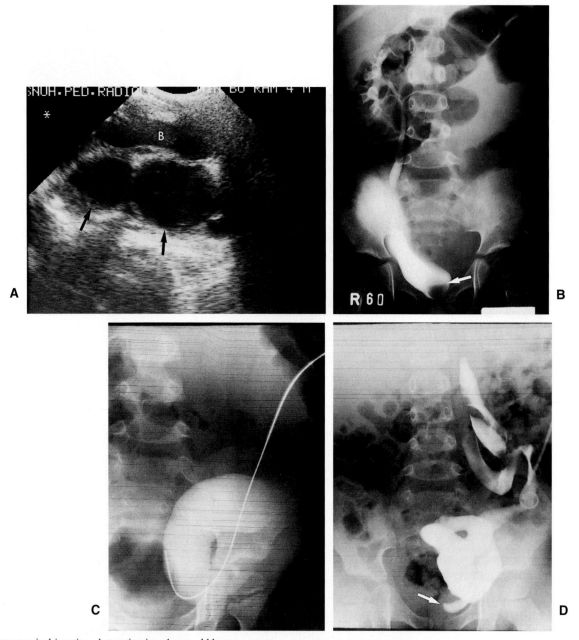

Fig. 1. Ureterovesical junction obstruction in a 4-year-old boy.
A. Longitudinal US of the pelvic cavity shows a large, tortuous, cystic structure, which is a severely dilated left ureter *(arrows)*, displacing the urinary bladder (B) anteriorly. **B.** A 1-hour IVU reveals nonvisualization of the left urinary system and the presence of a huge mass occupying the left abdomen and pelvis. The urinary bladder is displaced to the right side by the mass. Note an indentation on the bladder base by the dilated left distal ureter *(arrow)* mimicking a filling defect within the bladder. **C.** Percutaneous nephrostomy was tried. The tip of the guide wire is located in the dilated distal ureter. **D.** Antegrade urography through the catheter, which is malpositioned within the ureter, shows improved hydroureteronephrosis. The left ureter is obstructed at the ureterovesical junction *(arrow)*.

4. Hydronephrosis due to Vesicoureteral Reflux

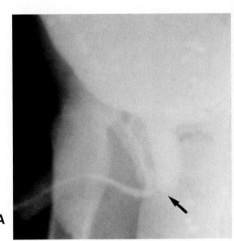

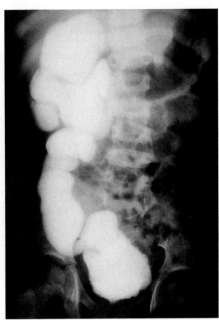

Fig. 1. Massive unilateral vesicoureteral reflux in a boy with posterior urethral valve. (Courtesy of Janet Strife, MD.) **A.** An oblique image of VCU shows distention of the posterior urethra and obstructing valve *(arrow)*. Note the thin stream of urine in the anterior urethra. **B.** Plain radiograph taken after VCU shows severe hydronephrosis and hydroureter due to vesicoureteral reflux in the right kidney. Note increased trabeculation of the urinary bladder.

A

B

5. **Multicystic Dysplastic Kidney**

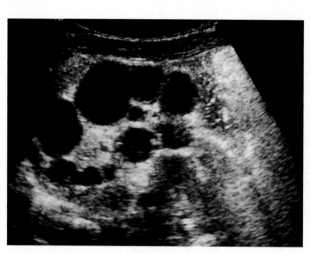

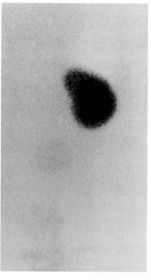

Fig. 1. Multicystic dysplastic kidney in a 1-month-old girl.
A. Longitudinal US of the right kidney shows multiple cysts of varying size and intervening hyperechoic area. Normal renal parenchyma is not demonstrated.
B. An anterior view of DMSA renal scintigraphy shows no uptake of radioisotope in the right kidney.

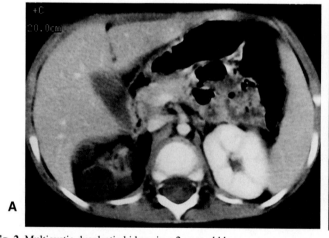

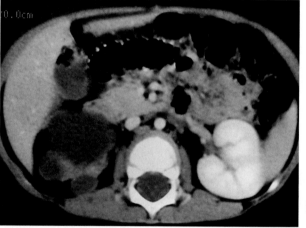

Fig. 2. Multicystic dysplastic kidney in a 2-year-old boy.
A, B. Contrast-enhanced CT scans show multiple, variable-sized cysts that are distributed randomly. Intervening dysplastic renal tissue shows no enhancement.

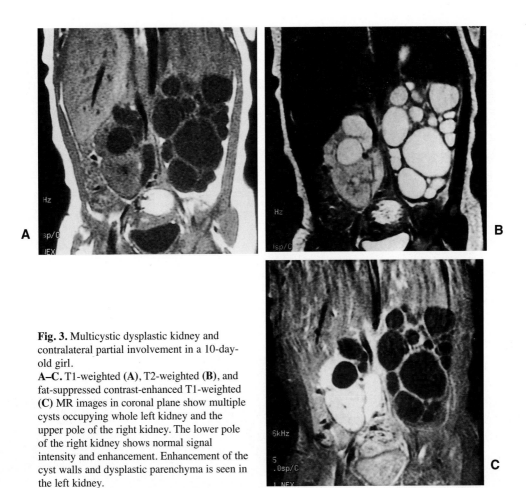

Fig. 3. Multicystic dysplastic kidney and contralateral partial involvement in a 10-day-old girl.
A–C. T1-weighted (**A**), T2-weighted (**B**), and fat-suppressed contrast-enhanced T1-weighted (**C**) MR images in coronal plane show multiple cysts occupying whole left kidney and the upper pole of the right kidney. The lower pole of the right kidney shows normal signal intensity and enhancement. Enhancement of the cyst walls and dysplastic parenchyma is seen in the left kidney.

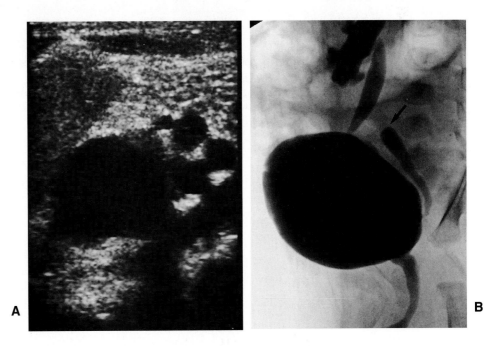

Fig. 4. Multicystic dysplastic kidney due to atresia of the distal ureter in a 2-month-old boy.
A. Longitudinal US of the left kidney shows multiple cysts without normal renal parenchyma. A cyst in the upper pole is the largest. **B.** VCU shows bilateral vesicoureteral reflux. Note the blind ending of the left distal ureter *(arrow)* indicating atresia of the ureter at that level.

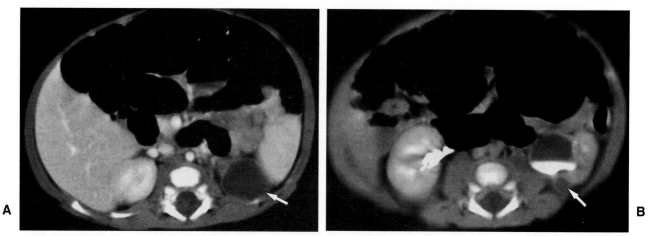

Fig. 5. Renal dysplasia in a 1-year-old boy with ureteropelvic junction obstruction.
A, B. Contrast-enhanced CT scans obtained 30 minutes after contrast injection show a larger cyst in the upper pole (*arrow* in **A**) and a smaller one (*arrow* in **B**) in the interpolar region of the left kidney. Layering of excreted contrast material is noted in the dilated left renal pelvis. Also note the small size of the left kidney.

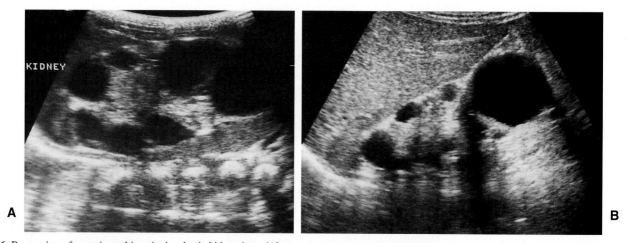

Fig. 6. Regression of cysts in multicystic dysplastic kidney in an infant.
A. Longitudinal US of the right kidney shows multiple, randomly distributed, cortical cysts of various sizes. **B.** Six months later, most of the cysts are decreased in size with the exception of a large cyst in the lower pole.

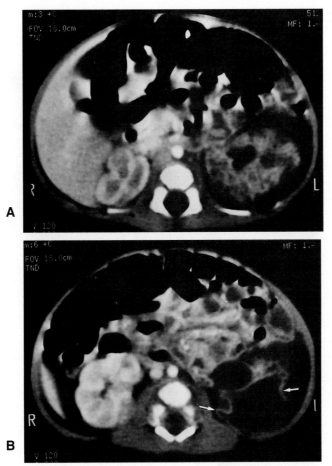

Fig. 7. Cyst rupture in multicystic dysplastic kidney in a 6-year-old boy. **A, B.** Contrast-enhanced CT scans show multiple cysts of varying size and poorly enhanced, dysplastic parenchyma in the left kidney. Note the wrinkled wall (*arrows* in **B**) of the largest cyst due to rupture. Also note the urine ascites and perirenal fluid collection.

6. Autosomal Recessive Polycystic Kidney Disease

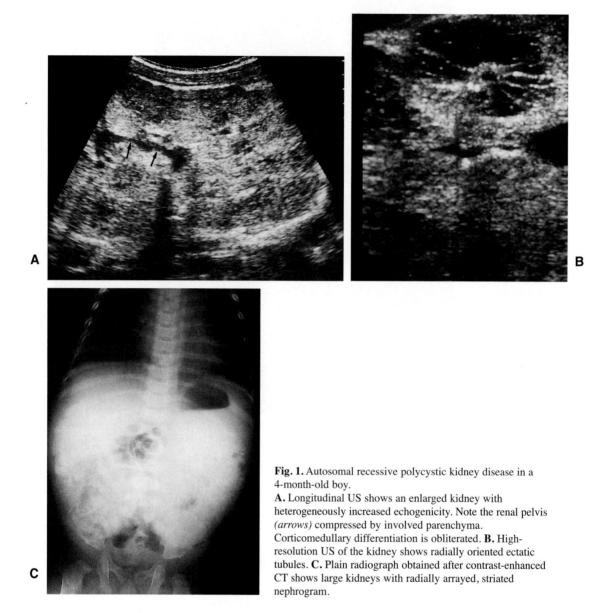

Fig. 1. Autosomal recessive polycystic kidney disease in a 4-month-old boy.
A. Longitudinal US shows an enlarged kidney with heterogeneously increased echogenicity. Note the renal pelvis *(arrows)* compressed by involved parenchyma. Corticomedullary differentiation is obliterated. **B.** High-resolution US of the kidney shows radially oriented ectatic tubules. **C.** Plain radiograph obtained after contrast-enhanced CT shows large kidneys with radially arrayed, striated nephrogram.

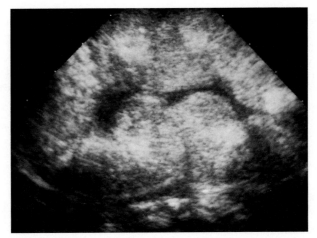

Fig. 2. Autosomal recessive polycystic kidney disease. Longitudinal US shows a large kidney with homogeneously increased echogenicity. Note that the peripheral renal cortex is relatively hypoechoic.

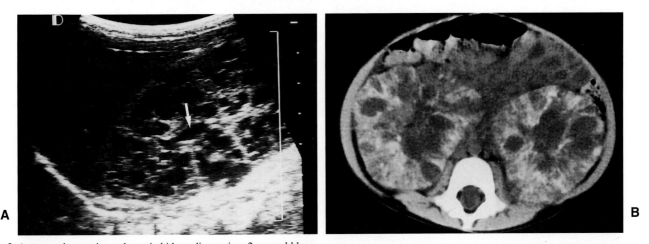

Fig. 3. Autosomal recessive polycystic kidney disease in a 2-year-old boy.
A. Longitudinal US shows numerous small cysts in the enlarged kidney. The intervening parenchyma is hyperechoic. The renal pelvis is seen *(arrow)*.
B. A 24-hour delayed CT scan after contrast enhancement shows innumerable cysts and contrast pooling in radially arrayed tubules in both kidneys.

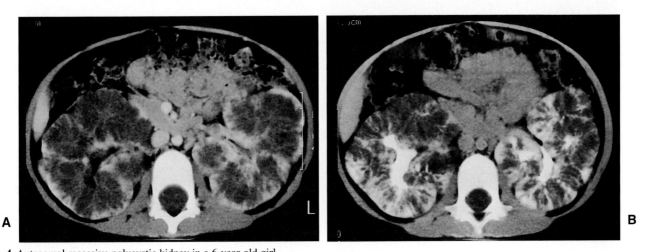

Fig. 4. Autosomal recessive polycystic kidney in a 6-year-old girl.
A. Contrast-enhanced CT shows nonopacification of ectatic tubules. The periphery of kidneys shows some enhancement. **B.** CT scan obtained 40 minutes after contrast enhancement shows pooling of contrast material in some of the involved tubules. Note that contrast material is excreted into the pelvocalyces.

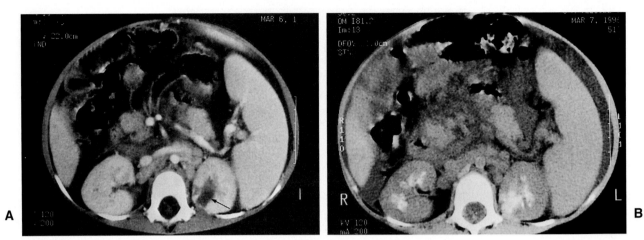

Fig. 5. Mild renal involvement of autosomal recessive polycystic kidney disease in a 7-year-old boy.
A. Contrast-enhanced CT shows poor enhancement of both kidneys. Nonenhancing lesion in the left kidney *(arrow)* and multiple, small, ill-defined radiations of low attenuation are seen in the medulla of both kidneys. Splenomegaly and ascites due to accompanied congenital hepatic fibrosis are present. **B.** CT scan obtained 24 hours after contrast enhancement shows contrast pooling in renal tubules in the low-attenuated lesions seen in **A.**

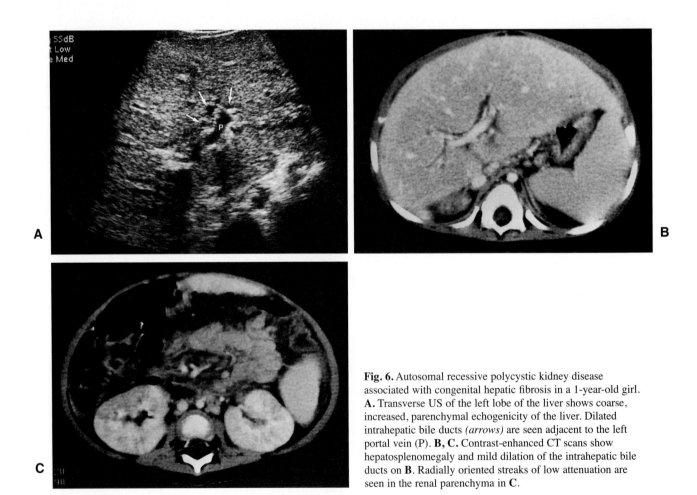

Fig. 6. Autosomal recessive polycystic kidney disease associated with congenital hepatic fibrosis in a 1-year-old girl. **A.** Transverse US of the left lobe of the liver shows coarse, increased, parenchymal echogenicity of the liver. Dilated intrahepatic bile ducts *(arrows)* are seen adjacent to the left portal vein (P). **B, C.** Contrast-enhanced CT scans show hepatosplenomegaly and mild dilation of the intrahepatic bile ducts on **B.** Radially oriented streaks of low attenuation are seen in the renal parenchyma in **C.**

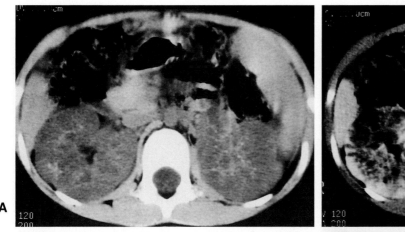

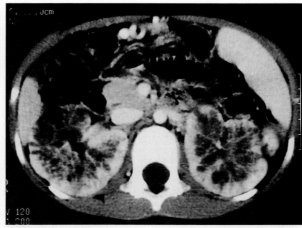

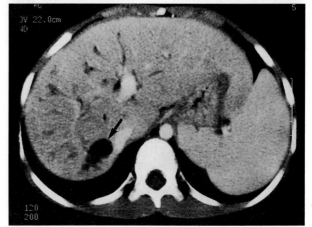

Fig. 7. Autosomal recessive polycystic kidney disease associated with Caroli's disease in a 7-year-old boy.
A. Nonenhanced CT shows multiple, tiny calcifications in both kidneys. **B, C.** Contrast-enhanced CT scan of the kidneys (**B**) shows radially oriented, ectatic tubules and small cysts. Uninvolved renal cortex shows enhancement. On liver CT (**C**), a cystic dilation of the intrahepatic bile duct *(arrow)* is seen in the right lobe of the liver. Other intrahepatic bile ducts are mildly dilated. Note the splenomegaly due to portal hypertension.

7. Wilms' Tumor

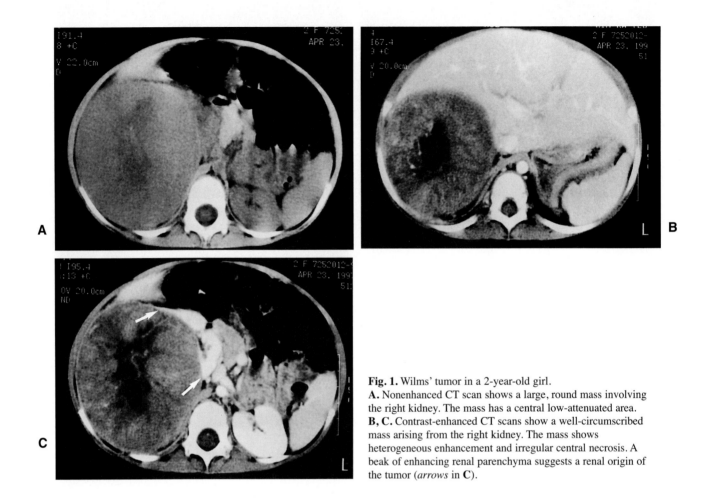

Fig. 1. Wilms' tumor in a 2-year-old girl.
A. Nonenhanced CT scan shows a large, round mass involving the right kidney. The mass has a central low-attenuated area.
B, C. Contrast-enhanced CT scans show a well-circumscribed mass arising from the right kidney. The mass shows heterogeneous enhancement and irregular central necrosis. A beak of enhancing renal parenchyma suggests a renal origin of the tumor (*arrows* in **C**).

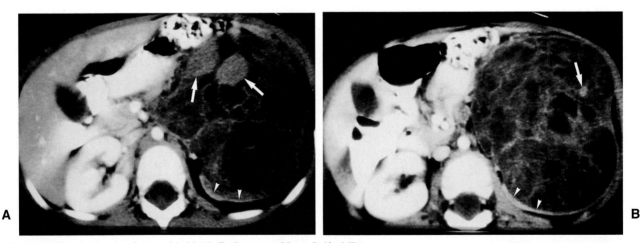

Fig. 2. Cystic Wilms' tumor in a 3-year-old girl. (**A, B,** Courtesy of Janet Strife, MD.)
A, B. Contrast-enhanced CT scans show a huge, multiloculated, cystic mass involving the left kidney. Some of the septa are thin, whereas others are thick and irregular. Note solid nodules (*arrows*) within the mass, which strongly suggests that the mass is more likely a nephroblastoma rather than a multilocular cystic renal tumor. Note the thin rim of the normal parenchyma (*arrowheads*).

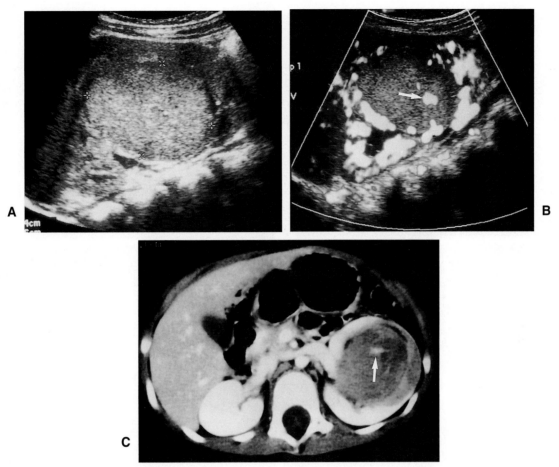

Fig. 3. Wilms' tumor involving the renal sinus.
A. Longitudinal US of the left kidney shows a homogeneously echogenic mass in the central region of the kidney. **B.** Power Doppler US of the mass shows an intratumoral vascular structure *(arrow)*. Note that tumor vascularity is far less than that of the normal renal parenchyma. **C.** Contrast-enhanced CT shows a heterogeneous mass involving the renal sinus. Note a strongly enhancing structure within the mass, which is probably a vessel *(arrow)* seen on power Doppler US.

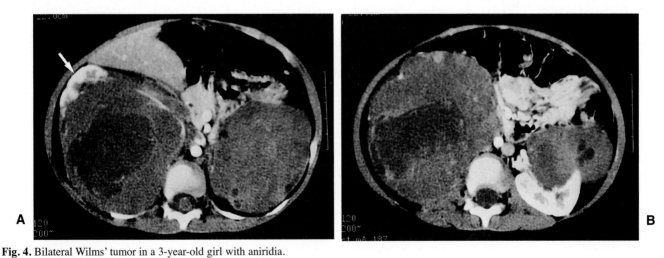

Fig. 4. Bilateral Wilms' tumor in a 3-year-old girl with aniridia.
A, B. Contrast-enhanced CT scans show large, low-attenuated, solid masses with a lobulated contour in both kidneys. The masses contain necrotic areas. The remaining renal parenchyma is displaced anteriorly in the right kidney *(arrow* in **A**).

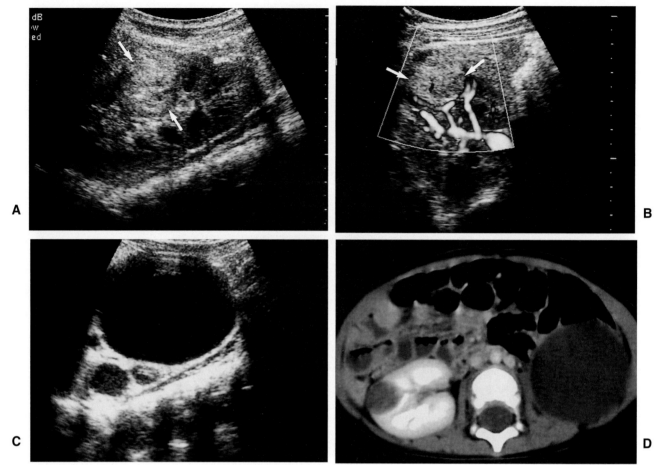

Fig. 5. Wilms' tumor and contralateral multicystic dysplastic kidney in a 1-year-old girl.
A. Coronal US of the left kidney shows an echogenic mass *(arrows)* in the interpolar region of the right kidney. **B.** Power Doppler US of the mass shows hypovascular nature of the mass *(arrows)*. **C.** Coronal US of the contralateral kidney shows a dominant cyst and multiple smaller cysts in the background of echogenic dysplastic parenchyma. **D.** Contrast-enhanced CT scan of the abdomen shows a round, low-attenuated mass in the right kidney, which was confirmed to be a Wilms' tumor. A dominant cyst of the multicystic dysplastic kidney is seen in the left kidney.

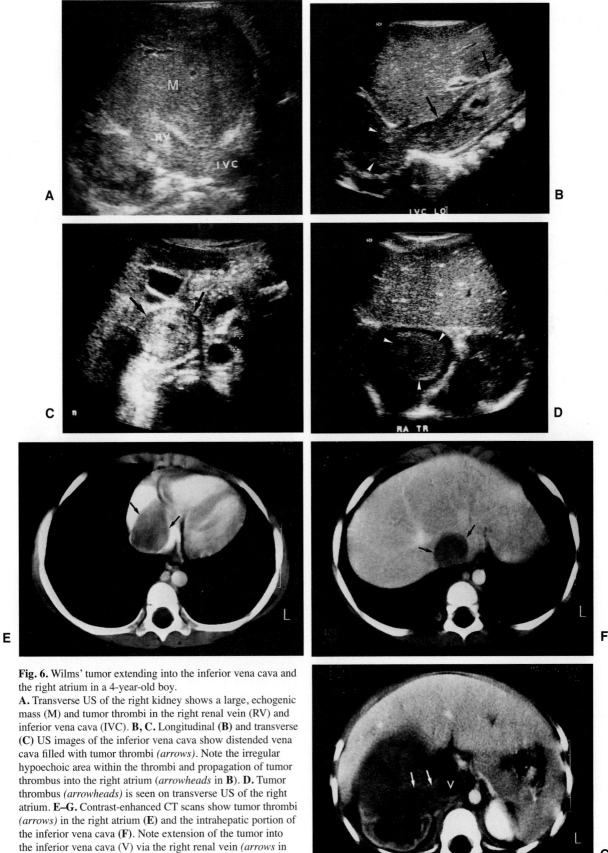

Fig. 6. Wilms' tumor extending into the inferior vena cava and the right atrium in a 4-year-old boy.
A. Transverse US of the right kidney shows a large, echogenic mass (M) and tumor thrombi in the right renal vein (RV) and inferior vena cava (IVC). **B, C.** Longitudinal (**B**) and transverse (**C**) US images of the inferior vena cava show distended vena cava filled with tumor thrombi *(arrows)*. Note the irregular hypoechoic area within the thrombi and propagation of tumor thrombus into the right atrium *(arrowheads in **B**)*. **D.** Tumor thrombus *(arrowheads)* is seen on transverse US of the right atrium. **E–G.** Contrast-enhanced CT scans show tumor thrombi *(arrows)* in the right atrium (**E**) and the intrahepatic portion of the inferior vena cava (**F**). Note extension of the tumor into the inferior vena cava (V) via the right renal vein *(arrows in **G**)*. Hydronephrosis and poor parenchymal enhancement of the right kidney are due to obstruction by the mass.

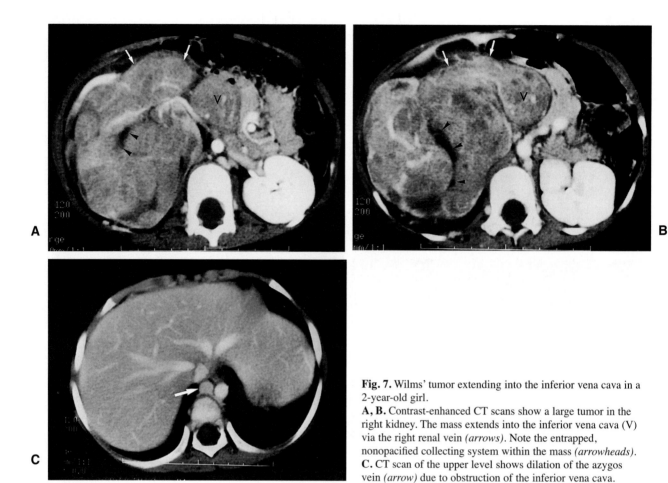

Fig. 7. Wilms' tumor extending into the inferior vena cava in a 2-year-old girl.
A, B. Contrast-enhanced CT scans show a large tumor in the right kidney. The mass extends into the inferior vena cava (V) via the right renal vein *(arrows)*. Note the entrapped, nonopacified collecting system within the mass *(arrowheads)*.
C. CT scan of the upper level shows dilation of the azygos vein *(arrow)* due to obstruction of the inferior vena cava.

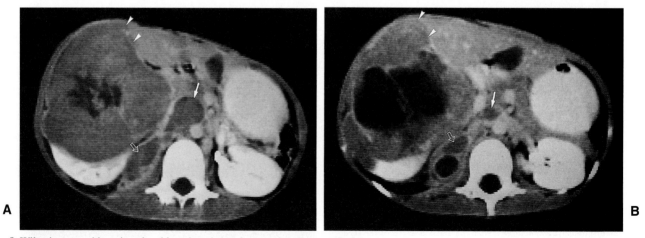

Fig. 8. Wilms' tumor with perirenal and lymph node involvement in a 9-year-old girl.
A, B. Contrast-enhanced CT scans show a large mass with central necrosis in the right kidney. The tumor invades adjacent perirenal space anteriorly *(arrowheads)*. Enlargement of a lymph node *(arrow)* with an attenuation similar to that of the mass is seen between the aorta and the inferior vena cava. A retroperitoneal mass along the right psoas muscle is also seen *(open arrow)*.

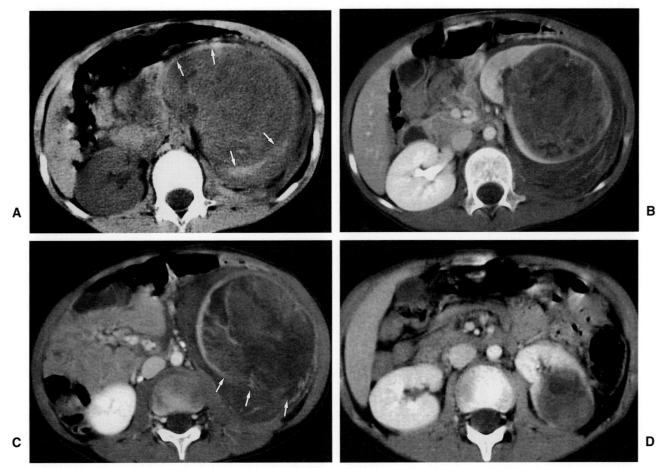

Fig. 9. Wilms' tumor with perirenal hematoma in a 7-year-old boy with signs of bleeding.
A–C. CT scans before (**A**) and after (**B**) contrast enhancement show a large left renal mass and fluid collection in the perirenal space. The perirenal hematoma (*arrows* in **A**) shows high attenuation on nonenhanced CT. Note disruption of the thin enhancing rim of the renal parenchyma in the posterior aspect of the tumor (*arrows* in **C**), which suggests the site of tumor rupture. **D.** CT scan after chemotherapy reveals a decrease in the size of the mass and disappearance of perirenal hematoma. After this examination, the patient underwent nephrectomy.

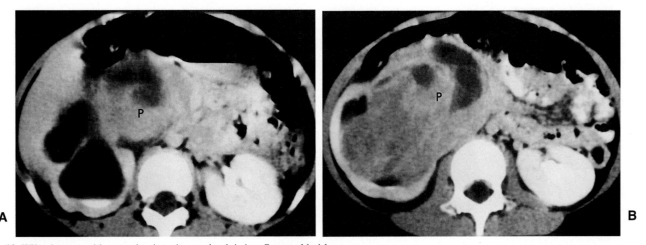

Fig. 10. Wilms' tumor with extension into the renal pelvis in a 7-year-old girl.
A, B. Contrast-enhanced CT scans show a large mass in the right kidney. The mass involves the central portion of the kidney and has grown mainly into the renal pelvis, which is markedly dilated (P). Calyces of the right kidney are dilated with a layering of contrast material within it. Renal parenchyma of the right kidney enhances less than that of the left kidney.

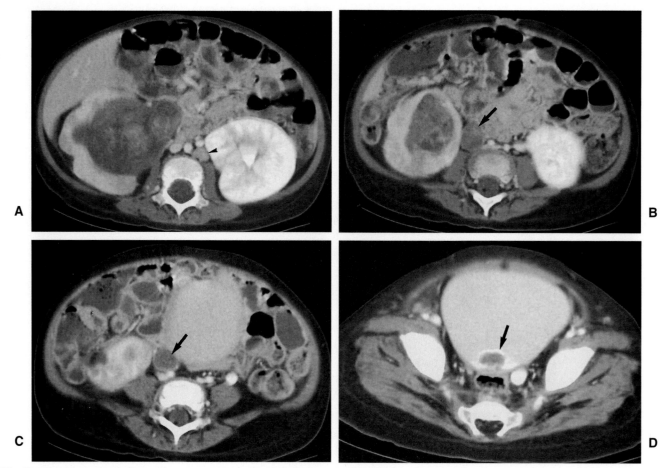

Fig. 11. Wilms' tumor extending to the ureter and the urinary bladder in botryoid fashion.
A–D. Contrast-enhanced CT scans show a renal mass involving the renal hilum (**A**). The mass extends into the right ureter *(arrow)* (**B, C**) and the urinary bladder (**D**). The right ureter is distended with tumor within it. A polypoid mass coated with contrast material is seen in the urinary bladder *(arrow)*. Note an enlarged para-aortic lymph node *(arrowhead* in **A**).

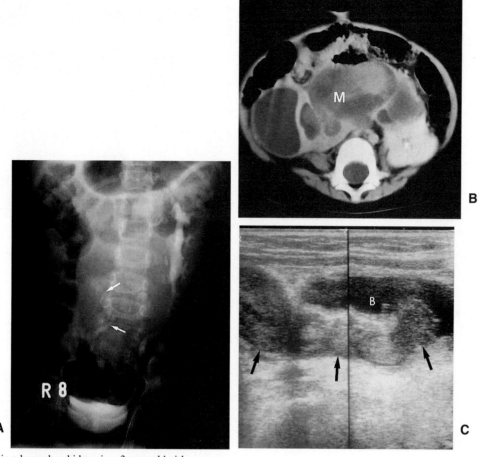

Fig. 12. Wilms' tumor in a horseshoe kidney in a 3-year-old girl.
A. An 8-minute IVU shows vertical orientation and rotation of the left kidney. Calyceal systems of the right kidney and the right ureter are demonstrated in the lower abdomen *(arrows)*. **B.** Contrast-enhanced CT scan performed 1 year after IVU shows a mass arising from the isthmus of the horseshoe kidney. The mass (M) is bridging the lower pole of the left kidney with malformed right kidney. The right kidney shows decreased enhancement and calyceal dilatation. **C.** Longitudinal US of the right ureter shows extension of the tumor *(arrows)* into the ureter and urinary bladder (B).

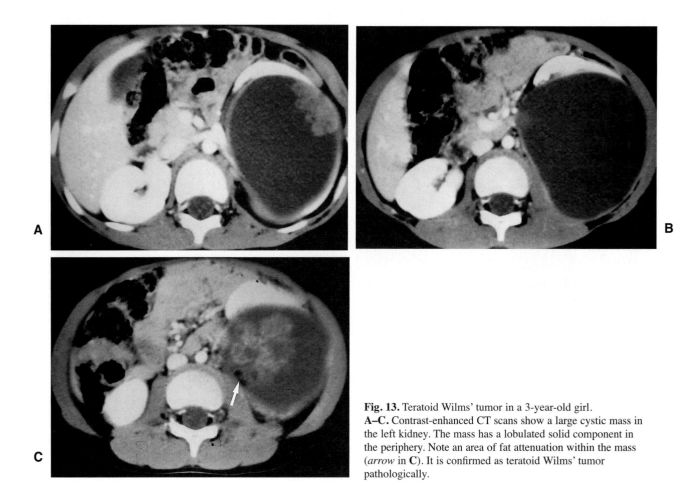

Fig. 13. Teratoid Wilms' tumor in a 3-year-old girl.
A–C. Contrast-enhanced CT scans show a large cystic mass in the left kidney. The mass has a lobulated solid component in the periphery. Note an area of fat attenuation within the mass (*arrow* in **C**). It is confirmed as teratoid Wilms' tumor pathologically.

8. Nephroblastomatosis

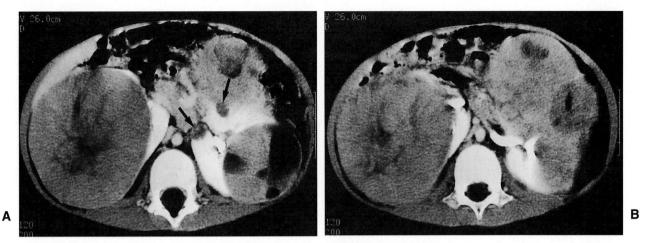

Fig. 1. Bilateral Wilms' tumor associated with nephroblastomatosis in a 7-year-old boy.
A, B. Contrast-enhanced CT scans show multiple renal masses of variable attenuation. Note that large tumors are superimposed on the background of multiple, peripheral, nephrogenic rests *(arrows in A)*. Also note severe cystic degeneration in the left renal mass.

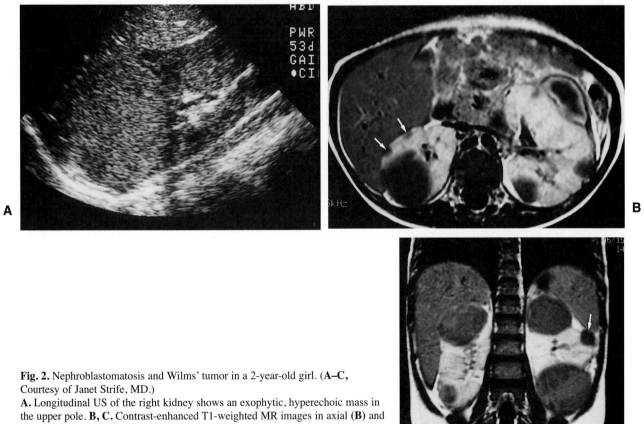

Fig. 2. Nephroblastomatosis and Wilms' tumor in a 2-year-old girl. (**A–C,** Courtesy of Janet Strife, MD.)
A. Longitudinal US of the right kidney shows an exophytic, hyperechoic mass in the upper pole. **B, C.** Contrast-enhanced T1-weighted MR images in axial (**B**) and coronal (**C**) planes show large, poorly enhancing masses and small, subcortical nodules *(arrows)*. Larger masses or nodules were detected by US but tiny nodules of nephrogenic rests were not.

9. Clear Cell Sarcoma

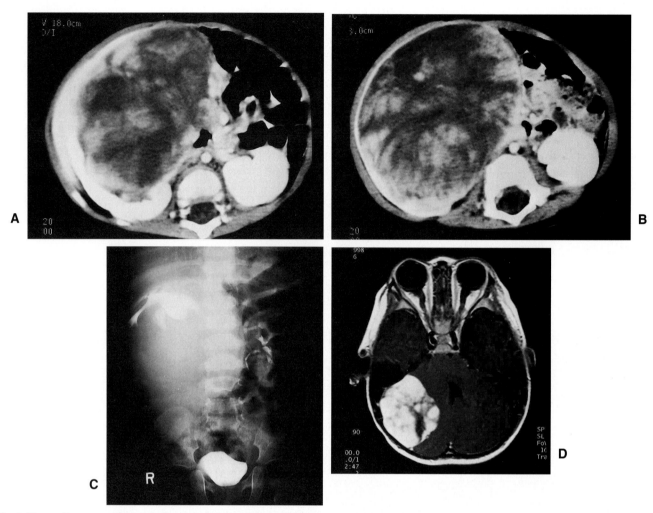

Fig. 1. Clear cell sarcoma with cerebellar metastasis in a 3-year-old boy.
A, B. Contrast-enhanced CT scans show a large heterogeneous mass and compressed renal parenchyma remainder in the right kidney. The mass shows enhancement of an irregular whirling pattern. **C.** Plain radiograph obtained after CT shows compression and displacement of the right pelvocalyceal system by the mass. **D.** Contrast-enhanced T1-weighted MR image of the brain shows a well-enhancing, solid mass in the right cerebellar hemisphere.

10. Rhabdoid Tumor

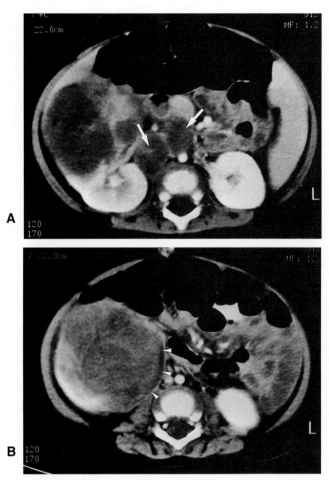

Fig. 1. Rhabdoid tumor of the kidney in a 1-year-old boy.
A, B. Contrast-enhanced CT scans show a large, heterogeneous mass in
the right kidney. There are multiple, low-attenuated areas within the
mass suggesting tumor necrosis. Note multiple, enlarged lymph nodes of
low attenuation in the renal hilum and the para-aortic area (*arrows* in **A**).
Subcapsular fluid collection, possibly hematoma, which is known to be a
characteristic finding in rhabdoid tumor, is seen (*arrowheads* in **B**). This
boy also had multiple metastases in the lungs and liver (not shown).

11. Congenital Mesoblastic Nephroma

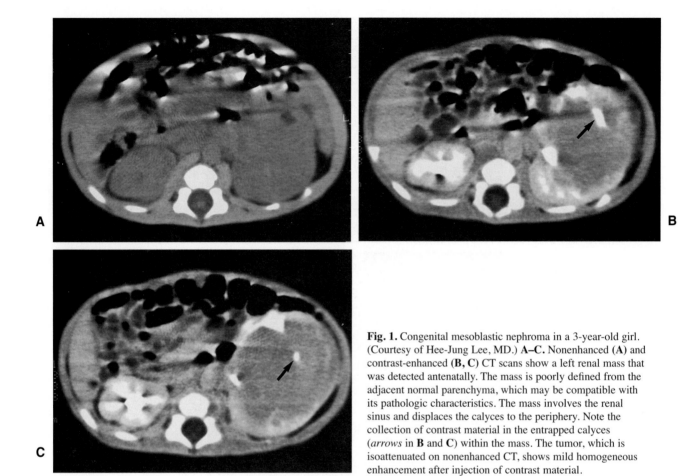

Fig. 1. Congenital mesoblastic nephroma in a 3-year-old girl. (Courtesy of Hee-Jung Lee, MD.) **A–C.** Nonenhanced (**A**) and contrast-enhanced (**B, C**) CT scans show a left renal mass that was detected antenatally. The mass is poorly defined from the adjacent normal parenchyma, which may be compatible with its pathologic characteristics. The mass involves the renal sinus and displaces the calyces to the periphery. Note the collection of contrast material in the entrapped calyces (*arrows* in **B** and **C**) within the mass. The tumor, which is isoattenuated on nonenhanced CT, shows mild homogeneous enhancement after injection of contrast material.

12. Renal Cell Carcinoma in Children

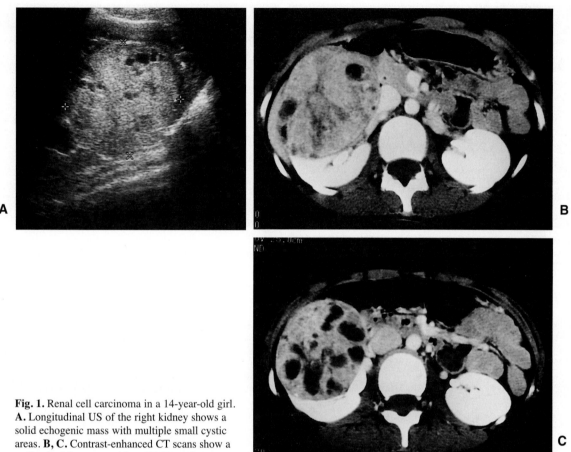

Fig. 1. Renal cell carcinoma in a 14-year-old girl. **A.** Longitudinal US of the right kidney shows a solid echogenic mass with multiple small cystic areas. **B, C.** Contrast-enhanced CT scans show a well-enhancing mass with multiple cystic areas.

13. **Multilocular Cystic Renal Tumor**

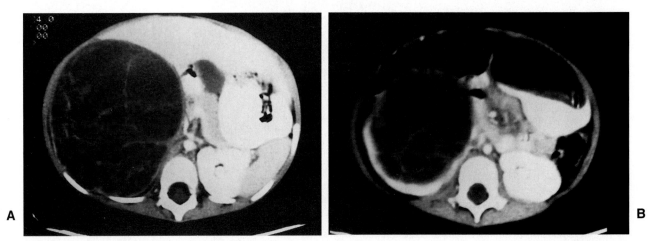

Fig. 1. Multilocular cystic nephroma in a 3-year-old girl.
A, B. Contrast-enhanced CT scans show a well-defined cystic mass in the right kidney. Note numerous fine septations without solid components. A crescent of compressed renal parenchyma is seen posteriorly.

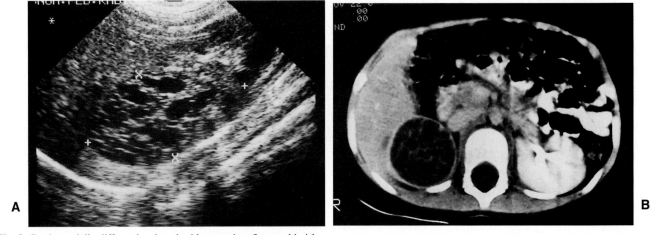

Fig. 2. Cystic partially differentiated nephroblastoma in a 5-year-old girl.
A. Longitudinal US of the right kidney shows a multilocular cystic mass. Septa appear relatively thick, presumably due to the presence of tiny cystic spaces, which are beyond the resolution ability of US. **B.** Contrast-enhanced CT scan shows a well-circumscribed cystic mass with thin septa.

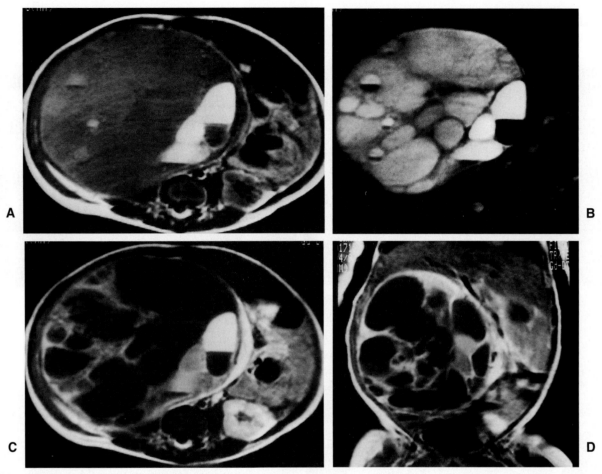

Fig. 3. Cystic partially differentiated nephroblastoma in a 4-month-old boy.
A–D. T1-weighted axial (**A**), T2-weighted axial (**B**), and contrast-enhanced T1-weighted axial (**C**) and coronal (**D**) MR images show huge septated cystic mass in the right kidney. Note multiple fluid-fluid levels due to hemorrhagic contents. Enhancement of the septa is seen, and some of them appear relatively thick.

14. Lymphoma and Leukemia

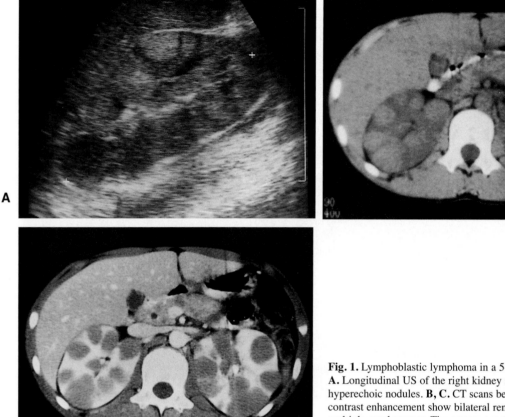

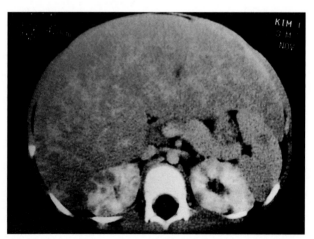

Fig. 1. Lymphoblastic lymphoma in a 5-year-old boy.
A. Longitudinal US of the right kidney shows multiple
hyperechoic nodules. **B, C.** CT scans before (**B**) and after (**C**)
contrast enhancement show bilateral renal enlargement with
multiple renal masses. The masses are slightly high attenuated
on nonenhanced CT and poorly enhanced on contrast-
enhanced CT.

Fig. 2. Burkitt's lymphoma in a 3-year-old boy. Contrast-enhanced CT
shows multiple, low-attenuated nodules in the kidneys, liver, and spleen.
Note massive hepatomegaly due to diffuse involvement.

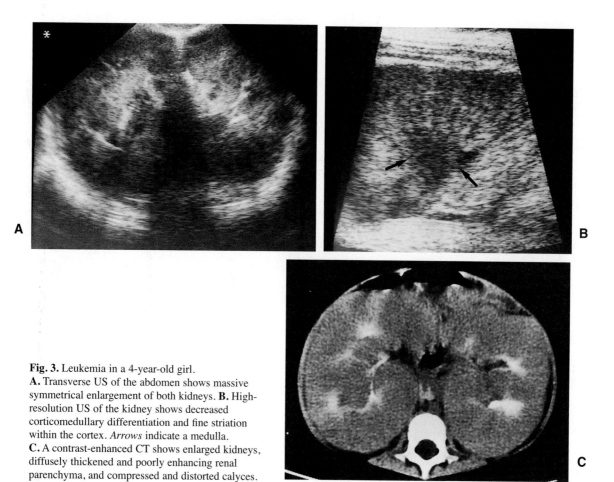

Fig. 3. Leukemia in a 4-year-old girl.
A. Transverse US of the abdomen shows massive symmetrical enlargement of both kidneys. **B.** High-resolution US of the kidney shows decreased corticomedullary differentiation and fine striation within the cortex. *Arrows* indicate a medulla.
C. A contrast-enhanced CT shows enlarged kidneys, diffusely thickened and poorly enhancing renal parenchyma, and compressed and distorted calyces.

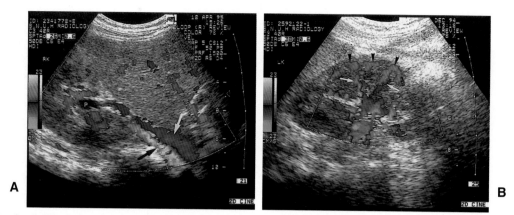

Chapter 1, Illustration 2, Fig. 3. Color Doppler US findings of the renal vessels: normal findings. **A.** Color Doppler US along the right renal vessels shows the right renal artery *(black arrow)* and the right renal vein *(white arrow)*. Anechoic structure without flow signal indicates the renal pelvis (p). **B.** Color Doppler US of the left kidney well demonstrates intrarenal vessels, including interlobar *(arrows)* and arcuate vessels *(arrowheads)*.

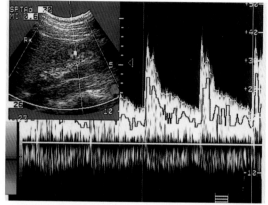

Chapter 1, Illustration 2, Fig. 4. Spectral Doppler US findings of the intrarenal arteries: normal findings. . . . **B.** Spectral Doppler US of the right kidney in another 25-year-old man shows a normal Doppler spectral pattern with a resistive index of 0.65. In this patient, early systolic compliance peak is not seen.

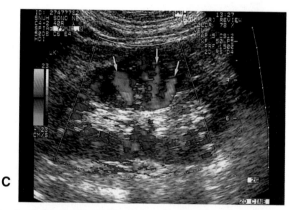

Chapter 1, Illustration 9, Fig. 2. Prominent column of Bertin in a 53-year-old man. . . . **C.** Color Doppler US shows flow signals *(arrows)* running through the column.

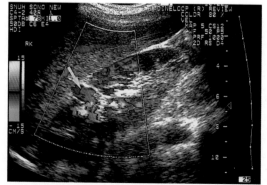

Chapter 1, Illustration 11, Fig. 2. Renal vein in a junctional parenchymal defect that mimics a cyst in a 41-year-old man. . . . **B.** Color Doppler US reveals that the anechoic structure seen on gray-scale US is a renal vessel *(arrow)*.

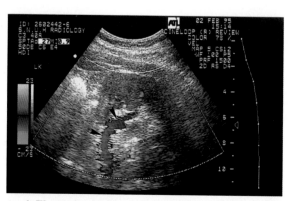

Chapter 1, Illustration 14, Fig. 1. US findings of pseudohydronephrosis by prominent renal vessels in a 27-year-old man. . . . **B.** Color Doppler US reveals flow signal in the tubular structure *(arrowheads)* confirming that the structure is a blood vessel and is not dilated pelvocalyces.

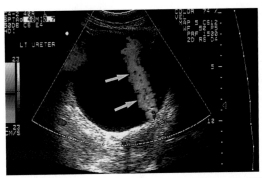

Chapter 1, Illustration 16, Fig. 2. Ureteral jet on color Doppler US in a 20-year-old woman. Color Doppler US of the bladder shows jetting of urine *(arrows)* from the left ureteral orifice. This finding of ureteral jet virtually excludes the possibility of significant obstruction of the urinary tract.

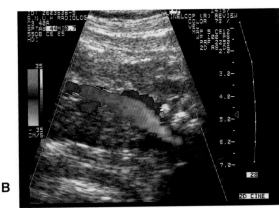

Chapter 2, Illustration 1, Fig. 2. Bilateral renal agenesis detected on prenatal US of a 28-week fetus. . . . **B.** Color Doppler US of the fetal abdomen in coronal plane well demonstrates the abdominal aorta, but renal arteries are not demonstrable.

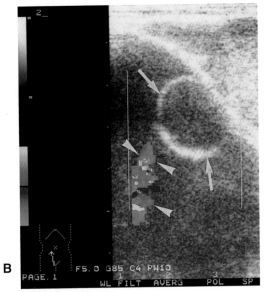

Chapter 2, Illustration 14, Fig. 3. Simple ureterocele in a 29-year-old man. . . . **B.** Color Doppler US in the same plane demonstrates urine flow *(arrowheads)* jetting from the top of the ureterocele *(arrows)*.

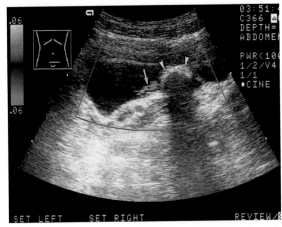

Chapter 2, Illustration 14, Fig. 6. US findings of ureterocele with a stone in a 34-year-old woman. . . . **B.** Color Doppler US shows color signal of urine flow *(arrow)* jetting from the ureterocele containing a stone *(arrowheads)*.

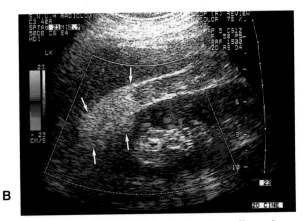

Chapter 3, Illustration 1, Fig. 1. Exophytic angiomyolipoma in a 45-year-old man. . . . **B.** Color Doppler US shows absence of flow signals within the mass *(arrows)*.

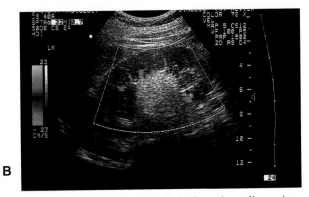

Chapter 3, Illustration 1, Fig. 2. Endophytic angiomyolipoma in a 46-year-old man. . . . **B.** No flow signals are demonstrated in the tumor on color Doppler US.

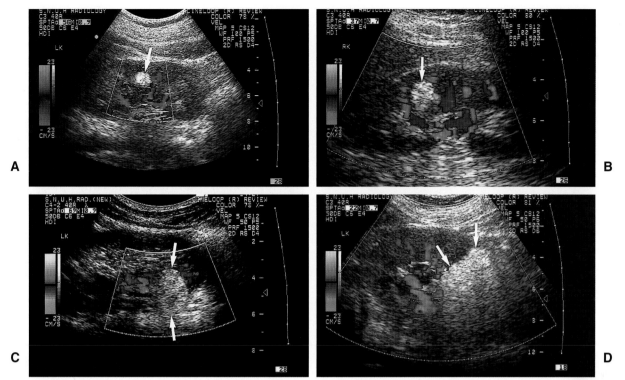

Chapter 3, Illustration 1, Fig. 4. Color Doppler US findings of angiomyolipoma. **A–D.** Color Doppler US images of four different cases of angiomyolipoma show no demonstrable flow signals in the mass *(arrows)* due to slow intratumoral blood flow even though most angiomyolipomas have vascular components by contrast-enhanced CT or angiography.

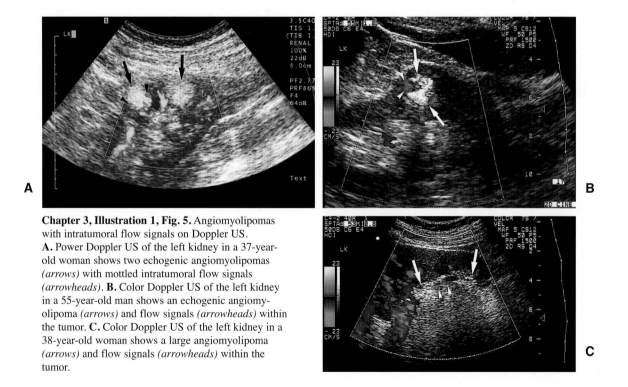

Chapter 3, Illustration 1, Fig. 5. Angiomyolipomas with intratumoral flow signals on Doppler US.
A. Power Doppler US of the left kidney in a 37-year-old woman shows two echogenic angiomyolipomas *(arrows)* with mottled intratumoral flow signals *(arrowheads)*. **B.** Color Doppler US of the left kidney in a 55-year-old man shows an echogenic angiomyolipoma *(arrows)* and flow signals *(arrowheads)* within the tumor. **C.** Color Doppler US of the left kidney in a 38-year-old woman shows a large angiomyolipoma *(arrows)* and flow signals *(arrowheads)* within the tumor.

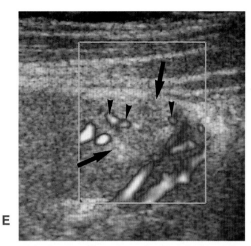

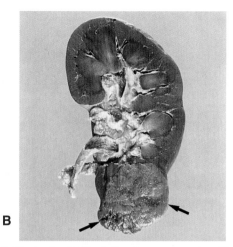

Chapter 3, Illustration 2, Fig. 2. Small angiomyolipoma appearing as a high-attenuated nodule on nonenhanced CT in a 37-year-old woman. . . . **E.** Power Doppler US of the kidney shows subtle flow signals *(arrowheads)* within the mass *(arrows)*. Therefore, imaging does not provide a specific diagnosis of angiomyolipoma.

Chapter 3, Illustration 7, Fig. 1. Renal oncocytoma in a 56-year-old man. . . . **B.** Photograph of the removed kidney shows a well-defined mass *(arrows)* with fibrous scar and focal hemorrhage in the lower pole of the left kidney.

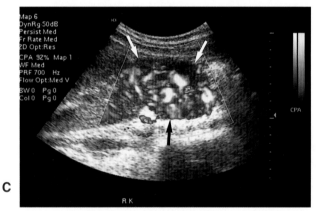

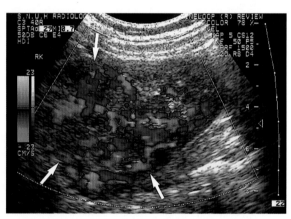

Chapter 3, Illustration 9, Fig. 3. Renal and pulmonary lymphangiomyomatosis in a 50-year-old woman without stigmata of tuberous sclerosis. . . . **C.** Power Doppler US shows hypervascularity of the mass *(arrows)*.

Chapter 4, Illustration 1, Fig. 2. Hypervascular renal cell carcinoma in a 47-year-old woman. Color Doppler US shows a large mass *(arrows)* in the upper pole of the right kidney. Note that the vascularity of the mass is higher than that of the remainder of the kidney.

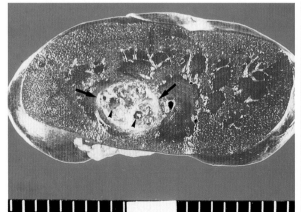

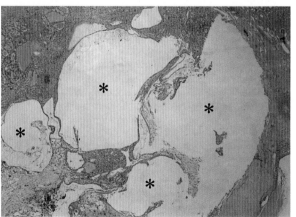

Chapter 4, Illustration 6, Fig. 1. Small renal cell carcinoma of clear cell type in a 39-year-old man. . . . **D.** Color photograph of the removed kidney shows the tumor *(arrows)* that contains small cysts (arrowheads). **E.** Color photomicrograph of the tumor shows intratumoral cysts *(asterisks)*.

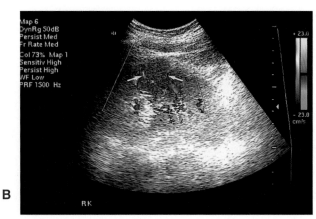

Chapter 4, Illustration 6, Fig. 4. Small renal cell carcinoma of clear cell type in a 65-year-old man with carcinoma of the common bile duct. . . . **B.** Color Doppler US shows vessels draping the tumor *(arrows)*.

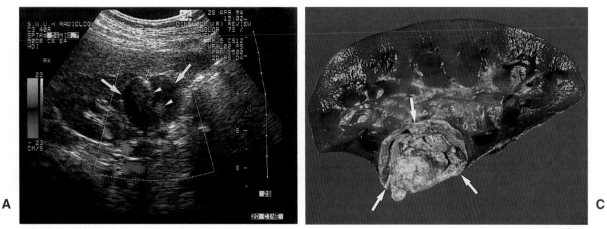

Chapter 4, Illustration 7, Fig. 1. Cystic renal cell carcinoma in a 36-year-old man. **A.** Color Doppler US of the right kidney shows a round cystic mass *(arrows)* that contains echogenic solid nodules *(arrowheads)*. But there is no demonstrable flow signal in the solid part of the mass. A small echogenic dot *(open arrow)* in the mass is probably a calcification. . . . **C.** Partial nephrectomy was performed and color photograph of the resected specimen shows the cystic mass with solid lesions *(arrows)*.

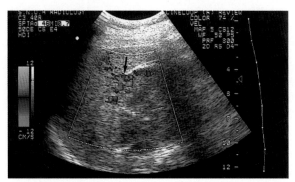

Chapter 4, Illustration 14, Fig. 6. Renal cell carcinoma of the right kidney with invasion of the liver in a 74-year-old man. . . . **C.** On US, the mass and the liver did not slide on their interface and color Doppler US shows prominent vessels *(arrow)* crossing the interface between the mass and the liver.

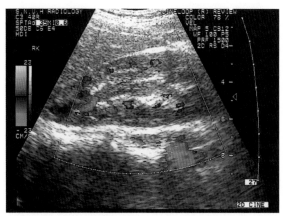

Chapter 5, Illustration 1, Fig. 6. Transitional cell carcinoma of the renal pelvocalyces in a 47-year-old man. . . . **B.** Color Doppler US shows hypovascular nature of the lesion.

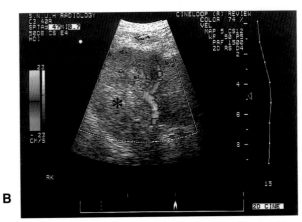

Chapter 5, Illustration 2, Fig 3. Transitional cell carcinoma with segmental arterial invasion in a 63-year-old man with history of colon cancer. . . . **B.** Color Doppler US of the right kidney in transverse plane with the patient in lateral decubitus position shows that the posterior aspect of the right kidney is poorly perfused *(asterisk)*.

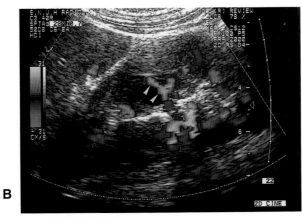

Chapter 6, Illustration 2, Fig. 3. Benign cyst with a pseudo-thick wall abutting renal sinus in a 40-year-old man. . . . **B.** Color Doppler US well demonstrates that the apparent irregularity of the cyst wall on gray-scale US was due to the vessels *(arrowheads)* in the renal sinus.

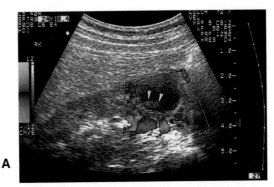

Chapter 6, Illustration 5, Fig. 3. Hemorrhagic cyst with clot mimicking a cystic renal cell carcinoma in a 26-year-old woman. **A.** Color Doppler US shows an avascular, cystic mass in the lower pole of the right kidney. The cystic mass contains echogenic materials *(arrowheads)*.

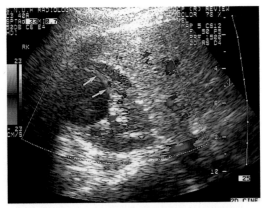

Chapter 6, Illustration 6, Fig. 1. Infected renal cyst in a 20-year-old woman. Color Doppler US shows a round cystic mass with a slightly thickened wall and low-level internal echoes. Note increased blood flow in the thickened wall *(arrows)*.

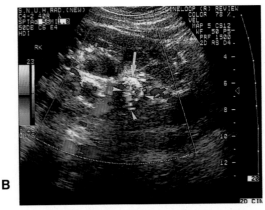

Chapter 6, Illustration 10, Fig. 2. Autosomal dominant polycystic kidney disease with a renal stone in a 42-year-old man. . . . **B.** Color Doppler US shows color twinkling artifacts *(arrowheads)* behind the echogenic lesion *(arrow)*, suggesting that the lesion is a stone.

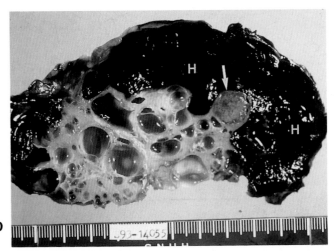

Chapter 6, Illustration 16, Fig. 4. Oncocytoma and perirenal hematoma associated with acquired cystic renal disease in a 48-year-old man. . . . **D.** Gross specimen of the removed left kidney shows multiple cysts and perirenal hematoma (H). Note a small solid mass *(arrow)* in the lower pole of the kidney which was confirmed as an oncocytoma.

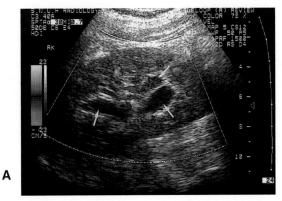

Chapter 6, Illustration 17, Fig. 2. Multiple parapelvic cysts in a 45-year-old man. **A.** Color Doppler US of the right kidney shows several ovoid, anechoic lesions *(arrows)* within the renal sinus, which may mimic dilated renal collecting system. Note that the cysts do not communicate with each other.

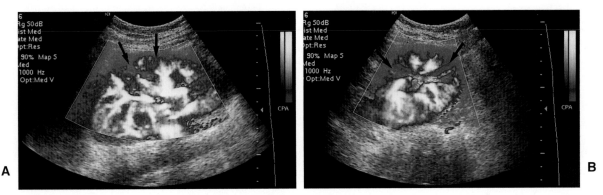

Chapter 8, Illustration 2, Fig. 3. Power Doppler US findings of acute pyelonephritis in a 50-year-old woman. **A, B.** Power Doppler US in longitudinal **(A)** and transverse **(B)** planes show decreased blood flow in the interpolar region *(arrows)* of the left kidney.

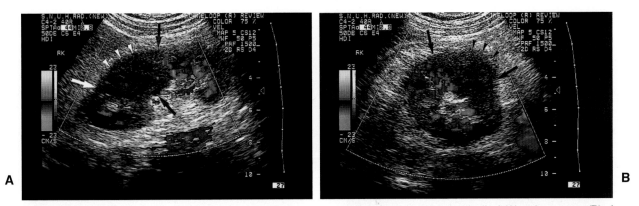

Chapter 8, Illustration 3, Fig. 5. Acute pyelonephritis in a 63-year-old man. **A, B.** Color Doppler US in longitudinal **(A)** and transverse **(B)** planes show decreased echogenicity and decreased blood flow in the interpolar area of the right kidney *(arrows)*. Note slight bulging of the renal contour *(arrowheads)*.

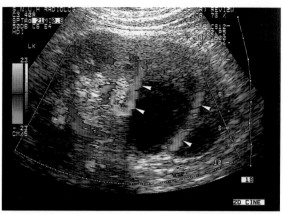

Chapter 8, Illustration 9, Fig. 3. Focal xanthogranulomatous pyelonephritis in a 63-year-old woman. . . . **B.** Color Doppler US shows stretched vessels *(arrowheads)* around the lesion, but there is no flow signal within the lesion. (From Han DH, Jung YG, Kim SH: Focal xanthogranulomatous pyelonephritis: Report of two cases. Korean J Radiol Soc 1996; 35:113–116.)

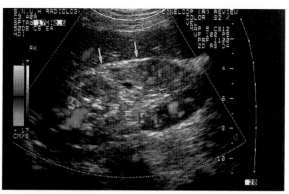

Chapter 9, Illustration 4, Fig. 1. Parenchymal fibrous scar caused by sequelae of renal tuberculosis in a 33-year-old man. . . . **C.** Color Doppler US shows decreased perfusion of the hyperechoic interpolar lesion *(arrows)* and a small cystic lesion representing a papillary cavity *(arrowhead)*. (From Kim SH: Urogenital tuberculosis. In Pollack HM, McClennan BL [eds]: Clinical Urography, 2nd ed, vol 1. Philadelphia, WB Saunders, 2000, pp 1193–1228.)

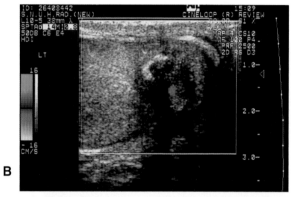

Chapter 9, Illustration 21, Fig. 1. Tuberculous epididymitis in a 35-year-old man. . . . **B.** On color Doppler US, the vascularity is not increased in the lesion.

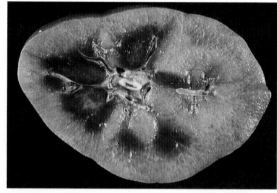

Chapter 11, Illustration 12, Fig. 4. Specimen MR imaging of the kidney of a 21-year-old man who succumbed to hemorrhagic fever with renal syndrome. . . . **C.** Specimen photograph of the kidney shows congestion and hemorrhage in the outer medullary region. (From Kim YS, Lee JS, Ahn C, et al: Magnetic resonance imaging of the kidney in hemorrhagic fever with renal syndrome: Its histopathologic correlation. Nephron 1997; 76:477–480.)

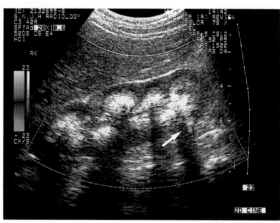

Chapter 12, Illustration 3, Fig. 1. Medullary nephrocalcinosis in a 34-year-old woman with renal tubular acidosis. . . . **C.** Color Doppler US of the right kidney shows the same findings. Note the echogenic lesion in the lower-polar region shows color twinkling artifacts *(arrow),* indicating the presence of calcifications.

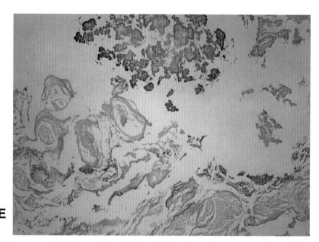

Chapter 13, Illustration 3, Fig. 1. Renal matrix stones with calcified center in a 55-year-old man. . . . **E.** Photomicrograph of the friable material surrounding calcified nidi shows amorphous and whorling appearance of fibrous matrix. (From Kim SH, Lee SE, Park IA: Case report: CT and US features of renal matrix stones with calcified center. J Comput Assist Tomogr 1996; 20:404–406.)

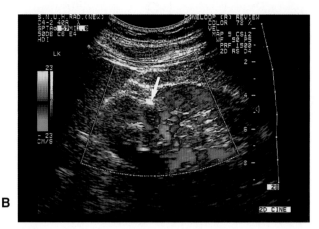

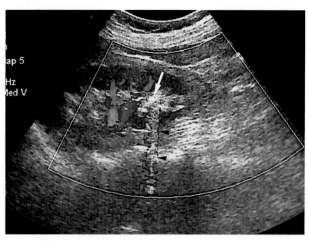

Chapter 13, Illustration 18, Fig. 3. Renal stone with parenchymal scar in a 64-year-old man. . . . **B.** Color Doppler US of the left kidney shows decreased vascularity around the stone *(arrow)* due to parenchymal scarring.

Chapter 13, Illustration 18, Fig. 5. Renal stone with color twinkling artifact in a 54-year-old woman with a renal stone. . . . **B.** Color Doppler US shows strong color twinkling artifact *(arrowheads)* posterior to the echogenic lesion *(arrow)* indicating that the echogenic lesion is a stone.

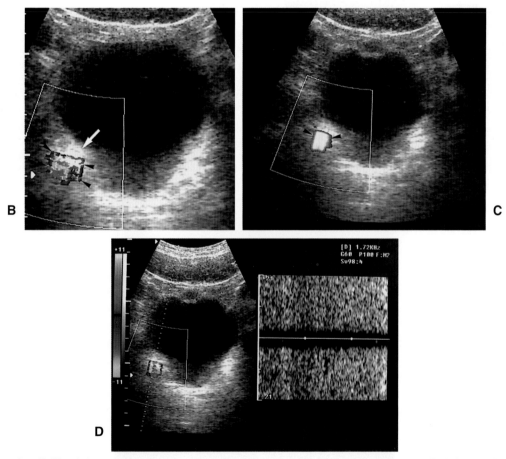

Chapter 13, Illustration 18, Fig. 6. A terminal ureter stone with color twinkling artifact in a 35-year-old man. . . . **B.** Color Doppler US shows prominent twinkling artifact *(arrowheads)* posterior to the echogenic lesion *(arrow)*. **C.** Power Doppler US also shows strong artifact *(arrowheads)*. **D.** Spectral Doppler US with the sample volume located in the echogenic lesion shows artifactual spectral signal. (**B, D,** From Lee JY, Kim SH, Cho JY, et al: Color and power Doppler twinkling artifacts from urinary stones: Clinical observations and phantom studies. AJR Am J Roentgenol 2001; 176:1441–1445.)

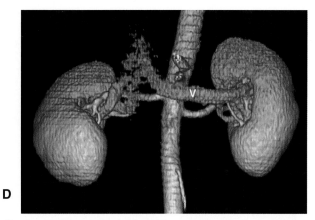

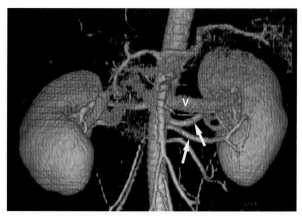

Chapter 15, Illustration 1, Fig. 2. Normal CT angiogram of the renal arteries in a 50-year-old man. . . . **D.** CT angiogram in shaded surface display well demonstrates normal renal arteries.

Chapter 15, Illustration 1, Fig. 3. Multiple renal arteries in a 30-year-old woman. CT angiogram in shaded surface display shows two renal arteries *(arrows)* in the right kidney. V, left renal vein.

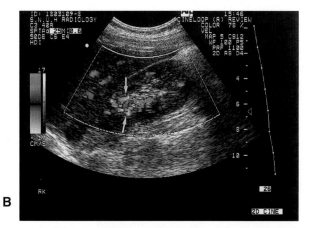

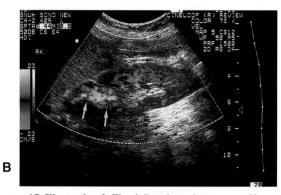

Chapter 15, Illustration 3, Fig. 1. Renal arteriovenous malformation in a 48-year-old woman who had a traffic accident with contusion on the right kidney seven years ago. . . . **B.** Color Doppler US shows hypervascular lesion with high frequency shift in the upper-polar region of the right kidney *(arrows)*.

Chapter 15, Illustration 3, Fig. 4. Renal arteriovenous malformation in a 57-year-old woman. . . . **B.** Color Doppler US shows hypervascular lesion *(arrows)* in the upper-polar area of the right kidney.

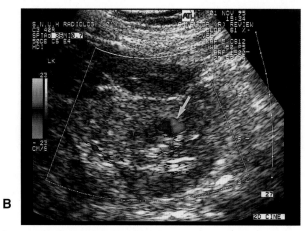

Chapter 15, Illustration 12, Fig. 1. Post-biopsy perirenal hematoma and pseudoaneurysm in a 50-year-old woman. . . . **B.** Color Doppler US well demonstrates the pseudoaneurysm *(arrow)*.

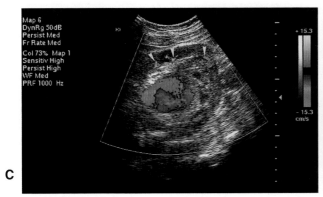

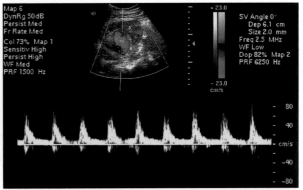

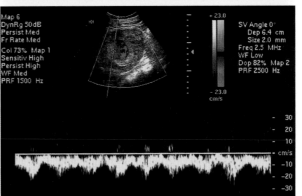

Chapter 15, Illustration 12, Fig. 2. Post-traumatic perirenal hematoma and pseudoaneurysm in a 47-year-old man. . . . **C.** Color Doppler US confirms that the cystic lesion is an aneurysm with whorling flow in it. Note that the soft tissue echogenicity surrounding the lesion is avascular, suggesting hematoma. The renal parenchyma that has intrarenal vessels *(arrowheads)* is displaced anteriorly. **D.** Spectral Doppler US obtained in the red portion of the lesion shows arterial spectral pattern. **E.** Spectral Doppler US obtained in the blue portion of the lesion shows mixed arterial and venous flow pattern.

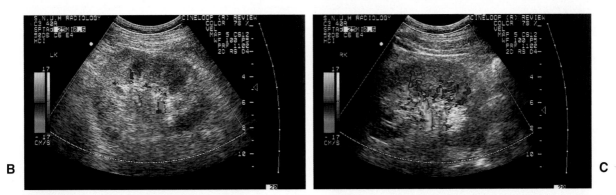

Chapter 15, Illustration 13, Fig. 2. Multifocal segmental infarction in a 57-year-old man. . . . **B, C.** Color Doppler US of the left kidney **(B)** shows markedly decreased blood flow as compared to the right kidney **(C)**. Note that blood flow is more decreased in the echogenic upper pole of the left kidney.

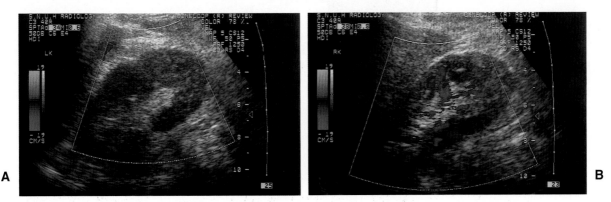

Chapter 15, Illustration 14, Fig. 1. Global renal infarction in a 70-year-old man. **A, B.** Color Doppler US of the left kidney **(A)** shows complete absence of flow signal while color Doppler US of the right kidney **(B)** shows normal blood flow.

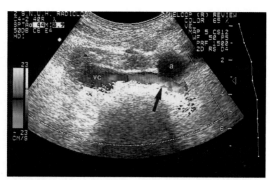

Chapter 15, Illustration 17, Fig. 2. Retroaortic left renal vein in a 69-year-old man with renal cell carcinoma of the left kidney. Color Doppler US in transverse plane shows left renal vein *(arrow)* coursing behind the abdominal aorta (a). vc, inferior vena cava.

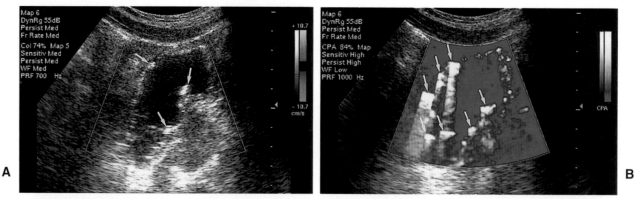

Chapter 17, Illustration 3, Fig. 3. Emphysematous cystitis in a 28-year-old man who underwent renal transplantation. **A.** Color Doppler US shows thickened bladder wall and dense echogenic lesions *(arrows)* in the bladder wall suggesting gas. **B.** Power Doppler US demonstrates reverberation artifacts *(arrows)* from the bladder wall suggesting the presence of gas in the bladder wall.

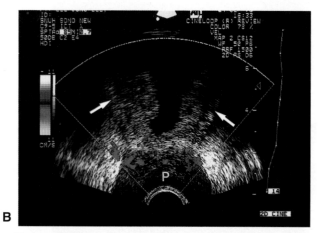

Chapter 17, Illustration 3, Fig. 8. Cystitis cystica in a 26-year-old man. . . . **B.** Transrectal color Doppler US in transverse plane shows markedly thickened bladder wall without prominent vessels *(arrows)*. P, prostate.

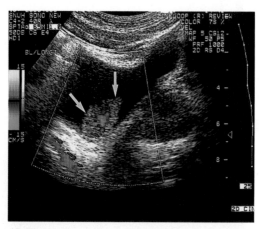

Chapter 17, Illustration 4, Fig. 5. Transitional cell carcinoma in a 47-year-old man. Color Doppler US of the bladder in longitudinal plane shows a fungating mass *(arrows)* in the posterior wall of the bladder with intratumoral vessels.

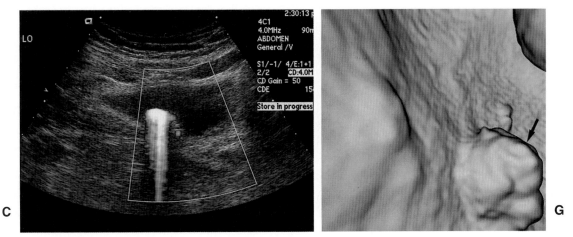

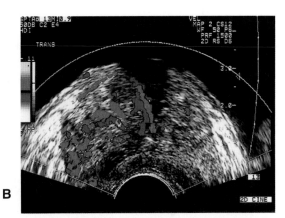

Chapter 17, Illustration 4, Fig. 11. Calcified bladder tumor in a 54-year-old man. . . . **C.** Power Doppler US shows strong twinkling artifact suggesting a calcified lesion. . . . **G.** Virtual CT cystoscopic image well demonstrates the mass *(arrow)*.

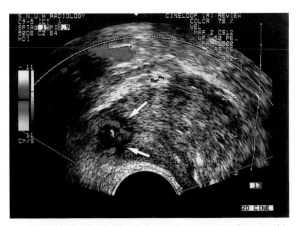

Chapter 19, Illustration 2, Fig. 1. Prostate cancer in a 68-year-old man. Color Doppler US shows a well-defined, hypoechoic lesion *(arrows)* in the right peripheral zone of the prostate. Note that the vascularity of the lesion is higher than that of the rest of the prostate.

Chapter 19, Illustration 2, Fig. 5. Prostate cancer involving peripheral and central glands in a 59-year-old man. . . . **B.** Color Doppler US well demonstrates that the lesion has marked hypervascularity. Note that the lesion involves not only the peripheral zone but also the central glands.

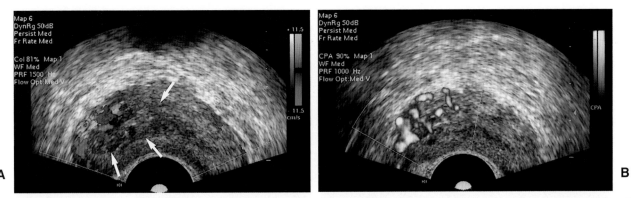

Chapter 19, Illustration 2, Fig. 7. Prostate cancer involving both peripheral and central glands in a 57-year-old man. **A, B.** Color Doppler **(A)** and power Doppler **(B)** US images of the prostate in axial plane show an ill-defined, hypoechoic lesion *(arrows)* in the central gland of the right prostate. Note that the vascularity is increased in the lesion.

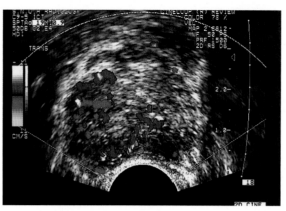 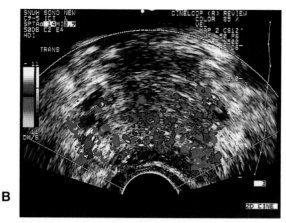

Chapter 19, Illustration 3, Fig. 4. Diffuse prostate cancer in a 68-year-old man. Color Doppler US shows ill-defined, diffuse, hypoechoic lesions with hypervascularity in the right and posterior peripheral zones of the prostate.

Chapter 19, Illustration 3, Fig. 5. Diffuse prostate cancer in a 65-year-old man. . . . **B.** On color Doppler US, vascularity is diffusely increased in the prostate. US-guided biopsy revealed diffuse prostate cancer with a Gleason's score of 8(4 + 4)/10.

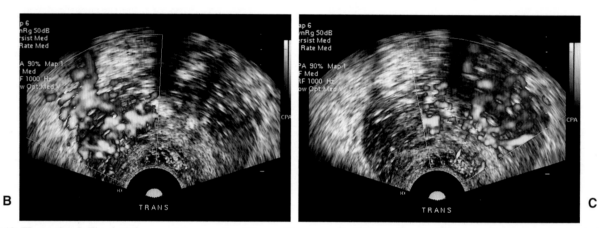

Chapter 19, Illustration 3, Fig. 6. Diffuse prostate cancer in a 77-year-old man. . . . **B, C.** Power Doppler US images of the prostate in axial plane show diffusely increased vascularity. US-guided biopsy revealed diffuse prostate cancer with a Gleason's score of 9(4 + 5)/10.

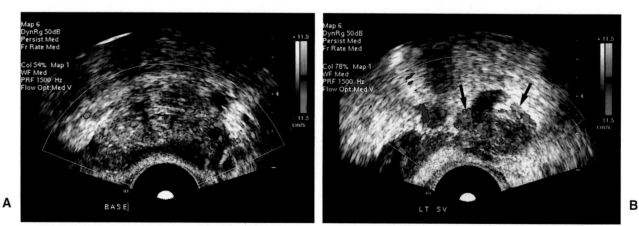

Chapter 19, Illustration 4, Fig. 4. Prostate cancer with involvement of the seminal vesicle in a 78-year-old man. **A.** Color Doppler US of the prostate in axial plane shows an ill-defined, hypoechoic lesion in the left posterolateral peripheral zone that has slight hypervascularity. **B.** Color Doppler US of the seminal vesicles in axial plane shows a slightly enlarged left seminal vesicle that has slight hypervascularity *(arrows)*. US-guided biopsy revealed prostate cancer with involvement of the left seminal vesicle.

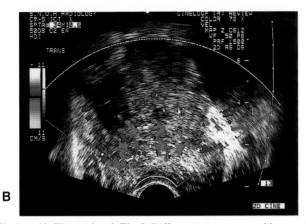

Chapter 19, Illustration 4, Fig. 9. Diffuse prostate cancer with extensive retroperitoneal nodal metastases in a 70-year-old man. . . . **B.** Color Doppler US shows diffusely increased vascularity of the prostate.

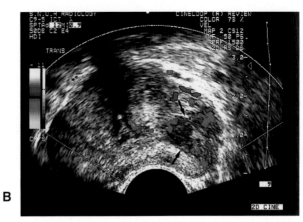

Chapter 19, Illustration 6, Fig. 1. Prostate cancer that was treated with bilateral orchiectomy in a 73-year-old man. . . . **B.** Color Doppler US demonstrates hypervascularity within the lesion *(arrows)*. Bilateral orchiectomy was performed.

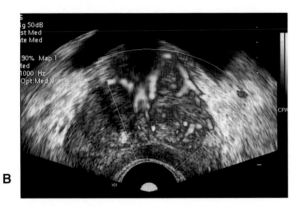

Chapter 19, Illustration 8, Fig. 4. Focal chronic inflammation of the prostate mimicking a prostate cancer in a 70-year-old man. . . . **B.** Power Doppler US shows that the vascularity of the lesion is lower than that of the rest of the prostate.

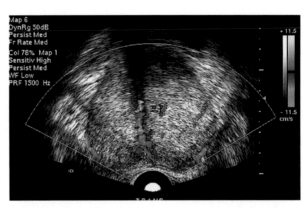

Chapter 19, Illustration 9, Fig. 3. Benign prostatic hyperplasia in a 56-year-old man. Color Doppler US shows large nodular masses in the central gland of the prostate and flow signals along the margin of the masses.

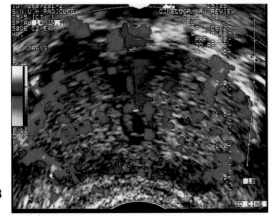

Chapter 19, Illustration 10, Fig. 1. Acute prostatitis in a 45-year-old man. . . . **B.** Color Doppler US of the prostate demonstrates diffusely increased vascularity of the prostate, especially in the peripheral portion.

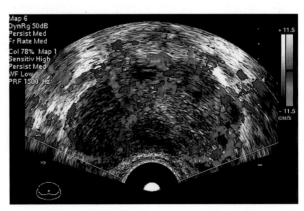

Chapter 19, Illustration 10, Fig. 2. Acute prostatitis in a 56-year-old man with diabetes. Color Doppler US of the prostate in axial plane shows an enlarged prostate with diffuse, heterogeneous hypoechogenicity. Note that the vascularity of the prostate is diffusely increased.

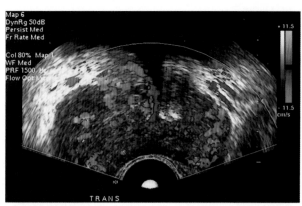

Chapter 19, Illustration 10, Fig. 3. Acute prostatitis in a 65-year-old man. Color Doppler US of the prostate in axial plane shows an enlarged prostate with diffuse hypoechogenicity. The prostate has diffuse hypervascularity.

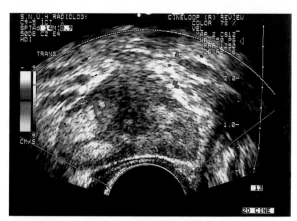

Chapter 19, Illustration 12, Fig. 1. Chronic prostatitis in a 47-year-old man. . . . **B.** Color Doppler US of the prostate shows no increased vascularity of the prostate.

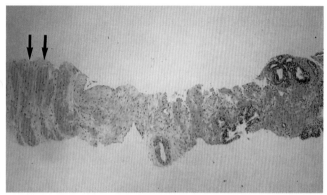

Chapter 19, Illustration 12, Fig. 4. A 64-year-old man with chronic prostatitis. . . . **B.** Transrectal US–guided biopsy was performed and a photomicrograph of the biopsy specimen at lower-power field (×40) reveals that the peripheral portion, seen at transrectal US as a hypoechoic rim, is composed of loose connective tissue with few prostatic glands and sparse infiltration of inflammatory cells *(arrows)*. (From Lee HJ, Choe GY, Seong CG, et al: Hypoechoic rim of the chronic prostatic inflammation: Histopathologic findings. Korean J Radiol 2001; 2:159–163.)

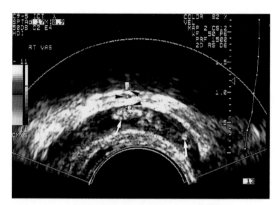

Chapter 20, Illustration 3, Fig. 3. Calcification of the vas deferens in a 69-year-old man. Color Doppler US of the right vas deferens shows echogenic lesions *(arrows)* that accompany color twinkling artifacts *(arrowheads)*, suggesting calcifications.

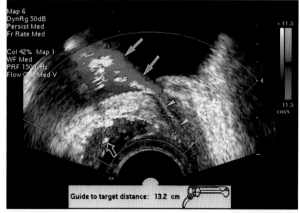

Chapter 20, Illustration 7, Fig. 2. Partial obstruction of the ejaculatory duct evaluated with transrectal US–guided aspiration in a 25-year-old man. . . . **B.** Transrectal US–guided aspiration was done, and contrast material was injected into the dilated ejaculatory duct. Color Doppler US in longitudinal plane, which was performed during the procedure, demonstrates flow of the fluid into the urethra *(arrowheads)* and bladder *(arrows)*. The *open arrow* indicates the tip of the needle in the dilated ejaculatory duct.

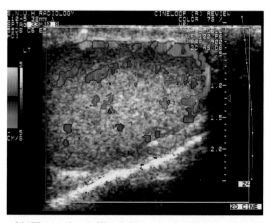

Chapter 21, Illustration 1, Fig. 4. Normal color Doppler US of the testis in a 51-year-old man. Longitudinal color Doppler US of the left testis shows normal capsular vessels and branching intratesticular vessels.

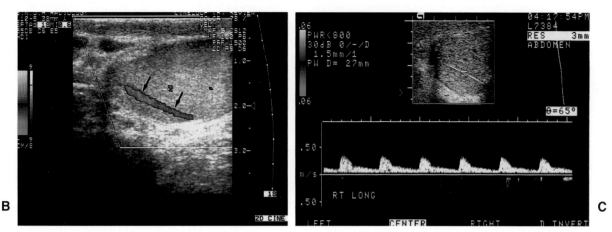

Chapter 21, Illustration 1, Fig. 5. Normal US of the testis showing prominent, linear, intratesticular vessels appearing as a hypoechoic band. . . . **B.** Color Doppler US demonstrates blood flow within the hypoechoic band *(arrows).* **C.** Spectral Doppler US from the hypoechoic band shows arterial flow.

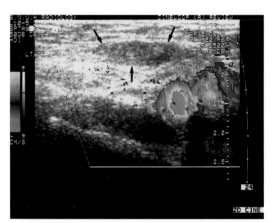

Chapter 21, Illustration 3, Fig. 2. Undescended testis in the superficial inguinal pouch in a 24-year-old man. Color Doppler US demonstrates a small, atrophic, undescended testis *(arrows)* anteromedial to the femoral vessels.

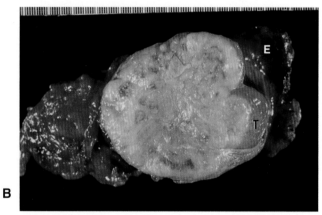

Chapter 21, Illustration 4, Fig. 1. Seminoma in a 32-year-old man. . . . **B.** Gross specimen of the removed testis and epididymis correlates well with the US findings. Note large tumor, remnant testis (T), and dilated epididymis (E).

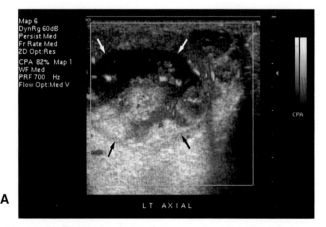

Chapter 21, Illustration 5, Fig. 2. Malignant teratoma in a 48-year-old man. **A.** Color Doppler US of the left testis in transverse plane shows a solid and cystic mass with heterogeneous echogenicity *(arrows).* The vascularity is slightly increased in the mass.

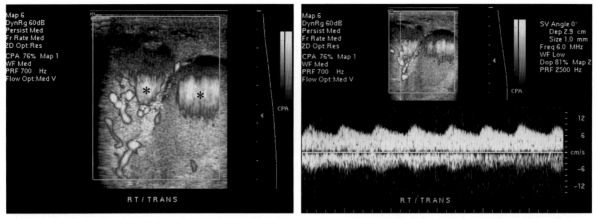

Chapter 21, Illustration 5, Fig. 4. Mixed germ cell tumor (embryonal cell carcinoma mixed with teratocarcinoma) in a 19-year-old man. . . . **B.** Color Doppler US shows increased vascularity in the solid component of the tumor. Color signals in the cystic components *(asterisks)* are due to blooming artifacts of color Doppler US. **C.** Spectral Doppler US obtained from the solid component shows low-resistance arterial flow.

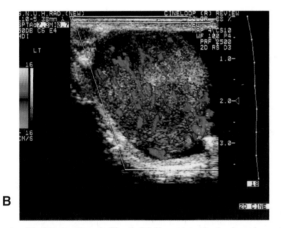

Chapter 21, Illustration 6, Fig. 1. Malignant testicular lymphoma in a 66-year-old man. . . . **B.** Color Doppler US of the left testis shows diffusely increased vascularity in the tumor.

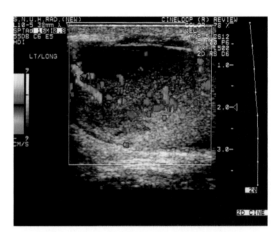

Chapter 21, Illustration 6, Fig. 2. Malignant lymphoma of the testis in a 60-year-old man. Color Doppler US of the left testis in longitudinal plane shows an enlarged testis with a poorly defined, hypoechoic lesion. Note increased vascularity in the mass.

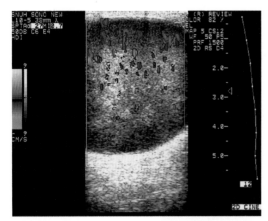

Chapter 21, Illustration 6, Fig. 3. Malignant lymphoma involving both testes in a 55-year-old man. Color Doppler US of the right testis in transverse plane shows an enlarged testis with poorly defined, hypoechoic areas and diffusely increased vascularity. The patient also had lymphomatous involvement of the nasal cavity and both adrenal glands.

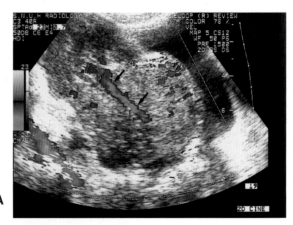

Chapter 21, Illustration 8, Fig. 4. Undescended left testis with seminoma in an 18-year-old man. **A.** Color Doppler US shows a lobulated pelvic mass with a linear, intratumoral vessel *(arrows)*.

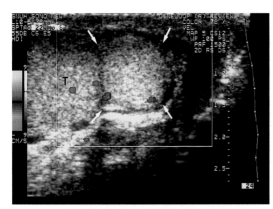

Chapter 21, Illustration 9, Fig. 1. Adenomatoid tumor of the epididymis in a 30-year-old man. Longitudinal color Doppler US of the left scrotum shows a round, solid mass *(arrows)* in the tail of the epididymis. Note that the echogenicity and vascularity of the mass are similar to those of the testis (T).

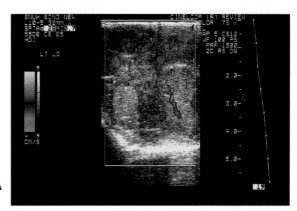

Chapter 21, Illustration 10, Fig. 2. Malignant mixed germ cell tumor with retroperitoneal lymph node metastases and tumor thrombus in the left renal vein and inferior vena cava in a 34-year-old man. **A.** Color Doppler US of the left testis shows enlarged, hypervascular testis occupied by multilobulated masses of heterogeneous echogenicity.

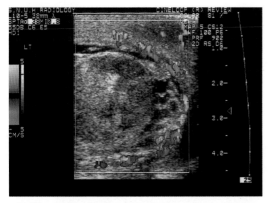

Chapter 21, Illustration 12, Fig. 1. Testicular torsion in a 16-year-old boy. Color Doppler US of the left scrotum shows swollen, heterogeneously hypoechoic testis. Note lack of blood flow in the testis and hypervascular rim in the scrotal wall.

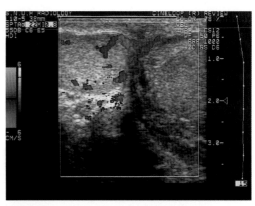

Chapter 21, Illustration 12, Fig. 2. Testicular torsion in a 30-year-old man. Color Doppler US of the scrotum in the transverse plane shows a markedly enlarged left testis with decreased echogenicity. Note the normal blood flow in the right testis but no demonstrable flow in the left testis.

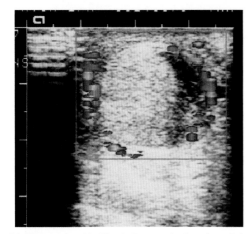

Chapter 21, Illustration 12, Fig. 3. Extravaginal torsion of the left testis in an infant. Transverse color Doppler US reveals enlarged, echogenic left testis. The blood flow is decreased in the testis but increased in the scrotal wall.

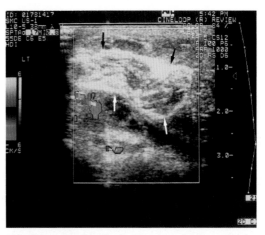

Chapter 21, Illustration 12, Fig. 5. Chronic testicular torsion in a 26-year-old man. . . . **B.** Longitudinal color Doppler US of the cranial portion of the left scrotum shows the twisted spermatic cord appearing as an echogenic mass *(arrows)*.

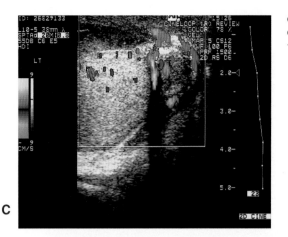

Chapter 21, Illustration 13, Fig. 1. Acute epididymitis in a 53-year-old man. . . . **C.** Longitudinal color Doppler US in caudal portion shows markedly increased vascularity in the epididymal tail.

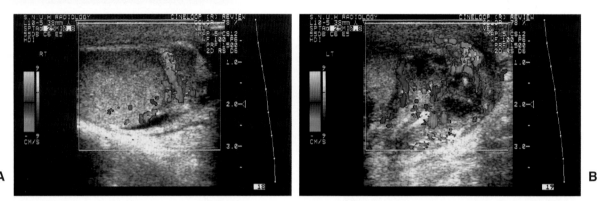

Chapter 21, Illustration 13, Fig. 3. Bilateral epididymitis in a 63-year-old man with acute scrotal pain. **A, B.** Longitudinal color Doppler US images of the right (**A**) and left (**B**) testes show swelling and increased vascularity in the enlarged epididymis at tail portion. Note diffuse thickening of the scrotal wall.

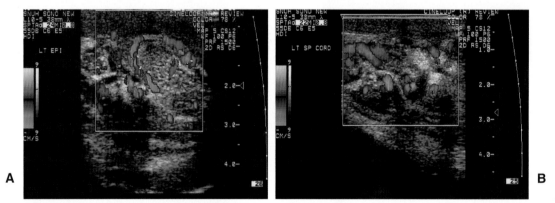

Chapter 21, Illustration 13, Fig. 5. Acute epididymitis in a 28-year-old man. **A.** Color Doppler US shows diffusely enlarged epididymis with increased vascularity. Note thickened scrotal wall. **B.** Color Doppler US along the left spermatic cord shows thickened spermatic cord with increased vascularity.

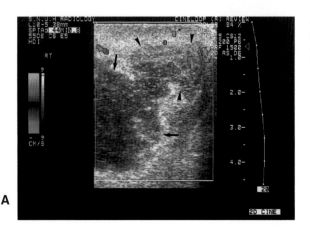

Chapter 21, Illustration 13, Fig. 6. Acute epididymitis with epididymal abscess in a 71-year-old man. **A.** Color Doppler US of the right scrotum shows enlarged epididymis with increased vascularity *(arrowheads)* and a large hypoechoic lesion suggesting an abscess cavity *(arrows)*.

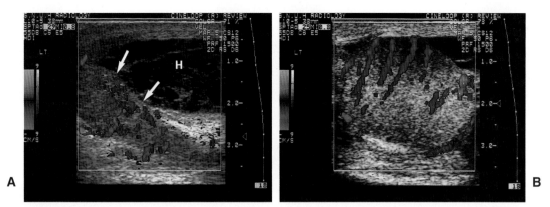

Chapter 21, Illustration 14, Fig. 1. Acute epididymo-orchitis in a 21-year-old man. **A.** Color Doppler US along the left epididymis shows diffusely enlarged epididymis with decreased echogenicity and increased vascularity *(arrows)*. Note septated hydrocele (H). **B.** Color Doppler US of the left testis shows markedly increased vascularity and slightly decreased echogenicity suggesting associated orchitis.

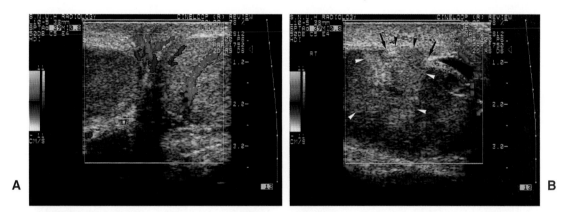

Chapter 21, Illustration 15, Fig. 1. A 20-year-old man with testicular rupture due to blunt scrotal trauma received four days ago. **A.** Transverse color Doppler US of the scrotum shows decreased echogenicity of the right testis with decreased vascularity. **B.** Color Doppler US of the right testis in longitudinal plane shows discontinuity of the tunica albuginea in the anterior aspect *(arrows)*. Note decreased echogenicity and decreased vascularity of the right testis. Also note ill-defined, increased echogenicity *(arrowheads)* across the tunical defect suggesting intratesticular and extratesticular hematoma.

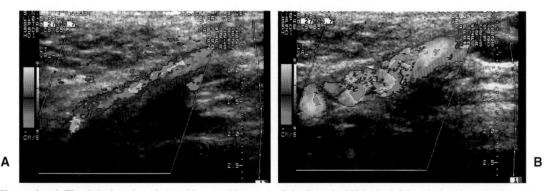

Chapter 22, Illustration 1, Fig. 1. Left varicocele in a 29-year-old man. **A.** Color Doppler US in the left inguinal region with the patient at rest shows a prominent left internal spermatic vein with the flow in the cranial direction. **B.** Color Doppler US with the Valsalva maneuver shows the markedly dilated internal spermatic vein with turbulent, reversed flow in the caudal direction.

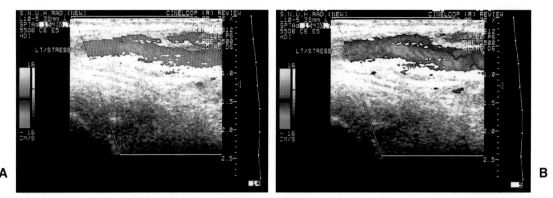

Chapter 22, Illustration 1, Fig. 2. Left varicocele in a 27-year-old man. **A, B.** Color Doppler US of the left inguinal region shows changing direction of blood flow with the Valsalva maneuver. Without the Valsalva maneuver (**A**), the vein is filled with red, representing the cranial direction of flow. With the Valsalva maneuver (**B**), the color signal changed to blue, representing the caudal direction of the flow.

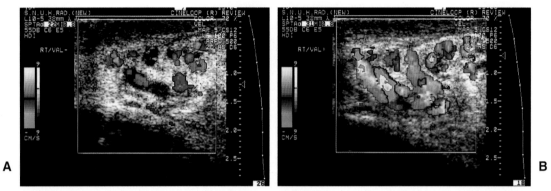

Chapter 22, Illustration 1, Fig. 3. Left varicocele in a 20-year-old man. **A, B.** Color Doppler US of the left scrotum in the region of the pampiniform plexus at rest (**A**) and with the Valsalva maneuver (**B**). Without the Valsalva maneuver, the vessels are dilated in the pampiniform plexus, and some of them show color flow signals. With the Valsalva maneuver, the venous channels are dilated and totally filled with prominent flow signals.

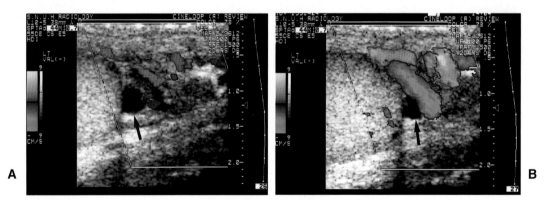

Chapter 22, Illustration 1, Fig. 4. Left varicocele in a 37-year-old man. **A.** Color Doppler US in the caudal portion of the left scrotum shows slightly dilated vessels with scanty flow signals in them. **B.** Color Doppler US with the Valsalva maneuver shows dilation of the vessels with prominent flow signals. Note a small cyst in the tail of the epididymis (*arrow* in **A, B**).

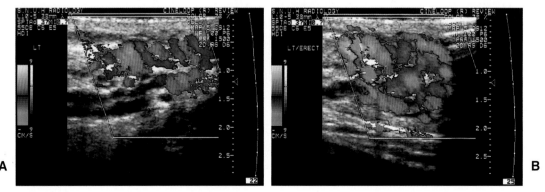

Chapter 22, Illustration 1, Fig. 5. A 22-year-old man with left varicocele shows changes of color Doppler findings with the changes in the patient's position. **A.** Color Doppler US with the patient in supine position shows tortuous, dilated vessels with flow signals in some of them. **B.** With the patient in erect position, the vessels are more dilated and all vessels are filled with flow signals of higher velocity.

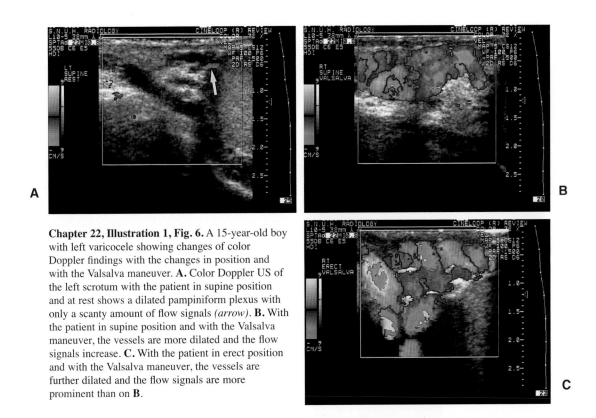

Chapter 22, Illustration 1, Fig. 6. A 15-year-old boy with left varicocele showing changes of color Doppler findings with the changes in position and with the Valsalva maneuver. **A.** Color Doppler US of the left scrotum with the patient in supine position and at rest shows a dilated pampiniform plexus with only a scanty amount of flow signals *(arrow)*. **B.** With the patient in supine position and with the Valsalva maneuver, the vessels are more dilated and the flow signals increase. **C.** With the patient in erect position and with the Valsalva maneuver, the vessels are further dilated and the flow signals are more prominent than on **B**.

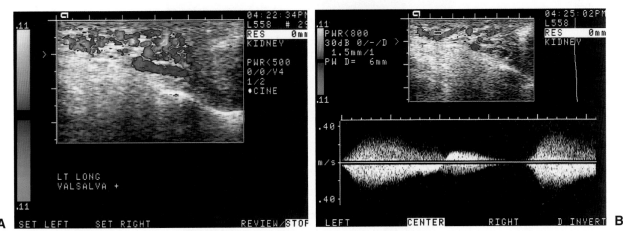

Chapter 22, Illustration 2, Fig. 1. Left varicocele in a 22-year-old man. **A.** Color Doppler US of the left scrotum with the Valsalva maneuver shows a dilated pampiniform plexus with flow signals. **B.** Spectral Doppler US obtained from the dilated plexus shows venous flow that changes its direction with Valsalva maneuvers.

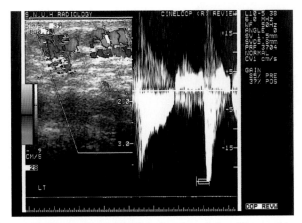

Chapter 22, Illustration 2, Fig. 2. Left varicocele in a 23-year-old man. Spectral Doppler US obtained from the dilated pampiniform plexus shows venous flow that changes its direction with Valsalva maneuvers.

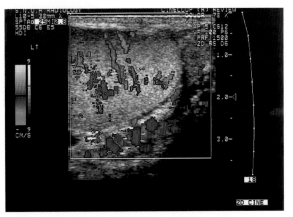

Chapter 22, Illustration 3, Fig. 1. Intratesticular varicocele in a 74-year-old man. Color Doppler US of the left scrotum shows dilated veins around the testis. Also note dilated vessels in the testis.

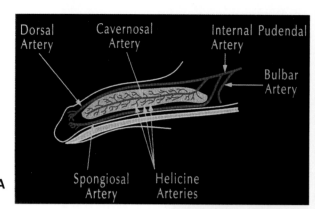

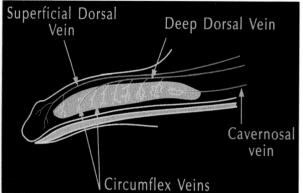

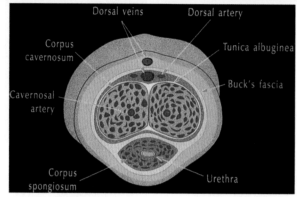

Chapter 23, Illustration 1, Fig 1. Diagram of the typical penile anatomy. (**A–C,** From Fitzgerald SW, Erickson SJ, Foley WD, et al: Color Doppler sonography in the evaluation of erectile dysfunction. Radiographics 1992; 12:3–17.) **A.** Penile arterial anatomy. Penile arteries arise as branches of the internal pudendal artery. The cavernosal arteries and their helicine branches supply the sinusoidal spaces of the corpora cavernosa. **B.** Penile venous anatomy. Superficial dorsal vein drains the distal corporal spaces, while most of the corporal sinusoidal outflow occurs through the deep dorsal vein. Proximal corporal spaces are drained by the cavernosal (crural) veins directly into the periprostatic venous plexus. Venous flow in the cavernosal veins is usually not visualized at Doppler US. **C.** Cross-sectional diagram of the penile shaft. Corpora cavernosa are enclosed with the tunica albuginea and Buck's fascia. The cavernosal arteries are located slightly medially in the center of the corpora cavernosa.

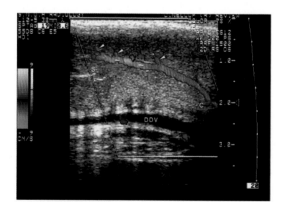

Chapter 23, Illustration 2, Fig. 2. Normal color Doppler US of the cavernosal artery. Longitudinal color Doppler US obtained through a plane including the right cavernosal artery and deep dorsal vein shows the right cavernosal artery running from the crus of the corpus cavernosum (C) to the penile shaft (S) and sending small helicine branches *(arrowheads)*. Note the absence of flow in the deep dorsal vein (DDV).

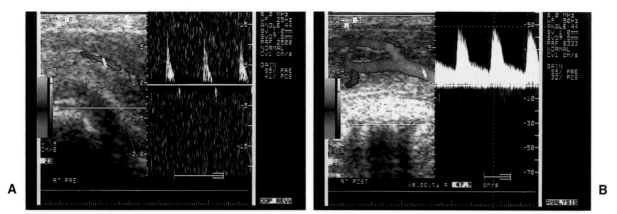

Chapter 23, Illustration 2, Fig. 3. Normal color Doppler US of cavernosal artery. (**A, B,** From Kim SH: Imaging for evaluation of erectile dysfunction. J Korean Soc Med US 2001; 20:1–13.) **A.** Longitudinal color and spectral Doppler US of the right cavernosal artery in the flaccid state. Color Doppler US shows the very small right cavernosal artery, and spectral Doppler US shows very weak flow with a low peak systolic velocity of about 10 cm/sec. **B.** Color and spectral Doppler US of the same artery obtained 3 minutes after an injection of 10 μg of prostaglandin E$_1$ shows the dilated artery and increased systolic and diastolic flow with a peak systolic velocity of 48 cm/sec. The right dorsal artery is not included in this image.

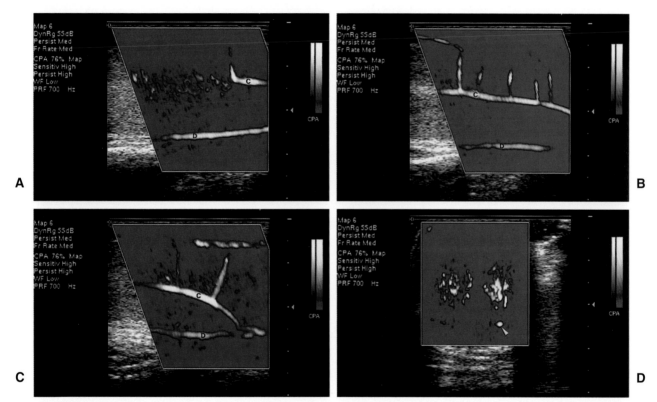

Chapter 23, Illustration 4, Fig. 4. Normal power Doppler US of the penis. **A–C.** Longitudinal power Doppler US images through distal (**A**), middle (**B**), and proximal (**C**) portions of the left corpus cavernosum well demonstrate the left cavernosal (C) and dorsal (D) arteries. Note the small helicine branches that are demonstrated better than on color Doppler US. **D.** Power Doppler US in transverse plane at the level of distal penile shaft shows prominent flow signals in the helicine branches of the cavernosal arteries. Note a prominent flow signal from the left dorsal penile artery *(arrowhead)*, but the right dorsal artery is not well demonstrated. This asymmetry of the right and left dorsal arteries is a common variation.

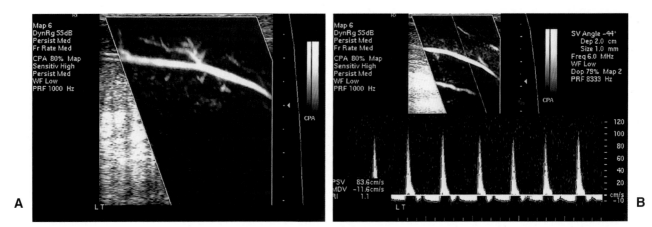

Chapter 23, Illustration 2, Fig. 5. Normal power Doppler US of the penis. **A.** Power Doppler US of the left cavernosal artery using a different color map clearly shows the left cavernosal artery and helicine branches. **B.** Power Doppler US with spectral Doppler shows the high-resistance pattern of the left cavernosal artery with a peak systolic velocity of 83 cm/sec. Note reversed end-diastolic flow (−11 cm/sec).

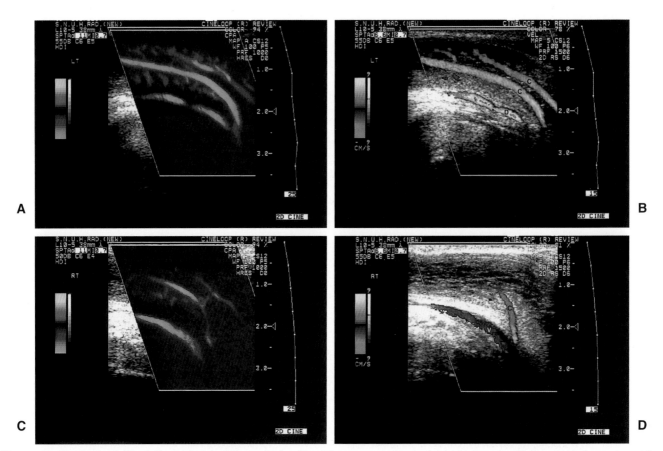

Chapter 23, Illustration 3, Fig. 1. Power Doppler US reveals slow blood flow more sensitively than color Doppler US does, but it does not provide directional information. Therefore, power Doppler US should be used in conjunction with color Doppler or spectral Doppler US. **A.** Power Doppler US of the left corpus cavernosum shows three vessels. **B.** Color Doppler US in the same patient as **A** shows two cavernosal arteries (C) and a dorsal artery (D). **C.** Power Doppler US of the right corpus cavernosum in another patient shows multiple vessels. **D.** Color Doppler US in the same patient as **C** shows a cavernosal artery (C) and venous flow in the deep dorsal vein (V).

Chapter 23, Illustration 4, Fig. 2. Time-velocity curves showing the progression of cavernosal arterial blood flow during erection. No specific time frame is shown because of the wide variation in temporal response to an intracavernosal injection of vasoactive agent. A–E correspond to the Doppler sampling time in **A–E** of Figure 1 (Chapter 23, Illustration 4). (Modified from Fitzgerald SW, Erickson SJ, Foley WD, et al: Color Doppler sonography in the evaluation of erectile dysfunction. Radiographics 1992; 12:3–17.)

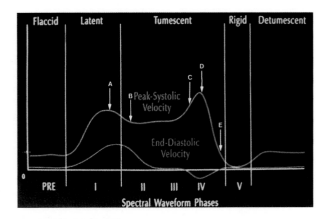

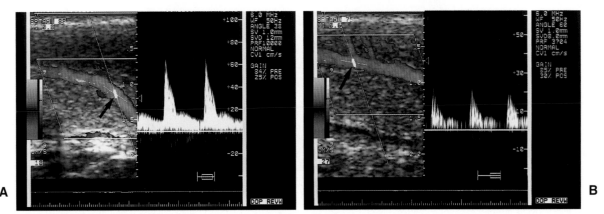

Chapter 23, Illustration 5, Fig. 1. The peak systolic velocity of the cavernosal artery varies significantly according to the sampling location. Doppler waveforms obtained at proximal and distal portions of a cavernosal artery in an early tumescent stage of erection. (**A, B,** From Kim SH, Paick JS, Lee SE, et al: Doppler sonography of deep cavernosal artery of the penis: Variation of peak systolic velocity according to sampling location. J Ultrasound Med 1994; 13:591–594.) **A.** Doppler waveform obtained at the base of the penis, where the vessel angles posteriorly *(arrow)*. Peak systolic velocity at this sampling location is 63 cm/sec. **B.** Doppler waveform of the same artery obtained immediately after **A** at the distal portion of the shaft, where the artery's course is straight *(arrow)*. Peak systolic velocity at this sampling location is 23 cm/sec.

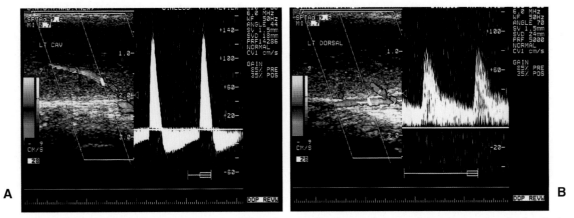

Chapter 23, Illustration 5, Fig. 3. Doppler waveforms are quite different between the cavernosal artery and dorsal artery since the dorsal artery is located outside the tunica albuginea. (**A, B,** From Kim SH: Imaging for evaluation of erectile dysfunction. J Korean Soc Med US 2001; 20:1–13.) **A.** Doppler waveform obtained at the left cavernosal artery shows a high-resistance pattern with reversed diastolic flow. **B.** Doppler waveform obtained at the left dorsal artery of the same patient immediately after **A** shows a low-resistance pattern with prominent, antegrade, diastolic flow.

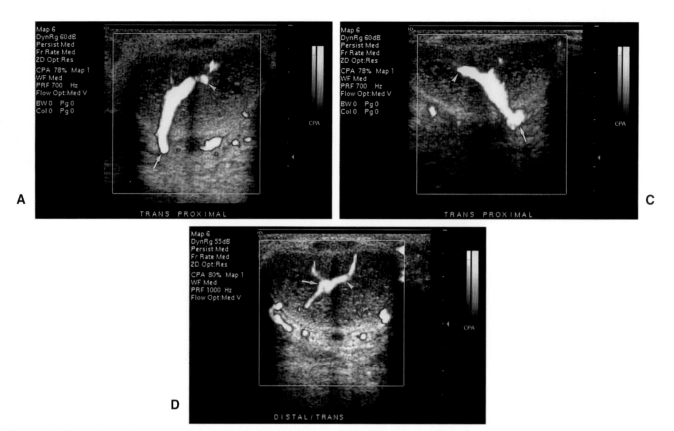

Chapter 23, Illustration 7, Fig. 2. A 32-year-old impotent man who received a left femur fracture due to a traffic accident 3 years earlier. Penile Doppler US revealed subnormal peak systolic velocities of both cavernosal arteries (right, 14.9 cm/sec; left, 25.2 cm/sec). Peak systolic velocities of right and left dorsal penile arteries were asymmetrical (right, 71.3 cm/sec; left, 28 cm/sec). **A.** Power Doppler US image of the penis in axial plane shows communication of the right dorsal penile artery *(arrow)* with the left cavernosal artery *(arrowhead)*. Doppler spectra have an upward direction, indicating that the flow direction is from the right dorsal artery to the left cavernosal artery. . . . **C.** Power Doppler US image in axial plane slightly distal to the level of **A** shows communication between the left dorsal penile artery *(arrow)* and right cavernosal artery *(arrowhead)*. **D.** Power Doppler US image in axial plane immediately distal to **C** shows communication between the right *(arrow)* and left *(arrowhead)* cavernosal arteries.

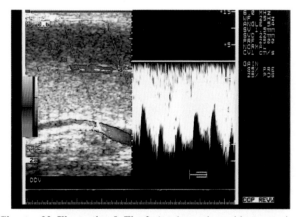

Chapter 23, Illustration 9, Fig. 2. Another patient with venogenic impotence. Color Doppler US shows a prominent venous leak with a pulsatile flow pattern.

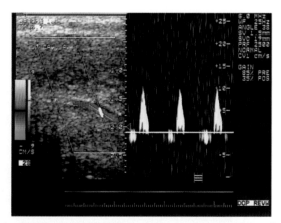

Chapter 23, Illustration 11, Fig. 1. A 49-year-old man with low-flow priapism. He complained of persistent painful erection for 4 days following an intracavernosal injection of a vasoactive agent. Doppler US of the left cavernosal artery without intracavernosal injection of vasoactive agent shows a weak flow signal with low peak systolic velocity (10 cm/sec) and high-resistance pattern. Aspiration of the corpus cavernosum revealed anoxic blood. Priapism was relieved after repeated aspiration of cavernosal blood, and follow-up Doppler US revealed restored cavernosal blood flow. (From Kim SH: Imaging for evaluation of erectile dysfunction. J Korean Soc Med US 2001; 20:1–13.)

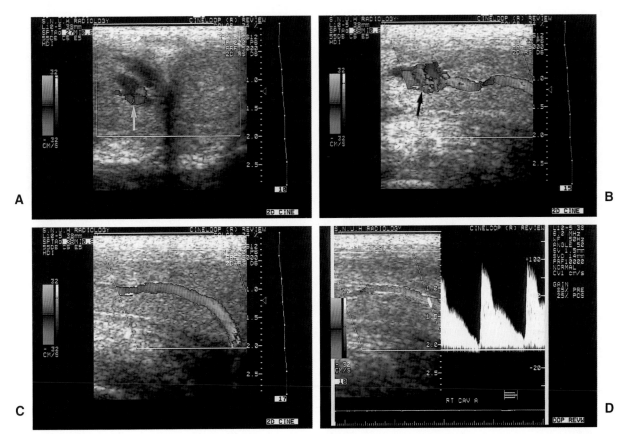

Chapter 23, Illustration 11, Fig. 2. A 30-year-old man with high-flow priapism. He complained of intermittent persistent erection and penile curvature to the right side following a blunt trauma to the penis that had occurred 3 years earlier. (**A–D,** From Kim SH: Imaging for evaluation of erectile dysfunction. J Korean Soc Med US 2001; 20:1–13.) **A.** Color Doppler US in transverse plane without intracavernosal injection of vasoactive agent shows prominent cavernosal vessels in the right corpus cavernosum *(arrows).* **B, C.** Color Doppler US images of the right corpus cavernosum in longitudinal plane at the region of distal **(B)** and proximal **(C)** shaft show prominent blood flow in the cavernosal artery forming an entangled vascular mass *(arrow)* in the distal penile shaft. **D.** Spectral Doppler US obtained in the proximal portion of the right cavernosal artery shows prominent blood flow with very high peak systolic velocity (100 cm/sec).

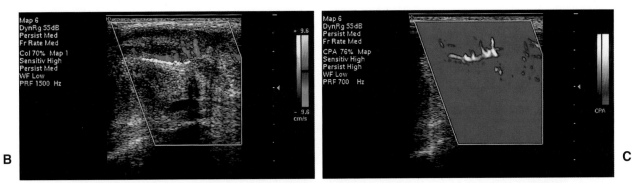

Chapter 23, Illustration 13, Fig. 1. Erectile dysfunction in a 60-year-old man with hypercholesterolemia. . . . **B, C.** Color **(B)** and power **(C)** Doppler US images of the same area reveal that the calcification is along the course of the cavernosal artery, indicating arterial wall calcification. (**B,** From Kim SH: Imaging for evaluation of erectile dysfunction. J Korean Soc Med US 2001; 20:1–13.)

Chapter 23, Illustration 13, Fig. 3. A 51-year-old man with penile sparganosis. . . . **B.** Photograph of the removed mass. A white live worm *(arrow)* was found. (From Kim SH: Imaging for evaluation of erectile dysfunction. J Korean Soc Med US 2001; 20:1–13.)

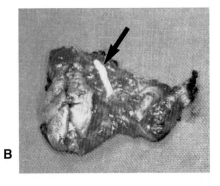

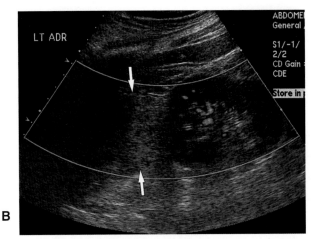

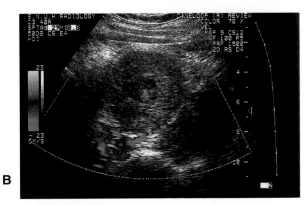

Chapter 25, Illustration 8, Fig. 3. Carcinoid tumor of the adrenal gland in a 41-year-old woman. . . . **B.** Color Doppler US shows the hypovascular nature of the tumor.

Chapter 25, Illustration 3, Fig. 2. Adrenal myelolipoma in a 46-year-old man. . . . **B.** Color Doppler US shows the hypovascular nature of the mass *(arrows).*

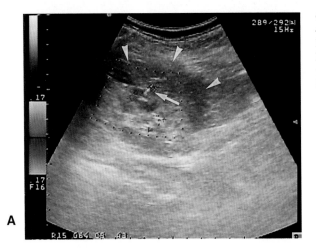

Chapter 26, Illustration 5, Fig. 1. Postbiopsy active bleeding in a 42-year-old woman with chronic renal parenchymal disease. **A.** Color Doppler US performed immediately after US-guided biopsy of the left kidney shows a developing perirenal hematoma *(arrowheads).* There were flow signals *(arrow)* crossing the renal capsule into the perirenal hematoma.

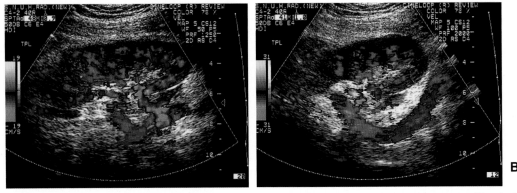

Chapter 27, Illustration 1, Fig. 1. Normal transplanted kidney in a 47-year-old man. **A, B.** Longitudinal **(A)** and transverse **(B)** color Doppler US of the transplant show normal flow in the main renal artery and vein and normal parenchymal vascularity throughout the transplanted kidney.

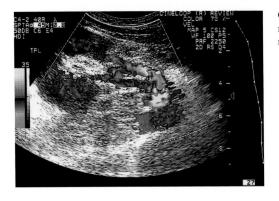

Chapter 27, Illustration 1, Fig. 2. Normal transplant in a 40-year-old man. Transverse color Doppler US of the renal hilum demonstrates normal blood flow in the main renal artery and vein.

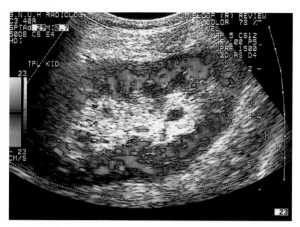

Chapter 27, Illustration 1, Fig. 3. Normal transplant in a 35-year-old man. Longitudinal color Doppler US demonstrates normal parenchymal vascularity.

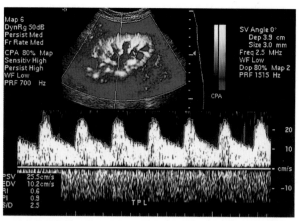

Chapter 27, Illustration 1, Fig. 4. Power Doppler and spectral Doppler US image of renal allograft in a 34-year-old man. Longitudinal power Doppler US shows normal parenchymal vascularity. Spectral Doppler US of interlobar artery demonstrates a normal resistive index of 0.6.

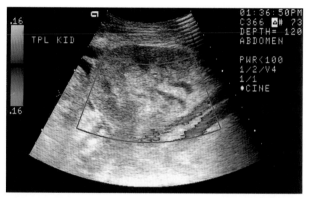

Chapter 27, Illustration 4, Fig. 2. Chronic renal allograft rejection in a 27-year-old man, who had undergone renal transplantation 6 years earlier. Transverse color Doppler US shows diffusely increased parenchymal echogenicity with markedly decreased vascularity, which is suggestive of chronic rejection.

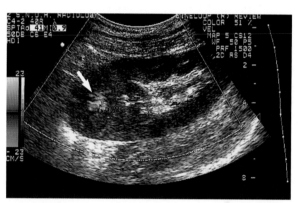

Chapter 27, Illustration 5, Fig. 2. Arteriovenous fistula in a 31-year-old man with transplant rejection, who had had renal biopsy 1 month earlier. Color Doppler US of renal allograft demonstrates a hypervascular lesion in the upper portion of the allograft *(arrow)*. Note the turbulence in the lesion shown as a mosaic pattern of flow signals.

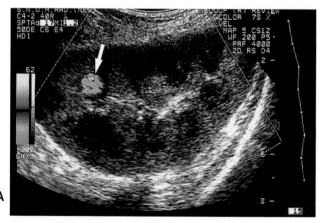

A

Chapter 27, Illustration 5, Fig. 3. Pseudoaneurysm in a 29-year-old woman with renal allograft, who had had allograft biopsy 1 year earlier. **A.** Color Doppler US reveals a focal area of high-velocity lesion with aliasing in the upper portion of the transplanted kidney *(arrow)*.

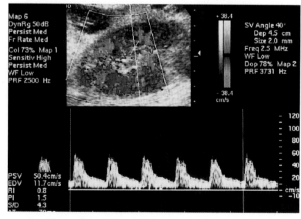

B

Chapter 27, Illustration 6, Fig. 3. Urinoma in a 60-year-old man who had received renal transplantation 18 days earlier. . . . **B.** Spectral Doppler US of the renal allograft shows an increased resistive index in the interlobar artery (0.8).

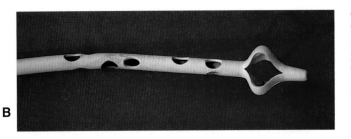

B

Chapter 29, Illustration 1, Fig. 3. Nephrostomy tube individually tailored to a patient with idiopathic retroperitoneal fibrosis. The renal sinus was diffusely infiltrated with retroperitoneal fibrosis and the renal pelvocalyceal systems are so narrowed that the usual pigtail-shaped catheter could not be accommodated in the pelvis. Therefore a Malecot catheter with multiple additional side-holes was used. . . . **B.** Photograph of the Malecot catheter with multiple side-holes.

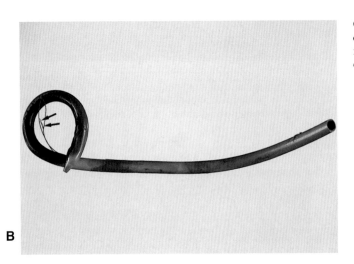

B

Chapter 29, Illustration 2, Fig. 1. Nephrostomy catheter locked by encrustation on the locking string. . . . **B.** The catheter was removed by introducing a sheath over the catheter. Photograph of the removed catheter shows encrustation on the string of the catheter *(arrows)*.

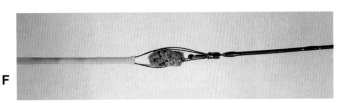

F

Chapter 29, Illustration 12, Fig. 1. Percutaneous retrieval of proximal ureteral stone under fluoroscopic guidance in a 47-year-old woman. . . . **F.** Photograph of the stone in the basket.

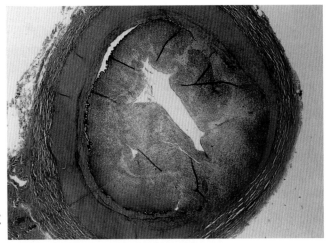

E

Chapter 30, Illustration 1, Fig. 2. Incomplete angioplasty and early restenosis in a 22-year-old woman with fibromuscular dysplasia of intimal hyperplasia type. . . . **E.** Photomicrograph of the resected renal artery shows prominent circumferential intimal hyperplasia.

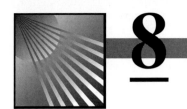

8

Renal Infection

JEONG YEON CHO AND LEE B. TALNER

ACUTE RENAL INFECTION

Acute pyelonephritis is the most common bacterial infection involving the kidney. It is an intense inflammation of the renal collecting system and parenchyma, which is usually multifocal. Bacteria, most commonly *Escherichia coli*, usually reach the kidney through the ureter. However, certain bacteria such as *Staphylococcus aureus* can reach the kidney by hematogenous seeding from a distant source. Conditions predisposing to acute pyelonephritis are vesicoureteral reflux, urinary tract obstruction, calculi, altered bladder function, altered host resistance, pregnancy, and congenital urinary tract anomalies. In most cases, the diagnosis can be made on the basis of typical symptoms and laboratory findings. Imaging studies including ultrasonography (US) and computed tomography (CT) are usually not needed in uncomplicated adult patients, but they are mandatory for early detection and follow-up in pediatric patients.

Acute pyelonephritis, uncomplicated

A variety of terms, including *bacterial nephritis, focal bacterial nephritis, lobar nephronia, renal cellulitis,* and *renal phlegmon,* have been coined to describe acute renal infection. In 1994, the Society of Uroradiology recommended a return to the term *acute pyelonephritis* to describe changes in the kidney caused by an acute renal infection.

Pathologic changes in acute pyelonephritis are well described. In ascending infection, inflammatory lesions begin in the pelvocalyceal system and papilla, and the inflammation spreads to the renal cortex through the tubules. Severe arterial constriction and edema cause multifocal, wedge-shaped lesions that extend from the papilla to the cortical surface with lobar or sublobar distribution. Hematogenous infection results in multiple peripheral lesions in the cortex with nonlobar distribution. However, it is difficult to distinguish a hematogenous infection from an ascending infection when the lesions progress.

Intravenous urography (IVU) is normal in 75% of patients with uncomplicated acute pyelonephritis. In the remainder, IVU may show diffuse renal enlargement, decreased patchy or striated nephrogram, focal renal mass, effacement of pelvocalyceal system, or delayed calyceal opacification.

US findings in patients with acute uncomplicated pyelonephritis are often normal, but the involved kidney may be enlarged with either decreased or increased renal parenchymal echogenicity. Power Doppler US may demonstrate triangular areas of decreased perfusion. New US techniques such as tissue harmonic imaging or pulse inversion harmonic imaging may help depict the renal parenchymal lesions in acute pyelonephritis.

CT is regarded as the most practical imaging study to estimate the severity and extent of acute pyelonephritis and to look for complications such as abscesses and obstruction. The characteristic CT findings are focal or diffuse renal enlargement, hypoenhanced regions in the renal parenchyma, impaired excretory function of the kidney, and renal or perirenal abscesses. Nonenhanced CT scan may show high-attenuated lesions if the lesion is hemorrhagic. On contrast-enhanced scans, striated foci of decreased enhancement are seen focally or diffusely depending on the degree of involvement. These striated regions probably reflect decreased excretion of contrast material due to slow flow of urine within the tubular lumen secondary to elevated interstitial pressure or tubular obstruction. With increasing severity of involvement, multiple wedge-shaped foci of decreased enhancement can be seen radiating from the papilla to the renal capsule. These wedge-shaped lesions may show contrast staining on delayed CT scans obtained without further injection of contrast material. The pathophysiologic mechanisms of these low-attenuated lesions are focal ischemia, obstruction of tubules, and extrinsic compression by interstitial edema. MR imaging does not have any advantages over US or CT in the evaluation of acute pyelonephritis.

In children, radionuclide scintigraphy is useful to document renal parenchymal involvement. However, it is of little use in adults, in whom the major issue is whether there is a complication such as abscess or obstruction.

Complications of acute pyelonephritis

Renal and perirenal abscesses

Acute pyelonephritis may progress to renal abscess if it is not treated successfully, especially in patients with diabetes mellitus, drug abuse, vesicoureteral reflux, and renal calculi. Renal abscess may be solitary or multiple. Multiple abscesses suggest hematogenous infection.

IVU may demonstrate decreased nephrogram of all or part of the kidney and decreased calyceal opacification with compression and displacement of the calyces in the affected area. Renal abscess appears as a thick-walled cystic lesion on US but contains internal echoes. As the abscess matures, internal echoes tend to disappear. CT is the imaging study of choice for

the diagnosis of renal abscess. The lesion appears as a low-attenuated, nonenhancing mass with thick, enhancing wall. In rare cases, gas may be present within the abscess. The renal fascia is often thickened, and soft tissue stranding is commonly found in the adjacent perirenal fat.

Renal abscess may cause perirenal abscess by extension through the renal capsule. Other causes of perirenal abscess are spread of infection from the adjacent retroperitoneal space and hematogenous spread from a distant focus. On plain radiographs, the renal margin and psoas shadow are indistinct. Scoliosis of the lumbar spine concave to the affected side also may be present. Air may be found within a large abscess. On IVU, the kidney shows changes of acute pyelonephritis, and the perirenal abscess may displace the kidney and obscure the renal margin. On US, perirenal abscess appears as a cystic mass of variable echogenicity adjacent to the kidney. Gas within the abscess causes dirty acoustic shadowing. The imaging study of choice for the detection of perirenal abscess is also CT. Extension into the psoas muscle, anterior or posterior pararenal spaces, and the true pelvis can be accurately delineated with CT. Malignant tumors with extrarenal extension, perirenal hematoma, and urinoma may appear similar to perirenal abscess on imaging studies.

Small, solitary renal abscesses (<2 cm) may be treated by antibiotic therapy. Larger intrarenal and all perirenal abscesses should be treated by drainage. Percutaneous catheter drainage is the preferred method and provides satisfactory results.

Emphysematous pyelonephritis

Emphysematous pyelonephritis is a rare, life-threatening form of pyelonephritis, characterized by gas formation within the renal parenchyma. The most common organism is *E. coli*, less frequently *Proteus* and *Klebsiella* species. Most of the cases occur in patients with diabetes mellitus. The gas develops by fermentation of glucose into carbon dioxide and hydrogen.

Emphysematous pyelonephritis can be classified into two types. Type I is the classic form in which gas is found diffusely within the renal parenchyma. Type II is a renal or perirenal fluid collection that contains bubbly or loculated gas. The type II lesion should be considered to be a form of renal or perirenal abscess and may be treated with percutaneous catheter drainage. The type I lesion, when extensive, should be treated by emergent nephrectomy. The early use of CT may detect milder type I cases that can be treated successfully with aggressive antibiotic therapy rather than nephrectomy.

Plain radiographic findings are characteristic. Streaks and bubbles of gas are seen within the renal parenchyma, radiating from the medulla to the cortex. Subcapsular and perirenal gas may also be present. US demonstrates dense echoes and dirty shadowing of gas in the kidney and perirenal area. CT delineates the exact location and extent of gas.

Pyonephrosis

The term *pyonephrosis* describes an obstructed and infected kidney. Parenchymal damage occurs and progresses quickly. The consequences are often grave if not treated promptly. Microabscesses and necrotizing papillitis develop early. Pyonephrosis is one of the few true urological emergencies. The obstruction is caused most frequently by a stone, less commonly by tumor, postoperative stricture, retroperitoneal fibrosis, or neurogenic bladder.

Classic US findings include a dilated pelvocalyceal system that contains fine echoes in the dependent portion, urine-debris levels that shift with changes in patient position, and gas in the collecting system. However, pyonephrosis often appears as simple hydronephrosis on US. On CT, the collecting system is dilated and may contain a urine-debris level or an air-fluid level. Thickening of the wall of the renal pelvis, heterogeneous nephrogram, streaky soft tissue attenuation in the perinephric and renal sinus fat, and thickening of renal fascia may be demonstrated on CT. Pyonephrosis may also look like simple hydronephrosis on CT, too. Percutaneous nephrostomy should be done emergently. The diagnostic nephrostogram should be delayed until urine becomes clear.

CHRONIC RENAL INFECTION

Chronic pyelonephritis

Chronic pyelonephritis, as a radiologic term, refers to renal parenchymal scarring that frequently results from vesicoureteral reflux severe enough to reflux infected urine back into the renal tubules, a process known as *intrarenal reflux*. Intrarenal reflux of infected urine causes an acute inflammatory reaction in the renal parenchyma. This ultimately results in parenchymal scarring, which typically involves the full thickness of the renal cortex and medulla and causes clubbing of the adjacent calyx. Scarring associated with reflux nephropathy more commonly occurs in early childhood, usually before the age of 4 years. Whether or not parenchymal scarring can result from reflux of uninfected urine is unsettled. The risk factors of chronic pyelonephritis in the adult are calculi, urinary tract obstruction, neurogenic bladder, and urinary diversion.

IVU demonstrates calyceal clubbing and retraction of the overlying renal parenchyma. Polar regions, especially the upper pole, are frequently involved. When there is a vesicoureteral reflux to the lower moiety of the duplicated system, the lower pole may be contracted resulting in a "nubbin sign" on IVU. US and CT demonstrate focal loss of renal parenchyma indicated by an irregularly indented contour of the kidney. Often clubbed calyces may be demonstrated on US or CT. In severe cases, scarring involves the entire kidney resulting in the atrophic or contracted kidney.

Xanthogranulomatous pyelonephritis

Xanthogranulomatous pyelonephritis, an uncommon chronic renal infection, has characteristic pathologic findings including scarring and contraction of the renal pelvis, renal parenchymal destruction, and yellowish granulomatous material containing lipid-laden macrophages and histiocytes. Renal obstruction by stone is present in 80% of cases. Xanthogranulomatous pyelonephritis frequently occurs in diabetic patients, and active infection with *E. coli*, *Proteus*, *Klebsiella*, or *Pseudomonas* is present in virtually every case.

In 85% of cases, the kidney is involved diffusely. The remainder takes a localized form that can be confused with a renal tumor on imaging studies. Most of the cases have extensive perirenal inflammation.

Plain radiograph usually demonstrates a faintly calcified, lamellated struvite stone and a poorly defined mass shadow in

the renal fossa. Usually the involved kidney does not opacify on IVU. US demonstrates diffuse renal enlargement with calculi and thick debris in the dilated calyces. Differentiation from tuberculosis can be difficult. CT demonstrates the enlarged kidney, calculi in a contracted renal pelvis, and the dilated calyces filled with low-attenuated pus. Contrast-enhanced CT demonstrates mild enhancement of the inflamed but nonfunctioning renal parenchyma around the calyces and the thickened renal fascia. Perirenal extension of the disease is well demonstrated on CT. Fistula may occur to nearby organs or to the skin.

Malacoplakia

Malacoplakia is a rare form of granulomatous inflammatory disease characterized histologically by distinctive histiocytes that contain Michaelis-Gutmann bodies. These inclusion bodies represent incomplete intracellular digestion of bacteria. Malacoplakia usually occurs in the urinary tract, most often in the urinary bladder. Renal involvement accounts for about 15% of the urinary tract cases. It occurs four times more frequently in women than in men. The peak age of renal malacoplakia is older than 50 years. Renal malacoplakia is multifocal in 75% and bilateral in 50% of cases. Solitary renal malacoplakia presents as a sharply demarcated mass that may be confused with a renal tumor.

The radiologic findings of renal malacoplakia depend on the pattern of involvement. US may demonstrate solitary or multiple, ill-defined masses of varying echogenicity. CT demonstrates mildly enhanced, solitary or multiple renal masses. Extension of the inflammatory process into the retroperitoneum is sometimes observed on CT.

FUNGAL INFECTION OF THE KIDNEY

Candidiasis is the most common fungal disease involving the kidney. Two patterns of renal candidiasis have been described. In systemic candidiasis, hematogenous spread to the kidney produces *Candida* pyelonephritis. CT may show multiple low-attenuated lesions in the liver, spleen, and kidney, representing microabscesses. Primary renal candidiasis occurs without hematogenous spread or other major organ involvement. IVU shows diminished excretion of the contrast material, papillary

necrosis, and hydronephrosis. Multiple filling defects in the collecting systems are caused by fungus balls.

References

1. Dunnick NR, Sandler CM, Amis ES, Newhouse JH: Renal inflammatory disease. In Textbook of Uroradiology, 3rd ed. Philadelphia, Lippincott Williams & Wilkins, 2001, pp 150–177.
2. Kim B, Lim HK, Choi MH, et al: Detection of parenchymal abnormalities in acute pyelonephritis by pulse inversion harmonic imaging with or without microbubble ultrasonographic contrast agent: Correlation with computed tomography. J Ultrasound Med 2001; 20:5–14.
3. Gold RP, McClennan BL: Acute infections of the renal parenchyma. In Pollack HM, McClennan BL (eds): Clinical Urography, 2nd ed, vol 1. Philadelphia, WB Saunders, 2000, pp 923–946.
4. Dacher JN, Pfster C, Monroc M, et al: Power Doppler sonographic pattern of acute pyelonephritis in children: Comparison with CT. AJR Am J Roentgenol 1996; 166:1451–1455.
5. Han DH, Jung YG, Kim SH: Focal xanthogranulomatous pyelonephritis: Report of two cases. Korean J Radiol Soc 1996; 35:113–116.
6. Wan YL, Lee TY, Bullard MJ, et al: Acute gas-producing bacterial renal infection: Correlation between imaging findings and clinical outcome. Radiology 1996; 198:433–438.
7. Oezcan H, Akyar S, Atassoy C: An unusual manifestation of xanthogranulomatous pyelonephritis: Bilateral focal solid renal masses. AJR Am J Roentgenol 1995; 165:1552–1553.
8. Gervais DA, Whitman GJ: Emphysematous pyelonephritis. AJR Am J Roentgenol 1994; 162:348.
9. Talner LB: Imaging in acute renal infection. In Syllabus for RSNA Categorical Course in Genitourinary Radiology. Oak Brook, Ill, Radiological Society of North America, 1994, pp 39–48.
10. Talner LB, Davison AJ, Levowitz RL, et al: Acute pyelonephritis: Can we agree on terminology? Radiology 1994; 192:297–305.
11. Fultz PJ, Hampton WR, Totterman SM: Computed tomography of pyonephrosis. Abdom Imaging 1993; 18:82–87.
12. Hayes WS, Hartman DS, Sesterhenn IA: Xanthogranulomatous pyelonephritis. Radiographics 1991; 11:485–498.
13. Kenney PJ: Imaging of chronic renal infections. AJR Am J Roentgenol 1990; 155:485–494.
14. Shirkhoda A: CT findings in hepatosplenic and renal candidiasis. J Comput Assist Tomogr 1987; 11:795–798.
15. Ishikawa I, Saito Y, Onouchi Z, et al: Delayed contrast enhancement in acute focal bacterial nephritis: CT features. J Comput Assist Tomogr 1985; 9:894–897.
16. Hodson CJ: Reflux nephropathy: A personal historical review. AJR Am J Roentgenol 1981; 137:451–462.
17. Stanton MJ, Maxted W: Malacoplakia: A study of the literature and current concepts of pathogenesis, diagnosis, and treatment. J Urol 1981; 125:139–146.
18. Hartman DS, Davis CJ Jr, Lichtenstein JE, et al: Renal parenchymal malacoplakia. Radiology 1980; 136:33–42.
19. Curtis JA, Pollack HM: Renal duplication with a diminutive lower pole: The nubbin sign. Radiology 1979; 131:327–331.

Illustrations • Renal Infection

1 • Acute pyelonephritis: IVU findings

2 • Acute pyelonephritis: US and Doppler US findings

3 • Acute pyelonephritis: CT findings

4 • Acute pyelonephritis: hematogenous origin

5 • Renal abscess

6 • Emphysematous pyelonephritis

7 • Pyonephrosis

8 • Chronic pyelonephritis

9 • Xanthogranulomatous pyelonephritis

10 • Malacoplakia

11 • Fungal infection

1. Acute Pyelonephritis: IVU Findings

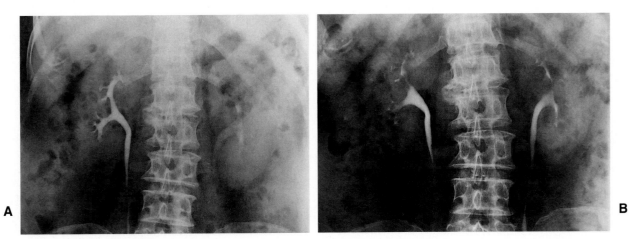

Fig. 1. Acute pyelonephritis in a 65-year-old woman.
A. IVU shows diminished opacification of pelvocalyceal system of the left kidney compared to the right kidney. **B.** Follow-up IVU obtained after 3 weeks of treatment shows normalized left urinary tract.

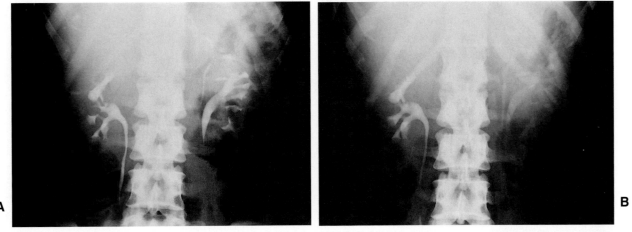

Fig. 2. Acute pyelonephritis in a 23-year-old woman with vesicoureteral reflux.
A. Baseline IVU when the patient was asymptomatic shows well-opacified pelvocalyceal systems of both kidneys. Note incomplete duplication of the left renal pelvis and ureter. **B.** IVU 1 year later, when the patient had symptoms of acute pyelonephritis, shows diminished opacification of duplicated pelvocalyceal system of the left kidney.

2. Acute Pyelonephritis: US and Doppler US Findings

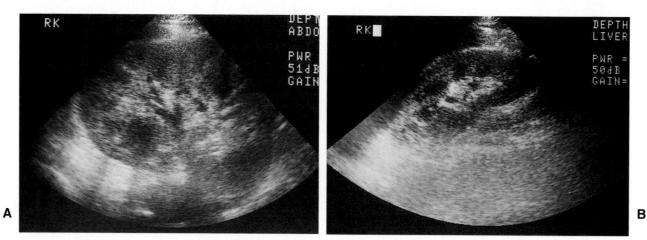

Fig. 1. US of acute pyelonephritis before and after treatment in a 45-year-old man.
A. US of the right kidney shows diffuse renal enlargement. The renal medullae are prominent and hypoechoic with slightly increased renal cortical echogenicity. **B.** Follow-up US obtained after 2 weeks of treatment shows normal size and echogenicity of the right kidney.

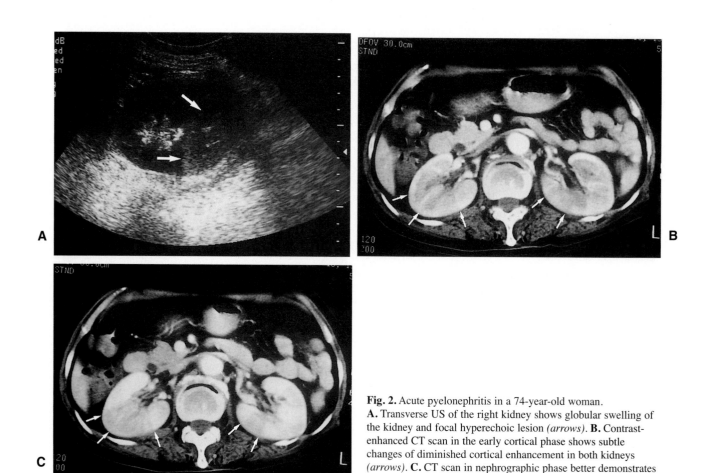

Fig. 2. Acute pyelonephritis in a 74-year-old woman.
A. Transverse US of the right kidney shows globular swelling of the kidney and focal hyperechoic lesion *(arrows)*. **B.** Contrast-enhanced CT scan in the early cortical phase shows subtle changes of diminished cortical enhancement in both kidneys *(arrows)*. **C.** CT scan in nephrographic phase better demonstrates wedge-shaped perfusion defects *(arrows)* in both kidneys.

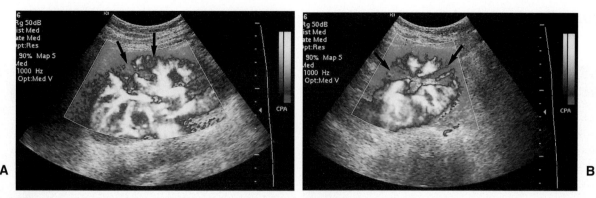

Fig. 3. Power Doppler US findings of acute pyelonephritis in a 50-year-old woman. (**A, B,** See also Color Section.)
A, B. Power Doppler US in longitudinal (**A**) and transverse (**B**) planes shows decreased blood flow in the interpolar region *(arrows)* of the left kidney.

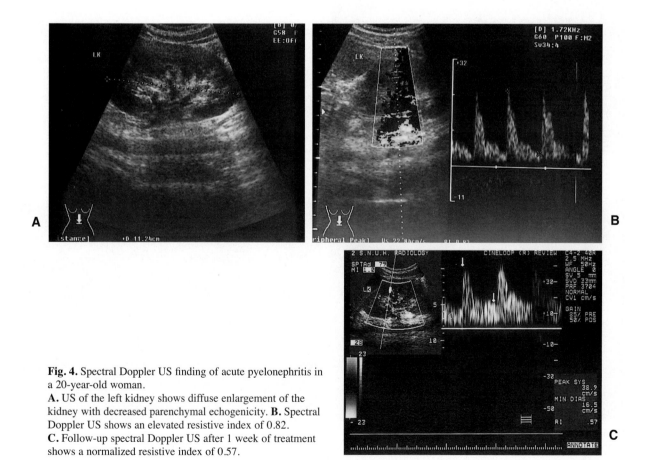

Fig. 4. Spectral Doppler US finding of acute pyelonephritis in
a 20-year-old woman.
A. US of the left kidney shows diffuse enlargement of the
kidney with decreased parenchymal echogenicity. **B.** Spectral
Doppler US shows an elevated resistive index of 0.82.
C. Follow-up spectral Doppler US after 1 week of treatment
shows a normalized resistive index of 0.57.

3. Acute Pyelonephritis: CT Findings

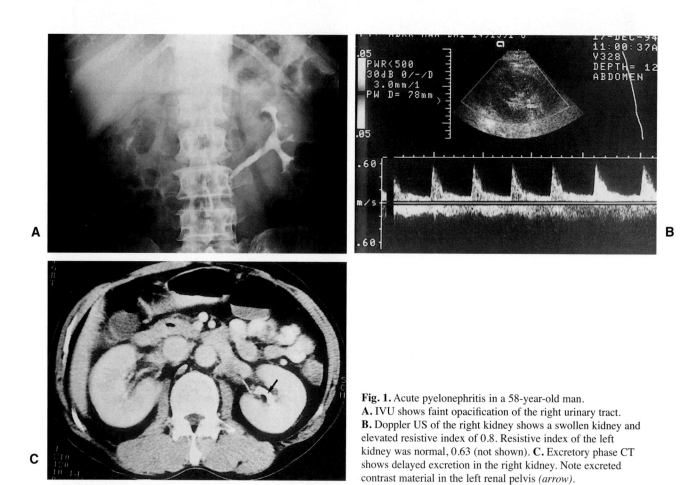

A

B

C

Fig. 1. Acute pyelonephritis in a 58-year-old man.
A. IVU shows faint opacification of the right urinary tract.
B. Doppler US of the right kidney shows a swollen kidney and elevated resistive index of 0.8. Resistive index of the left kidney was normal, 0.63 (not shown). C. Excretory phase CT shows delayed excretion in the right kidney. Note excreted contrast material in the left renal pelvis *(arrow)*.

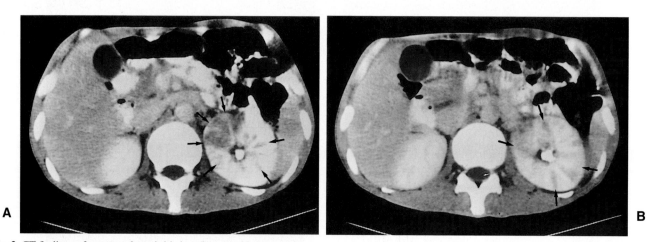

A

B

Fig. 2. CT findings of acute pyelonephritis in a 51-year-old man.
A, B. Contrast-enhanced CT scans show diffuse enlargement of the left kidney with multiple, striated, low-attenuated lesions *(arrows)*.

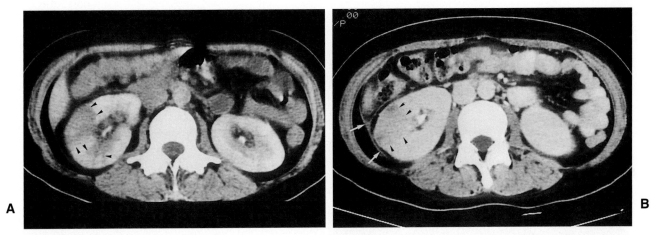

Fig. 3. Acute pyelonephritis in a 29-year-old woman.
A. Contrast-enhanced CT in cortical phase shows wedge-shaped, streaky *(arrowheads)*, low-attenuated lesions in the enlarged right kidney. **B.** CT scan in excretory phase shows lesions that are less well-defined *(arrowheads)* in the right kidney. Note the thickened renal fasciae *(arrows)* around the right kidney.

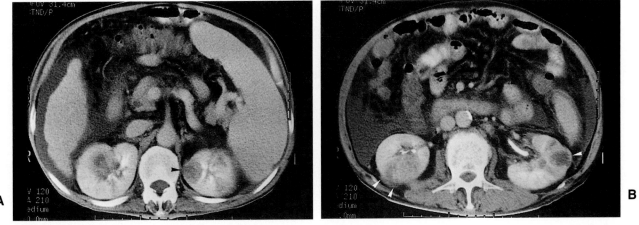

Fig. 4. Acute pyelonephritis in a 63-year-old man with diabetes.
A, B. Contrast-enhanced CT scans in excretory phase show multiple, round or wedge-shaped, low-attenuated lesions in both kidneys. Note that some lesions accompany contour bulging and perirenal changes *(arrowheads)*.

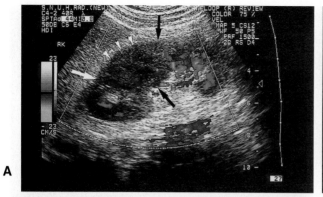

A

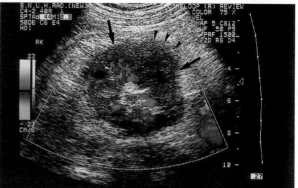

B

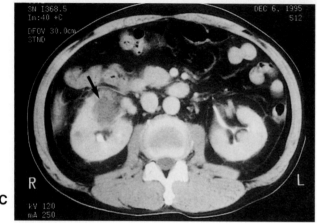

C

Fig. 5. Acute pyelonephritis in a 63-year-old man. (**A, B,** See also Color Section.)
A, B. Color Doppler US in longitudinal (**A**) and transverse (**B**) planes shows decreased echogenicity and decreased blood flow in the interpolar area of the right kidney *(arrows)*. Note slight bulging of the renal contour *(arrowheads)*. **C.** Contrast-enhanced CT scan shows ill-defined, round, low-attenuated lesion *(arrow)* in the anterior aspect of the right kidney.

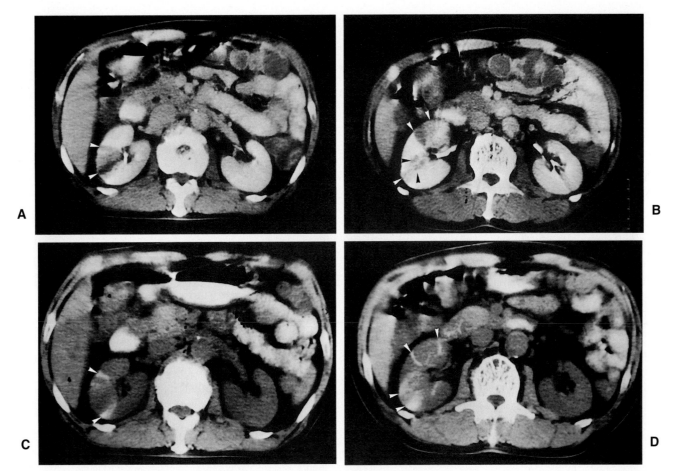

Fig. 6. Findings of acute pyelonephritis on delayed CT in a 65-year-old man.
A, B. Contrast-enhanced CT scans show enlarged right kidney with multiple, wedge-shaped lesions of low attenuation *(arrowheads)*. **C, D.** Delayed CT scans taken 12 hours later without further injection of contrast material show retained contrast material *(arrowheads)* in the area of poor enhancement at initial CT.

4. Acute Pyelonephritis: Hematogenous Origin

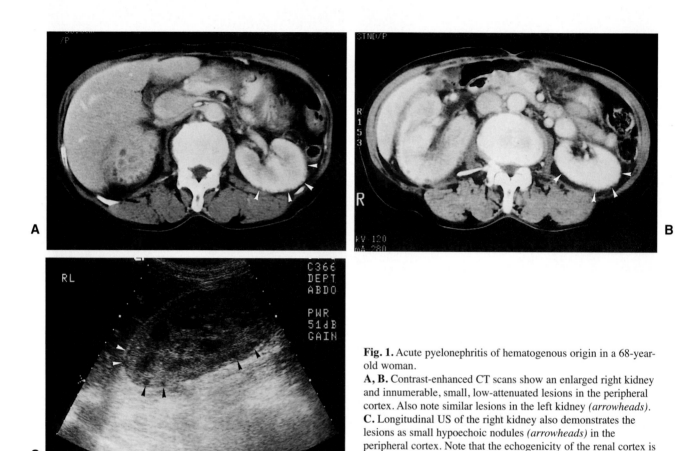

Fig. 1. Acute pyelonephritis of hematogenous origin in a 68-year-old woman.
A, B. Contrast-enhanced CT scans show an enlarged right kidney and innumerable, small, low-attenuated lesions in the peripheral cortex. Also note similar lesions in the left kidney *(arrowheads)*.
C. Longitudinal US of the right kidney also demonstrates the lesions as small hypoechoic nodules *(arrowheads)* in the peripheral cortex. Note that the echogenicity of the renal cortex is diffusely increased. *Escherichia coli* was found in the urine and blood.

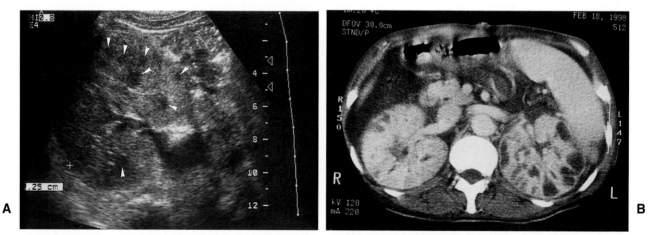

Fig. 2. Acute pyelonephritis of hematogenous origin with multiple small abscesses in a 55-year-old man with recurrent rectal cancer.
A. US of the left kidney in transverse plane shows diffuse renal enlargement and multiple hypoechoic lesions *(arrowheads)* in the peripheral renal parenchyma. **B.** Contrast-enhanced CT shows diffuse enlargement of both kidneys and multiple, low-attenuated lesions in the peripheral renal cortex.

5. Renal Abscess

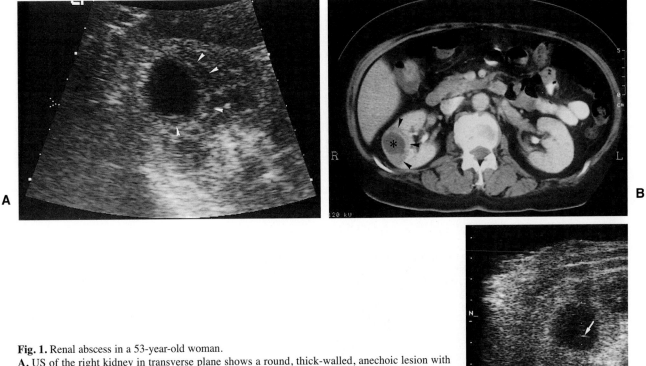

Fig. 1. Renal abscess in a 53-year-old woman.
A. US of the right kidney in transverse plane shows a round, thick-walled, anechoic lesion with posterior sonic enhancement. Note ill-defined hypoechogenicity *(arrowheads)* around the lesion, suggesting surrounding inflammatory changes. **B.** Contrast-enhanced CT shows a round, low-attenuated, nonenhancing lesion *(asterisk)* in the right kidney. Note the faint hypoechoic rim *(arrowheads)* around the lesion, representing surrounding inflammation (pyelonephritis).
C. US-guided aspiration was done by using an 18-gauge needle, and 8 mL of pus was aspirated from the lesion. Note a bright echo within the lesion representing the tip of the needle *(arrow)*.

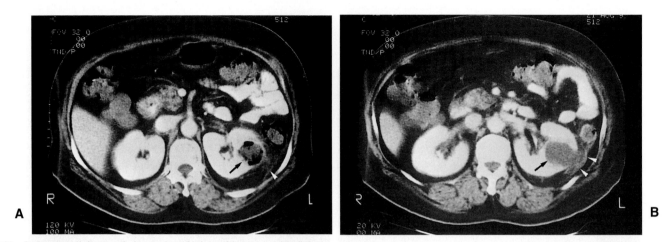

Fig. 2. Gas-containing renal abscess in a 64-year-old woman with diabetes.
A, B. Contrast-enhanced CT scans show a gas-containing, low-attenuated, nonenhancing lesion *(arrow)* in the left kidney. Note streaky infiltrations in the perirenal space and thickened renal fascia *(arrowheads)*.

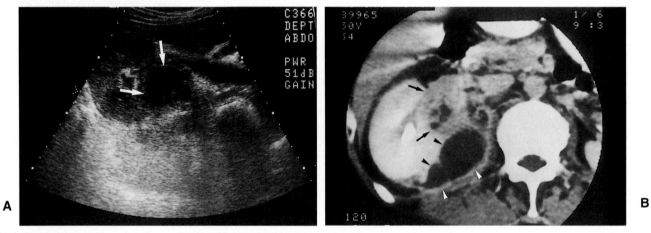

Fig. 3. Renal abscess with perirenal extension in a 59-year-old man.
A. US of the right kidney in transverse plane shows an ill-defined, hypoechoic lesion *(arrows)* in the posteromedial aspect of the right kidney.
B. Contrast-enhanced CT shows a low-attenuated abscess *(arrows)* in the right kidney. Note fluid collection *(arrowheads)* in the perirenal space adjacent to the renal abscess.

6. Emphysematous Pyelonephritis

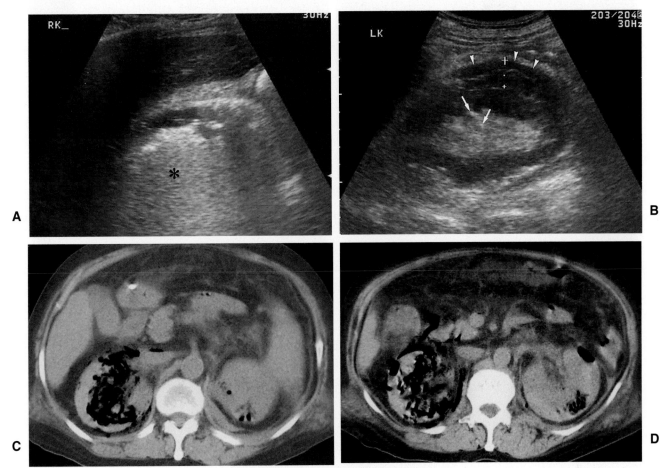

Fig. 1. Bilateral emphysematous pyelonephritis in a 80-year-old woman with diabetes.
A. Longitudinal US of the right kidney shows poor delineation of the right kidney due to dense echoes accompanying posterior sonic shadowing *(asterisk)* due to gas in the kidney. **B.** Longitudinal US of the left kidney shows perirenal fluid collection *(arrowheads)* and small, dense echoes *(arrows)* in the kidney representing gas. **C, D.** Nonenhanced CT scans show extensive gas collection in the parenchyma of both kidneys and perirenal spaces.

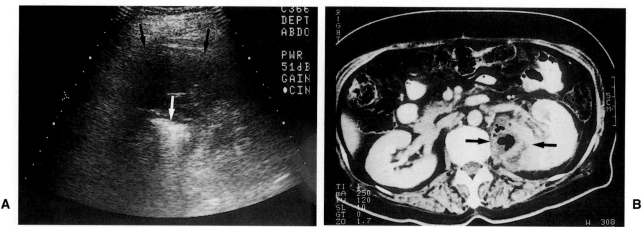

Fig. 2. Emphysematous pyelonephritis in a 60-year-old woman with diabetes.
A. On longitudinal US, the left kidney is swollen and hypoechoic *(black arrows)*. Note a dense echo *(white arrow)* with dirty sonic shadowing representing intrarenal gas. **B.** Contrast-enhanced CT shows an ill-defined, low-attenuated lesion *(arrows)* that contains mottled gas in the left kidney.

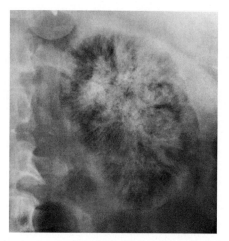

Fig. 3. Emphysematous pyelonephritis. Plain radiograph of the abdomen shows characteristic streaks of gas radiating from the center to the periphery of the kidney. A thin crescent of subcapsular gas is also present. No gas is visible in the pyelocalyceal system. (From Talner LB: Imaging in acute renal infection. In Syllabus for RSNA Categorical Course in Genitourinary Radiology. Oak Brook, Ill, Radiological Society of North America, 1994, pp 39–48.)

7. Pyonephrosis

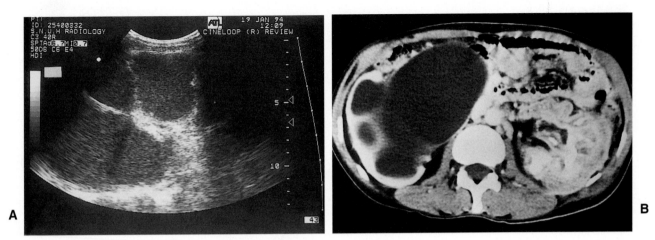

Fig. 1. Pyonephrosis in a 37-year-old woman with renal tuberculosis.
A. US of the right kidney shows markedly dilated calyces filled with echogenic debris. **B.** Contrast-enhanced CT shows markedly dilated pelvocalyces of the right kidney. Also note the deformed and calcified left kidney due to tuberculosis.

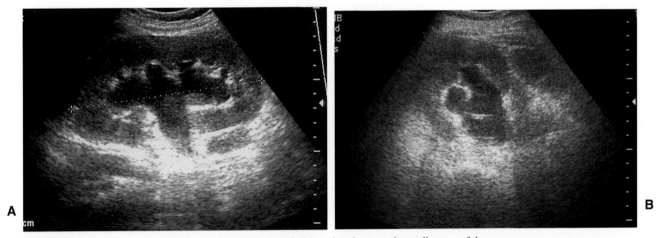

Fig. 2. Pyonephrosis in a 45-year-old woman with bilateral ureteral obstruction due to a giant cell tumor of the sacrum.
A, B. Longitudinal (**A**) and transverse (**B**) US of the right kidney shows echogenic debris in dependent portion of the dilated pelvocalyces.

8. Chronic Pyelonephritis

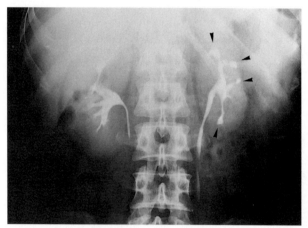

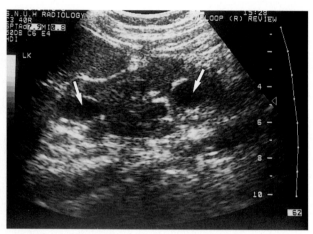

Fig. 1. Chronic pyelonephritis in a 40-year-old woman. IVU shows small left kidney with parenchymal scars *(arrowheads)*. Note clubbing of the calyces adjacent to the parenchymal scars.

Fig. 2. Chronic pyelonephritis in a 35-year-old woman with neurogenic bladder. Longitudinal US of the left kidney shows dilated calyces *(arrows)* in the upper and lower poles with thinning of overlying renal parenchyma.

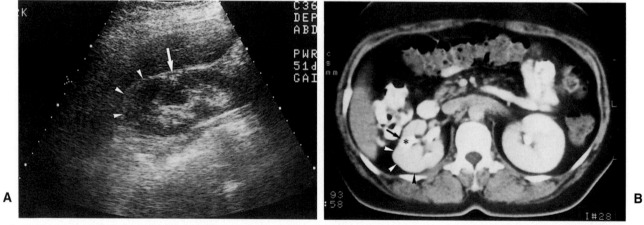

Fig. 3. Chronic pyelonephritis in a 50-year-old woman.
A. Longitudinal US of the right kidney shows an echogenic scar of the renal parenchyma *(arrow)* and focal compensatory hypertrophy in the upper pole *(arrowheads)*. **B.** Contrast-enhanced CT shows focal thinning of the renal parenchyma *(arrow)* with clubbing of the adjacent calyx *(asterisk)*. Note hypertrophied parenchyma due to compensatory hypertrophy *(arrowheads)* that may mimic a tumor.

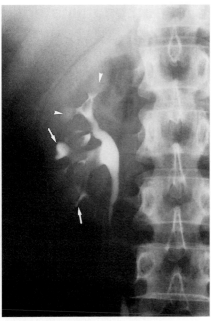

Fig. 4. Chronic pyelonephritis with echogenic parenchymal scar in a 43-year-old woman. **A.** Longitudinal US of the right kidney shows loss of normal renal parenchyma replaced by echogenic scars *(arrows)* in the interpolar and lower-polar regions of the kidney. Note that the lower-polar lesion may mimic an echogenic tumor such as angiomyolipoma. **B.** IVU reveals surface indentation and blunted calyces *(arrows)* in the interpolar and lower-polar regions of the right kidney. Note normal papillary blush in the upper pole *(arrowheads).*

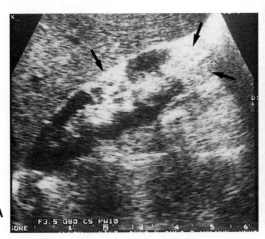

Fig. 5. A 41-year-old woman with chronic pyelonephritis due to vesicoureteral reflux to the lower moiety of duplicated urinary system.
A. IVU shows faint opacification of the lower pole of the duplicated right kidney where renal parenchyma is thinned *(arrows)*, producing a "nubbin sign." **B.** VCU shows vesicoureteral reflux to the lower-moiety urinary tract *(arrows)* with calyceal blunting *(arrowheads).* **C.** Longitudinal US of the right kidney shows thinned renal parenchyma with increased echogenicity in the lower half of the right kidney *(arrows).*

9. Xanthogranulomatous Pyelonephritis

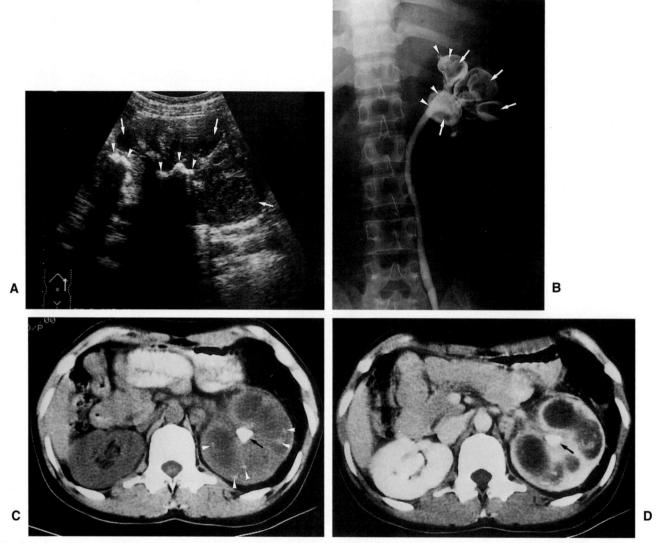

Fig. 1. Xanthogranulomatous pyelonephritis in a 36-year-old woman.
A. Longitudinal US of the left kidney shows enlarged kidney with dilated calyces *(arrows)* filled with heterogeneous echogenic material. There are large stones *(arrowheads)* in the renal pelvis and upper-polar calyx. **B.** RGP shows dilated calyces with filling defects *(arrows)*. Note the stones *(arrowheads)* in the renal pelvis and upper-pole calyx. **C, D.** Nonenhanced **(C)** and contrast-enhanced **(D)** CT scans show an enlarged left kidney and dilated calyces filled with low-attenuated material and small calcifications *(arrowheads* in **C)**. Note a large stone in the renal pelvis *(arrow)*.

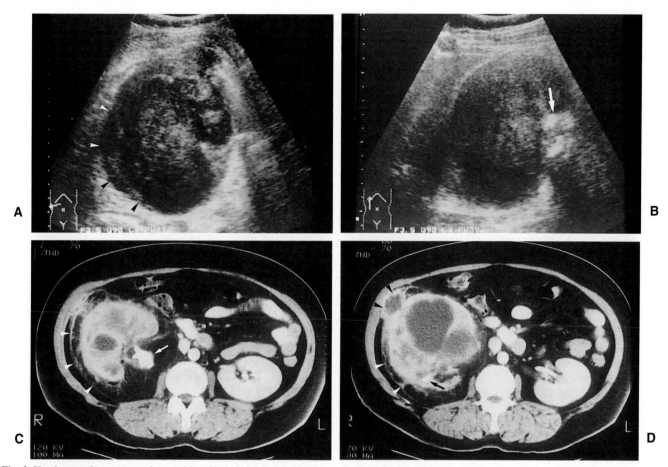

Fig. 2. Xanthogranulomatous pyelonephritis with perinephric extension in a 40-year-old woman.
A, B. US of the right kidney in transverse (**A**) and longitudinal (**B**) planes shows enlarged kidney and dilated calyces filled with heterogeneous echogenic material. Note a stone in the renal pelvis (*arrow* in **B**) and perirenal extension of the lesion (*arrowheads* in **A**). **C, D.** Contrast-enhanced CT scans show enlarged right kidney and dilated calyces. There are stones in the renal pelvis (*white arrow* in **C**) and calyx (*black arrow* in **D**). Note perirenal extension of the lesion (*black arrowheads* in **D**) and streaky perirenal infiltration and thickening of the renal fasciae *(white arrowheads)*.

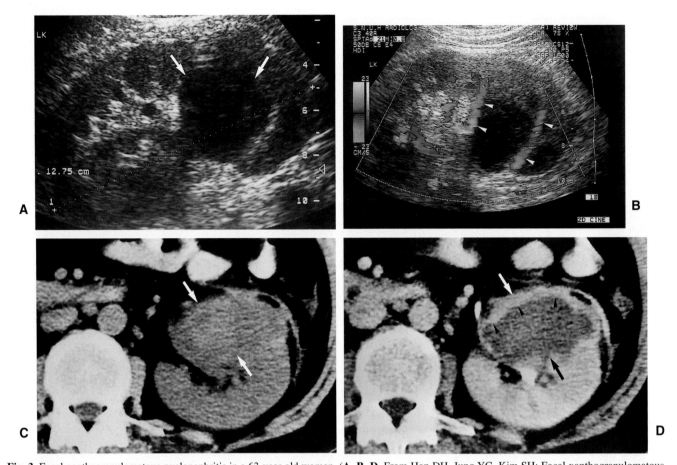

Fig. 3. Focal xanthogranulomatous pyelonephritis in a 63-year-old woman. (**A, B, D,** From Han DH, Jung YG, Kim SH: Focal xanthogranulomatous pyelonephritis: Report of two cases. Korean J Radiol Soc 1996; 35:113–116.)
A. Longitudinal US of the left kidney shows a round hypoechoic lesion *(arrows)* in the lower pole. **B.** Color Doppler US shows stretched vessels *(arrowheads)* around the lesion, but there is no flow signal within the lesion. (**B,** See also Color Section.) **C, D.** Nonenhanced (**C**) and contrast-enhanced (**D**) CT scans show an ill-defined lesion in the anterior aspect of the left kidney *(arrows)*. The lesion has a slightly higher attenuation than the noninvolved kidney on nonenhanced CT and has low attenuation with a thick rim *(arrowheads* in **D**) on contrast-enhanced CT.

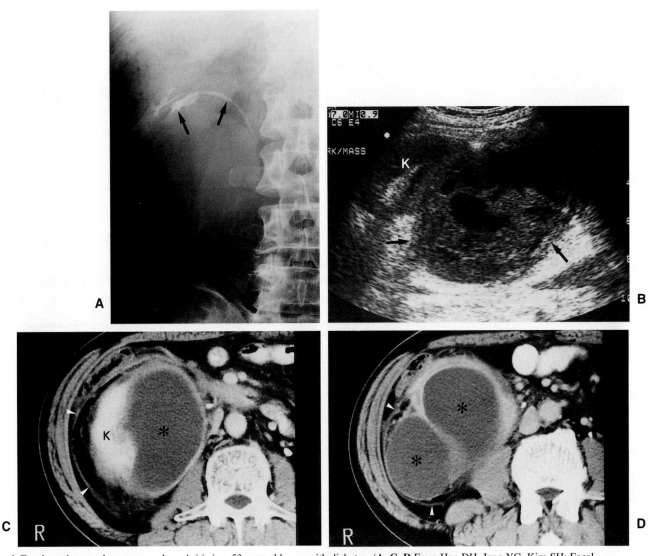

Fig. 4. Focal xanthogranulomatous pyelonephritis in a 53-year-old man with diabetes. (**A, C, D** From Han DH, Jung YG, Kim SH: Focal xanthogranulomatous pyelonephritis: Report of two cases. Korean J Radiol Soc 1996; 35:113–116.)
A. IVU shows right pelvocalyceal system and proximal ureter *(arrows)* displaced upward by a large mass. **B.** Longitudinal US shows a large mass of heterogeneous echogenicity *(arrows)* caudal to the right kidney (K). **C, D.** Contrast-enhanced CT scans show exophytic, thick-walled, low-attenuated, nonenhancing mass *(asterisks)* in the caudal and medial aspect of the right kidney (K). Note thickened renal fasciae *(arrowheads)*.

10. Malacoplakia

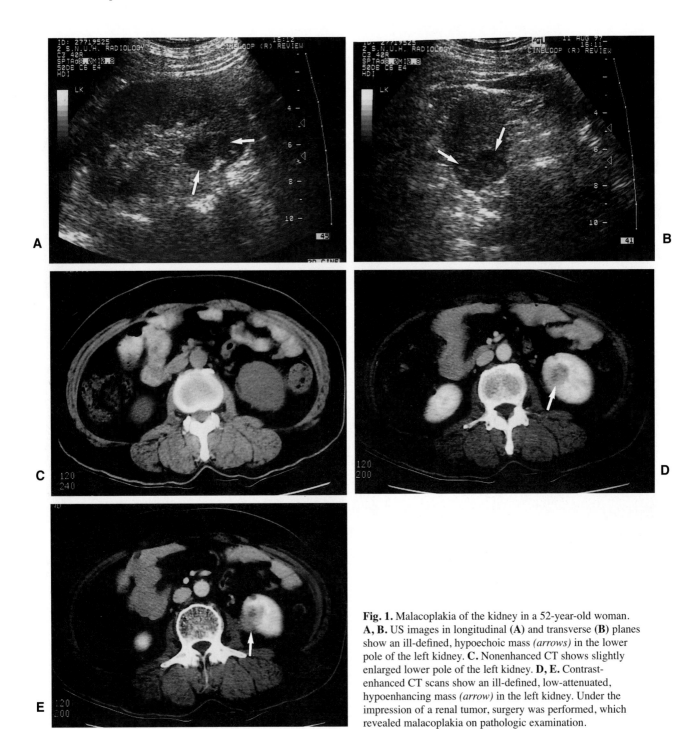

Fig. 1. Malacoplakia of the kidney in a 52-year-old woman. **A, B.** US images in longitudinal (**A**) and transverse (**B**) planes show an ill-defined, hypoechoic mass *(arrows)* in the lower pole of the left kidney. **C.** Nonenhanced CT shows slightly enlarged lower pole of the left kidney. **D, E.** Contrast-enhanced CT scans show an ill-defined, low-attenuated, hypoenhancing mass *(arrow)* in the left kidney. Under the impression of a renal tumor, surgery was performed, which revealed malacoplakia on pathologic examination.

11. Fungal Infection

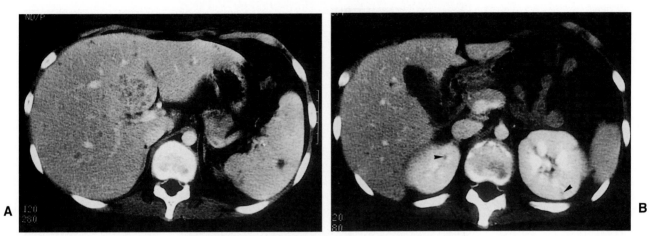

Fig. 1. Candidiasis involving the kidneys, liver, and spleen in a 20-year-old man.
A, B. Contrast-enhanced CT scans show multiple, tiny, low-attenuated lesions in the liver, spleen, and both kidneys (*arrowheads* in **B**) representing microabscesses caused by *Candida* infection.

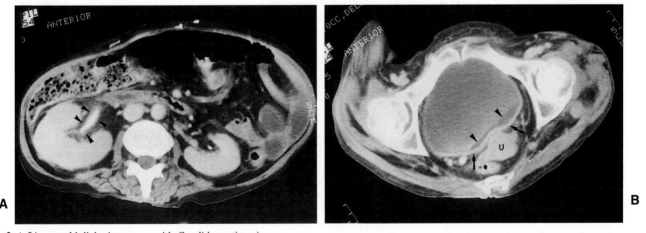

Fig. 2. A 54-year-old diabetic woman with *Candida* septicemia.
A. Contrast-enhanced CT scan shows enlarged right kidney and diffuse thickening of the wall of the renal pelvis *(arrowheads)*. **B.** CT scan of the pelvic cavity shows a thickened bladder wall *(arrows)* and debris layered in the dependent portion of the bladder *(arrowheads)*. U, uterus.

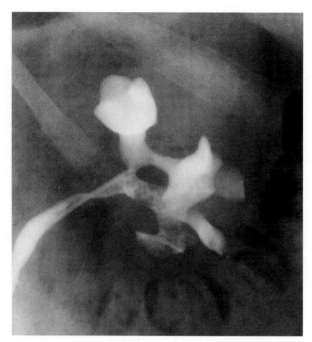

Fig. 3. *Candida* fungus ball. RGP shows irregular filling defects in the renal pelvis and lower calyces. The patient had received antibiotics for several months following left pyelolithotomy for a staghorn stone. (From Talner LB: Imaging in acute renal infection. In Syllabus for RSNA Categorical Course in Genitourinary Radiology. Oak Brook, Ill, Radiological Society of North America, 1994, pp 39–48.)

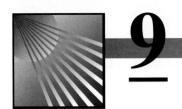

9

Urogenital Tuberculosis

SEUNG HYUP KIM

Nearly 15% to 20% of all new cases of tuberculosis involve sites outside the lung, and approximately 30% of cases of extrapulmonary tuberculosis involve the urogenital tract. The initial manifestations of urogenital tuberculosis occur most commonly in the 20- to 50-year age group with a slight male predominance. Fewer than 5% of patients with urogenital tuberculosis have concomitant active pulmonary tuberculosis, and only 30% to 50% have evidence of a lung abnormality on chest radiographs. Recent resurgence of tuberculosis is related to the spread of human immunodeficiency virus infection and acquired immunodeficiency syndrome. The risk of urogenital tuberculosis is also increased in patients who received intravesical bacillus Calmette-Guérin therapy for transitional cell carcinoma of the urinary bladder.

PATHOPHYSIOLOGY

The kidneys are thought to be inoculated with *Mycobacterium tuberculosis* at the time of the initial pulmonary infection. The bacilli are trapped in the periglomerular capillaries and cause formation of numerous small abscesses in both kidneys. If cellular immunity of the host is intact, the organisms stay confined to the cortex with subsequent formation of multiple small healed granulomas.

When host immunity is compromised, reactivation may occur. Initial cortical foci reactivate with extension of the lesions down the loops of Henle to the renal pyramids. The disease is often unilateral and tends to be polar. The papillary foci caseate and cavitate, producing ulcerocavernous lesions of papillary necrosis with subsequent rupture into the calyceal system. Then the disease spreads distally by seeding through the urothelial submucosa and the lymphatics to the infundibula, renal pelvis, ureter, and urinary bladder. The uroepithelium becomes inflamed and ulcerated, and multiple tiny granulomas form in the mucosa and submucosa.

During the healing phase, fibrosis and secondary obstruction can destroy additional renal tissue. Depending on the location of obstruction and the amount of collecting system isolated, considerable renal damage may occur. Massive parenchymal destruction may produce large coalescent granulomas containing caseous or calcific material. If the hydronephrotic kidney becomes nonfunctioning, extensive dystrophic calcification may form a cast of the kidney, referred to as an *autonephrectomized kidney*. Perirenal and pararenal extension may create fistulas to the skin or gastrointestinal tract.

IMAGING

Imaging studies neither confirm nor exclude the presence of urinary tract tuberculosis. Early findings are best detected on intravenous urography (IVU) or retrograde pyelography (RGP). Ultrasonography (US), computed tomography (CT), and magnetic resonance (MR) imaging do not have spatial resolution to demonstrate minor papillary and urothelial changes that are features of early renal tuberculosis. Late or chronic changes are optimally evaluated with US and CT, especially when the kidneys are nonvisualized at IVU. CT is the best imaging study to evaluate the extent of retroperitoneal involvement and involvement of other organs.

RENAL TUBERCULOSIS

During the initial stage of dissemination, cortical lesions, unless calcified, are usually too small to be imaged. During the early stage of reactivation, US or CT may reveal the lesions, with CT being more sensitive than US. When a calyx is involved, we may notice a slight loss of sharpness of the calyx, which probably represents mucosal edema. Progressive enlargement of the tuberculoma and its caseation and rupture into the adjacent calyx result in an irregular cavity with resultant findings of renal papillary necrosis. It has been suggested that the erosion of the papillae from tuberculosis is more ragged and irregular than that from other causes of papillary necrosis. If appropriate antituberculous medication is given in the early stage of the disease, only slight calyceal deformity or minor parenchymal scars may be formed.

Involvement of the calyceal infundibulum and renal pelvis begins with mucosal tubercles and ulcerations and then progresses to fibrosis with infundibular narrowing and scarring of the renal pelvis, resulting in uneven caliectasis. When a dilated or diseased calyx is not opacified on IVU, it is referred to as a "phantom calyx."

Renal tuberculosis may spread into the perirenal area and cause an extrarenal tuberculous abscess, which may in turn cause fistulous communication with other retroperitoneal or intraperitoneal organs or even may drain spontaneously to the skin or bowel.

URETERAL TUBERCULOSIS

Ureteral involvement with tuberculosis is rarely found in the absence of more severe renal changes. Mucosal nodules and

ulceration occur with thickening of the ureteral wall, fibrosis, and calcification. The earliest changes most commonly occur distally. The ureter is dilated initially, but later it becomes strictured and eventually forms a straight, rigid tube. The process of destruction followed by fibrotic healing causes the characteristic beaded, corkscrew, or pipe-stem appearance of the ureter. The ureterovesical orifice may become gaping, leading to reflux from the bladder. Renal damage secondary to urinary tract obstruction may be more severe than the effect of the original parenchymal involvement.

The fibrosis causing the strictures represents healing of tuberculous ulcerations, and this may also develop during appropriate chemotherapy. Early scarring may be reversible by steroid therapy, but late fibrotic strictures are irreversible with medical treatment. Dilation and stenting of ureteral strictures may regain or retain ureteral patency and salvage a kidney. We found that antegrade dilation of the urinary tract combined with ureteral stenting is an effective technique for the management of tuberculous strictures of the urinary tract.

TUBERCULOSIS OF URINARY BLADDER AND URETHRA

Cystitis develops in about one third of patients with tuberculosis of the upper urinary tract, usually late in the course of the disease. Coalescence of mucosal tubercles produces superficial ulcerations that are usually shallow and irregular with undermined edges. If untreated, the inflammation progresses to involve the muscularis layer, and mural fibrosis causes the bladder to become markedly thickened and contracted. A faint, irregular rim or nodular calcification may outline the bladder wall. Urethral tuberculosis is uncommon and usually occurs secondary to prostatic or renal infection. It may result in nonspecific stricture, fistula, and urinary incontinence.

MALE GENITAL TUBERCULOSIS

The epididymis and prostate are the most common sites for tuberculous involvement of the male genital tract. Epididymal infection can occur from hematogenous seeding, lymphatic spread, or retrograde canalicular spread via the vas deferens. In tuberculous epididymitis, US shows an enlarged epididymis with heterogeneous echogenicity, often predominantly in the tail portion. US findings of associated testicular involvement consist of a diffusely enlarged hypoechoic testis, multiple intratesticular hypoechoic nodules, ill-defined focal intratesticular hypoechoic areas, or an irregular margin between the testis and epididymis.

Prostatic tuberculosis appears as focal areas of nonspecific changes of echogenicity, attenuation, and signal intensity on US, CT, and MR imaging, respectively. In early stage of prostate tuberculosis, the lesion appears as a well-demarcated hypoechoic lesion that mimics prostate cancer. Later the lesion may become contracted and calcified. Seminal vesicles and vas deferens involved with tuberculosis may demonstrate internal debris, wall thickening, contraction, or calcification.

FEMALE GENITAL TUBERCULOSIS

In women, genital tuberculosis is an important cause of infertility and often occurs without urinary tract involvement.

Although the usual route of infection is hematogenous from pulmonary foci, lymphatic spread from peritoneal implants or direct extension from an intestinal lesion may be the source. The fallopian tubes are most frequently involved, resulting in multiple strictures, hydrosalpinx, pyosalpinx, or calcifications. Rupture of a tuberculous pyosalpinx into an adherent intestine may cause tubointestinal fistula. Tubal patency is preserved in about half of patients, but normal salpingograms are rare. Tuberculosis is most likely when calcified pelvic or mesenteric lymph nodes are associated with bilaterally occluded, rigid tubes. The ovary may be involved by direct extension of a tubal lesion, resulting in tubo-ovarian mass, which may also contain adherent omentum and intestine. Uterine endometrium is involved in 50% of patients who have tubal tuberculosis. Endometrial tuberculosis results in a shrunken cavity due to intrauterine adhesions and intravasation of contrast material on hysterosalpingography.

PERITONEAL TUBERCULOSIS

Peritoneal tuberculosis is often associated with female genital tuberculosis. On CT, free or loculated ascitic fluid is commonly seen that may have high attenuation. Strands or fine septa and debris within the fluid are characteristic but are better appreciated on US. On CT, the peritoneum is diffusely thickened. Omental thickening or mesenteric infiltration may be associated.

Similar imaging findings may be seen in peritoneal carcinomatosis. On CT, smoothly thickened peritoneum and pronounced enhancement suggest tuberculous peritonitis, whereas nodular implants and irregular peritoneal thickening suggest peritoneal carcinomatosis.

References

1. Kim SH: Urogenital tuberculosis. In Pollack HM, McClennan BL (eds): Clinical Urography, 2nd ed, vol 1. Philadelphia, WB Saunders, 2000, pp 1193–1228.
2. Moon MH, Seong CK, Lee KH, et al: BCG-induced granulomatous prostatitis: A case report. J Korean Radiol Soc 2000; 42:675–677.
3. Yang DM, Chang MS, Oh YH, et al: Chronic tuberculous epididymitis: Color Doppler US findings with histopathologic correlation. Abdom Imaging 2000; 25:559–562.
4. Naik KS, Carey BM: The transrectal ultrasound and MRI appearances of granulomatous prostatitis and its differentiation from carcinoma. Clin Radiol 1999; 54:173–175.
5. Ravery V, de la Taille A, Hoffmann P, et al: Balloon catheter dilatation in the treatment of ureteral and ureteroenteric stricture. J Endourol 1998; 12:335–340.
6. Chung JJ, Kim MJ, Lee T, et al: Sonographic findings in tuberculous epididymitis and epididymo-orchitis. J Clin Ultrasound 1997; 25:390–394.
7. Crowley JJ, Ramji FG, Amundson GM: Genital tract tuberculosis with peritoneal involvement: MR appearance. Abdom Imaging 1997; 22:445–447.
8. Jadvar H, Mindelzun RE, Olcott EW, et al: Still the great mimicker: Abdominal tuberculosis. AJR Am J Roentgenol 1997; 168:1455–1460.
9. Terris MK, Macy M, Freiha FS: Transrectal ultrasound appearance of prostatic granulo mas secondary to bacillus Calmette-Guérin instillation. J Urol 1997; 158:126–127.
10. Demirkazik FB, Akhan O, Oezmen N, et al: US and CT findings in the diagnosis of tuberculous peritonitis. Acta Radiol 1996; 37:517–520.
11. Ha HK, Jung JI, Lee MS, et al: CT differentiation of tuberculous peritonitis and peritoneal carcinomatosis. AJR Am J Roentgenol 1996; 167:743–748.
12. Rodriguez E, Pombo F: Peritoneal tuberculosis versus peritoneal carcinomatosis: Distinction based on CT findings. J Comput Assist Tomogr 1996; 20:269–272.

13. Wasserman NF: Inflammatory diseases of the ureter. Radiol Clin North Am 1996; 34:1131–1156.
14. Kim SH, Kim SH, Kim WH: Imaging makes progress in urinary tract tuberculosis. Diagn Imaging Asia Pacific 1995; 2:22–28.
15. Kim SH, Yoon HK, Park JH, et al: Tuberculous stricture of the urinary tract: Antegrade balloon dilation and ureteral stenting. Abdom Imaging 1993; 18:186–190.
16. Kim SH, Pollack HM, Cho KS, et al: Tuberculous epididymitis and epididymo-orchitis: Sonographic findings. J Urol 1993; 150:81–84.
17. Asch MR, Toi A: Seminal vesicles: Imaging and intervention using transrectal ultrasound. J Ultrasound Med 1991; 10:19–23.
18. Birnbaum BA, Friedman JP, Lubat E, et al: Extrarenal genitourinary tuberculosis: CT appearance of calcified pipe-stem ureter and seminal vesicle abscess. J Comput Assist Tomogr 1990; 14:653–655.
19. Kenny PJ: Imaging of chronic renal infections. AJR Am J Roentgenol 1990; 155:485–494.
20. Becker JA: Renal tuberculosis. Urol Radiol 1988; 10:25–30.

Illustrations • Urogenital Tuberculosis

1 • Renal tuberculosis: initial dissemination and healed granulomas

2 • Renal tuberculosis: early reactivation demonstrated on US and CT

3 • Renal tuberculosis: early IVU findings

4 • Renal tuberculosis: healing with scar formation

5 • Renal tuberculosis: extensive destruction

6 • Renal tuberculosis: a cause of papillary necrosis

7 • Renal tuberculosis: infundibular narrowing and pelvic contraction

8 • Renal tuberculosis: uneven caliectasis

9 • Renal tuberculosis: evolution of infundibular narrowing and pelvic contraction

10 • Renal tuberculosis: phantom calyx

11 • Renal tuberculosis: hiked-up pelvis

12 • Renal tuberculosis: calcified

13 • Renal tuberculosis: calcified autonephrectomy

14 • Renal tuberculosis: US-guided aspiration

15 • Ureteral tuberculosis

16 • Ureteral tuberculosis with vesicoureteral reflux

17 • Ureteral tuberculosis: percutaneous ureteroplasty

18 • Bladder tuberculosis: early changes

19 • Bladder tuberculosis: late changes

20 • Urethral tuberculosis

21 • Tuberculous epididymitis and epididymo-orchitis

22 • Tuberculosis of the prostate and seminal tracts

23 • Tuberculosis of the retroperitoneum and lymph nodes

24 • Peritoneal tuberculosis

1. Renal Tuberculosis: Initial Dissemination and Healed Granulomas

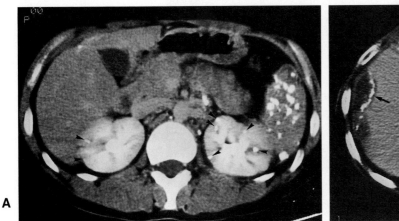
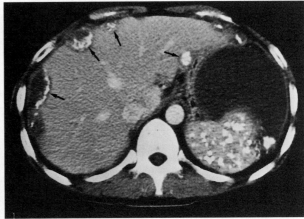

Fig 1. Calcified, healed renal granulomas in a 23-year-old woman with a history of pulmonary tuberculosis.
A. CT scan at the level of kidneys shows multiple tiny nodular calcifications *(arrowheads)* in both kidneys, suggesting calcified cortical granulomas that were formed in the initial stage of dissemination. Also note calcifications in the spleen and lymph nodes. (**A,** From Kim SH, Kim SH, Kim WH: Imaging makes progress in urinary tract tuberculosis. Diagn Imaging Asia Pacific 1995; 2:22–28.) **B.** CT scan at the level cranial to **A** shows low-attenuated lesions with calcification in the peripheral portion of the liver *(arrows)*. Also note mottled, dense calcifications in the spleen. (**B,** From Kim SH: Urogenital tuberculosis. In Pollack HM, McClennan BL [eds]: Clinical Urography, 2nd ed, vol 1. Philadelphia, WB Saunders, 2000, pp 1193–1228.)

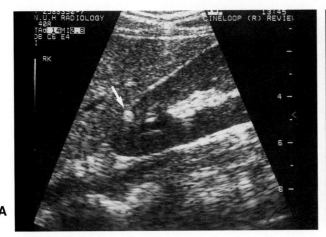
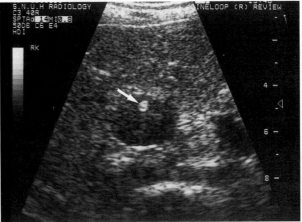

Fig 2. Healed renal granuloma in a 31-year-old man with history of pulmonary tuberculosis.
A, B. Longitudinal (**A**) and transverse (**B**) US images of the right kidney show a small, echogenic lesion in the peripheral cortex *(arrow)*, which is probably a healed tuberculous granuloma.

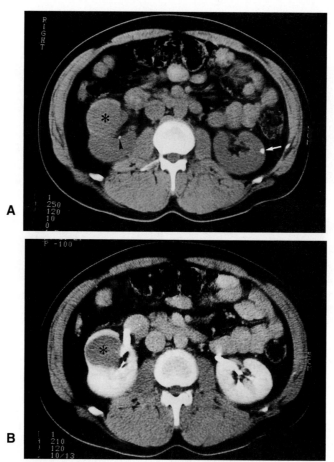

Fig 3. Calcified, healed renal granuloma in a 33-year-old man.
A, B. Nonenhanced (**A**) and contrast-enhanced (**B**) CT scans show a
round, calcified nodule in the peripheral cortex of the left kidney (*arrow*
in **A**). Right kidney has a dilated calyx *(asterisk)* due to renal
tuberculosis. Also note a small calcification in a papillary region of the
right kidney (*arrowhead* in **A**).

2. Renal Tuberculosis: Early Reactivation Demonstrated on US and CT

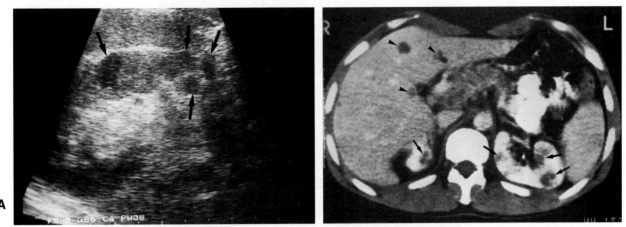

Fig 1. Early reactivation tuberculosis in a 39-year-old man with mild fever for several days. (**A, B,** From Kim SH, Kim SH, Kim WH: Imaging makes progress in urinary tract tuberculosis. Diagn Imaging Asia Pacific 1995; 2:22–28.)
A. US shows multiple small hypoechoic cortical nodules *(arrows)* in the right kidney. **B.** Contrast-enhanced CT shows multiple, low-attenuated nodules in both kidneys *(arrows)* and liver *(arrowheads)*. US-guided aspiration of the hepatic lesion demonstrated acid-fast bacilli.

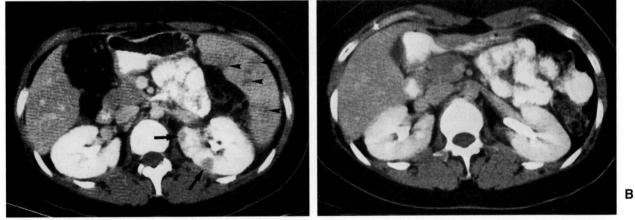

Fig 2. Early reactivation tuberculosis in a 19-year-old woman with miliary tuberculosis of the lung, tuberculous meningitis, and tuberculous chorioretinitis. (**A, B,** From Kim SH: Urogenital tuberculosis. In Pollack HM, McClennan BL [eds]: Clinical Urography, 2nd ed, vol 1. Philadelphia, WB Saunders, 2000, pp 1193–1228.)
A. Contrast-enhanced CT shows multiple, round, low-attenuated lesions in left renal cortex *(arrows)* and spleen *(arrowheads)*. **B.** Follow-up CT scan taken 18 months after antituberculous medication shows complete disappearance of the renal and splenic lesions. The spleen is not shown due to decreased size.

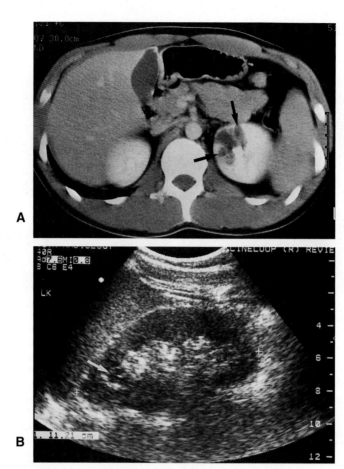

Fig. 3. Early reactivation tuberculosis in a 15-year-old male patient with positive acid-fast bacilli in sputum and urine. Renal lesion was demonstrated on CT but not on US. (**A, B,** From Kim SH: Urogenital tuberculosis. In Pollack HM, McClennan BL [eds]: Clinical Urography, 2nd ed, vol 1. Philadelphia, WB Saunders, 2000, pp 1193–1228.) **A.** Contrast-enhanced CT scan shows well-defined, irregular, low-attenuated lesion in the upper pole of the left kidney *(arrows)*. **B.** The lesion is not demonstrated on US and barely distorts the renal sinus echo in the upper pole *(arrow)*.

3. Renal Tuberculosis: Early IVU Findings

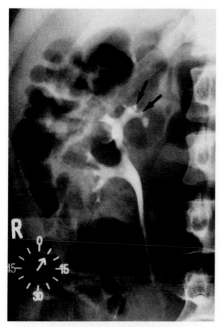

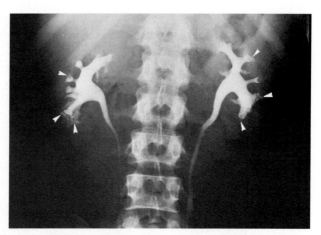

Fig. 2. Renal tuberculosis mimicking medullary sponge kidney in a 19-year-old man with positive urine acid-fast bacilli. IVU shows an irregular margin of the calyces with papillary cavities in both kidneys *(arrowheads)*. (From Kim SH: Urogenital tuberculosis. In Pollack HM, McClennan BL [eds]: Clinical Urography, 2nd ed, vol 1. Philadelphia, WB Saunders, 2000, pp 1193–1228.)

Fig. 1. Earliest IVU finding of renal tuberculosis in a 25-year-old man with tuberculosis of the kidney and epididymis. A 5-minute IVU shows irregular and moth-eaten appearance of the upper pole calyx of the right kidney *(arrows)*. (From Kim SH, Kim SH, Kim WH: Imaging makes progress in urinary tract tuberculosis. Diagn Imaging Asia Pacific 1995; 2:22–28.)

4. Renal Tuberculosis: Healing with Scar Formation

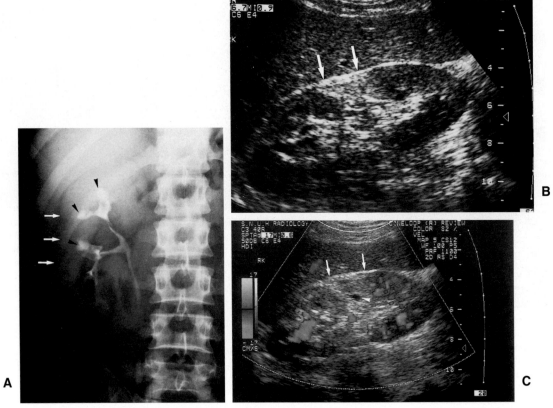

Fig. 1. Parenchymal fibrous scar caused by sequelae of renal tuberculosis in a 33-year-old man. (**A, C,** From Kim SH: Urogenital tuberculosis. In Pollack HM, McClennan BL [eds]: Clinical Urography, 2nd ed, vol 1. Philadelphia, WB Saunders, 2000, pp 1193–1228.)
A. IVU shows calyceal deformities caused by papillary cavities *(arrowheads)* and cortical scarring *(arrows)* in the right kidney. **B.** US shows increased parenchymal echogenicity in the interpolar area of the right kidney *(arrows)*. **C.** Color Doppler US shows decreased perfusion of the hyperechoic interpolar lesion *(arrow)* and a small cystic lesion representing a papillary cavity *(arrowhead)*. (**C,** See also Color Section.)

5. Renal Tuberculosis: Extensive Destruction

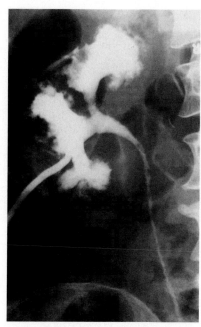

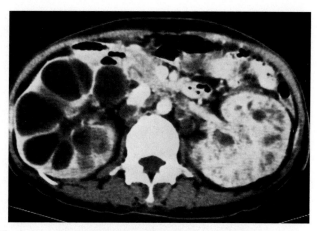

Fig. 2. Parenchymal destruction of left kidney due to tuberculosis in a 47-year-old woman. This patient also had pelvic contraction and caliectasis in the right kidney. Contrast-enhanced CT shows severe parenchymal destruction in the left kidney and severe caliectasis with contracted renal pelvis in the right kidney. (From Kim SH, Kim SH, Kim WH: Imaging makes progress in urinary tract tuberculosis. Diagn Imaging Asia Pacific 1995; 2:22–28.)

Fig. 1. Nonfunctioning left kidney and hydronephrotic right kidney in a 55-year-old woman. Percutaneous nephrostomy was performed on the right kidney, and nephrostogram shows severe irregularities of the calyces due to extensive papillary necrosis. Also note irregularities and fine nodularities along the renal pelvis and ureter. (From Kim SH, Kim SH, Kim WH: Imaging makes progress in urinary tract tuberculosis. Diagn Imaging Asia Pacific 1995; 2:22–28.)

6. Renal Tuberculosis: A Cause of Papillary Necrosis

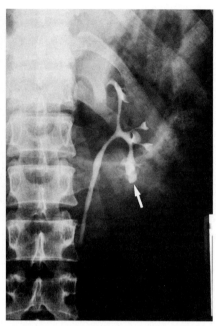

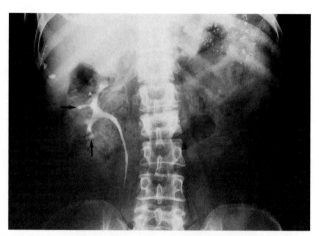

Fig. 2. Renal tuberculosis with findings of papillary necrosis in a 57-year-old woman. A 15-minute IVU shows papillary cavities in the interpolar and lower pole of the right kidney *(arrows)*. The left kidney was removed 10 years previously due to tuberculosis. Also note calcifications in the spleen. (From Kim SH: Urogenital tuberculosis. In Pollack HM, McClennan BL [eds]: Clinical Urography, 2nd ed, vol 1. Philadelphia, WB Saunders, 2000, pp 1193–1228.)

Fig. 1. Renal tuberculosis with findings of papillary necrosis in a 45-year-old man. A 5-minute IVU shows large papillary cavities in the lower pole of the left kidney *(arrow)*. (From Kim SH: Urogenital tuberculosis. In Pollack HM, McClennan BL [eds]: Clinical Urography, 2nd ed, vol 1. Philadelphia, WB Saunders, 2000, pp 1193–1228.)

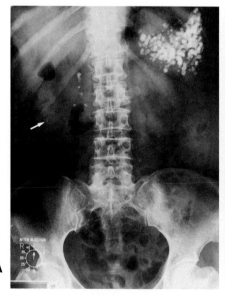

A

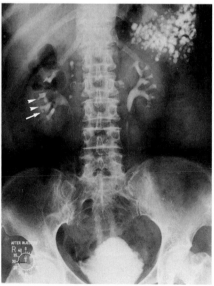

B

Fig. 3. Renal tuberculosis with papillary necrosis and calcification in situ in a 60-year-old woman.
A. Plain radiograph shows multiple calcifications in the spleen, paravertebral region, and right renal area *(arrow)*. **B.** A 30-minute IVU shows multiple papillary cavities in both kidneys. Note a small calcification in a papillary cavity of the right kidney *(arrow)*. Also note lesions of papillary necrosis due to tuberculosis *(arrowheads)*.

7. Renal Tuberculosis: Infundibular Narrowing and Pelvic Contraction

Fig. 1. Contracted renal pelvis with calcification in a 24-year-old man.
A. Plain radiograph shows irregular calcifications *(arrow)* in the left renal area.
B. A 15-minute IVU shows contracted renal pelvis and narrowed infundibula with calcifications.

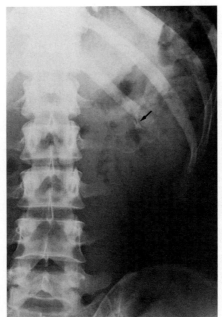

A

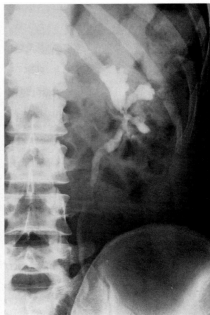

B

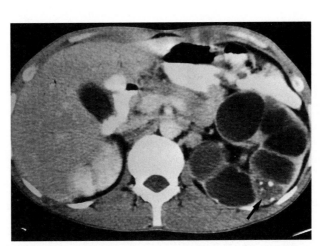

Fig. 2. Dilated calyces and contracted renal pelvis in a 24-year-old man with tuberculosis involving the left kidney, ureter, prostate, and seminal vesicles. Contrast-enhanced CT shows markedly dilated calyces with thinned parenchyma of the left kidney due to contracted renal pelvis and infundibular stenoses. Also note mottled calcifications in a calyx *(arrow)*.

8. Renal Tuberculosis: Uneven Caliectasis

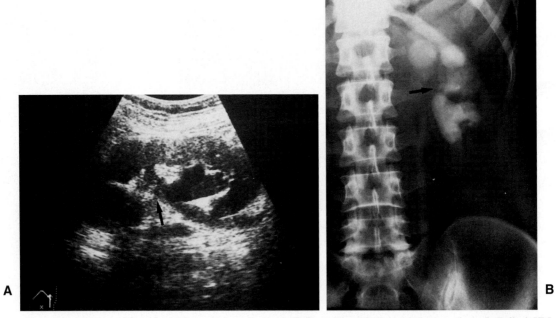

Fig. 1. Uneven caliectasis in a 36-year-old woman with renal tuberculosis. (**A, B,** From Kim SH: Urogenital tuberculosis. In Pollack HM, McClennan BL [eds]: Clinical Urography, 2nd ed, vol 1. Philadelphia, WB Saunders, 2000, pp 1193–1228.)
A. US shows marked calyceal dilation with parenchymal loss in the upper-pole area, relatively preserved interpolar area, moderate caliectasis in the lower-pole area, and contracted renal pelvis *(arrow)*. **B.** IVU shows diffuse calyceal dilation due to infundibular stenoses and contracted pelvis *(arrow)*.

9. Renal Tuberculosis: Evolution of Infundibular Narrowing and Pelvic Contraction

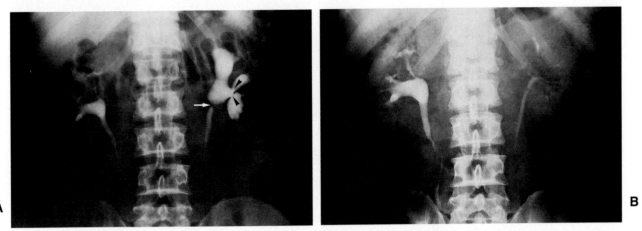

Fig. 1. Markedly improved infundibular stenosis and pelvic contraction after antituberculous medication in a 50-year-old man.
A. IVU shows narrowing of the infundibula *(arrowheads)* and ureteropelvic junction *(arrow)* with dilation of the pelvocalyces. **B.** After treatment with antituberculous medication, follow-up IVU taken 3 years later shows marked improvement.

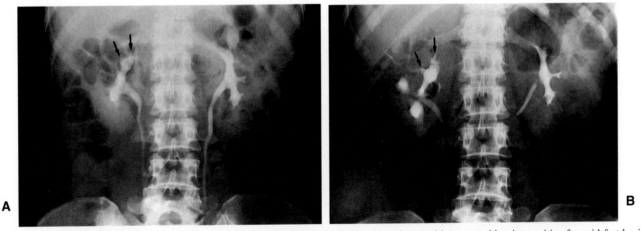

Fig. 2. Progression of pelvic contraction during a course of antituberculous medication in a 43-year-old woman with urine positive for acid-fast bacilli. **A.** IVU shows calyceal irregularities in the upper pole of the right kidney *(arrows)*. **B.** After treatment with antituberculous medication, follow-up IVU taken 6 months later shows marked progression of pelvic contraction and infundibular narrowing with calyceal dilation. Note findings of papillary necrosis in the upper-polar calyces *(arrows)*.

10. Renal Tuberculosis: Phantom Calyx

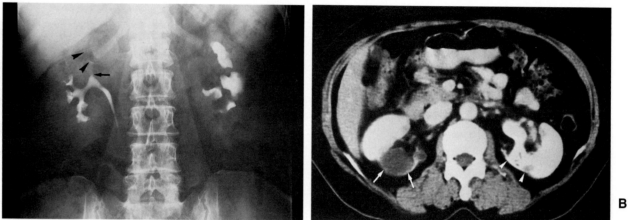

Fig. 1. Phantom calyx in a 61-year-old woman with bilateral renal tuberculosis.
A. IVU shows faint opacification of a dilated calyx *(arrowheads)* with infundibular obstruction *(arrow)* in the upper pole of the right kidney. Also note uneven caliectasis in the left kidney. (**A,** From Kim SH, Kim SH, Kim WH: Imaging makes progress in urinary tract tuberculosis. Diagn Imaging Asia Pacific 1995; 2:22–28.) **B.** Contrast-enhanced CT shows dilated, nonopacified, posterior calyx with calcified parenchymal rim *(arrows)*. Also note parenchymal loss in the left kidney due to tuberculosis *(arrowheads)*.

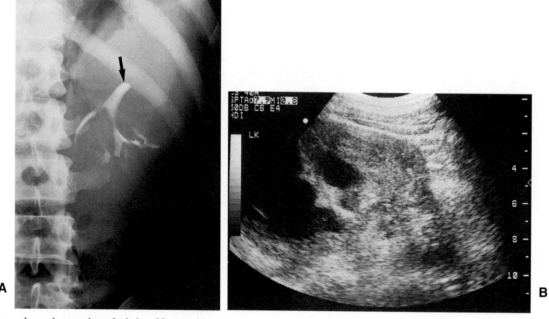

Fig. 2. Phantom calyces due to tuberculosis in a 22-year-old man.
A. Another patient with phantom calyx *(arrow)* in the upper pole of the left kidney. Note smooth margin of the amputated infundibulum. (**A,** From Kim SH: Urogenital tuberculosis. In Pollack HM, McClennan BL [eds]: Clinical Urography, 2nd ed, vol 1. Philadelphia, WB Saunders, 2000, pp 1193–1228.) **B.** US shows dilated upper pole calyces that were not opacified on IVU.

11. Renal Tuberculosis: Hiked-Up Pelvis

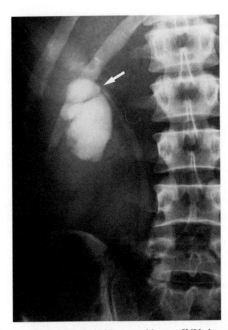

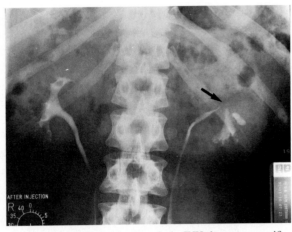

Fig. 2. A 30-year-old man with tuberculosis. IVU shows nonopacification of the upper-pole calyx and hiked-up appearance of the renal pelvis *(arrow)*.

Fig. 1. Hiked-up renal pelvis in a 32-year-old man. IVU shows narrowing and contraction of upper calyceal infundibulum, and renal pelvis with dilated lower pole calyx, causing hiked-up appearance of the renal pelvis *(arrow)*. (From Kim SH: Urogenital tuberculosis. In Pollack HM, McClennan BL [eds]: Clinical Urography, 2nd ed, vol 1. Philadelphia, WB Saunders, 2000, pp 1193–1228.)

12. Renal Tuberculosis: Calcified

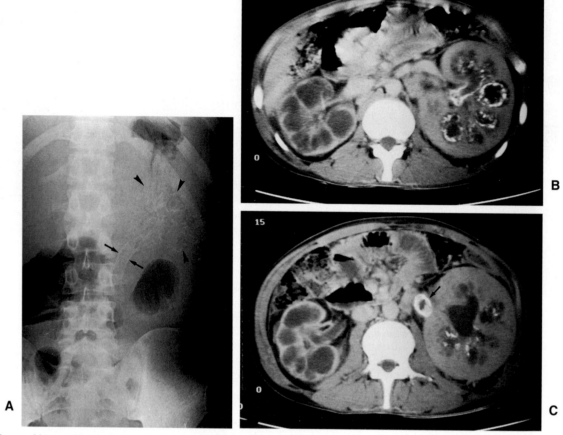

Fig. 1. A 45-year-old man with tuberculosis involving both kidneys and ureters.
A. Plain radiograph shows irregular branching calcifications in the left renal area *(arrowheads)* and tubular calcifications in the course of the left ureter *(arrows)*. **B.** Contrast-enhanced CT shows dilated calyces and contracted renal pelvis in both kidneys. Also note extensive calcifications along the inner margin of the dilated calyces in the left kidney. **C.** CT scan at lower level shows calcifications along the inner margin of the dilated calyces and ureter *(arrow)* on the left side. Also note infundibular stenosis and contracted pelvis due to tuberculosis in the right kidney.

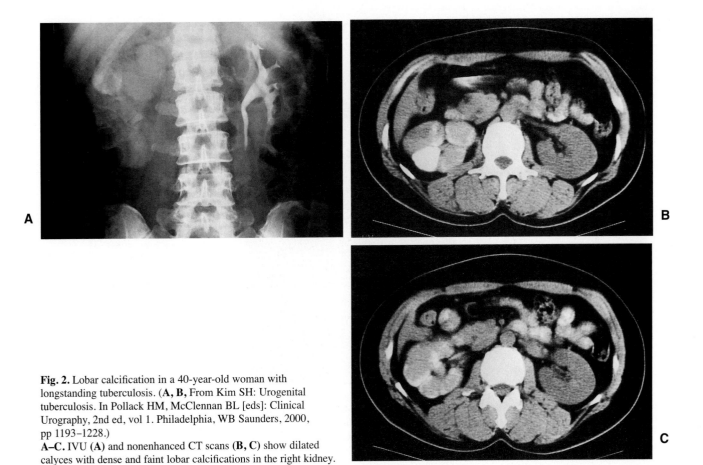

Fig. 2. Lobar calcification in a 40-year-old woman with longstanding tuberculosis. (**A, B,** From Kim SH: Urogenital tuberculosis. In Pollack HM, McClennan BL [eds]: Clinical Urography, 2nd ed, vol 1. Philadelphia, WB Saunders, 2000, pp 1193–1228.)
A–C. IVU (**A**) and nonenhanced CT scans (**B, C**) show dilated calyces with dense and faint lobar calcifications in the right kidney.

Fig. 3. Lobar calcification in tuberculosis. (**A, B,** From Kim SH: Urogenital tuberculosis. In Pollack HM, McClennan BL [eds]: Clinical Urography, 2nd ed, vol 1. Philadelphia, WB Saunders, 2000, pp 1193–1228.)
A. IVU in a 62-year-old man with longstanding tuberculosis shows dilated calyces with flocculent calcifications in the upper pole of the left kidney *(arrows)*.
B. IVU in a 52-year-old man demonstrates mottled lobar calcification in the lower-pole area of the left kidney *(arrows)*. Also note small papillary cavities in the interpolar area *(arrowheads)*.

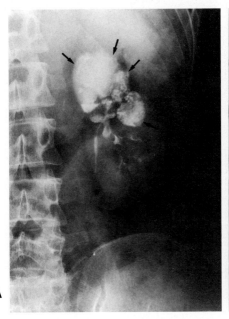

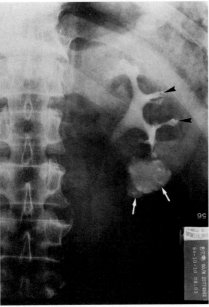

13. Renal Tuberculosis: Calcified Autonephrectomy

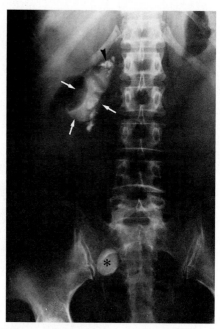

Fig. 1. Calcified autonephrectomy state of the right kidney in a 44-year-old woman. Plain radiograph shows small, totally calcified right kidney *(arrows)*. Also note calcifications in the right adrenal gland *(arrowhead)* and right ureter *(asterisk)*.

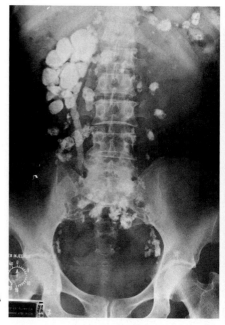

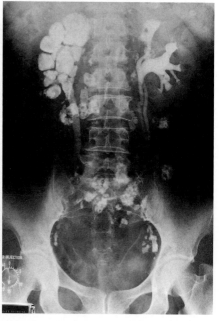

A

B

Fig. 2. Calcified autonephrectomy state in a 55-year-old woman. **A, B.** Plain radiograph (**A**) and a 15-minute IVU (**B**) show densely calcified, nonfunctioning right kidney and ureter. The left kidney has pyeloureteral duplication and is normally functioning. Also note extensive lymph node calcifications.

14. Renal Tuberculosis: US-Guided Aspiration

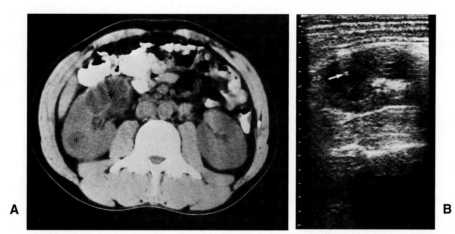

Fig. 1. Localized caliectasis due to tuberculosis in a 26-year-old man with hematuria, in whom the diagnosis was made by US-guided aspiration. **A.** Nonenhanced CT shows large right kidney with low-attenuated lesions that probably represent dilated calyces *(asterisks)*. **B.** Multiple urine cultures were negative for acid-fast bacilli. Therefore, US-guided aspiration was performed and culture of aspirated material revealed acid-fast bacilli. Note an echogenic dot representing the needle tip *(arrow)* in the hypoechoic renal lesion. (**B,** From Kim SH: Urogenital tuberculosis. In Pollack HM, McClennan BL [eds]: Clinical Urography, 2nd ed, vol 1. Philadelphia, WB Saunders, 2000, pp 1193–1228.)

15. Ureteral Tuberculosis

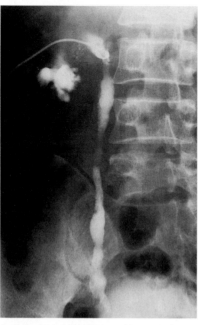

Fig. 1. Ureteral tuberculosis in a 47-year-old man. AGP obtained during percutaneous nephrostomy shows dilated ureter with ragged and irregular margin representing fine mucosal nodules and ulcerations. (From Kim SH: Urogenital tuberculosis. In Pollack HM, McClennan BL [eds]: Clinical Urography, 2nd ed, vol 1. Philadelphia, WB Saunders, 2000, pp 1193–1228.)

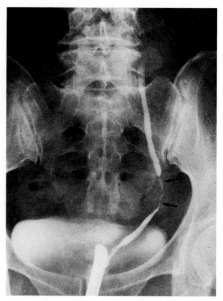

Fig. 2. Ureteral tuberculosis with focal stricture in a 50-year-old woman. RGP shows a focal stenosis with relatively smooth margin *(arrows)*. Segmental resection and anastomosis was performed, and pathologic diagnosis was ureteral tuberculosis. (From Kim SH: Urogenital tuberculosis. In Pollack HM, McClennan BL [eds]: Clinical Urography, 2nd ed, vol 1. Philadelphia, WB Saunders, 2000, pp 1193–1228.)

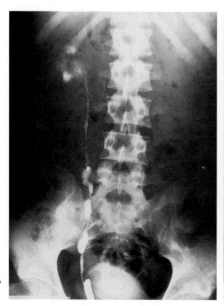

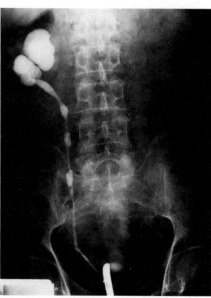

A　　　　　　　　　　　　　　　　　　　　　**B**

Fig. 3. Tuberculous strictures of the ureter with beaded appearance in two different patients.
A. RGP in a 20-year-old man shows diffuse irregularity of the ureter with a beaded appearance at the distal portion. (**A,** From Kim SH, Kim SH, Kim WH: Imaging makes progress in urinary tract tuberculosis. Diagn Imaging Asia Pacific 1995; 2:22–28.) **B.** RGP in a 51-year-old man shows diffuse stenosis of the right ureter with characteristic beaded and pipe-stem appearance. Note nonopacification of the lower-pole calyces due to infundibular obstruction. (**B,** From Kim SH: Urogenital tuberculosis. In Pollack HM, McClennan BL [eds]: Clinical Urography, 2nd ed, vol 1. Philadelphia, WB Saunders, 2000, pp 1193–1228.)

16. Ureteral Tuberculosis with Vesicoureteral Reflux

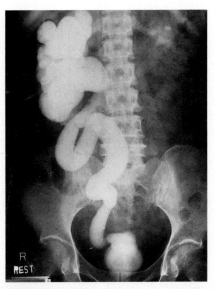

Fig. 1. Contracted urinary bladder with vesicoureteral reflux due to tuberculosis. VCU shows contracted urinary bladder with severe vesicoureteral reflux on the right side due to old tuberculosis.

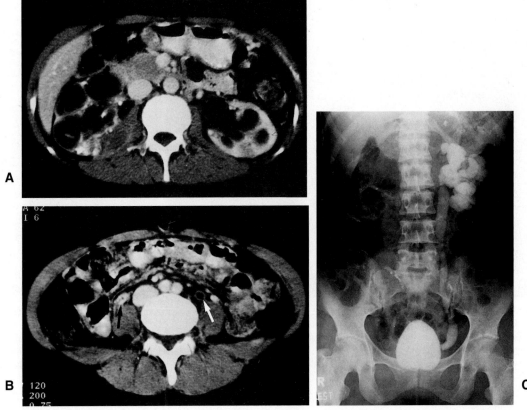

Fig. 2. Tuberculosis of the right urinary tract and urinary bladder with contralateral vesicoureteral reflux in a 34-year-old woman.
A. Contrast-enhanced CT scan at the level of the kidney shows bilateral hydronephrosis, more severe on the right. Note that the right renal pelvis is contracted, whereas the left renal pelvis is dilated. **B.** CT scan at lower level shows narrowed right ureter with thickened enhancing wall *(black arrow)* and dilated left ureter *(white arrow)*. **C.** VCU shows severe vesicoureteral reflux on the left side, which is probably not due to tuberculosis on the left urinary tract but to tuberculosis of the bladder.

17. Ureteral Tuberculosis: Percutaneous Ureteroplasty

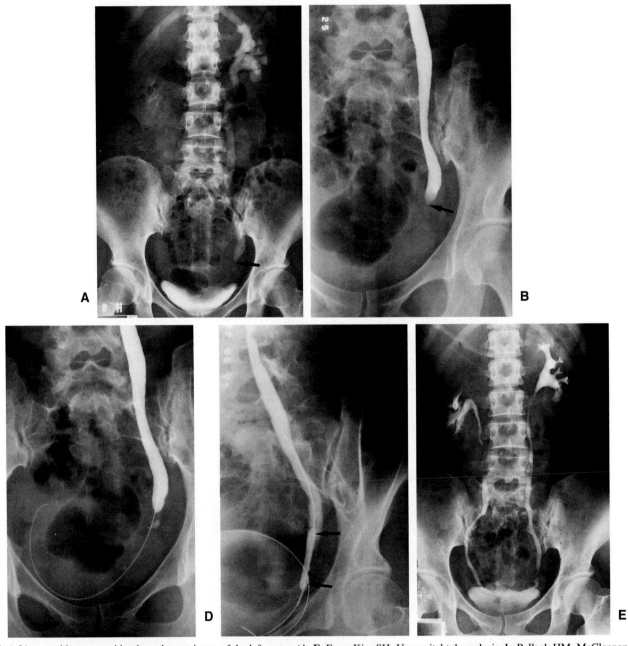

Fig. 1. A 31-year-old woman with tuberculous stricture of the left ureter. (**A–E,** From Kim SH: Urogenital tuberculosis. In Pollack HM, McClennan BL [eds]: Clinical Urography, 2nd ed, vol 1. Philadelphia, WB Saunders, 2000, pp 1193–1228.)
A. Initial IVU shows hydronephrosis and hydroureter on the left side with distal ureteral stricture *(arrow)*. **B.** Tubogram obtained following percutaneous nephrostomy shows complete obstruction of the left distal ureter *(arrow)*. **C.** Occluded ureter was negotiated with a guide wire and a catheter. **D.** Narrowed portion of the ureter was dilated with a balloon *(arrows)*, and a ureteral stent was placed for 4 weeks. **E.** Follow-up IVU taken 6 months later shows marked improvement.

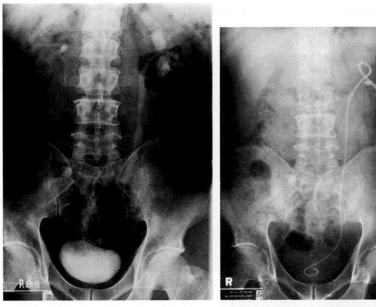

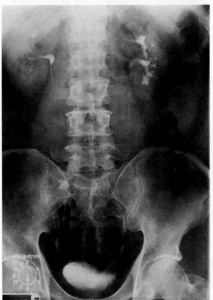

Fig. 2. A 48-year-old man with tuberculosis of the left kidney with ureteral stricture.
A. Initial IVU shows caliectasis, infundibular narrowing, contracted pelvis, and hydroureter on the left side.
B. Antituberculous medication was started. At the same time percutaneous nephrostomy was performed and distal ureteral stricture was dilated with a balloon. Then an internal-external ureteral stent was inserted and kept until 3 months after completion of antituberculous medication. **C.** Follow-up IVU taken 2 years later shows marked improvement with subtle residual changes of renal tuberculosis in the left kidney.

18. Bladder Tuberculosis: Early Changes

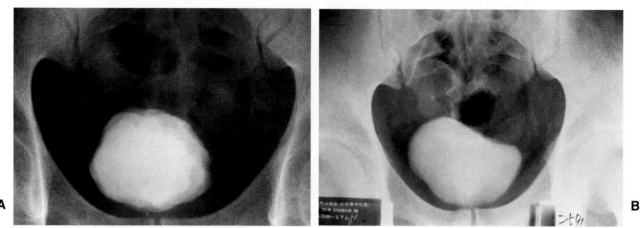

Fig. 1. Tuberculous cystitis in a 24-year-old man. (**A, B,** From Kim SH: Urogenital tuberculosis. In Pollack HM, McClennan BL [eds]: Clinical Urography, 2nd ed, vol 1. Philadelphia, WB Saunders, 2000, pp 1193–1228.)
A. IVU at the time of diagnosis shows thickened bladder wall with nodularities and irregularities. **B.** Follow-up IVU taken 7 months later with antituberculous medication shows marked improvement.

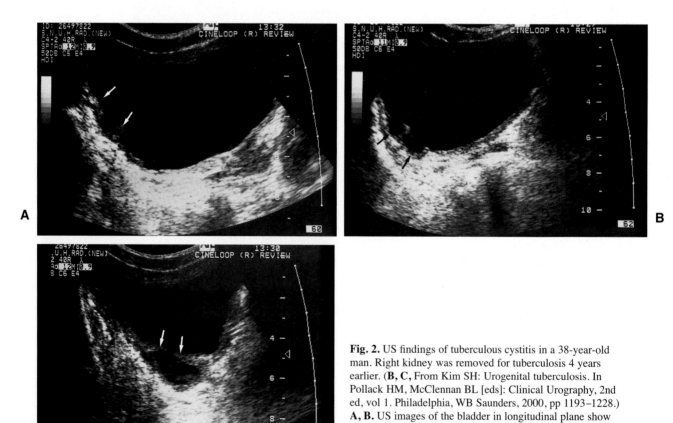

Fig. 2. US findings of tuberculous cystitis in a 38-year-old man. Right kidney was removed for tuberculosis 4 years earlier. (**B, C,** From Kim SH: Urogenital tuberculosis. In Pollack HM, McClennan BL [eds]: Clinical Urography, 2nd ed, vol 1. Philadelphia, WB Saunders, 2000, pp 1193–1228.)
A, B. US images of the bladder in longitudinal plane show thickening of the bladder wall with nodularities *(white arrows)* and ulcerations *(black arrows)*. **C.** US of the bladder at parasagittal plane shows thick adhesive band *(arrows)*.

19. Bladder Tuberculosis: Late Changes

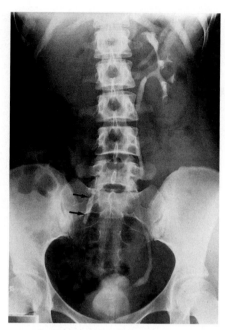

Fig. 1. Late-stage tuberculosis of the right urinary tract and urinary bladder in a 25-year-old woman. IVU shows contracted, dumbbell-shaped urinary bladder and normal-appearing left urinary tract. The right kidney was removed for tuberculosis 3 years earlier. Note calcification in the remnant right ureter *(arrows)*.

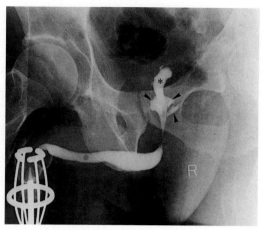

Fig. 2. Bilateral renal tuberculosis in a 51-year-old man who underwent left nephrectomy and right ureteral diversion using ileal conduit. RGU shows markedly contracted bladder *(asterisk)* and reflux of contrast material into the prostate *(arrowheads)*.

20. Urethral Tuberculosis

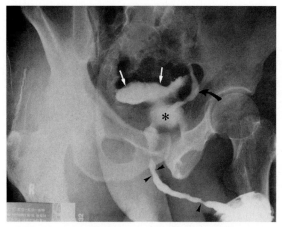

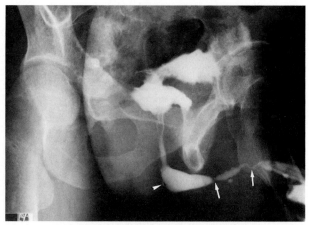

Fig. 1. A 35-year-old man who underwent augmentation cystoplasty for bladder tuberculosis. RGU shows contracted native bladder *(asterisk)*, augmented bladder *(arrows)*, and refluxing left ureter *(curved arrow)*. Also note irregularities in the pendulous and bulbous portions of the urethra *(arrowheads)* due to urethral tuberculosis.

Fig. 2. Urethral tuberculosis in a 39-year-old man with a history of renal tuberculosis and tuberculous cystitis. RGU shows multiple strictures in the pendulous urethra *(arrows)*. Note deformed urinary bladder due to tuberculosis and opacification of Cowper's gland duct *(arrowhead)*.

21. Tuberculous Epididymitis and Epididymo-orchitis

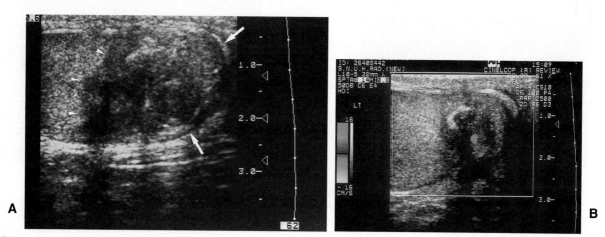

Fig. 1. Tuberculous epididymitis in a 35-year-old man.
A. Longitudinal US of the left scrotum shows enlargement of the tail portion of the left epididymis with heterogeneous hypoechogenicity *(arrows).* Note that the margin between the epididymal lesion and the testis is irregular *(arrowheads),* suggesting testicular involvement. **B.** On color Doppler US, the vascularity is not increased in the lesion. (**B**, See also Color Section.)

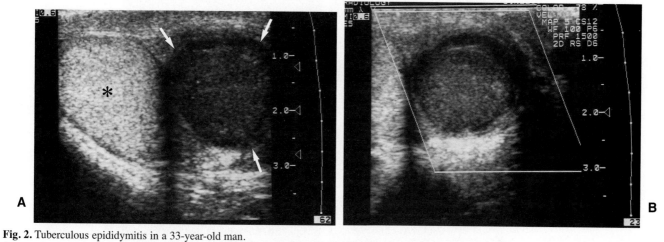

Fig. 2. Tuberculous epididymitis in a 33-year-old man.
A. Longitudinal US of the left scrotum shows a round hypoechoic mass *(arrows)* in the tail portion of the left epididymis. Note the normal appearance of the left testis *(asterisk).* (**A,** From Kim SH: Urogenital tuberculosis. In Pollack HM, McClennan BL [eds]: Clinical Urography, 2nd ed, vol 1. Philadelphia, WB Saunders, 2000, pp 1193–1228.) **B.** Doppler US shows absent flow signal in and around the mass. At surgery, the lesion was found to be an abscess cavity filled with caseous material, and pathologic examination confirmed tuberculous epididymitis.

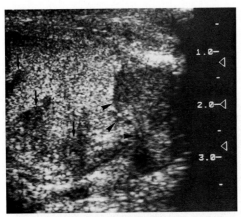

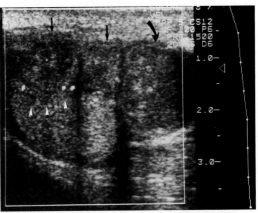

Fig. 3. Tuberculous epididymo-orchitis in a 26-year-old man. Longitudinal US of the right scrotum shows an enlarged tail portion of the right epididymis with heterogeneous hypoechogenicity. The margin between the involved epididymis and testicle is irregular *(arrowheads).* Also note ill-defined multifocal hypoechoic lesions in the testicle *(arrows).* (From Kim SH, Kim SH, Kim WH: Imaging makes progress in urinary tract tuberculosis. Diagn Imaging Asia Pacific 1995; 2:22–28.)

Fig. 4. Tuberculous epididymo-orchitis in a 44-year-old man with history of left nephrectomy for tuberculosis. Doppler US of the right scrotum shows diffusely enlarged epididymis with heterogeneous hypoechogenicity and lobulated contour *(arrows).* Note that the epididymal enlargement is most prominent in the tail portion *(curved arrow).* The margin between the epididymis and testis is ill-defined and irregular *(arrowheads).*

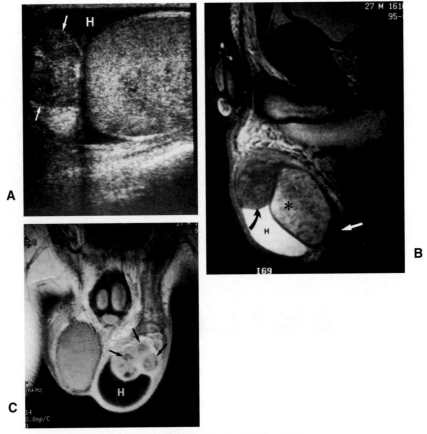

Fig. 5. Tuberculous epididymo-orchitis in a 27-year-old man. (**A, C,** Courtesy of Kyung Sik Cho, MD.)
A. Longitudinal US of the left scrotum shows enlarged hypoechoic epididymis in head portion *(arrows)* and multiple hypoechoic nodules in the testicle. H, hydrocele. **B.** T2-weighted sagittal MR image of the left scrotum shows enlarged head *(curved arrow)* and tail *(arrow)* portions of the left epididymis with marked low signal intensity. Also note hydrocele (H) and mottled low-intensity lesions in the left testicle *(asterisk).* (**B,** From Kim SH: Urogenital tuberculosis. In Pollack HM, McClennan BL [eds]: Clinical Urography, 2nd ed, vol 1. Philadelphia, WB Saunders, 2000, pp 1193–1228.) **C.** Contrast-enhanced T1-weighted MR image in coronal plane shows nodular, low-intensity lesions *(arrows)* in the enlarged epididymal head. H, hydrocele.

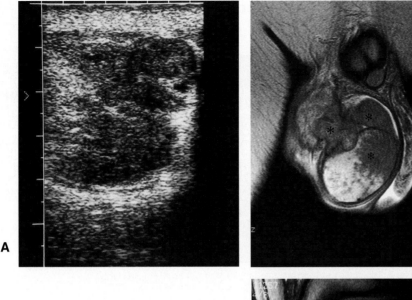

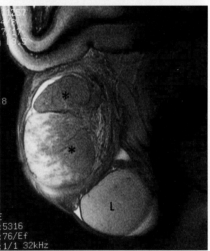

Fig. 6. Tuberculous epididymo-orchitis in a 38-year-old man. (**A–C**, Courtesy of Bohyun Kim, MD.)
A. Longitudinal US of the right scrotum shows diffusely enlarged epididymis and testis with heterogeneously decreased echogenicity. Note that the testis and epididymis are not well demarcated.
B, C. T2-weighted MR images in coronal (**B**) and sagittal (**C**) planes show enlarged right testis and epididymis with markedly decreased signal intensity *(asterisks)*. L, left testis.

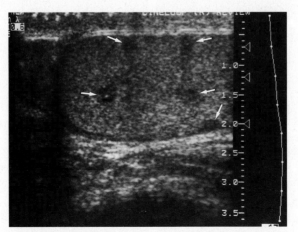

Fig. 7. Testicular tuberculosis in a 30-year-old man with acquired immunodeficiency syndrome. US of the left scrotum in longitudinal plane shows multiple hypoechoic nodules in the testicle *(arrows)*.

22. Tuberculosis of the Prostate and Seminal Tracts

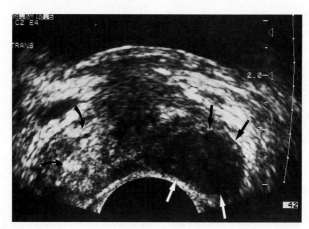

Fig. 1. Tuberculosis of the prostate in a 40-year-old man. Transrectal US in transverse plane shows a large, ill-defined hypoechoic lesion in left aspect of the prostate *(arrows)*. Also note increased echogenicity in the right aspect of the prostate *(curved arrows)*. Transrectal US-guided biopsy revealed tuberculosis.

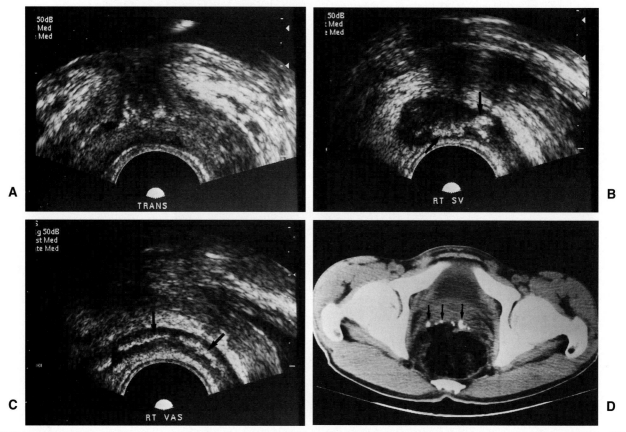

Fig. 2. Tuberculosis of the prostate and seminal vesicles in a 24-year-old man with tuberculosis in the left kidney and ureter. (**B–D,** From Kim SH: Urogenital tuberculosis. In Pollack HM, McClennan BL [eds]: Clinical Urography, 2nd ed, vol 1. Philadelphia, WB Saunders, 2000, pp 1193–1228.) **A.** Transrectal US in transverse plane shows heterogeneously increased echogenicity of the prostate. **B, C.** Transrectal US images of the right seminal vesicle (**B**) and right vas deferens (**C**) show thickened wall of seminal vesicles and vas with intraluminal calcifications *(arrows)*. **D.** CT scan shows irregular intraluminal calcifications in both seminal vesicles *(arrows)*.

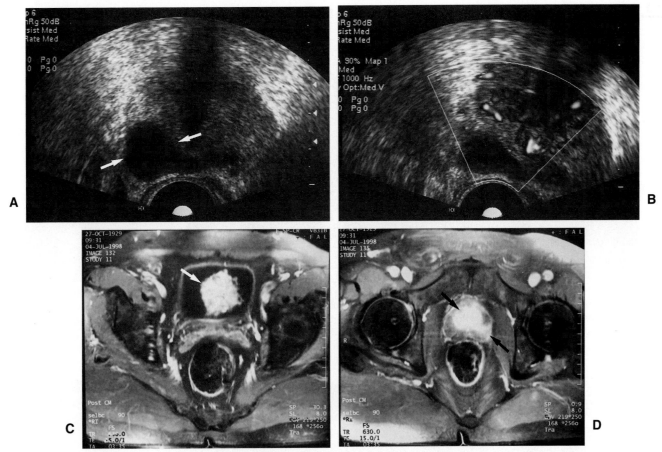

Fig. 3. Tuberculosis of the prostate caused by intravesical instillation of bacillus Calmette-Guérin for bladder cancer in a 69-year-old man. (**A–D,** From Moon MH, Seong CK, Lee KH, et al: BCG-induced granulomatous prostatitis: A case report. J Korean Radiol Soc 2000; 42:675–677.) **A.** Transrectal US of the prostate in transverse plane shows a well-defined, hypoechoic lesion *(arrows)* in the right aspect of the prostate. **B.** Doppler US demonstrates hypovascular nature of the lesion. **C.** Contrast-enhanced T1-weighted MR image shows a strongly enhancing mass in the bladder indicating bladder cancer *(arrow)*. **D.** Contrast-enhanced T1-weighted MR image at the level of the prostate shows strong enhancement of the central gland and left posterior peripheral gland of the prostate indicating invasion of the prostate by bladder cancer *(arrows)*. Note that the lesion in the right prostate seen on transrectal US does not enhance well.

23. Tuberculosis of the Retroperitoneum and Lymph Nodes

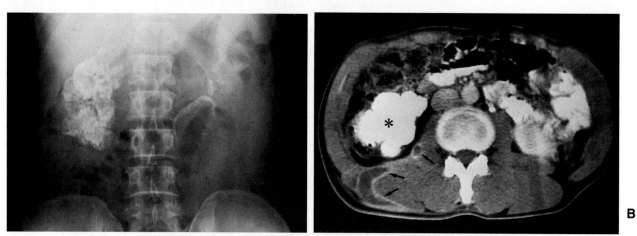

A   **B**

Fig. 1. A 47-year-old man with calcified autonephrectomy state of the right kidney and extension of tuberculous abscess to the right back muscle. **A.** IVU shows nonfunctioning right kidney with amorphous calcification forming a cast of the kidney. **B.** Contrast-enhanced CT shows densely calcified right kidney *(asterisk)* with retroperitoneal extension forming tuberculous abscess cavities *(arrows)*. (**B,** From Kim SH: Urogenital tuberculosis. In Pollack HM, McClennan BL [eds]: Clinical Urography, 2nd ed, vol 1. Philadelphia, WB Saunders, 2000, pp 1193–1228.)

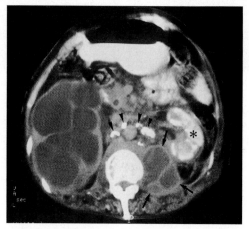

Fig. 2. Bilateral renal tuberculosis and left psoas abscess in a 36-year-old woman. Contrast-enhanced CT shows hydronephrotic right kidney and calcified autonephrectomized left kidney *(asterisk)*. Note a large psoas abscess with enhancing wall *(arrows)* and calcified lymph nodes in the retroperitoneum *(arrowheads)*.

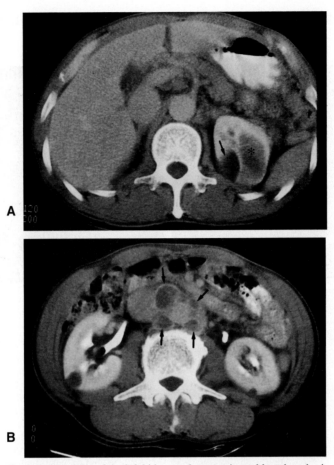

Fig. 3. Tuberculosis of the left kidney and retroperitoneal lymph nodes in a 61-year-old man.
A. CT scan at the level of upper pole of the left kidney shows dilated calyces due to tuberculosis *(asterisk)*. Also note a cortical cyst medially *(arrow)*. **B.** CT scan at lower level shows multiple low-attenuated para-aortic lymph nodes with enhancing rim *(arrows)*. Also note multiple, small, cortical cysts in both kidneys.

24. Peritoneal Tuberculosis

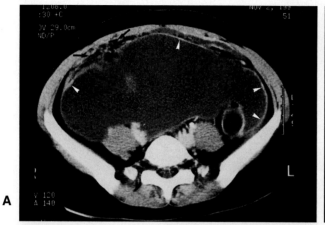

A

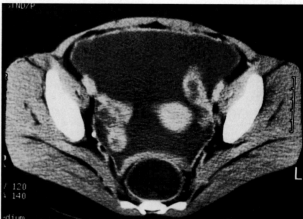

B

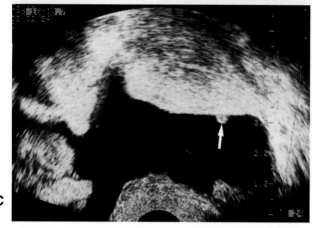

C

Fig. 1. A 14-year-old girl with peritoneal tuberculosis.
A. Contrast-enhanced CT shows diffuse thickening of
peritoneum with strong enhancement *(arrowheads)*. Note
diffuse infiltration of the omentum forming an omental cake
(arrows). **B.** CT scan in pelvic level shows no abnormal
finding in the uterus and ovaries. Also note diffuse thickening
of the pelvic peritoneum. (**B,** From Kim SH: Urogenital
tuberculosis. In Pollack HM, McClennan BL [eds]: Clinical
Urography, 2nd ed, vol 1. Philadelphia, WB Saunders, 2000,
pp 1193–1228.) **C.** Transvaginal US at the level of cul-de-sac
shows peritoneal fluid containing fine echogenic debris and a
small nodule *(arrow)* attached to the peritoneal surface.

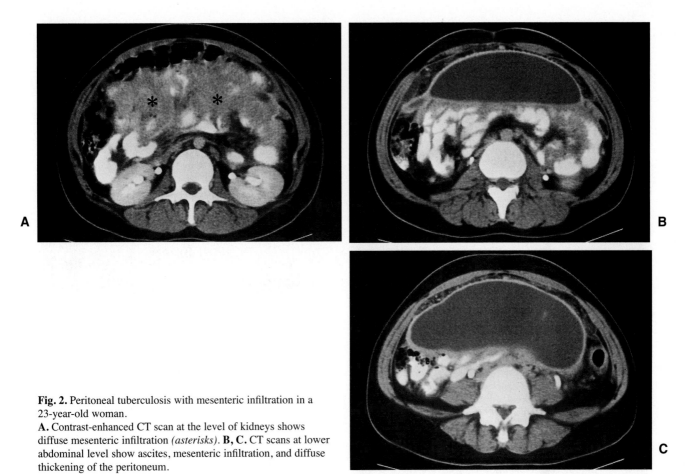

Fig. 2. Peritoneal tuberculosis with mesenteric infiltration in a 23-year-old woman.
A. Contrast-enhanced CT scan at the level of kidneys shows diffuse mesenteric infiltration *(asterisks)*. **B, C.** CT scans at lower abdominal level show ascites, mesenteric infiltration, and diffuse thickening of the peritoneum.

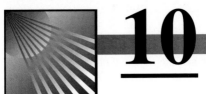

10

Renal Papillary Necrosis

SEUNG HYUP KIM

Renal papillary necrosis is not a pathologic entity but a descriptive term for the disorders causing necrosis of the renal papillae. Renal papillary necrosis develops in a variety of diseases that cause chronic tubulointerstitial nephropathy in which the lesion is predominant in the inner medulla. Major underlying causes of renal papillary necrosis can be remembered by the word "POSTCARD": Pyelonephritis, Obstructive uropathy, Sickle cell disease, Tuberculosis, Calculi, Analgesics, Renal vein thrombosis, and Diabetes mellitus. Other causes include acute tubular necrosis, chronic alcoholism, and severe infantile diarrhea. In many cases, the cause is multifactorial. Transplanted kidneys, particularly cadaveric allografts, appear to be susceptible to renal papillary necrosis.

The basic lesion in renal papillary necrosis is regarded as impairment of the vascular supply and subsequent focal or diffuse ischemic necrosis of the distal segments of the renal pyramids. In the affected papilla, the sharp demarcation of the lesion and coagulative necrosis seen in the early stages of the disease closely resemble those of infarction.

COMMON CAUSES OF PAPILLARY NECROSIS

Diabetes mellitus is the most common condition associated with renal papillary necrosis, accounting for more than 50% of all cases, and renal papillary necrosis has been reported in about 25% of patients with insulin-dependent diabetes mellitus. It is often associated with urinary tract infection and impaired renal function but can be seen in patients without evidence of apparent diabetic nephropathy. The kidneys are enlarged in earlier stages but become small and scarred in later stages. In diabetic patients, acute bacterial infection within the renal pyramids and the impaired circulation to the papilla caused by vascular sclerosis induce an infarct-like necrosis of the distal segment of the renal pyramid.

Analgesic nephropathy is caused by excessive intake of analgesics, usually more than 1 kg. Analgesic nephropathy is most common in middle-aged women. Urinary tract infection accompanies in about 50% of patients, and pyuria and urinary tract obstruction due to sloughed papillae are also common. Histologically, analgesic nephropathy is characterized by chronic tubulointerstitial nephropathy and renal papillary necrosis. In milder cases, the disease may be limited to one or several papillae and the kidneys are usually normal sized. In advanced cases, however, the kidneys eventually become shrunken due to diffuse fibrosis and atrophy.

S hemoglobinopathy is another well-known cause of renal papillary necrosis. Medullary ischemia caused by sickling is the main cause of the disease. Papillary necrosis can be seen in both homozygous and heterozygous-S hemoglobinopathies but is more common in heterozygous-S disease. Homozygous-S disease is commonly associated with occlusion of small vessels resulting in lobar infarcts, tubular obliteration, and fibrosis, but heterozygous-S hemoglobinopathies often manifest as papillary necrosis without association with renal failure. The kidneys are enlarged in earlier stages but become small and scarred later. Calcifications in the renal papillae or cortex and perinephric hematoma can be accompanying features.

Pyelonephritis can result in papillary necrosis, and infection is present in most cases of renal papillary necrosis. However, its exact prevalence as the cause of renal papillary necrosis is difficult to determine because infection may develop secondary to obstruction or diabetes, which remain the primary causes of renal papillary necrosis.

IMAGING FINDINGS

Radiologic findings of renal papillary necrosis are independent of its etiology. More severe changes are common in the presence of urinary tract infection or obstruction, and the involvement is usually minimal with heterozygous-S hemoglobinopathy. Although renal papillary necrosis can involve both kidneys, unilateral involvement is often seen in patients with pyelonephritis, obstructive uropathy, tuberculosis, and renal vein thrombosis. Radiologically renal papillary necrosis can be best evaluated on intravenous urography (IVU) or retrograde pyelography (RGP). Iodinated contrast material should be given carefully since higher incidence of contrast material–associated nephrotoxicity is associated with diabetes mellitus and sickling may occur in the presence of contrast material in patients with S hemoglobinopathy.

Renal papillae may undergo necrosis totally or partially. Three types of parenchymal involvement can be seen: medullary (usually partial), papillary (usually total), and necrosis in situ. In the medullary form, cavitation occurs in the central portion of the papillae extending from the fornix. In the papillary form, necrosis and cavitation develop at the periphery of the papillae eventually resulting in sloughing of them. If a necrotic papilla is surrounded by contrast material on IVU or RGP, a urographic ring shadow may be observed. A sloughed papilla can be seen as a triangular filling defect within a pelvocalyceal system or ureter, occasionally with ring-shaped

peripheral calcifications. It may cause acute ureteral obstruction. The third type, necrosis in situ, refers to necrotic papillae that remain attached, shrink, and frequently calcify. These papillary calcifications may pass as small stones. Shrinkage of the kidney with reduction of parenchymal thickness is a common sequela in papillary necrosis. This has been attributed to secondary atrophy of the nephrons caused by necrosis of the loops of Henle that pass deeply into the medulla.

Ultrasonography (US) is not commonly used for the diagnosis of renal papillary necrosis, and only a few studies have reported US findings of this condition. In the early stage of papillary necrosis, renal papillae may appear as echogenic foci surrounded by sonolucent rims that represent fluid dissecting around necrotic papillae. In advanced disease with sloughing of the necrotic papillae, US may demonstrate cavities in the renal medullary areas, which are continuous with the calyces. In these cases, other causes of cystic lesions in the areas of renal medulla or sinus should be differentiated. These lesions include hydronephrosis, congenital megacalyces, parapelvic cysts, and calyceal diverticula. The location of the arcuate artery relative to the cystic lesions may be helpful in this differentiation. US can demonstrate calcifications in the necrosis in situ type with a typical garland pattern.

Computed tomography (CT) may demonstrate small contracted kidneys, ring-shaped medullary calcifications, contrast-filled clefts in the renal parenchyma, or filling defect with ring shadow of excreted contrast material. In cases of sloughed papillae, CT may demonstrate hydronephrosis and filling defects in the renal pelvis or ureter that may contain calcification.

References

1. Kim SH, Kim B: Renal parenchymal disease. In Pollack HM, McClennan BL (eds): Clinical Urography, 2nd ed, vol 3. Philadelphia, WB Saunders, 2000, pp 2673–2676.
2. Sekine H, Mine M, Ohya K, et al: Renal papillary necrosis caused by urinary calculus-induced obstruction alone. Urol Int 1995; 54:112–114.
3. Segasothy M, Abdul Samad S, Zulfiqar A, et al: Computed tomography and ultrasonography: A comparative study in the diagnosis of analgesic nephropathy. Nephron 1994; 66:62–66.
4. Cheung H, Chan PSF, Metreweli C: Case report: Echogenic necrotic renal papillae simulating calculi. Clin Radiol 1992; 46:61–62.
5. Braden GL, Kozinn DR, Hampf FE Jr, et al: Ultrasound diagnosis of early renal papillary necrosis. J Ultrasound Med 1991; 10:401–403.
6. Saifuddin A, Bark M: Case report: Computed tomography demonstration of renal papillary necrosis. Clin Radiol 1991; 44:275–276.
7. Shapeero LG, Vordermark JS: Papillary necrosis causing hydronephrosis in the renal allograft: Sonographic findings. J Ultrasound Med 1989; 8:579–581.
8. Eknoyan G: Chronic tubulointerstitial nephropathies. In Schrier RW, Gottschalk CW (eds): Diseases of the Kidney, 4th ed. Boston, Little, Brown, 1988, pp 2209–2212.
9. Andriole GL, Bahnson RR: Computed tomographic diagnosis of ureteral obstruction caused by sloughed papilla. Urol Radiol 1987; 9:45–46.
10. Hoffman JC, Schnur MJ, Koenigsberg M: Demonstration of renal papillary necrosis by sonography. Radiology 1982; 145:785–787.
11. Poynter JD, Hare WSC: Necrosis in situ: A form of renal papillary necrosis seen in analgesic nephropathy. Radiology 1974; 111:69–76.

Illustrations • Renal Papillary Necrosis

1 • Diffuse bilateral papillary necrosis

2 • Unilateral papillary necrosis

3 • Focal papillary necrosis

4 • Papillary necrosis with calcification

5 • Sloughed papilla

6 • Papillary necrosis manifesting as a ureteral stone

7 • Papillary necrosis: US and CT demonstration

1. Diffuse Bilateral Papillary Necrosis

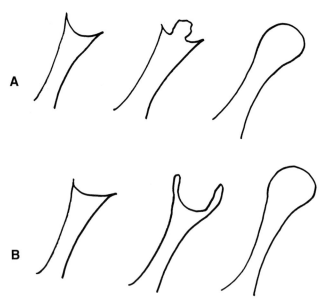

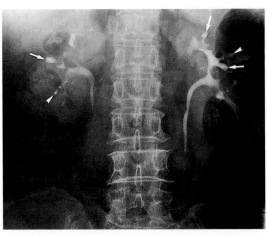

Fig. 2. Diffuse bilateral papillary necrosis in an 80-year-old woman with history of diabetes for 20 years. IVU shows papillary necroses in both kidneys. Some lesions show an ovoid pool of contrast material *(arrowheads)*, whereas others show complete excavation of the papillae with calyceal clubbing *(arrows)*.

Fig. 1. Schematic drawing of two types of renal papillary necrosis: medullary type (**A**) and papillary type (**B**). Papillary necrosis of the papillary type may cause sloughing of the papilla.

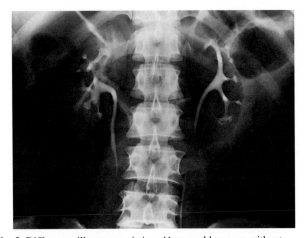

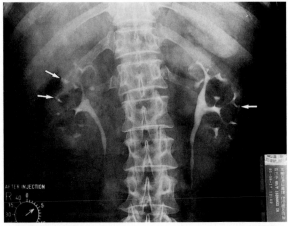

Fig. 3. Diffuse papillary necrosis in a 41-year-old woman without specific history. IVU shows papillary cavities of varying appearances in both kidneys.

Fig. 4. Diffuse papillary necrosis in a 60-year-old woman who suffered from hemorrhagic fever with renal syndrome 14 years earlier. IVU shows multiple papillary cavities of varying appearance in both kidneys *(arrows)*. Papillary necrosis in this patient is probably a sequela of hemorrhagic fever with renal syndrome.

2. Unilateral Papillary Necrosis

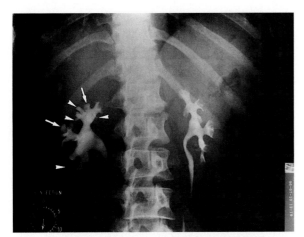

Fig. 1. Focal papillary necrosis involving the right kidney in a 38-year-old woman without specific history. IVU shows round *(arrow)* and linear *(arrowheads)* pools of contrast material due to the medullary type of papillary necrosis in the right kidney.

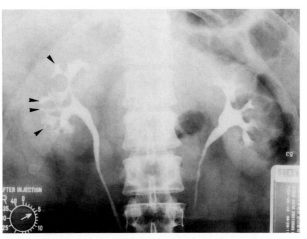

Fig. 2. Unilateral papillary necrosis in a 42-year-old man with liver cirrhosis. IVU shows multiple papillary cavities of varying appearance in the right kidney *(arrowheads)*.

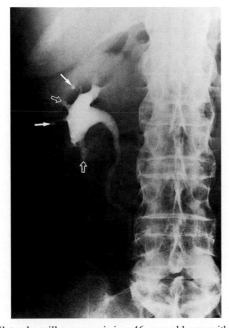

Fig. 3. Unilateral papillary necrosis in a 46-year-old man with ankylosing spondylitis. He had taken analgesics for several years. IVU shows multiple papillary cavities *(arrows)* in the right kidney. Some of them have mottled appearance *(open arrows)* similar to the findings of medullary sponge kidney.

3. Focal Papillary Necrosis

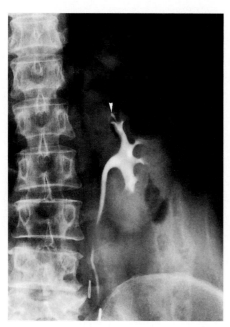

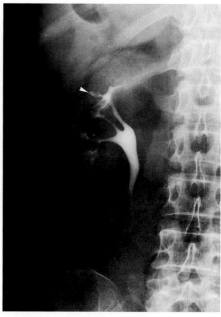

Fig. 1. Focal papillary necrosis of medullary type in a 69-year-old woman. IVU shows a teardrop-shaped papillary cavity in the upper-polar calyx of the left kidney *(arrowhead)*.

Fig. 2. Focal papillary necrosis of medullary type in a 62-year-old woman with diabetes mellitus. IVU shows an oval-shaped papillary cavity in the upper-polar calyx of the right kidney *(arrowhead)*.

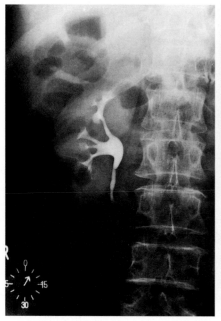

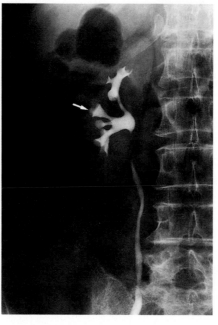

A

B

Fig. 3. Focal papillary necrosis in a 63-year-old woman, which is not evident at a 5-minute IVU film but is well demonstrated at a 15-minute IVU film. **A.** A 5-minute IVU shows no definite abnormality. **B.** A 15-minute IVU clearly demonstrates a round papillary cavity *(arrow)* in the interpolar calyx of the right kidney. This is probably an early stage of papillary necrosis of the medullary type.

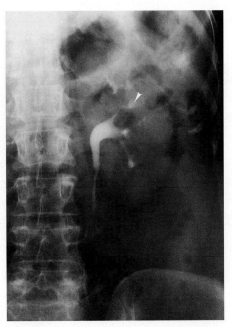

Fig. 4. Small papillary cavity seen on IVU in a 60-year-old woman who had a history of analgesic abuse. A small necrotic papilla was discovered in the urine. IVU shows a small dotlike collection of contrast material in the center of a calyceal fornix seen on end *(arrowhead)*.

4. Papillary Necrosis with Calcification

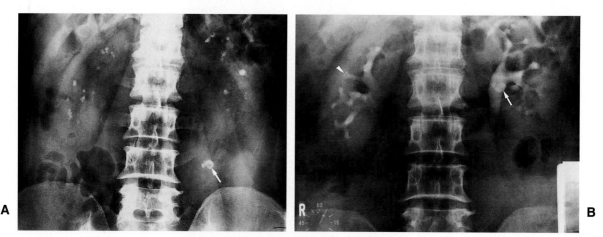

Fig. 1. Diffuse papillary necrosis with calcification in a 47-year-old man with a history of prolonged intake of analgesics. (**A, B,** From Kim SH, Kim B: Renal parenchymal disease. In Pollack HM, McClennan BL [eds]: Clinical Urography, 2nd ed, vol 3. Philadelphia, WB Saunders, 2000, pp 2673–2676.) **A.** Plain radiograph shows multiple calcifications in the region of the renal medulla in both kidneys. Note an extrarenal calcification *(arrow)*, which is probably a calcified lymph node. **B.** IVU confirms that the calcifications that were seen on plain radiograph are located in the tip of the clubbed calyces suggesting calcified necrotic papillae. Note a small filling defect in the tip of the right interpolar calyx *(arrowhead)*. Also note an extrarenal calcification *(arrow)*.

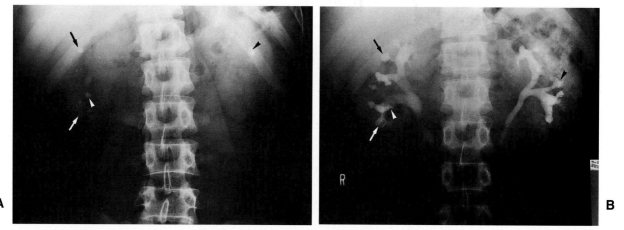

Fig. 2. Diffuse papillary necrosis with calcification in a 30-year-old man. Compare the location of the calcifications by *arrows* and *arrowheads*. **A.** Plain radiograph shows multiple calcifications of varying size in both kidneys. **B.** IVU shows clubbing of calyces in both kidneys that contain calcifications in their tips.

5. Sloughed Papilla

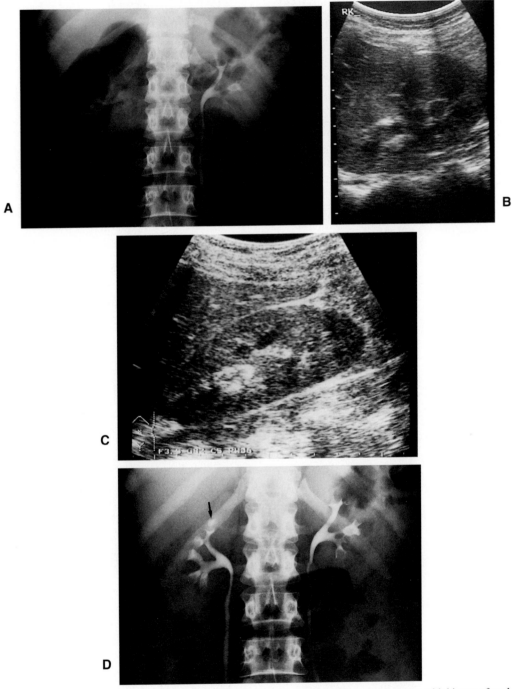

Fig. 1. Focal papillary necrosis with acute urinary obstruction due to a sloughed papilla in a 27-year-old woman with history of analgesic abuse.
A. IVU obtained at the time of acute right flank pain shows nonopacification of the right urinary tract. **B.** US of the right kidney obtained at the same time as **A** shows dilated pelvocalyces. **C.** US of the right kidney obtained on the following day shows disappeared hydronephrosis. **D.** IVU taken on the next day shows a well-opacified right urinary tract and a collection of contrast material in the region of the renal papilla in the upper pole of the right kidney *(arrow)*. (**D,** From Kim SH, Kim B: Renal parenchymal disease. In Pollack HM, McClennan BL [eds]: Clinical Urography, 2nd ed, vol 3. Philadelphia, WB Saunders, 2000, pp 2673–2676.)

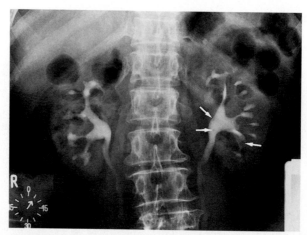

Fig. 2. Diffuse papillary necrosis in a 63-year-old woman who had taken analgesics for a long time. IVU shows papillary cavities with calyceal clubbing in both kidneys. Also note pelvocalyceal filling defects *(arrows)* in the left kidney indicating sloughed papillae.

6. Papillary Necrosis Manifesting as a Ureteral Stone

Fig. 1. Focal papillary necrosis with a distal ureteral stone in a 36-year-old man.
A. Plain radiograph shows a small, faint radiopacity in the left pelvic cavity *(arrow)*.
B. IVU confirms a distal ureter stone with mild obstruction *(arrow)*. Also note two small papillary cavities *(arrowheads)* in the left kidney representing the origin of the stone.

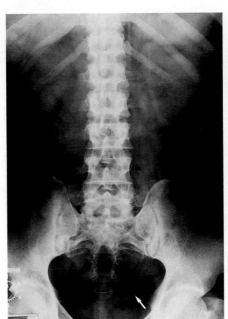

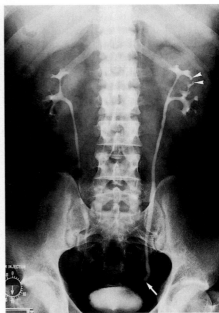

A

B

7. Papillary Necrosis: US and CT Demonstration

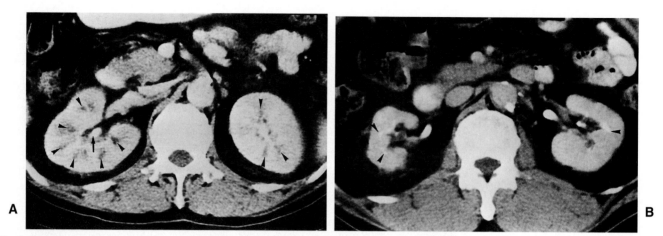

Fig. 1. Diffuse renal papillary necrosis in a 67-year-old man with clinical findings of recurrent urinary tract infection.
A. Contrast-enhanced CT scan in excretory phase shows multiple triangular-shaped, low-attenuated lesions *(arrowheads)* in the papillary regions of the swollen kidneys. Note that the contrast material is excreted into the renal pelvis *(arrow)*. This is probably an early stage of renal papillary necrosis associated with infection, so-called necrotizing papillitis. **B.** Follow-up CT scan obtained 1 year later shows both kidneys markedly contracted and clubbing of the calyces *(arrowheads)*.

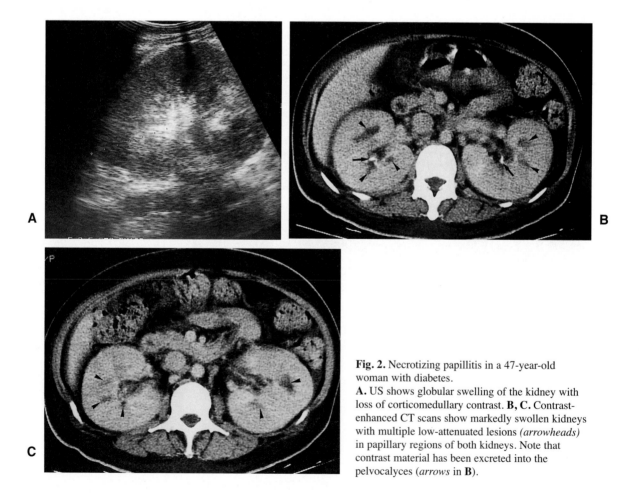

Fig. 2. Necrotizing papillitis in a 47-year-old woman with diabetes.
A. US shows globular swelling of the kidney with loss of corticomedullary contrast. **B, C.** Contrast-enhanced CT scans show markedly swollen kidneys with multiple low-attenuated lesions *(arrowheads)* in papillary regions of both kidneys. Note that contrast material has been excreted into the pelvocalyces *(arrows in B)*.

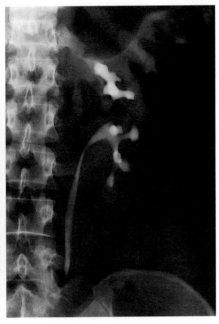

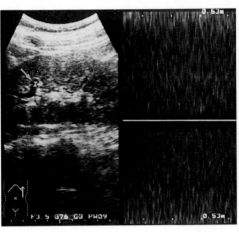

Fig. 3. Papillary necrosis demonstrated by US in a 25-year-old woman. **A.** Doppler US shows a clubbed calyx *(arrow)* in the upper pole of the left kidney. There was no evidence of flow signal from the lesion at Doppler US. **B.** IVU shows diffuse papillary necrosis with calyceal clubbing in the left kidney.

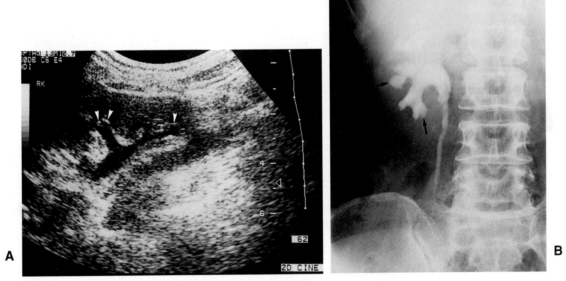

Fig. 4. Papillary necrosis demonstrated by US in a 50-year-old woman.
A. Longitudinal US shows clubbed calyces in the interpolar and lower-polar calyces marginated by linear echoes representing arcuate vessels *(arrowheads).* **B.** IVU demonstrates clubbing of those calyces *(arrows)* by papillary necrosis.

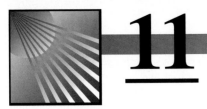

11

Renal Parenchymal Disease

BOHYUN KIM

DEFINITION AND CLASSIFICATION

Renal parenchymal disease refers to a disease affecting the renal parenchyma, that is, the glomeruli, tubules, interstitium, or blood vessels of the kidney. It also includes the systemic diseases that involve the kidneys. Renal parenchymal diseases can be classified into three categories: glomerular, tubulointerstitial, and vascular.

Glomerular diseases

Glomerular disease is the major cause of end-stage renal disease. The pathologic process is either confined to the kidney (primary glomerulopathies) or associated with systemic or hereditary diseases (secondary glomerulopathies).

Primary glomerulopathies

Acute poststreptococcal glomerulonephritis is quite a common disorder worldwide, which usually develops 10 to 14 days following pharyngitis or skin infection. Minimal change disease (lipoid nephrosis), focal segmental glomerulosclerosis, membranous nephropathy, and membranoproliferative glomerulonephritis are the main causes of idiopathic nephrotic syndrome.

Secondary glomerulopathies

Many systemic diseases of immunologic, metabolic, or hereditary causes associated with glomerular injury are called *secondary glomerulopathies*. Diabetes mellitus is a major cause of end-stage renal disease, which first affects the glomerulus but eventually involves all components of the kidney. Lupus nephritis is another common systemic disease, which commonly affects the glomeruli.

Other causes of secondary glomerulopathies include Goodpasture's syndrome, various forms of vasculitis (Henoch-Schönlein purpura, polyarteritis nodosa, hypersensitivity angitis, Wegener's granulomatosis), deposition diseases (amyloidosis, Waldenström's macroglobulinemia), hereditary diseases (Alport's syndrome, Fabry's disease, nail-patella syndrome), infectious diseases (hepatitis, human immuno-deficiency virus infection, bacterial endocarditis), and neoplastic diseases (lymphoma, leukemia).

Tubulointerstitial diseases

The major components of tubulointerstitial diseases include acute tubular necrosis, tubulointerstitial nephritis, and the dis-orders causing intratubular obstruction such as multiple myeloma and uric acid and oxalate nephropathy.

Acute tubular necrosis is the major cause of acute renal failure and is a reversible tubular damage caused by either ischemia or various exogenous and endogenous toxins. Tubulointerstitial nephritis is an inflammatory disease of the tubules and interstitium of various causes and different mechanism of tissue damage. Tubulointerstitial nephritis is often classified according to the causes of the disease, such as hypersensitivity interstitial nephritis, analgesic nephropathy, or radiation nephritis.

Vascular diseases

Benign and malignant nephrosclerosis, renal artery stenosis, renal vein thrombosis, and atheroembolic disease are the main constituents of renal vascular diseases. Thrombotic microangiopathies (hemolytic uremic syndrome and thrombotic thrombocytopenic purpura), which are characterized by thrombosis of small arteries and glomeruli with necrosis of vessel wall, sickle cell nephropathy, and scleroderma (progressive systemic sclerosis), are other components of vascular diseases.

SYSTEMIC APPROACH TO RADIOLOGIC DIAGNOSIS

For radiologic evaluation, most useful morphologic criteria include renal size, contour, and laterality of involvement. Most of renal parenchymal diseases in their early phase cause smooth, bilateral and symmetric enlargement of the kidneys, and chronic renal diseases usually cause bilaterally small, contracted kidneys. Vascular diseases, however, can cause unilateral or bilateral, small or large kidneys depending on the underlying pathology.

Renal size is the most important diagnostic clue. Small kidneys often result from a loss of renal substance due to hypoplasia, necrosis, atrophy, or fibrosis of the kidney. Large kidneys result from accumulation of fluid, deposition of abnormal proteins, inflammatory or neoplastic infiltrates, glomerular or microvascular proliferation, or cellular hypertrophy.

Renal contour and laterality are other important clues. Smooth renal contour and uniform parenchymal thickness associated with renal size change represent a global disease process affecting the whole kidney, and bilateral lesions are either a result of global renal process or a part of multisystem disorders.

RADIOLOGIC MODALITIES

Although the diagnosis of renal parenchymal diseases still largely depends on renal biopsy, imaging studies have important roles in the evaluation of the patients. The aims of the renal imaging in the evaluation of renal parenchymal disease are to measure renal size, to exclude urinary tract obstruction, and, finally, to evaluate the morphologic changes in the renal parenchyma.

Plain radiography and urography

In evaluating patients with renal parenchymal disease, a plain radiograph may offer valuable information such as renal size and presence of parenchymal calcifications. Although different nephrographic patterns may be useful in the differentiation of renal parenchymal diseases, excretory urography is not commonly used for the evaluation of renal parenchymal diseases except the ones primarily affecting the renal pelvocalyceal system such as renal papillary necrosis.

Ultrasonography

Ultrasonography (US) is often the first-line imaging modality for the evaluation of the renal parenchymal diseases. Renal US is used fairly routinely in patients with azotemia to exclude possible obstructive uropathy, to measure the size of the kidneys, and to evaluate renal parenchymal echoes particularly with respect to cortical echogenicity and the distinctness of the corticomedullary differentiation.

The change in renal parenchymal echogenicity is the most commonly used clue for the US diagnosis of renal parenchymal disease. Normal renal cortical echogenicity is less than that of the liver or spleen in adults. If the echogenicity of the renal cortex is higher than that of the liver or spleen in adults, it is assumed that renal parenchymal disease is present. When it is equal to the liver, the renal function is normal in 70% of cases.

Renal corticomedullary differentiation is another important parameter in the US evaluation of the kidney. Renal medullary echogenicity is normally slightly lower than that of the renal cortex. In cases of renal parenchymal disease, renal corticomedullary differentiation may be preserved, obliterated, or accentuated.

Doppler ultrasonography

Doppler US is an easy and noninvasive technique for the evaluation of renal blood vessels and the hemodynamic changes of the kidney. Power Doppler US is known to be superior to color Doppler US in the demonstration of fine intrarenal vasculature.

In Doppler spectral analysis, resistive index (RI) is the most commonly used index. Interlobar and arcuate arteries are commonly used to obtain Doppler spectra, but interlobar arteries are preferred to arcuate arteries since the Doppler signals are stronger due to smaller Doppler angles, especially in the interpolar areas of the kidney. Doppler spectra are obtained at least in three regions (upper polar, lower polar, and interpolar regions) of each kidney and the average value is taken. The upper normal limit of RI is considered 0.7, and the mean normal values reported in various studies range between 0.59 and 0.63. Certain factors such as age and systemic blood pressure may affect the RI of the intrarenal arteries.

The diseases involving the tubulointerstitial or vascular compartments generally result in an elevated RI, whereas RI is usually normal range in diseases limited to the glomeruli. Diabetic nephropathy, hepatorenal syndrome, and hemolytic uremic syndrome are examples in which elevated RI was reported to correlate well with the severity of the disease.

For patients with acute renal failure, Doppler US findings may reflect the status of renal hemodynamics, which is different among the types of acute renal failure. In a study by Platt and colleagues, elevated RI was observed in 91% of patients with renal type failure accompanying acute tubular necrosis, whereas only 20% of patients with prerenal type failure showed an elevated RI.

Computed tomography

The role of computed tomography (CT) in renal parenchymal disease is limited, but it may be useful in selected cases. Noncontrast CT is useful in detecting renal parenchymal calcifications.

For patients with renal parenchymal disease, contrast enhancement should be avoided if possible. Contrast-enhanced spiral CT scan, if performed, may provide useful information regarding the pattern of contrast enhancement and excretion in patients with impaired renal function. In a study that correlated the degree of renal cortical enhancement on spiral CT with the serum level of creatinine, there was a significant correlation between the two, and the degree of cortical enhancement was different between those with renal parenchymal disease and the normal group. Globally absent nephrogram is due to pedicle trauma in most cases, and segmental absence may be due to focal infarction, pyelonephritis, or acute renal failure secondary to renal vasoconstriction.

Magnetic resonance imaging

Recent advances in magnetic resonance (MR) imaging such as breath-holding rapid-imaging technique and dynamic contrast-enhanced studies extended the role of MR imaging in the evaluation of renal parenchymal diseases. Gadolinium-based contrast media (most commonly, gadopentetate dimeglumine) are used routinely for MR imaging of the kidney. Although a case of fatal reaction to gadopentetate dimeglumine has been reported, it is generally accepted that the agent is safe and tolerable at the usual dose in patients with impaired renal function.

Most of the normal kidneys show distinct contrast between the renal cortex and medulla on T1-weighted images, whereas the signal intensities of the renal cortex and medulla are similar on T2-weighted images. Obliteration of the corticomedullary contrast on T1-weighted spin-echo image is regarded as a sensitive but nonspecific finding of the renal parenchymal disease. The parenchymal enhancement pattern is more clearly demonstrated on gradient-echo imaging than on T1-weighted spin-echo imaging. It was reported that there is a correlation between the distinctness of corticomedullary differentiation and serum creatinine levels.

Angiography

The role of angiography in evaluation of the patients with renal parenchymal disease is limited. However, it may be useful in patients with secondary glomerulopathies such as polyarteritis nodosa, Wegener's granulomatosis, and systemic lupus erythematosus. It is also useful in the evaluation of renal vascular diseases, including renal artery stenosis, arteriosclerosis, atheroembolic disease, and various forms of vasculitis.

Renal biopsy

Renal biopsy is an invasive but irreplaceable tool for the diagnosis of renal parenchymal diseases. It helps establish an accurate diagnosis, assess prognosis, and guide treatment in many renal parenchymal diseases. US is now widely used to locate the kidney and to guide biopsy.

Major indications include idiopathic nephrotic syndrome, systemic lupus erythematosus, Wegener's granulomatosis, rapid progressive glomerulonephritis, acute renal failure of an unknown cause, and renal transplant dysfunction. Renal biopsy is rarely indicated for patients with chronic renal failure or typical diabetic nephropathy. Renal biopsy is essential for adult patients with idiopathic nephrotic syndrome. However, for pediatric patients with nephrotic syndrome in whom the renal disease is often due to minimal change disease and responds well with empirical steroid treatment, biopsy is not recommended in most cases.

Percutaneous renal biopsy is usually performed in the lower pole of the left kidney. Various biopsy needles can be used including the TruCut disposable, Franklin-Silverman, Vim-Silverman, and automated gun biopsy needle. Compared with the classic 14-gauge hand-driven system, an 18-gauge spring-driven biopsy gun carries a comparable number of glomeruli per core and is associated with a lower risk of significant bleeding.

RADIOLOGIC FINDINGS

Diabetic nephropathy

Diabetic nephropathy is the single most important disorder leading to renal failure in adults. Diabetic nephropathy develops in 40% to 45% of insulin-dependent patients and 20% of non-insulin-dependent diabetic patients. Diabetic nephropathy is more commonly seen in males and is associated with a higher mortality rate.

Diabetes mellitus is one of the common causes of bilaterally enlarged kidneys. Imaging studies may reveal renal enlargement in the early stage of diabetic nephropathy and shrunken kidneys in the late stage. For demonstration of the changes of renal size, US is the best imaging modality available. Papillary necrosis that is occasionally associated can be demonstrated on intravenous urography (IVU).

In the early stage of the disease, US may show an enlarged kidney with normal parenchymal echogenicity. In advanced stage, renal US may show a shrunken kidney with increased renal parenchymal echogenicity and variable corticomedullary differentiation, which is not different from the findings of end-stage renal disease due to other causes.

Doppler US of the kidney with measurement of RI from intrarenal arteries may well demonstrate the peripheral renal vascular resistance. RI obtained from the interlobar artery correlates well with functional parameters of the kidney such as serum creatinine or creatinine clearance levels.

Lupus nephritis

Systemic lupus erythematosus is an autoimmune disease involving multiple organs. The kidneys are most commonly affected, causing significant morbidity and mortality. Although renal biopsy reveals evidence of renal involvement in almost all cases, specific imaging findings have not been reported.

Gray-scale US shows nonspecific changes of renal size and parenchymal echogenicity. It may demonstrate multiple variable-sized cortical hypoechoic areas, which may represent regions of active edema. However, similar findings can be seen in cases of multifocal processes such as acute pyelonephritis, abscesses, or tumors.

The correlation between Doppler spectral changes and the severity of lupus nephritis determined by laboratory findings and histopathologic changes is not certain. In one report Doppler parameters were normal in all nine patients and no significant correlation was found among the Doppler parameters and laboratory or histopathologic findings. In another report, RI correlated with creatinine level, chronicity index, and presence of interstitial disease.

Amyloidosis

Amyloidosis is a systemic disease characterized by deposition of a pathologic proteinaceous substance between cells in various organs. Amyloidosis can occur without any associated disease (primary amyloidosis) or in association with chronic destructive diseases such as chronic osteomyelitis, rheumatoid arthritis, tuberculosis, or various malignancies (secondary amyloidosis). Renal involvement is more common with secondary amyloidosis. Glomeruli are involved in 75% to 90% of the patients. Isolated involvement of the ureter, bladder, urethra, prostate, and seminal vesicles has been reported. Renal vein thrombosis may occur.

Amyloidosis is more common in men than in women. The patients may present with heavy proteinuria, nephrotic syndrome, and/or impaired glomerular filtration. Characteristically, the kidney is normal in size or slightly enlarged. IVU may demonstrate smooth bilateral enlargement of the kidneys with faint nephrogram. US may show both kidneys enlarged with increased cortical echogenicity. Renal infarction, perirenal lesion, and abdominal visceral calcification including the kidney were reported to be associated with primary or secondary amyloidosis involving the kidneys.

Renal diseases in patients with AIDS

The most common renal abnormality in patients with acquired immunodeficiency syndrome (AIDS) is nephropathy that is manifested by deterioration of renal function and proteinuria. Other renal abnormalities associated with AIDS include acute tubular necrosis, intrarenal infections, focal nephrocalcinosis, and renal neoplasms.

In patients with AIDS-associated nephropathy, the kidneys may be enlarged or normal sized. On pathologic examinations, glomerular lesions, particularly focal glomerulosclerosis, are

dominant. Other changes including acute tubular necrosis, focal interstitial nephritis, nephrocalcinosis, and tubular atrophy have also been reported.

On US, renal cortical echogenicity is increased in more than half of the patients, and the tubular changes including focal dilation are considered the main factor responsible for increased cortical echogenicity.

Acute and chronic renal failure

Acute renal failure is due to insufficient renal perfusion (prerenal), intrinsic renal disease (renal), or urinary tract obstruction (postrenal). Among these, intrinsic renal parenchymal disease is the most common cause of acute renal failure.

US is commonly used in evaluating the kidneys in acute renal failure. The primary role of US is to rule out urinary tract obstruction. In acute renal failure due to primary renal parenchymal disease, gray-scale US may reveal globular renal enlargement. Renal parenchymal echogenicity is variable but is frequently hypoechoic due to edema. The degree of renal corticomedullary differentiation is also variable. Renal medulla is often prominent and hypoechoic resulting in increased corticomedullary differentiation.

RI obtained in intrarenal arteries is usually elevated, and end-diastolic velocity of the Doppler spectrum is frequently zero (RI is 1.0). In a study of children with acute renal failure secondary to hemolytic uremic syndrome, Doppler RI improved before clinical improvement. In an experimental study of acute renal failure in rabbits, the change in the RI preceded the change in serum creatinine levels in recovery phase.

Chronic renal failure refers to irreversible loss of renal function. Radiologically it is characterized by bilaterally small kidneys. On US, parenchymal echogenicity may be variable depending on the etiology of renal failure but most often is diffusely increased. CT may demonstrate bilaterally small kidneys with parenchymal thinning. Occasionally, parenchymal calcifications can be seen on nonenhanced CT.

Acute renal failure secondary to rhabdomyolysis

Rhabdomyolysis is a condition in which injury to the skeletal muscle results in leakage of myoglobin from myocytes into the plasma. Myoglobinuric renal failure accounts for 5% to 8% of all cases of acute renal failure. The major causes of rhabdomyolysis include trauma, ischemic or thermal muscle injury, exposure to drugs and toxins, and extreme muscular activity.

The diagnosis of rhabdomyolysis and associated acute renal failure is easily made by detection of urinary myoglobin and elevated creatinine phosphokinase, but myoglobin is absent in the urine in about 30% of the patients.

IVU and CT may demonstrate enlarged kidneys and a striate nephrogram. However, these findings are nonspecific and can be seen in any condition that may alter renal blood flow, including hypotension and renal vein thrombosis. Common US findings of the kidneys include renal enlargement, increased cortical echogenicity, and prominent renal medulla. On MR imaging, unlike other renal parenchymal diseases, corticomedullary contrast is preserved on T1-weighted MR images.

Exercise-induced nonmyoglobinuric acute renal failure

Acute nonmyoglobinuric renal failure with severe loin pain and patchy renal vasoconstriction is a clinical syndrome that usually occurs in young and previously healthy persons following strenuous exercise such as a track race, swimming, or skiing. Most of the patients have a history of taking analgesics prior to exercise. Several cases of this syndrome have been reported since it was first described in 1981. The pathophysiology of this syndrome is thought to be renal vasoconstriction at the level of the arcuate or interlobar arteries.

US findings are nonspecific. Immediate contrast-enhanced CT demonstrates multiple patchy areas of poor contrast enhancement. These areas of poor contrast enhancement at initial CT scan appear as patchy or wedge-shaped areas of enhancement on delayed scans obtained several hours later without further injection of contrast media. Although delayed patchy nephrogram is a characteristic finding of exercise-induced nonmyoglobinuric acute renal failure, it can also be seen in the hepatorenal syndrome, the recovery phase of rhabdomyolysis-related acute renal failure or hemorrhagic fever with renal syndrome, or the focal form of acute pyelonephritis.

Contrast material–induced acute renal failure

Acute renal failure is a serious complication following the use of intravascular radiographic contrast material. The exact incidence and mechanism of contrast material–induced renal failure are unknown, but like other nephrotoxins, acute tubular necrosis is considered to be a major mechanism of the renal failure. The diagnosis of contrast material–induced renal failure is made when azotemia develops more than 24 hours after the use of contrast material. Most of the patients are nonoliguric, except those with preexisting renal diseases.

Careful observation of the pattern of nephrographic density on IVU can allow the radiologist to predict subsequent renal functional impairment. Persistently dense nephrogram on IVU may be a clue to the detection of contrast material–induced acute renal failure. When a 30-minute nephrogram is denser than a 5-minute nephrogram and no evidence of obstruction is seen on IVU, contrast material–induced renal failure should be suspected.

Paroxysmal nocturnal hemoglobinuria

Paroxysmal nocturnal hemoglobinuria is an acquired hemolytic disorder characterized by acute or chronic intravascular hemolysis. Major clinical features include hemoglobinuria, iron deficiency anemia, and venous thrombosis. The basic pathophysiology of the disease is an increased sensitivity to complement-mediated erythrocyte lysis. Intravascular hemolysis results in release of hemoglobin into the plasma. When the amount of released hemoglobin exceeds the binding capacity of plasma haptoglobin, hemoglobin is filtered through the glomerulus into the urine and is reabsorbed and stored as hemosiderin in the epithelial cells of the proximal convoluted tubules.

MR imaging may demonstrate characteristic findings caused by paramagnetic effect of hemosiderin. The signal intensity of the renal cortex is markedly decreased on both T1- and T2-weighted MR images, but the finding is more prominent on T2-weighted images than on T1-weighted images. On contrast-enhanced CT, hemosiderin pigments deposited in the renal cortex may reveal slightly high attenuation. Similar radiologic findings may be seen in any conditions that cause severe intravascular hemolysis and deposition of hemosiderin in the

renal cortex. The examples of such conditions are sickle cell disease and longstanding mechanical hemolysis due to malfunctioning cardiac valves.

Hemorrhagic fever with renal syndrome

Hemorrhagic fever with renal syndrome is an acute infectious disease caused by Hantavirus and clinically characterized by fever, visceral hemorrhage, and a variable degree of renal failure. Hemorrhagic fever with renal syndrome occurs primarily in Asia and Europe. The most prominent pathologic features of the disease are hemorrhage in the renal medulla, right atrium of the heart, and anterior lobe of the pituitary gland.

Plain radiography, US, and CT of the kidney show nonspecific findings of acute renal failure, that is, globular renal swelling and impaired renal perfusion. US findings include swollen kidneys, compressed renal sinus, increased cortical echogenicity, and prominent renal medulla. Doppler spectrum obtained at intrarenal arteries may demonstrate elevated RI. Contrast-enhanced CT demonstrates delayed washout of contrast media from the kidney with a cart-wheel pattern.

The constant and characteristic MR imaging finding of the severe disease is low signal intensity along the medulla, especially outer medulla, on T2-weighted images, probably representing medullary congestion and hemorrhage. This may be due to paramagnetic effect of deoxyhemoglobin or methemoglobin within intact erythrocytes at the region of outer medulla where hemorrhage and congestion are most severe.

References

1. Kim SH, Kim B: Renal parenchymal disease. In Pollack HM, McClennan BL (eds): Clinical Urography, 2nd ed, vol 3. Philadelphia, WB Saunders, 2000, pp 2652–2687.
2. Lee JW, Kim SH, Yoon CJ: Hemosiderin deposition on the renal cortex by mechanical hemolysis due to malfunctioning prosthetic cardiac valve: Report of MR findings in two cases. J Comput Assist Tomogr 1999; 23:445–447.
3. Kim YS, Lee JS, Ahn C, et al: Magnetic resonance imaging of the kidney in hemorrhagic fever with renal syndrome: Its histopathologic correlation. Nephron 1997; 76:477–480.
4. Platt JF, Rubin JM, Ellis JH: Lupus nephritis: Predictive value of conventional and Doppler US and comparison with serologic and biopsy parameters. Radiology 1997; 203:82–86.
5. Arias M, Abreu JA, Iglesias A, et al: Primary amyloidosis presenting as renal infarction. Eur Radiol 1996; 6:346–348.
6. Kettritz U, Semelka RC, Brown ED, et al: MR findings in diffuse renal parenchymal disease. J Magn Res Imaging 1996; 6:136–144.
7. Kim YS, Ahn C, Han JS, Kim S, et al: Hemorrhagic fever with renal syndrome caused by the Seoul virus. Nephron 1995; 71:419–427.
8. Özbek SS, Büyükberber S, Tolunay Ö, et al: Image-directed color Doppler ultrasonography of kidney in systemic lupus nephritis. J Clin Ultrasound 1995; 23:17–20.
9. Yoon DY, Kim SH, Kim HD, et al: Doppler sonography in experimentally induced acute renal failure in rabbits: Resistive index versus serum creatinine levels. Invest Radiol 1995; 30:168–172.
10. Bude RO, Rubin JM, Adler R: Power versus conventional color Doppler sonography: Comparison in the depiction of normal intrarenal vasculature. Radiology 1994; 192:777–780.
11. Davidson AJ, Hartman DS: A systemic approach to the radiologic diagnosis of parenchymal disease of the kidney. In Davidson AJ, Hartman DS (eds): Radiology of the Kidney and Urinary Tract, 2nd ed. Philadelphia, WB Saunders, 1994, pp 99–107.
12. Gollub MJ, Yee JM: Unusual pattern of reversible renal hyperechogenicity associated with acute myoglobinuric renal failure. J Clin Ultrasound 1994; 22:279–281.
13. Semelka RC, Corrigan K, Ascher SM, et al: Renal corticomedullary differentiation: Observation in patients with differing serum creatinine levels. Radiology 1994; 190:149–152.
14. Kay CJ: Renal diseases in patients with AIDS: Sonographic findings. AJR A J Roentgenol 1992; 159:551–554.
15. Kim SH, Han MC, Kim S, et al: Acute renal failure secondary to rhabdomyolysis: MR imaging of the kidney. Acta Radiol 1992; 33:573–576.
16. Kim SH, Kim WH, Choi BI, et al: Duplex Doppler US in patients with medical renal disease: Resistive index versus serum creatinine level. Clin Radiol 1992; 45:85–87.
17. Kim SH, Kim SM, Lee HK, et al: Diabetic nephropathy: Duplex Doppler ultrasound findings. Diabetes Res Clin Pract 1992; 18:75–81.
18. Han JS, Kim YG, Kim S, et al: Bone scintigraphy in acute renal failure with severe loin pain and patchy renal vasoconstriction. Nephron 1991; 59:254–260.
19. Kim SH, Han MC, Han JS, et al: Exercise-induced acute renal failure and patchy renal vasoconstriction: CT and MR findings. J Comput Assist Tomogr 1991; 15:985–988.
20. Kim SH, Han MC, Lee JS, et al: Paroxysmal nocturnal hemoglobinuria: Case report of MR imaging and CT findings. Acta Radiol 1991; 32:315–316.
21. Platt JF, Rubin JM, Ellis JH: Acute renal failure: Possible role of duplex Doppler US in distinction between acute prerenal failure and acute tubular necrosis. Radiology 1991; 179:419–423.
22. Kim SH, Kim S, Lee JS, et al: Hemorrhagic fever with renal syndrome: MR imaging of the kidney. Radiology 1990; 175:823–825.
23. Platt JF, Ellis JH, Rubin JM, et al: Intrarenal arterial Doppler sonography in patients with nonobstructive renal disease: Correlation of resistive index with biopsy findings. AJR Am J Roentgenol 1990; 154:1223–1227.
24. Hamper UM, Goldblum LE, Hutchins GM, et al: Renal involvement in AIDS: Sonographic-pathologic correlation. AJR Am J Roentgenol 1988; 150:1321–1325.
25. Ozaki I, Sakemi T, Sanai T, et al: Patchy renal vasoconstriction in rhabdomyolysis-related acute renal failure. Nephron 1988; 48:136–137.
26. Patriquin HB, O'Regan S, Robitaille P, et al: Hemolytic-uremic syndrome: Intrarenal arterial Doppler patterns as a useful guide to therapy. Radiology 1989; 172:625–628.
27. Platt JF, Rubin JM, Bowerman RA, et al: The inability to detect kidney disease on the basis of echogenicity. AJR Am J Roentgenol 1988; 151:317–319.
28. Ishikawa I, Saito Y, Shinoda A, et al: Evidence for patchy renal vasoconstriction in man: Observation by CT scan. Nephron 1981; 27:31–34.

Illustrations • Renal Parenchymal Disease

1 • Renal parenchymal disease: US findings

2 • Diabetic nephropathy

3 • Lupus nephritis

4 • Scleroderma

5 • Polyarteritis nodosa

6 • Acute renal failure

7 • Shock nephrogram

8 • Renal cortical necrosis

9 • Exercise-induced acute renal failure

10 • Rhabdomyolysis-associated acute renal failure

11 • Hepatorenal syndrome

12 • Hemorrhagic fever with renal syndrome

13 • Paroxysmal nocturnal hemoglobinuria

14 • Other causes of iron deposition in the kidney

15 • Chronic renal failure

16 • Renal osteodystrophy

1. Renal Parenchymal Disease: US Findings

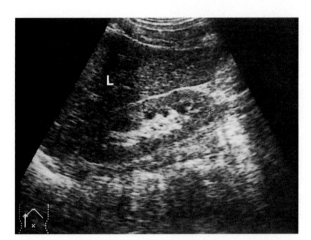

Fig. 1. Renal parenchymal disease in a 47-year-old man. Longitudinal US of the right kidney shows normal size but increased cortical echogenicity. Note that the renal cortical echogenicity *(asterisks)* is higher than that of the liver (L). Corticomedullary differentiation is preserved.

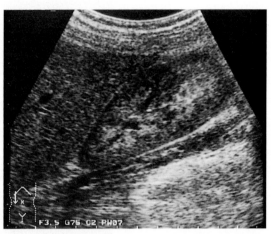

Fig. 2. A 27-year-old woman with nephrotic syndrome. Longitudinal US of the right kidney shows increased echogenicity of renal parenchyma with obliteration of corticomedullary contrast. Note that there is an ill-defined hypoechoic rim along the subcapsular cortex. Renal biopsy revealed mesangiopathic glomerulopathy with focal segmental glomerulosclerosis. (From Kim SH, Kim B: Renal parenchymal disease. In Pollack HM, McClennan BL [eds]: Clinical Urography, 2nd ed, vol 3. Philadelphia, WB Saunders, 2000, pp 2652–2687.)

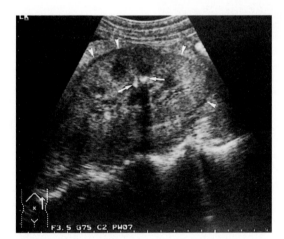

Fig. 3. Renal parenchymal disease in a 60-year-old man with diabetes and pituitary adenoma with acromegaly. Longitudinal US of the left kidney shows increased cortical echogenicity with preserved corticomedullary differentiation. Note a thin hypoechoic rim *(arrowheads)* beneath the outer margin of the kidney, which is often seen in patients with renal parenchymal disease. Also note small calcifications in the tip of the renal papilla *(arrows)*.

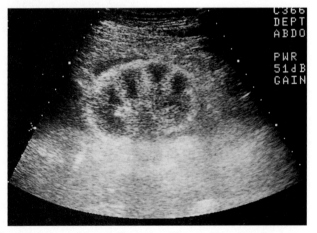

Fig. 4. Renal parenchymal disease in a 54-year-old woman. On longitudinal US, the kidney is small with a hyperechoic cortex and hypoechoic medulla causing accentuation of corticomedullary contrast. (From Kim SH, Kim B: Renal parenchymal disease. In Pollack HM, McClennan BL [eds]: Clinical Urography, 2nd ed, vol 3. Philadelphia, WB Saunders, 2000, pp 2652–2687.)

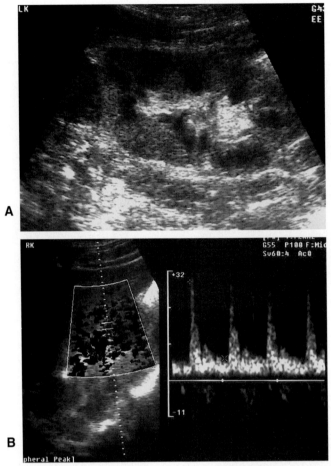

Fig. 5. Amyloidosis of the kidney associated with multiple myeloma in a 59-year-old man. (**A, B,** Courtesy of Se Hyung Kim, MD.)
A. US shows large kidney with increased renal cortical echogenicity.
B. Spectral Doppler US of the right kidney shows elevated resistive index of 0.77.

2. Diabetic Nephropathy

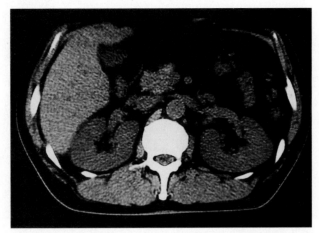

Fig. 1. Chronic renal failure due to diabetic nephropathy in a 46-year-old man. Nonenhanced CT scan shows normal size and shape of the kidneys in spite of end-stage renal disease. This finding is characteristic of diabetic nephropathy.

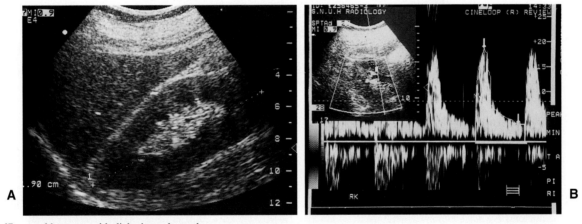

Fig. 2. A 67-year-old woman with diabetic nephropathy.
A. On gray-scale US, the right kidney appears normal in size and echogenicity. **B.** Spectral Doppler US performed at interlobar artery of the right kidney demonstrates decreased end-diastolic frequency shift and elevated resistive index (0.81).

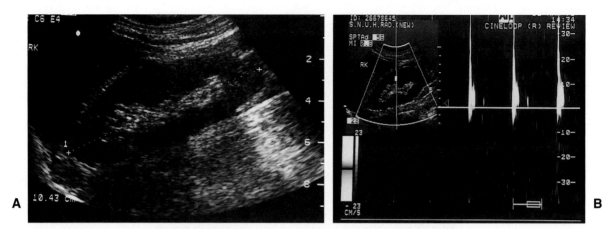

Fig. 3. A 62-year-old man with severe diabetic nephropathy.
A, B. Although the kidneys appeared normal on gray-scale US (**A**), spectral Doppler US (**B**) shows markedly decreased renal blood flow and absent end-diastolic flow with resistive index of 1.0.

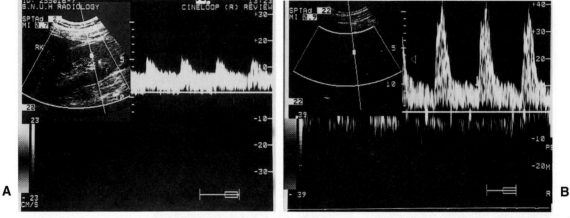

Fig. 4. A 28-year-old woman with progressing diabetic nephropathy.
A. Spectral Doppler US of the right kidney shows normal spectral pattern and normal resistive index. **B.** Spectral Doppler US taken 3 years later demonstrates markedly changed spectral pattern with an elevated resistive index (0.8).

2. Diabetic Nephropathy

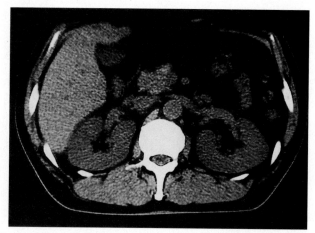

Fig. 1. Chronic renal failure due to diabetic nephropathy in a 46-year-old man. Nonenhanced CT scan shows normal size and shape of the kidneys in spite of end-stage renal disease. This finding is characteristic of diabetic nephropathy.

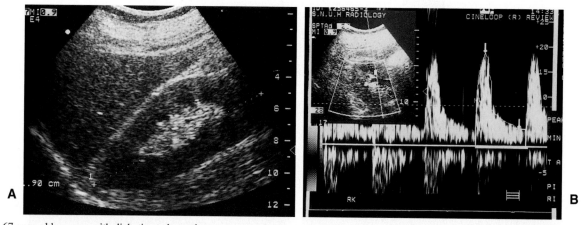

Fig. 2. A 67-year-old woman with diabetic nephropathy.
A. On gray-scale US, the right kidney appears normal in size and echogenicity. **B.** Spectral Doppler US performed at interlobar artery of the right kidney demonstrates decreased end-diastolic frequency shift and elevated resistive index (0.81).

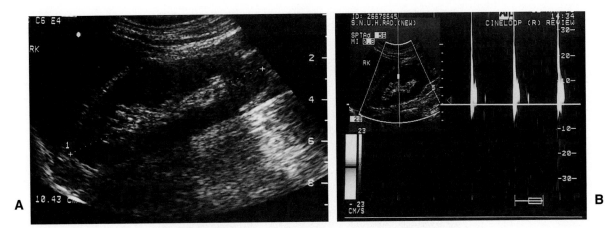

Fig. 3. A 62-year-old man with severe diabetic nephropathy.
A, B. Although the kidneys appeared normal on gray-scale US (**A**), spectral Doppler US (**B**) shows markedly decreased renal blood flow and absent end-diastolic flow with resistive index of 1.0.

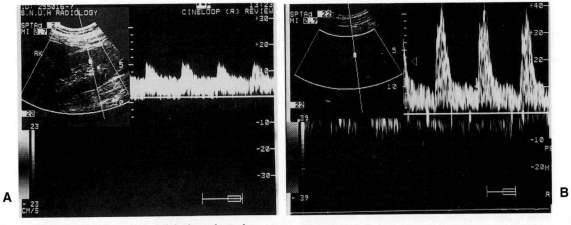

Fig. 4. A 28-year-old woman with progressing diabetic nephropathy.
A. Spectral Doppler US of the right kidney shows normal spectral pattern and normal resistive index. **B.** Spectral Doppler US taken 3 years later demonstrates markedly changed spectral pattern with an elevated resistive index (0.8).

3. Lupus Nephritis

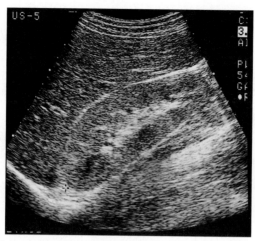

Fig. 1. Systemic lupus erythematosus in a 31-year-old man. Longitudinal US of the right kidney shows diffusely increased parenchymal echogenicity. Note that the cortical echogenicity is higher than that of the liver.

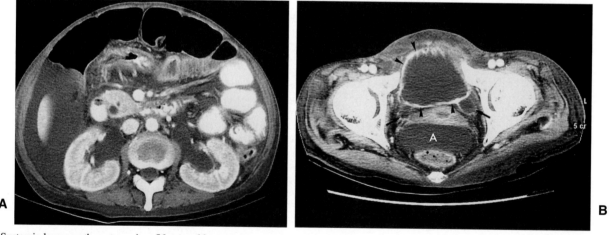

Fig. 2. Systemic lupus erythematosus in a 56-year-old woman.
A. Contrast-enhanced CT shows bilateral hydronephrosis and ascites. Note that the renal cortex is thin and poorly enhanced. **B.** On CT scan at a lower level, bladder wall strongly enhances *(arrowheads)*. Terminal ureters *(arrows)* are dilated without obstructive lesion at the ureterovesical junctions. Note ascites (A) in rectouterine pouch.

4. Scleroderma

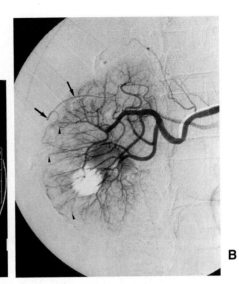

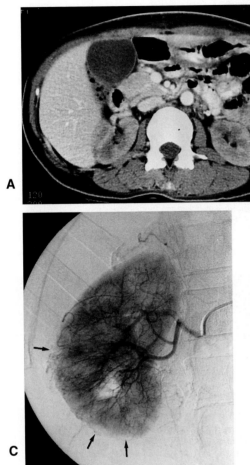

Fig. 1. Renal failure caused by scleroderma in a 46-year-old woman. (**A–C,** From Kim SH, Kim B: Renal parenchymal disease. In Pollack HM, McClennan BL [eds]: Clinical Urography, 2nd ed, vol 3. Philadelphia, WB Saunders, 2000, pp 2652–2687.) **A.** Contrast-enhanced CT shows small kidneys with poor parenchymal enhancement. **B.** Renal arteriogram in early arterial phase shows diffuse irregularity of small arterial branches. Note that some arteries are cut off at interlobar levels *(arrowheads)*. Also note collateral circulation through prominent capsular arteries *(arrows)*. **C.** Renal arteriogram in nephrographic phase shows multiple perfusion defects *(arrows)* in the periphery of interpolar and lower-polar regions of the right kidney.

5. Polyarteritis Nodosa

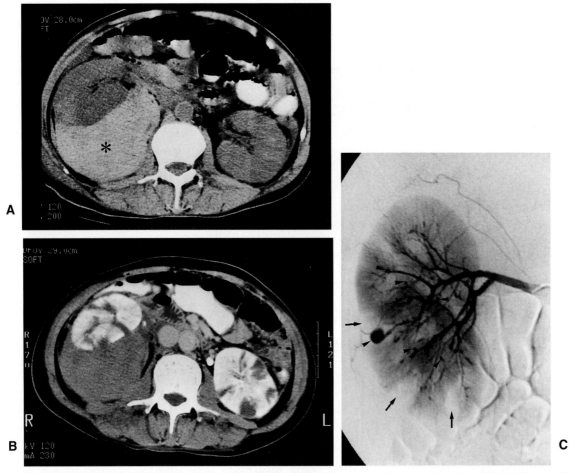

Fig. 1. Polyarteritis nodosa in a 42-year-old man. (**A, C,** From Kim SH, Kim B: Renal parenchymal disease. In Pollack HM, McClennan BL [eds]: Clinical Urography, 2nd ed, vol 3. Philadelphia, WB Saunders, 2000, pp 2652–2687.)
A. Nonenhanced CT shows a large, high-attenuated hematoma *(asterisk)* in the right perirenal space, displacing the right kidney anteriorly.
B. Contrast-enhanced CT shows multiple perfusion defects in both kidneys representing multifocal renal infarcts. **C.** Right renal arteriogram shows multiple aneurysms *(arrowheads)* of the intrarenal arteries. Also note multifocal wedge-shaped perfusion defects *(arrows)* in both kidneys representing infarcts.

6. Acute Renal Failure

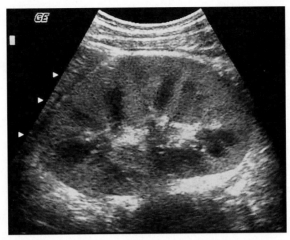

Fig. 1. Acute renal failure developed following strenuous exercise in a 19-year-old man. Longitudinal US of the right kidney shows globular renal swelling, increased cortical echogenicity, and accentuated corticomedullary contrast.

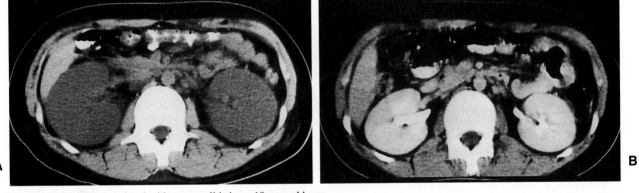

Fig. 2. Acute renal failure associated with enterocolitis in an 18-year-old man.
A. Nonenhanced CT shows globular renal swelling and obliteration of renal sinus fat in both kidneys. (**A,** From Kim SH, Kim B: Renal parenchymal disease. In Pollack HM, McClennan BL [eds]: Clinical Urography, 2nd ed, vol 3. Philadelphia, WB Saunders, 2000, pp 2652–2687.) **B.** Contrast-enhanced CT scan taken 2 weeks after **A** when renal failure resolved shows decreased renal size and regained renal excretory function.

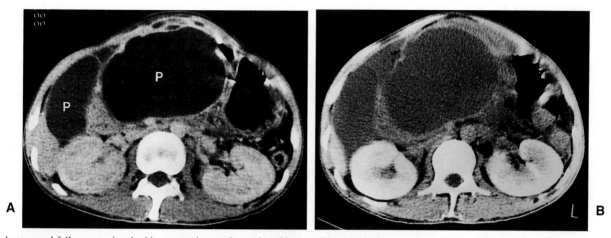

Fig. 3. Acute renal failure associated with pancreatic pseudocyst in a 30-year-old man. (**A, B,** From Kim SH, Kim B: Renal parenchymal disease. In Pollack HM, McClennan BL [eds]: Clinical Urography, 2nd ed, vol 3. Philadelphia, WB Saunders, 2000, pp 2652–2687.)
A. Contrast-enhanced CT shows multiple, large pseudocysts of the pancreas (P) and both kidneys poorly enhancing. **B.** A 24-hour-delayed CT scan shows prolonged dense nephrogram of both kidneys.

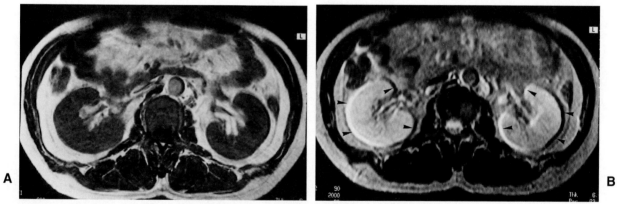

Fig. 4. Acute renal failure in a 50-year-old man. (**A, B,** From Kim SH, Kim B: Renal parenchymal disease. In Pollack HM, McClennan BL [eds]: Clinical Urography, 2nd ed, vol 3. Philadelphia, WB Saunders, 2000, pp 2652–2687.)
A, B. T1-weighted (**A**) and T2-weighted (**B**) MR images of the kidney show both kidneys swollen and obliterated corticomedullary contrast on T1-weighted image. Note chemical shift artifacts on T2-weighted image *(arrowheads)*.

7. Shock Nephrogram

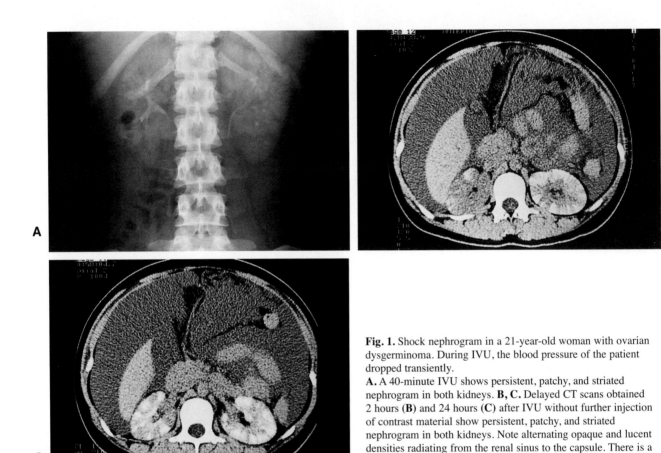

Fig. 1. Shock nephrogram in a 21-year-old woman with ovarian dysgerminoma. During IVU, the blood pressure of the patient dropped transiently.
A. A 40-minute IVU shows persistent, patchy, and striated nephrogram in both kidneys. **B, C.** Delayed CT scans obtained 2 hours (**B**) and 24 hours (**C**) after IVU without further injection of contrast material show persistent, patchy, and striated nephrogram in both kidneys. Note alternating opaque and lucent densities radiating from the renal sinus to the capsule. There is a large amount of ascites due to peritoneal seeding of ovarian dysgerminoma.

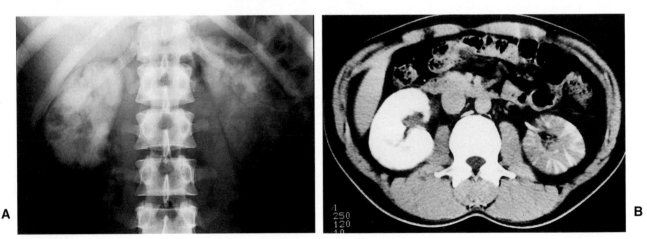

Fig. 2. Shock nephrogram in a 25-year-old man with right ureter stone.
A. A 2-hour delayed IVU shows dense striated nephrogram of the right kidney due to obstruction by a ureteral stone. Note striated and patchy nephrogram of the left kidney due to patchy renal vasoconstriction. The patient did not have any symptoms during IVU. **B.** CT scan obtained 30 minutes after **A** without further injection of contrast material demonstrates dense nephrogram of the right kidney due to obstruction and patchy and striated nephrogram of the left kidney due to renal vasoconstriction.

8. Renal Cortical Necrosis

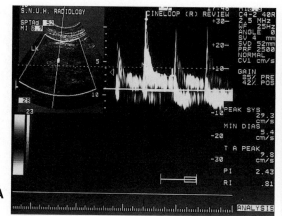

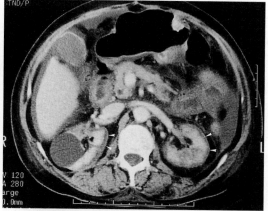

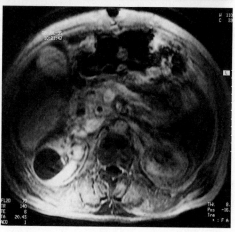

Fig. 1. Acute renal cortical necrosis developed following gastrectomy for stomach cancer in a 73-year-old man.
A. Spectral Doppler US of the left kidney shows elevated resistive index (0.81). **B.** Contrast-enhanced CT shows lack of contrast enhancement selectively in the renal cortex with preserved enhancement of the renal medulla. Note a thin, enhancing rim of subcapsular cortex *(arrowheads)*. There is a renal cyst in the right kidney. **C.** Contrast-enhanced T1-weighted MR image similarly shows lack of enhancement in the renal cortex.

9. Exercise-induced Acute Renal Failure

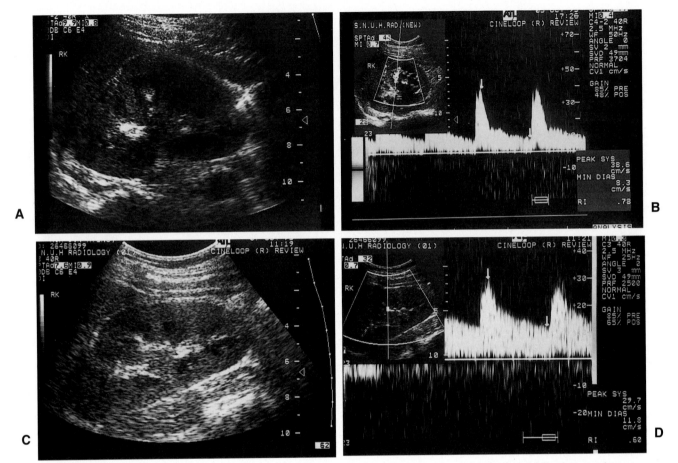

Fig. 1. Exercise-induced acute renal failure in an 18-year-old man. The patient presented with anuria, which developed following a track race. (**A–D,** From Kim SH, Kim B: Renal parenchymal disease. In Pollack HM, McClennan BL [eds]: Clinical Urography, 2nd ed, vol 3. Philadelphia, WB Saunders, 2000, pp 2652–2687.)
A. US of the right kidney shows globular swelling, slightly increased cortical echogenicity, and preserved corticomedullary contrast. **B.** Spectral Doppler US shows decreased end-diastolic frequency shift and elevated resistive index (0.78). **C.** US of the right kidney taken 2 days later shows decreased renal swelling. **D.** Spectral Doppler US obtained at the same time as **C** shows a normalized Doppler spectral waveform with normal resistive index (0.60).

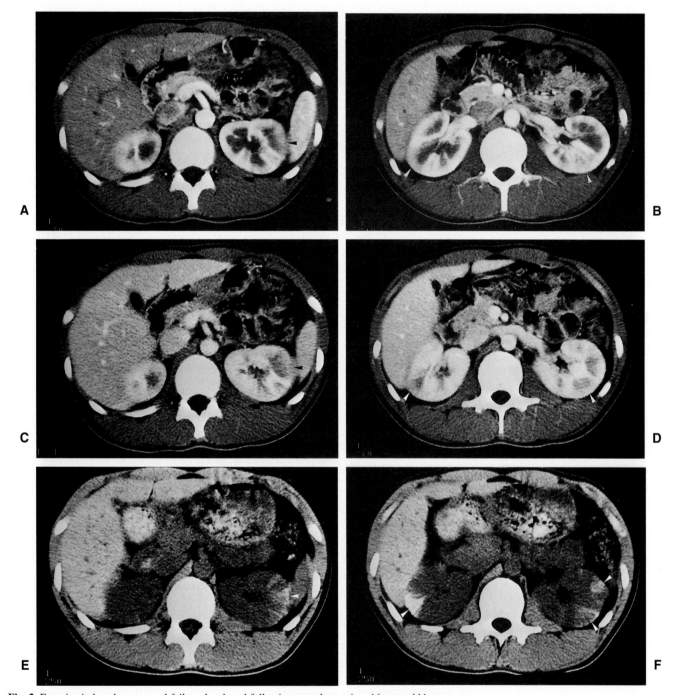

Fig. 2. Exercise-induced acute renal failure developed following a track race in a 16-year-old boy.
A, B. Contrast-enhanced CT scans in early cortical phase demonstrate ill-defined perfusion defects *(arrowheads)* in the renal cortex. **C, D.** On nephrographic phase CT scans, the perfusion defects *(arrowheads)* are better demonstrated. **E, F.** Nonenhanced CT scans obtained 24 hours later demonstrate patchy areas of delayed enhancement *(arrowheads)*. These areas correlate well with the perfusion defects seen on **A–D.**

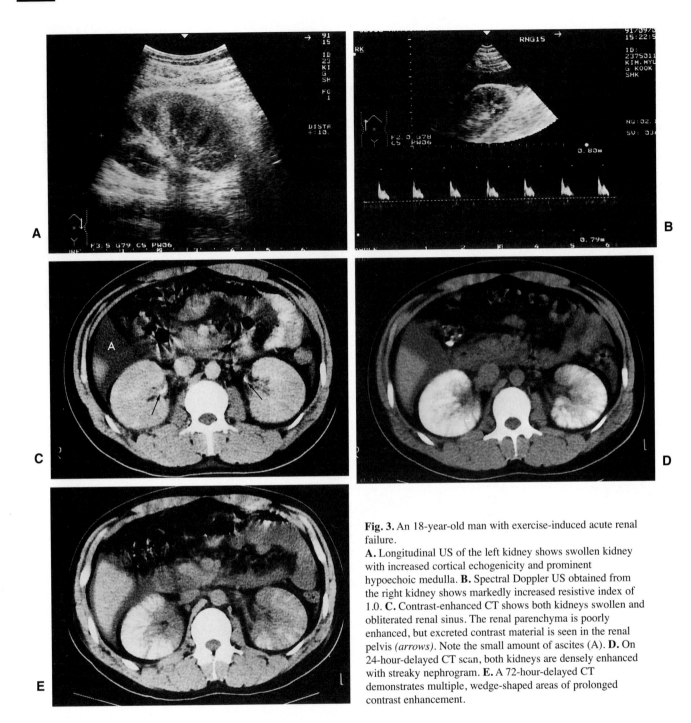

Fig. 3. An 18-year-old man with exercise-induced acute renal failure.
A. Longitudinal US of the left kidney shows swollen kidney with increased cortical echogenicity and prominent hypoechoic medulla. **B.** Spectral Doppler US obtained from the right kidney shows markedly increased resistive index of 1.0. **C.** Contrast-enhanced CT shows both kidneys swollen and obliterated renal sinus. The renal parenchyma is poorly enhanced, but excreted contrast material is seen in the renal pelvis *(arrows)*. Note the small amount of ascites (A). **D.** On 24-hour-delayed CT scan, both kidneys are densely enhanced with streaky nephrogram. **E.** A 72-hour-delayed CT demonstrates multiple, wedge-shaped areas of prolonged contrast enhancement.

10. Rhabdomyolysis-associated Acute Renal Failure

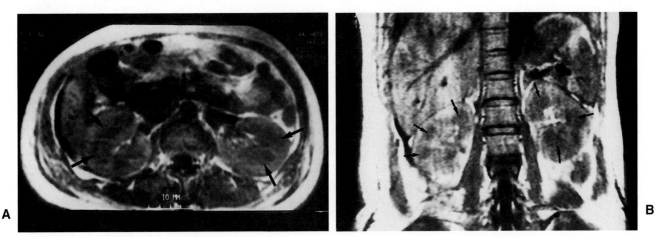

A   B

Fig. 1. Rhabdomyolysis-associated acute renal failure that occurred following a snake bite in a 48-year-old woman. (**A, B,** From Kim SH, Han MC, Kim S, et al: Acute renal failure secondary to rhabdomyolysis: MR imaging of the kidney. Acta Radiol 1992; 33:573–576.)
A, B. T1-weighted MR images in axial (**A**) and coronal (**B**) planes show globular swelling of both kidneys and relatively preserved low signal intensity of the renal medullae *(arrows)* and resultant preserved corticomedullary contrast. Renal biopsy revealed acute tubular necrosis.

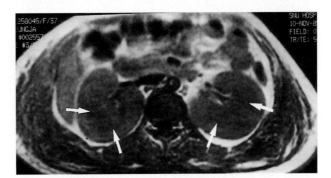

Fig. 2. A 38-year-old woman with acute renal failure secondary to rhabdomyolysis caused by carbon monoxide poisoning. T1-weighted MR image shows swollen kidneys with relatively preserved corticomedullary contrast by low signal intensity of renal medullae *(arrows)*.

11. Hepatorenal Syndrome

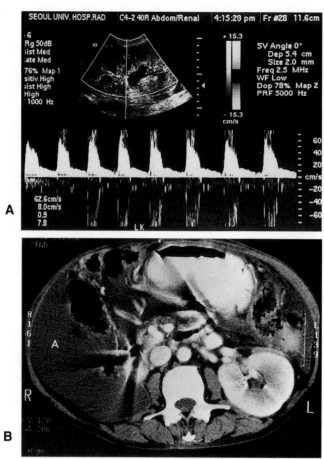

Fig. 1. Hepatorenal syndrome in a 70-year-old woman who had liver cirrhosis and hepatocellular carcinoma. She underwent right nephrectomy for arteriovenous malformation 20 years earlier.
A. Spectral Doppler US of the left kidney shows decreased end-diastolic frequency shift and elevated resistive index (0.9). **B.** Contrast-enhanced CT obtained for evaluation of the liver shows swelling of the left kidney with poor contrast enhancement. Note that the right kidney is absent due to previous nephrectomy and there is a large amount of ascites (A).

12. Hemorrhagic Fever with Renal Syndrome

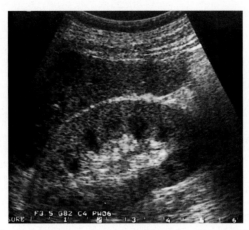

Fig. 1. Hemorrhagic fever with renal syndrome in a 45-year-old man. Longitudinal US of the right kidney shows an enlarged kidney and increased renal cortical echogenicity. Renal medullae are prominent, and corticomedullary contrast is preserved.

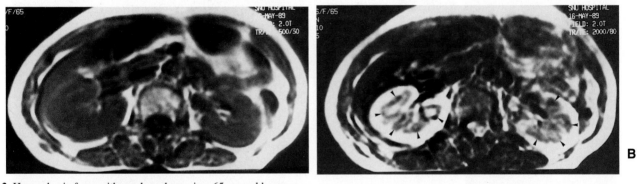

Fig. 2. Hemorrhagic fever with renal syndrome in a 65-year-old woman.
A. T1-weighted MR image shows globular renal swelling. **B.** T2-weighted MR image shows low-intensity bands along the outer medulla *(arrowheads)* due to congestion and hemorrhage. (**B,** From Kim SH, Kim S, Lee JS, et al: Hemorrhagic fever with renal syndrome: MR imaging of the kidney. Radiology 1990; 175:823–825.)

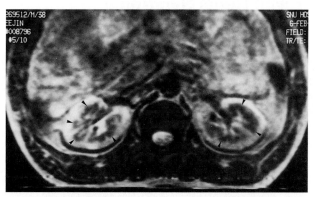

Fig. 3. Hemorrhagic fever with renal syndrome in a 38-year-old man. T2-weighted MR image well demonstrates the low-intensity lesions along the outer medulla *(arrowheads)*. (From Kim SH, Kim B: Renal parenchymal disease. In Pollack HM, McClennan BL [eds]: Clinical Urography, 2nd ed, vol 3. Philadelphia, WB Saunders, 2000, pp 2652–2687.)

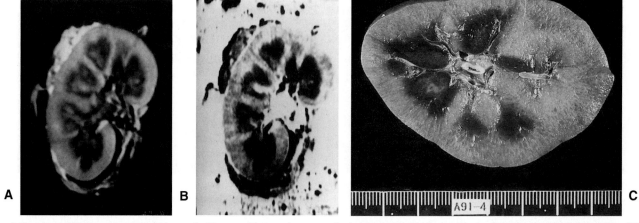

Fig. 4. Specimen MR imaging of the kidney of a 21-year-old man who succumbed to hemorrhagic fever with renal syndrome. (**A–C**, From Kim YS, Lee JS, Ahn C, et al: Magnetic resonance imaging of the kidney in hemorrhagic fever with renal syndrome: Its histopathologic correlation. Nephron 1997; 76:477–480.)
A, B. T1-weighted (**A**) and T2-weighted (**B**) MR images of the autopsy specimen of the kidney clearly show low-intensity lesions along the outer medulla. **C.** Specimen photograph of the kidney shows congestion and hemorrhage in the outer medullary region. (**C,** See also Color Section.)

13. Paroxysmal Nocturnal Hemoglobinuria

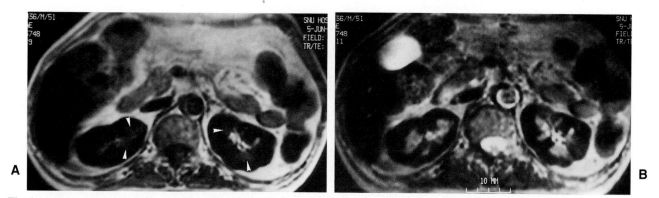

Fig. 1. Paroxysmal nocturnal hemoglobinuria in a 61-year-old man.
A. T1-weighted MR image shows that the signal intensity of the renal cortex is lower than that of the medulla *(arrowheads)*. **B.** T2-weighted MR image well demonstrates the low signal intensity of the renal cortex and normal high intensity of the renal medulla.

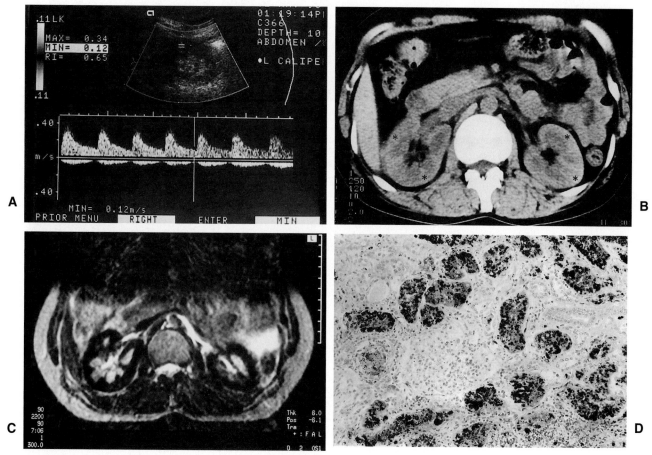

Fig. 2. Paroxysmal nocturnal hemoglobinuria in a 36-year-old woman.
A. Renal Doppler US shows normal gray-scale US findings and normal Doppler spectral patterns. **B.** Nonenhanced CT scan shows slightly high attenuation of the renal cortex *(asterisks)* as compared to the medulla due to iron deposition in the cortex. **C.** T2-weighted MR image clearly demonstrates the low signal intensity of the renal cortex. **D.** Photomicrograph of the renal biopsy specimen with iron staining shows extensive deposition of hemosiderin in the epithelial cells of the proximal convoluted tubules, which appears as dark spots in this photograph.

14. Other Causes of Iron Deposition in the Kidney

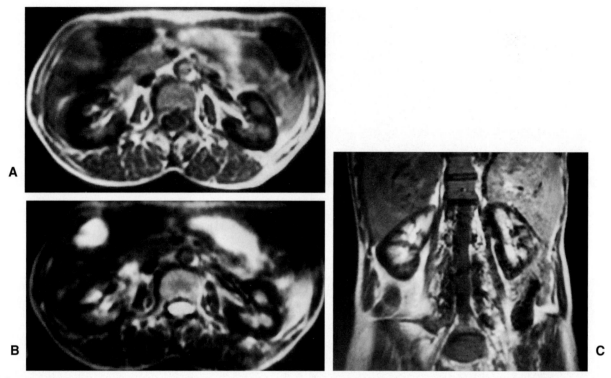

Fig. 1. Iron deposition in the renal cortex caused by intravascular hemolysis due to malfunctioning prosthetic cardiac valves in a 50-year-old woman who received mitral and tricuspid valve replacements 7 years earlier. (**A–C,** From Lee JW, Kim SH, Yoon CJ: Hemosiderin deposition on the renal cortex by mechanical hemolysis due to malfunctioning prosthetic cardiac valve: Report of MR findings in two cases. J Comput Assist Tomogr 1999; 23:445–447.)
A–C. T1-weighted axial (**A**), T2-weighted axial (**B**), and enhanced T1-weighted coronal (**C**) MR images show diffuse low signal intensity of the renal cortex with preserved medullary signal intensity. These MR imaging findings are basically the same as the findings of paroxysmal nocturnal hemoglobinuria.

15. Chronic Renal Failure

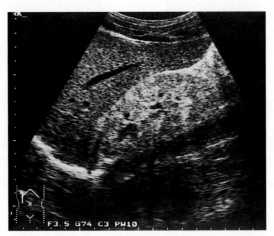

Fig. 1. Chronic renal failure in a 30-year-old man. Longitudinal US shows a small right kidney with markedly increased renal parenchymal echogenicity and obliterated corticomedullary contrast. (From Kim SH, Kim B: Renal parenchymal disease. In Pollack HM, McClennan BL [eds]: Clinical Urography, 2nd ed, vol 3. Philadelphia, WB Saunders, 2000, pp 2652–2687.)

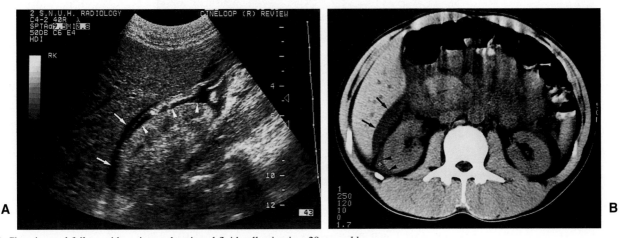

Fig. 2. Chronic renal failure with ascites and perirenal fluid collection in a 28-year-old man.
A. Longitudinal US of the right kidney shows ascites *(arrows)* and fluid collection in the perirenal space *(arrowheads)*. **B.** Nonenhanced CT scan well demonstrates ascites *(arrows)* and perirenal fluid *(arrowheads)*.

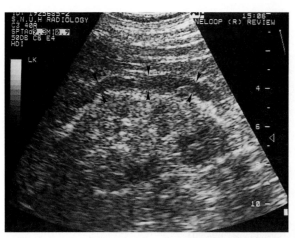

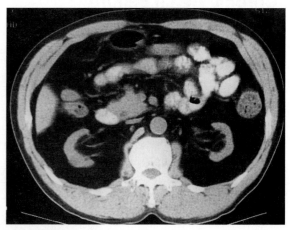

Fig. 3. Chronic renal failure with prominent perirenal fat in a 63-year-old man. Longitudinal US of the left kidney shows a contracted kidney with a lobulated margin. Note the prominent hypoechoic perirenal fat *(arrowheads)* that surrounds the echogenic kidney.

Fig. 4. End-stage renal disease in a 77-year-old man. Nonenhanced CT shows both kidneys to be small and contracted with prominent fatty tissues in the renal sinus and perirenal space. (From Kim SH, Kim B: Renal parenchymal disease. In Pollack HM, McClennan BL [eds]: Clinical Urography, 2nd ed, vol 3. Philadelphia, WB Saunders, 2000, pp 2652–2687.)

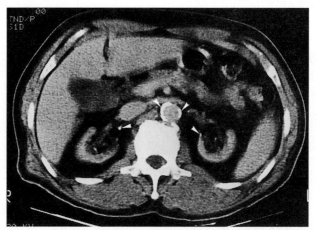

Fig. 5. End-stage renal disease in a 73-year-old man. Contrast-enhanced CT demonstrates contracted kidneys with poor contrast enhancement. Note calcifications in walls of the aorta and renal arteries *(arrowheads)*. (From Kim SH, Kim B: Renal parenchymal disease. In Pollack HM, McClennan BL [eds]: Clinical Urography, 2nd ed, vol 3. Philadelphia, WB Saunders, 2000, pp 2652–2687.)

16. Renal Osteodystrophy

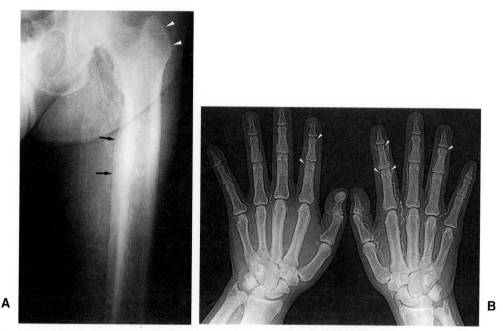

A

B

Fig. 1. Renal osteodystrophy in a 38-year-old woman with chronic renal failure and secondary hyperparathyroidism.
A, B. Plain radiographs of the left thigh (**A**) and both hands (**B**) demonstrate extensive vascular calcifications and bony resorptions *(arrowheads)*. Note periosteal neostosis of the medial aspect of the left femur *(arrows in* **A***)*.

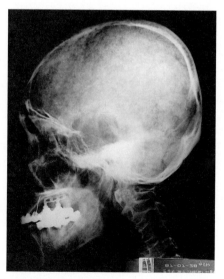

Fig. 2. Renal osteodystrophy in a 62-year-old woman. Plain radiograph of the skull in lateral projection shows a typical salt-and-pepper appearance due to subperiosteal resorption.

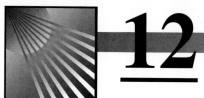

12

Nephrocalcinosis

HAK JONG LEE AND WILLIAM H. BUSH, JR.

Nephrocalcinosis represents calcifications in the renal parenchyma. It can be divided with respect to the locations of calcification. Calcification confined to, or predominantly located in, the renal cortex is known as *cortical nephrocalcinosis*. When the cortex is spared and calcium salts are deposited only in the medullary interstitium or tubular lumina, the condition is known as *medullary nephrocalcinosis*. Medullary nephrocalcinosis is much more common.

CORTICAL NEPHROCALCINOSIS

Cortical nephrocalcinosis is characterized by the peripheral location of the parenchymal calcifications. Most common causes of cortical nephrocalcinosis are renal cortical necrosis and chronic glomerulonephritis.

Renal cortical necrosis, which represents death of the renal cortex with sparing of the medulla, results from any condition that causes an acute and prolonged shock. It occurs often in pregnant women with third-trimester bleeding secondary to abruptio placentae or placenta previa. Renal cortical necrosis can also occur in conditions of sepsis, transfusion reaction, dehydration, and shock.

Cortical nephrocalcinosis also has been seen in chronic glomerulonephritis, rejected renal transplants, hereditary nephropathy with deafness (Alport's syndrome), severe forms of primary hyperoxaluria, chronic paraneoplastic hypercalcemia, and infections associated with acquired immunodeficiency syndrome caused by cytomegalovirus, *Mycobacterium avium-intracellulare*, or *Pneumocystis carinii*.

Radiographic findings of cortical nephrocalcinosis include a single thin peripheral band of calcification, often with perpendicular extensions into the Bertin's septa, parallel calcific tracks showing tram-line appearance, or diffuse distribution of punctate calcific densities representing necrotic calcified cortical glomeruli and tubules. US shows increased cortical echogenicity that may produce acoustic shadowing. CT scans demonstrate increased CT attenuation values in the renal cortex. CT scan is sensitive and can detect nephrocalcinosis before it can be detected on plain radiography. MR imaging findings of cortical nephrocalcinosis reveal low signal intensity on T1- and T2-weighted images representing the calcified renal cortex.

MEDULLARY NEPHROCALCINOSIS

The most common causes of medullary nephrocalcinosis are hyperparathyroidism, renal tubular acidosis, and renal tubular ectasia (medullary sponge kidney). Approximately 40% of cases of medullary nephrocalcinosis are attributable to primary hyperparathyroidism and 20% to renal tubular acidosis. Renal tubular acidosis may be the result of excessive urinary loss of bicarbonate ions, impaired excretion of hydrogen ions, or both. Impaired tubular reabsorption of bicarbonate ions followed by urinary loss of bicarbonate ions is a proximal tubular defect, while impaired ability of secreting hydrogen ions in the distal nephrons is a distal tubular defect. Most of the patients with renal tubular acidosis showing nephrocalcinosis have distal tubular defects. The other causes of medullary nephrocalcinosis are any conditions showing hypercalcemia such as malignancy, bone metastasis, Cushing's syndrome, milk-alkali syndrome, sarcoidosis, hypervitaminosis D, and amphotericin B toxicity. Nephrolithiasis can be caused by the same conditions in which medullary nephrocalcinosis occurs.

The typical plain radiographic finding of medullary nephrocalcinosis is bilateral, stippled calcifications involving the renal pyramids. CT may show uniform deposition of calcium or asymmetrical calcification in renal medullae characterized by calcifications in the dilated collecting ducts of renal tubular ectasia.

On US, medullary nephrocalcinosis appears as increased echogenicity of the renal medullae resulting in reversal of the normal corticomedullary echogenicity. The medullary pyramids may become more echogenic than the adjacent cortex. Small echogenic foci at the tips of medullary pyramids can be observed, which represent the US demonstration of the calcific medullary plaques and foci as the precursors of renal calculi.

Increased medullary echoes on US, so-called hyperechoic medullae, are most often found in premature infants treated with furosemide to prevent pulmonary congestion of bronchopulmonary dysplasia. Furosemide causes hypercalciuria and nephrocalcinosis. Other causes of hyperechoic medullae include polycystic kidney disease, Cushing's syndrome with increased fat, abnormal protein deposition disorder, and renal vein thrombosis.

The patterns of medullary nephrocalcinosis are different according to the underlying diseases. In the case of hyper-

parathyroidism or renal tubular acidosis, diffuse or uniform calcification usually occurs. On the other hand, in the case of medullary sponge kidney, the calcifications are often asymmetrical, segmental, or unilateral.

COMBINED MEDULLARY AND CORTICAL NEPHROCALCINOSIS

Primary and secondary oxalosis characteristically demonstrate both cortical and medullary calcifications. The pattern of calcifications in oxalosis is diffuse and regular. Although renal oxalosis produces increased cortical echogenicity early in its course, it eventually results in diffusely echogenic kidneys without corticomedullary differentiation. CT reveals global calcification of the cortex and medulla.

Nephrocalcinosis caused by infection with *M. avium-intracellulare*, *P. carinii*, or *Histoplasma* may asymmetrically involve the renal cortex and medulla in patients with acquired immunodeficiency syndrome. Partial cortical and medullary nephrocalcinosis may be caused by dystrophic calcification secondary to infection by an atypical *Mycobacterium* or other organisms in these patients. US shows focal areas of increased echogenicity within the kidney. CT in these patients shows increased attenuation in some pyramids and interrupted cortical calcifications.

References

1. Kim SH, Kim B: Renal parenchymal disease. In Pollack HM, McClennan BL (eds): Clinical Urography, 2nd ed, vol 3. Philadelphia, WB Saunders, 2000, pp 2652–2687.
2. Ramchandani P: Radiologic evaluation of renal calculous disease. In Pollack HM, McClennan BL (eds): Clinical Urography, 2nd ed, vol 2. Philadelphia, WB Saunders, 2000, pp 2147–2200.
3. Schepens D, Verswijvel G, Kuypers D, et al: Renal cortical nephrocalcinosis. Nephrol Dial Transplant 2000; 15:1080–1082.
4. Kemper MJ, Muller-Wiefel DE: Nephrocalcinosis in a patient with primary hyperoxaluria type 2. Pediatr Nephrol 1996; 10:442–444.
5. Slovis TL, Bernstein J, Gruskin A: Hyperechoic kidneys in the newborn and young infant. Pediatr Nephrol 1993; 7:294–302.
6. Kay CJ: Renal diseases in patients with AIDS: Sonographic findings. AJR Am J Roentgenol 1992; 159:551–554.
7. Kim SH, Han MC, Lee JS: MR imaging of acute renal cortical necrosis. Acta Radiol 1992; 33:431–433.
8. Falkoff GE, Rigsby CM, Rosenfield AT: Partial, combined cortical and medullary nephrocalcinosis: US and CT patterns in AIDS-associated MAI infection. Radiology 1987; 162:343–344.
9. Day DL, Scheinman JI, Mahan J: Radiological aspects of primary hyperoxaluria. AJR Am J Roentgenol 1986; 146:395–401.
10. Patriquin H, Robitaille P: Renal calcium deposition in children: Sonographic demonstration of Anderson-Carr progression. AJR Am J Roentgenol 1986; 146:1253–1256.
11. Shuman WP, Mack LA, Rogers JV: Diffuse nephrocalcinosis: Hyperechoic sonographic appearance. AJR Am J Roentgenol 1981; 136:830–832.

Illustrations • Nephrocalcinosis

1 • Cortical nephrocalcinosis due to renal cortical necrosis

2 • Medullary nephrocalcinosis due to renal tubular ectasia (medullary sponge kidney)

3 • Medullary nephrocalcinosis due to renal tubular acidosis

4 • Medullary nephrocalcinosis due to other causes

5 • Hyperechoic medullae on US

6 • Cortical and medullary nephrocalcinosis

1. Cortical Nephrocalcinosis due to Renal Cortical Necrosis

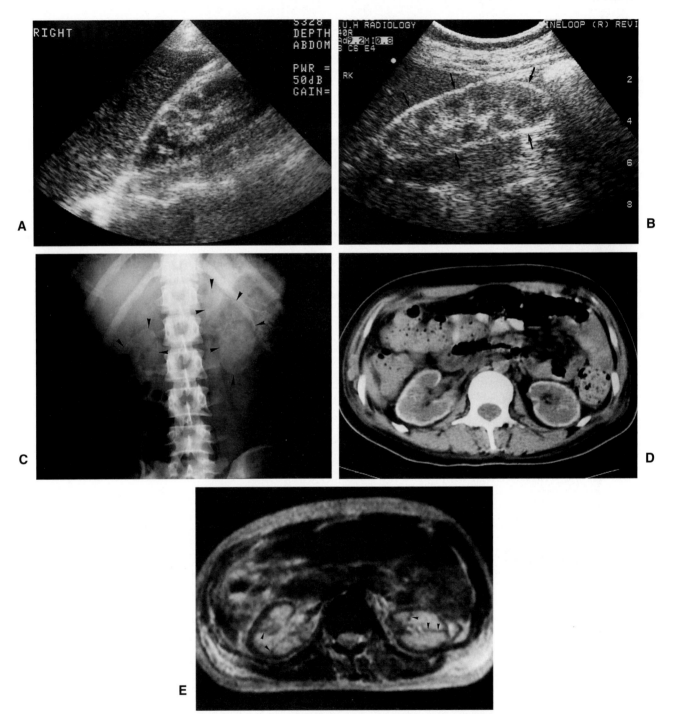

Fig. 1. Cortical nephrocalcinosis due to renal cortical necrosis caused by massive bleeding and shock after abortion in a 28-year-old woman. (**C,** From Kim SH, Kim B: Renal parenchymal disease. In Pollack HM, McClennan BL [eds]: Clinical Urography, 2nd ed, vol 3. Philadelphia, WB Saunders, 2000, pp 2652–2687. **D, E,** From Kim SH, Han MC, Lee JS: MR imaging of acute renal cortical necrosis. Acta Radiol 1992; 33:431–433.)
A. Longitudinal US of the right kidney performed 1 week after the incident shows no morphologic abnormality.
B. Longitudinal US of the right kidney obtained 1 month later shows increased parenchymal echogenicity, especially along the outer margin of the kidney *(arrows)*. **C.** Plain radiograph shows egg-shell calcification outlining both kidneys *(arrowheads)*. **D.** Nonenhanced CT clearly demonstrates calcification of the outer cortex. **E.** T2-weighted MR image demonstrates low-intensity renal cortex due to calcifications. Note that the cortical columns *(arrowheads)* also show low signal intensity.

2. Medullary Nephrocalcinosis due to Renal Tubular Ectasia (Medullary Sponge Kidney)

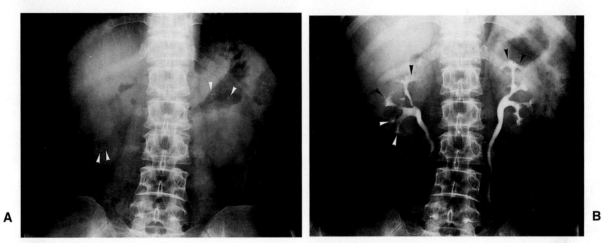

Fig. 1. Renal tubular ectasia (medullary sponge kidney) with medullary nephrocalcinosis in a 61-year-old woman.
A. Plain radiograph shows mottled calcifications asymmetrically distributed in the medullary regions of both kidneys *(arrowheads)*. **B.** IVU shows mottled and brush appearance of the renal medulla due to contrast material in the dilated collecting ducts *(arrowheads)*, some of which contain calcifications. The characteristic finding in renal tubular ectasia is "blooming" of the calculi on IVU as the dilated collecting ducts fill with contrast material around the calculi in the ducts.

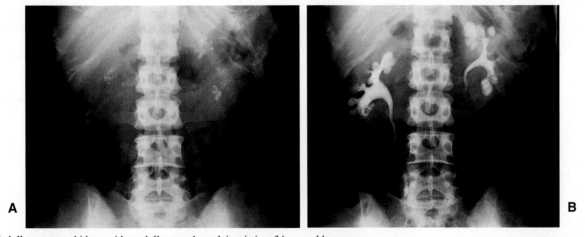

Fig. 2. Medullary sponge kidney with medullary nephrocalcinosis in a 34-year-old woman.
A. Plain radiograph shows multiple small calcifications asymmetrically distributed in the renal medullary regions. **B.** IVU shows mottled and brush appearance of the renal medulla with opacified dilated collecting ducts causing the preexisting calculi to appear to "bloom" and become more prominent.

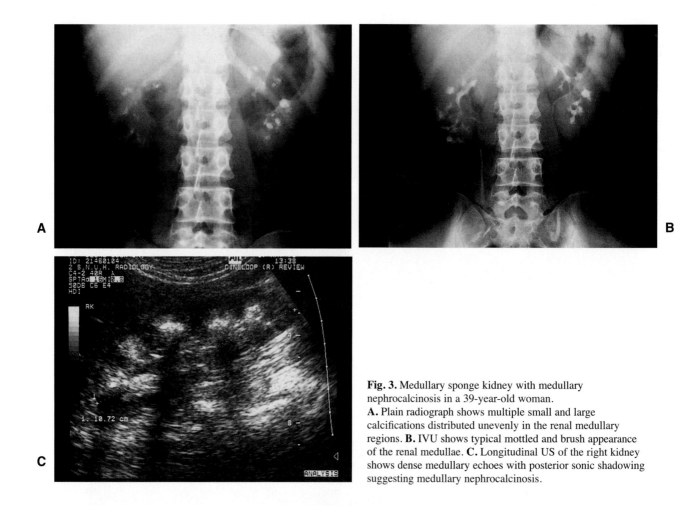

Fig. 3. Medullary sponge kidney with medullary nephrocalcinosis in a 39-year-old woman.
A. Plain radiograph shows multiple small and large calcifications distributed unevenly in the renal medullary regions. **B.** IVU shows typical mottled and brush appearance of the renal medullae. **C.** Longitudinal US of the right kidney shows dense medullary echoes with posterior sonic shadowing suggesting medullary nephrocalcinosis.

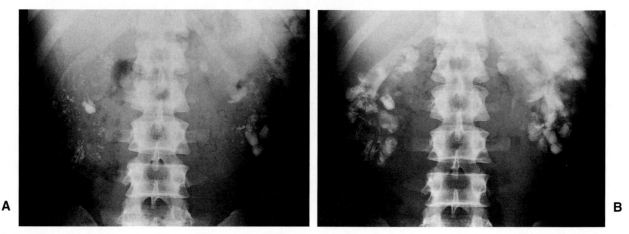

Fig. 4. Medullary nephrocalcinosis in a 33-year-old man with medullary sponge kidney.
A. Plain radiograph shows large and small calcifications scattered in both kidneys, predominantly in the medullary regions. **B.** IVU shows cystic and linear spaces representing dilated collecting ducts opacified with contrast material in the regions where calcifications were seen on plain radiograph.

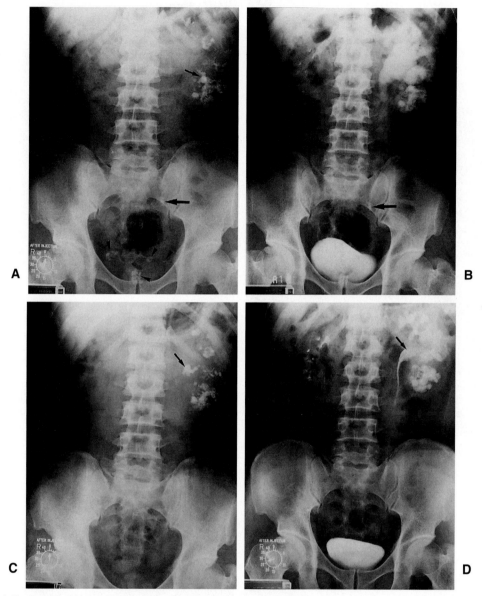

Fig. 5. Unilateral medullary sponge kidney with urinary tract stones in a 42-year-old man.
A, B. Plain radiograph (**A**) and IVU (**B**) show enlarged left renal shadow with innumerable calcifications in the medullary regions. Note a stone in the left distal ureter causing obstruction *(large arrow)*. Also note multiple stones in the urinary bladder and dilated prostatic urethra *(arrowheads* in **A**).
C, D. Plain radiograph (**C**) and IVU (**D**) obtained 18 months later show clearance of stones from the left ureter and urinary bladder and relieved ureteral obstruction. Note a calcification that was in the lower pole of the left kidney on **A** *(small arrow* in **A**) moved to the renal pelvis *(arrow)*.

3. Medullary Nephrocalcinosis due to Renal Tubular Acidosis

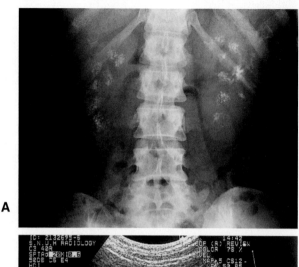

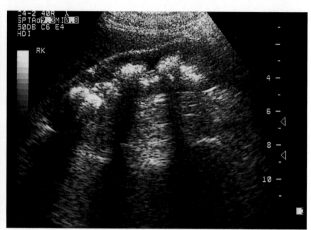

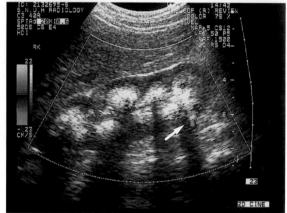

Fig. 1. Medullary nephrocalcinosis in a 34-year-old woman with renal tubular acidosis. (**A, B,** From Kim SH, Kim B: Renal parenchymal disease. In Pollack HM, McClennan BL [eds]: Clinical Urography, 2nd ed, vol 3. Philadelphia, WB Saunders, 2000, pp 2652–2687.) **A.** Plain radiograph shows mottled calcifications occupying entire medullary regions of both kidneys. The calcifications are small and uniform in size and show a relatively symmetrical distribution. **B.** Longitudinal US of the right kidney shows dense echoes with posterior sonic shadowing in the medullary regions. **C.** Color Doppler US of the right kidney shows the same findings. Note the echogenic lesion in the lower-polar region shows color twinkling artifacts (*arrow*) indicating the presence of calcifications. (**C,** See also Color Section.)

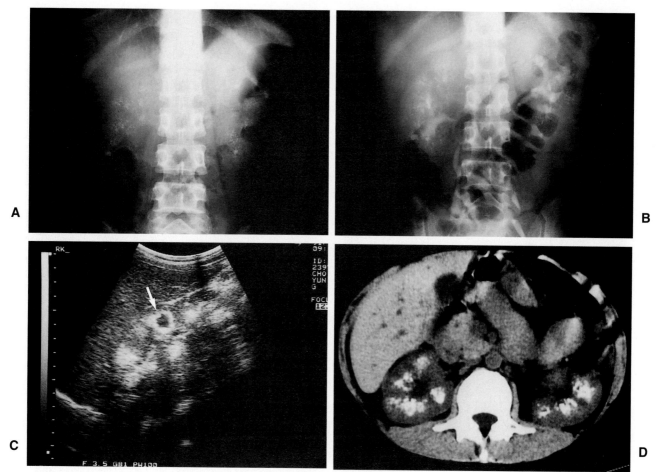

Fig. 2. Medullary nephrocalcinosis due to distal renal tubular acidosis in a 34-year-old woman.
A, B. Plain radiograph (**A**) and a 15-minute IVU (**B**) show innumerable calcifications distributed quite uniformly in the medullary regions of both kidneys. After injection of contrast material, note the absence of papillary brush or calculus "blooming" to suggest medullary sponge kidney.
C. Longitudinal US of the right kidney shows hyperechoic renal medullae. Most of the medullae are totally echogenic, but one of them shows hyperechogenicity in the outer medulla resulting in a ring-shaped echo (*arrow*). **D.** Nonenhanced CT shows multiple calcifications in the medullae of both kidneys.

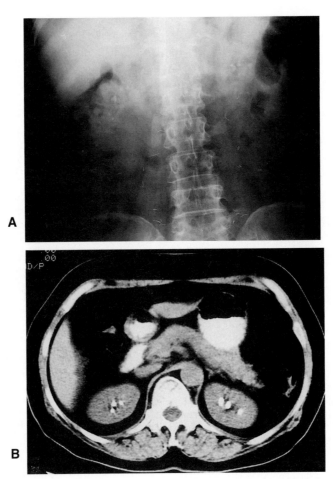

Fig. 3. Medullary nephrocalcinosis due to distal renal tubular acidosis in a 60-year-old woman with repeated history of stone passage.
A. Plain radiograph shows multiple calcifications of varying size in the medullary regions of both kidneys. **B.** Nonenhanced CT shows multiple calcifications in the medullae of both kidneys.

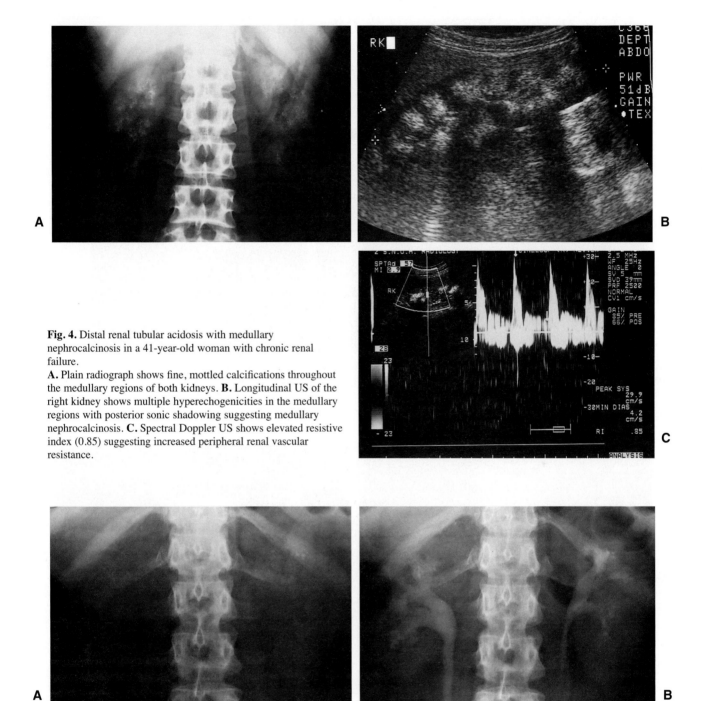

Fig. 4. Distal renal tubular acidosis with medullary nephrocalcinosis in a 41-year-old woman with chronic renal failure.
A. Plain radiograph shows fine, mottled calcifications throughout the medullary regions of both kidneys. **B.** Longitudinal US of the right kidney shows multiple hyperechogenicities in the medullary regions with posterior sonic shadowing suggesting medullary nephrocalcinosis. **C.** Spectral Doppler US shows elevated resistive index (0.85) suggesting increased peripheral renal vascular resistance.

Fig. 5. Medullary nephrocalcinosis due to renal tubular acidosis in a 47-year-old woman.
A. Plain radiograph shows bilateral, relatively symmetrical calcifications in the medullary regions of both kidneys. **B.** IVU shows the bilateral medullary calcifications, and they have a similar appearance as on the plain radiograph. There is no additional filling of collecting ducts in the medullae as one would see in medullary sponge kidney; in other words, there is no "blooming" of the calcifications. Mild right hydronephrosis is due to a partially obstructing distal right ureteral calculus (not shown).

4. Medullary Nephrocalcinosis due to Other Causes

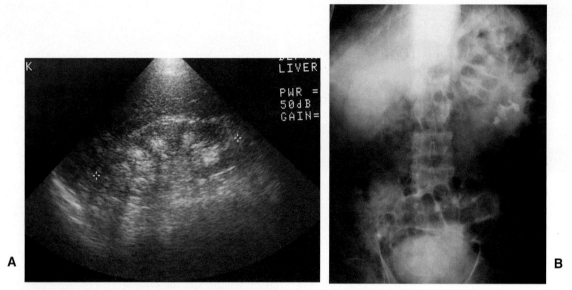

Fig. 1. Hyperechoic medullae in a 37-year-old man with hyperparathyroidism due to parathyroid adenoma.
A. Longitudinal US of the right kidney shows diffuse hyperechogenicity in the renal medullae. **B.** Plain radiograph shows mottled calcifications in the renal medullae and large stones in the left renal collecting system.

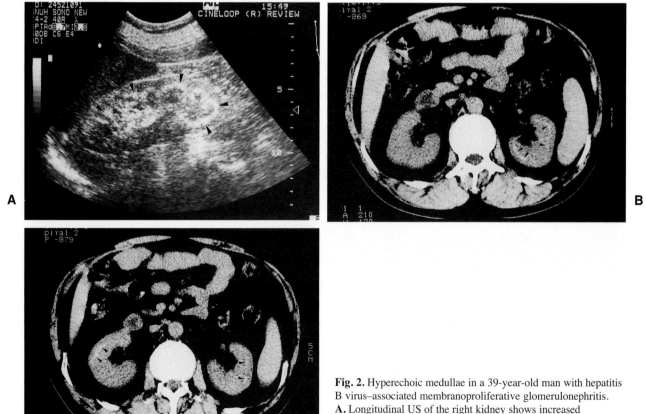

Fig. 2. Hyperechoic medullae in a 39-year-old man with hepatitis B virus–associated membranoproliferative glomerulonephritis.
A. Longitudinal US of the right kidney shows increased echogenicity along the outer medullae *(arrowheads)*.
B, C. Nonenhanced CT scans show faint, curvilinear calcifications along the outer medullae *(arrowheads)*.

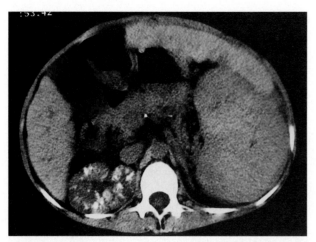

Fig. 3. Medullary nephrocalcinosis associated with autosomal recessive polycystic kidney disease in a 23-year-old woman. Nonenhanced CT shows mottled calcifications in the renal medullae of both kidneys. The left kidney is not included in this image due to splenomegaly.

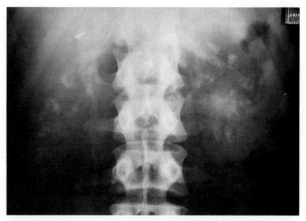

Fig. 4. Medullary nephrocalcinosis in a 26-year-old woman with hyperparathyroidism due to parathyroid adenoma. Plain radiograph shows numerous, dense calcifications distributed quite symmetrically throughout the medullary regions of both kidneys.

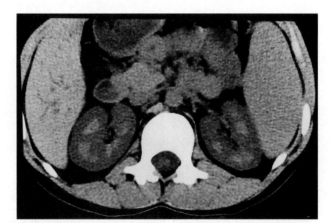

Fig. 5. Medullary nephrocalcinosis in a 14-year-old boy with cystinosis. Nonenhanced CT scan shows diffuse, mildly increased attenuation throughout the medullary regions due to sulfur-containing cystine deposits.

5. Hyperechoic Medullae on US

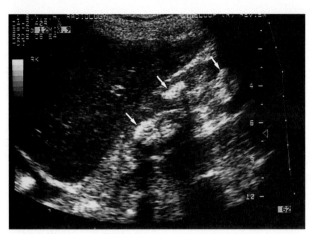

Fig. 1. Medullary nephrocalcinosis in a 67-year-old man with gout. Longitudinal US of the right kidney shows hyperechoic renal medullae *(arrows)*. Note that some of the echogenic medullae show posterior sonic shadowing.

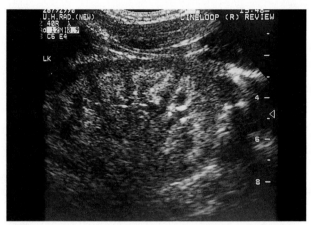

Fig. 2. Hyperechoic medullae in a 29-year-old man without history of using diuretics. The patient did not have hypokalemia and the renal function was normal. Longitudinal US of the left kidney shows hyperechoic medullae along the outer medulla.

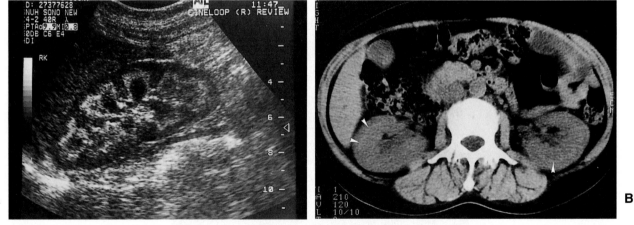

A   B

Fig. 3. Hyperechoic medullae in a 44-year-old woman with history of taking furosemide for 10 years.
A. Longitudinal US of the right kidney shows hyperechoic rims along the outer medullae, which do not accompany posterior sonic shadowing.
B. Nonenhanced CT demonstrates a layer of subtle high attenuation in the outer medullary regions *(arrowheads)*.

6. Cortical and Medullary Nephrocalcinosis

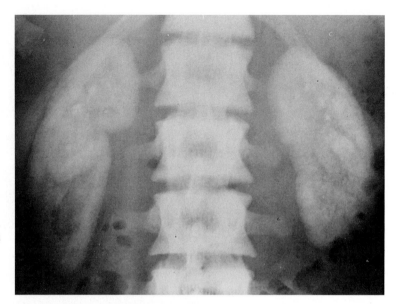

Fig. 1. Cortical and medullary nephrocalcinosis in oxalosis. Note the diffusely dense kidneys, bilateral renal calculi, and skeletal abnormalities. (From Ramchandani P: Radiologic evaluation of renal calculous disease. In Pollack HM, McClennan BL [eds]: Clinical Urography, 2nd ed, vol 2. Philadelphia, WB Saunders, 2000, p 2190.)

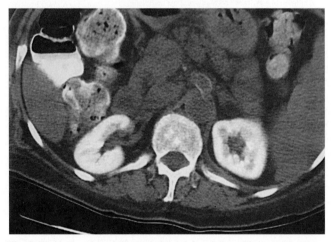

Fig. 2. Cortical and medullary nephrocalcinosis in a 55-year-old woman with oxalosis maintained by hemodialysis. Nonenhanced CT shows heterogeneously dense kidneys caused by diffuse cortical and medullary nephrocalcinosis. (From Ramchandani P: Radiologic evaluation of renal calculous disease. In Pollack HM, McClennan BL [eds]: Clinical Urography, 2nd ed, vol 2. Philadelphia, WB Saunders, 2000, p 2189.)

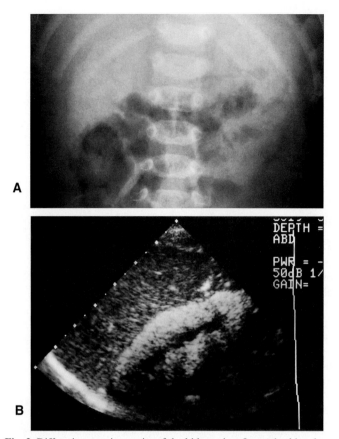

Fig. 3. Diffuse increase in opacity of the kidneys in a 3-month-old male infant due to oxalosis.
A. Plain radiograph shows bilaterally enlarged kidneys that have a uniform increase in opacity. **B.** Longitudinal US of the right kidney shows diffuse, uniformly increased echogenicity of the renal parenchyma with prominent posterior sonic shadowing caused by oxalosis.

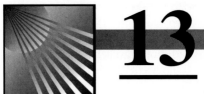

13

Urolithiasis

HAK JONG LEE

GENERAL CONSIDERATIONS

Incidence and epidemiology

Urolithiasis is the most common cause of calcification in the kidney and a common cause of obstructive uropathy. The prevalence of urinary stones increases with age. Stones are two or three times more common in men than in women. Bilateral stones occur in about 10% to 15% of patients with a stone.

The predisposing factors of stone formation include heredity, food, occupation, and life style. Climate and weather can affect the incidence of stone disease. In hot weather and during summer, stones form more frequently due to dehydration, increased urine concentration, and increased endogenous production of vitamin D during summer months. Factory workers working in hot environments are also at increased risk for urolithiasis.

Mechanisms of stone formation

Theories of calculogenesis include precipitation crystallization theory, stone matrix theory, and inhibitors of crystallization theory, but the exact mechanism is not known. Randall observed two types of papillary calcifications known as *Randall's plaque*: calcium deposition on the basement membrane of the collecting tubules and calcium deposition in the collecting tubule or papillary duct. Sometimes it is difficult to differentiate the Randall's plaque located in papilla from a small stone in the calyx.

CLINICAL MANIFESTATIONS

The usual clinical manifestations of urolithiasis are ureteral colic and hematuria. Renal colic is abrupt in onset, most frequently begins in the flank, and radiates to the groin. Men may complain of testicular pain, whereas women feel discomfort radiating to the labia majora. The pain frequently radiates to the lateral flank and abdomen and may be accompanied by nausea and vomiting. Due to the distribution of the autonomic nervous system and combined innervations of the kidneys and stomach by the celiac ganglion, it is common for ureteral colic to be accompanied by nausea and vomiting. Hematuria is one of the most common symptoms of urolithiasis. However, hematuria may be absent in 15% of patients, particularly in cases of complete obstruction. Sometimes, the symptoms may not disappear completely after the passage of stone and the patient may com-

plain of persistent flank pain or discomfort, hematuria, and/or persistent urinary tract infection.

COMPOSITION AND CLASSIFICATIONS OF CALCULI

The analysis of the mineral contents of stone is important for the determination of etiology and treatment modality. The frequencies and mineral compositions of stone are shown in Table 13–1.

Calcium stones

Calcium stones are the most common stones formed in the urinary tract. They are commonly composed of a mixture of calcium oxalate and calcium phosphate with oxalate predominating. Calcium oxalate is a radiopaque crystal that usually occurs in uninfected urine, and two forms of these crystals may be seen in calculi: a monohydrate and a dihydrate. Pure calcium oxalate monohydrate calculi are usually small, smooth or mamillated, and densely opaque. Grossly, such a stone resembles a mulberry. Calcium oxalate dihydrate infrequently forms a pure stone but commonly combines with other crystals, most frequently with monohydrate. As dihydrate crystallizes in a spiculated fashion, mixed oxalate calculi have a jagged or irregular shape. These stones are known as *jackstone*. Calcium oxalate monohydrate stones are more resistant to extracorporeal shock wave lithotripsy than are dihydrate stones. Calcium oxalate stones are frequently mixed with calcium phosphate, uric acid, and magnesium ammonium phosphate.

The next common substance is calcium phosphate. Calcium phosphate stones are often multiple and associated with primary hyperparathyroidism. Calcium phosphate rarely forms

Table 13–1	Stone Composition and Frequency
Composition	**Frequency (%)***
Calcium	70–70
Calcium phosphate	5–10
Calcium oxalate-phosphate	30–40
Calcium oxalate	20–30
Struvite	15–20
Cystine	1–3
Uric acid	5–10

*In order of decreasing radiographic opacity.

a pure calculus but commonly combines with either calcium oxalate or magnesium ammonium phosphate, causing a laminated appearance of these mixed stones. Calcium phosphate is an important constituent of calculi present in infected, alkaline urine.

Magnesium ammonium phosphate hexahydrate (struvite) stones

Struvite or infection-induced stones account for 15% to 20% of all renal calculi and occur with a female-to-male ratio of 2:1. These stones are usually associated with an alkaline urine and are almost always accompanied by urinary tract infection caused by urea-splitting bacteria such as *Proteus* species, *Klebsiella*, and *Pseudomonas*.

Pure struvite stones are of relatively low radiopacity and quite rare. More often struvite stones are laminated with more dense calcium salts, usually calcium phosphate. These laminations in struvite stones suggest repeated urinary tract infection and frequent changes in urinary pH. They often have the shape of staghorn or coral calculi.

Uric acid stones and other radiolucent stones

Humans lack the enzyme urease that converts uric acid into allantoin. In urine, uric acid exists either free or as sodium urate. Acidic urine contributes to an increased concentration of the less soluble free uric acid.

Uric acid stones account for 5% to 10% of all calculi. Pure uric acid stones are radiolucent. Patients with uric acid stones have hyperuricosuria and acidic concentrated urine. Pure uric acid stone tends to be relatively small and smooth and is often disc shaped. Conditions predisposing to uric acid stone formation include acidic and strongly concentrated urine, excess urinary excretion of uric acid, distal small bowel disease or resection, ileostomy, myeloproliferative disorders treated with chemotherapy, and inadequate caloric or fluid intake.

Radiolucent stones other than uric acid stone include xanthine and matrix stones. Matrix stones are soft, mushy, poorly mineralized urinary mucoid concretions. The matrix is organic substance such as mucoprotein or mucopolysaccharide.

RADIOLOGIC FINDINGS

Plain radiography is the primary tool for detection of urinary tract calculi, since about 90% of them are radiopaque. The differential diagnosis of radiopaque renal stones includes calcified costal cartilage, gallstone, vascular calcification, calcified mesenteric lymph node, enterolith, calcified granulomas in basal lung or spleen, and pancreatic or adrenal calcifications. The conditions that may be confused with radiopaque ureter stones include pelvic phlebolith, bony islands in the sacrum, and dense cortical margin of a vertebral transverse process.

Pelvic phleboliths can sometimes resemble a distal ureter stone, and intravenous urography (IVU) is often needed for diagnosis. In general, phleboliths are multiple, round or oval shaped, and may have radiolucent centers. Phleboliths are most often located lateral to the sacrum and below the ischial spines. On the other hand, ureteral calculi are usually single and homogeneously dense and have an angular appearance. Rarely, it is possible to confuse phleboliths of the gonadal veins or appendicoliths with midureter stones. Radiolucent stones of the urinary tract should be distinguished from urothelial tumors, blood clots, sloughed papillae, and fungus balls.

The common sites of the ureter stones are the narrowest sites in the ureter, including the ureteropelvic junction, the site where the ureter crosses the iliac vessels, and the ureterovesical junction. The stones are also common in the areas of ureteral stricture due to prior ureteral surgery or secondary to an extrinsic fibrotic process.

Ureteral stone usually causes ureteral spasm, which manifests as narrowing of the ureter just distal to the stone. On the other hand, ureteral tumors, by nature of their slow growing within the ureteral lumen, tend to demonstrate ureteral widening just distal to a tumor's lower margin, which is known as *Bergman's sign*. It also has been reported that focal ureteral widening around tumor often allowed a ureteral catheter to coil within the dilated ureteral segment if it could not be passed beyond the tumor. Detritus plug is deposition of debris on urinary stones. On IVU, detritus plug appears as an ill-defined radiolucent lesion above the stone.

US is helpful in detecting radiolucent renal calculi and differentiating them from other pyelocalyceal filling defects. It is not easy but usually possible to demonstrate ureter stones with US if ureteral dilation is present proximal to the stones. US with bladder filling or transrectal US may be helpful in detecting distal ureteral stones. The overall sensitivity for detection of urinary tract stones with US is around 95%. Sometimes, detection of urinary stones with US may be difficult when they are obscured by sonic-attenuating tissue such as renal sinus fat, mesenteric fat, or bowel or when their posterior shadowing is weak. Color Doppler twinkling artifacts from urinary stones occur frequently and may be helpful in determining the presence of urinary stones. Differential diagnosis of renal stones on US includes intrarenal gas, renal arterial calcification, and calcified transitional cell carcinoma.

Nonenhanced computed tomography (CT) is now accepted as a highly accurate modality to detect urinary tract stones. The advantage of CT is not only in revealing the radiolucent stones but also in differentiating radiolucent stones from blood clots or urothelial tumors in patients having filling defect on urography.

CT numbers may be helpful to differentiate ureteral lesions. These values are as follows:

Calcium oxalate stones—500 to 1000 Hounsfield units (HU)
Uric acid stones—300 to 500 HU
Transitional cell carcinoma or blood clot—20 to 75 HU

Several articles reported the value of spiral CT in differentiating between the pelvic phlebolith and calculi and in predicting the clinical outcome of ureteral stones based on the degree of perirenal fat stranding and extent of perirenal fluid collection.

CONDITIONS RELATED TO CALCULI

Calyceal diverticulum is an outpouching lesion from the calyceal fornix. It is a thin-walled cystic cavity lined by transitional epithelium. The diagnosis of calyceal diverticulum is established by demonstrating a thin channel from a calyceal fornix to the diverticular pouch. Calyceal diverticula frequently contain stones, reportedly in 36%.

Milk of calcium consists of numerous small calcific granules, usually composed of calcium carbonate, suspended in the fluid

contained within the cyst or diverticulum. This suspension of precipitated calcium salts layers in the dependent portion of the cavity or diverticulum, producing a characteristic fluid-granule layer.

About 35% of ureteroceles contain calculi. Although the incidence of ureterocele is more common in females, the incidence of associated stone is more common in males. The ureterocele must be differentiated from pseudoureterocele caused by edema of the ureteral orifice associated with passed stone, or parameatal bladder neoplasm. The true ureterocele is surrounded by a thin, regular, radiolucent halo within the contrast-filled bladder, whereas in the case of pseudoureterocele, the halo is uneven, asymmetrical, or of variable thickness.

The frequency of stone formation increases in cases of immobilization, because immobilization induces hypercalcemia and hypercalciuria as the results of bone resorption. In addition, bedridden patients may have an intake of less fluid and a low urine output. When immobilized patients or patients with paraplegia and other neuromuscular disorders develop a urinary tract infection, the frequency of stone formation increases markedly. Rarely, bladder stones may form over foreign bodies introduced through the urethra or surgical staples used in formation of the neobladder.

References

1. Dunnick NR, Sandler CM, Newhouse JH, Amis S Jr: Nephrocalcinosis and nephrolithiasis. In Textbook of Uroradiology, 2nd ed. Philadelphia, Lippincott Williams & Wilkins, 2001, pp 178–104.
2. Lee JY, Kim SH, Cho JY, et al: Color and power Doppler twinkling artifacts from urinary stones: Clinical observations and phantom studies. AJR Am J Roentgenol 2001; 176:1441–1445.
3. Lee HJ, Kim SH: Characteristic plain radiographic and intravenous urographic findings of bladder calculi formed over a hair nidus: A case report. Korean J Radiol 2001; 2:61–62.
4. Ramchandani P: Radiologic evaluation of renal calculous disease. In Pollack HM, McClennan BL (eds): Clinical Urography, 2nd ed, vol 2. Philadelphia, WB Saunders, 2000, pp 2147–2200.
5. Mostafavi MR, Ernst RD, Saltzman B: Accurate determination of chemical composition of urinary calculi by spiral computerized tomography. J Urol 1998; 159:673–675.
6. Kim SH, Lee SE, Park IA: Case report: CT and US features of renal matrix stones with calcified center. J Comput Assist Tomogr 1996; 20:404–406.
7. Middleton WD, Dodds WJ, Lawson TL, et al: Renal calculi: Sensitivity for detection with US. Radiology 1988; 167:239–244.
8. Golomb J, Korezak D, Lindner A: Giant obstructing calculus in the distal ureter secondary to obstruction by a ureterocele. Urol Radiol 1987; 9:168–170.
9. Hillman BJ, Drach GW, Tracey P, et al: Computed tomographic analysis of renal calculi. AJR Am J Roentgenol 1984; 142:549–552.
10. Newhouse JH, Prien EL, Amis ES, et al: Computed tomographic analysis of urinary calculi. AJR Am J Roentgenol 1984; 142:545–548.
11. Van Arsdalen KN: Pathogenesis of renal calculi. Urol Radiol 1984; 6:65–73.
12. Parienty RA, Ducellier R, Pradel J, et al: Diagnostic value of CT numbers in pelvocalyceal filling defects. Radiology 1982; 145:743–748.
13. Federle MP, McAninch JW, Kaiser JA, et al: Computed tomography of urinary calculi. AJR Am J Roentgenol 1981; 136:255–258.
14. Pollack HM, Arger PH, Banner MP, et al: Computed tomography of renal pelvic filling defects. Radiology 1981; 138:645–651.
15. Bergman H, Friedenberg RM, Sayegh V: New roentgenologic signs of carcinoma of the ureter. AJR Am J Roentgenol 1961; 86:707–717.

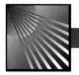

Illustrations • Urolithiasis

1 • Calcium stones

2 • Uric acid stones

3 • Matrix stones

4 • Staghorn stones

5 • Stones in renal papilla

6 • Calyceal diverticulum with stone

7 • Obstructing stones

8 • Ureter stone without obstruction

9 • Ureter stone with papillary cavity

10 • Ureter stone with detritus plug

11 • Ureter stone with distal dilation

12 • Migration of ureter stone during IVU

13 • Stone in ureterocele

14 • Ureter stone with bladder edema

15 • Pseudoureterocele due to stone

16 • Ureter stone: other findings

17 • Ureter stone versus phlebolith

18 • Urolithiasis: US findings

19 • Urolithiasis: CT findings

1. Calcium Stones

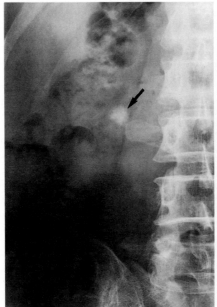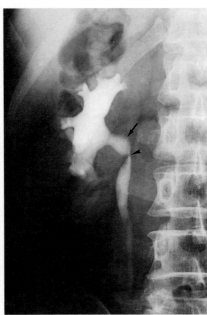

Fig. 1. Calcium oxalate stone in a 56-year-old man.
A. Plain radiograph shows a radiopaque stone *(arrow)* in the right kidney. Note spiculated margin of the stone. **B.** IVU demonstrates that this stone is located in the ureteropelvic junction *(arrow)*. Note focal narrowing of the ureter distal to the stone due to spasm *(arrowhead)*.

A   **B**

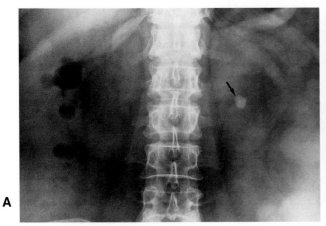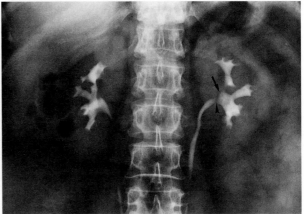

A   **B**

Fig. 2. Calcium oxalate stone in a 45-year-old man.
A. Plain radiograph shows a radiopaque stone with fine spiculated margin in the left kidney *(arrow)*. **B.** IVU demonstrates the stone in the left renal pelvis *(arrow)* and spasm *(arrowhead)* distal to the stone.

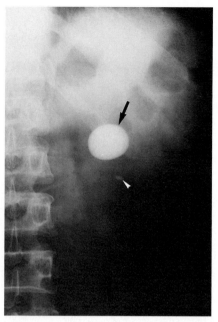

Fig. 3. Renal stone composed of calcium oxalate and magnesium in a 46-year-old man. Plain radiograph shows a round, homogeneously dense radiopacity in the left renal region *(arrow)*. Also note a small stone *(arrowhead)* in the lower-polar region of the left kidney.

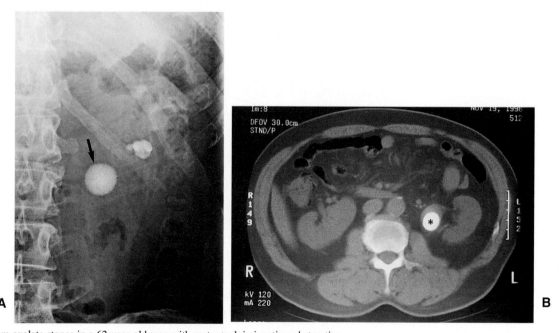

Fig. 4. Calcium oxalate stones in a 62-year-old man with ureteropelvic junction obstruction.
A. Plain radiograph shows two stones in the left kidney. Lower medial one *(arrow)* shows a fine, spiculated margin. **B.** Nonenhanced CT shows the stone *(asterisk)* in the dilated left renal pelvis. The spiculated margin is not well demonstrated on this CT.

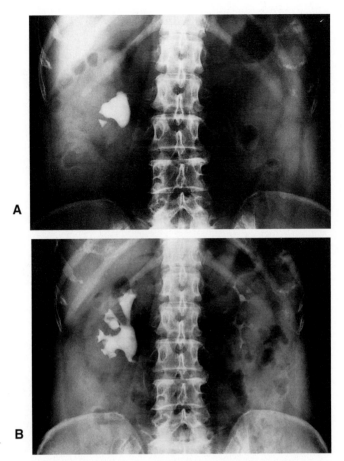

Fig. 5. Calcium oxalate and phosphate stones in a 66-year-old woman.
A, B. Plain radiograph (**A**) and a 5-minute IVU (**B**) show stones in the
right pelvocalyces. Note that the stones are homogeneously dense and
have a smooth surface.

2. Uric Acid Stones

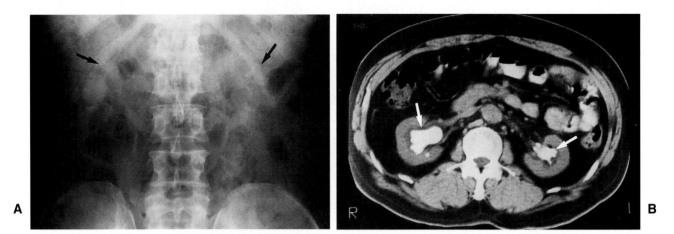

Fig. 1. Uric acid stones in a 56-year-old man with gout.
A. Plain radiograph shows suspicious radiopacities in the renal regions *(arrows)*. **B.** Nonenhanced CT reveals stones filling both renal pelvises *(arrows)*, which were confirmed as uric acid stones.

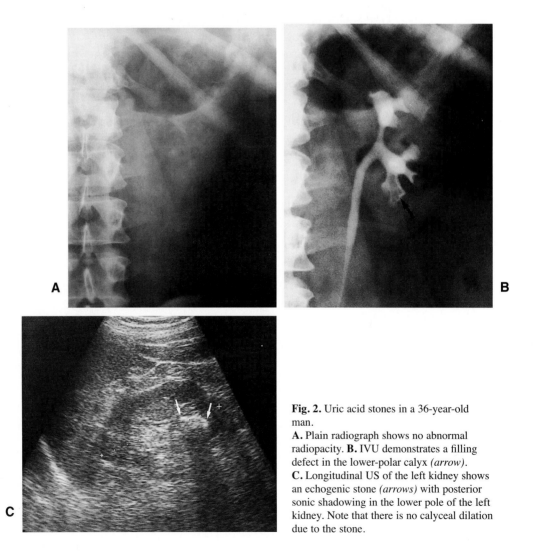

Fig. 2. Uric acid stones in a 36-year-old man.
A. Plain radiograph shows no abnormal radiopacity. **B.** IVU demonstrates a filling defect in the lower-polar calyx *(arrow)*.
C. Longitudinal US of the left kidney shows an echogenic stone *(arrows)* with posterior sonic shadowing in the lower pole of the left kidney. Note that there is no calyceal dilation due to the stone.

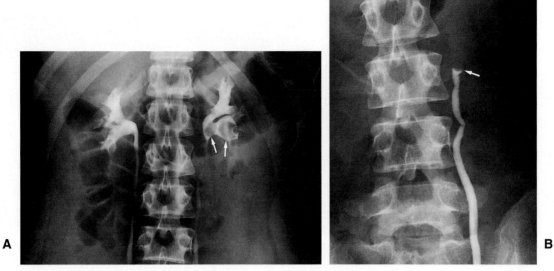

Fig. 3. Multiple uric acid stones in a 21-year-old woman.
A. IVU shows two round, smooth-margined filling defects *(arrows)* in the pelvocalyces of the left kidney. **B.** Six months later, the patient complained of severe pain on her left flank. RGP shows obstruction of the left proximal ureter by distal migration of the stone. Note the absence of spasm and slight widening of the ureter just distal to the obstruction *(arrow)*, which may suggest a finding of ureteral tumor rather than a stone if the history of the stone is not considered. The stone was composed of ammonium and urate.

3. Matrix Stones

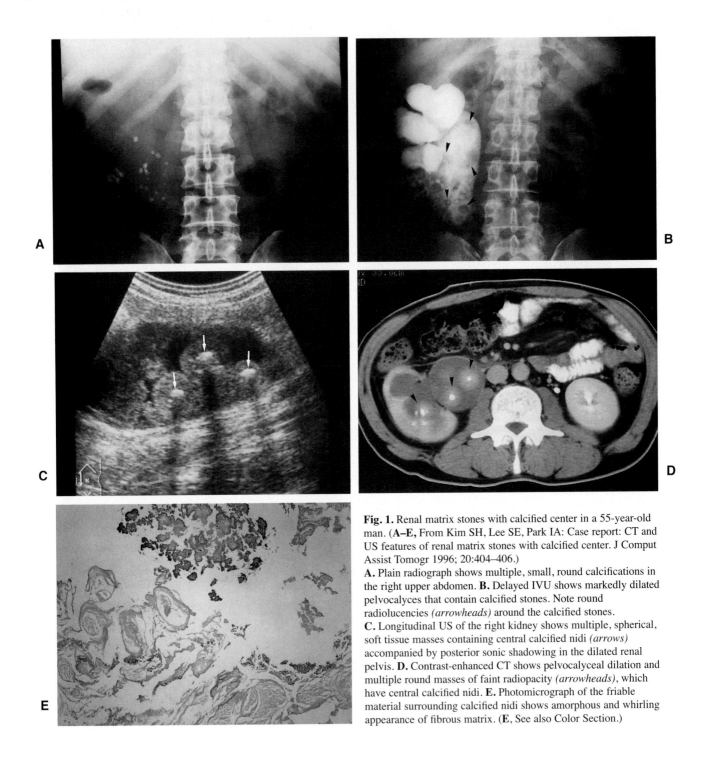

Fig. 1. Renal matrix stones with calcified center in a 55-year-old man. (**A–E,** From Kim SH, Lee SE, Park IA: Case report: CT and US features of renal matrix stones with calcified center. J Comput Assist Tomogr 1996; 20:404–406.)
A. Plain radiograph shows multiple, small, round calcifications in the right upper abdomen. **B.** Delayed IVU shows markedly dilated pelvocalyces that contain calcified stones. Note round radiolucencies *(arrowheads)* around the calcified stones.
C. Longitudinal US of the right kidney shows multiple, spherical, soft tissue masses containing central calcified nidi *(arrows)* accompanied by posterior sonic shadowing in the dilated renal pelvis. **D.** Contrast-enhanced CT shows pelvocalyceal dilation and multiple round masses of faint radiopacity *(arrowheads)*, which have central calcified nidi. **E.** Photomicrograph of the friable material surrounding calcified nidi shows amorphous and whirling appearance of fibrous matrix. (**E,** See also Color Section.)

4. Staghorn Stones

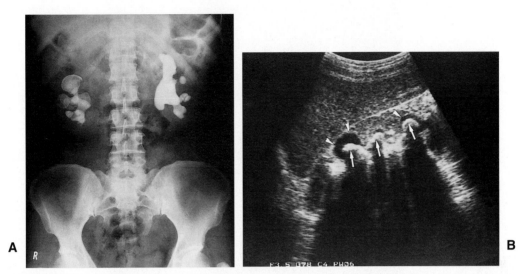

Fig. 1. Staghorn stones in both kidneys in a 60-year-old woman. The stones were composed of calcium phosphate and magnesium ammonium phosphate.
A. Plain radiograph shows large staghorn stones filling the pelvocalyces of both kidneys. Note lamellated appearance of the stone in the right kidney suggesting recurrent infections and frequent changes in urinary pH. **B.** Longitudinal US of the right kidney shows densely echogenic surface of the staghorn stone *(arrows)* with posterior sonic shadowing. Note slightly dilated calyces *(arrowheads)*.

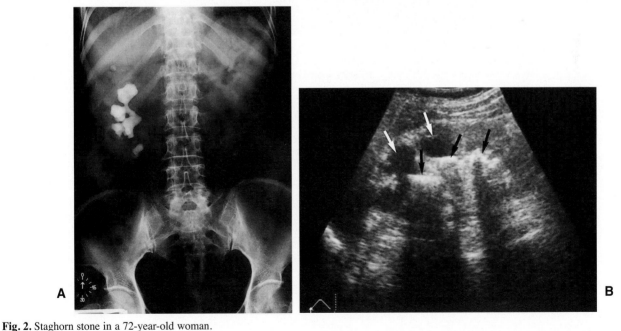

Fig. 2. Staghorn stone in a 72-year-old woman.
A. Plain radiograph shows a large staghorn stone in the renal pelvis and small stones in the lower-polar calyx. **B.** Longitudinal US of the right kidney demonstrates the staghorn stone by dense echoes *(black arrows)* with posterior sonic shadowing. Note dilated calyces *(white arrows)* around the stone.

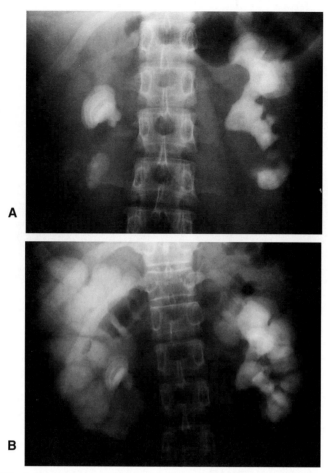

Fig. 3. Staghorn stones with severe caliectasis in a 36-year-old man.
A. Plain radiograph shows large, lamellated stones in both kidneys. **B.** A
6-hour-delayed IVU shows markedly dilated calyces due to the stones.

5. Stones in Renal Papilla

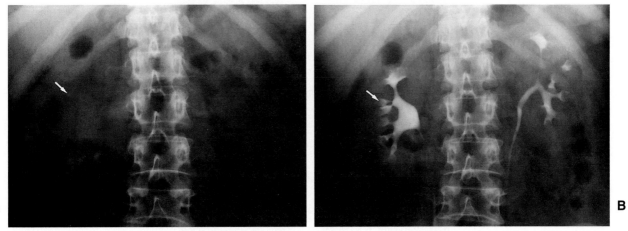

Fig. 1. A small stone in the renal papilla in a 46-year-old woman.
A. Plain radiograph shows a small calcification *(arrow)* in the right kidney. **B.** IVU shows that the calcification is located in the renal papilla *(arrow)* of an interpolar calyx.

Fig. 2. A small stone in the renal papilla in a 50-year-old woman.
A. Plain radiograph shows a small, ovoid calcification *(arrow)* in the upper-polar region of the left kidney. **B.** IVU reveals that the calcification is located in the renal papilla *(arrow)*.

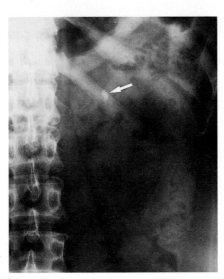

A

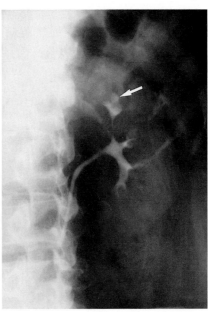

B

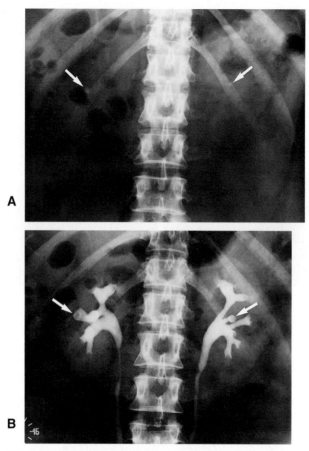

Fig. 3. Small stones in the renal papillae in a 41-year-old woman.
A. Plain radiograph shows small calcifications *(arrows)* in both
kidneys. **B.** A 5-minute IVU shows that the calcifications are located
in the papillae of the interpolar regions of both kidneys *(arrows)*.

6. Calyceal Diverticulum with Stone

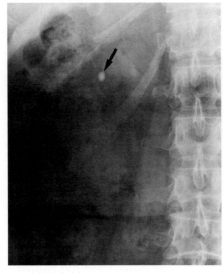
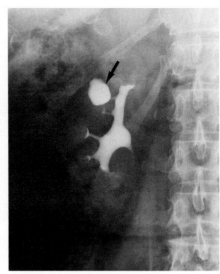

Fig. 1. Calyceal diverticulum with a stone in a 68-year-old woman.
A. Plain radiograph shows a round calcification *(arrow)* in the upper-polar region of the right kidney. **B.** IVU shows a large calyceal diverticulum *(arrow)* that contains the stone.

A

B

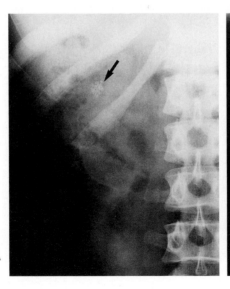
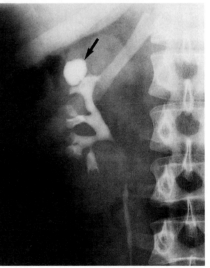

Fig. 2. Calyceal diverticulum with multiple small stones in a 35-year-old man.
A. Plain radiograph shows multiple small calcifications *(arrow)* in the upper-polar region of the right kidney. **B.** IVU shows a round calyceal diverticulum *(arrow)* that contains the stones.

A

B

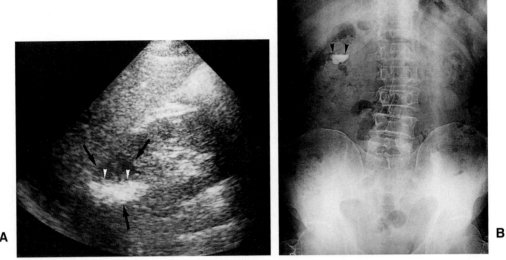

Fig. 3. Calyceal diverticulum containing sandy stones in a 64-year-old man.
A. Longitudinal US of the right kidney shows a cystic lesion *(arrows)* that has echogenic materials *(arrowheads)* layered in the dependent portion.
B. Plain radiograph in upright position shows sandy stones *(arrowheads)* layered in the dependent portion of a calyceal diverticulum.

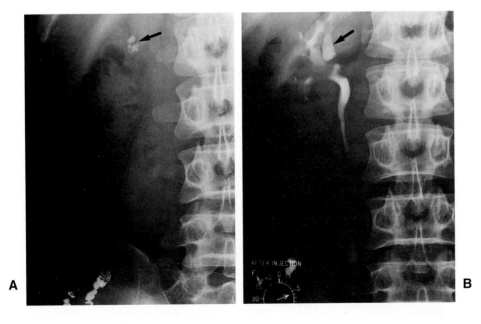

Fig. 4. Calyceal diverticulum with multiple stones in a 37-year-old man. **A.** Plain radiograph shows multiple calcifications in the upper-polar region of the right kidney *(arrow)*. **B.** IVU shows an oval-shaped calyceal diverticulum *(arrow)* containing multiple stones.

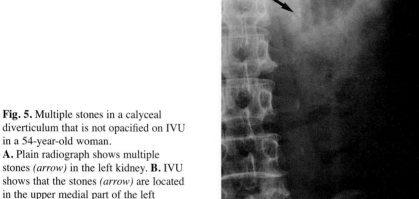

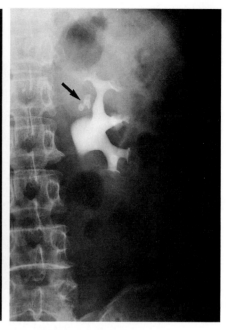

Fig. 5. Multiple stones in a calyceal diverticulum that is not opacified on IVU in a 54-year-old woman.
A. Plain radiograph shows multiple stones *(arrow)* in the left kidney. **B.** IVU shows that the stones *(arrow)* are located in the upper medial part of the left kidney. The stones are probably within a calyceal diverticulum that was not opacified on IVU.

A

B

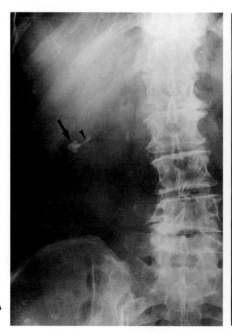

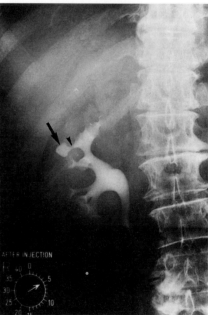

Fig. 6. Calyceal diverticulum with stones growing in the neck of diverticulum in a 69-year-old woman.
A. Plain radiograph shows calcifications *(arrow)* with a stalk *(arrowhead)* in the right kidney.
B. IVU reveals that the stones are located in a calyceal diverticulum *(arrow)* and its neck *(arrowhead)*.

A

B

7. Obstructing Stones

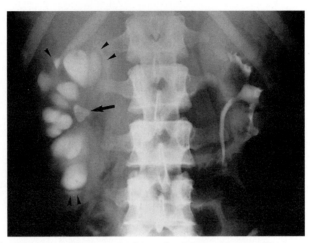

Fig. 1. An obstructing stone in the renal pelvis in a 23-year-old man. IVU shows a triangular stone *(arrow)* in the right renal pelvis with marked dilation of the renal calyces. Note calyceal crescents *(arrowheads)* caused by collection of contrast material in the collecting ducts.

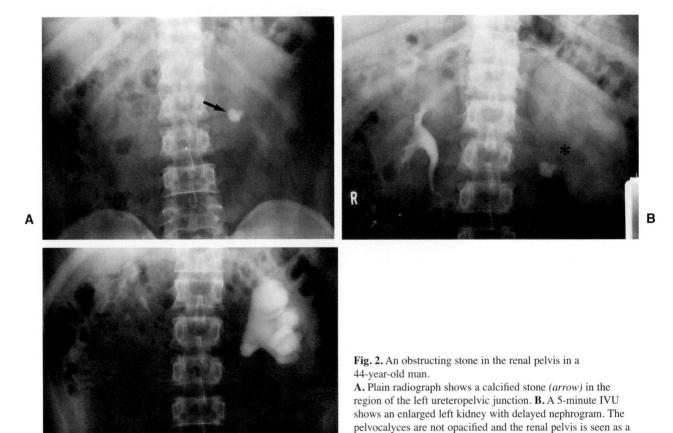

Fig. 2. An obstructing stone in the renal pelvis in a 44-year-old man.
A. Plain radiograph shows a calcified stone *(arrow)* in the region of the left ureteropelvic junction. **B.** A 5-minute IVU shows an enlarged left kidney with delayed nephrogram. The pelvocalyces are not opacified and the renal pelvis is seen as a radiolucent area *(asterisk)* producing the finding of negative pyelogram. **C.** A 2-hour-delayed IVU well demonstrates the stone and dilated pelvocalyces.

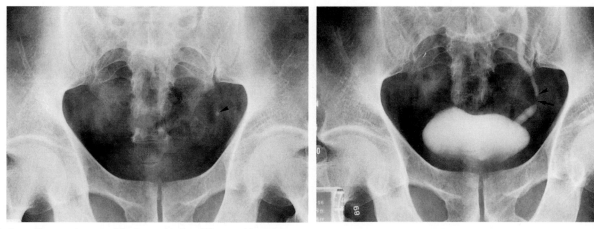

A   B

Fig. 3. A small ureteral stone with obstruction in a 56-year-old man.
A. Plain radiograph shows a small, round calcification in the left pelvic cavity *(arrowhead)*. **B.** IVU demonstrates the stone in the left distal ureter *(arrowhead)* with dilation and stagnation of excreted contrast material proximal to the stone. Note severe spasm *(arrow)* of the ureter distal to the stone.

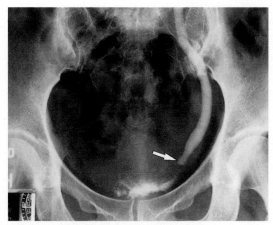

Fig. 4. A distal ureteral stone with obstruction in a 60-year-old woman. A 1-hour postvoiding IVU shows an obstructing stone *(arrow)* in the distal ureter with dilation of the ureter proximal to the stone.

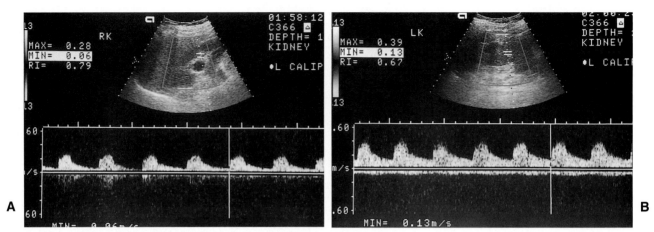

Fig. 5. Doppler US findings of the kidney in a 62-year-old woman with an obstructing stone.
A. Doppler US of the right kidney shows decreased diastolic frequency shift and increased resistive index of 0.79 due to obstruction. **B.** Doppler US of the normal left kidney shows a normal resistive index of 0.67.

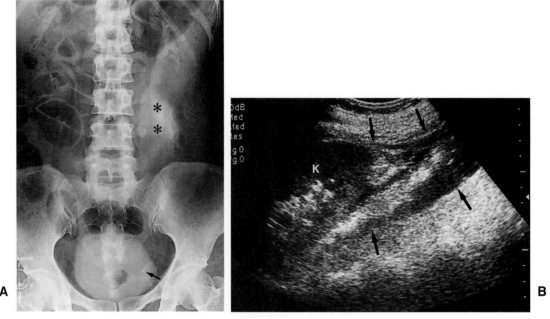

Fig. 6. Forniceal rupture due to an obstructing ureteral stone in a 43-year-old woman.
A. A 15-minute IVU shows extravasation of contrast material in the perirenal space *(asterisks)* probably due to forniceal rupture secondary to an obstructing stone in the distal ureter *(arrow)*. **B.** Longitudinal US of the left flank shows an ill-defined lesion of fluid collection with heterogeneous echogenicity *(arrows)* below the left kidney (K). This lesion probably represents urinoma due to forniceal rupture by an obstructing ureteral stone.

8. Ureter Stone without Obstruction

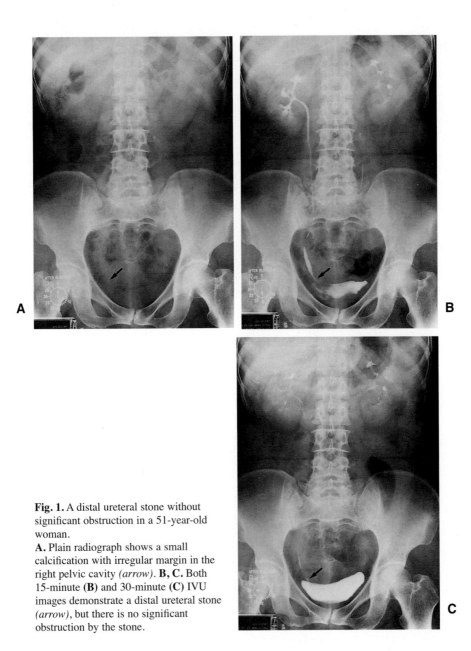

Fig. 1. A distal ureteral stone without significant obstruction in a 51-year-old woman.
A. Plain radiograph shows a small calcification with irregular margin in the right pelvic cavity *(arrow)*. **B, C.** Both 15-minute **(B)** and 30-minute **(C)** IVU images demonstrate a distal ureteral stone *(arrow)*, but there is no significant obstruction by the stone.

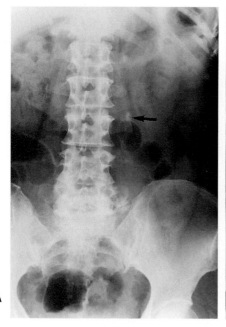

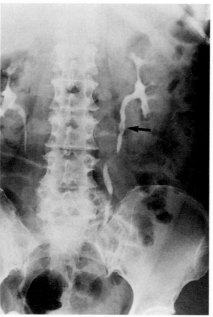

A

B

Fig. 2. A ureteral stone without significant obstruction in a 56-year-old woman. **A.** Plain radiograph shows a calcification in the left paravertebral region *(arrow)*. **B.** IVU shows that the calcification is a stone *(arrow)* in the left proximal ureter. Note that the upper urinary tract is not dilated, and excreted contrast material is passing well into the distal ureter.

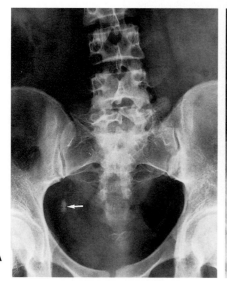

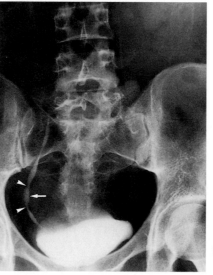

A

B

Fig. 3. A ureteral stone with mild spasm in a 29-year-old woman. **A, B.** Plain radiograph **(A)** and IVU **(B)** show an elongated, irregularly margined stone *(arrow)* in the right distal ureter. The stone staying in the ureter for some time often has an elongated shape along the course of the ureter. Note that there is no significant obstruction by the stone and only mild spasm *(arrowheads)* is seen in the ureter adjacent to the stone.

9. Ureter Stone with Papillary Cavity

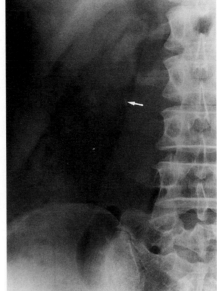 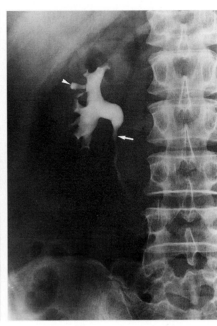

Fig. 1. A small ureteral stone and a papillary cavity that is probably the origin of the stone in a 52-year-old man. **A.** Plain radiograph shows a small ovoid calcification in the right paravertebral region *(arrow)*. **B.** A 30-minute IVU shows the stone in the right ureteropelvic junction *(arrow)* and mild dilation of the pelvocalyces. Also note a papillary cavity *(arrowhead)* in the upper-polar calyx that probably is the origin of the stone.

A

B

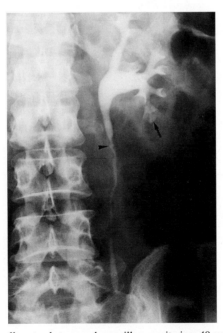

Fig. 2. A small ureteral stone and a papillary cavity in a 49-year-old woman. IVU shows a small stone in the left proximal ureter *(arrowhead)* and a small papillary cavity in the lower-polar calyx *(arrow)*, which is probably the origin of the stone.

10. Ureter Stone with Detritus Plug

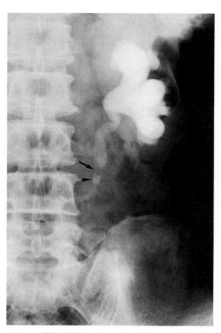

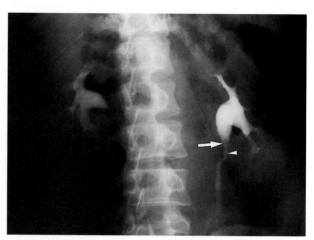

Fig. 2. Ureter stone with detritus plug in a 33-year-old man. A 15-minute IVU in oblique projection shows radiolucency *(arrow)* above a ureteral stone *(arrowhead),* suggesting a detritus plug.

Fig. 1. Ureter stone with detritus plug in a 60-year-old man. IVU shows an irregularly margined stone *(arrowhead)* in the left midureter and dilation of the proximal ureter and pelvocalyces. Note a radiolucent gap *(arrow)* between the stone and opacified ureter. This radiolucency, known as *detritus plug,* represents a plug composed of detached urothelium, blood cells, and mucoid materials.

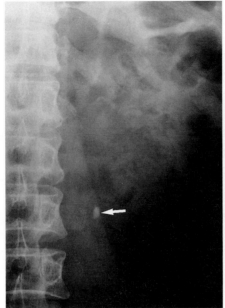

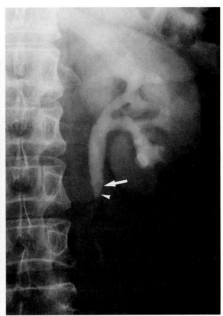

A   B

Fig. 3. Ureter stone with a detritus plug in a 48-year-old man. **A.** Plain radiograph shows a left ureteral stone *(arrow)*. **B.** A 15-minute IVU shows a radiolucent cap *(arrow)* above the stone *(arrowhead)* representing a detritus plug.

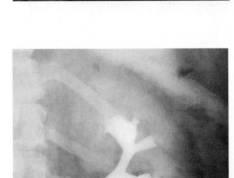

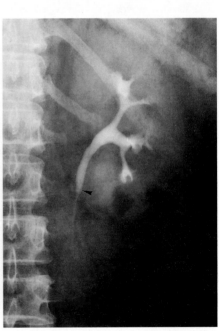

A   B

Fig. 4. Ureter stone with a detritus plug in a 50-year-old woman. **A.** A 15-minute IVU shows a ureteral stone *(arrowhead)* in the left proximal ureter and a thin radiolucent cap *(arrow)* above the stone indicating a detritus plug. **B.** On a 30-minute IVU, the radiolucent lesion above the stone *(arrowhead)* is no longer seen.

11. Ureter Stone with Distal Dilation

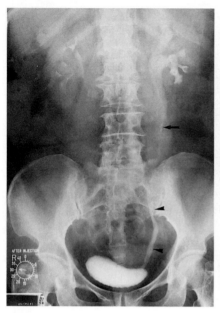
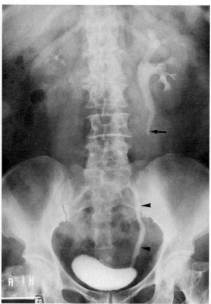

Fig. 1. Ureter stone with dilation of the ureter distal to the stone in a 52-year-old woman.
A, B. A 30-minute (**A**) and a 1-hour (**B**) IVU image show a small stone *(arrow)* in the left midureter with dilation of the proximal ureter and pelvocalyces. Note that the left distal ureter is persistently dilated *(arrowheads)* down to the ureterovesical junction. There was no obstruction in the left ureterovesical junction, and the dilation of the ureter distal to the stone is probably due to decreased peristalsis, so-called ureteral ileus.

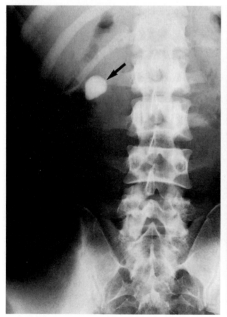
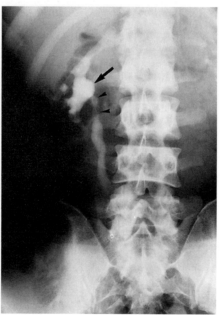

Fig. 2. A stone in the renal pelvis with ureteral dilation in a 22-year-old man.
A. Plain radiograph shows a large radiopaque stone *(arrow)* in the right kidney. **B.** IVU shows dilated calyces due to the stone in the renal pelvis *(arrow)*. Note that the right ureter is dilated in spite of the obstructing stone in the renal pelvis. Also note irregularities and fine nodularities in the proximal ureter *(arrowheads)* just distal to the stone, suggesting urothelial edema.

12. Migration of Ureter Stone during IVU

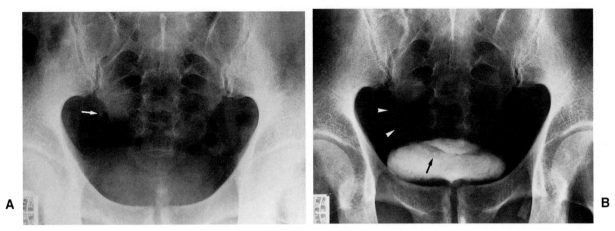

Fig. 1. Ureter stone that moved during IVU in a 60-year-old man.
A. Plain radiograph shows a small calcification in the right pelvic cavity *(arrow)*. **B.** During IVU, the stone moved to the ureterovesical junction *(arrow)*. Note dilation of the ureter *(arrowheads)* above the stone.

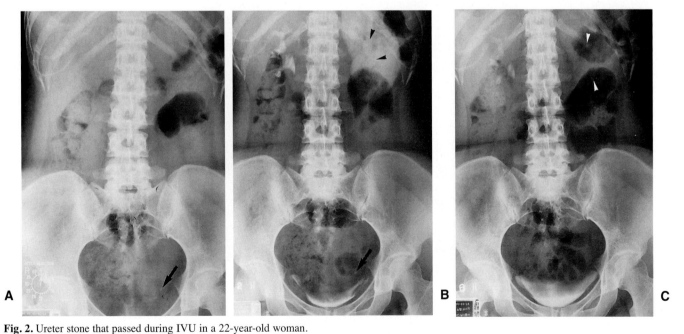

Fig. 2. Ureter stone that passed during IVU in a 22-year-old woman.
A. Plain radiograph shows a small calcification in the left pelvic cavity *(arrow)*. **B.** A 2-hour IVU shows severe obstruction of the left urinary tract with delayed dense nephrogram due to a stone *(arrow)* in the pelvic cavity. Note that the dilated left pelvocalyces are faintly opacified *(arrowheads)*. After taking this radiograph, the patient complained of severe flank pain, which was suddenly improved. **C.** On a 6-hour IVU, the calcified density in the left pelvic cavity disappeared and contrast material had been already excreted. Note that the calyces are collapsed in the left kidney *(arrowheads)*.

13. Stone in Ureterocele

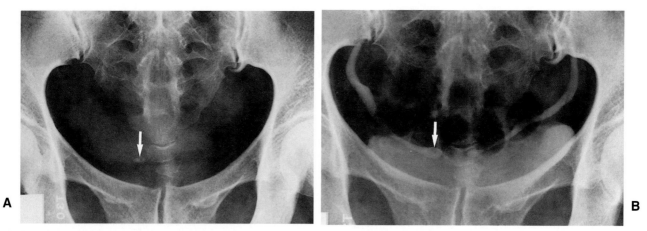

Fig. 1. Stone in ureterocele in a 60-year-old woman.
A. Plain radiograph shows an ovoid calcification with an irregular margin in the right pelvic cavity *(arrow)*. **B.** IVU shows bilateral ureterocele and a stone in the right ureterocele appearing as a filling defect *(arrow)*.

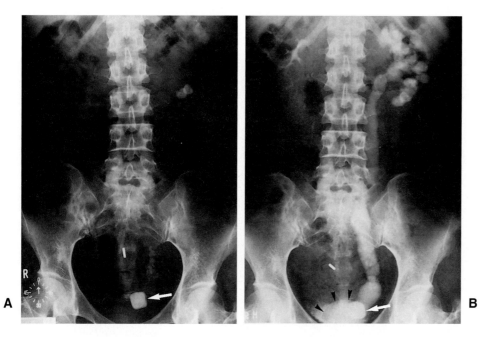

Fig. 2. Stones in ureterocele in a 34-year-old woman.
A, B. Plain radiograph (**A**) and IVU (**B**) show a rectangular stone *(arrow)* in the left pelvic cavity, which is in the ureterocele *(arrowheads* in **B**). Also note multiple stones in the dilated ureter and calyx of the left urinary tract.

12. Migration of Ureter Stone during IVU

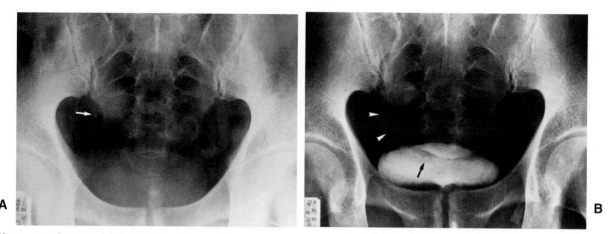

Fig. 1. Ureter stone that moved during IVU in a 60-year-old man.
A. Plain radiograph shows a small calcification in the right pelvic cavity *(arrow)*. **B.** During IVU, the stone moved to the ureterovesical junction *(arrow)*. Note dilation of the ureter *(arrowheads)* above the stone.

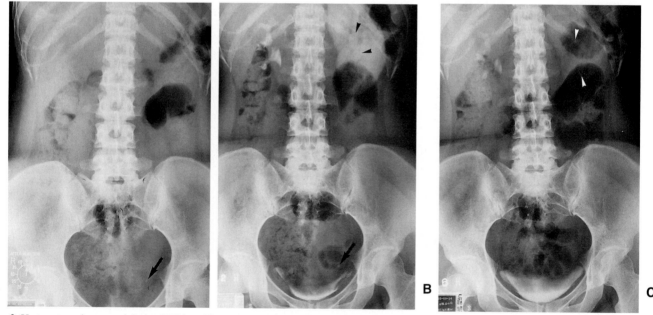

Fig. 2. Ureter stone that passed during IVU in a 22-year-old woman.
A. Plain radiograph shows a small calcification in the left pelvic cavity *(arrow)*. **B.** A 2-hour IVU shows severe obstruction of the left urinary tract with delayed dense nephrogram due to a stone *(arrow)* in the pelvic cavity. Note that the dilated left pelvocalyces are faintly opacified *(arrowheads)*. After taking this radiograph, the patient complained of severe flank pain, which was suddenly improved. **C.** On a 6-hour IVU, the calcified density in the left pelvic cavity disappeared and contrast material had been already excreted. Note that the calyces are collapsed in the left kidney *(arrowheads)*.

13. Stone in Ureterocele

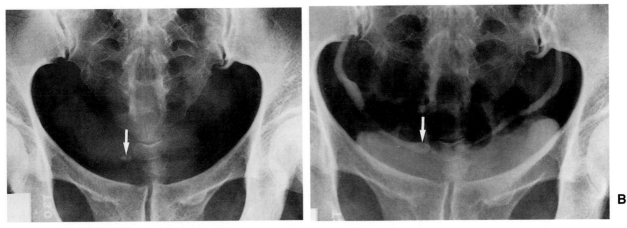

Fig. 1. Stone in ureterocele in a 60-year-old woman.
A. Plain radiograph shows an ovoid calcification with an irregular margin in the right pelvic cavity *(arrow)*. **B.** IVU shows bilateral ureterocele and a stone in the right ureterocele appearing as a filling defect *(arrow)*.

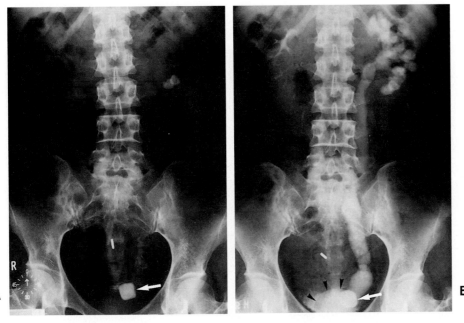

Fig. 2. Stones in ureterocele in a 34-year-old woman.
A, B. Plain radiograph (**A**) and IVU (**B**) show a rectangular stone *(arrow)* in the left pelvic cavity, which is in the ureterocele (*arrowheads* in **B**). Also note multiple stones in the dilated ureter and calyx of the left urinary tract.

14. Ureter Stone with Bladder Edema

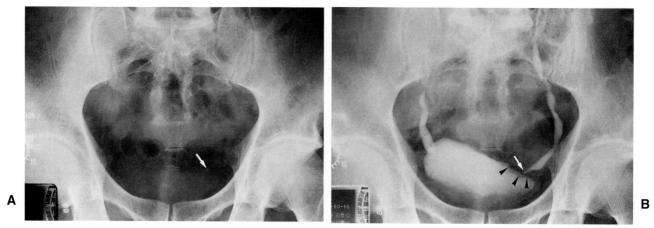

Fig. 1. A small stone in the ureteropelvic junction causing edema in a 57-year-old man.
A. Plain radiograph shows a small, round radiopacity *(arrow)* in the left pelvic cavity below the ischial spine. **B.** IVU shows a distal ureteral stone *(arrow)* with edematous swelling of the adjacent bladder wall *(arrowheads)*.

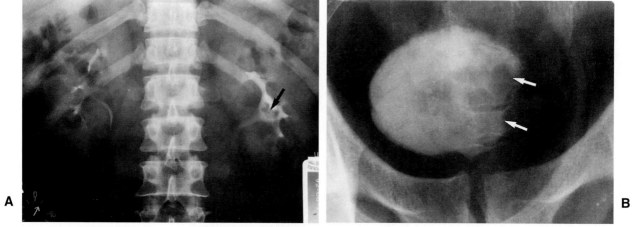

Fig. 2. Severe edema of the bladder after stone passage in a 40-year-old man.
A. IVU shows a filling defect *(arrow)* that was a uric acid stone. **B.** The stone was passed and follow-up IVU obtained 3 days later shows severe edema on the left aspect of the bladder *(arrows)*.

15. Pseudoureterocele due to Stone

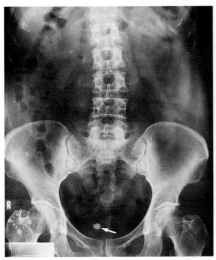

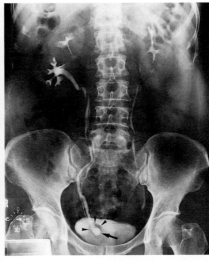

Fig. 1. A stone in the ureterovesical junction with pseudoureterocele in a 60-year-old woman.
A. Plain radiograph shows a round calcification with an irregular margin in the right pelvic cavity *(arrow)*. **B.** A 15-minute IVU shows duplication of the right urinary tract with a stone in the ureterovesical junction *(arrow)*. Note a thick, radiolucent halo *(arrowheads)* representing edema around the stone, which is called *pseudoureterocele*.

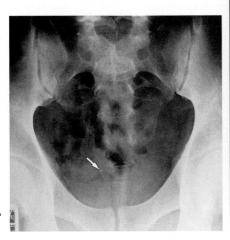

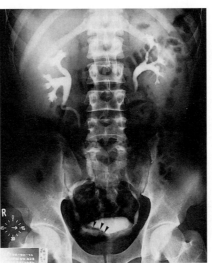

Fig. 2. A stone in the ureterovesical junction with pseudoureterocele in a 32-year-old man.
A. Plain radiograph shows a small calcification *(arrow)* in the right pelvic cavity. **B.** A 15-minute IVU shows the finding of pseudoureterocele by dilation of the distal ureter and edema *(arrowheads)* on the right ureterovesical junction due to the stone.

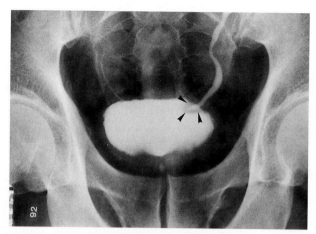

Fig. 3. Pseudoureterocele due to edema of the ureterovesical junction after stone passage in a 59-year-old woman. IVU shows thick, asymmetrical halo *(arrowheads)* due to edema of the ureterovesical junction after passage of a stone.

16. Ureter Stone: Other Findings

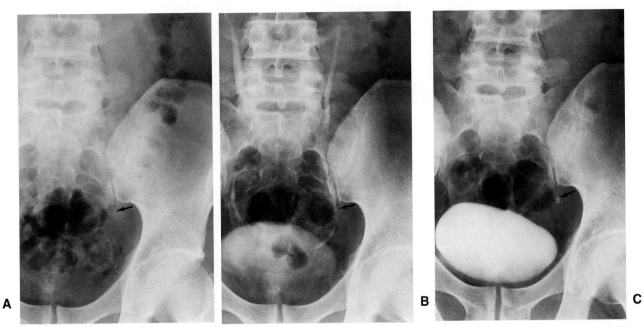

Fig. 1. A small, faintly radiopaque stone in the distal ureter, which becomes more radiopaque during IVU due to coating with contrast material in a 26-year-old man.
A. Plain radiograph shows a small faint radiopacity *(arrow)* in the left pelvic cavity. **B.** IVU confirms that the radiopacity is a stone in the left distal ureter *(arrow)*. **C.** On delayed IVU, stone appears more radiopaque *(arrow)* as compared to **A**, probably due to coating of the stone surface with contrast material.

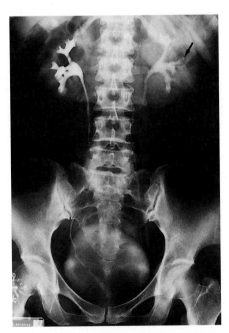

Fig. 2. A 39-year-old man who passed a small stone from the left urinary tract 1 day before IVU. A 15-minute IVU shows decreased concentration of contrast material on the left urinary tract as compared to the right urinary tract. Note a small papillary cavity *(arrow)* in the interpolar calyx of the left kidney that is probably the origin of the stone.

17. Ureter Stone versus Phlebolith

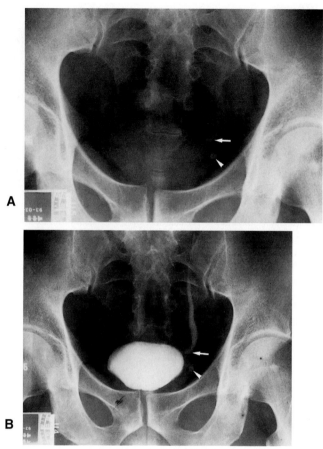

Fig. 1. A distal ureteral stone and a phlebolith in a 39-year-old man.
A. Plain radiograph shows two radiopacities in the left pelvic cavity. The
upper one *(arrow)*, located above the ischial spine, has irregular margin,
whereas the lower one *(arrowhead)*, located below the ischial spine, is
round and has central radiolucency. **B.** IVU reveals that the upper
radiopacity is a distal ureteral stone *(arrow)* and the lower one is a
phlebolith *(arrowhead)*.

18. Urolithiasis: US Findings

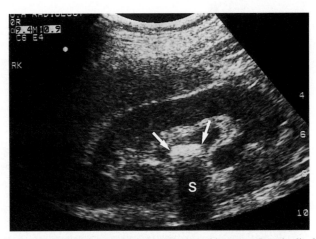

Fig. 1. A stone in the renal pelvis in a 40-year-old woman. Longitudinal US of the right kidney shows slightly dilated renal pelvis and an echogenic stone *(arrows)* within it. Note dense sonic shadowing (S) posterior to the stone.

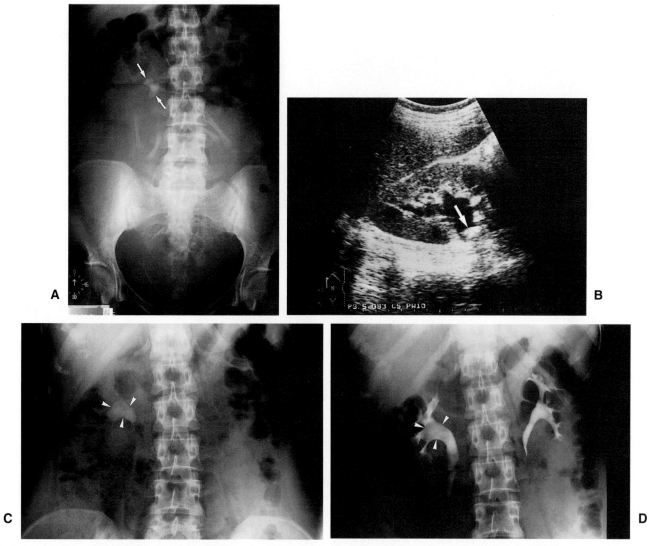

Fig. 2. A renal stone in a 29-year-old woman with a 26-week pregnancy.
A. Plain radiograph shows the fetus and a large stone *(arrows)* in the right renal region. **B.** Longitudinal US of the right kidney shows hydronephrosis and a stone *(arrow)* in the renal pelvis. **C, D.** Plain radiograph **(C)** and IVU **(D)** taken after delivery of the fetus show the stone *(arrowheads)* in the right renal pelvis. The stone was removed by percutaneous nephrostolithotomy.

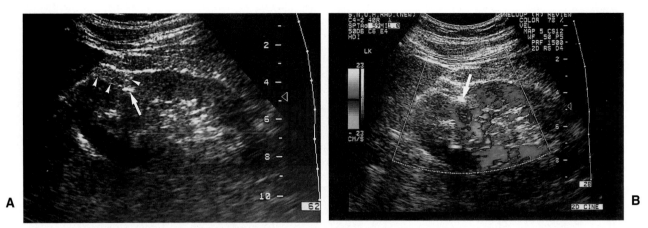

Fig. 3. Renal stone with parenchymal scar in a 64-year-old man.
A. Longitudinal US of the left kidney shows a stone *(arrow)* with posterior sonic shadowing in the upper polar region. Note parenchymal scar *(arrowheads)* adjacent to the stone. **B.** Color Doppler US of the left kidney shows decreased vascularity around the stone *(arrow)* due to parenchymal scarring. (**B,** See also Color Section.)

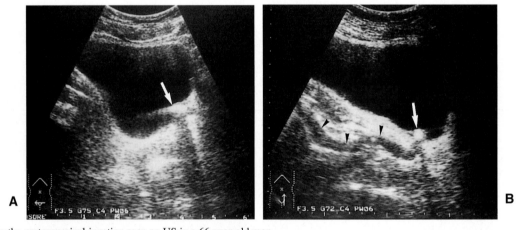

Fig. 4. A stone in the ureterovesical junction seen on US in a 66-year-old man.
A. US of the bladder in transverse plane shows a stone *(arrow)* in the region of the left ureterovesical junction. **B.** Longitudinal US along the course of the left ureter shows the stone *(arrow)* in the ureterovesical junction and dilated distal ureter *(arrowheads)*.

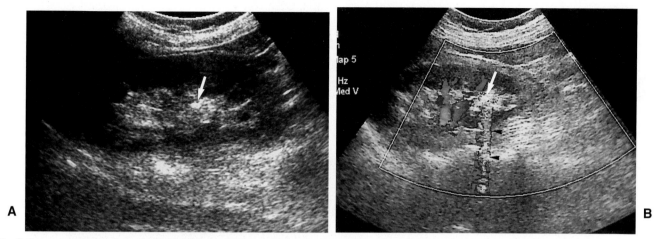

Fig. 5. Renal stone with color twinkling artifact in a 54-year-old woman.
A. Longitudinal US of the right kidney shows an echogenic lesion *(arrow)* in the renal sinus suspicious of a stone. Sonic shadowing is not evident posterior to the echogenic lesion. **B.** Color Doppler US shows strong color twinkling artifact *(arrowheads)* posterior to the echogenic lesion *(arrow)* indicating that the echogenic lesion is a stone. (**B,** See also Color Section.)

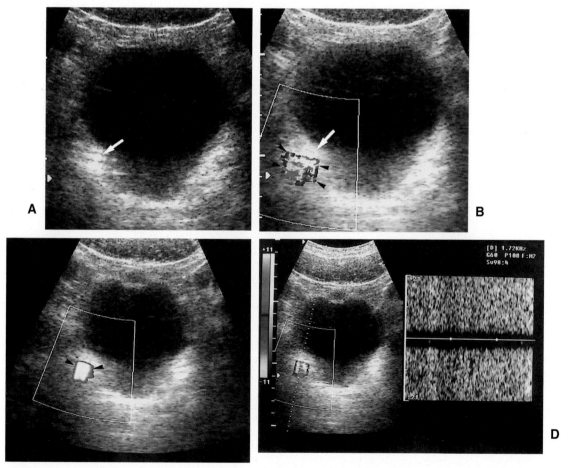

Fig. 6. A terminal ureter stone with color twinkling artifact in a 35-year-old man. (**A, B, D,** From Lee JY, Kim SH, Cho JY, et al: Color and power Doppler twinkling artifacts from urinary stones: Clinical observations and phantom studies. AJR Am J Roentgenol 2001; 176:1441–1445.) (**B–D,** See also Color Section.)
A. Transverse US shows an echogenic lesion in the right ureterovesical junction *(arrow)* with faint posterior sonic shadowing. **B.** Color Doppler US shows prominent twinkling artifact *(arrowheads)* posterior to the echogenic lesion *(arrow)*. **C.** Power Doppler US also shows strong artifact *(arrowheads)*. **D.** Spectral Doppler US with the sample volume located in the echogenic lesion shows artifactual spectral signal.

19. Urolithiasis: CT Findings

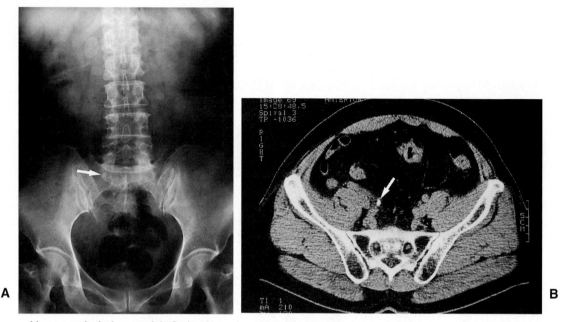

Fig. 1. A 50-year-old woman who had severe right flank pain.
A. Plain radiograph shows a suspicious stone *(arrow)* over the sacrum. **B.** Nonenhanced CT clearly shows a stone in the right ureter with a slightly thickened ureteral wall *(arrow)*. The stone was not well demonstrated on plain radiograph owing to the presacral location of the stone. In cases of a ureter stone located in front of the sacrum, the stone is often difficult to detect; therefore this area is called the *graveyard of stone*.

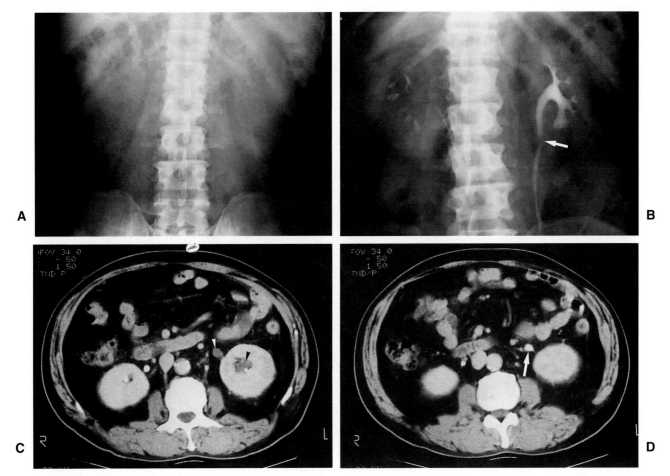

Fig. 2. Radiolucent ureteral stone in a 62-year-old man.
A. Plain radiograph shows no radiopaque stone. **B.** IVU shows a filling defect *(arrow)* in the left proximal ureter. **C, D.** Contrast-enhanced CT scans show a high-attenuated stone *(arrow* in **D**) in the left proximal ureter and mild dilation of proximal ureter and pelvocalyces *(arrowheads* in **C**).

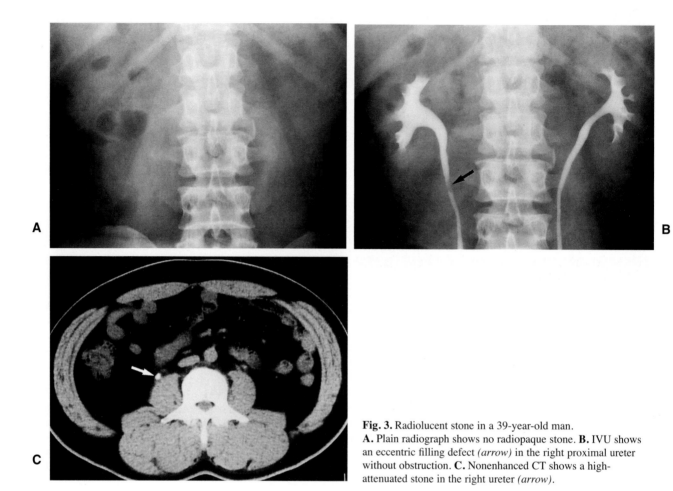

A

B

C

Fig. 3. Radiolucent stone in a 39-year-old man.
A. Plain radiograph shows no radiopaque stone. **B.** IVU shows
an eccentric filling defect *(arrow)* in the right proximal ureter
without obstruction. **C.** Nonenhanced CT shows a high-
attenuated stone in the right ureter *(arrow)*.

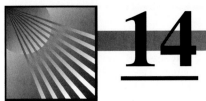

14

Obstructive Uropathy

HAK JONG LEE

DEFINITION

Hydronephrosis is the dilation of the renal pelvis and calyces. It is synonymous with pyelocaliectasis and may or may not be associated with parenchymal thinning. Whitaker, a British urologist, defined obstruction as a narrowing such that the proximal pressure must be raised to transmit the usual flow through it. In the patients with obstruction, anatomic narrowing may be demonstrated in a specific point (anatomic obstruction), but sometimes anatomic narrowing may not be demonstrated (functional obstruction). The examples of functional obstruction are primary obstructive megaureter, ureteropelvic junction obstruction, and detrusor–bladder neck and detrusor–external sphincter dyssynergia.

Most of the significant obstruction causes hydronephrosis, but not all hydronephrosis is caused by obstruction. Therefore, hydronephrosis can be classified into obstructive and nonobstructive hydronephrosis. Nonobstructive hydronephrosis includes congenital megacalyces, postobstructive dilation, vesicoureteral reflux, and high-flow states.

PATHOPHYSIOLOGY

The normal pressure of the intrarenal collecting system is estimated to be 8 to 12 cm H_2O. Pressures higher than 15 cm H_2O are abnormal and indicate obstruction. In an experimental study, renal blood flow increases for several hours after obstruction, falls back to baseline thereafter, and subsequently declines steadily with continued obstruction. Unlike the biphasic pattern of renal blood flow, glomerular filtration rate falls immediately after the onset of obstruction and continues to fall. The increase in renal vascular resistance and progressive deterioration of glomerular filtration rate are not dependent on increased intrapelvic pressure. It is reported that the declines in glomerular filtration rate and renal blood flow are mainly the results of preglomerular vasoconstriction. The increase of renal vascular resistance is followed by the decrease in the diastolic blood flow. Renal lymphatic drainage increases up to five times the normal rate and drains excess fluid from the interstitial tissues.

Long periods of obstruction cause progressive nephron loss resulting in medullary and cortical atrophy, a series of events called *obstructive atrophy*.

IVU FINDINGS OF ACUTE OBSTRUCTION

The most common etiology of acute obstruction is urinary calculus. The typical intravenous urography (IVU) findings of acute obstruction are increasingly dense nephrogram, modest kidney enlargement, delayed calyceal opacification, minimal to moderate dilation of the collecting system, forniceal rupture, and spontaneous pyelosinous extravasation. Other IVU findings that may be seen in urinary tract obstruction are mucosal striations of the renal pelvis and ureter and heterotopic excretion of contrast material.

An increasingly dense nephrogram, or obstructive nephrogram, means that IVU shows increased opacity of renal shadow without visualization of the pelvocalyces and ureter long after contrast material injection. This pattern of nephrogram indicates acute high-grade ureteral obstruction.

The ability of the kidney to develop a dense nephrogram depends on the condition in which renal blood flow and renal tubules are normal. In the cases of severe renal infection or other underlying parenchymal disease, an obstructive nephrogram may not develop in spite of acute obstruction. An increasingly dense nephrogram may also be observed with systemic hypotension, arterial stenosis, acute renal failure, and renal vein thrombosis.

Sometimes, fine, radiopaque, and radiolucent lines arranged radially in the parenchyma and perpendicular to the renal margin are observed within the obstructive nephrogram. These striations are thought to represent contrast material within bundles of proximal tubules and collecting ducts in the medullary rays.

The gallbladder is sometimes opacified on delayed IVU in patients with acute urinary obstruction. This finding is called *heterotopic* or *vicarious excretion of contrast material*. Infrequently this finding is noted in patients without urinary tract obstruction. When the plasma levels of the contrast material elevate above threshold because of decreased glomerular filtration, hepatic extraction and excretion into the bile occur.

IVU FINDINGS OF CHRONIC OBSTRUCTION

With chronic partial obstruction, nephrographic density is often normal, but the nephrogram is distorted by the dilated pyelocalyceal system. The IVU findings of chronic obstruction

include negative pyelogram, calyceal crescents, dilated papillary duct, soap-bubble nephrogram, and ball pyelogram.

Negative pyelogram is the finding that the parenchyma is seen as a radiopaque mantle outside a radiolucent urine-filled collecting system. Calyceal crescents are thin, semilunar collections of contrast material, which have denser radiopacity than that of medulla. Calyceal crescents represent compressed and realigned collecting ducts located at right angles to their usual orientation. Sometimes these dilated collecting ducts may appear as dots of contrast material just outside the dilated calyces. These dots should be distinguished from lacunae representing spaces in the renal sinus that communicate with the collecting system via forniceal tears.

The soap-bubble nephrogram represents bubble-like, curved, white densities of thin thickness that appear after the intravenous or intra-arterial injection of contrast material. Each bubble represents a dilated calyx.

IVU obtained with the patient supine often shows round puddles of contrast material with unsharp edges known as a *ball pyelogram*. It may appear separated from the nephrogram by radiolucent boundaries of nonopaque urine. Because the upper-polar calyces are located in more dependent position than the lower-polar calyces, these ball pyelograms appear mainly in the upper-polar calyces. On CT, this finding is seen as a urine-contrast level in the pelvocalyces.

Marked dilation of renal pelvis may be caused by congenital ureteropelvic junction obstruction, in which the renal pelvis is markedly enlarged, but the ureter is normal size. Severe dilation of the renal pelvis can also result from tuberculosis and other acquired obstructions near the ureteropelvic junction.

Certain degree of ureteral obstruction is usually present after surgery for pelvic malignancies, especially when the distal ureters are stripped off during the surgery and postoperative radiation therapy is applied. Usually this obstruction is transient but may progress. Therefore these patients should be followed up carefully.

Mucosal striations are sometimes observed in renal pelvis or ureter of the patients with reflux, obstruction, and infection. In adults, striations are most often seen following episodes of ureterolithiasis, whereas in children striations are usually associated with reflux and infection. Even in some normal infants and children, it is also possible to see fine striations, since the mucosa of the normal renal pelvis and ureter is longitudinally plicated. The cause of striations in obstruction or reflux is still incompletely understood, but it is likely that the normal folds of the pelvis or ureter become deepened owing to dilation or intermittent stretching. In the presence of infection, these longitudinal ridges may be exaggerated and stiffened by edema, cellular infiltration, and mucosal hypertrophy.

ULTRASONOGRAPHY

Ultrasonography (US) is a noninvasive, excellent method in anatomic evaluation of the lesion. US diagnosis of urinary tract obstruction depends on the presence of dilation in the collecting system. In the diagnosis of obstruction with US, it was reported that the sensitivity and the specificity are 98% and 75%, respectively. The causes of false-positive findings include extrarenal pelvis, renal cystic disease, vesicoureteral reflux, and vessels crossing renal sinus. The causes of false-negative findings include small intrarenal pelvis, hyperacute obstruction, obstruction due to tumor infiltration, severe dehydration, and decompression state due to backflow or tear.

Color Doppler US helps distinguish collecting systems from renal sinus vessels by confirming blood flow in the vessels. The resistive index (RI) ([peak systolic velocity − end-diastolic velocity]/peak systolic velocity) can help the diagnosis of obstruction. RI is measured in the interlobar artery and can be affected by measurement location, age, blood pressure, and heart rate. According to some reports about RI, RI higher than 0.7 or difference of RI (dRI) higher than 0.1 can be the criteria in the diagnosis of urinary obstruction. However, elevated RI is not observed in cases of obstruction except those that are acute and severe. RI measurement after furosemide administration is reported in clinical and experimental study as a more accurate method in the diagnosis of obstruction.

COMPUTED TOMOGRAPHY

Nonenhanced computed tomography (CT) helps the diagnosis of hydronephrosis, especially in patients who have allergy to contrast material or azotemia or in the cases in which US findings are not definite. CT has advantages over other examinations in evaluating the etiology of obstruction. CT made it possible to detect not only intrinsic lesions such as stones or urothelial tumor that are not demonstrated in simple radiograph but also extrinsic lesions such as retroperitoneal mass or fibrosis. Urine-contrast level, which is shown in dilated collecting system because of the difference between urine and contrast material, helps the diagnosis of urinary obstruction. In general, CT contributed to exact diagnosis of various diseases, but contrast-enhanced CT in early cortical phase may cause confusion in the diagnosis of hydronephrosis.

References

1. Lee HJ, Cho JY, Kim SH: Resistive index in rabbits with experimentally induced hydronephrosis: Effect of furosemide. Acad Radiol 2001; 8:987–992.
2. Talner LB, O'Reilly PH, Roy C: Urinary obstruction. In Pollack HM, McClennan BL (eds): Clinical Urography, 2nd ed, vol 2. Philadelphia, WB Saunders, 2000, pp 1846–1966.
3. Lee KH, Kim SH, Kim YJ, et al: Pseudohydronephrosis in two-phase spiral CT of the abdomen. J Korean Radiol Soc 1997; 37:889–892.
4. Lee HJ, Kim SH, Jeong YK, et al: Doppler sonographic resistive index in obstructed kidneys. J Ultrasound Med 1996; 15:613–618.
5. Platt JF, Rubin JM, Ellis JH, et al: Duplex Doppler US of the kidney: Differentiation of obstructive from nonobstructive dilatation. Radiology 1989; 171:515–517.
6. Klahr S: Pathophysiology of obstructive nephropathy. Kidney Int 1983; 23:414–426.
7. McCrory WW: Regulation of renal functional development. Urol Clin North Am 1980; 7:243–264.
8. Whitaker R: Clinical application of upper urinary tract dynamics. Urol Clin North Am 1979; 6:137–141.
9. Bigongiari LR, Davis RM, Novak WG, et al: Visualization of the medullary rays on excretory urography in experimental ureteric obstruction. AJR Am J Roentgenol 1977; 129:89–93.
10. Sokoloff J, Talner LB: The heterotopic excretion of sodium iothalamate. Br J Radiol 1973; 46:571–577.

Illustrations • Obstructive Uropathy

1 • Dense striated nephrogram

2 • Calyceal crescent

3 • Forniceal rupture and leak of contrast material

4 • Ball pyelogram and urine-contrast level

5 • Negative pyelogram

6 • Soap-bubble nephrogram

7 • Mucosal striation

8 • Doppler US findings of obstructive uropathy

9 • Various causes of obstruction

10 • Nonobstructive hydronephrosis

11 • Postobstructive atrophy

12 • Vicarious excretion of contrast material

1. Dense Striated Nephrogram

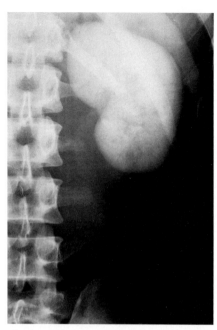

Fig. 1. Delayed striated nephrogram in a 30-year-old woman with a ureter stone. IVU demonstrates fine, radiopaque, and radiolucent lines arranged radially in the renal parenchyma. These striations represent contrast material within bundles of proximal tubules and collecting ducts in the medullary rays.

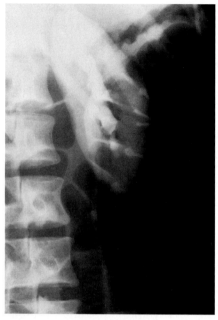

Fig. 2. Striated nephrogram in a 21-year-old man with a ureteral stone. IVU shows streaks composed of alternating radiopaque and radiolucent lines arranged radially in the renal parenchyma.

2. Calyceal Crescent

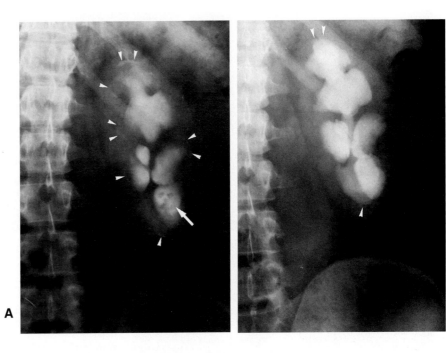

Fig. 1. Hydronephrosis with a crescent sign in a 17-year-old boy with congenital ureteropelvic junction obstruction. **A.** A 15-minute IVU shows a dilated collecting system and peripherally located curvilinear radiopacities *(arrowheads)*. These calyceal crescents represent compressed and realigned collecting ducts containing contrast material. Note filling defects in the lower-polar calyx *(arrow)* due to small stones. **B.** A 25-minute IVU shows dilated calyces filled with dense contrast material. Note still demonstrable calyceal crescents *(arrowheads)*.

A

B

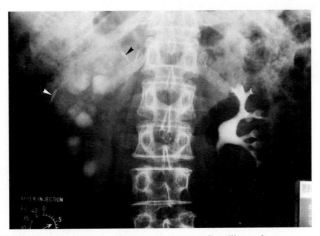

Fig. 2. Crescent sign in a 50-year-old woman. Curvilinear dense radiopacities are noted in peripheral portion of the calyces *(arrowheads)*.

3. Forniceal Rupture and Leak of Contrast Material

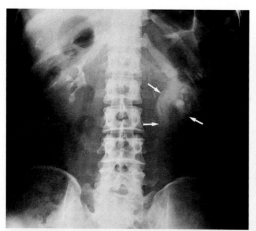

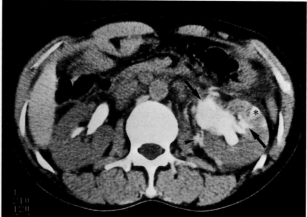

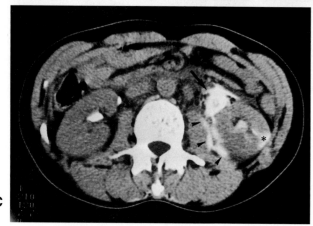

Fig. 1. Leak of contrast material due to ureteral obstruction in a 40-year-old woman with retroperitoneal metastasis from unknown primary tumor.
A. A 15-minute IVU shows leak of contrast material around the pelvocalyces and ureter *(arrows)*. **B, C.** CT scans taken 2 hours after IVU without further injection of contrast material demonstrate leak of contrast material around the pelvocalyces *(arrows)*. Note leaked contrast material in the perirenal space *(arrowheads)*. Also note focally retained contrast material in the renal parenchyma of the left kidney *(asterisks)*.

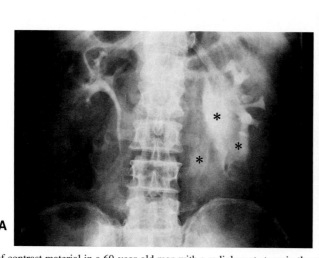

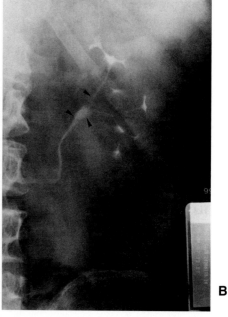

Fig. 2. Leak of contrast material in a 60-year-old man with a radiolucent stone in the ureter.
A. IVU shows dilated calyces and leak of contrast material in the renal hilar region *(asterisks)*. **B.** After passage of the stone, hydronephrosis is relieved and fine longitudinal striations *(arrowheads)* are noted in the pelvocalyces and proximal ureter.

4. Ball Pyelogram and Urine-Contrast Level

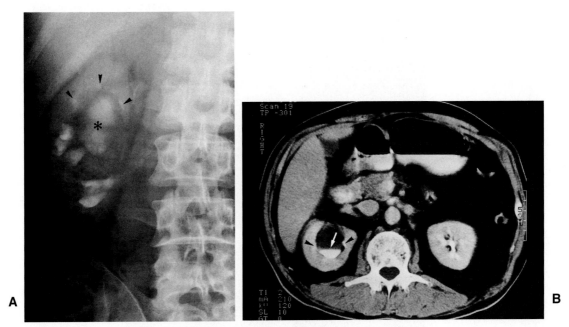

A

B

Fig. 1. Ureteropelvic junction obstruction with ball pyelogram and crescent sign in a 63-year-old man.
A. IVU demonstrates curvilinear, dense radiopacities outlining the dilated calyces producing the finding of calyceal crescents *(arrowheads)*. Note that excreted contrast material is collected in the dependent portion of the dilated collecting systems, producing the finding of ball pyelogram *(asterisk)*.
B. Contrast-enhanced CT scan of the same patient shows ureteropelvic junction obstruction with dilated collecting systems containing urine-contrast level *(arrow)*. The curvilinear opacities displaced by dilated collecting systems represent calyceal crescents *(arrowheads)*.

5. Negative Pyelogram

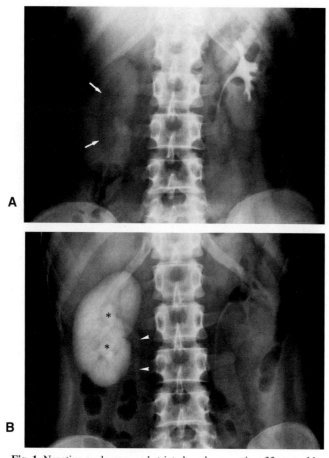

Fig. 1. Negative pyelogram and striated nephrogram in a 33-year-old man with a stone in the ureterovesical junction.
A. A 15-minute IVU shows delayed excretion of contrast material in the right urinary tract. Note that the right renal parenchyma is seen as radiopacity surrounding urine-filled, radiolucent renal pelvis *(arrows)*.
B. A 5-hour-delayed IVU shows dense, striated nephrogram and faint opacification of the dilated pelvocalyces *(asterisks)* and ureter *(arrowheads)*.

6. Soap-bubble Nephrogram

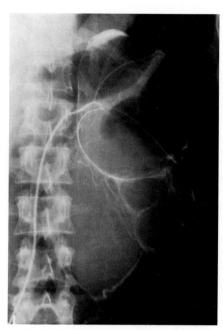

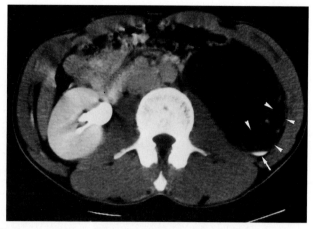

Fig. 2. Congenital UPJ obstruction in a 36-year-old man. Contrast-enhanced CT shows severe hydronephrosis of the left kidney. There is marked thinning of the renal parenchyma *(arrowheads)*, which is a CT finding of soap-bubble nephrogram. Note the small amount of excreted contrast material in the dilated renal calyx *(arrow)*.

Fig. 1. Soap-bubble nephrogram demonstrated on renal arteriogram in a 50-year-old woman with congenital ureteropelvic junction obstruction. Left renal arteriogram shows soap-bubble appearance due to severe hydronephrosis and paper-thin renal parenchyma.

7. Mucosal Striation

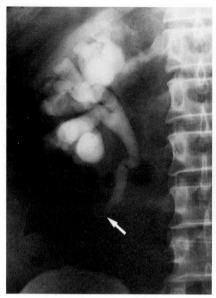

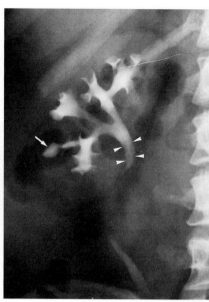

A

B

Fig. 1. Longitudinal striations in the renal pelvis after passage of a ureteral stone in a 39-year-old man.
A. IVU shows hydronephrosis of the right kidney caused by a ureteral stone *(arrow)*.
B. After stone passage, the dilated renal pelvis has been decompressed. Note the longitudinal striations of the ureter *(arrowheads)* due to previous dilation and stretching. Note a papillary cavity in the lower-polar calyx that probably is the origin of the stone *(arrow)*.

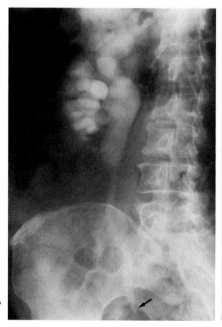

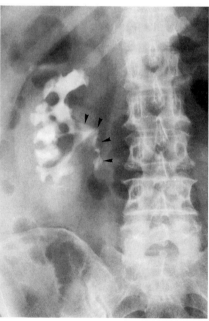

A

B

Fig. 2. Wrinkling of renal pelvic mucosa after relief of obstruction by a ureteral stone in a 54-year-old woman.
A. IVU shows hydronephrosis and hydroureter due to a distal ureteral stone *(arrow).* **B.** After passage of the stone, the renal pelvis is collapsed and shows wrinkling *(arrowheads).*

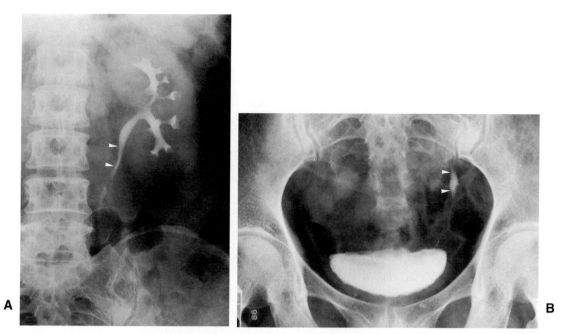

Fig. 3. Ureteral striations due to previous obstruction in a 59-year-old woman with bladder tumor.
A, B. IVU images show longitudinal striations in the proximal and distal parts of the left ureter *(arrowheads)*. This patient had hydronephrosis of the left urinary tract due to a bladder tumor that was treated by transurethral resection.

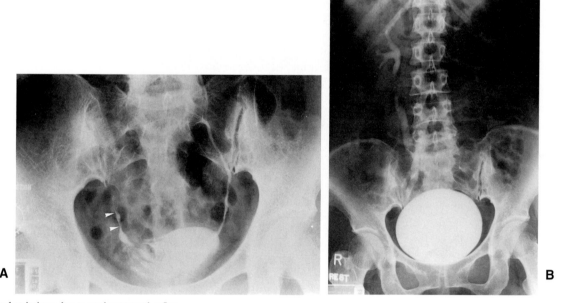

Fig. 4. Ureteral striations due to vesicoureteral reflux.
A. IVU shows fine longitudinal striations in the distal portion of the right ureter *(arrowheads)*. **B.** VCU reveals vesicoureteral reflux on the right side.

8. Doppler US Findings of Obstructive Uropathy

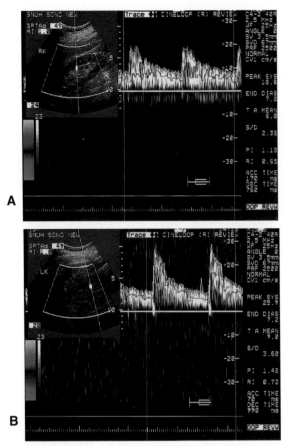

Fig. 1. Renal Doppler US in a 30-year-old woman with a stone in the left distal ureter.
A. Spectral Doppler US of the right kidney shows normal resistive index (0.65). **B.** The resistive index of the left kidney that is obstructed by a ureteral stone is elevated (0.72).

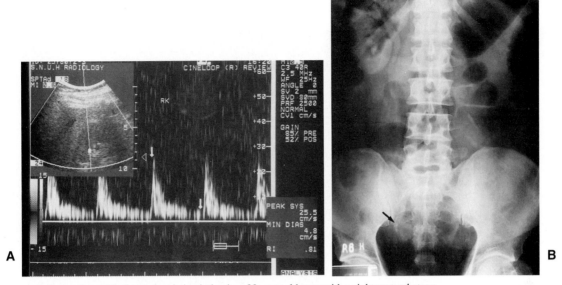

Fig. 2. Acute ureteral obstruction with elevated resistive index in a 32-year-old man with a right ureteral stone.
A. Spectral Doppler US of the right kidney shows markedly elevated resistive index (0.81). **B.** A 6-hour-delayed IVU shows a right ureter stone *(arrow)* with delayed excretion of contrast material. Note that dilation of the urinary tract proximal to the stone is not severe.

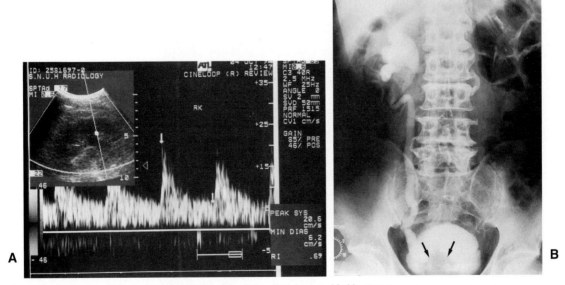

Fig. 3. Normal resistive index in a 59-year-old man with chronic obstruction due to a bladder tumor.
A. Spectral Doppler US of the hydronephrotic right kidney shows a normal resistive index (0.69). Resistive index of the left kidney was 0.61. **B.** A 30-minute IVU reveals marked dilation of the right urinary tract. There is a large filling defect with irregular margin in the urinary bladder indicating a tumor *(arrows)*.

9. Various Causes of Obstruction

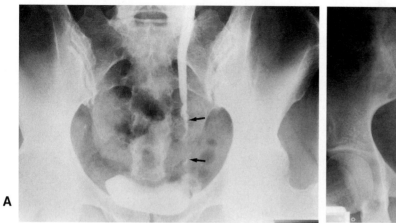
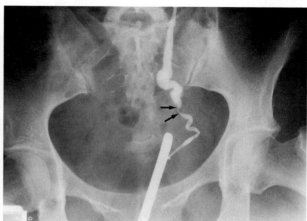

Fig. 1. Ureteral obstruction due to endometriosis.
A. IVU in a 42-year-old woman with endometriosis shows irregular narrowing of the left distal ureter *(arrows)* with proximal dilation. **B.** RGP in a 32-year-old woman with endometriosis shows distal ureteral obstruction with a corkscrew appearance *(arrows)*.

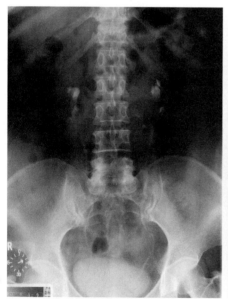
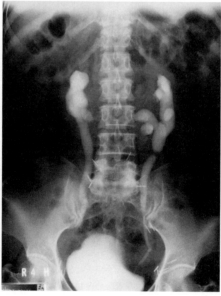

Fig. 2. Transient bilateral hydronephrosis following radical hysterectomy and pelvic node dissection for uterine cervical carcinoma in a 53-year-old woman with horseshoe kidney.
A. Preoperative 10-minute IVU shows vertical axes of the kidneys due to horseshoe kidney and normal excretion of contrast material in the urinary tract.
B. A 4-hour-delayed IVU taken 2 weeks after surgery shows bilateral hydronephrosis and hydroureter. Note multiple surgical clips and deformity of the urinary bladder. On follow-up IVU hydronephrosis in both urinary tracts was improved.

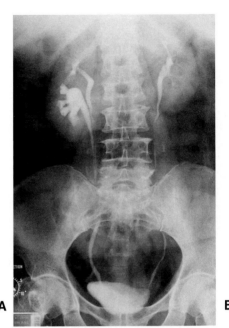 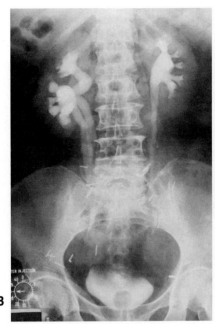 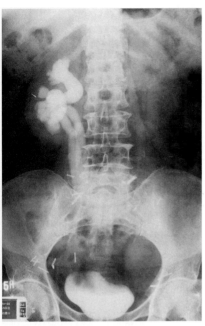

A   **B**   **C**

Fig. 3. Bilateral hydronephrosis following radical hysterectomy and pelvic node dissection in a 59-year-old woman with uterine cervical carcinoma. **A.** Preoperative 10-minute IVU shows normal excretion of contrast material in both urinary tracts. Note incomplete duplication of the collecting system in the right urinary tract. **B.** A 30-minute IVU taken 2 weeks after surgery shows bilateral hydronephrosis and hydroureter due to distal ureteral obstruction. Note multiple surgical clips in the pelvic cavity. **C.** A 5-hour-delayed IVU taken 1 month later shows progressed hydronephrosis on the right side. Contrast material has been already excreted on the normalized left urinary tract.

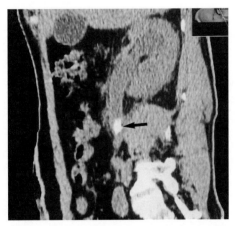

Fig. 4. Ureter stone demonstrated by three-dimensional reformation CT in a 63-year-old man. Maximal intensity projection image of nonenhanced spiral CT shows hydronephrosis due to a ureteral stone *(arrow)*.

10. Nonobstructive Hydronephrosis

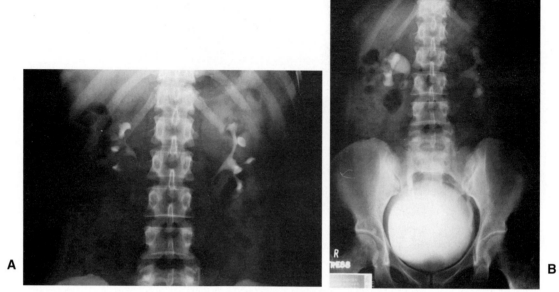

A
B

Fig. 1. Nonobstructive hydronephrosis due to vesicoureteral reflux in a 32-year-old woman with history of repeated pyelonephritis. **A.** IVU shows mild dilation of the renal calyces with clubbing. **B.** VCU reveals vesicoureteral reflux on both sides.

11. Postobstructive Atrophy

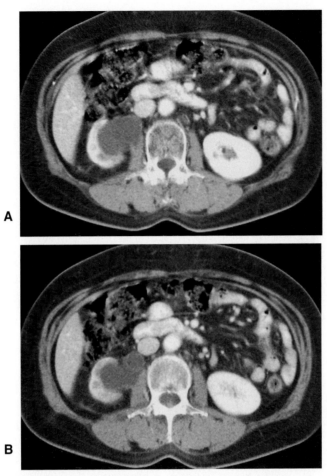

Fig. 1. Renal atrophy due to longstanding hydronephrosis in a
53-year-old woman with postoperative stricture of the ureter that
occurred following radical hysterectomy and pelvic lymph node
dissection for uterine cervical carcinoma.
A, B. Contrast-enhanced CT scans show small right kidney with poor
perfusion and dilated pelvocalyces and ureter.

12. Vicarious Excretion of Contrast Material

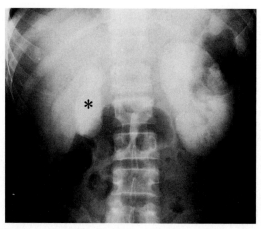

Fig. 1. Vicarious hepatobiliary excretion of contrast material in a 13-year-old boy with leukemia in whom left distal ureter was obstructed by a stone. IVU taken 4 hours after injection of contrast material shows delayed, dense, streaky nephrogram of the left kidney due to obstruction. Contrast material has been already excreted from the right urinary tract. Note that the gallbladder *(asterisk)* is densely opacified with contrast material.

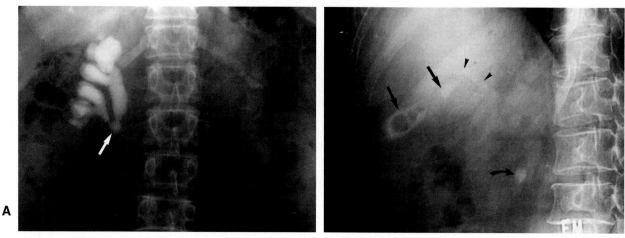

Fig. 2. Vicarious biliary excretion of contrast material in a 63-year-old woman with a stone in the ureteropelvic junction.
A. IVU shows an obstructing stone *(arrow)* in the ureteropelvic junction of the right kidney. The right renal pelvis is bifid. **B.** Plain radiograph in an oblique projection obtained 24 hours later shows the gallbladder *(arrows)* and common bile ducts *(arrowheads)* opacified by vicarious excretion of contrast material. Note that the gallbladder has multiple stones appearing as filling defects. *Curved arrow* indicates the stone in the right ureteropelvic junction.

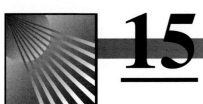

15

Vascular Diseases of the Kidney

SEUNG HYUP KIM

RENAL VASCULAR EMBRYOLOGY, ANATOMY, AND NORMAL VARIATIONS

Renal arterial system

Knowledge of the normal renal vascular development and its variations is important in understanding the imaging findings of the normal kidneys and kidneys with renal vascular diseases. As the kidneys ascend from the pelvic cavity, they receive their blood supply from the network of multiple mesonephric arteries. Initially renal arteries are branches of the common iliac arteries. As they ascend further, the kidneys receive their blood supply from the distal abdominal aorta. When they reach a higher level, they receive new branches from the aorta, and the inferior branches normally undergo involution and disappear. The kidneys come into contact with the adrenal gland in the 9th week and the ascent stops. The right renal artery is longer and often more superior than the left renal artery.

A single renal artery to each kidney is present in about 75% of people, and about 25% of adult kidneys have two or more renal arteries. Half of these have two or more renal arteries entering at the hilum and the other half have one entering at the hilum and the other entering directly into the renal tissue in the polar region. Multiplicity of renal arteries and more distal points of origin are more common with renal ectopy and malrotation.

The renal artery branches into an anterior and posterior division. The anterior division supplies the anterior parenchyma and usually lower-polar region whereas the posterior division supplies the posterior parenchyma and usually the upper-polar region. The anterior branch lies between the renal vein and renal pelvis and the posterior branch lies behind the renal pelvis. Renal arteries and veins can cause an extrinsic impression on the pelvocalyceal system and possibly obstruct the upper-pole infundibulum resulting in Fraley's syndrome. The arborizing anterior and posterior vessels leave a relatively avascular region at the true mid-coronal plane of the kidney. This is the ideal area for percutaneous approach to the kidney.

Renal venous system

The cardinal veins are the important system of embryonic venous drainage. The posterior cardinal veins, which arise dorsal to the mesonephros, appear first and regress as the mesonephros disappears. They persist caudally as the common iliac veins and their confluence and cranially as the root of the azygos vein. The subcardinal veins, which arise ventral to the mesonephros, develop next. The supracardinal veins, which arise dorsal and medial to the posterior cardinal veins, develop last. The subcardinal and supracardinal veins anastomose in mid-body (supracardinal-subcardinal anastomosis). The right supracardinal vein becomes most of the infrarenal inferior vena cava (IVC) and the right subcardinal vein becomes the suprarenal IVC. The subcardinal veins remain as the gonadal veins, adrenal veins, and a portion of the left renal vein.

The supracardinal veins are interrupted at the level of the renal veins. Cranially, they become the azygos and hemiazygos veins. The metanephric renal veins end at the subcardinal-supracardinal anastomosis. The right side of the anastomosis contributes directly to the formation of the IVC at the renal vein level. Thus the right renal vein drains directly into the IVC. The left renal vein develops from the left subcardinal vein and continues across the aorta via the subcardinal-supracardinal anastomosis. Thus the right gonadal vein comes to enter the IVC directly and the left gonadal vein drains into the left renal vein.

Fourteen percent of kidneys have multiple renal veins, more commonly on the right. The subcardinal-supracardinal anastomosis, which passes on both sides of the aorta, may persist and result in a retroaortic or circumaortic renal vein in 6% of people. The retroaortic component typically inserts more caudally into the IVC. Persistence of the left supracardinal vein leads to the presence of another vena cava to the left of the aorta.

Persistence of a caudal subcardinal vein as the infrarenal IVC segment leads to retrocaval or circumcaval ureter. The right renal artery normally passes behind the portion of the IVC formed by the ventral right subcardinal vein as it passes across the midline to its kidney. If the artery originates lower than normal at the level of the posteriorly located right supracardinal vein, the artery will course anterior to the infrarenal IVC. Thus, supernumerary lower-pole vessels or arteries supplying ectopic kidneys may lie anterior to the IVC.

RENAL ARTERIOVENOUS MALFORMATIONS AND FISTULA

Renal arteriovenous malformations (AVMs) and arteriovenous fistulas (AVFs) are different types of pathologic arteriovenous communications. *AVM* is commonly used to describe congenital abnormalities of the vascular system, whereas *AVF* represents acquired lesions seen following trauma, after biopsy,

or in the presence of neoplasm. An AVF consists of a single communication between an artery and a vein, whereas an AVM is a complex network of arteriovenous communications. Congenital AVM is rare, and 75% of arteriovenous communications are acquired AVF. Congenital AVMs can be classified into cirsoid or aneurysmal. In cirsoid AVM, there are multiple arteriovenous communications resulting in a cluster of tortuous arterial and venous structures.

The most common cause of AVF is trauma, usually penetrating trauma from biopsy, although many such fistulas close spontaneously. The patient usually presents with hematuria or hypertension, although large lesions may produce high-flow congestive heart failure. Hypertension is related to an internal steal that renders renal tissue distal to the lesion ischemic and results in excessive renin secretion. The most definite diagnosis is made by renal arteriography, but other imaging studies such as color Doppler ultrasonography (US), computed tomography (CT), or magnetic resonance (MR) imaging may suggest the presence of such vascular lesions. In a kidney with AVF, Doppler US shows increased flow velocity, decreased resistive index, and arterialization of the venous waveform.

RENAL ARTERY ANEURYSM

Renal artery aneurysms may be congenital, inflammatory, traumatic, or atherosclerotic, or they may occur in conjunction with renal artery stenoses of various causes. Acquired aneurysm is also called *pseudoaneurysm*. Traumatic pseudoaneurysms are most common and frequently are the result of renal biopsy. Many renal artery aneurysms are asymptomatic, but they often cause hypertension. Surgical treatment should be considered when there is a risk of rupture or aneurysm-related hypertension. This consideration becomes important when the aneurysm is greater than 2 cm and noncalcified or when the patient is likely to be in a physiologic state of higher than normal blood pressure or flow, such as pregnancy. Renal artery aneurysm may be diagnosed by using CT, color Doppler US, or MR imaging, but angiography is usually required prior to surgery. Color Doppler US demonstrates a hypoechoic mass with flow signal along the course of the renal artery. Spectral Doppler US shows turbulent flow within the aneurysm.

RENAL ARTERY STENOSIS

Renal artery stenosis is the most important cause of renovascular hypertension. Atherosclerosis, fibromuscular dysplasia, and Takayasu's arteritis are the important underlying pathology of renal artery stenosis. Renal artery stenosis may be suspected with excretory urography (rapid-sequence pyelography), renal scintigraphy with use of captopril, and renal vein renin sampling, but the most definite diagnosis is made with arteriography. Although captopril-enhanced renal scintigraphy can detect significant renal arterial disease, it can neither localize the arterial lesion nor characterize the severity of the stenosis. The role of arteriography has been extended with the popular use of percutaneous transluminal angioplasty.

Recently there has been extensive research on the use of Doppler US as a screening test to detect renal artery stenosis, but controversies exist with regard to the value of this study in detecting renal artery stenosis. Initial efforts at detecting renal artery stenosis were focused on Doppler spectral changes at the main renal arteries. With this technique, criteria proposed for the detection of hemodynamically significant stenosis included high peak systolic velocity (>100 cm/sec), spectral broadening, increased ratio of peak systolic velocity of renal artery to that of the aorta (>3.5), and no detectable renal arterial flow when the stenosis is severe. However, this Doppler technique examining the main renal artery was never widely embraced as a screening test for renal artery stenosis mainly because of the technical difficulties in visualizing the main renal arteries and the high incidence of accessory renal arteries, which are even more difficult to visualize.

Hemodynamically significant stenosis of a main renal artery causes a dampened pulse in the downstream arterial network, producing an intrarenal arterial waveform of decreased amplitude and slowed systolic upstroke (pulsus parvus and tardus). With this intrarenal approach, the proposed criteria for detecting proximal renal artery stenosis are prolonged acceleration time (>0.07 seconds), which is the time from the start of systole to the systolic peak; diminished acceleration index (<3.0 m/sec^2), which is the slope of the systolic upstroke; decreased resistive index (<0.56); and the loss of normal early systolic compliance peak. With this technique and these criteria, Doppler US has a fairly high technical success rate, short examination time, and high sensitivity (72% to 100%) and specificity (62% to 100%) for detection of renal artery stenosis. However, some recommend simple pattern recognition, which has better sensitivity and specificity than these indexes. Similar Doppler spectral changes may be seen in patients with dissecting aneurysm involving the abdominal aorta. To ensure detection of a stenosis at a segmental artery or an accessory renal artery, intrarenal Doppler spectrum should be obtained in at least three regions in each kidney: upper, lower, and interpolar. The use of microbubble-based intravenous contrast agent may enhance Doppler signal intensity and may facilitate Doppler examination.

MR angiography or CT angiography may also be used to demonstrate renal artery stenosis but are not appropriate as a screening technique. CT angiography requires a relatively large amount of intravenous contrast material, which is undesirable in patients with renal insufficiency, and it seems to underestimate the severity of some renal artery stenosis.

RENAL INFARCTION

The diagnosis of renal infarction can usually be made on the basis of patient history, clinical manifestations, and specific CT findings including a sharply marginated, wedge- or hemispheric-shaped area of poor contrast enhancement and a high-attenuation cortical rim peripheral to the lesion. These CT findings of renal infarction are so distinctive that confirmatory renal arteriography is usually unnecessary. This finding, the so-called cortical rim sign, represents 2- to 3-mm-thick, dense, outer nephrogram of the preserved subcapsular cortex supplied by capsular arteries. However, this sign is neither sensitive nor specific for renal infarction. The cortical rim sign is reported to be present in about 50% of renal infarcts and may be absent at the very early stage of infarction. Other conditions that may accompany the cortical rim sign include renal vein thrombosis, acute tubular necrosis, and acute pyelonephritis. Renal medulla can be enhanced in a vermiform or spoke-wheel pattern in renal infarction. This medullary enhancement does not represent

functioning renal tissue but rather blood flow through peripelvic collaterals.

US findings of renal infarction are usually nonspecific changes of renal parenchymal echoes. Color Doppler or power Doppler US may demonstrate the extent of renal infarction. Doppler US enhanced with contrast material containing microbubbles may well demonstrate renal parenchymal perfusion defect. MR imaging, especially contrast-enhanced MR imaging, may demonstrate the extent of the infarction with accuracy comparable to CT or angiography without the danger of iodinated contrast material, to which damaged kidneys are more susceptible. The changes of the signal intensity on MR imaging may represent the renal parenchymal changes caused by infarction. Most of the renal infarcts appear as low-intensity lesions on both T1- and T2-weighted images. These changes of the signal intensity are due to lack of blood perfusion in the early phase and organization of the infarcts in the late phase. Sometimes the infarcts have high signal intensities on T1- and T2-weighted images, which may be related to the hemorrhagic component of the infarcts. Sometimes it is difficult to differentiate renal infarction from renal tumor or renal infection.

POLYARTERITIS NODOSA

Renal vasculitis is a diverse group of disorders affecting mostly the medium and small vessels within the renal parenchyma. They are mostly of autoimmune origin. There is considerable variability within disease entities and also overlap among the manifestations of the various conditions, clinically and radiologically.

The disorder that may serve as the prototype of the angiitis is polyarteritis nodosa. Other immune and autoimmune conditions may present with vascular findings similar to those encountered in polyarteritis nodosa. These conditions include scleroderma, systemic lupus erythematosus, Churg-Strauss syndrome (allergic granulomatosis and angiitis), other necrotizing angiitis including Wegener's granulomatosis, multiple drug abuse, bacterial endocarditis, and Behçet's disease.

Polyarteritis nodosa results in usually bilateral, but often asymmetrical, transmural fibrinoid necrosis and surrounding inflammation of medium and small vessels. Progression of inflammation with scarring produces vascular irregularity, angulation, truncation, and small areas of infarction. The disease may manifest as spontaneous perirenal and subcapsular hemorrhage or hypertension. Progressive destruction of renal tissues results in renal failure. The arteriographic findings correlate well with the pathologic abnormalities. The most striking arteriographic finding is the appearance of aneurysms that are probably related to the rupture of the vessel wall. Although previously considered pathognomonic of polyarteritis nodosa, it is now recognized that aneurysms can occur with any of the necrotizing arteritides. Contrast-enhanced CT scan well demonstrates multiple, small, wedge-shaped, low-attenuated areas of infarcts. The microaneurysms are usually not demonstrable with CT.

TRAUMATIC INJURY OF RENAL ARTERY

Traumatic main renal artery occlusion is detected on CT by a normal sized, nonenhancing kidney, usually with little perirenal hemorrhage. A hematoma surrounding the renal hilum is not uncommon. A rim of cortical tissue may be perfused by capsular collateral vessels. The enhanced renal artery may show an abrupt cutoff, and retrograde filling of the renal vein can be seen.

RENAL VEIN THROMBOSIS

The causes of the renal vein thrombosis are either neoplastic or non-neoplastic. Non-neoplastic causes include dehydration and febrile illness in children and nephrotic syndrome, hypercoagulable states, and postpartum state in adults. Despite its invasiveness, renal venography remains the principal radiologic technique used for diagnosis. Less invasive techniques, including intravenous urography (IVU), US, CT, and MR imaging, have been used. Contrast-enhanced CT with thin section can demonstrate thrombus as a filling defect and MR imaging, especially gradient-echo imaging, can well demonstrate thrombus without injection of contrast material. However, thrombi in the renal vein are often difficult to demonstrate, and renal parenchymal changes are not specific enough for the diagnosis.

In the acute stage, the kidneys are enlarged with decreased nephrographic density. US may demonstrate hyperechoic interlobular streaks, which probably result from vascular congestion and edema. Doppler US may demonstrate increased resistance pattern with peaked systolic flow and absent or reversed end-diastolic flow. This change of Doppler spectrum is known to be specific for renal vein thrombosis in transplanted kidneys but not in the native kidneys. This difference may be explained by the different ability of native and transplanted kidneys to form collateral circulation. Without collateral circulation, the kidney will be totally infarcted. When collateral vessels are developed, renal perfusion regains and pelvic and ureteral notching and cobwebs in perirenal space may be seen. Cortical rim sign may also be seen in renal vein thrombosis. Thrombi in renal vein may calcify. T2-weighted MR image may demonstrate low signal intensity in the renal medulla that probably represents medullary congestion and hemorrhage secondary to renal vein obstruction. We reproduced these MR imaging findings through an experimental study in rabbits following ligation of the renal vein. In renal vein thrombosis associated with renal cell carcinoma, imaging studies may demonstrate tumor neovascularity within the thrombi.

NUTCRACKER SYNDROME

Nutcracker syndrome refers to compression of the left renal vein (LRV) between the aorta and superior mesenteric artery, which results in elevation of the pressure of the LRV and development of collateral venous channels. Nutcracker syndrome occurs in relatively young and previously healthy patients and causes intermittent gross hematuria secondary to LRV hypertension. Nutcracker syndrome can be suspected from the clinical history, urine erythrocyte morphology of predominant isomorphic erythrocytes, and cystoscopic finding of left-sided hematuria.

US or CT may demonstrate compression of LRV at aortomesenteric angle and venous collaterals. Color Doppler US in conjunction with flow-velocity measurement may demonstrate high-flow velocity of the LRV at aortomesenteric angle due to compression between the aorta and superior mesenteric artery. In our Doppler study comparing nutcracker patients and normal

controls, we found that the peak velocity of LRV at the aorto-mesenteric portion usually exceeded 80 cm/sec in nutcracker patients, whereas it was usually less than that velocity in normal controls. MR or CT angiography can demonstrate the compression also, but the diagnosis of a nutcracker syndrome cannot be made with the finding of compression alone. In the case of retroaortic LRV, it can be compressed between the aorta and vertebra, resulting in a so-called posterior nutcracker syndrome.

References

1. Seong CK, Kim SH, Sim JS: Detection of segmental branch renal artery stenosis by Doppler US: A case report. Korean J Radiol 2001; 2:57–60.

2. Choo SW, Kim SH, Jeong YG, et al: MR imaging of segmental renal infarction: An experimental study. Clin Radiol 1997; 52:65–68.

3. Helenon O, Melki P, Correas JM, et al: Renovascular disease: Doppler ultrasound. Semin Ultrasound CT MR 1997; 18:136–146.

4. Melani ML, Grant EG: Clinical experience with sonographic contrast agents. Semin Ultrasound CT MR 1997; 18:3–12.

5. Beregi J, Elkohen M, Dekunder G, et al: Helical CT angiography compared with arteriography in the detection of renal artery stenosis. AJR Am J Roentgenol 1996; 167:495–501.

6. Kamel IR, Berkowitz JF: Assessment of the cortical rim sign in posttraumatic renal infarction. J Comput Assist Tomogr 1996; 20:803–806.

7. Kim SH, Cho SW, Kim HD, et al: Nutcracker syndrome: Diagnosis with Doppler US. Radiology 1996; 198:93–97.

8. Fukuda T, Hayashi K, Sakamoto I, et al: Acute renal infarction caused by Behçet's disease. Abd Imaging 1995; 20:264–266.

9. Garel L, Dubios J, Robitaille P, et al: Renovascular hypertension in children: Curability predicted with negative intrarenal Doppler US results. Radiology 1995; 195:401–405.

10. Gottlieb RH, Lieberman JL, Pabico RC, et al: Diagnosis of renal artery stenosis in transplanted kidneys: Value of Doppler waveform analysis of the intrarenal arteries. AJR Am J Roentgenol 1995; 165:1441–1446.

11. Halpern EJ, Needleman L, Nack TL, et al: Renal artery stenosis: Should we study the main renal artery or segmental vessels? Radiology 1995; 195:799–804.

12. Helenon O, El Rody F, Correas JM, et al: Color Doppler US of renovascular disease in native kidneys. Radiographics 1995; 15:833–854.

13. Bude RO, Rubin JM, Platt JF, et al: Pulsus tardus: Its cause and potential limitations in detection of arterial stenosis. Radiology 1994; 190:779–784.

14. Kim SH, Byun HS, Park JH, et al: Renal parenchymal abnormalities associated with renal vein thrombosis: Correlation between MR imaging and pathologic findings in rabbits. AJR Am J Roentgenol 1994; 162:1361–1365.

15. Platt JF, Ellis JH, Rubin JM: Intrarenal arterial Doppler sonography in the detection of renal vein thrombosis of the native kidney. AJR Am J Roentgenol 1994; 162:1367–1370.

16. Kliewer MA, Tupler RH, Carroll BA, et al: Renal artery stenosis: Analysis of Doppler waveform parameters and tardus-parvus pattern. Radiology 1993; 189:779–787.

17. Moore KL: The urogenital system. In Moore KL, Persaud TVN (eds): The Developing Human: Clinically Oriented Embryology, 5th ed. Philadelphia, WB Saunders, 1993, pp 269–275.

18. Moore KL: The cardiovascular system. In Moore KL, Persaud TVN (eds): The Developing Human: Clinically Oriented Embryology, 5th ed. Philadelphia, WB Saunders, 1993, pp 304–309.

19. Kim SH, Park JH, Han JK, et al: Infarction of the kidney: Role of contrast-enhanced MRI. J Comput Assist Tomogr 1992; 16:924–928.

20. Malmed AS, Love L, Jeffrey RB: Medullary CT enhancement in acute renal artery occlusion. J Comput Assist Tomogr 1992; 16:107–109.

21. Stavros AT, Parker SH, Wayne FY, et al: Segmental stenosis of the renal artery: Pattern recognition of tardus and parvus abnormalities with duplex sonography. Radiology 1992; 184:487–492.

22. Derchi L, Saffioti S, DeCaro G, et al: Arteriovenous fistula of the native kidney: Diagnosis by duplex Doppler ultrasound. J Ultrasound Med 1991; 10:595–597.

23. Soulen MC, Benenati JF, Sheth S, et al: Changes in renal artery Doppler indexes following renal angioplasty. J Vasc Interv Radiol 1991; 2:457–462.

24. Middleton WD, Kellman GH, Melson GL, et al: Postbiopsy renal transplant arteriovenous fistulas: Color Doppler US characteristics. Radiology 1989; 171:253–257.

25. Reuter G, Wanjura D, Bauer H: Acute renal vein thrombosis in renal allografts: Detection with duplex Doppler US. Radiology 1989; 170:557–558.

26. Hekali P, Kivisaari L, Standertskjoeld-Nordenstam CG, et al: Renal complications of polyarteritis nodosa: CT findings. J Comput Assist Tomogr 1985; 9:333–338.

27. Hann L, Pfister RC: Renal subcapsular rim sign: New etiologies and pathogenesis. AJR Am J Roentgenol 1982; 138:51–54.

Illustrations • Vascular Diseases of the Kidney

1 • Normal renal artery

2 • Normal renal vein

3 • Renal arteriovenous malformation

4 • Renal arteriovenous fistula

5 • Polyarteritis nodosa

6 • Renal artery stenosis: unilateral stenosis

7 • Renal artery stenosis: bilateral stenosis

8 • Renal artery stenosis: segmental artery stenoses

9 • Renal artery stenosis: changes following percutaneous transluminal angioplasty

10 • Aortic dissection involving renal artery

11 • Renal artery aneurysm

12 • Pseudoaneurysm of renal artery

13 • Renal infarction: segmental infarction

14 • Renal infarction: global infarction

15 • Renal infarction: associated diseases

16 • Renal infarction: MR imaging findings

17 • Renal vein anomalies

18 • Renal vein thrombosis

19 • Renal vein thrombosis: MR imaging findings

20 • Nutcracker syndrome

1. Normal Renal Artery

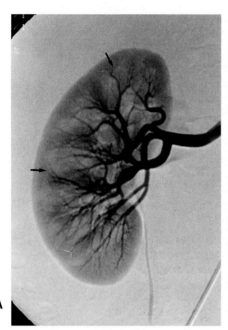

A

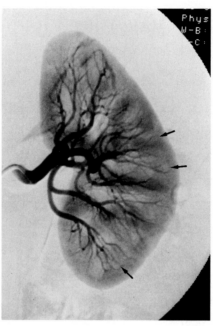

B

Fig. 1. Normal renal arteriogram in a 46-year-old woman.

A, B. Late arterial-phase images of right (**A**) and left (**B**) renal arteriograms show anterior and posterior division arteries and their distal branches. The anterior division artery supplies the anterior parenchyma and lower-polar area and the posterior division artery supplies the posterior parenchyma and upper-polar area. Also note that the posterior division arteries are opacified more densely than the anterior division arteries in the arteriograms taken in supine position. These arteriograms well demonstrate segmental and interlobar arteries. Arcuate arteries can be identified in some areas *(arrows)*.

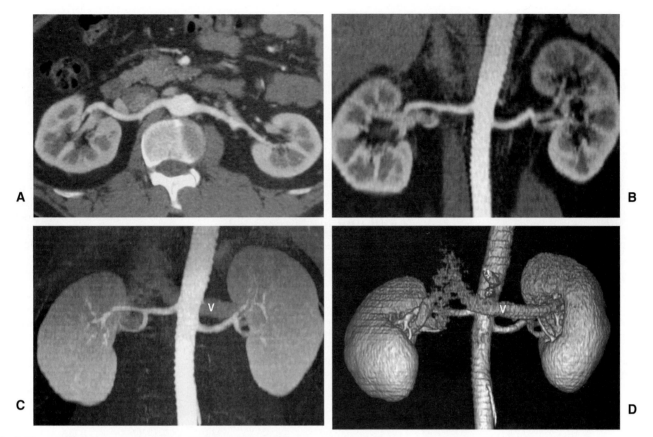

Fig. 2. Normal CT angiogram of the renal arteries in a 50-year-old man.
A. Contrast-enhanced CT in early arterial phase shows both renal arteries coming from the abdominal aorta. **B–D.** CT angiograms in coronal reformation (**B**), maximal intensity projection (**C**), and shaded surface display (**D**) well demonstrate normal renal arteries. V, left renal vein. (**D,** See also Color Section.)

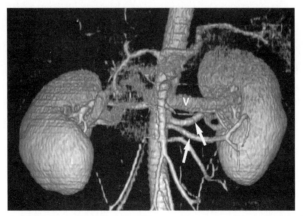

Fig. 3. Multiple renal arteries in a 30-year-old woman. CT angiogram in shaded surface display shows two renal arteries *(arrows)* in the left kidney. V, left renal vein. (See also Color Section.)

2. Normal Renal Vein

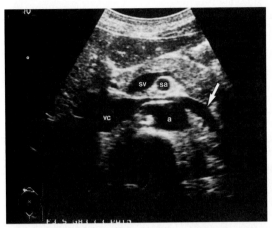

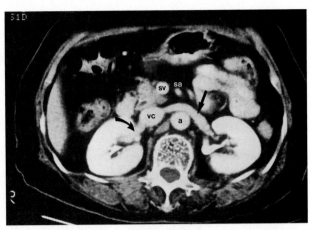

Fig. 1. Normal renal vein in a 68-year-old man. US in transverse plane shows left renal vein *(arrow)* coursing between the aorta (a) and superior mesenteric artery (sa) into the inferior vena cava (vc). sv, superior mesenteric vein merging with splenic vein.

Fig. 2. Normal renal vein in a 75-year-old woman. Contrast-enhanced CT well demonstrates the left *(arrow)* and right *(curved arrow)* renal veins draining into the inferior vena cava (vc). a, aorta; sa, superior mesenteric artery; sv, superior mesenteric vein.

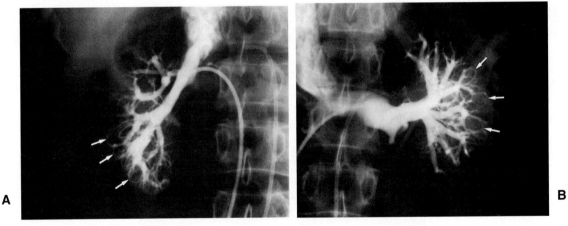

Fig. 3. Normal renal venogram in a 50-year-old woman.
A, B. Selective right (**A**) and left (**B**) renal venograms show main renal veins, segmental and interlobar veins, and arcuate veins *(arrows)*. Interlobular veins are not well demonstrated.

3. Renal Arteriovenous Malformation

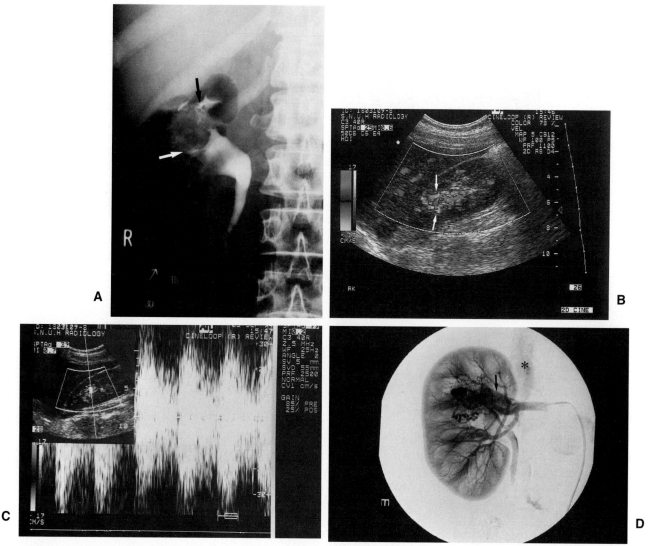

Fig. 1. Renal arteriovenous malformation in a 48-year-old woman who had had a traffic accident with contusion on the right kidney 7 years earlier. **A.** IVU shows irregular filling defects in the upper-polar and interpolar calyces *(arrows)* suggesting blood clots. **B.** Color Doppler US shows hypervascular lesion with high-frequency shift in the upper-polar region of the right kidney *(arrows)*. (**B,** See also Color Section.) **C.** Spectral Doppler US obtained from the lesion shows turbulent flow with high velocity. **D.** Selective right renal arteriogram shows tortuous, entangled vessels in the upper-polar region with early opacification of the renal vein *(arrow)* and inferior vena cava *(asterisk)*.

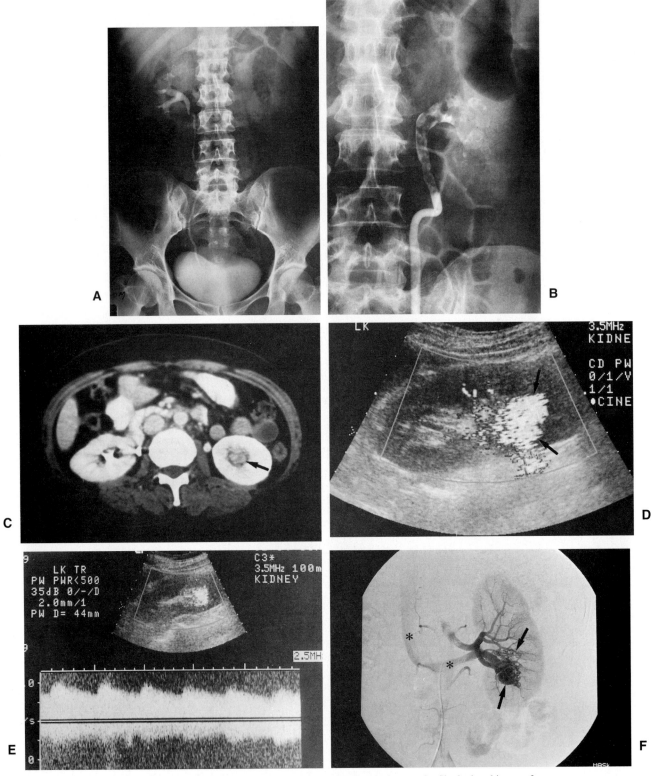

Fig. 2. Renal arteriovenous malformation in a 43-year-old woman with intermittent gross hematuria. She had no history of trauma.
A. Initial IVU at the time of hematuria shows large left kidney with faint nephrogram and no pelvocalyceal opacification. **B.** RGP obtained on the next day shows multiple filling defects in the renal pelvis and proximal ureter indicating the presence of blood clots. **C.** CT scan obtained on the next day shows ill-defined, small, low-attenuated lesion *(arrow)* in the lower pole of the left kidney. **D.** Doppler US shows hypervascular lesion in the lower-polar region of the left kidney *(arrows)*. **E.** Spectral Doppler US reveals strong flow signals of low-resistance pattern from the lesion.
F. Selective left renal arteriogram shows entangled vascular lesion *(arrows)* with early drainage to the renal vein and inferior vena cava *(asterisks)*.

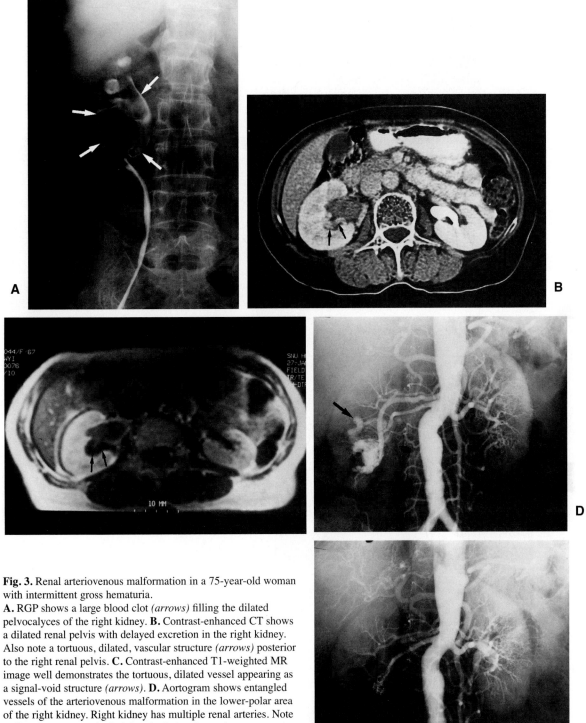

Fig. 3. Renal arteriovenous malformation in a 75-year-old woman with intermittent gross hematuria.
A. RGP shows a large blood clot *(arrows)* filling the dilated pelvocalyces of the right kidney. **B.** Contrast-enhanced CT shows a dilated renal pelvis with delayed excretion in the right kidney. Also note a tortuous, dilated, vascular structure *(arrows)* posterior to the right renal pelvis. **C.** Contrast-enhanced T1-weighted MR image well demonstrates the tortuous, dilated vessel appearing as a signal-void structure *(arrows)*. **D.** Aortogram shows entangled vessels of the arteriovenous malformation in the lower-polar area of the right kidney. Right kidney has multiple renal arteries. Note a dilated, tortuous vein draining the lesion *(arrow)*.
E. Aortogram obtained following embolization by using coils reveals that the lesion is no longer opacified.

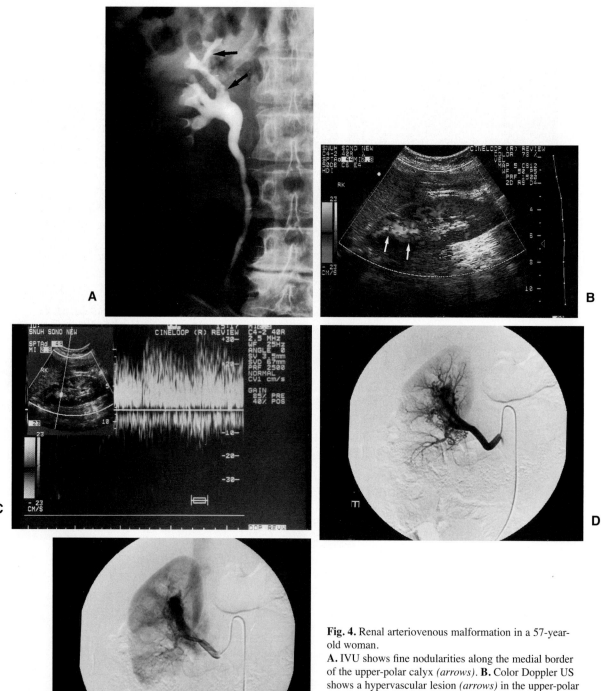

Fig. 4. Renal arteriovenous malformation in a 57-year-old woman.
A. IVU shows fine nodularities along the medial border of the upper-polar calyx *(arrows)*. **B.** Color Doppler US shows a hypervascular lesion *(arrows)* in the upper-polar area of the right kidney. (**B,** See also Color Section.) **C.** Spectral Doppler US shows noisy, turbulent flow signals from the lesion. **D, E.** Selective right renal arteriograms in early (**D**) and late (**E**) arterial phases show tortuous vascular lesion in the upper-polar area.

4. Renal Arteriovenous Fistula

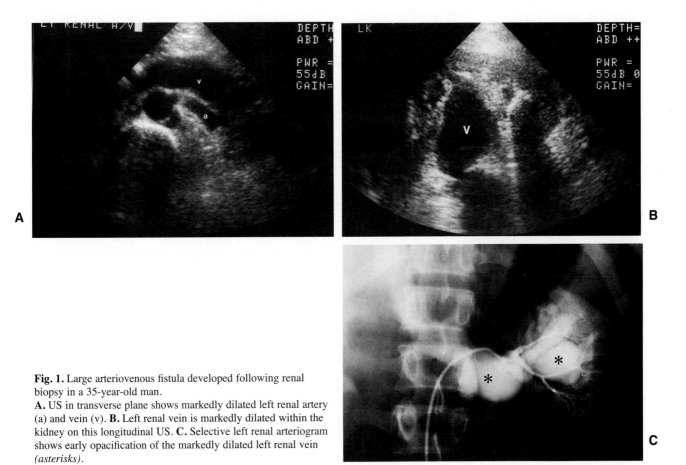

Fig. 1. Large arteriovenous fistula developed following renal biopsy in a 35-year-old man.
A. US in transverse plane shows markedly dilated left renal artery (a) and vein (v). **B.** Left renal vein is markedly dilated within the kidney on this longitudinal US. **C.** Selective left renal arteriogram shows early opacification of the markedly dilated left renal vein (*asterisks*).

5. Polyarteritis Nodosa

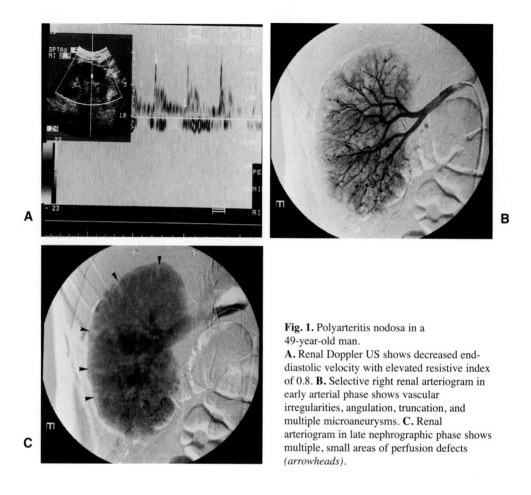

Fig. 1. Polyarteritis nodosa in a 49-year-old man.
A. Renal Doppler US shows decreased end-diastolic velocity with elevated resistive index of 0.8. **B.** Selective right renal arteriogram in early arterial phase shows vascular irregularities, angulation, truncation, and multiple microaneurysms. **C.** Renal arteriogram in late nephrographic phase shows multiple, small areas of perfusion defects (*arrowheads*).

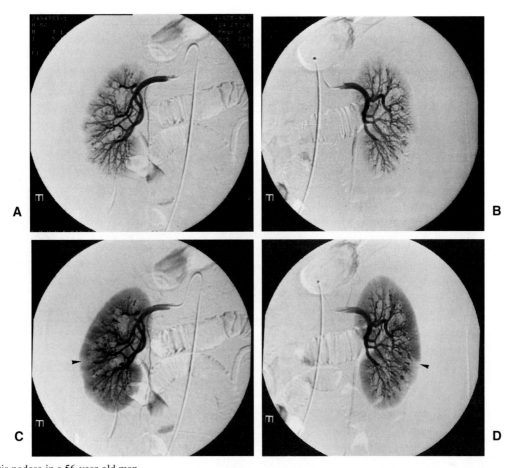

Fig. 2. Polyarteritis nodosa in a 56-year-old man.
A–D. Renal arteriograms of the right (**A, C**) and left (**B, D**) kidneys at early arterial (**A, B**) and nephrographic (**C, D**) phases show irregularities and truncation of arterial branches, multiple microaneurysms, and focal areas of decreased perfusion (*arrowheads* in **C** and **D**).

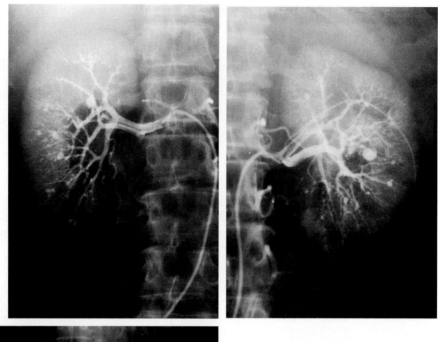

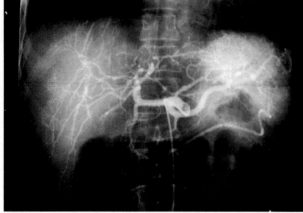

Fig. 3. Churg-Strauss syndrome in a 53-year-old man showing arteriographic findings identical to those of polyarteritis nodosa. **A, B.** Renal arteriograms of the right (**A**) and left (**B**) kidneys show multiple, small and large aneurysms with irregularities of arterial branches. **C.** Hepatosplenic arteriogram shows irregularity and truncation of hepatic arterial branches.

6. Renal Artery Stenosis: Unilateral Stenosis

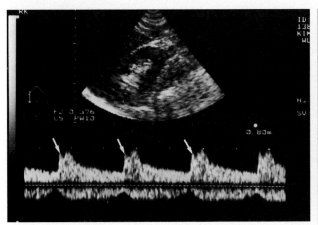

A

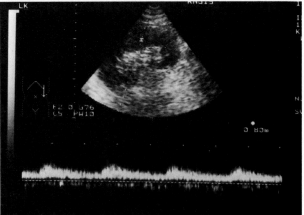

B

Fig 1. Left renal artery stenosis in a 50-year-old hypertensive man. **A.** Spectral Doppler US of the right kidney shows typical normal spectrum of rapid systolic upstroke and early systolic compliance peak *(arrows)*. **B.** Spectral Doppler US of the left kidney shows typical finding of pulsus parvus and tardus with low amplitude and slowed systolic upstroke. Note that normal early systolic compliance peak is not seen. **C.** Aortogram shows stenosis of the left renal artery *(arrow)*.

C

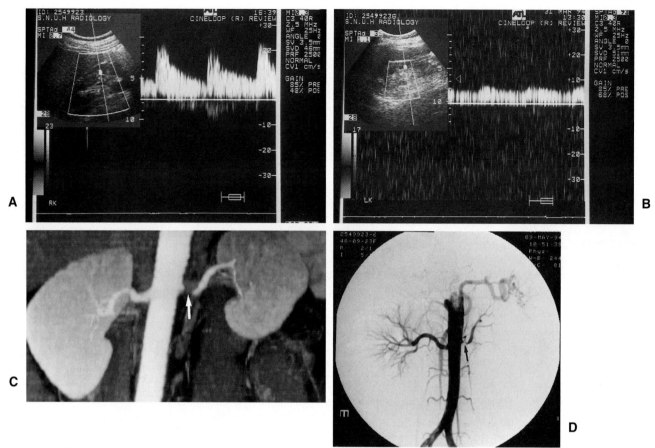

Fig. 2. Left renal artery stenosis in a 47-year-old hypertensive woman.
A. Spectral Doppler US of the right kidney shows normal spectral pattern. **B.** Spectral Doppler US of the left kidney shows very weak and slow-rising spectral pattern (pulsus tardus and parvus). **C.** CT angiogram well demonstrates a high-grade stenosis of the left main renal artery *(arrow)*.
D. Aortogram confirms the stenosis of the left renal artery *(arrow)*.

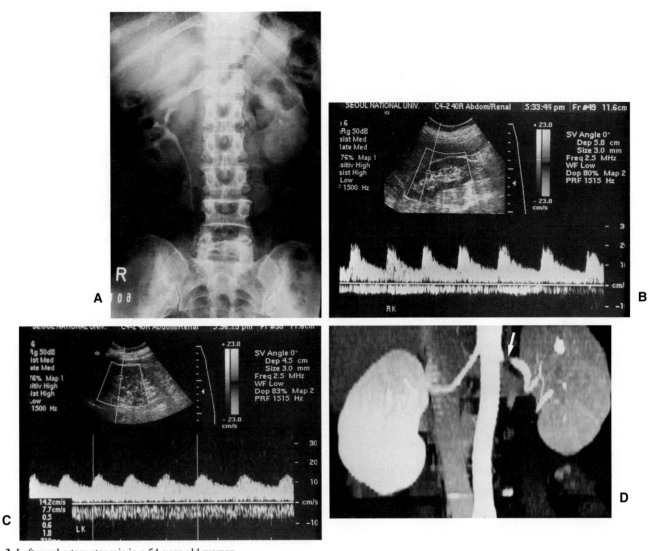

Fig. 3. Left renal artery stenosis in a 54-year-old woman.
A. IVU shows normal-sized left kidney with delayed nephrogram. **B.** Spectral Doppler US of the right kidney shows a normal spectral pattern.
C. Spectral Doppler US of the left kidney shows a slightly weak but definitely slow-rising spectral pattern. **D.** CT angiogram in maximal intensity projection shows severe, focal stenosis of the left main renal artery *(arrow)*.

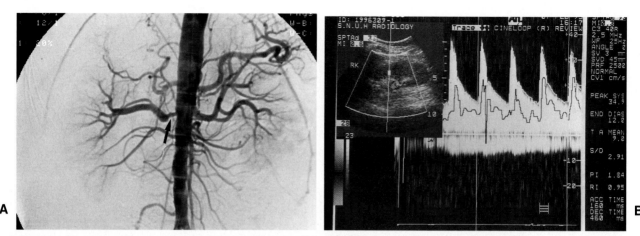

Fig. 4. Stenosis of the right renal artery demonstrated on angiography without Doppler spectral changes in a 53-year-old man. This patient was not hypertensive, and the discrepancy between angiographic and Doppler US findings probably indicates that the stenosis is not hemodynamically significant.
A. Aortogram shows more than 50% stenosis in the right renal artery *(arrow)*. **B.** Spectral Doppler US of the right kidney shows a normal spectral pattern.

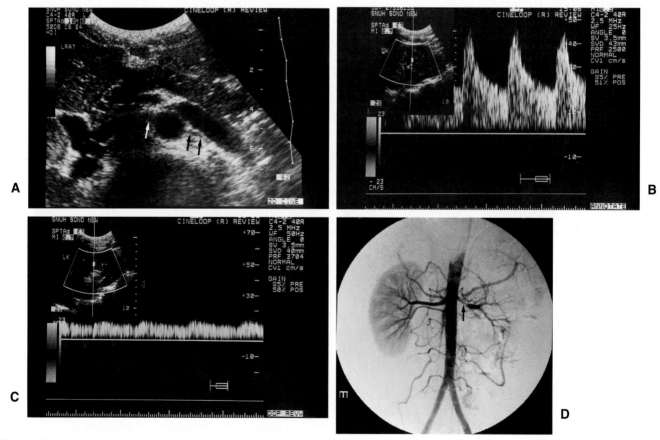

Fig. 5. Left renal artery stenosis demonstrated on gray-scale US in a 16-year-old boy.
A. Gray-scale US well demonstrates the orifice of the normal right renal artery *(white arrow)* but the left renal artery appears very small *(black arrows)*. **B.** Spectral Doppler US of the right kidney shows normal spectral pattern. **C.** Spectral Doppler US of the left kidney shows severe pulsus tardus and parvus pattern. **D.** Aortogram shows a long-segment stenosis of the left renal artery *(arrow)*.

7. Renal Artery Stenosis: Bilateral Stenosis

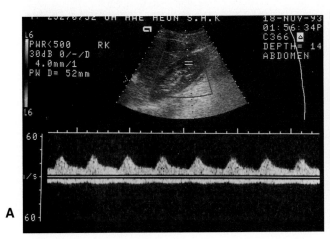

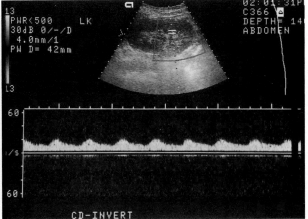

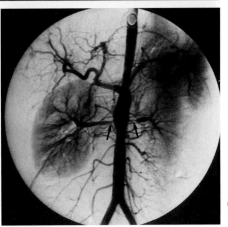

Fig. 1. Bilateral renal artery stenosis in an 18-year-old woman with Takayasu's arteritis.
A. Spectral Doppler US of the right kidney shows slowed systolic upstroke.
B. Spectral Doppler US of the left kidney shows more severe pattern of pulsus tardus and parvus. **C.** Aortogram shows bilateral renal artery stenoses *(arrows)*, more severe on the left side.

8. Renal Artery Stenosis: Segmental Artery Stenoses

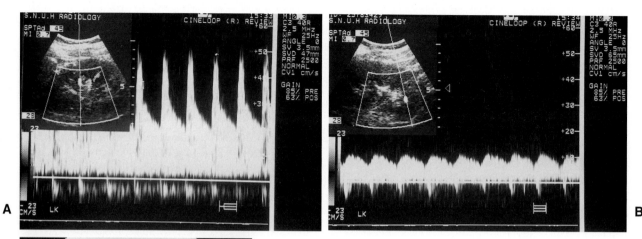

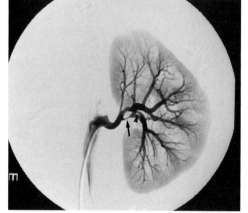

Fig. 1. Stenoses of segmental renal arteries in a 27-year-old hypertensive woman. (**A–C,** From Seong CK, Kim SH, Sim JS: Detection of segmental branch renal artery stenosis by Doppler US: A case report. Korean J Radiol 2001; 2:57–60.)
A. Spectral Doppler US performed in the interpolar region of the left kidney shows normal Doppler spectral pattern. **B.** Spectral Doppler US performed in the lower-polar region of the left kidney shows weak and slow-rising pulse.
C. Selective left renal arteriogram shows a tight stenotic lesion in the posterior division artery *(arrow)*. Note another stenotic lesion in the lower segmental branch of the anterior division artery *(arrowhead)*.

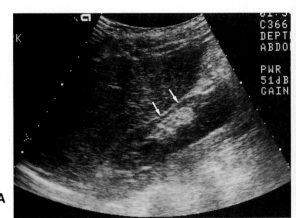

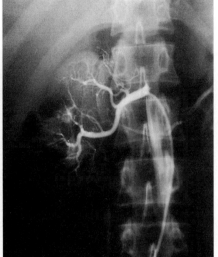

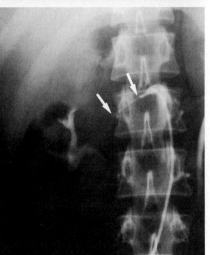

Fig. 2. Stenosis of one of double right renal arteries in a 25-year-old hypertensive woman.
A. Gray-scale US shows small right kidney with thinning of anterior renal parenchyma *(arrows)*. **B.** Selective arteriogram of the one renal artery, which is probably a posterior division artery, shows normal appearance without stenosis.
C. There was another right renal artery that was almost completely occluded due to very severe stenosis *(arrows)*.

9. Renal Artery Stenosis: Changes Following Percutaneous Transluminal Angioplasty

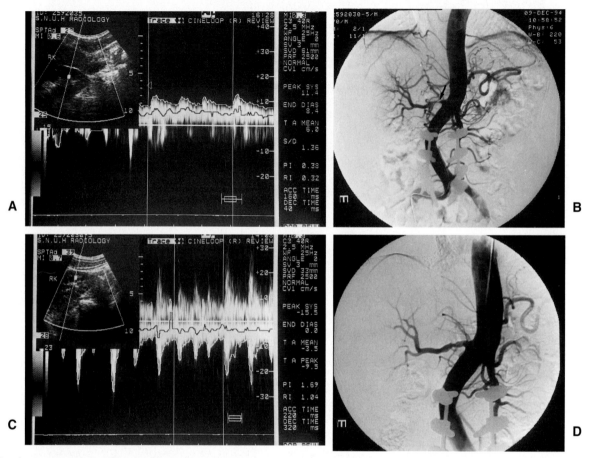

Fig. 1. Renal artery stenosis in a 71-year-old man.
A. Spectral Doppler US of the right kidney shows pulsus tardus and parvus pattern. **B.** Aortogram shows stenosis of the right renal artery *(arrow)*. Percutaneous transluminal angioplasty was performed. **C.** Follow-up Doppler US shows improved Doppler spectral pattern. This patient has an arrhythmia. **D.** Follow-up aortogram shows improved stenosis in the right renal artery.

10. Aortic Dissection Involving Renal Artery

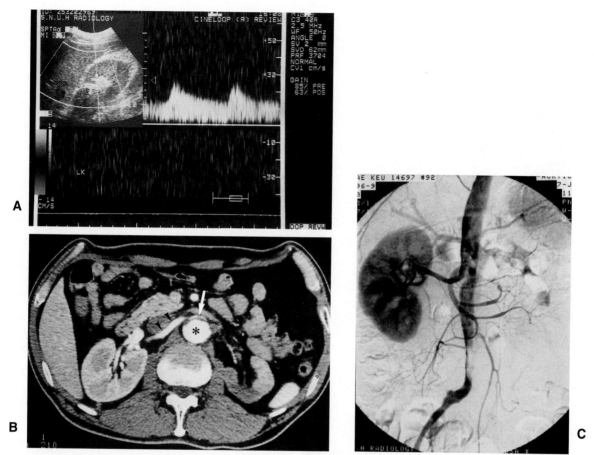

Fig. 1. Aortic dissection involving renal artery with Doppler US findings mimicking those of renal artery stenosis in a 63-year-old man. **A.** Spectral Doppler US of the left kidney shows weak and slow-rising pulse suggesting renal artery stenosis. **B.** Contrast-enhanced CT scan at an early arterial phase shows an aortic dissection with an intimal flap dividing the anterior true lumen *(arrow)* that supplies the right renal artery *(arrowheads)* and the large posterior false lumen *(asterisk)*. Both kidneys are poorly perfused, and the left kidney is small. **C.** Aortogram with a catheter in the true lumen shows that the right renal artery originates in the true lumen, and the left renal artery is not opacified.

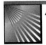

11. Renal Artery Aneurysm

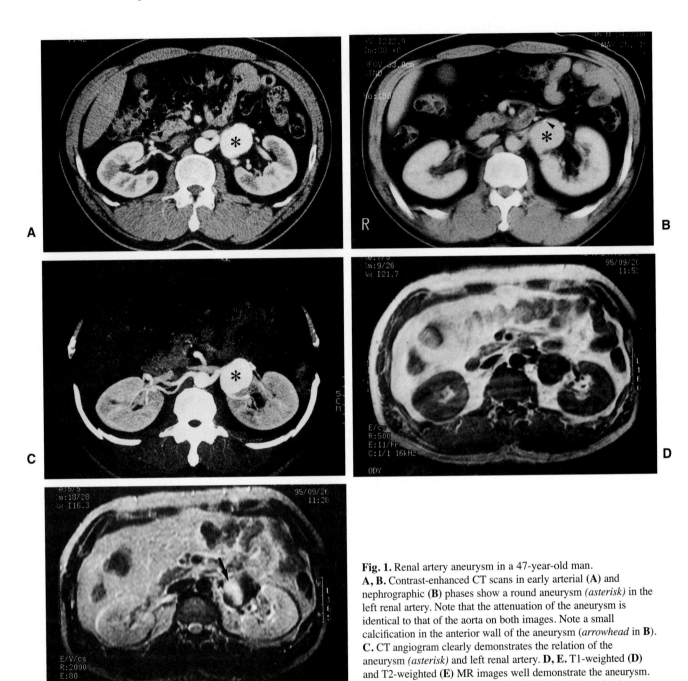

Fig. 1. Renal artery aneurysm in a 47-year-old man.
A, B. Contrast-enhanced CT scans in early arterial (**A**) and nephrographic (**B**) phases show a round aneurysm *(asterisk)* in the left renal artery. Note that the attenuation of the aneurysm is identical to that of the aorta on both images. Note a small calcification in the anterior wall of the aneurysm *(arrowhead in* **B**). **C.** CT angiogram clearly demonstrates the relation of the aneurysm *(asterisk)* and left renal artery. **D, E.** T1-weighted (**D**) and T2-weighted (**E**) MR images well demonstrate the aneurysm. The medial part of the aneurysm has high signal intensity *(arrow in* **E**) on T2-weighted image due to turbulent flow.

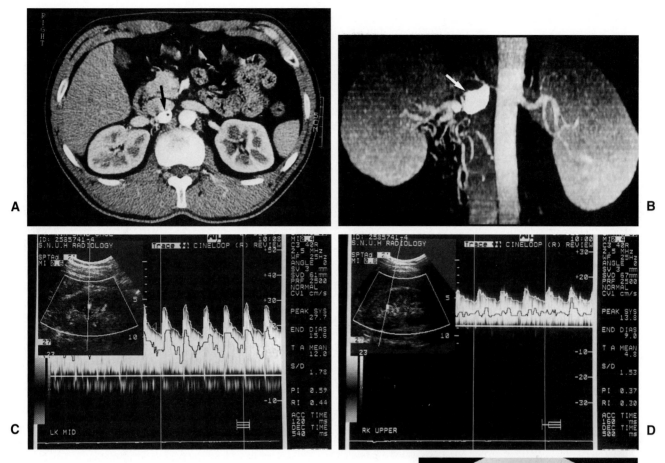

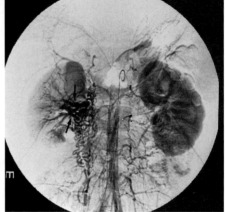

Fig. 2. Calcified aneurysm with arterial occlusion and collateral circulation in the right renal artery in a 31-year-old man.
A. Contrast-enhanced CT scan in arterial phase shows densely calcified aneurysm *(arrow)* in the right renal artery. The right kidney is well perfused on this CT image. **B.** CT angiogram demonstrates calcified aneurysm *(arrow)* and collateral vessels supplying the right kidney. **C.** Spectral Doppler US of the left kidney shows normal spectral pattern. **D.** Spectral Doppler US of the right kidney shows slightly low-amplitude spectrum with slightly slowed systolic upstroke mimicking pulsus tardus and parvus pattern. **E.** Abdominal aortogram in the late nephrographic phase shows complete occlusion of the right renal artery with abundant collateral vessels reconstructing intrarenal arteries *(arrows)*.

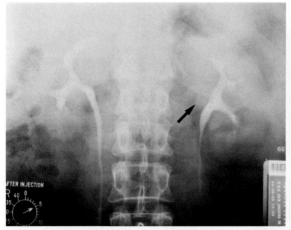

A

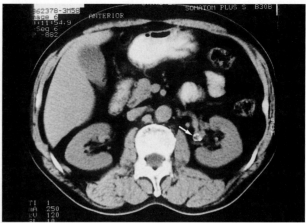

B

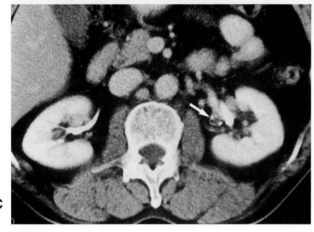

C

Fig. 3. Small calcified aneurysm of the left renal artery in a 58-year-old man.
A. IVU shows a small ring-shaped calcification *(arrow)* just medial to the left renal pelvis. **B, C.** Nonenhanced **(B)** and contrast-enhanced **(C)** CT scans show a small calcified aneurysm *(arrow)* of the left renal artery without perfusion disturbance to the left kidney.

12. Pseudoaneurysm of Renal Artery

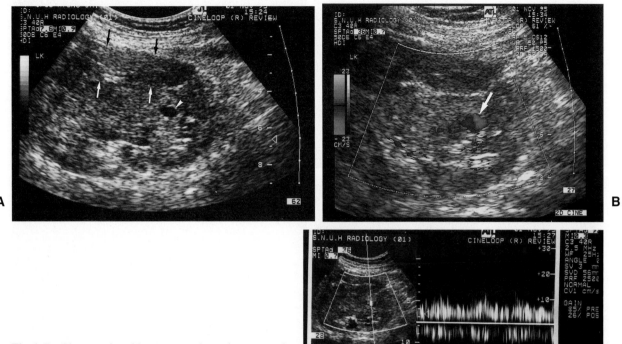

Fig. 1. Postbiopsy perirenal hematoma and pseudoaneurysm in a 50-year-old woman.
A. Gray-scale US shows large perirenal hematoma *(arrows)* and a small, round anechoic lesion in the lower-polar region *(arrowhead)*. **B.** Color Doppler US well demonstrates the pseudoaneurysm *(arrow)*. (**B,** See also Color Section.)
C. Spectral Doppler US obtained in the lesion shows turbulent flow signal.

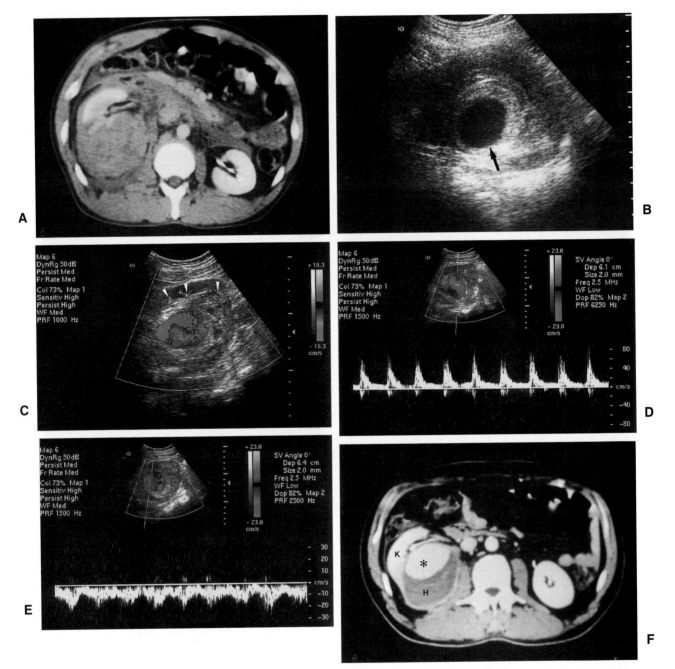

Fig. 2. Post-traumatic perirenal hematoma and pseudoaneurysm in a 47-year-old man. (**C–E,** See also Color Section.)
A. Initial contrast-enhanced CT scan at the time of trauma shows renal parenchymal laceration and a large perirenal and subcapsular hematoma in the right kidney. **B.** Longitudinal US of the right kidney shows a round cystic lesion *(arrow)* with surrounding soft tissue echogenicity. **C.** Color Doppler US confirms that the cystic lesion is an aneurysm with whirling flow in it. Note that the soft tissue echogenicity surrounding the lesion is avascular suggesting hematoma. The renal parenchyma that has intrarenal vessels *(arrowheads)* is displaced anteriorly. **D.** Spectral Doppler US obtained in the red portion of the lesion shows arterial spectral pattern. **E.** Spectral Doppler US obtained in the blue portion of the lesion shows mixed arterial and venous flow pattern. **F.** Contrast-enhanced CT shows a large pseudoaneurysm *(asterisk)*, subcapsular hematoma (H), and anteriorly displaced renal parenchyma (K).

13. Renal Infarction: Segmental Infarction

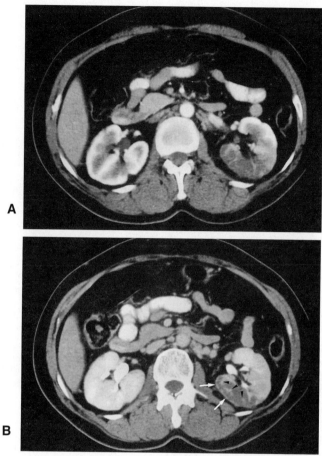

Fig. 1. Segmental infarction of the left kidney in a 57-year-old woman. **A, B.** Contrast-enhanced CT scans in early arterial (**A**) and late excretory (**B**) phases shows well-demarcated area of perfusion defect in the posterior aspect of the left kidney. Note that the enhancement of a thin layer of cortical rim (*arrows* in **B**) and medullary islands (*arrowheads* in **B**) is demonstrated better on **B** than on **A**.

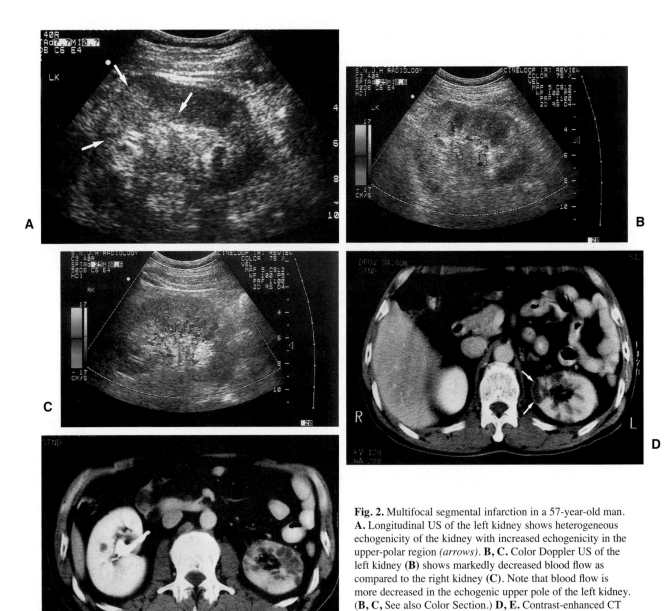

Fig. 2. Multifocal segmental infarction in a 57-year-old man. **A.** Longitudinal US of the left kidney shows heterogeneous echogenicity of the kidney with increased echogenicity in the upper-polar region *(arrows)*. **B, C.** Color Doppler US of the left kidney **(B)** shows markedly decreased blood flow as compared to the right kidney **(C)**. Note that blood flow is more decreased in the echogenic upper pole of the left kidney. **(B, C,** See also Color Section.) **D, E.** Contrast-enhanced CT scans of the kidney show multifocal perfusion defects in the left kidney. Cortical rim sign is clearly seen in one of the lesions *(arrows in* **D**).

14. Renal Infarction: Global Infarction

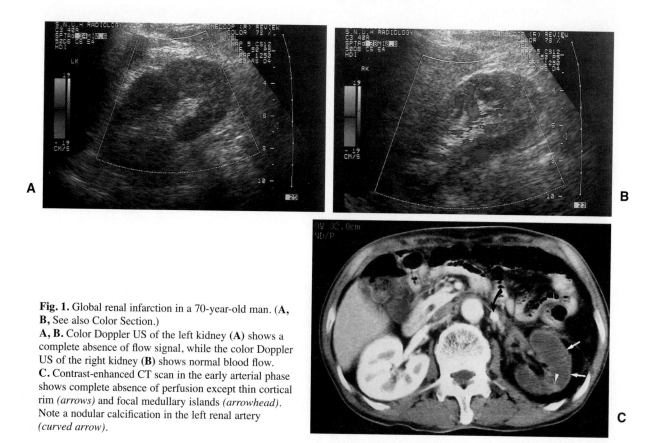

Fig. 1. Global renal infarction in a 70-year-old man. (**A, B,** See also Color Section.)
A, B. Color Doppler US of the left kidney (**A**) shows a complete absence of flow signal, while the color Doppler US of the right kidney (**B**) shows normal blood flow.
C. Contrast-enhanced CT scan in the early arterial phase shows complete absence of perfusion except thin cortical rim *(arrows)* and focal medullary islands *(arrowhead).* Note a nodular calcification in the left renal artery *(curved arrow).*

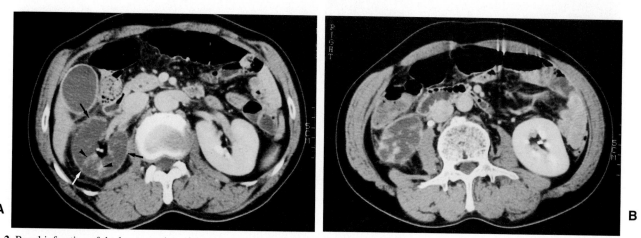

Fig. 2. Renal infarction of the lower portion of the right kidney in a 62-year-old man.
A, B. Contrast-enhanced CT scans show global infarction of the right kidney with enhancing cortical rim *(arrows* in **A**) and medullary islands *(arrowheads* in **A**).

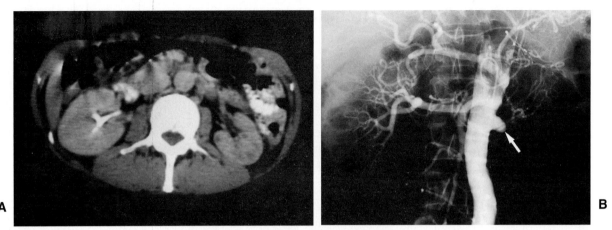

Fig. 3. Complete occlusion of the left renal artery with an old global infarction in a 52-year-old man.
A. Contrast-enhanced CT scan at late excretory phase shows absence of excretion of contrast material from the contracted left kidney. **B.** Abdominal aortogram shows total occlusion of the left renal artery *(arrow)* without collateral circulation.

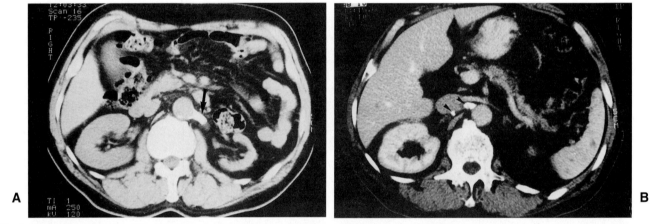

Fig. 4. Old, global infarction of the left kidney with calcification of main renal artery in a 66-year-old man.
A, B. Contrast-enhanced CT scans in a delayed phase show contracted left kidney due to old, global infarction and a large calcified plaque in the origin of the left renal artery *(arrow in **A**)*. Also note small calcifications *(arrowheads in **B**)* in the proximal portion of the right renal artery.

15. Renal Infarction: Associated Diseases

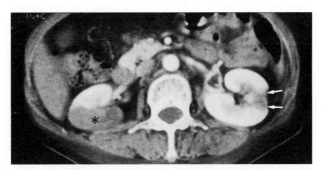

Fig. 1. Renal infarction in a 53-year-old woman with amyloidosis.
Contrast-enhanced CT shows absence of perfusion in the posterior half
of the right kidney *(asterisk)*. The cortical rim sign is not evident in the
lesion. Also note a wedge-shaped, low-attenuated lesion with cortical
depression in the left kidney suggesting an old infarction *(arrows)*.

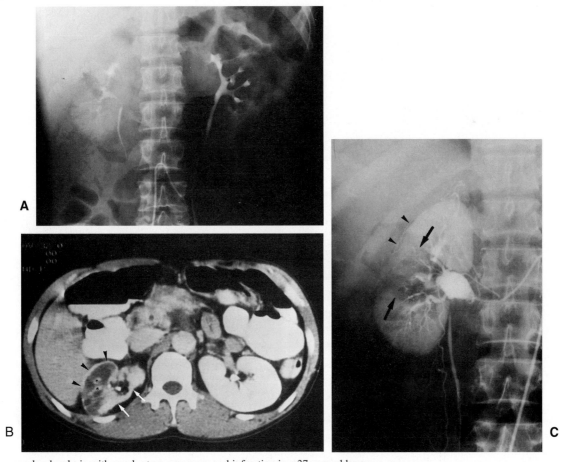

Fig. 2. Fibromuscular dysplasia with renal artery aneurysm and infarction in a 37-year-old man.
A. IVU shows delayed nephrogram and faint opacification of the pelvocalyceal system in the right kidney. **B.** Contrast-enhanced CT shows the
findings of old and fresh infarcts in the same kidney. The posterior part of the right kidney shows parenchymal loss due to old infarction *(arrows)* and
the lateral part of the same kidney shows cortical rim sign *(arrowheads)* and enhancing medullary islands *(asterisks)* due to fresh infarction.
C. Selective right renal arteriogram demonstrates a prominent capsular artery *(arrowheads)* that is the basis of the cortical rim sign seen on contrast-
enhanced CT. Also note the area of poor perfusion in the interpolar region of the right kidney *(arrows)*.

16. Renal Infarction: MR Imaging Findings

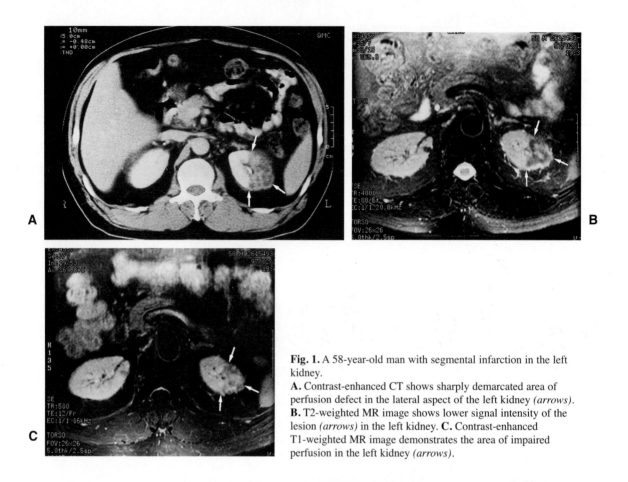

Fig. 1. A 58-year-old man with segmental infarction in the left kidney.
A. Contrast-enhanced CT shows sharply demarcated area of perfusion defect in the lateral aspect of the left kidney *(arrows)*.
B. T2-weighted MR image shows lower signal intensity of the lesion *(arrows)* in the left kidney. **C.** Contrast-enhanced T1-weighted MR image demonstrates the area of impaired perfusion in the left kidney *(arrows)*.

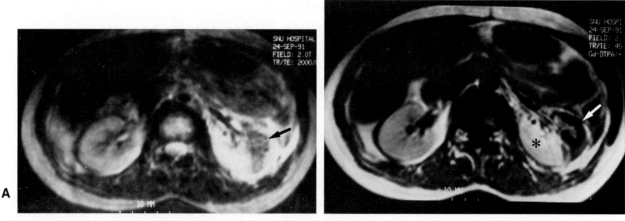

Fig. 2. Segmental renal infarction in a 25-year-old woman who underwent aortic valvular replacement and complained of severe left flank pain 2 days before MR imaging.
A. T2-weighted MR image shows an ill-defined, low-intensity lesion in the lateral portion of the left kidney *(arrow)*. **B.** Contrast-enhanced T1-weighted MR image shows nonenhanced, infarcted area in lateral portion of the left kidney *(arrow)*. Note that the signal intensity of the noninfarcted medial portion of the left kidney *(asterisk)* is much higher than that of the noninvolved right kidney. (**B,** From Kim SH, Park JH, Han JK, et al: Infarction of the kidney: Role of contrast-enhanced MRI. J Comput Assist Tomogr 1992; 16:924–928.)

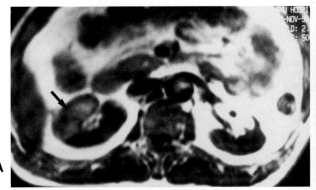

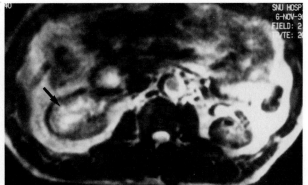

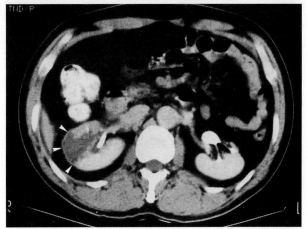

Fig. 3. Hemorrhagic infarction in a 40-year-old man who had undergone aortic valvular replacement 11 years earlier. He had left flank pain 2 years earlier and severe right flank pain 9 days before MR imaging. (**A–C,** From Kim SH, Park JH, Han JK, et al: Infarction of the kidney: Role of contrast-enhanced MRI. J Comput Assist Tomogr 1992; 16:924–928.)
A. T1-weighted MR image shows a small left kidney due to old infarction and high signal intensity lesion in the anterior portion of the right kidney *(arrow)*, suggesting hemorrhagic infarction.
B. T2-weighted MR image shows increased signal intensity of the infarcted area in the right kidney *(arrow)*. **C.** Contrast-enhanced CT shows a wedge-shaped infarction in the right kidney with cortical rim sign *(arrowheads)*. Note the small, contracted left kidney due to old infarction.

17. Renal Vein Anomalies

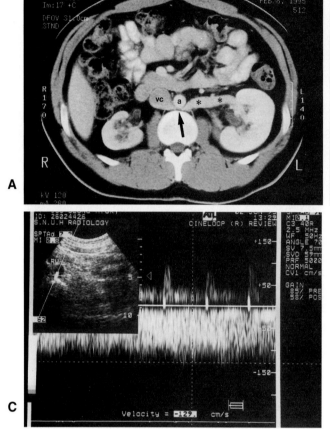

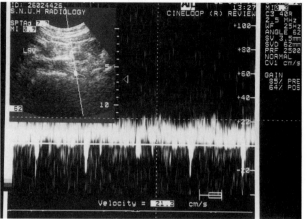

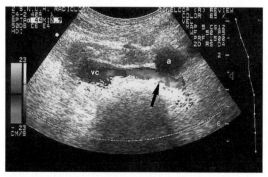

Fig. 1. Retroaortic left renal vein with posterior nutcracker syndrome in a 26-year-old man.
A. Contrast-enhanced CT shows hypoplastic right kidney and compensatory hypertrophy of the left kidney. Left renal vein *(asterisks)* courses between the vertebra and aorta (a) with severe compression between them *(arrow)*. vc, inferior vena cava. **B, C.** Spectral Doppler US of the left renal vein at hilar portion **(B)** and retroaortic portion **(C)** shows normal flow velocity at hilar portion (21.3 cm/sec) and markedly increased flow velocity at retroaortic portion (129 cm/sec), suggesting the so-called posterior nutcracker syndrome.

Fig. 2. Retroaortic left renal vein in a 69-year-old man with renal cell carcinoma of the left kidney. Color Doppler US in transverse plane shows left renal vein *(arrow)* coursing behind the abdominal aorta (a). vc, inferior vena cava. (See also Color Section.)

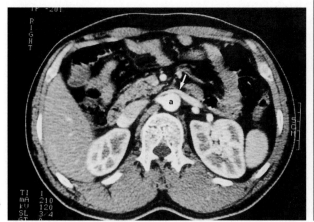

A

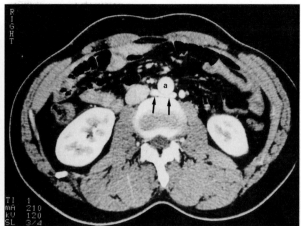

B

Fig. 3. Circumaortic left renal vein in a 53-year-old man.
A. Contrast-enhanced CT in axial plane shows normal course of the left renal vein *(arrow)* anterior to the abdominal aorta (a).
B. CT scan at a lower level shows another left renal vein *(arrows)* coursing behind the abdominal aorta (a). **C.** Three-dimensional CT with maximal intensity projection technique well demonstrates circumaortic left renal vein with upper vein *(asterisk)* coursing normally and lower vein *(arrows)* coursing behind the aorta (a). Note that the left gonadal vein *(arrowheads)* is connected to the lower renal vein. ra, renal arteries.

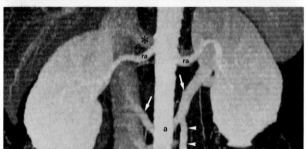

C

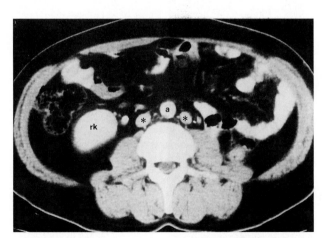

Fig. 4. Double inferior vena cava in a 51-year old man who received left radical nephrectomy for a renal cell carcinoma. Contrast-enhanced CT shows double inferior vena cava *(asterisks)* on both sides of the abdominal aorta (a). This anomaly is caused by persistence of left supracardinal vein and may be confused with retroperitoneal lymphadenopathy. rk, lower pole of the right kidney.

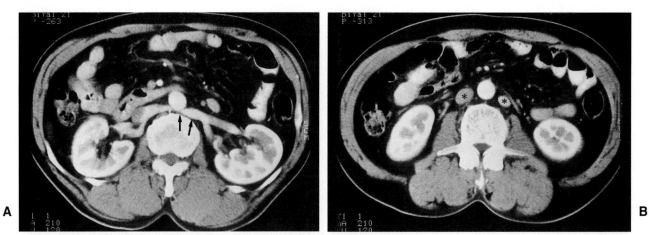

Fig. 5. Double inferior vena cava with retroaortic left renal vein in a 66-year-old man.
A, B. Contrast-enhanced CT scans show double inferior vena cava at infrarenal level (*asterisks* on **B**) with left inferior vena cava connected to the retroaortic left renal vein (*arrows* on **A**).

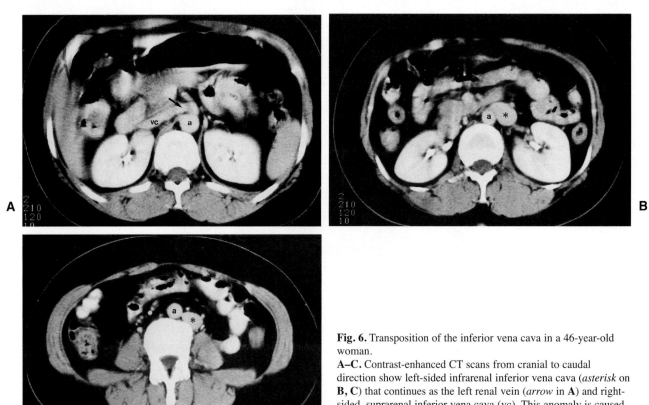

Fig. 6. Transposition of the inferior vena cava in a 46-year-old woman.
A–C. Contrast-enhanced CT scans from cranial to caudal direction show left-sided infrarenal inferior vena cava (*asterisk* on **B, C**) that continues as the left renal vein (*arrow* in **A**) and right-sided, suprarenal inferior vena cava (vc). This anomaly is caused by regression of the right supracardinal vein instead of normal regression of the left supracardinal vein at the infrarenal level. a, abdominal aorta.

18. Renal Vein Thrombosis

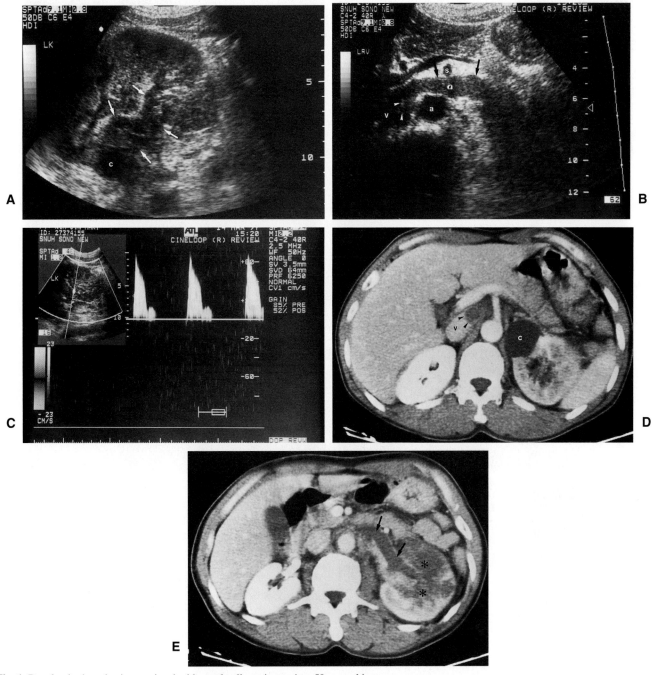

Fig. 1. Renal vein thrombosis associated with renal cell carcinoma in a 59-year-old man.
A. US shows swollen left kidney and dilated renal vein filled with echogenic thrombi *(arrows)*. Note a small cyst (c) in the left kidney. **B.** Transverse US well demonstrates the dilated left renal vein filled with echogenic thrombi *(arrows)*. The end of the thrombus *(arrowheads)* bulges into the inferior vena cava (v). a, aorta; s, superior mesenteric artery. **C.** Spectral Doppler US obtained in the intrarenal artery shows a very high resistance pattern with a resistive index of 1.0. **D, E.** Contrast-enhanced CT scans show a swollen left kidney with decreased perfusion; an ill-defined, low-attenuated lesion representing renal cell carcinoma *(asterisks in* **E***)*; and a dilated left renal vein filled with low-attenuated thrombi *(arrows in* **E***)*. Also note the end of the thrombi *(arrowheads in* **D***)* bulging into the inferior vena cava (v). A renal cyst (c) is seen in the left kidney.

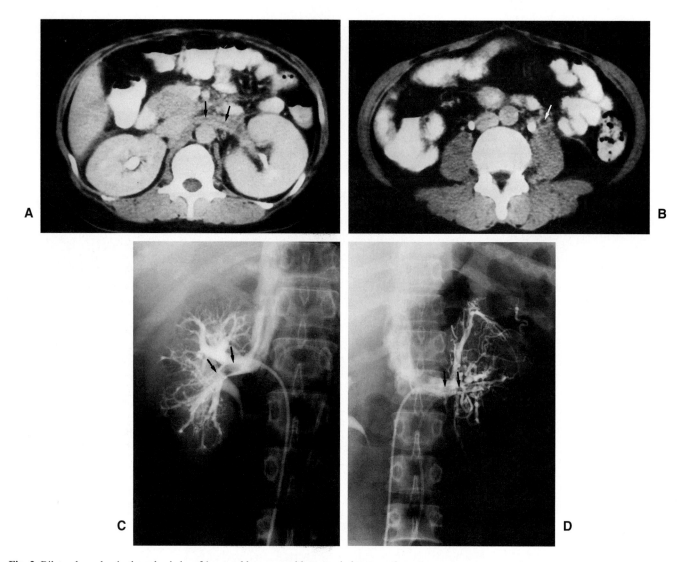

Fig. 2. Bilateral renal vein thrombosis in a 31-year-old woman with systemic lupus erythematosus.
A. Contrast-enhanced CT shows large kidneys and a suspicious linear filling defect suggesting thrombus *(arrows)* in the left renal vein. **B.** Lower level CT shows thrombus in the left ovarian vein *(arrow)*. **C, D.** Selective right **(C)** and left **(D)** renal venograms show linear filling defects *(arrows)* in both renal veins representing thrombi. Note intrarenal veins are occluded in the left kidney with abundant collateral vessels.

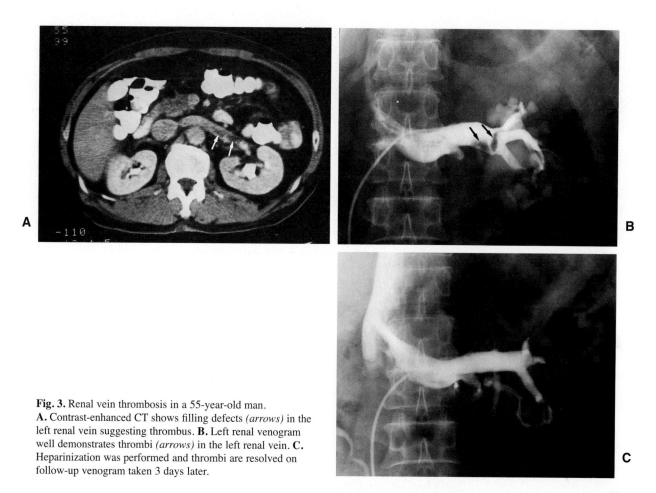

Fig. 3. Renal vein thrombosis in a 55-year-old man.
A. Contrast-enhanced CT shows filling defects *(arrows)* in the left renal vein suggesting thrombus. **B.** Left renal venogram well demonstrates thrombi *(arrows)* in the left renal vein. **C.** Heparinization was performed and thrombi are resolved on follow-up venogram taken 3 days later.

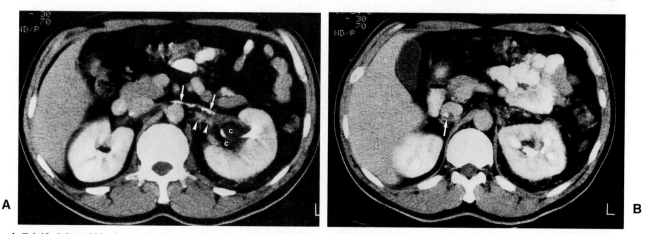

Fig. 4. Calcified thrombi in the renal vein and inferior vena cava in a 39-year-old man.
A. Contrast-enhanced CT shows calcified thrombi in the left renal vein *(arrows)*. Left renal excretion is preserved due to collateral circulation *(arrowheads)*. Note parapelvic cysts (c) in the left renal hilar region. **B.** CT scan at upper level shows calcified thrombus *(arrow)* in the inferior vena cava.

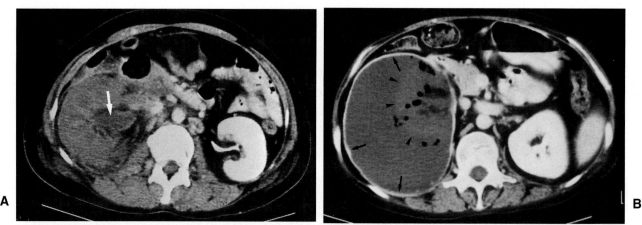

Fig. 5. Renal vein thrombosis with venous infarction in a 35-year-old woman with membranous nephropathy.
A. Contrast-enhanced CT shows a swollen, nonperfused right kidney with a large thrombus in the dilated right renal vein *(arrow)*. **B.** CT scan obtained 3 months later shows venous infarction with gas formation in the right kidney. Note large amount of perirenal fluid collection surrounded by a thick enhancing rim *(arrows)* and faint outline of the kidney *(arrowheads)*.

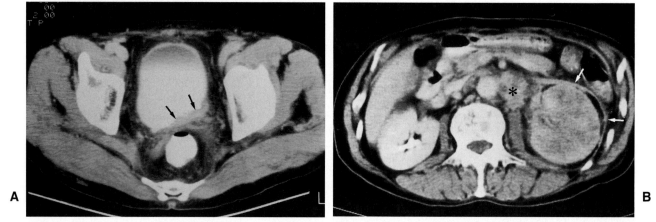

Fig. 6. A 70-year-old man with squamous cell carcinoma of the urinary bladder and retroperitoneal lymph node metastases and acute renal vein thrombosis. This patient complained of severe flank pain on the left side with fever. To relieve these intractable symptoms, the left renal artery was embolized with coils, and there was symptomatic relief.
A. Contrast-enhanced CT shows infiltrating lesion in the posterior wall of the bladder *(arrows)*. **B.** Contrast-enhanced CT scan at the kidney level shows a swollen left kidney with decreased perfusion and thickened renal fascia *(arrows)*. Note that there is a large metastatic lymph node *(asterisk)* in the para-aortic region with infiltration into the renal hilar area. The left renal vein is not demonstrated and is probably occluded by the infiltration of the metastatic lymph node.

19. Renal Vein Thrombosis: MR Imaging Findings

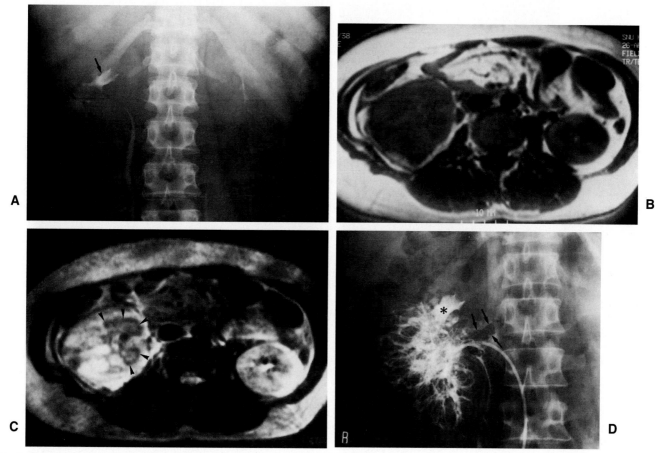

Fig. 1. A 38-year-old woman with double right renal veins and thrombosis of the lower renal vein associated with lupus nephritis. (**B–D,** From Kim SH, Byun HS, Park JH, et al: Renal parenchymal abnormalities associated with renal vein thrombosis: Correlation between MR imaging and pathologic findings in rabbits. AJR Am J Roentgenol 1994; 162:1361–1365.)
A. IVU shows swollen right kidney nonopacification of the lower part of the right kidney. Only upper-polar calyces are opacified *(arrows)*.
B. T1-weighted MR image shows swollen right kidney with diminished corticomedullary contrast. **C.** T2-weighted MR image shows wavy rim of low signal intensity *(arrowheads)* along the outer part of medulla. Areas of low signal intensity around the right side of both kidneys are due to chemical shift artifact. **D.** Venogram of the lower renal vein shows filling defect *(arrows)*, suggestive of renal vein thrombosis. Note the excreted contrast material in the upper-polar calyx *(asterisk)*.

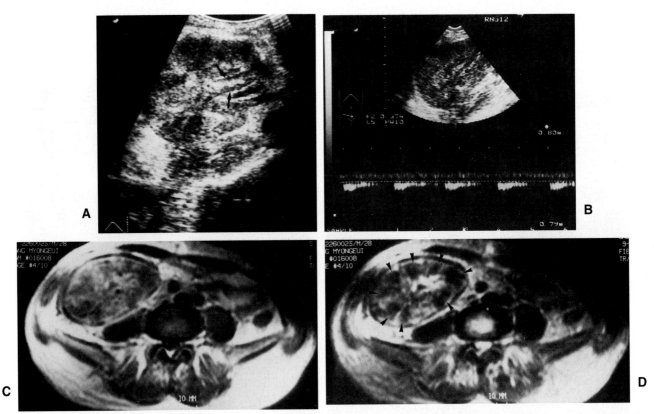

Fig. 2. A 29-year-old man with renal vein thrombosis in a transplanted kidney. (**C, D,** From Kim SH, Byun HS, Park JH, et al: Renal parenchymal abnormalities associated with renal vein thrombosis: Correlation between MR imaging and pathologic findings in rabbits. AJR Am J Roentgenol 1994; 162:1361–1365.)

A. US shows swollen transplanted kidney with prominent renal medulla. Note renal vein filled with echogenic thrombi *(arrows)*. **B.** Spectral Doppler US shows very weak flow signal with absent diastolic flow suggesting high resistance of the kidney to arterial inflow. **C.** T1-weighted MR image shows swollen transplanted kidney with poorly defined, low-intensity medulla. **D.** T2-weighted MR image shows prominent areas of low signal intensity in the renal medulla *(arrowheads)*.

20. Nutcracker Syndrome

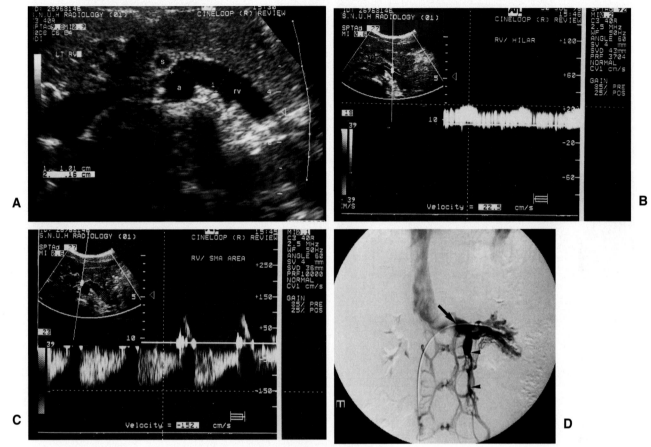

Fig. 1. Nutcracker syndrome in a 16-year-old boy with intermittent gross hematuria.

A. US of the left renal vein in transverse plane shows a dilated left renal vein (rv) that is compressed between the aorta (a) and superior mesenteric artery (s). The diameter of the left renal vein at hilar portion is 10.1 mm, whereas that of the aortomesenteric portion is 1.6 mm. **B.** Spectral Doppler US at hilar portion of the left renal vein shows a normal flow velocity of 22.5 cm/sec. **C.** Spectral Doppler US at the aortomesenteric portion of the left renal vein demonstrates high flow velocity of 152 cm/sec. **D.** Left renal venogram shows evidence of compression of the left renal vein *(arrow)* between the aorta and superior mesenteric artery. Also note prominent collateral circulations, including the gonadal vein *(arrowheads)*. There was a significant pressure gradient (6 mm Hg) between the left renal vein and inferior vena cava.

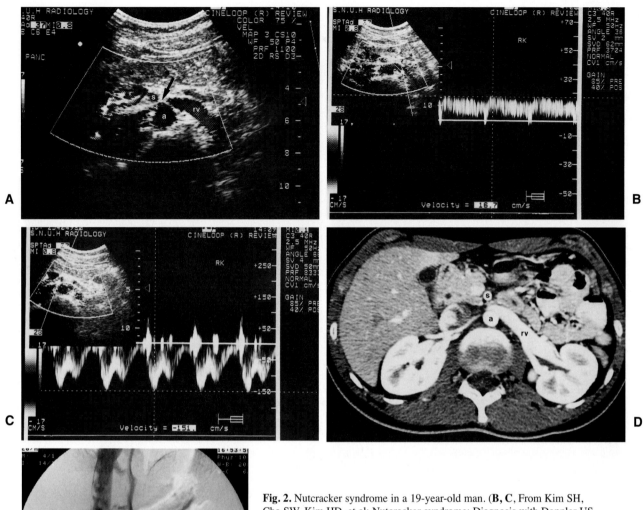

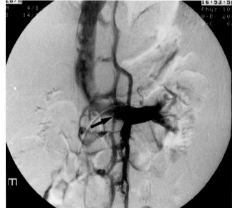

Fig. 2. Nutcracker syndrome in a 19-year-old man. (**B, C**, From Kim SH, Cho SW, Kim HD, et al: Nutcracker syndrome: Diagnosis with Doppler US. Radiology 1996; 198:93–97.) **A.** Doppler US of the left renal vein in transverse plane shows severe compression *(arrow)* of the left renal vein (rv) between the aorta (a) and superior mesenteric artery (s). **B.** Spectral Doppler US at the hilar portion of left renal vein shows normal flow velocity (16.7 cm/sec). **C.** Spectral Doppler US at aortomesenteric portion of the left renal vein shows high flow velocity (151 cm/sec). **D.** Contrast-enhanced CT well demonstrates dilated left renal vein (rv) with compression of the vein between the aorta (a) and superior mesenteric artery (s). **E.** Left renal venogram shows compression of the left renal vein *(arrow)*. Also note the abundant retroperitoneal collateral vessels. The pressure gradient between the left renal vein and inferior vena cava was 3.5 mm Hg.

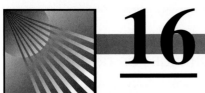

16

Renal Pelvis and Ureter

JUNG SUK SIM AND WILLIAM H. BUSH, JR.

URETERITIS

Primary inflammatory disease of the ureter is rare. Ureteral inflammation may be caused by spread from the upper urinary tract via urine, hematogenous spread, or direct extension from lesions in adjacent organs. Regardless of the origin of inflammation, ureteral responses include loss of peristalsis, dilation and striation due to redundancy, gas formation, mural infiltration, ulceration, pseudodiverticulation, edema, and/or fibrosis.

Bacteria itself or endotoxin can decrease ureteral peristalsis. Dilation results from poor emptying of the paralyzed ureter, so-called ureteral ileus. Mucosal striations are usually due to redundancy of the dilated ureter, but longitudinal striations due to mucosal edema are occasionally seen without dilation.

Focal ureteral stricture can be caused by instrumentation, irradiation, calculi, or infection. Secondary inflammation after extraurinary infection, such as appendicitis, pelvic inflammatory disorders, diverticulitis, or inflammatory bowel disease, can also cause ureteral stricture. Idiopathic segmental ureteritis or nonspecific granulomatous ureteritis, an intrinsic inflammatory disease of the ureter with no history of previous related disease, results in focal ureteral stricture that can be multiple.

Intramural or intraluminal gas-forming infection, such as ureteritis emphysematosa, is usually associated with infection of the kidney or bladder, so-called emphysematous pyelonephritis and emphysematous cystitis. Common organisms are *Escherichia coli* and *Aerobacter aerogenes*, and these infections are most often found in patients with diabetes mellitus. Fistula formation from adjacent organs by Crohn's disease or carcinoma of the bowel or uterus may cause ureteral gas.

PYELOURETERITIS CYSTICA

Pyelouteritis cystica is a condition in which subepithelial cysts filled with proteinaceous fluid are formed. The cyst wall consists of inflamed epithelium. Pyelouteritis cystica is usually associated with chronic urinary tract infection.

Typical urographic findings of pyelouteritis cystica are multiple, small, sharply marginated, smooth, uniform filling defects in the renal pelvis and ureter. Most of the lesions are only a few millimeters in diameter, but rarely they can reach several centimeters.

SUBUROTHELIAL HEMORRHAGE

Suburothelial or intramural hemorrhage of the ureter is usually secondary to trauma or excessive administration of anticoagulant. Radiologic appearance consists of multiple smooth filling defects of the ureter or sometimes the renal pelvis resembling pyelouteritis cystica. A few days after correction of coagulopathy, the radiologic abnormality disappears. On computed tomography (CT) or other cross-sectional studies, the wall of the ureter or renal pelvis is thickened.

URETERAL PSEUDODIVERTICULOSIS

Chronic inflammatory irritation causes the ureteral mucosa to become hyperplastic, which can then invaginate into the loose lamina propria of the ureter. This results in formation of pseudodiverticula. The outpouched areas of lumen are seen during urography as multiple, small diverticula. They are usually multiple, and there are conflicting reports about an increased risk of ureteral transitional cell carcinoma. Congenital ureteral diverticulum is rare and usually large and single and has all layers of the ureter.

MALACOPLAKIA

Malacoplakia is a rare granulomatous inflammatory disease, presumed to be associated with bacterial infection, especially *E. coli*. The histologic hallmark of malacoplakia is Michaelis-Gutmann bodies within the urothelial cells representing partially digested bacterial fragments. As the name indicates, the gross appearance of malacoplakia is a soft (Greek *malakos*) and yellowish mucosal elevation (*plakos*). Ureteral malacoplakia is usually coincident with malacoplakia of the kidney or urinary bladder. Radiologically, malacoplakia of the ureter is seen as smooth elevations of the mucosal surface, which can be solitary or multiple.

RADIATION URETERITIS

Radiation therapy for malignancies of the pelvic organs, such as uterine cervix and urinary bladder, can cause ureteral change. An early change is subepithelial inflammatory infiltration; late change is fibrosis. The typical radiologic finding of

radiation fibrosis of the ureter is smooth narrowing of the lumen in the distal one third.

MESENCHYMAL TUMORS OF URINARY TRACT

The urinary tract is covered by transitional cells, and its wall is composed of mesenchymal tissues. Although they are rare, various tumors can arise from the wall of the renal pelvis and ureter. They include hemangioma, leiomyoma, neurofibroma, fibroepithelial polyp, and lymphoma.

Among them fibroepithelial polyps are relatively common and have a unique morphology. They are benign tumors of the ureter, composed of a fibrovascular core covered by transitional epithelium. Their shapes are long and slender, ranging from 1 to 13 cm in length. They can arise anywhere in the course of the ureter, even in the proximity of ureteropelvic junction. Having a long pedicle, they can move freely, and about half of them cause urinary obstruction.

PERIURETERAL METASTASIS

There are several ways tumors can reach the ureters: hematogenous metastasis to the submucosa, direct invasion from the adjacent organs such as uterine cervix and sigmoid colon, and scirrhous spread to the periureteral tissues, especially from the organs of the upper abdomen such as stomach or pancreas. On intravenous urography (IVU), scirrhous periureteral metastasis appears as a long, irregular stricture of the ureter. On CT, the wall of the ureter is thickened and occasionally enhancing after injection of contrast material.

POSTOPERATIVE CHANGES OF THE URETER

Nonurologic surgical procedures involving the lower abdomen and pelvis can result in various changes of the urinary tract. Among them, medial deviation of ureters, transient hydronephroureter due to adynamic ileus of the ureters, and posterior displacement of bladder and seminal vesicles are most common. Most of the fistulas involving the ureters occur in association with surgery. In these cases, fistulas to the skin and gynecologic organs are common. In cases of chronic inflammation, such as Crohn's disease, a ureterointestinal fistula can be formed.

References

1. Wasserman NF: Inflammatory disease of the ureter. Radiol Clin North Am 1996; 34:1131–1156.
2. Lee JY, Kim SH, Kim TS, et al: CT findings of ureteral metastases. J Korean Radiol Soc 1995; 33:785–791.
3. Wasserman NF, Posalaky IP, Dykoski R: The pathology of ureteral pseudodiverticulosis. Invest Radiol 1988; 23:592–598.
4. Wasserman NF, La Pointe S, Posalaky IP: Ureteral pseudodiverticulosis. Radiology 1985; 155:561–566.
5. Goodman M, Dalton JR: Ureteral strictures following radiotherapy: Incidence, etiology, and treatment guidelines. J Urol 1982; 128:21–24.
6. Imray TJ, Huberty LH: Isolated ureteritis emphysematosa simulating pneumatosis intestinalis. AJR Am J Roentgenol 1980; 135:1082–1083.
7. Bissada NK, Finkbeiner AE: Idiopathic segmental ureteritis. Urology 1978; 12:64–66.
8. Sklaroff DM, Gnaneswaran P, Sklaroff RB: Postirradiation ureteric stricture. Gynecol Oncol 1978; 6:538–545.
9. Dahl DS: Segmental ureteritis: A report of four surgical cases. J Urol 1971; 105:642–646.
10. Wright FW: Mucosal edema of the ureter and renal pelvis. Radiology 1969; 93:1309–1312.

Illustrations • Renal Pelvis and Ureter

1. Nonspecific Ureteritis

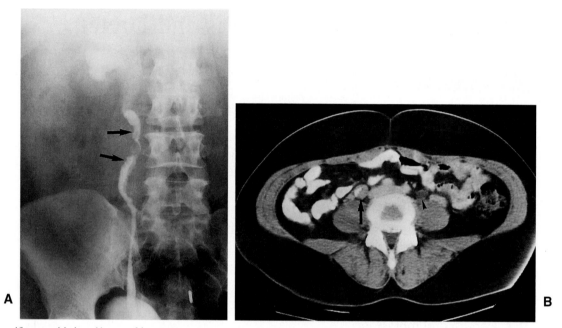

Fig. 1. Nonspecific ureteritis in a 41-year-old woman.
A. RGP shows irregular nodular elevated lesions in the right midureter *(arrows)*. Ureteroscopic biopsy revealed nonspecific inflammation and the patient's symptoms improved without specific treatment. **B.** Contrast-enhanced CT shows eccentric thickening of the right ureteral wall *(arrow)* and excreted contrast material in the ureteral lumen. Also note the dilated left ureter *(arrowhead)*.

2. Pyelouereteritis Cystica

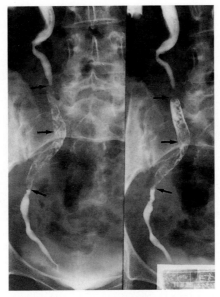

Fig. 1. Ureteritis cystica in a 28-year-old woman. RGP images show innumerable linear and nodular filling defects in the distal portion of the right ureter without significant obstruction *(arrows)*.

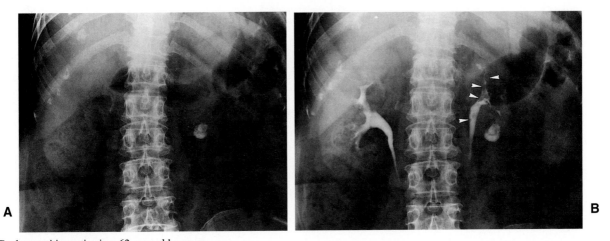

Fig. 2. Pyelouereteritis cystica in a 62-year-old woman.
A. Plain radiograph shows a round calcification in the left abdomen. **B.** IVU shows that the calcification is a stone in a calyceal diverticulum in the lower-polar region of the left kidney. Also note nodular lesions *(arrowheads)* in the left pelvocalyces and proximal ureter due to pyelouereteritis cystica.

3. Pyelouteral Striation

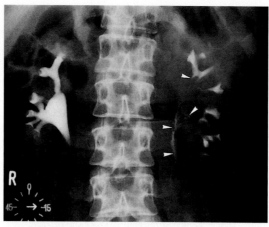

Fig. 1. Pyelouteral striation in a 29-year-old woman who had left ureteral obstruction due to uterine cervical carcinoma, which was relieved after radiation therapy. IVU shows severe striation in the left renal pelvis and proximal ureter *(arrowheads)* due to previous obstruction.

4. Suburothelial Hemorrhage

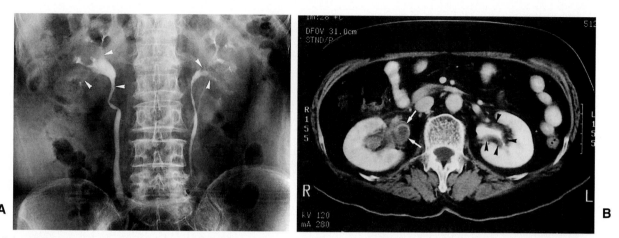

Fig. 1. Suburothelial hemorrhage in a 64-year-old woman who was receiving anticoagulation therapy for atrial fibrillation and had severe hematuria in the preceding 10 days.
A. IVU shows mucosal irregularities and nodularities in the infundibula, renal pelvis, and the ureters *(arrowheads)*. **B.** The patient developed gross hematuria. Contrast-enhanced CT performed on the next day shows delayed excretion in the right kidney with clot-filled, dilated pelvocalyces and thickened wall *(arrows)*. Also note thickened wall of the left renal pelvis *(arrowheads)* due to suburothelial hemorrhage.

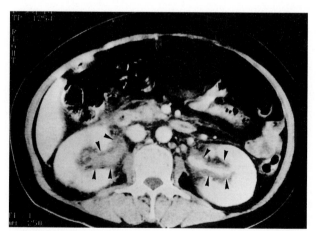

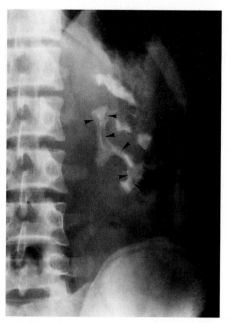

Fig. 2. Suburothelial hemorrhage in a 57-year-old woman who was receiving anticoagulation therapy for 2 years following mitral valve replacement for mitral regurgitation. The patient had gross hematuria during the preceding week. Contrast-enhanced CT shows thickened wall of the renal pelvis *(arrowheads)* in both kidneys due to suburothelial hemorrhage.

Fig. 3. Suburothelial hemorrhage in a 16-year-old boy who was receiving anticoagulation therapy for ventricular septal defect. IVU shows prominent irregularities and nodularities in the left pelvocalyceal wall *(arrowheads)* due to suburothelial hemorrhage.

5. Diverticulum and Pseudodiverticulosis of the Ureter

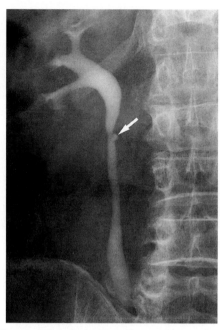

Fig. 1. Small ureteral diverticulum in a 64-year-old woman. IVU shows a small, saccular diverticulum in the right proximal ureter *(arrow)*. This may be either a true or false diverticulum.

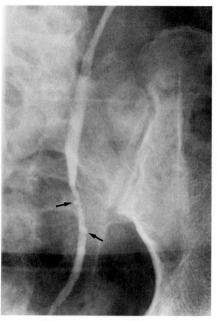

Fig. 2. Pseudodiverticulosis in a 65-year-old woman with ureteral obstruction due to uterine cervical carcinoma. Percutaneous nephrostomy was performed, and the nephrostogram shows multiple diverticular projections in the left distal ureter *(arrows)*.

6. Air in the Collecting System

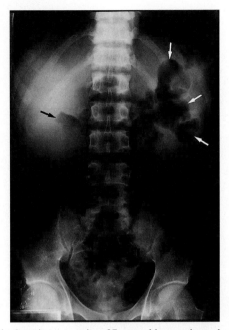

Fig. 1. Air in the urinary tract in a 27-year-old man who underwent ureterosigmoidostomy for contracted bladder due to tuberculosis. Plain radiograph shows a large amount of air *(arrows)* in the dilated pelvocalyces and ureter.

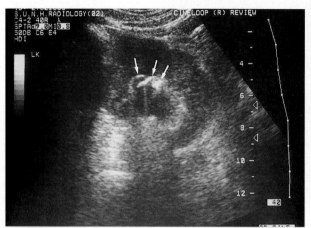

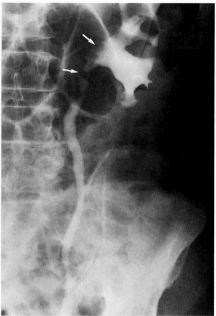

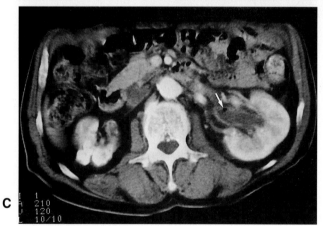

Fig. 2. Air in the urinary tract due to vesicoureteral reflux of the air, which was introduced through a Foley catheter in a 72-year-old woman with tuberculosis of the right urinary tract and urinary bladder. **A.** Longitudinal US of the left kidney shows prominent echoes *(arrows)* in the nondependent portion of the dilated renal pelvis with accompanying posterior sonic shadowing. **B.** VCU shows reflux of contrast material and air *(arrows)* into the left urinary tract. **C.** Contrast-enhanced CT shows dilated left renal pelvis containing air bubbles in the nondependent portion *(arrow)*. Also note the contracted right kidney with calcification due to tuberculosis.

7. Fibroepithelial Polyp

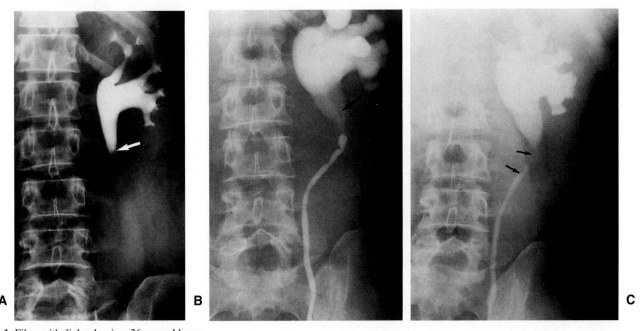

Fig. 1. Fibroepithelial polyp in a 26-year-old man.
A. A 25-minute IVU shows mild hydronephrosis of the left kidney and a linear filling defect *(arrow)* in the proximal ureter. **B.** RGP shows narrowing of the left proximal ureter and a linear filling defect *(arrow)* in the dilated ureter proximal to the narrowing. Note that the filling defect appears to be attached to the narrowed portion of the ureter. **C.** Delayed image of RGP shows that the filling defect *(arrows)* moved distally but still appears attached to the narrowed portion of the ureter.

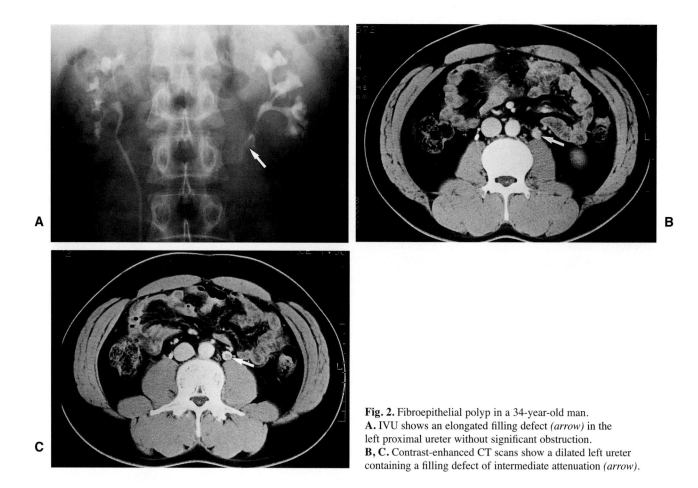

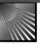

Fig. 2. Fibroepithelial polyp in a 34-year-old man.
A. IVU shows an elongated filling defect *(arrow)* in the left proximal ureter without significant obstruction.
B, C. Contrast-enhanced CT scans show a dilated left ureter containing a filling defect of intermediate attenuation *(arrow)*.

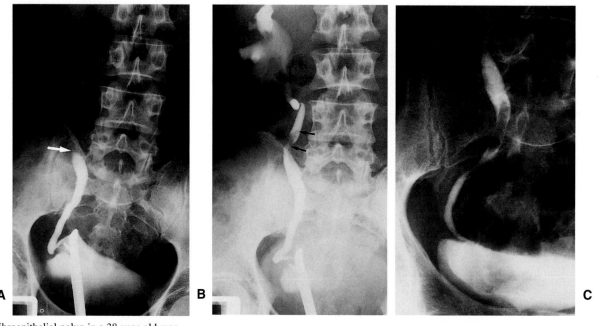

Fig. 3. Fibroepithelial polyp in a 38-year-old man.
A. RGP initially showed obstruction in the right distal ureter *(arrow)*. **B.** RGP with further injection shows passage of contrast material into the upper urinary tract and a polypoid and linear filling defect *(arrows)* in the midureter. **C.** An additional image demonstrates an elongated polypoid, intraluminal filling defect, which moved distally. The shape, intraluminal location, and restricted movement are indicative of an attached polypoid lesion.

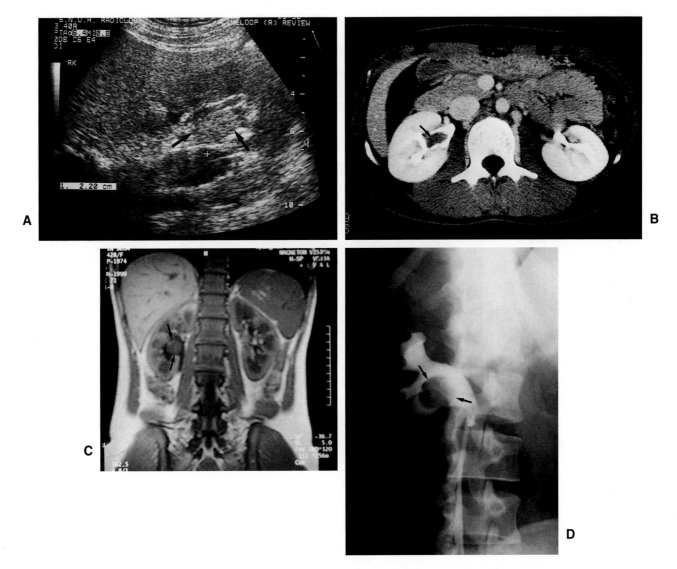

Fig. 4. Fibroepithelial polyp in the renal pelvis in a 24-year-old woman.
A. US of the right kidney shows a round, slightly echogenic mass *(arrows)* in the renal sinus region. **B.** Contrast-enhanced CT shows a filling defect *(arrow)* in the right renal pelvis. **C.** T1-weighted coronal MR image demonstrates a mass *(arrows)* in the right renal pelvis. **D.** RGP shows a large mass *(arrows)* in the right renal pelvis.

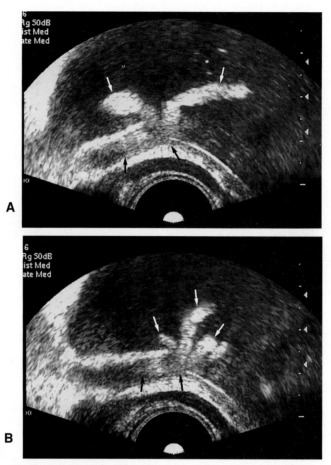

Fig. 5. Fibroepithelial polyp of the distal ureter protruding into the bladder. (**A, B,** Courtesy of Dal Mo Yang, MD.)
A, B. US of the right aspect of the urinary bladder in transverse plane shows hyperechoic vermiform masses in the right terminal ureter protruding into the bladder *(arrows)*.

8. Hemangioma of the Renal Pelvis

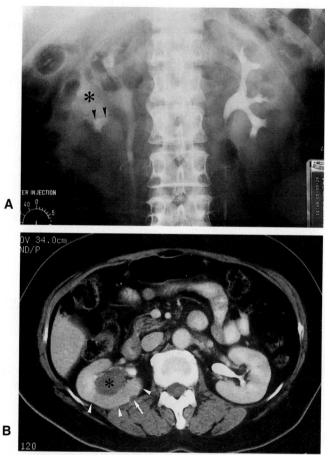

Fig. 1. Cavernous hemangioma of the kidney in a 62-year-old woman. **A.** IVU shows nonopacification of the interpolar calyx of the right kidney *(asterisk)* and compression effect on the lower-polar calyx *(arrowheads)*. **B.** Contrast-enhanced CT shows a low-attenuated mass *(asterisk)* in the renal sinus region of the right kidney with poor enhancement of the posterior renal parenchyma *(arrowheads)*. Note a small cyst in the posteromedial aspect of the right kidney *(arrow)*. At pathologic examination, the tumor was composed of dilated vessels with organizing thrombi and was consistent with cavernous hemangioma.

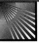
9. Periureteral Metastasis

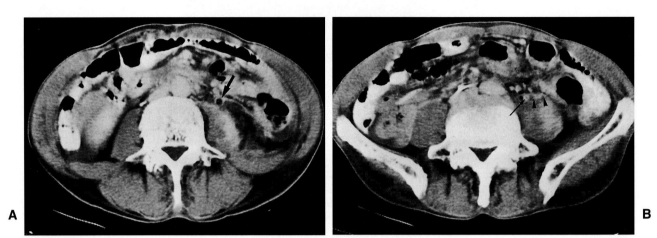

Fig. 1. Periureteral metastasis in a 71-year-old man who underwent partial gastrectomy for gastric cancer 2 years earlier.
A. Contrast-enhanced CT shows a dilated left ureter *(arrow)*. **B.** CT scan at a lower level shows a thickened ureteral wall *(arrow)* and fine, nodular, enhancing tissue *(arrowheads)* along the anterior margin of the left psoas muscle.

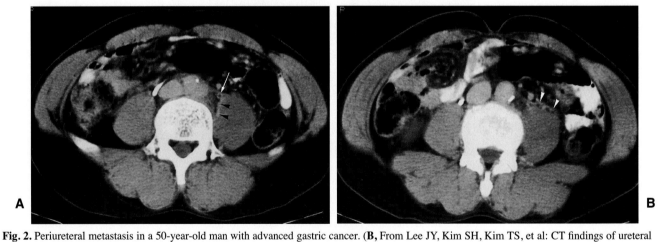

Fig. 2. Periureteral metastasis in a 50-year-old man with advanced gastric cancer. (**B,** From Lee JY, Kim SH, Kim TS, et al: CT findings of ureteral metastases. J Korean Radiol Soc 1995; 33:785–791.)
A, B. Contrast-enhanced CT scans show thickened left ureteral wall *(arrow in* **A***)* and enhancing tissue *(arrowheads)* along the anteromedial margin of the left psoas muscle.

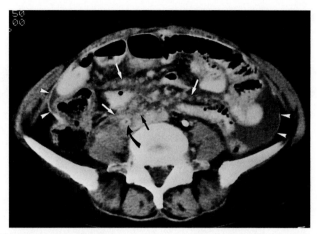

Fig. 3. Periureteral metastasis in a 58-year-old woman who underwent radical subtotal gastrectomy for advanced gastric cancer 5 years earlier. Contrast-enhanced CT shows extensive infiltration *(black and white arrows)* around the right ureter *(curved arrow)* and along the mesentery. Also note ascites and peritoneal thickening *(arrowheads)* due to peritoneal carcinomatosis.

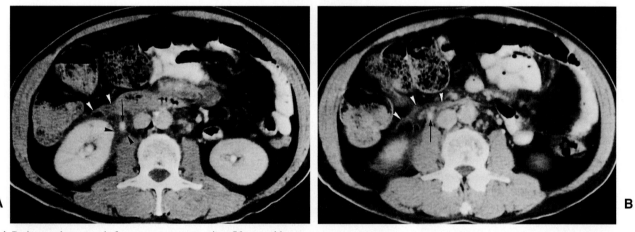

A   B

Fig. 4. Periureteral metastasis from pancreas cancer in a 56-year-old man.
A, B. Contrast-enhanced CT scans show soft tissue infiltration *(arrowheads)* around the right ureter *(arrow)* due to periureteral metastasis.

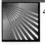

10. Miscellaneous Conditions of the Ureter

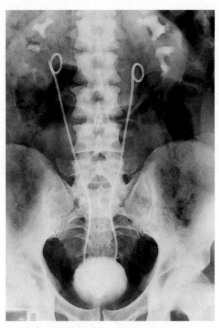

Fig. 1. Medial deviation of the lower ureters in a 43-year-old man who underwent Miles' operation for rectal cancer. IVU shows bilateral ureteral stents that are medially displaced over the sacrum. Ureteral stents were introduced to relieve bilateral ureteral obstruction due to postoperative strictures.

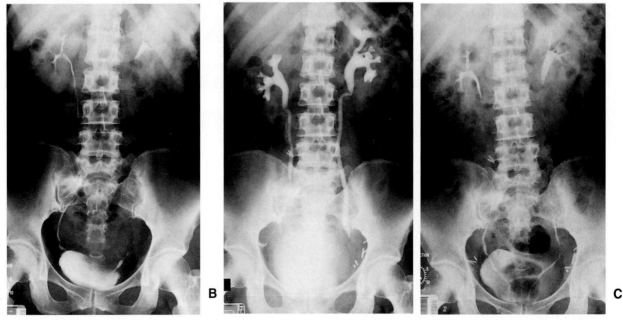

Fig. 2. Transient postoperative hydronephrosis in a 50-year-old woman who underwent radical hysterectomy and lymph node dissection for uterine cervical carcinoma.
A. Preoperative IVU shows normal findings. Left ureter is incompletely opacified due to peristalsis. **B.** IVU obtained 2 weeks after the surgery shows mild bilateral hydronephrosis and hydroureter due to impaired peristalsis of the distal ureters. **C.** Follow-up IVU obtained 2 months later shows return of normal peristalsis.

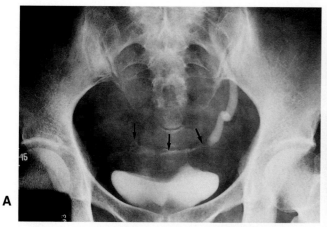
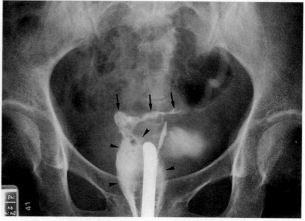

Fig. 3. Ureterovaginal fistula that occurred following hysterectomy for uterine myoma in a 50-year-old woman.
A. IVU shows a dilated left ureter and a linear leak of contrast material *(arrows)* from the distal portion of the left ureter. **B.** RGP demonstrates a ureterovaginal fistula *(arrows)* and opacification of the vagina *(arrowheads)*.

Fig. 4. A 28-year-old man with history of active inflammatory bowel disease (Crohn's disease) and increasing right flank pain over the previous 2 weeks.
A. IVU image taken 1 hour after injection of contrast material shows moderate hydronephrosis with tapered narrowing of the ureter *(arrow)* in the right lower abdomen. Distally the ureter is not dilated *(open arrow)*. **B.** Small bowel barium study shows changes of active inflammatory bowel disease with narrowings, ulcerations, and skip areas *(arrows)*. The associated inflammatory changes are affecting the right ureter as it crosses the iliac vessels and causing partial obstruction, as seen on IVU.

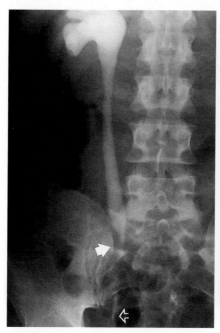
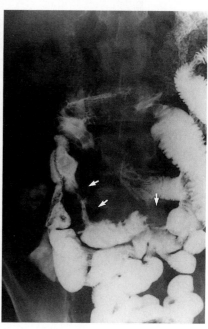

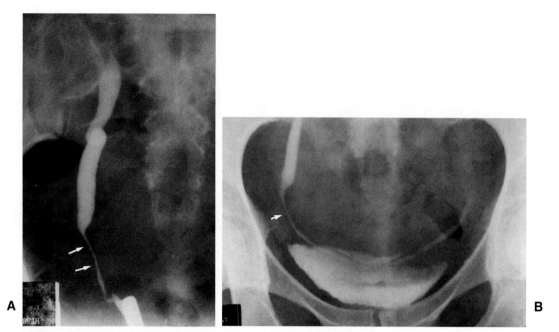

Fig. 5. A 25-year-old woman who 2 years previously had a hysterectomy for endometriosis. Now she has right flank pain and episodic vaginal bleeding. Clinical examination revealed a small endometrial implant at the vaginal cuff.
A. Right RGP shows a long, smooth narrowing of the right distal ureter *(arrows)* with moderate hydronephrosis proximal to the narrowing. Hormonal therapy was begun. **B.** IVU done 2 years after the RGP shows some persistent smooth narrowing of the distal right ureter *(arrow)*. However, the patient was asymptomatic and the hydronephrosis had resolved considerably. The pelvocalyces were no longer dilated (not shown).

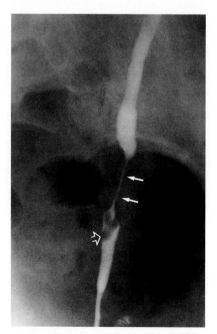

Fig. 6. Endometriosis (transmural involvement) in a 24-year-old woman who presented with hematuria. Left RGP shows an area of smooth, tight ureteral narrowing *(arrows)* with mild shelf configuration superiorly. Below the narrowed area are small intraluminal filling defects due to blood clots *(open arrow)*.

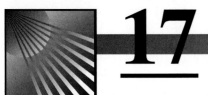

17

Urinary Bladder

CHANG KYU SEONG

ANATOMY

The urinary bladder is a distensible muscular organ that changes in size as it distends with urine. Its wall consists of mucosa, submucosa, lamina propria, and smooth muscle. The bladder wall musculature consists of three layers: an inner longitudinal, a middle circular, and an outer longitudinal. Its base is anchored inferiorly by the urogenital diaphragm. Ventrally, it borders with the symphysis pubis, dorsally with the rectum or vagina, and laterally with the paravesical fat and connective tissue. The dome of the bladder is covered by peritoneum. The trigone is a triangular area between the two ureteral orifices and the internal urethral opening. Between the ureteral orifices, the musculature of the bladder floor is hypertrophied, forming the interureteric ridge.

CONGENITAL ANOMALIES

Bladder exstrophy

Bladder exstrophy is a rare congenital anomaly. It is often referred to as the *exstrophy-epispadias complex*. It occurs as a spectrum of anterior abdominal wall defects caused by varying degrees of failure of midline fusion of the mesodermal tissue below the umbilicus. In classic exstrophy, the bladder lies open and everted on the anterior abdominal wall. The urethra is epispadic, and there is a concomitant wide separation of the symphysis pubis with outward rotation of the innominate bone and squaring of the iliac notch. Intravenous urography (IVU) usually demonstrates normal upper urinary tracts, but the most distal portion of the ureters may have a bulbous angulation.

Urachal remnants

The urachus is a normal embryonic structure that extends from the umbilicus to the anterior superior surface of the bladder. The obliterated urachus is known as the *median umbilical ligament*. However, multiple anomalies of urachal closure may occur anywhere from the bladder dome to the umbilicus. They include a patent urachus, urachal cyst, urachal sinus, and urachal diverticulum. Urachal cyst is developed from the closure at both ends of the urachal lumen with incomplete obliteration. Urachal cyst may become infected. Urachal sinus and diverticulum represent incomplete closure of umbilical and vesical ends of the urachus, respectively. Adenocarcinoma of the urachus is a rare tumor found in the midline, intramuscular portion of the bladder dome.

INFECTIONS AND INFLAMMATIONS OF THE BLADDER

Acute bacterial cystitis

Bacterial cystitis is most commonly caused by *Escherichia coli*. It is primarily a disease of women and is sometimes related to sexual intercourse. In men, it is usually associated with lower urinary tract obstruction or bacterial prostatitis. The radiologic findings of bacterial cystitis are nonspecific. The major finding is that of bladder edema. Diffuse irregularity and thickening of mucosal folds may be seen. These findings are often more prominent at the bladder base and trigone but may involve the entire bladder wall. The bladder may have a decreased capacity due to edema and irritation.

Emphysematous cystitis

Emphysematous cystitis is an unusual manifestation of bladder infection in which gas is present within the wall of the bladder. It is most commonly seen in patients with longstanding and poorly controlled diabetes mellitus. Other cases are related to longstanding urinary stasis secondary to outlet obstruction, neurogenic bladder, or bladder diverticulum. The offending organism is usually *E. coli*, but a variety of other bacteria and yeast infections have also been reported. In addition to gas within the bladder wall, gas collection can be seen within the bladder lumen or perivesical space. Infection with luminal gas, but without mural gas, is described as a separate entity (primary pneumocystitis). Gas in the lumen of the bladder may also result from fistula or instrumentation, but the gas in the wall is almost always attributable to infection.

Radiation cystitis

Intracavitary or external radiation therapy may cause either immediate or delayed radiation cystitis. Radiographic changes are nonspecific and may show an irregular bladder outline due to edema and hemorrhage, followed by mucosal ulceration, fibrosis, and a small-capacity bladder. Rarely calcification is seen in the bladder wall.

Cyclophosphamide cystitis

Cyclophosphamide cystitis is a drug-induced cystitis. It is probably due to prolonged contact of the bladder mucosa with

primary and secondary metabolites of cyclophosphamide. Radiographically, bladder wall thickening and mucosal irregularities due to hemorrhage and edema can be seen. In the chronic stage, depending on the extent of the damage, bladder wall fibrosis may ensue, resulting in a small-capacity bladder. Occasionally, calcification of the bladder wall appears.

Cystitis cystica and cystitis glandularis

Two benign proliferative lesions of the urinary bladder that are frequently confused with bladder tumors are cystitis cystica and cystitis glandularis. The etiology is unknown, but there is a clear relationship to recurrent or chronic urinary tract infection, and both lesions are believed to represent metaplastic changes in the bladder epithelium induced by various noxious stimuli. Cystitis cystica appear histologically as a submucosal nest of epithelial cells surrounding a central liquefied region of cellular degeneration. They are more frequent in women and children with chronic urinary tract infection and are most common at the trigone and base of the bladder. Cystitis glandularis is similar to cystitis cystica except that the Brunn's nests have undergone glandular metaplasia. The urographic appearance of these two types of cystitis varies from a single large tumor-like mass to multiple, discrete, nodular filling defects. On cross-sectional image they can be seen as areas of focal or diffuse thickening of the bladder wall or a well-defined fungating lesion.

Malacoplakia

Malacoplakia is a rare granulomatous lesion characterized by mucosal plaques involving the bladder or, less commonly, the kidney, retroperitoneum, testis, and prostate. It is more frequent in women and is usually associated with chronic urinary tract infection. It often present as a tumor-like mass of the bladder wall, which may be impossible to differentiate radiographically from invasive bladder neoplasms.

Schistosomiasis

Schistosomiasis of the urinary bladder is caused by *Schistosoma haematobium*. It is a parasitic infection, which is endemic in some countries. The ova are excreted in urine and often entrapped in the mucosa and penetrate the submucosa of the ureter and bladder, causing granulomatous reaction, fibrosis, and death of the eggs. Hematuria is the most common symptom. The dead eggs calcify, causing fine, linear calcifications in the wall of the ureter and bladder. Large conglomerations of eggs in the bladder wall cause masses, which eventually calcify.

BLADDER INJURIES

Injury of the bladder may occur as a result of blunt, penetrating, or iatrogenic trauma. It is related not only to the mechanism of injury but also to the degree of filling of the bladder at the time of injury. A full or obstructed bladder or one that is in fixed position by scar or tumor is most likely to be injured.

Bladder contusion is the most common form of bladder injury, and its radiographic findings are usually normal. Intraperitoneal bladder rupture occurs when there is sudden rise in intravesical pressure as a result of a blow to the lower abdomen in patients who have a distended bladder. The rupture usually occurs at the weakest portion of the bladder wall, the dome, where the bladder is in contact with the peritoneal surface. Unlike intraperitoneal rupture, extraperitoneal rupture of the bladder is almost invariably associated with pelvic fracture, in which bony spicules from pelvic fracture may directly puncture the bladder. In intraperitoneal rupture of the bladder, there is leakage of contrast material that is free flowing, fills the cul-de-sac and paracolic gutters, and outlines the abdominal viscera and loops of bowel. In extraperitoneal rupture of the bladder, leaked contrast material is not free flowing and tends to streak in a flamelike fashion adjacent to the bladder. Extravasation of contrast material may extend beyond the confines of the perivesical space. Combined intraperitoneal and extraperitoneal rupture of the bladder may occur, and it will demonstrate both sets of findings. Penetrating injury of the bladder may occur as a result of stab or gunshot wound. It may result in intraperitoneal, extraperitoneal, or combined bladder injury.

Injury of the bladder may also occur in any type of pelvic surgery and iatrogenic instrumentation. Obstetric bladder injury may result from laceration of the bladder during cesarean section, injury secondary to trauma from obstetric forceps, or from pressure necrosis of the bladder wall during labor. Vesicouterine fistula is a rare, delayed complication of cesarean section. Such patients may present with menouria, which is called *Youssef's syndrome*.

BLADDER TUMORS

Urothelial tumors of the bladder

Benign urothelial tumors in the urinary bladder are rare. Malignant bladder tumors, however, are the most common malignancies of the urinary tract. Most of them are transitional cell carcinomas, accounting for 90% of all primary malignant lesions. Men are affected at least three times more often than women. The peak age is between 50 and 80 years. The most common clinical symptom is painless gross hematuria. About one third of bladder cancers are multifocal at the time of diagnosis. Synchronous tumors of the upper urinary tract occur in 2.3% of patients with bladder transitional cell carcinoma. There is also an increased prevalence (3.9%) of upper urinary tract tumors after the initial diagnosis and treatment of bladder cancer. Between 23% and 40% of patients with upper urinary tract tumors at some time will develop bladder cancer.

Transitional cell carcinomas arise most commonly in the region of the trigone or bladder base or on the lateral walls. They manifest a variety of patterns of tumor growth, including papillary, infiltrative, papillary and infiltrative, or nonpapillary and noninfiltrative (carcinoma in situ). They often have calcification that is due to dystrophic calcification within tumor necrosis. Lymphatic drainage is to the external iliac and hypogastric lymph nodes. The tumor stage (Table 17–1) and grade determine the prognosis. On computed tomographic (CT) scan, isolated bladder wall thickening and/or papillary tumor growth may be seen. Fuzzy external borders of the bladder may suggest the presence of invasion of the tumor into extravesical fat tissue.

Squamous cell carcinomas represent 5% of bladder cancers. They are usually associated with chronic irritation from urinary calculi, long-term indwelling catheters, chronic or recurrent infection, and schistosomiasis. Although they are radiologi-

Table 17–1	Jewett-Strong-Marshall Staging System and TNM Classification of Bladder Tumors	

Jewett-Strong-Marshall	TNM	Histopathologic Findings
0	Tis	Carcinoma in situ
	Ta	Papillary noninvasive carcinoma
A	T1	Tumor invades subepithelial connective tissue (lamina propria)
B1	T2	Tumor invades superficial muscle
B2	T3a	Tumor invades deep muscle
C	T3b	Tumor invades perivesical fat
D1	T4a	Tumor invades neighboring structures (prostate, uterus, or vagina)
D1	T4b	Tumor invades pelvic or abdominal wall
D1	N1	Single homolateral regional lymph node metastasis
D1	N2	Contralateral, bilateral, or multiple regional lymph node metastases
D1	N3	Fixed regional lymph node packages
D2	N4	Juxtaregional lymph node metastases
D2	M1	Distant metastases

cally similar to some transitional cell carcinomas, they usually appear as sessile masses with or without extravesical extension. Papillary tumors or predominantly intravesical growth patterns are not typical. Because of the tendency of these lesions to show early infiltration, the patients have a poor prognosis.

Adenocarcinomas account for less than 2% of bladder cancers. They are classified into three groups: primary vesical, urachal, and metastatic. Calcification within the tumor is more commonly seen in adenocarcinomas than in other tumors.

Nonurothelial tumors of the bladder

Leiomyomas are the most common nonepithelial benign bladder tumors. About two thirds of the tumors grow intravesically, one third extravesically, and only about 7% purely intramurally. They are characterized by slow and noninvasive growth, without destruction of the overlying mucosa. Other benign nonepithelial tumors of the bladder include paragangliomas, hemangiomas, and neurofibromas.

Leiomyosarcomas, fibrosarcomas, and osteosarcomas are rare malignant bladder tumors. The radiologic findings are nonspecific, and differentiation among them or from a large invasive transitional cell carcinoma is difficult. The urinary bladder and prostate are the most common locations of rhabdomyosarcoma, following the head and neck region. They are the most common pelvic malignancy in the pediatric group and may arise in the bladder wall itself or from adjacent structures and secondarily involve the bladder. Differentiating between a rhabdomyosarcoma arising in the bladder and one arising in the prostate or vagina may be difficult. Large, cauliflower-like tumors with a locally invasive growth pattern and early hematogenous and lymphatic metastasis are typical findings of rhabdomyosarcomas.

Primary bladder lymphoma is extremely rare, and secondary involvement of systemic lymphoma is more common. Radiographically they are indistinguishable from transitional cell carcinoma. Irregularities, thickening, and nodular pattern of the bladder wall are nonspecific radiologic findings.

The urinary bladder may be invaded directly by primary malignancies of adjacent pelvic organs including rectosig-moid colon, prostate, seminal vesicle, uterine cervix, uterine corpus, and ovary. Carcinoma of the uterine cervix or uterine corpus is the most common cause of direct bladder invasion in women, whereas carcinoma of the rectosigmoid colon is the most common cause in men. The cystographic findings of direct bladder invasion include smooth indentation, irregular spiculated deformity, or fistulous communication between the primary site and urinary bladder. These findings may vary with the depth of invasion of the vesical wall, and these findings are not specific for neoplastic invasion, because the extension of inflammatory conditions can show identical findings.

MISCELLANEOUS CONDITIONS OF THE BLADDER

Bladder hernia

Bladder hernia is an uncommon condition, and it can occur with any type of hernia in the groin. It may be seen in 1% to 3% of all inguinal hernias. The bladder may also be involved in incisional, femoral, ischiorectal, and obturator hernias. The most common type of vesicoinguinal hernia is paraperitoneal, with the peritoneum over the dome of the bladder herniating adjacent to the bladder into the inguinal canal. Less common are the intraperitoneal and extraperitoneal types. Small bladder hernias are better visualized in the upright or prone position during IVU and cystography.

Bladder ear

A significant number of infants younger than 1 year of age show protrusion of the inferolateral aspect of the bladder into the inguinal ring. These protrusions, which have been termed *bladder ears*, represent transitory extraperitoneal hernias of the bladder because of still incompetent inguinal rings. They can be unilateral or bilateral and usually disappear on distention of the bladder. Bladder ear is a normal variation during bladder development and usually disappears by 1 year of age. Persistence of bladder ears in older children usually means true inguinal hernia.

Bladder stones

Bladder stones can be classified as migrant, primary idiopathic endemic, or secondary. Secondary bladder stones are the stones related to urinary stasis or foreign bodies. The causes of urinary stasis include bladder outlet obstruction such as prostatic hypertrophy, neurogenic bladder, urethral stricture, urethral or bladder diverticulum, or cystocele. This may be further complicated by superimposed infection. Bladder stones may also form on a nonabsorbable suture, sponge, catheter, or other foreign bodies that serve as a nidus for stone formation. Radiopacity of the bladder stones varies from very dense to radiolucent. They may be obscured by feces and gas in the rectosigmoid colon or by the sacrum. They may be single or multiple and are occasionally laminated.

Bladder diverticulum

Bladder diverticulum is a round outpouching of the bladder wall connected to the bladder by a neck. It may be

congenital or acquired, single or multiple. Congenital bladder diverticula are rare and usually single. Most are located paraureterally along the posterolateral margin of the bladder (Hutch diverticulum). Another example of a congenital diverticulum is a vesicourachal diverticulum, which is located at the bladder apex.

Acquired diverticula are often multiple and result from the chronically raised intravesical pressure in association with anatomic or neuropathic bladder outflow obstruction. As the outflow bladder obstruction continues, the mucosal layer invaginates through a focal weakness in bladder muscle and protrudes outward. Small outpouchings between the hypertrophied muscle bundles are called *cellules* or *saccules*. Although the distinction is somewhat arbitrary and subjective, it is convenient to consider cellules, saccules, and diverticula, in that order, as increasingly severe manifestations of a chronically raised intravesical pressure.

A wide-necked diverticulum empties readily when the bladder empties. A narrow-necked diverticulum empties slowly as the bladder empties and is therefore more likely to have residual urine and urinary stasis. Retention of urine in the diverticulum results in infection and stone formation. The neck of the diverticulum can occasionally obliterate, resulting in the radiographic appearance of a paravesical space-occupying lesion. Bladder diverticula may be complicated by neoplasm.

Urine leak in unused bladder

Two groups of patients may have unused bladder for prolonged periods: patients who for various reasons have been diverted but whose bladder was left in place, and those anephric patients maintained on dialysis. To evaluate bladder volume, bladder outflow tract, and vesicoureteral reflux, unused bladder may be examined by cystography prior to undiversion or renal transplantation. Intramural or extraperitoneal extravasation of contrast material during cystography may occur on occasion but is apparently an inconsequential finding.

Pelvic lipomatosis

Pelvic lipomatosis is a rare disorder of unknown etiology characterized by the benign overgrowth of histologically normal fat within the pelvic cavity and compression of the bladder and rectum. On cystography, the bladder is elongated with cephalad displacement and narrowing of the bladder base. The abnormal configuration of the bladder is described as teardrop or pear shaped. CT or magnetic resonance (MR) imaging well demonstrates excessive fatty tissue in the pelvic cavity.

Vesical fistula

Vesical fistula is an abnormal communication between the urinary bladder and the other organs as a result of an inflammation or malignancy. It may cause involuntary loss of urine. The causes include surgical complication, penetrating trauma, bladder cancer, colon cancer, sigmoid diverticulitis, Crohn's disease, and radiation therapy for pelvic malignancy. Vesicovaginal fistula is most commonly iatrogenic, due to

bladder injury during obstetric or gynecologic procedures. The fistulous tracts are usually demonstrated at voiding cystourethrography (VCU).

Bladder outlet obstruction

Prolonged bladder outflow obstruction results in hypertrophy of the detrusor muscle, thickening of the bladder wall, and bladder diverticula or cellule formation. The causes of bladder outflow obstruction include prostatic hypertrophy or carcinoma, neurogenic bladder dysfunction, bladder stones or neoplasms, and urethral strictures. Increased intravesical pressure is transmitted to the upper urinary tract system resulting in hydronephrosis, hydroureter, and vesicoureteral reflux, eventually leading to renal function deterioration. When the residual volume exceeds the physiologic capacity of the bladder, the bladder is enlarged, sometimes markedly, due to deterioration of detrusor function. Bladder stones are a frequent complication of chronic intravesical urinary stasis.

Stress urinary incontinence

Urinary incontinence is defined as the inability to store urine and can be due to bladder or urethral dysfunction. Stress urinary incontinence is the most frequent form of urethral insufficiency. In this condition sudden increase in intra-abdominal pressure caused by stress such as laughing, coughing, or change of posture results in involuntary urine leakage without detrusor contraction and without an urge to urinate. It is caused by weak pelvic floor muscles, mostly related to delivery trauma. It is commonly associated with a cystocele. The method of assessing stress incontinence is videourodynamic VCU, chain cystourethrography, transperineal or transvaginal ultrasonography (US), and MR imaging. Stress incontinence must be distinguished from bladder-related incontinence clinically.

Cystocele

Cystocele is defined radiologically as any bladder that drops below the inferior margin of the symphysis pubis during straining when the patient is in the standing position. It is a prolapse of the anterior vaginal wall with descent of the base of the bladder, trigone, and urethra into the vagina. In severe cases there may be complete uterine prolapse or obstructive findings of upper urinary tract. Cystocele may be associated with stress incontinence.

Neurogenic bladder

Neurogenic bladder refers to neuromuscular dysfunction of the detrusor muscle and the urethral sphincter. Both storage and emptying functions of the bladder require complex, neurologically regulated synergistic cooperation between the detrusor, sphincter, and pelvic floor muscles. If a lesion affects the central neurons, a spastic neurogenic bladder results. If a lesion affects the peripheral neuron, a flaccid bladder is the usual outcome. The usual findings are small capacity, trabeculation, and "Christmas tree" appearance of the bladder.

References

1. Dunnick NR, Sandler CM, Newhouse JH, Amis ES Jr: Textbook of Uroradiology, 3rd ed. Philadelphia, Lippincott Williams & Wilkins, 2001, pp 352–393.
2. Kim HC, Kim SH, Hwang SI, et al: Isolated bladder metastases from stomach cancer: CT demonstration. Abdom Imaging 2001; 26:333–335.
3. Lee HJ, Kim SH: Characteristic plain radiographic and intravenous urographic findings of bladder calculi formed over a hair nidus: A case report. Korean J Radiol 2001; 2:61–62.
4. Moon SG, Kim SH, Lee HJ, et al: Pelvic fistulas complicating pelvic surgery or diseases: Spectrum of imaging findings. Korean J Radiol 2001; 2:97–104.
5. Friedland GW, deVries PA, Nino-Murcia M: Congenital anomalies of the urachus and bladder. In Pollack HM, McClennan BL (eds): Clinical Urography, 2nd ed, vol 1. Philadelphia, WB Saunders, 2000, pp 826–851.
6. Saluja S, Lazzarini KM, Smith RC: Inflammation of the urinary bladder. In Pollack HM. McClennan BL (eds): Clinical Urography, 2nd ed, vol 1. Philadelphia, WB Saunders, 2000, pp 1019–1039.
7. Park BK, Kim SH, Cho JY, et al: Vesicouterine fistula after cesarean section: Ultrasonographic findings in two cases. J Ultrasound Med 1999; 18:441–443.
8. Amendila MA: Imaging of benign conditions of the bladder: Urography/cystography/ultrasound/CT. In Jafri SZH, Diokno AC, Amendola MA (eds): Lower Genitourinary Radiology: Imaging and Intervention. New York, Springer, 1998, pp 35–79.
9. Brooks JD: Anatomy of the lower urinary tract and male genitalia. In Walsh PC, Retik AB, Vaughan ED Jr, Wein AJ (eds): Campbell's Urology, 7th ed, vol 1. Philadelphia, WB Saunders, 1998, pp 89–128.
10. Wong-You-Cheong JJ, Wagner BJ, Davis CJ Jr: Transitional cell carcinoma of the urinary tract: Radiologic-pathologic correlation. Radiographics 1998; 18:123–142.
11. Kim SH, Han MC: Invasion of the urinary bladder by uterine cervical carcinoma: Evaluation with MR imaging. AJR Am J Roentgenol 1997; 168:393–397.
12. Fernbach SK, Feinstein KA: Abnormalities of the bladder in children: Imaging findings. AJR Am J Roentgenol 1994; 162:1143–1150.
13. Hayes WS: The urinary bladder. In Davidson AJ, Hartman DS, Choyke PL, Wagner BJ (eds): Radiology of the Kidney and Genitourinary Tract, 3rd ed. Philadelphia, WB Saunders, 1994, pp 485–515.
14. Kim B, Semelka RC, Ascher SM, et al: Bladder tumor staging: Comparison of contrast-enhanced CT, T1- and T2-weighted MR imaging, dynamic gadolinium-enhanced imaging, and late gadolinium-enhanced imaging. Radiology 1994; 193:239–245.
15. Izes BA, Larsen CR, Izes JK, et al: Computerized tomographic appearance of hernias of the bladder. J Urol 1993; 149:1002–1005.
16. Kim SH, Han MC: Reversed-contrast urine levels in urinary bladder: CT findings. Urol Radiol 1992; 13:249–252.
17. Kim SH, Na DG, Choi BI, et al: Direct invasion of urinary bladder from sigmoid colon cancer: CT findings. J Comput Assist Tomogr 1992; 16:709–712.
18. Moon WK, Kim SH, Lee SJ, et al: Case report. Paraffinoma in the bladder: CT findings. J Comput Assist Tomogr 1992; 16:308–310.
19. Quint HJ, Drach GW, Rappaport WD, et al: Emphysematous cystitis: A review of the spectrum of disease. J Urol 1992; 147:134–137.
20. Barbaric ZL: Principles of Genitourinary Radiology. New York, Thieme, 1991, pp 358–386.
21. Elster AD, Sobol WT, Hinson WH: Pseudolayering of Gd-DTPA in the urinary bladder. Radiology 1990; 174:379–381.
22. Amis ES Jr, Newhouse JH, Olsson CA: Continent urinary diversions: Review of current surgical procedures and radiologic imaging. Radiology 1988; 168:395–401.
23. Yousem DM, Gatewood OM, Goldman SM, et al: Synchronous and metachronous transitional cell carcinoma of the urinary tract: Prevalence, incidence, and radiographic detection. Radiology 1988; 167:613–618.
24. Bidwell JK, Dunne MG: Computed tomography of bladder malakoplakia. J Comput Assist Tomogr 1987; 11:909–910.
25. Amendola MA, Glazer GM, Grossman HB, et al: Staging of bladder carcinoma: MRI-CT-surgical correlation. AJR Am J Roentgenol 1986; 146:1179–1183.
26. Bonavita JA, Pollack HM: Trauma of the adult bladder and urethra. Semin Roentgenol 1983; 18:299–306.
27. Imray TJ, Kaplan P: Lower urinary tract infections and calculi in the adult. Semin Roentgenol 1983; 18:276–287.
28. Lang EK: Neoplasms of the bladder, prostate, and urethra. Semin Roentgenol 1983; 18:288–298.
29. Yoder IC, Pfister RC: Congenital anomalies of the adult bladder and urethra. Semin Roentgenol 1983; 18:267–275.

Illustrations • Urinary Bladder

1. Congenital Anomalies of the Bladder

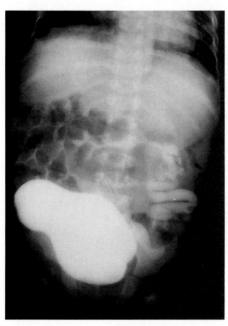

Fig. 1. Prune-belly syndrome in a 3-year-old boy. VCU shows a huge bladder and vesicoureteral reflux into the tortuous, dilated left ureter.

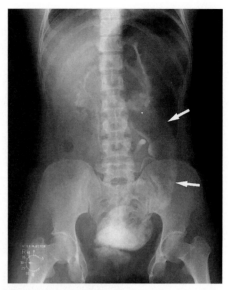

Fig. 2. Bladder exstrophy in a 27-year-old woman who underwent ureterocolostomy. A 30-minute IVU shows both urinary tracts and excretion of contrast material into the colon *(arrows)*. Note wide separation of the symphysis pubis.

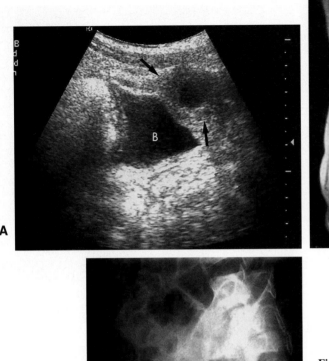

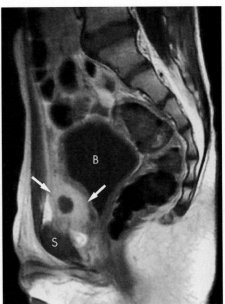

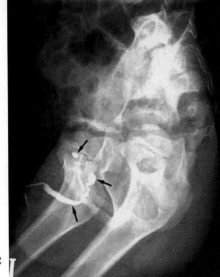

Fig. 3. Duplicated bladder and urethra in a 7-year-old boy with a history of suprapubic pain and fever. (**A–C,** Courtesy of Joo Won Lim, MD.)
A. Longitudinal US of the pelvis shows a thick-walled cystic mass *(arrows)* in the lower pelvis, anterior and inferior to the bladder (B).
B. Contrast-enhanced T1-weighted MR image in sagittal plane shows the mass with thick enhancing wall *(arrows).* B, urinary bladder; S, symphysis pubis. **C.** Injection of contrast material into a small opening in the dorsal surface of the penis demonstrates a duplicated urethra and bladder *(arrows).*

2. Urachal Anomalies

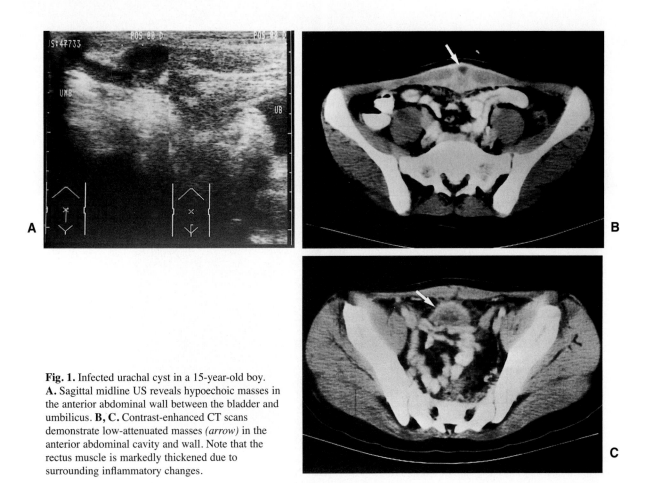

Fig. 1. Infected urachal cyst in a 15-year-old boy.
A. Sagittal midline US reveals hypoechoic masses in the anterior abdominal wall between the bladder and umbilicus. **B, C.** Contrast-enhanced CT scans demonstrate low-attenuated masses *(arrow)* in the anterior abdominal cavity and wall. Note that the rectus muscle is markedly thickened due to surrounding inflammatory changes.

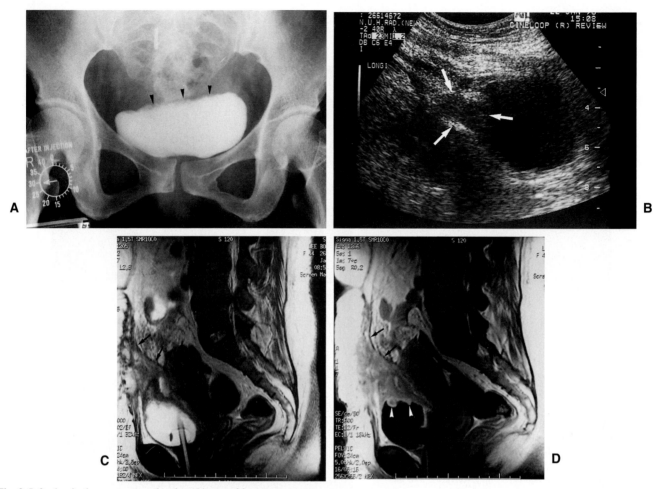

Fig. 2. Infection in the remnant urachus in a 44-year-old woman.
A. IVU shows fine irregularity in the dome of the urinary bladder *(arrowheads)*. **B.** Longitudinal US of the pelvis shows a soft tissue mass *(arrows)* in the dome of the urinary bladder, which has a cone shape and tapers cranially. **C.** T2-weighted MR image shows a cone-shaped, soft tissue mass in the region of the urachus with heterogeneous signal intensity *(arrows)*. **D.** Contrast-enhanced T1-weighted MR image demonstrates heterogeneous enhancement of the lesion *(arrows)* and bullous edema in the surface of the bladder *(arrowheads)*.

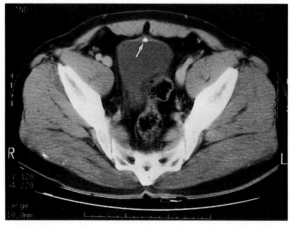

Fig. 3. Stone in the urachal diverticulum in a 50-year-old man. CT scan shows a dense calcification in the anterior wall of the bladder in the midline *(arrow)*.

3. Infections and Inflammatory Conditions of the Bladder

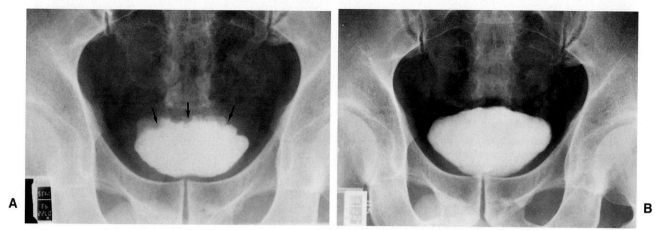

Fig. 1. Acute cystitis in a 45-year-old man.
A. Bladder image from an IVU shows irregular, scalloped contour of the dome of the bladder *(arrows)*. These findings represent mucosal edema and fold thickening due to inflammation. **B.** Follow-up IVU obtained 2 months later with treatment shows normalized contour of the bladder.

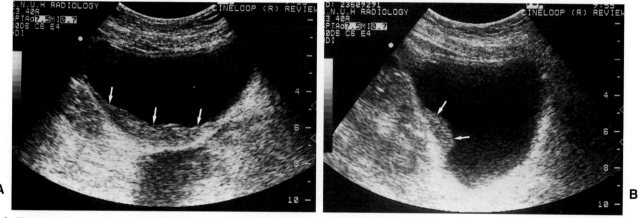

Fig. 2. Chronic active cystitis mimicking bladder tumor in a 47-year-old woman who had undergone radiation therapy for uterine cervical carcinoma 3 years earlier.
A, B. Transabdominal US images in transverse **(A)** and longitudinal **(B)** planes show focal thickening *(arrows)* of the posterior bladder wall mimicking a broad-based tumor.

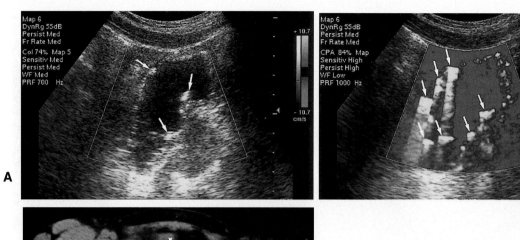

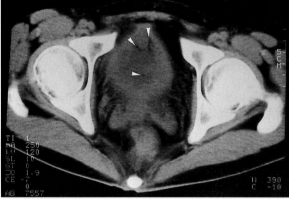

Fig. 3. Emphysematous cystitis in a 28-year-old man who underwent renal transplantation. (**A, B,** See also Color Section.)
A. Color Doppler US shows thickened bladder wall and dense echogenic lesions *(arrows)* in the bladder wall suggesting gas.
B. Power Doppler US demonstrates reverberation artifacts *(arrows)* from the bladder wall, suggesting the presence of gas in the bladder wall.
C. Nonenhanced CT shows mottled gas in the bladder wall *(arrowheads)*.

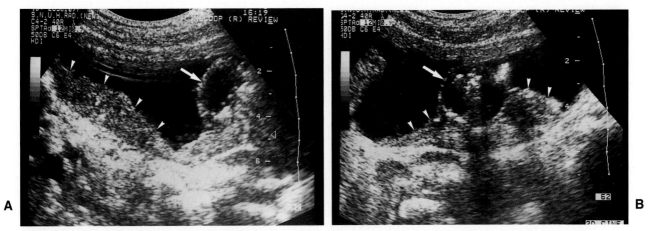

Fig. 4. Hemorrhagic cystitis in a 69-year-old man with diabetes.
A, B. US of the urinary bladder in longitudinal (**A**) and transverse (**B**) planes shows diffuse thickening of the posterior wall of the urinary bladder *(arrowheads)*. Note a Foley catheter balloon *(arrow)* in the bladder.

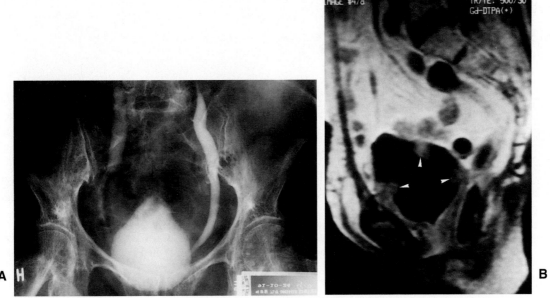

Fig. 5. Radiation-induced hemorrhagic cystitis in a 71-year-old woman who underwent radiation therapy for uterine cervical cancer.
A. Bladder image from an IVU shows reduced bladder capacity particularly in the dome region. Both ureters are slightly dilated. **B.** Contrast-enhanced T1-weighted MR image in sagittal plane shows multiple, enhancing, nodular lesions *(arrowheads)* in the bladder wall. Cystoscopy revealed that these lesions represent focal bullous edema and hemorrhage.

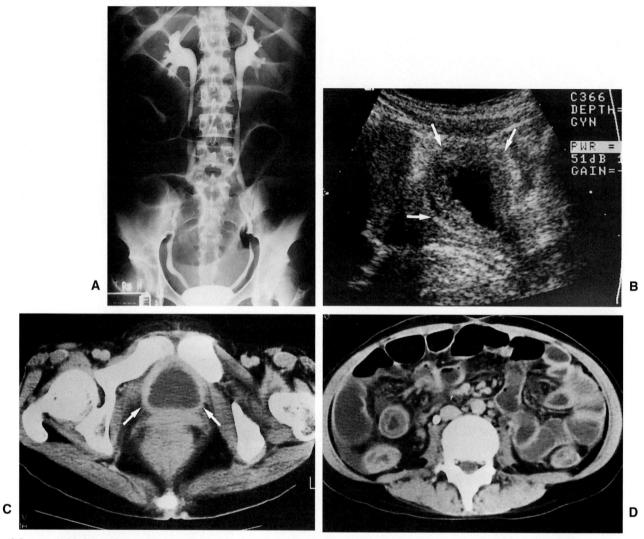

Fig. 6. Lupus cystitis in an 18-year-old woman.
A. A 3-hour-delayed IVU shows delayed excretion of contrast material in both urinary tracts and small bladder. Note markedly dilated, gas-filled bowel loops. **B.** Longitudinal US of the pelvis shows markedly thickened wall of the bladder *(arrows)*. **C.** Contrast-enhanced CT shows small capacity of the bladder with markedly thickened wall *(arrows)*. **D.** CT scan at the upper level shows dilated bowel loops with thickened, edematous wall.

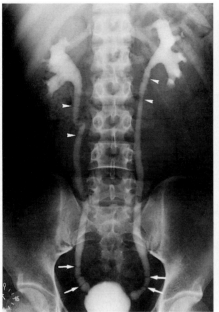
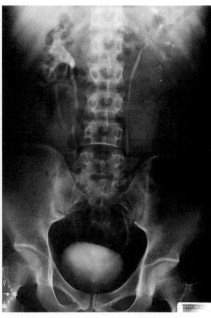
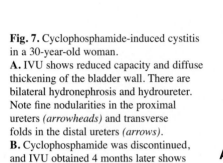

Fig. 7. Cyclophosphamide-induced cystitis in a 30-year-old woman.
A. IVU shows reduced capacity and diffuse thickening of the bladder wall. There are bilateral hydronephrosis and hydroureter. Note fine nodularities in the proximal ureters *(arrowheads)* and transverse folds in the distal ureters *(arrows)*.
B. Cyclophosphamide was discontinued, and IVU obtained 4 months later shows normalized urinary tracts.

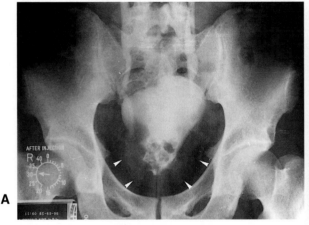
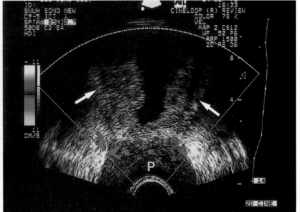
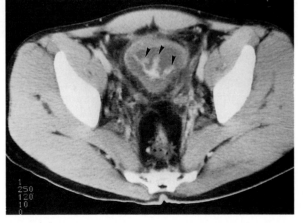

Fig. 8. Cystitis cystica in a 26-year-old man.
A. Bladder image from an IVU shows multiple, nodular masses and markedly thickened wall in the inferior part of the bladder. *Arrowheads* indicate outer margin of the bladder in the inferior part. Note that both ureters are dilated.
B. Transrectal color Doppler US in transverse plane shows markedly thickened bladder wall without prominent vessels *(arrows)*. P, prostate. (**B,** See also Color Section.) **C.** Contrast-enhanced CT shows irregular thickening of the inferior wall of the bladder. Note strong enhancement of the bladder mucosa in this part of the bladder *(arrowheads)*. Cystoscopic biopsy revealed cystitis cystica.

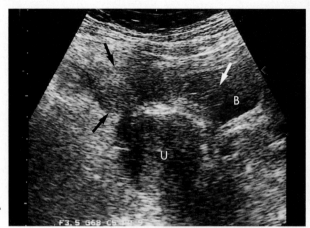

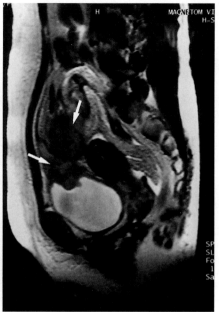

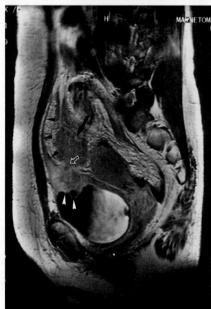

Fig. 9. Malacoplakia of the urachus in a 47-year-old woman.
A. Longitudinal US of the lower abdomen shows ill-defined, hypoechoic masses *(arrows)* superior to the bladder (B). U, uterus. **B.** T2-weighted MR image in sagittal plane shows ill-defined supravesical masses of low signal intensity *(arrows)* that are continuous with the dome of the bladder. **C.** Contrast-enhanced T1-weighted sagittal MR image demonstrates the masses with various enhancements. There is a triangular, enhancing mass in the dome of the bladder, which is continuous with the urachus *(black arrowheads)*. Note the changes of bullous edema *(white arrowheads)* in the dome of the urinary bladder. The mass in the cranial site *(arrow)* does not enhance and is probably caused by rupture *(open arrow)* of the urachal mass. Both US-guided and cystoscopic biopsies revealed malacoplakia. After treatment with antibiotics, the lesions nearly disappeared.

4. Transitional Cell Carcinoma of the Bladder

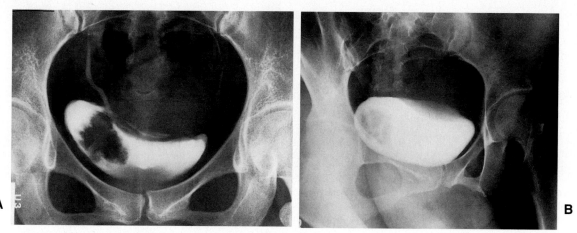

Fig. 1. Transitional cell carcinoma of the bladder in a 33-year-old woman.
A. Bladder image from an IVU demonstrates a large filling defect with irregular papillary surface in the bladder. **B.** On right anterior oblique view, the stipple sign is well demonstrated, which represents entrapped contrast material in the surface of the papillary tumor.

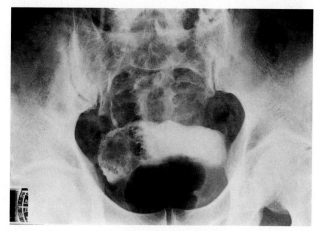

Fig. 2. Bladder tumor in a 64-year-old man. Bladder image from an IVU shows a large filling defect in the bladder with stippling of contrast material suggesting papillary surface of the tumor.

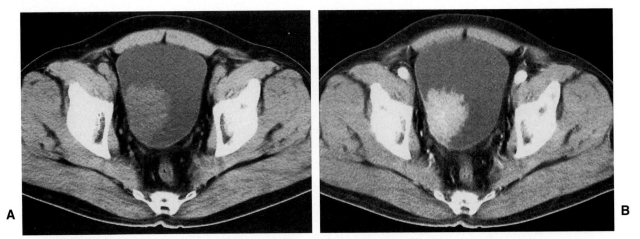

Fig. 3. Transitional cell carcinoma of the bladder in a 58-year-old man.
A, B. Nonenhanced (**A**) and contrast-enhanced (**B**) CT scans show a large, papillary tumor in the right posterior aspect of the bladder. The tumor enhances well with contrast material. Bladder contour is smooth, and there is no perivesical tumor spread.

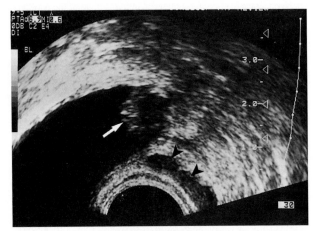

Fig. 4. Bladder cancer incidentally found on transrectal US of the prostate in a 71-year-old man. Transrectal US in transverse plane shows a soft tissue mass (*arrow*) in the left aspect of the urinary bladder. *Arrowheads* indicate right seminal vesicle.

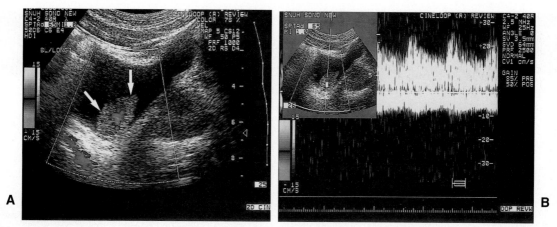

Fig. 5. Transitional cell carcinoma in a 47-year-old man.
A. Color Doppler US of the bladder in longitudinal plane shows a fungating mass *(arrows)* in the posterior wall of the bladder with intratumoral vessels. (**A,** See also Color Section.) **B.** Spectral Doppler US performed on the intratumoral vessels shows low-resistance arterial flow.

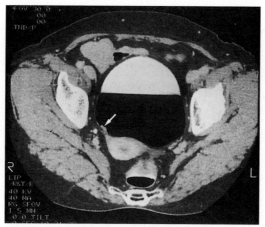

Fig. 6. Small transitional cell carcinoma in a 46-year-old man. CT scan obtained following instillation of diluted contrast material and air with the patient in prone position demonstrates a small sessile lesion *(arrow)* in right posterolateral wall of the bladder. Negative contrast by air depicts the lesion clearly.

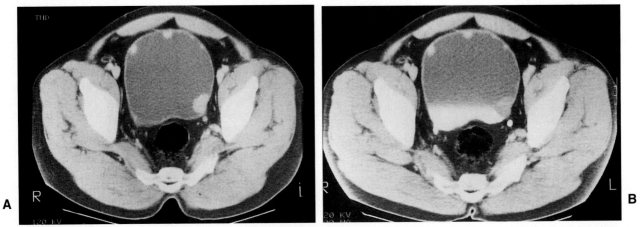

Fig. 7. Multiple transitional cell carcinomas of the bladder in a 62-year-old man.
A, B. Contrast-enhanced CT scans in early vascular (**A**) and late excretory (**B**) phases show multiple fungating tumors in the bladder. Note that the tumors are well enhancing in early vascular phase, and there is no evidence of extravesical tumor spread.

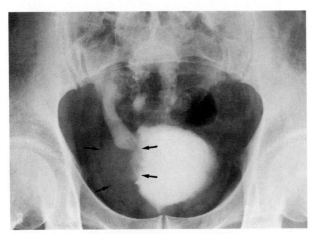

Fig. 8. A 59-year-old man with an infiltrating transitional cell carcinoma of the bladder. IVU shows a large, irregularly margined mass *(arrows)* involving the right side of the bladder and dilation of the right terminal ureter.

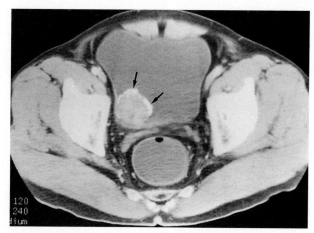

Fig. 9. Transitional cell carcinoma of the bladder with surface calcification in a 62-year-old man. Contrast-enhanced CT shows a round, soft tissue mass that protrudes into the bladder lumen. There are curvilinear calcifications *(arrows)* on the surface of the mass. The outer margin of the bladder is smooth, representing no extravesical extension.

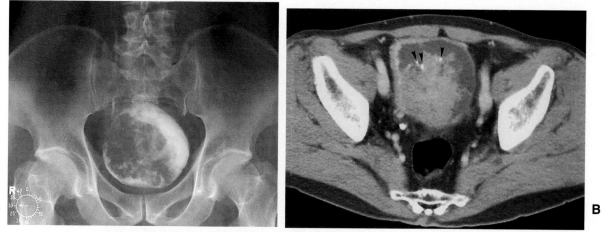

Fig. 10. Large transitional cell carcinoma of the bladder in a 55-year-old man.
A. Bladder image from IVU shows a large tumor with a papillary surface showing stipple sign in the bladder. **B.** Contrast-enhanced CT shows a large bladder tumor with mottled calcifications *(arrowheads)* in the surface of the tumor. The outer margin of the bladder is smooth, suggesting the absence of perivesical invasion.

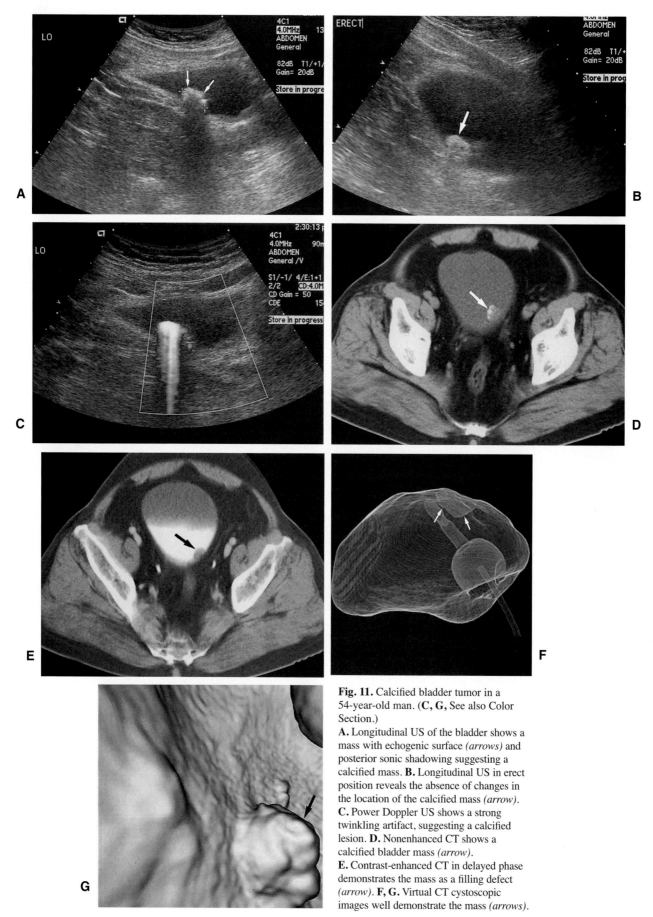

Fig. 11. Calcified bladder tumor in a 54-year-old man. (**C, G,** See also Color Section.)
A. Longitudinal US of the bladder shows a mass with echogenic surface *(arrows)* and posterior sonic shadowing suggesting a calcified mass. **B.** Longitudinal US in erect position reveals the absence of changes in the location of the calcified mass *(arrow)*. **C.** Power Doppler US shows a strong twinkling artifact, suggesting a calcified lesion. **D.** Nonenhanced CT shows a calcified bladder mass *(arrow)*.
E. Contrast-enhanced CT in delayed phase demonstrates the mass as a filling defect *(arrow)*. **F, G.** Virtual CT cystoscopic images well demonstrate the mass *(arrows)*.

5. Transitional Cell Carcinoma of the Bladder: Perivesical Tumor Spread

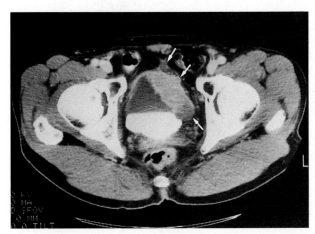

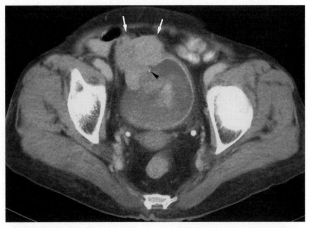

Fig. 1. Transitional cell carcinoma with squamous differentiation in the bladder with perivesical extension in a 63-year-old man. Contrast-enhanced CT shows a flat, infiltrating tumor in the left anterior wall of the bladder with extension of the tumor into the perivesical region *(arrows)*.

Fig. 2. Transitional cell carcinoma of the bladder with perivesical tumor extension in a 77-year-old man. Contrast-enhanced CT shows a large tumor in the anterior wall of the bladder. The tumor has an extensive perivesical invasion with an irregular infiltrating margin *(arrows)*. Note a small calcification in the surface of the tumor *(arrowhead)*.

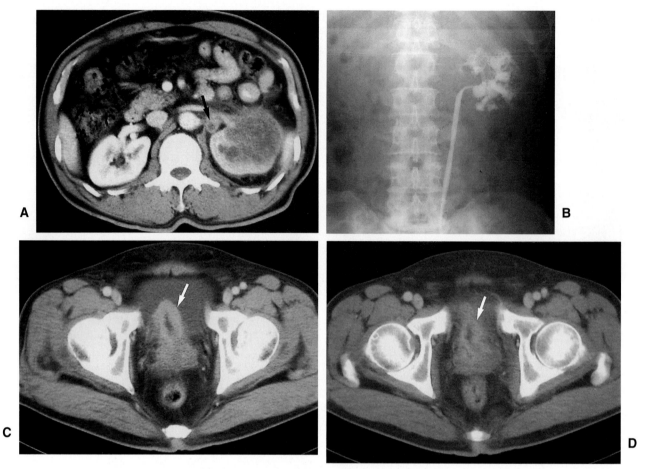

Fig. 3. Transitional cell carcinoma of the bladder with invasion of the prostate in a 54-year-old man who also has transitional cell carcinoma of the renal pelvis.
A. Contrast-enhanced CT of the kidney shows a large, low-attenuated, infiltrating tumor in the left kidney that was proved to be a transitional cell carcinoma of the renal pelvis with renal parenchymal invasion. Also note a necrotic lymph node *(arrow)* in the renal hilar region. **B.** Left RGP shows poor opacification of the renal pelvis and upper-polar calyx. Note puddling of contrast material, which is probably an insinuation of contrast material into the tumor. **C, D.** CT scans of the bladder show an enhancing tumor *(arrow)* in the neck of the bladder with invasion of the prostate and seminal vesicles.

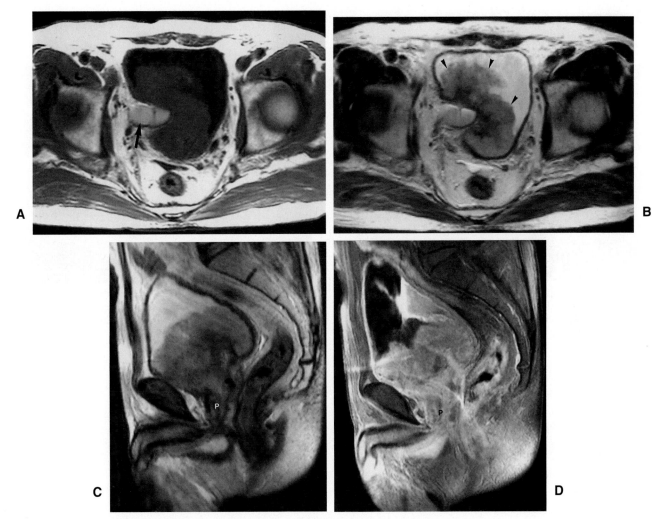

Fig. 4. Transitional cell carcinoma of the bladder with invasion of the prostate in a 64-year-old man.
A. T1-weighted MR image in transverse plane shows a large tumor in the bladder with involvement of the right ureterovesical junction causing dilation of the right ureter *(arrow)*. Note that the dilated right distal ureter has high-intensity, bloody content. **B.** T2-weighted MR image in transverse plane well demonstrates the tumor *(arrowheads)* in the bladder. **C, D.** T2-weighted **(C)** and contrast-enhanced T1-weighted **(D)** MR images in the sagittal plane well demonstrate the extent of the tumor, which involves the prostate (P).

6. Squamous Cell Carcinoma of the Bladder

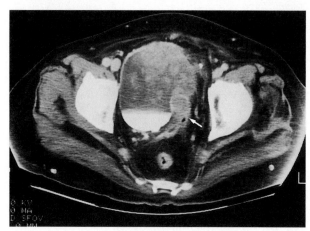

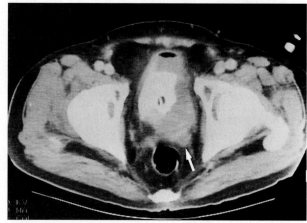

Fig. 1. Squamous cell carcinoma of the urinary bladder in a 65-year-old woman. Contrast-enhanced CT shows broad-based tumor masses in the left wall of the urinary bladder with perivesical spread and invasion of the sigmoid colon *(arrow)*.

Fig. 2. Squamous cell carcinoma of the urinary bladder in a 66-year-old man. Contrast-enhanced CT shows diffuse thickening of the bladder wall on the left side with perivesical tumor spread and invasion of the left seminal vesicle *(arrow)*.

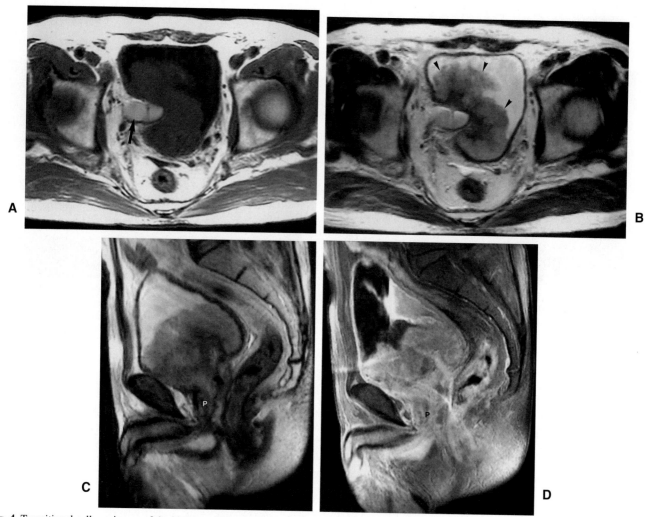

Fig. 4. Transitional cell carcinoma of the bladder with invasion of the prostate in a 64-year-old man.
A. T1-weighted MR image in transverse plane shows a large tumor in the bladder with involvement of the right ureterovesical junction causing dilation of the right ureter *(arrow)*. Note that the dilated right distal ureter has high-intensity, bloody content. **B.** T2-weighted MR image in transverse plane well demonstrates the tumor *(arrowheads)* in the bladder. **C, D.** T2-weighted **(C)** and contrast-enhanced T1-weighted **(D)** MR images in the sagittal plane well demonstrate the extent of the tumor, which involves the prostate (P).

6. Squamous Cell Carcinoma of the Bladder

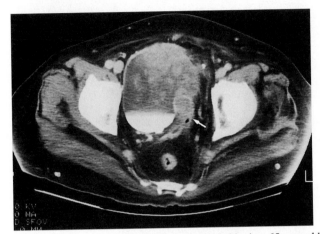

Fig. 1. Squamous cell carcinoma of the urinary bladder in a 65-year-old woman. Contrast-enhanced CT shows broad-based tumor masses in the left wall of the urinary bladder with perivesical spread and invasion of the sigmoid colon *(arrow)*.

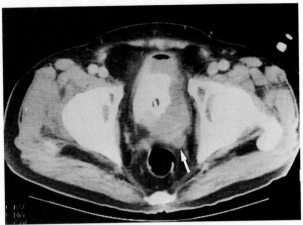

Fig. 2. Squamous cell carcinoma of the urinary bladder in a 66-year-old man. Contrast-enhanced CT shows diffuse thickening of the bladder wall on the left side with perivesical tumor spread and invasion of the left seminal vesicle *(arrow)*.

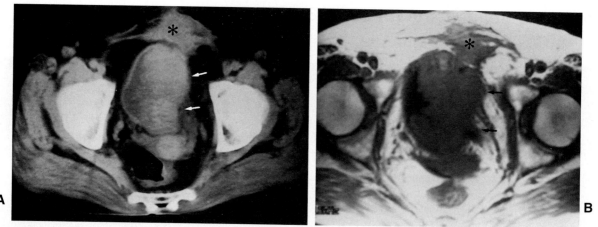

Fig. 3. Squamous cell carcinoma of the bladder in a 56-year-old woman.
A. Contrast-enhanced CT shows a large mass in the left aspect of the bladder with deformed contour. Note irregular outer margin of the bladder *(arrows)* and infiltrating mass in the abdominal wall *(asterisk)*. **B.** T1-weighted MR image well demonstrates the bladder tumor, perivesical tumor spread *(arrows)*, and extension of the tumor in the anterior abdominal wall *(asterisk)*.

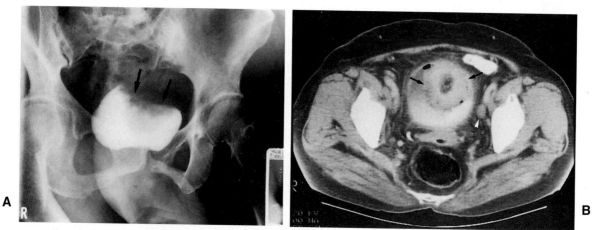

Fig. 4. Squamous cell carcinoma of the bladder in a 66-year-old woman.
A. Bladder image from an IVU shows a large, irregularly margined mass *(arrows)* in the dome of the urinary bladder. **B.** Contrast-enhanced CT demonstrates a large polypoid mass *(arrows)* arising from the anterior wall of the bladder. There is a low-attenuated area within the mass, suggesting central necrosis. Note an enlarged lymph node in the left pelvic cavity *(arrowhead)*.

7. Adenocarcinoma of the Bladder

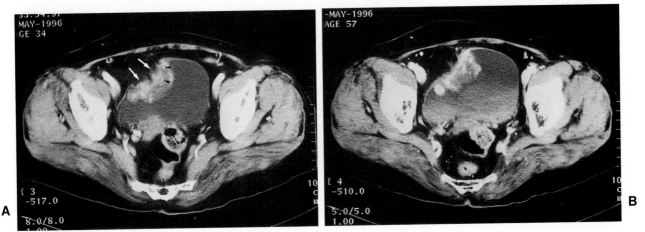

Fig. 1. Adenocarcinoma of the bladder in a 65-year-old woman.
A, B. Contrast-enhanced CT scans show a well-enhancing mass arising in the right anterolateral wall of the bladder. Bladder contour is deformed, and there are irregularities in the outer margin of the bladder *(arrows* in **A***)* indicating perivesical extension of the tumor. Note mottled calcifications *(arrowheads* in **A***)* in the tumor.

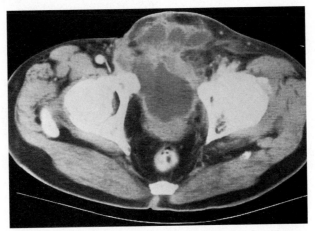

Fig. 2. Mucinous adenocarcinoma of the bladder in a 54-year-old man who had suprapubic cystostomy for 30 years. Contrast-enhanced CT shows irregular thickening of the bladder wall and extensive perivesical spread of the tumor in the anterior abdominal wall.

8. Other Tumors of the Bladder

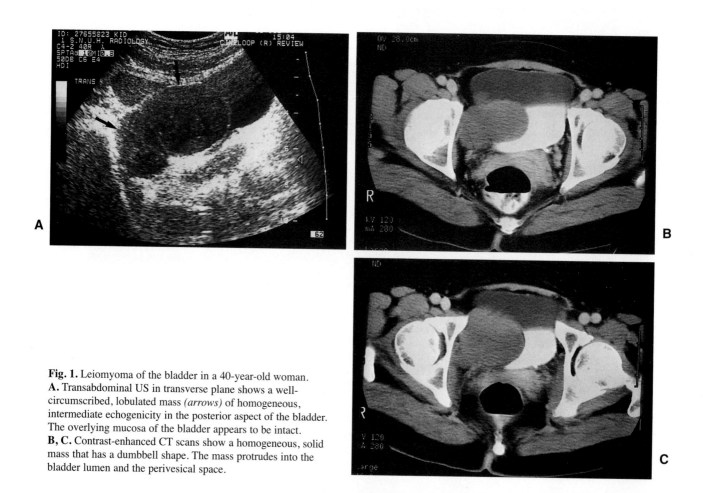

Fig. 1. Leiomyoma of the bladder in a 40-year-old woman.
A. Transabdominal US in transverse plane shows a well-circumscribed, lobulated mass *(arrows)* of homogeneous, intermediate echogenicity in the posterior aspect of the bladder. The overlying mucosa of the bladder appears to be intact.
B, C. Contrast-enhanced CT scans show a homogeneous, solid mass that has a dumbbell shape. The mass protrudes into the bladder lumen and the perivesical space.

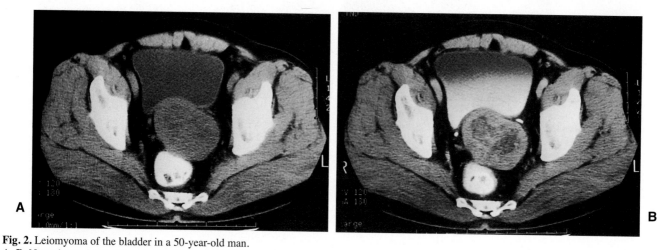

Fig. 2. Leiomyoma of the bladder in a 50-year-old man.
A, B. Nonenhanced (**A**) and contrast-enhanced (**B**) CT scans show a smooth-margined, soft tissue mass in the space between the bladder and rectum. The mass is relatively homogeneous on nonenhanced CT but shows heterogeneous enhancement on contrast-enhanced CT. At surgery the mass was arising in the posterior wall of the urinary bladder.

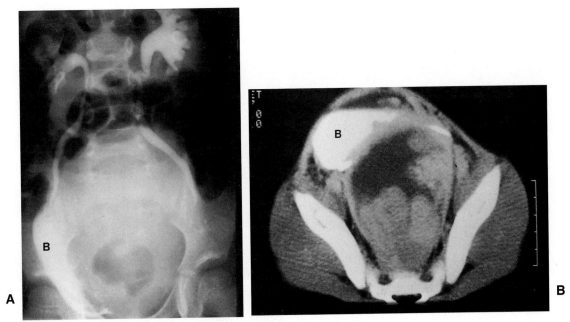

Fig. 3. Embryonal rhabdomyosarcoma in a 5-year-old girl.
A. IVU demonstrates a huge mass in the pelvic cavity with displacement of the remnant bladder lumen (B) and distal ureters. **B.** Contrast-enhanced CT in axial plane demonstrates a bulky, soft tissue mass with extensive necrosis. Bladder lumen (B) is displaced anteriorly and partially filled with the tumor. The large size of the bladder mass in a young patient is a typical feature of rhabdomyosarcoma.

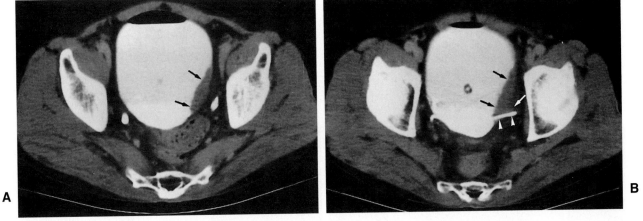

Fig. 4. Small cell carcinoma of the bladder in a 65-year-old man.
A, B. Contrast-enhanced CT scans show a broad-based, flat mass *(black arrows)* in the left wall of the urinary bladder. Note that the mass extends into the perivesical adipose tissue *(white arrow* in **B)** in front of the left terminal ureter *(arrowheads* in **B).**

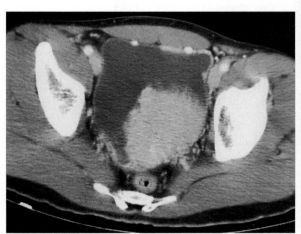

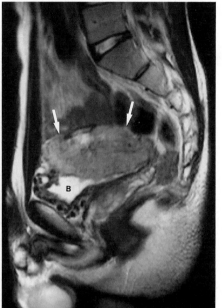

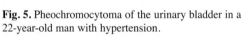

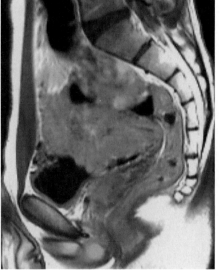

Fig. 5. Pheochromocytoma of the urinary bladder in a 22-year-old man with hypertension.
A. Contrast-enhanced CT shows a large, enhancing mass in the posterior aspect of the bladder. Note prominent vessels around the mass supplying the mass. **B.** T2-weighted sagittal MR image shows a large mass *(arrows)* in the dome of the urinary bladder. Note that low-intensity wall of the bladder is not defined in the dome, suggesting the mural origin of the mass. B, lumen of the bladder. **C.** Contrast-enhanced T1-weighted MR image in sagittal plane shows strong enhancement of the mass.

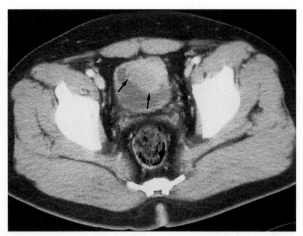

Fig. 6. Neurofibroma of the bladder in a 23-year-old man. Contrast-enhanced CT shows a soft tissue mass *(arrows)* in the anterior wall of the bladder. This finding is indistinguishable from the findings of other bladder tumors.

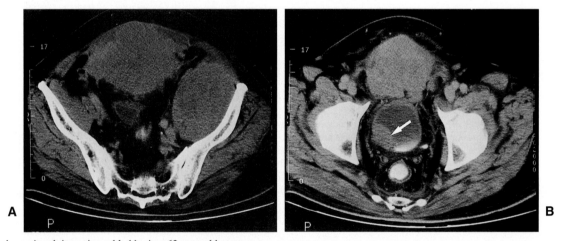

Fig. 7. Lymphoma involving urinary bladder in a 62-year-old man.
A. Contrast-enhanced CT shows large, homogeneous, soft tissue masses in the anterior and left aspects of the pelvic cavity. **B.** CT scan at lower level shows a mass in the urinary bladder *(arrow)*. US-guided biopsy of the pelvic mass and urine cytology revealed malignant lymphoma of anaplastic large cell type.

9. Metastasis and Direct Invasion to the Bladder

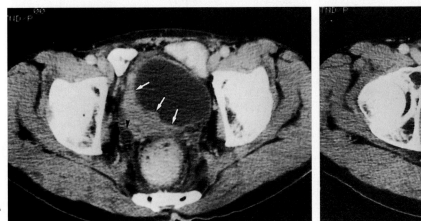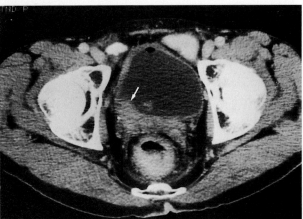

A **B**

Fig. 1. Isolated bladder metastasis from stomach cancer in a 52-year-old man who had undergone total gastrectomy 3 years earlier.
A, B. Contrast-enhanced CT scans show diffuse thickening of the right and posterior wall of the urinary bladder *(arrows)* with perivesical infiltration. Note the dilated right ureter *(arrowhead* in **A**) just before entering the bladder.

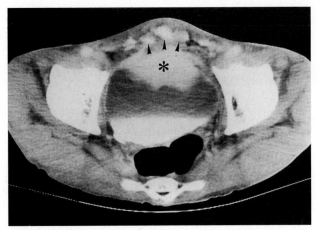

Fig. 2. Isolated bladder metastasis from stomach cancer in a 60-year-old man who had undergone total gastrectomy 1 year earlier. Contrast-enhanced CT shows a broad-based, homogeneous, soft tissue mass in the anterior wall of the bladder *(asterisk)*. Also note the multiple nodular masses in the anterior abdominal wall *(arrowheads)*. Cystoscopic biopsy revealed metastatic adenocarcinoma from stomach cancer. (From Kim HC, Kim SH, Hwang SI, et al: Isolated bladder metastases from stomach cancer: CT demonstration. Abdom Imaging 2001; 26:333–335.)

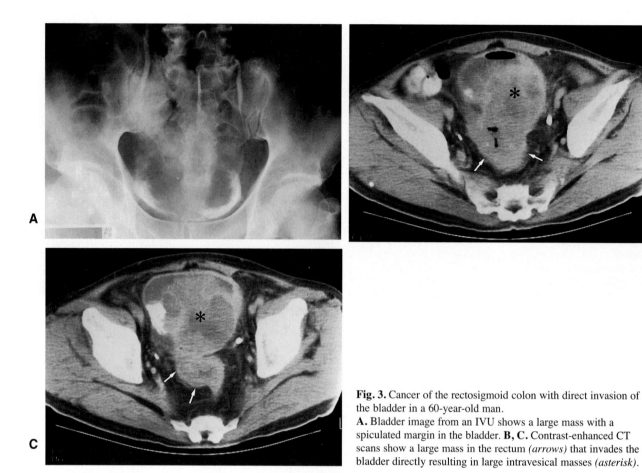

Fig. 3. Cancer of the rectosigmoid colon with direct invasion of the bladder in a 60-year-old man.
A. Bladder image from an IVU shows a large mass with a spiculated margin in the bladder. **B, C.** Contrast-enhanced CT scans show a large mass in the rectum *(arrows)* that invades the bladder directly resulting in large intravesical masses *(asterisk)*.

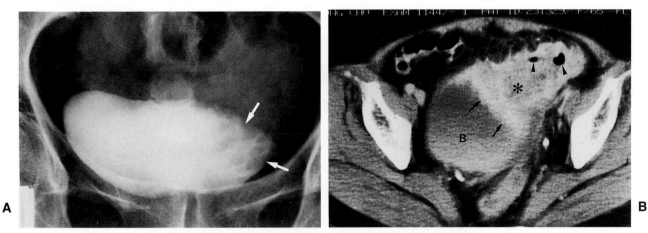

Fig. 4. Sigmoid colon cancer with direct invasion of the bladder in a 65-year-old woman. (**A, B,** From Kim SH, Na DG, Choi BI, et al: Direct invasion of urinary bladder from sigmoid colon cancer: CT findings. J Comput Assist Tomogr 1992; 16:709–712.)
A. Bladder image of an IVU shows irregular nodular indentations *(arrows)* on the left dome and left side-wall of the bladder. **B.** Contrast-enhanced CT demonstrates a large soft tissue mass *(asterisk)* contiguous with the bladder wall *(arrows)* and sigmoid colon that contains irregular luminal air *(arrowheads)*. B, bladder lumen.

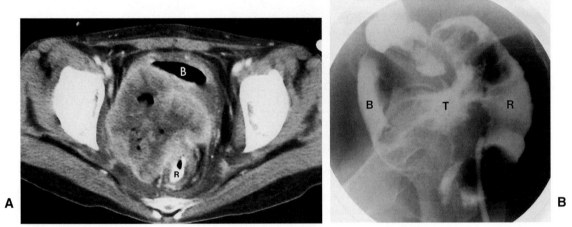

Fig. 5. Recurrent uterine cervical carcinoma with invasion of the bladder and rectum in a 28-year-old woman.
A. Contrast-enhanced CT shows a large recurrent tumor in the pelvic cavity, which has extensive necrosis and air. Also note air in the urinary bladder (B). The mass has poor demarcation with the bladder and rectum, suggesting direct invasion of those organs. R, rectum. **B.** Instillation of contrast material into the rectum (R) demonstrates a fistulous communication with the recurrent tumor (T) and bladder (B).

10. Tumors of the Urachus

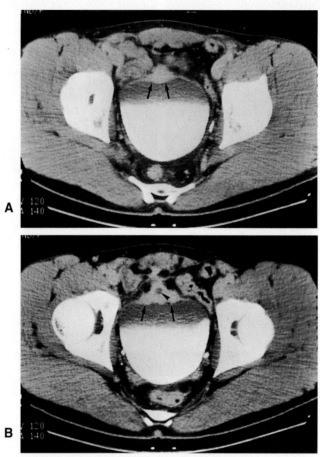

Fig. 1. Urachal adenocarcinoma in a 33-year-old man.
A, B. Contrast-enhanced CT scans show a midline mass in the anterior wall of the urinary bladder *(arrows)*. The mass is predominantly exophytic and contains a small cystic lesion *(arrowhead* in **B**).

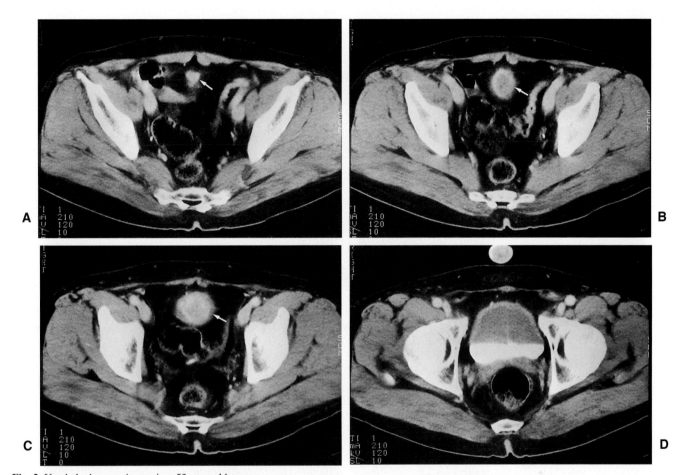

Fig. 2. Urachal adenocarcinoma in a 53-year-old man.
A–D. Consecutive images of contrast-enhanced CT from cranial to caudal direction show an elongated soft tissue mass (*arrow* in **A–C**) in the course of the urachus. Note that the mass has a spiculated margin suggesting periurachal infiltration. The mass does not protrude into the bladder lumen on **D**.

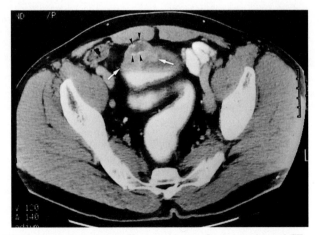

Fig. 3. Urachal cancer in a 53-year-old man. Contrast-enhanced CT shows an ill-defined mass (*arrows*) in the anterior wall of the dome of the bladder. Note that the mass contains punctuate calcifications (*arrowheads*).

11. Bladder Stones

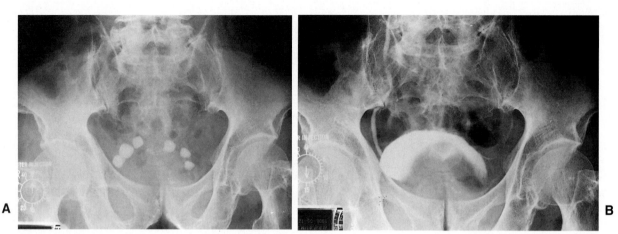

Fig. 1. Multiple bladder stones in an 81-year-old man with severe prostatic hyperplasia.
A. Plain radiograph shows multiple, homogeneously dense stones in the pelvic cavity. The stones are arranged in a line with superior convexity. **B.** On a bladder image from IVU, the stones are obscured by excreted contrast material, indicating an intravesical location of the stones. The base of the bladder is elevated due to benign prostatic hyperplasia.

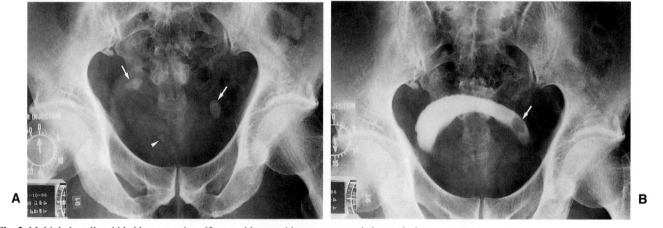

Fig. 2. Multiple lamellated bladder stones in a 62-year-old man with severe prostatic hyperplasia.
A. Plain radiograph shows two radiopaque, lamellated stones *(arrows)*. A small prostatic calcification is also seen *(arrowhead)*. **B.** On a bladder image from IVU, one stone is seen as a filling defect *(arrow)*, whereas the other is obscured by excreted contrast material. Note the markedly elevated base of the bladder due to large prostate.

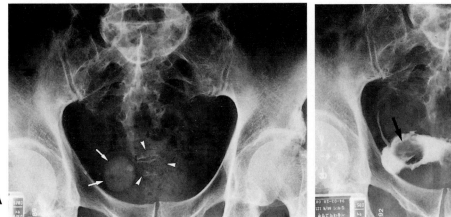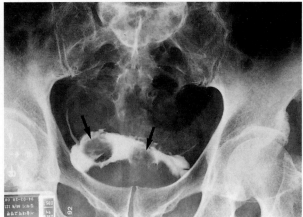

Fig. 3. Bladder stones in an 86-year-old man with benign prostatic hyperplasia.
A. Plain radiograph shows a round, faintly opaque stone in the right side of the pelvic cavity *(arrows)*. Another faintly opaque stone *(arrowheads)* is difficult to detect due to overlying bowel gas and sacrum. **B.** Bladder image from an IVU well demonstrates two stones appearing as filling defects *(arrows)* and elevated bladder base due to prostatic hyperplasia.

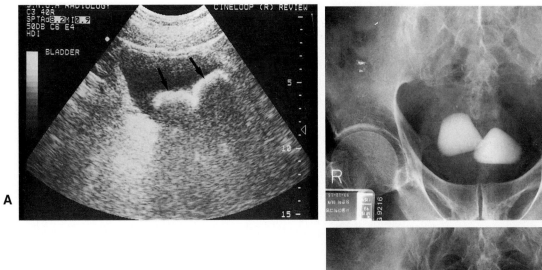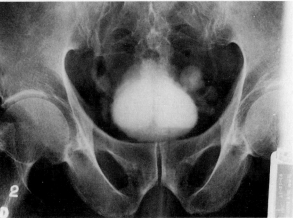

Fig. 4. Large bladder stones in a 59-year-old man with neurogenic bladder.
A. Transabdominal US shows two large stones appearing as curvilinear, echogenic lesions *(arrows)* accompanying posterior sonic shadowing. **B.** Plain radiograph shows two large faceted bladder stones with homogeneous radiopacity. **C.** Bladder image from an IVU confirmed intravesical location of the stones. Note multiple diverticular projections of the bladder due to neurogenic bladder.

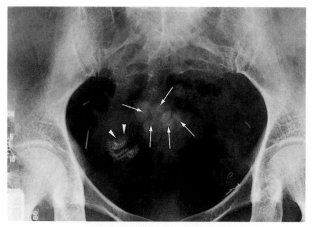

Fig. 5. Bladder stones formed over surgical staples in a 37-year-old woman who had undergone partial cystectomy and augmentation cystoplasty for bladder cancer 3 years earlier. Plain radiograph shows multiple stones of faint radiopacity. Each stone contains a surgical staple in its center *(arrows)*. Note a small stone *(arrowheads)* forming on the staples that were used to make an intussuscepted afferent nipple valve of the ileal reservoir to prevent reflux.

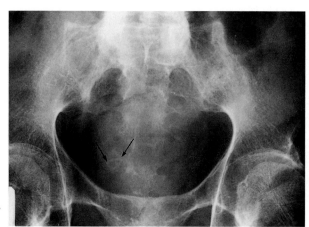

A

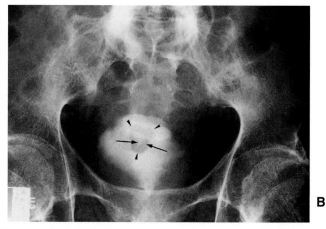

B

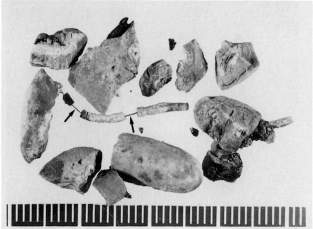

C

Fig. 6. Bladder calculi formed over a hair nidus in a 66-year-old quadriplegic man in whom intermittent catheterization was done due to neurogenic bladder. (**A–C,** From Lee HJ, Kim SH: Characteristic plain radiographic and intravenous urographic findings of bladder calculi formed over a hair nidus: A case report. Korean J Radiol 2001; 2:61–62.)
A. Plain radiograph shows a ringlike radiopacity in the pelvic cavity *(arrows)*. **B.** Bladder image of an IVU shows a round filling defect *(arrowheads)* that contains the ringlike radiopacity *(arrows)* that was seen on plain radiograph.
C. Photograph of fragmented and removed stones shows that the ringlike radiopacity was a linear calcification formed over a hair *(arrows)*. The radiolucent part of the stone was formed over the linear radiopaque calcification.

12. Bladder Injury

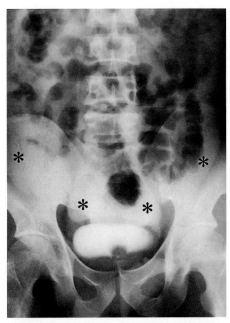

Fig. 1. Intraperitoneal rupture of the bladder in a 29-year-old man who received blunt trauma on the lower abdomen. IVU demonstrates intraperitoneal leak of contrast material *(asterisks)*.

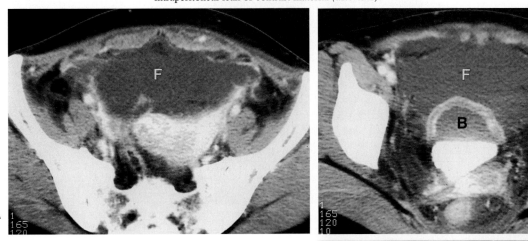

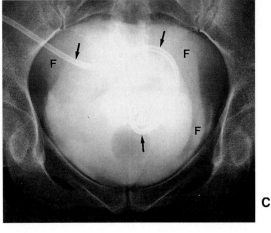

Fig. 2. Extraperitoneal bladder rupture in a 45-year-old woman who fell down. (**A–C,** Courtesy of Dae Hee Han, MD.)
A. Contrast-enhanced CT through upper pelvis shows a low-attenuated fluid collection (F) in the prevesical space.
B. Contrast-enhanced CT through the urinary bladder demonstrates molar tooth configuration, typical of prevesical fluid collection (F). B, urinary bladder. **C.** Cystogram obtained with contrast material instilled through Foley catheter shows leak of contrast material into the perivesical fluid collection (F). No intraperitoneal leak is seen. A pigtail catheter *(arrows)* was inserted into the perivesical urinoma.

13. Fistulas of the Bladder

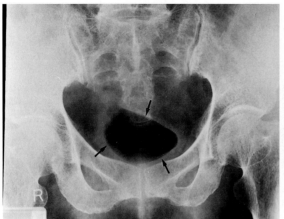

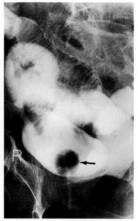

A

B

Fig. 1. Vesicoenteric fistula in a 60-year-old woman with advanced uterine cervical carcinoma.
A. Plain radiograph shows gas-filled urinary bladder *(arrows)*. **B.** Cystogram demonstrates opacification of ileal loops of small bowel. Note the balloon of the Foley catheter *(arrow)* in the bladder.

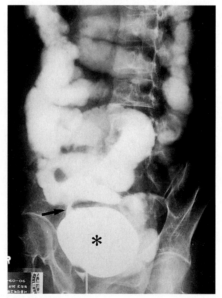

Fig. 2. Vesicoenteric fistula in a 24-year-old woman with Crohn's disease. Cystography opacifies the bladder *(asterisk)* and then contrast material flows freely into the ileum through the fistula *(arrow)*.

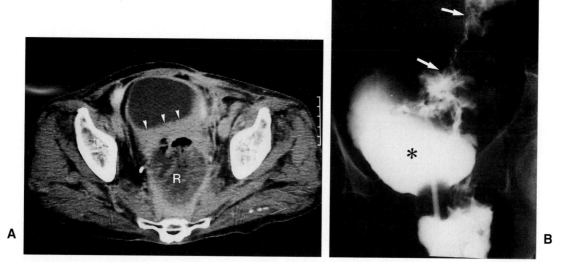

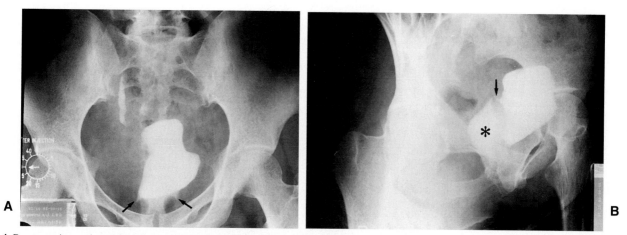

Fig. 3. Vesicocolic fistula in a 60-year-old man with colon cancer.
A. Contrast-enhanced CT demonstrates a circumferentially thickened wall of the rectosigmoid colon (R) and irregularly thickened posterior wall of the urinary bladder *(arrowheads)*. The fat plane between the rectosigmoid colon and bladder is obliterated. Intraluminal air is absent in the bladder.
B. Cystography opacifies the bladder *(asterisk)* and leak of contrast material into the rectosigmoid colon, which has an annuloconstricting lesion *(arrows)*.

Fig. 4. Postoperative vesicovaginal fistula in a 27-year-old woman.
A. IVU shows deformed urinary bladder and suspicious extravesical collection of contrast material *(arrows)*. **B.** Radiograph obtained with the patient in right anterior oblique projection well demonstrates collection of contrast material in the vagina *(asterisk)*. Note the fistulous tract *(arrow)* between the bladder and vagina.

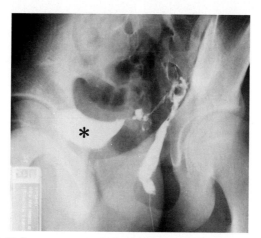

Fig. 5. Vesicocutaneous fistula in a 19-year-old man who had a history of trauma. Fistulography demonstrates a long fistulous tract and opacification of the bladder *(asterisk)*.

14. Bladder Diverticulum

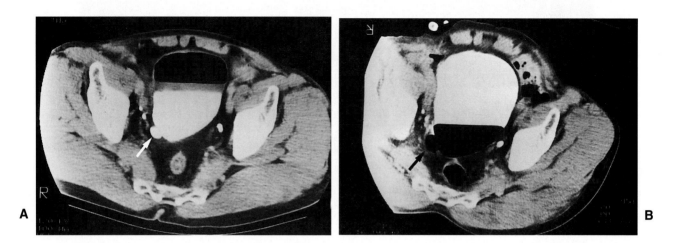

Fig. 1. Small diverticulum of the urinary bladder in a 78-year-old man.
A. CT scan with double contrast in the bladder with the patient in supine position shows a small diverticulum in the right posterior wall of the bladder filled with contrast material *(arrow)*. Note that the diverticulum is close to the right ureterovesical junction. **B.** CT scan obtained with the patient in prone position demonstrates the diverticulum filled with air *(arrow)*.

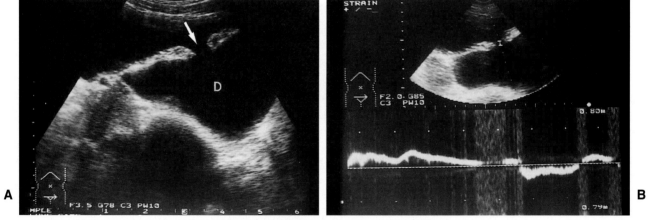

Fig. 2. Large diverticulum of the bladder in a 75-year-old man.
A. US of the bladder shows a large diverticulum (D) connected to the bladder through a narrow neck *(arrow)*. **B.** Spectral Doppler US obtained in the neck of the diverticulum with the patient performing straining and relaxing shows to-and-fro flow of urine through the neck of the diverticulum.

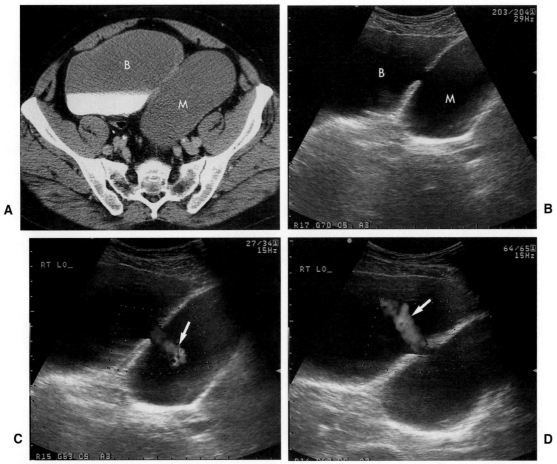

Fig. 3. Large diverticulum of the bladder in a 67-year-old man.
A. Contrast-enhanced CT shows a large cystic mass (M) in the left pelvic cavity, posterolateral to the urinary bladder (B). There is a suspicious small window between the mass and bladder. **B.** US of the pelvis in transverse plane well demonstrates the window between the bladder (B) and mass (M). **C, D.** Power Doppler US of the bladder with the patient straining (**C**) and relaxing (**D**) shows to-and-fro movement of urine *(arrow)* through the window between the bladder and mass.

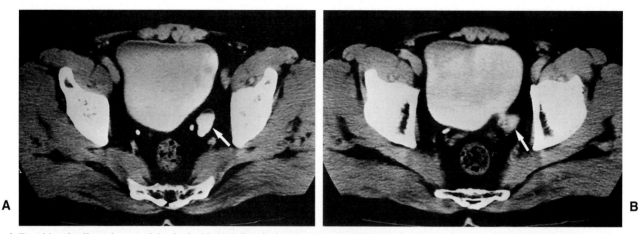

Fig. 4. Transitional cell carcinoma arising in the bladder diverticulum in a 50-year-old man.
A. Contrast-enhanced CT shows a small diverticulum filled with contrast material in the left posterior aspect of the bladder *(arrow)*. **B.** CT scan at the immediately lower level shows that the diverticulum is filled with a soft tissue mass *(arrow)*.

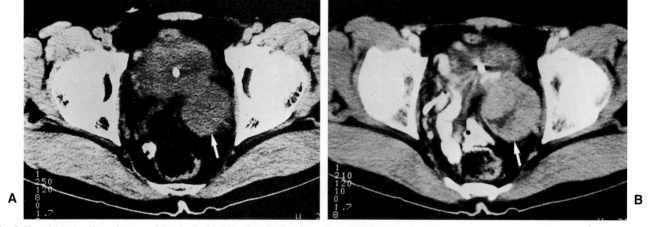

Fig. 5. Transitional cell carcinoma arising in the bladder diverticulum in a 45-year-old man.
A, B. Nonenhanced and contrast-enhanced CT scans of the pelvis show a large soft tissue mass *(arrow)* in the left pelvic cavity that is continuous with the left posterior wall of the bladder. Note that the mass has low-attenuated central necrosis on contrast-enhanced CT.

15. Cystocele

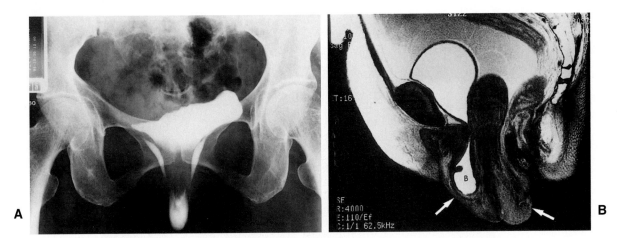

Fig. 1. Cystocele and uterine prolapse in a 57-year-old woman.
A. Bladder image from an IVU shows prolapse of the base and trigone of the bladder, and distal ureters. **B.** T2-weighted MR image in sagittal plane well demonstrates protruding perineal mass *(arrows)* containing the bladder (B), vagina, uterus, and anterior rectal wall.

16. Stress Urinary Incontinence

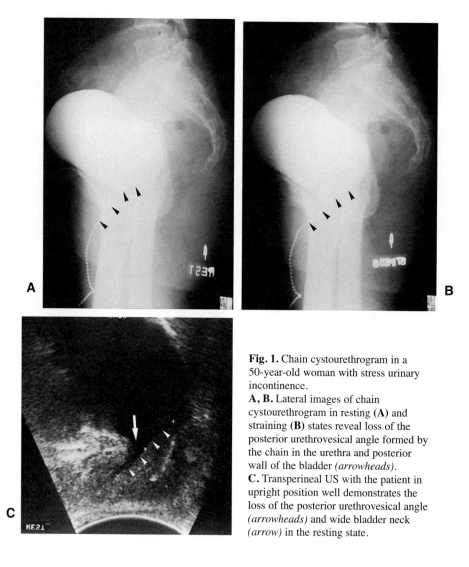

Fig. 1. Chain cystourethrogram in a 50-year-old woman with stress urinary incontinence.
A, B. Lateral images of chain cystourethrogram in resting (**A**) and straining (**B**) states reveal loss of the posterior urethrovesical angle formed by the chain in the urethra and posterior wall of the bladder *(arrowheads)*.
C. Transperineal US with the patient in upright position well demonstrates the loss of the posterior urethrovesical angle *(arrowheads)* and wide bladder neck *(arrow)* in the resting state.

17. Neurogenic Bladder

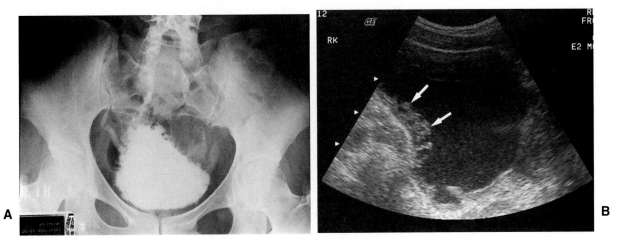

Fig. 1. Neurogenic bladder in a patient who underwent surgery for meningomyelocele.
A. Bladder image of an IVU shows triangular-shaped bladder with its apex directed cranially and markedly increased trabeculation. Note bony defect of the sacrum associated with meningomyelocele. **B.** Longitudinal US of the bladder shows markedly increased trabeculation in the bladder, especially in the dome region *(arrows)*.

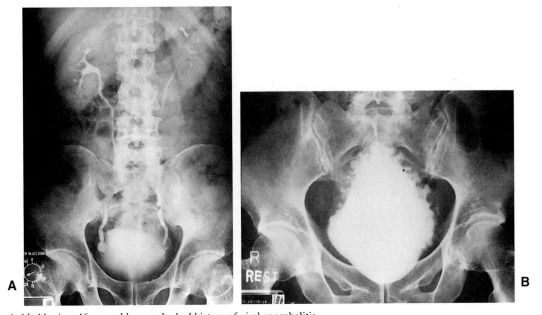

Fig. 2. Neurogenic bladder in a 46-year-old man who had history of viral encephalitis.
A. IVU shows normal upper urinary tract but faint opacification of the bladder. **B.** Cystogram reveals a typical "Christmas tree" appearance of the bladder with increased trabeculation.

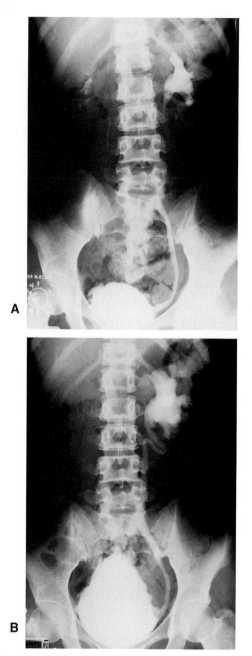

Fig. 3. Neurogenic bladder with vesicoureteral reflux in a 28-year-old woman.
A. IVU shows mild hydronephrosis and hydroureter on the left side. The urinary bladder has prominent trabeculation and multiple small diverticula. **B.** VCU shows a "Christmas tree" appearance of the bladder and vesicoureteral reflux on the left side.

18. Unused Urinary Bladder

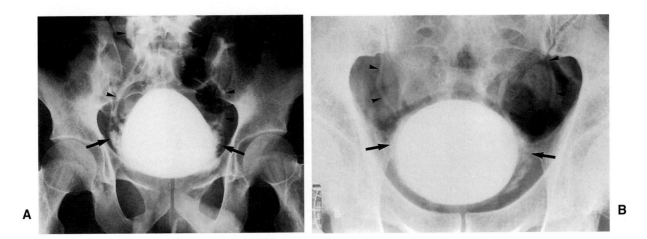

A   B

Fig. 1. Perivesical leak of contrast material from unused bladder due to chronic renal failure.
A. A 27-year-old man with chronic renal failure. VCU shows decreased capacity of the bladder and bilateral vesicoureteral reflux *(arrowheads)*. Note perivesical leak of contrast material *(arrows)*. **B.** A 37-year-old woman with chronic renal failure. VCU shows bilateral vesicoureteral reflux *(arrowheads)* and perivesical leak of contrast material *(arrows)*.

19. Layering of Contrast Material in the Bladder

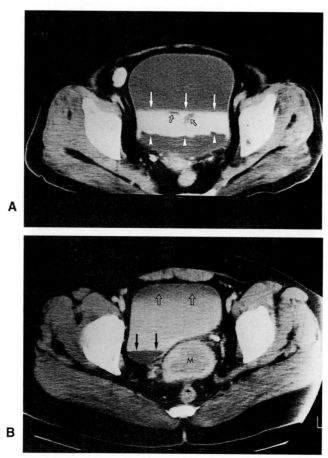

Fig. 1. Reversed urine-contrast level in the bladder on contrast-enhanced CT. (**A, B,** From Kim SH, Han MC: Reversed-contrast urine levels in urinary bladder: CT findings. Urol Radiol 1992; 13:249–252.)
A. A 69-year-old diabetic woman with repeated urinary tract infection. Contrast-enhanced CT shows three layers in the bladder. Note straight anterior fluid-fluid level (*arrows*), irregular posterior fluid-fluid level (*arrowheads*), and low-attenuated materials (*open arrows*) floating in the opacified middle layer. This unusual urine-contrast level is presumably caused by high specific gravity of the infected debris. **B.** A 36-year-old woman with uterine cervical carcinoma. Contrast-enhanced CT shows a reversed urine-contrast level in the bladder (*arrows*). Note supernatant unopacified urine in the top (*open arrows*) because of poor mixing of the urine with excreted contrast material in the bladder. Also note a mass in the uterine cervix (M).

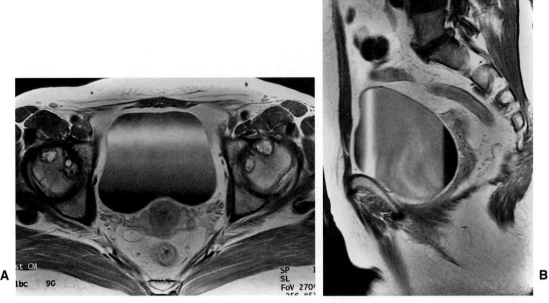

Fig. 2. Pseudolayering in the bladder on contrast-enhanced MR imaging in a 48-year-old woman with uterine cervical carcinoma.
A, B. Contrast-enhanced T1-weighted axial **(A)** and sagittal **(B)** MR images demonstrate multiple layers with various signal intensities in the bladder. This layering is artifactual and is caused by different concentrations of excreted contrast material in the urine. The low-intensity bottom layer represents high concentration of gadolinium contrast material; the middle, high-intensity layer represents lower concentration of contrast material; and the upper, low-intensity top layer represents urine not mixed with contrast material.

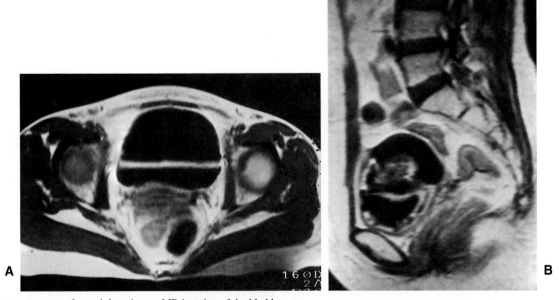

Fig. 3. Various appearance of pseudolayering on MR imaging of the bladder.
A. Contrast-enhanced T1-weighted MR image shows three sharply defined layers in the bladder. **B.** In another patient, contrast-enhanced T1-weighted MR image in sagittal plane shows whirling, high-intensity layers, probably due to active ureteral jetting.

20. Miscellaneous Conditions of the Bladder

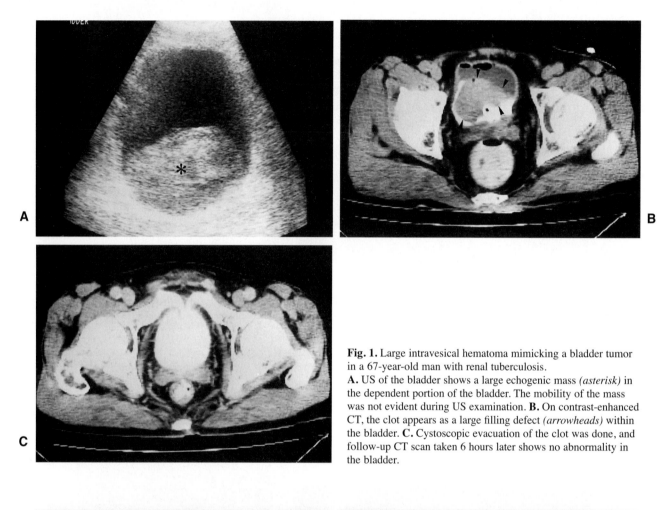

Fig. 1. Large intravesical hematoma mimicking a bladder tumor in a 67-year-old man with renal tuberculosis.
A. US of the bladder shows a large echogenic mass *(asterisk)* in the dependent portion of the bladder. The mobility of the mass was not evident during US examination. **B.** On contrast-enhanced CT, the clot appears as a large filling defect *(arrowheads)* within the bladder. **C.** Cystoscopic evacuation of the clot was done, and follow-up CT scan taken 6 hours later shows no abnormality in the bladder.

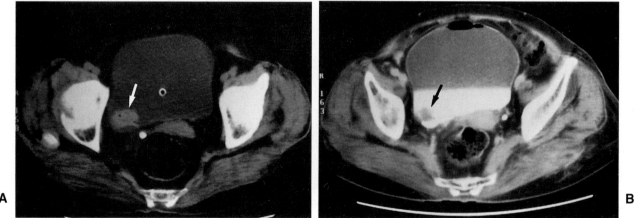

Fig. 2. Blood clot mimicking a bladder tumor in a 78-year-old woman.
A. Nonenhanced CT shows a high-attenuated clot in the right posterior aspect of the bladder *(arrow)*. **B.** Contrast-enhanced CT demonstrates the clot as a filling defect *(arrow)*.

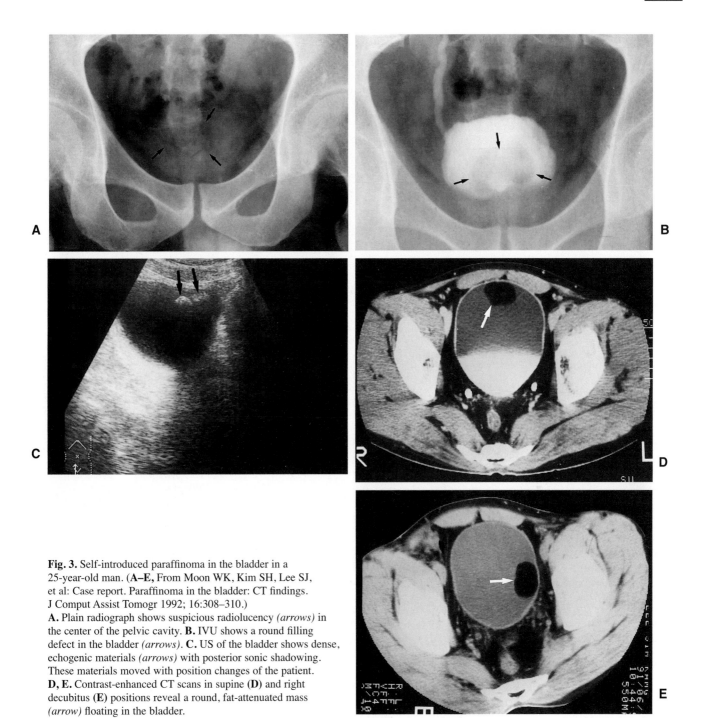

Fig. 3. Self-introduced paraffinoma in the bladder in a
25-year-old man. (**A–E,** From Moon WK, Kim SH, Lee SJ,
et al: Case report. Paraffinoma in the bladder: CT findings.
J Comput Assist Tomogr 1992; 16:308–310.)
A. Plain radiograph shows suspicious radiolucency *(arrows)* in
the center of the pelvic cavity. **B.** IVU shows a round filling
defect in the bladder *(arrows)*. **C.** US of the bladder shows dense,
echogenic materials *(arrows)* with posterior sonic shadowing.
These materials moved with position changes of the patient.
D, E. Contrast-enhanced CT scans in supine (**D**) and right
decubitus (**E**) positions reveal a round, fat-attenuated mass
(arrow) floating in the bladder.

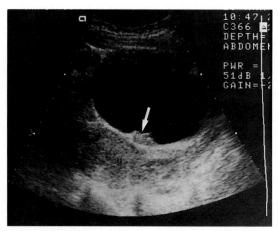

Fig. 4. Endometriosis of the bladder in a 43-year-old woman. Longitudinal US of the pelvis shows small, nodular, elevated lesion *(arrow)* in the bladder. This lesion is indistinguishable from a bladder tumor. U, uterus.

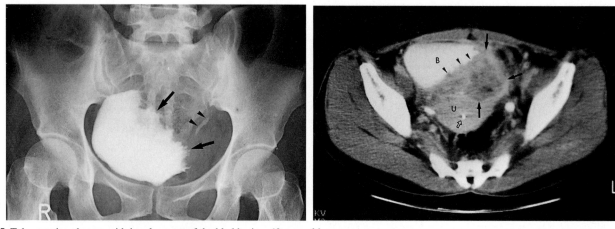

Fig. 5. Tubo-ovarian abscess with involvement of the bladder in a 40-year-old woman.
A. IVU shows large masses with irregular margin in the left aspect of the bladder *(arrows)*. Left ureter *(arrowheads)* is not dilated. **B.** Contrast-enhanced CT shows a large, low-attenuated mass *(arrows)* between the uterus (U) and bladder (B). Note the irregular margin of the bladder *(arrowheads)*. Also note an intrauterine device *(open arrow)* in the uterine cavity.

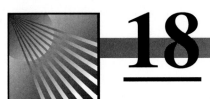

18

Urethral Diseases

CHANG KYU SEONG AND LEE B. TALNER

ANATOMY OF THE URETHRA

Male urethra

The male urethra is divided into two portions, posterior and anterior, each of which is subdivided into two parts. The posterior urethra extends from the bladder neck to the inferior aspect of the urogenital diaphragm and is divided into the prostatic and membranous urethras. The prostatic urethra is approximately 3.5 cm long and traverses the anterior portion of the prostate. The membranous urethra is approximately 1 to 1.5 cm in length and passes through the urogenital diaphragm. It is the narrowest part of the urethra, even during voiding. The verumontanum is a protuberance at the posterior wall of the prostatic urethra, and its distal end marks the beginning of the membranous urethra. Two ejaculatory ducts and utricle have their openings in the verumontanum. The prostatic glands drain into the prostatic urethra through multiple small openings.

The male anterior urethra extends from the urogenital diaphragm to the external meatus and is subdivided into bulbous and pendulous (or penile) portions. The bulbous part of the urethra runs through the bulb of the penis, where the urethra shows a fusiform dilation and is surrounded by the bulbocavernosus muscle. The pendulous urethra extends from the penoscrotal junction to the external meatus and lies entirely within the penis. Penoscrotal junction can be identified by a mild angulation of the anterior urethra on urethrograms. Fossa navicularis is a 1-cm-long bulbous dilation of the very distal pendulous urethra. Cowper's glands are paired structures that lie within the urogenital diaphragm. Their ducts, often 4 to 5 cm long, enter the proximal bulbous urethra. Numerous, small periurethral glands of Littre open into the anterior urethra, and they are more numerous in the bulbous urethra.

On urethrograms, normal indentations or narrowings may be seen in the male urethra. Incisura intermuscularis is an anterior indentation on the posterior urethra due to pressure from the urogenital diaphragm. Other indentations are caused by constrictor nudae muscle and Cobb's collar.

Female urethra

The female urethra is approximately 4 cm long, nearly equivalent to the length of the posterior urethra in the male. It passes downward and forward from the bladder neck to the urogenital diaphragm. On voiding cystourethrography (VCU), its width is variable and depends on the urine flow rate. During voiding, the distal segment dilates less. Numerous submucosal periurethral glands surround the distal urethra.

Normal structures opacified during urethrography

Various periurethral structures may be opacified normally during urethrography. Cowper's duct and the prostatic utricle are common examples. However, strictures may cause reflux of contrast material into Cowper's ducts and glands. Opacification of the prostatic glands and/or glands of Littre is normally associated with chronic periurethral infection or urethral strictures. After prostatic resections, contrast material may reflux into the prostatic ducts, ejaculatory ducts, vas deferens, and seminal vesicles. If the integrity of the urethral mucosa is breached by high-injection pressures during a retrograde urethrography (RGU), corpus cavernosum, corpus spongiosum, and draining veins may be opacified by intravasated contrast material.

CONGENITAL ANOMALIES

Posterior urethral valves

Posterior urethral valves are the most common congenital anomaly of the male urethra and produce moderate to severe outflow obstruction. There are three types of valves. Type I valves are the most common and consist of thin sheets of tissue extending from the distal verumontanum to the wall of the prostatic urethra. Type II valves are mucosal folds that extend from the verumontanum to the bladder neck. Although in the past these were considered to be true valves, it is now generally acknowledged that these are nonobstructive. Type III valve occurs at the distal prostatic urethra in the form of a diaphragm or concentric ring with a central opening.

Posterior urethral valves may be associated with vesicoureteral reflux, dilation of the upper urinary tract, and hypertrophy of the bladder wall. VCU shows marked dilation of the posterior urethra proximal to the valves. The urethra distal to the valve is of normal caliber but may appear narrowed on VCU because of underfilling. It is continuous with the dilated portions along its posterior border.

Anterior urethral valves

Anterior urethral valves are obstructive mucosal flaps in the pendulous urethra. The urethra proximal to the valve may dilate

significantly. Congenital diverticulum of the anterior urethra may also create outflow obstruction with proximal dilation by valvelike action of the distal lip of the diverticulum. Radiologically it may be difficult to differentiate between anterior urethral valve and congenital diverticulum.

Urethral duplication

There are variations and degrees of urethral duplication, including short blind-ending channel, accessory urethra joining the main urethra with or without a bladder opening, and complete urethral duplication. Whether one or both channels is opacified during VCU or RGU depends on the anatomy. Urethral duplication may accompany duplication of the bladder or penis, or both. Penile deformity such as hypoplasia of the corpora may be associated.

Epispadias and hypospadias

Epispadias is an anomaly of the dorsally located urethral meatus on the penile shaft with urethral shortening. It is usually associated with bladder exstrophy. Isolated epispadias is a partial failure of fusion of the dorsal wall of the urethra, and the pubic bones are less separated than in exstrophy. In hypospadias, the urethral meatus is located anywhere along the ventral aspect of the penis proximal to the glans. A chordee, or fibrous band, causing downward curvature of the penis is frequently associated.

INFLAMMATORY DISEASES

Gonorrhea

The most common cause of urethral stricture is inflammatory disease of the urethra. Gonococcal urethritis is one of the most common etiologies of the postinflammatory stricture of the urethra. The infection starts in the distal urethra and proceeds proximally into the bulb where the external urethral sphincter inhibits more proximal spread. In the late stages, fibrous scarring and stricturing may occur. Although posttraumatic stricture is usually short and focal, postinflammatory stricture tends to involve longer segments of the urethra. Urethrography shows opacification of the periurethral glands as a result of patulous ostia. The stricture often has a beaded or irregular contour and is more commonly seen in the bulbous than in the pendulous urethra. In severe cases, the entire anterior urethra may become narrowed.

Nongonococcal urethritis

Urethral infection may be caused by pathogens other than *Gonococcus*. *Chlamydia trachomatis* is believed to be the most common etiology of urethritis. Nongonococcal urethritis rarely causes urethral stricture, but it is uncertain because the possibility of a previous gonococcal infection can seldom be excluded.

Condyloma acuminatum

Condyloma acuminatum is a common viral venereal disease, manifested by squamous papillomas occurring on the moist, mucocutaneous regions of the external genitalia and perineal and perianal regions. It can extend into the urethra. On urethrography, characteristic multiple intraurethral filling defects

are more numerous in the anterior than in the posterior urethra. Generally, strictures and ulcerations are absent.

URETHRAL TRAUMA

Posterior urethral injuries

The prostatomembranous junction in the posterior urethra is the most common area injured in patients with pelvic fractures. Because of the relative differences in fixation of the membranous and prostatic portions of the urethra, tears of the prostatomembranous urethra are usually the result of shearing forces rather than direct penetration by bony spicules.

Three classic types of posterior urethral injury have been proposed based on retrograde urethrographic patterns of extravasation. In type I injury, posterior urethra is stretched without extravasation of contrast material. In type II, there is rupture of the urethra at the prostatomembranous junction above the urogenital diaphragm. On RGU, contrast material leaks above an intact urogenital diaphragm into the pelvic extraperitoneal space. In type III, there is disruption of the urethra and the urogenital diaphragm, and contrast extravasation is seen both above and below the urogenital diaphragm. The presence of a bony pelvic fracture raises the chance of a posterior urethral injury, especially if the pubic symphysis is wider or free floating. Strictures of the urethra in the area of injury are common.

Recently, bladder neck laceration extending into the proximal prostatic urethra has been called *type IV urethral injury*.

Anterior urethral injuries

The anterior urethra is much less commonly injured than the posterior urethra. The usual mechanism of injury is a direct blow to the perineum such as straddle injury, which results in compression of the bulbous urethra between the object and the inferior margin of the pubic bones. The injury of the anterior urethra may be classified as contusion, or partial or complete tear. Partial or complete pure anterior urethral injury is called *type V injury* in recent classification. Urethral stricture is a common late complication and is usually a short, well-defined narrowing in middle or proximal bulbous urethra. Urethral surgery, instrumentation such as cystoscopy, insertion of foreign bodies, or indwelling urethral catheter may also produce anterior urethral injury.

Iatrogenic urethral injuries

Indwelling urethral catheters, traumatic urethral catheterization, radiation, and transurethral surgery or procedure may cause urethral injury. Stricture is the most common late complication. Although urethral inflammation associated with long-term catheterization can cause strictures in any part of the urethra, most occur at the penoscrotal junction, where the catheter can cause pressure ischemia or necrosis.

URETHRAL TUMORS

Urethral polyp

Most urethral polyps originate in the male posterior urethra and have a stalk attached to the verumontanum. They are

usually discovered at a young age and consist of a fibrovascular core covered by transitional cell epithelium. Urethrography demonstrates an elongated or oval filling defect in the posterior urethra. Ultrasonography (US) may be used to differentiate a polyp from a urethral calculus or a clot.

Urethral carcinoma

Squamous cell carcinoma is the most common malignant urethral tumor, usually developing in the anterior urethra in an area of pre-existing, postinflammatory urethral stricture. Transitional cell carcinoma tends to occur in the posterior urethra. Adenocarcinoma of the urethra is thought to originate from either Cowper's glands or the periurethral glands of Littre.

Urethrography demonstrates filling defects or irregular strictures. However, because most cancers of the urethra develop at the site of inflammatory stricture, it is often difficult to differentiate radiologically between urethral cancer and benign stricture.

Urethral metastasis

Metastatic tumor to the urethra is not infrequent. Transitional cell carcinoma of the bladder and adenocarcinoma of the prostate are the most common tumors to secondarily involve the urethra, usually by direct extension. Urethral metastases from distant malignancies also can occur.

MISCELLANEOUS DISEASES OF THE URETHRA

Urethral stones

Most urethral stones are migrant stones that originated in the upper urinary tract or bladder and became trapped in the urethra because of urethral stricture or small caliber of the urethra. Native urethral stones typically do not cause acute symptoms because they grow slowly, but migrant stones can cause acute obstruction. Native urethral stones are usually associated with chronic urine stasis, infection, stricture, or urethral diverticulum. In women, urethral stones may be seen in a urethral diverticulum.

Urethral fistula

Urethral fistulas may be postinfectious, traumatic, surgical, or congenital. They may be blind or open into the skin, into adjacent hollow organs, or into another urethral segment. Urethrovaginal fistulas in the female are characterized by the opacification of the vagina during VCU. This cause of vaginal opacification must be distinguished from the reflux of contrast material into the vagina, a common physiologic phenomenon in young girls during voiding.

Urethral diverticulum

Urethral diverticulum is sometimes congenital, but most cases are acquired as a complication of infection or injury. It may result from rupture or fistulization of a pyogenic periurethral abscess into the urethra. Most occur in women and may be multiloculated or multiple, and contain stones. Benign or malignant tumor may arise from the lining. Urethral diverticula may opacify during VCU, and opacification persists on the postvoid radiograph. However, some diverticula do not fill on VCU. Perineal or endovaginal US or magnetic resonance (MR) imaging can be helpful in such cases.

References

1. Disantis DJ: Inflammatory conditions of the urethra. In Pollack HM, McClennan BL (eds): Clinical Urography, 2nd ed, vol 1. Philadelphia, WB Saunders, 2000, pp 1041–1057.
2. Friedland GW, Nino-Murcia M, deVries PA: Congenital anomalies of the urethra. In Pollack HM, McClennan BL (eds): Clinical Urography, 2nd ed, vol 1. Philadelphia, WB Saunders, 2000, pp 852–868.
3. Older RA, Hertz M: Cystourethrography. In Pollack HM, McClennan BL (eds): Clinical Urography, 2nd ed, vol 1. Philadelphia, WB Saunders, 2000, pp 303–355.
4. Talner LB, O'Reilly PH, Wasserman NF: Specific causes of obstruction. In Pollack HM, McClennan BL (eds): Clinical Urography, 2nd ed, vol 2. Philadelphia, WB Saunders, 2000, pp 1967–2136.
5. Sandler CM, McCallum RW: Urethral trauma. In Pollack HM, McClennan BL (eds): Clinical Urography, 2nd ed, vol 2. Philadelphia, WB Saunders, 2000, pp 1819–1838.
6. Goldman SM, Sandler CM, Corriere JN Jr, et al: Blunt urethral trauma: A unified, anatomical mechanical classification. J Urol 1997; 157:85–89.
7. Amis ES Jr: The urethra. RSNA Categorical Course in Genitourinary Radiology. Oak Brook, IL, Radiological Society of North America, 1994, pp 147–157.
8. Kim B, Hricak H, Tanagho EA: Diagnosis of urethral diverticula in women: Value of MR imaging. AJR Am J Roentgenol 1993; 161:809–815.
9. Rimon U, Hertz M, Jonas P: Diverticula of the male urethra: A review of 61 cases. Urol Radiol 1992; 14:49–55.
10. Amis ES Jr, Newhouse JH, Cronan JJ: Radiology of male periurethral structures. AJR Am J Roentgenol 1988; 151:321–324.
11. MacPherson RI, Leithiser RE, Gordon L, et al: Posterior urethral valves: An update and review. Radiographics 1986; 6:753–791.
12. Lee RA: Diverticulum of the urethra: Clinical presentation, diagnosis, and management. Clin Obstet Gynecol 1984; 27:490–498.
13. Bonavita JA, Pollack HM: Trauma of the adult bladder and urethra. Semin Roentgenol 1983; 18:299–306.
14. Friedenberg RM: Abnormalities affecting structure and function of the bladder and urethra. Semin Roentgenol 1983; 18:307–321.
15. Imray TJ, Kaplan P: Lower urinary tract infections and calculi in the adult. Semin Roentgenol 1983; 18:276–287.
16. Yoder IC, Pfister RC: Congenital anomalies of the adult bladder and urethra. Semin Roentgenol 1983; 18:267–275.
17. Sandler CM, Harris JH Jr, Corriere JN Jr, et al: Posterior urethral injuries after pelvic fractures. AJR Am J Roentgenol 1981; 137:1233–1237.

Illustrations • Urethral Diseases

1 • Normal urethra

2 • Opacified periurethral structures during urethrography

3 • Inflammatory diseases of the urethra

4 • Urethral injury

5 • Urethral stricture

6 • Urethral stone

7 • Urethral tumors

8 • Miscellaneous conditions of the urethra

1. Normal Urethra

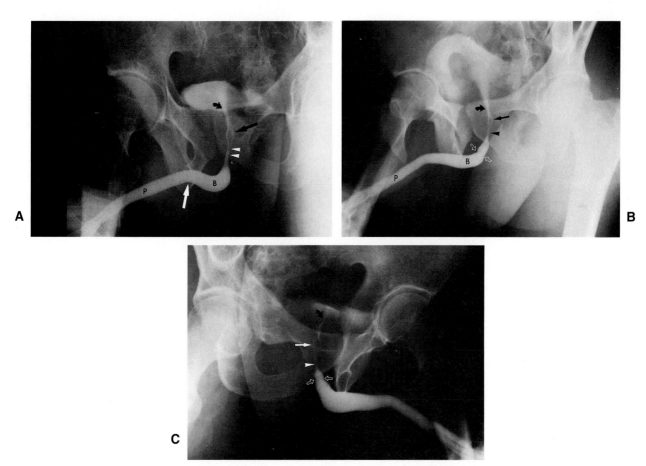

Fig. 1. Normal urethra on RGU.
A. Normal RGU in a 33-year-old man. Verumontanum *(black arrow)* is seen as an ovoid filling defect in the prostatic urethra. Membranous urethra *(arrowheads)* is the narrowest portion of the urethra, between the distal end of the verumontanum and the conical end of the bulbous urethra. Note slight angulation of the urethra at the penoscrotal junction *(white arrow)*. The bladder neck *(curved arrow)* can be identified by beginning of jet of contrast material into the bladder. It is usual for the posterior urethra to be undistended on RGU. P, pendulous urethra; B, bulbous urethra. **B, C.** Normal RGUs in two other patients. Normal pendulous urethra (P), bulbous urethra (B), membranous urethra *(arrowhead)*, and verumontanum *(arrow)* in the prostatic urethra. Slight indentation *(open arrows)* on the proximal bulbous urethra is a normal finding related to the constrictor nudae muscle, a musculotendinous sling of the bulbocavernosus muscle. The bladder neck *(curved arrow)* can be identified by the beginning of a jet of contrast material into the bladder.

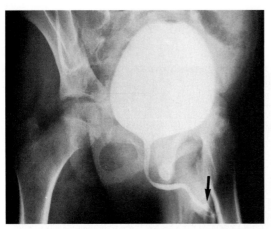

Fig. 2. Normal urethra on VCU in a 15-year-old boy. On normal voiding study, prostatic and membranous portions of the urethra are distended. Fossa navicularis is seen as a bulbous dilation of the most distal part of the pendulous urethra *(arrow)*.

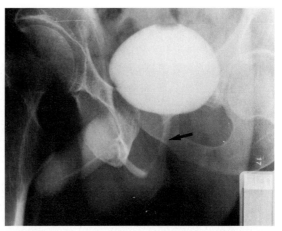

Fig. 3. Normal urethra on VCU in a 19-year-old man. On voiding study, posterior urethra is normally distended. Anterior urethra is less distended, especially distal to the kink at the penoscrotal junction. Verumontanum *(arrow)* is less well demonstrated than on RGU and can be identified as a faint indentation on posterior aspect of the prostatic urethra.

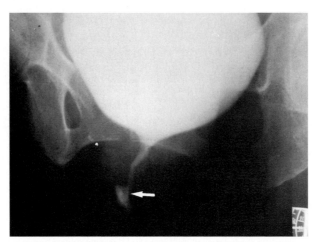

Fig. 4. Normal female urethra on VCU in a 50-year-old woman. The female urethra is short and courses obliquely downward and forward from the bladder neck to the external urethral meatus *(arrow)*. Proximal part of the urethra dilates in a fusiform shape during voiding.

2. Opacified Periurethral Structures during Urethrography

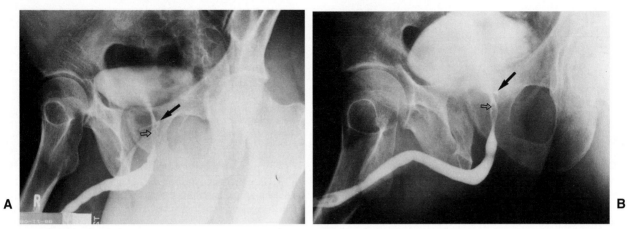

A

B

Fig. 1. The utricle opacified during RGU.
A. RGU in a 30-year-old man shows opacification of the normal utricle *(arrow)*, which opens in the center of the verumontanum *(open arrow)*.
B. RGU in a 43-year-old man shows opacification of prominent utricle *(arrow)* and its opening in the center of the verumontanum *(open arrow)*.

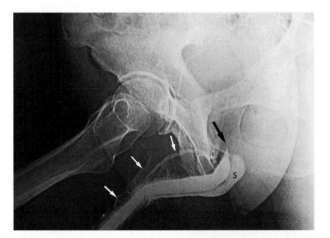

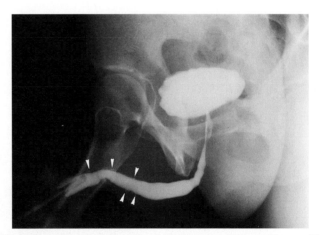

Fig. 2. Opacification of corpus spongiosum and penile veins during RGU in a 50-year-old man. RGU shows tight membranous urethra *(black arrow)* caused by spasm or voluntary contraction. Extravasated contrast material opacifies the corpus spongiosum (s) and draining penile veins *(white arrows)*.

Fig. 3. Opacification of the periurethral glands in a 33-year-old man with history of nongonococcal urethritis. RGU shows opacification of the periurethral glands *(arrowheads)* in the anterior urethra. It usually suggests the presence of inflammation of the urethra.

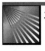

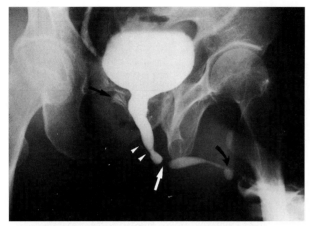

Fig. 4. Opacification of the Cowper's gland and prostatic ducts in a 44-year-old man with post-traumatic urethral stricture. Contrast material was introduced into the urinary bladder through a suprapubic cystostomy, and simultaneous RGU was performed with the patient straining. The urethra is discontinuous at the bulbous portion *(white arrow)*, and contrast material is refluxed into the prostatic ducts *(black arrow)* and Cowper's gland duct *(arrowheads)*. Note bilateral vesicoureteral reflux, diffuse narrowing of the pendulous urethra, and a saccular diverticulum *(curved arrow)* on the ventral aspect of the pendulous urethra.

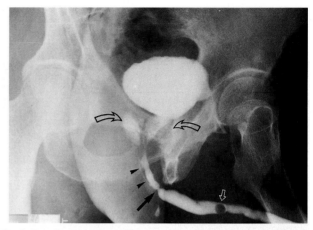

Fig. 5. Opacification of the Cowper's gland duct in a 66-year-old man with urethral stricture. RGU show a severe stricture in the proximal bulbous urethra *(arrow)* and opacification of the Cowper's gland duct *(arrowheads)*. Note an air bubble in the pendulous urethra *(open arrow)* and diffuse calcifications in the prostate *(curved open arrows)*.

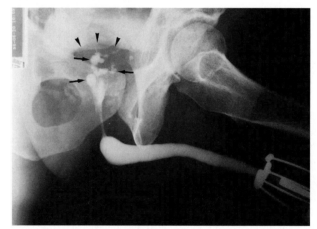

Fig. 6. Opacification of the seminal vesicles during RGU in a 65-year-old man who had undergone laser prostatectomy for benign prostatic hyperplasia. Note narrowing and elongation of the prostatic urethra and elevated base of the bladder *(arrowheads)* due to enlarged prostate. Note opacification of the seminal vesicles *(arrows)*.

3. Inflammatory Diseases of the Urethra

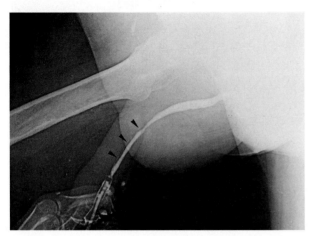

Fig. 1. Urethral stricture in a 60-year-old man with history of syphilis. This patient also had an aortic aneurysm due to syphilis. RGU shows diffuse narrowing of the anterior urethra. Note opacified periurethral glands *(arrowheads)* in the pendulous urethra.

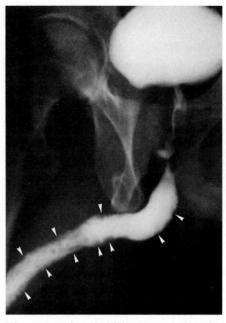

Fig. 2. Condylomata acuminata involving the urethra in a 34-year-old man. RGU shows multiple, small nodularities *(arrowheads)* in the pendulous and bulbous urethra.

4. Urethral Injury

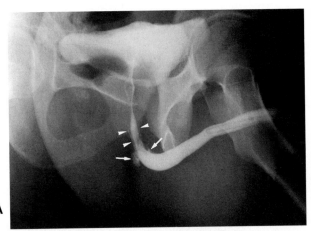

Fig. 1. Minor laceration of the urethra due to straddle injury in a 25-year-old man.
A. RGU shows leak of small amount of contrast material from the bulbous urethra *(arrows)*. Also note opacification of Cowper's gland ducts *(arrowheads)*. **B.** Follow-up RGU obtained 2 weeks later after conservative management shows normal urethra.

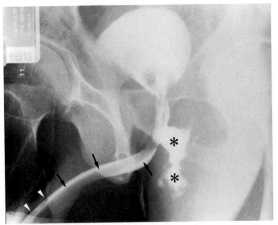

Fig. 2. Urethral injury during Miles' operation for rectal cancer in a 36-year-old man. Pericatheter RGU shows leak of contrast material into the perineum *(asterisks)* from region of distal prostatic urethra. Note a catheter for RGU *(arrowheads)*, which is inserted alongside the bladder catheter *(arrows)*.

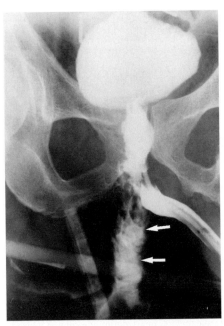

Fig. 3. Urethral injury with a urethrocutaneous fistula that occurred following Miles' operation for rectal cancer in a 57-year-old man. RGU shows leak of contrast material from the posterior urethra with opacification of wide fistulous tract *(arrows)*.

5. Urethral Stricture

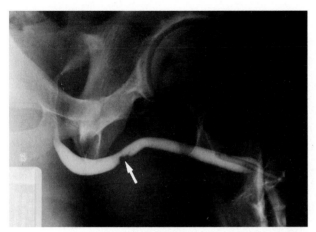

Fig. 1. Urethral stricture in a 32-year-old man who received a straddle injury 7 years earlier. RGU shows a focal eccentric stricture in the distal bulbous urethra *(arrow)*.

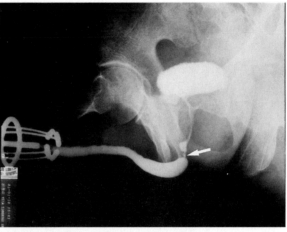

Fig. 2. Urethral stricture following a straddle injury in a 42-year-old man. RGU performed 2 months after trauma shows a short, tight stricture in the proximal bulbous urethra *(arrow)*.

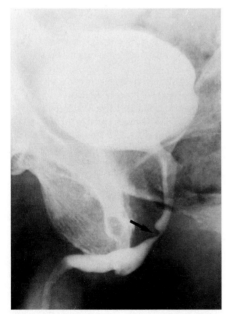

Fig. 3. Iatrogenic urethral injury during insertion of a bladder catheter in a 79-year-old man. VCU shows a focal, eccentric stricture in the proximal bulbous urethra *(arrow)*.

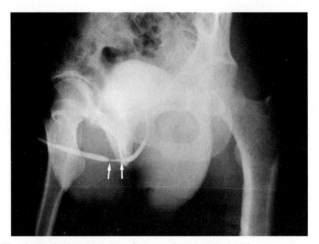

Fig. 4. Urethral stricture in a 20-year-old man who had long-term indwelling bladder catheter when he underwent surgery for ventricular septal defect 18 years earlier. RGU shows a segmental urethral stricture near the penoscrotal junction *(arrows)*.

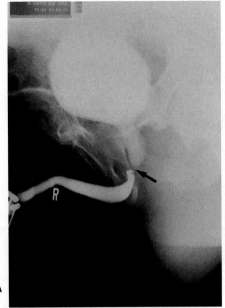

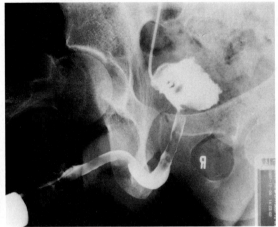

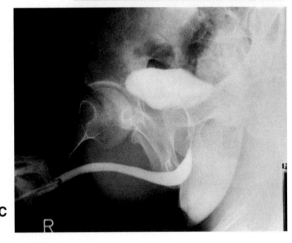

Fig. 5. Urethral obstruction in a 28-year-old man who received a urethral injury in a motorcycle crash 10 years earlier.
A. Urinary bladder was filled with contrast material through suprapubic cystostomy, and simultaneous RGU was performed with the patient straining. There is a discontinuity in the short segment at the membranous urethra *(arrow)*.
B. Pericatheter RGU performed 3 weeks after surgical repair shows a reconstructed urethra without leak of contrast material. **C.** Follow-up RGU performed 4 months after surgery shows normal appearance of the urethra.

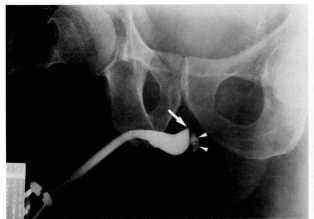

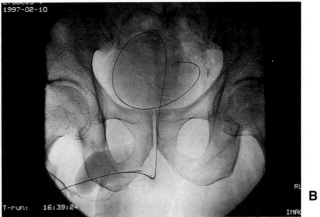

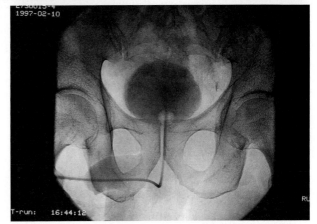

Fig. 6. Insertion of a Foley catheter under fluoroscopic guidance in a 71-year-old man.
A. There was a difficulty in insertion of a bladder catheter, and RGU was performed. RGU shows obstruction of the urethra in the bulbomembranous junction *(arrow)* and leak of contrast material *(arrowheads)*. **B.** A floppy guide wire was inserted into the bladder under fluoroscopic guidance. **C.** A bladder catheter was inserted easily over the guide wire.

6. Urethral Stone

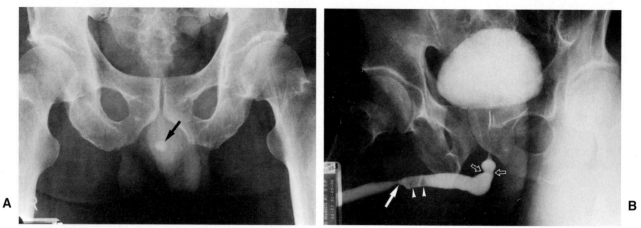

Fig. 1. Urethral stone in a 58-year-old man with a urethral stricture.
A. Anteroposterior plain radiograph shows a round calcification *(arrow)* projecting below the symphysis pubis. **B.** Oblique RGU reveals a focal concentric stricture *(white arrow)* in the pendulous urethra and stones seen as filling defects *(arrowheads)* in the urethra just proximal to the stricture. Note concentric narrowing in proximal bulbous urethra *(open arrows)*, which is a normal finding called *Cobb's collar*.

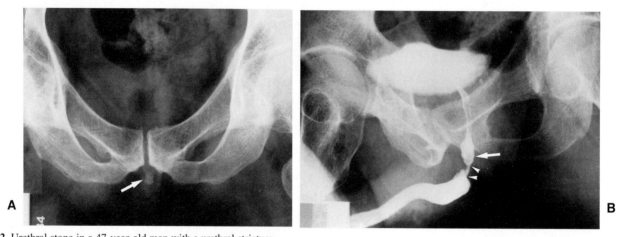

Fig. 2. Urethral stone in a 47-year-old man with a urethral stricture.
A. Plain radiograph shows a calcification *(arrow)* below the symphysis pubis. **B.** RGU shows a stone *(arrow)* proximal to a stricture *(arrowheads)* in the proximal bulbous urethra.

7. Urethral Tumors

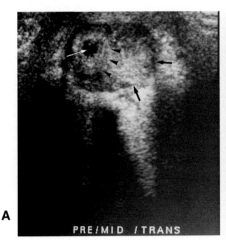

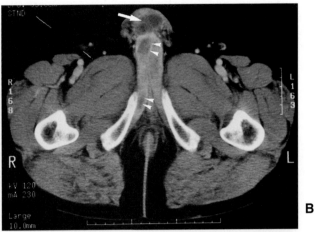

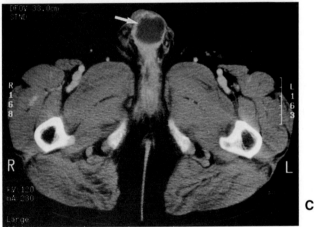

Fig. 1. Papillary transitional cell carcinoma of the urethra with invasion of the corpus cavernosum in a 77-year-old man.
A. US of the urethra in transverse plane shows a round, solid, echogenic mass *(arrows)* in the penile shaft. Note focal obliteration of normal hypoechoic wall of the urethra where the mass arises *(arrowheads)*. The *white arrow* indicates a Foley catheter in the urethral lumen. **B, C.** Contrast-enhanced CT scans show a low-attenuated mass *(arrow)* in the penile shaft. Also note ill-defined, low-attenuated lesions in the right corpus cavernosum *(arrowheads in **B**)*.

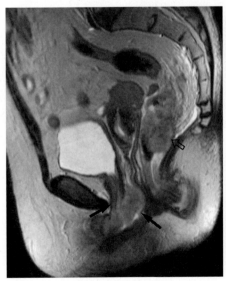

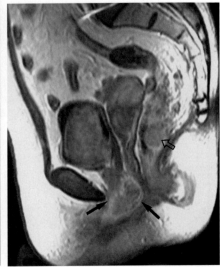

Fig. 2. Squamous cell carcinoma of the urethra in a 79-year-old woman.
A, B. T2-weighted **(A)** and contrast-enhanced T1-weighted **(B)** MR images show a large, soft tissue mass involving the urethra *(arrows)*. The mass has slightly high intensity on T2-weighted image and nonenhancing central necrosis on contrast-enhanced T1-weighted image. Also note a mass in the rectum *(open arrow)*, which was found to be a metastatic squamous cell carcinoma.

8. Miscellaneous Conditions of the Urethra

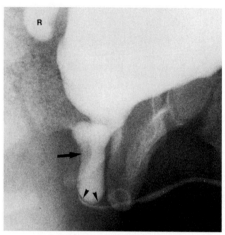

Fig. 1. Posterior urethral valve in a 3-year-old boy. VCU shows characteristic features of type I posterior urethral valve: elongation and dilation of the posterior urethra, downward ballooning of the valve leaflets *(arrowheads)*, underfilling of the urethra distal to the valves, prominent posterior indentation at the bladder neck, and a large verumontanum *(arrow)*. Reflux is occurring into the distal end of the right ureter (R). (From Talner LB, O'Reilly PH, Wasserman NF: Specific causes of obstruction. In Pollack HM, McClennan BL [eds]: Clinical Urography, 2nd ed, vol 2. Philadelphia, WB Saunders, 2000, pp 1967–2136.)

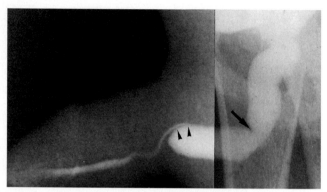

Fig. 2. Anterior urethral valve in a 6-year-old boy viewed by composite VCU. The urethra is dilated proximal to the obstructing valve *(arrowheads)*. Note how the urethra balloons at the site of the valve and compresses and displaces the adjacent portion of the distal segment of the urethra. The valve obstructs sufficiently to cause poor distention of the distal portion of the urethra. The dorsal infolding *(arrow)* at the urogenital diaphragm is normal. (From Talner LB, O'Reilly PH, Wasserman NF: Specific causes of obstruction. In Pollack HM, McClennan BL [eds]: Clinical Urography, 2nd ed, vol 2. Philadelphia, WB Saunders, 2000, pp 1967–2136.)

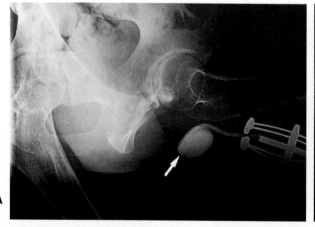

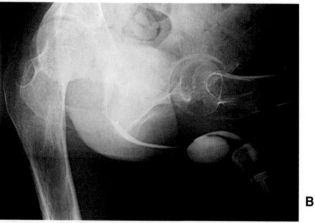

A

B

Fig. 3. Anterior urethral diverticulum in a 22-year-old paraplegic man with history of prolonged catheterization.
A. RGU shows a large diverticulum *(arrow)* connected to the pendulous urethra near the penoscrotal junction. **B.** With further injection of contrast material, the whole urethra is opacified and the connection to the diverticulum is well demonstrated. The patient complained of discharge of urine when the penile mass was compressed.

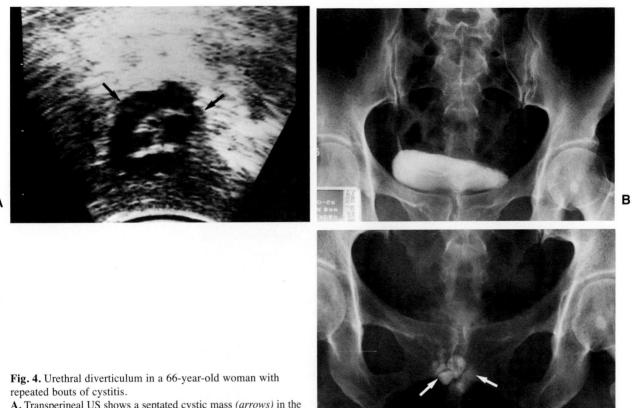

Fig. 4. Urethral diverticulum in a 66-year-old woman with repeated bouts of cystitis.
A. Transperineal US shows a septated cystic mass *(arrows)* in the periurethral region. **B.** IVU shows no abnormal finding.
C. Postvoiding radiograph shows residual contrast material in a multiloculated urethral diverticulum *(arrows)*.

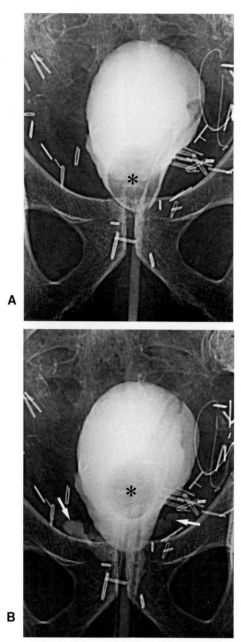

A

B

Fig. 5. Leak of contrast material at urethral anastomosis site in a 65-year-old man who underwent radical prostatectomy for prostate cancer. **A.** Cystogram obtained with a Foley catheter balloon *(asterisk)* in the bladder neck shows no evidence of leak of contrast material. **B.** Cystogram obtained with a Foley catheter advanced *(asterisk)* shows leak of contrast material *(arrows)*.

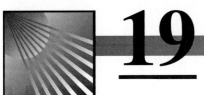

19

Prostate

JEONG YEON CHO

The major advances that have improved our understanding of prostatic disease are a significant revision of prostatic anatomy, the development of serum assays for prostate-specific antigen, and an improvement in imaging techniques, specifically transrectal ultrasonography (US) and magnetic resonance (MR) imaging.

PROSTATE ANATOMY

The prostate is located inferior to the urinary bladder with a shape like an inverted cone. The cephalic end of the prostate is called the *base* and the caudal end the *apex*.

In 1912, Lowsley described the anatomy of the prostate, which divided the prostate into anterior, posterior, middle, and two lateral lobes. McNeal proposed a zonal concept of prostate anatomy that considers the different histologic components of the gland. In McNeal's zonal concept, the prostate is composed of glandular zones (peripheral zone, central zone, transition zone, and periurethral glandular tissue) and a nonglandular region (anterior fibromuscular stroma).

The transition zone constitutes about 5% of prostatic glandular tissue. It is located on both sides of the prostatic urethra and ends at the verumontanum. It is in this zone that most of benign prostatic hyperplasia (BPH) develops. The central zone constitutes approximately 25% of prostatic glandular tissue in the young adult and is located around the base of the prostate in a pyramidal shape. The ejaculatory ducts pass through this zone to reach the verumontanum. The confluence of the vas deferens and the seminal vesicles forms a beak, which is an anatomically weak area for the spread of cancer. The peripheral zone constitutes 70% of prostatic glandular tissue and is located at the posterior, lateral, and apical aspects of the gland. Its ducts drain into the distal urethra, distal to the verumontanum. Seventy percent to 80% of the prostate cancers originate in the peripheral zone. The anterior fibromuscular stroma is a nonglandular region that forms the anterior surface of the prostate gland.

The term *central gland* is often used to refer to the combination of the central zone and the transition zone since those zones usually could not be separated from each other on either transrectal US or MR imaging.

TRANSRECTAL ULTRASONOGRAPHY OF THE PROSTATE

Transrectal US is a useful imaging modality of the prostate. Transrectal US with state-of-the-art transducers has the capa-

bility to demonstrate the zonal anatomy of the prostate, seminal vesicles, the ejaculatory ducts, and urethra. The texture of the gland can be assessed for focal lesions, BPH, or cancer.

The anterior fibromuscular stroma is usually hypoechoic. The transition zone is hypoechoic surrounding the urethra. The echogenicity may become heterogeneous with aging. The peripheral zone is homogeneously isoechoic or hyperechoic. The central zone and peripheral zone cannot be differentiated on US. The seminal vesicle and vas deferens are symmetrical and hypoechoic with a thin wall.

Transrectal US can also determine glandular volume accurately. The most commonly used method to measure prostatic or tumor volume is the formula for a prolate ellipse: length × width × height × 0.523. Volumes can then be easily converted to weight because 1 mL of prostatic tissue is equivalent to 1 g.

MAGNETIC RESONANCE IMAGING OF THE PROSTATE

MR imaging is considered to be the imaging method of choice for preoperative staging with regard to the local spread of the tumor beyond the prostate. Both T1- and T2-weighted spin-echo sequences are required to evaluate the prostate adequately. Standard T2-weighted sequences are replaced by T2-weighted fast spin-echo sequences, which can be performed in a shorter scan time while improving resolution. Various coils are used to image the prostate, including body coil, external surface coil, and balloon-mounted endorectal surface coil. Endorectal coil is used for higher-resolution evaluation of the prostate, prostate capsule, and neurovascular bundles. When an endorectal coil is used to image the prostate, supplemental body coil imaging of the abdomen and pelvis is still required to detect lymphadenopathy.

T1-weighted images are helpful in imaging the periprostatic fat, periprostatic veins, neurovascular bundles, perivesical tissues, and lymph nodes. The high contrast between the periprostatic fat and water-containing structures such as the prostate, seminal vesicles, and blood vessels aids in the detection of extraprostatic spread of tumor.

T2-weighted images demonstrate the internal architecture of the prostate and seminal vesicles better than T1-weighted images. The peripheral zone is of high signal intensity on the T2-weighted images because of its high fluid content. The central gland is of intermediate signal intensity on this sequence.

PROSTATE CANCER

Prostate cancer occurs in up to 50% of all men by age 50, and almost all men by age 80 have at least microscopic evidence of prostate cancer. Serum level of prostate-specific antigen is being used for screening of prostate cancer. Its sensitivity is between 73% and 96%, but its specificity is limited.

The imaging modality most commonly used in the diagnosis of prostate cancer is transrectal US. The classic appearance of prostate cancer on transrectal US is a hypoechoic lesion in the peripheral zone of the prostate. However, not all cancers are hypoechoic and not all hypoechoic lesions are cancers. Approximately 60% of prostate cancers are hypoechoic on transrectal US, and only 20% to 30% of hypoechoic lesions are cancers. The hypoechoic lesions that mimic prostate cancer include inflammation, atrophy, infarction, and benign hyperplasia.

Prostate cancers that locate in the transition or central zone and diffuse cancers infiltrating the entire peripheral zone or the entire gland do not appear with classic findings on transrectal US. The secondary characteristics of prostate cancers may help detect prostate cancers with transrectal US in these cases. The criteria include capsular bulge, asymmetry of echogenicity, periprostatic fat irregularity, and loss of normal echo of the seminal vesicle.

Color or power Doppler US is a simple technique to demonstrate the vascularity of a lesion. In malignant tumors, which are usually hypervascular, the vascularity of the tumors can be demonstrated with color or power Doppler US. Most prostate cancers have hypervascularity as compared to benign prostatic diseases. Therefore, color or power Doppler US may be helpful in differentiating prostate cancers from benign prostatic lesions by demonstrating a hypervascular nature of the lesion. Color or power Doppler US also may help identify an appropriate site for biopsy. Some investigators, however, indicate that the increase in positive predictive value achieved is not sufficient.

On T2-weighted MR images, prostate cancer typically appears as a low-intensity lesion within the high signal intensity of the normal peripheral zone. Not all cancers, however, appear as a low-intensity lesion. Prostate cancers located in the transition or central zone may be obscured by the normal low or heterogeneous signal intensity of those zones. The secondary changes such as asymmetry, contour bulge, irregular outer margin, and the change of the seminal vesicles should be searched for in these cases. As on transrectal US, not all low-intensity lesions on T2-weighted MR images are prostate cancers. Detection of prostate cancers may be hindered by postbiopsy hemorrhage. MR imaging should be performed at least 3 weeks after biopsy to avoid the effect of postbiopsy hemorrhage.

The value of MR imaging of the prostate is in local staging of prostate cancer, especially in detecting extracapsular spread of the tumor. Prostate cancers confined to the prostate appear as low-intensity lesions located in the peripheral zone. Although the lateral margin of the prostate can bulge, the contour is usually smooth. MR imaging findings of extracapsular spread include an irregular bulge of the prostate, contour deformity, and evidence of direct extension of the tumor beyond the capsule. Findings on T2-weighted MR image suggesting invasion of the seminal vesicles include low-intensity tumor in the seminal vesicle, decreased signal intensity of the seminal vesicles, and thickening or obliteration of the seminal vesicle wall. High signal intensity of the seminal vesicle on T1-weighted image indicates hemorrhage and therefore suggests tumor invasion. However, this finding is often seen following prostate biopsy without tumor invasion. The accuracy of staging of prostate cancer with MR imaging was reported to be higher than 80%.

OTHER MALIGNANT TUMORS OF THE PROSTATE

Lymphoma

Prostate lymphomas are rare, and most of them are secondary lymphomas. Primary lymphoma of the prostate is less than 0.2% of extranodal non-Hodgkin's lymphoma. The clinical symptoms and signs are similar to prostate cancer. Transrectal US finding of the prostate lymphoma is not specific. The prostate is usually enlarged, and focal or diffuse hypoechoic lesions may be identified.

Rhabdomyosarcoma

Rhabdomyosarcoma usually occurs in the first decade of life. At the time of diagnosis, the tumors are usually large. They may cause obstructive uropathy and may involve the rectum producing bloody stool and constipation. The radiologic findings are markedly enlarged prostate and tumor invasion of adjacent organs.

Leiomyosarcoma

Leiomyosarcoma is the second most common sarcoma to involve the prostate. It usually occurs between 40 and 70 years of age and presents as a bulky tumor with diffuse infiltration of surrounding tissue. The typical symptoms are frequency, urgency, and dysuria. It often metastasizes to the lung, liver, and genitourinary tract. The radiologic findings of leiomyosarcoma are not distinguishable from those of rhabdomyosarcoma.

BENIGN PROSTATIC HYPERPLASIA

Enlargement of the prostate is present in most elderly men. Approximately 95% of cases of BPH arise in the transition zone and 5% from periurethral glandular tissue. BPH presents with variable voiding symptoms such as reduction in force of urine stream, feeling of residual urine, nocturia, and hesitancy.

Transrectal US findings of BPH vary depending on histopathologic changes. BPH may appear as distinct nodules or diffuse enlargement of the prostate. Typically, the central gland enlarges in BPH. Often with BPH, the central gland remains hypoechoic compared with the peripheral gland. However, depending on admixture of glandular and stromal elements, the echotexture may become heterogeneous or even hyperechoic.

Occasionally, BPH compresses the central zone as well as the peripheral zone to only a few millimeters in thickness. The surgical capsule is the line of demarcation between the central BPH and the compressed peripheral gland. On transrectal US, this surgical capsule appears as a hypoechoic halo, and often calcifications are seen along this capsule. BPH nodules can bulge the capsule of the prostate or compress the lateral margins, but they should not disrupt the capsule or periprostatic fat.

MR imaging findings of BPH are variable. The signal characteristics in BPH are variable and depend on the amount of glandular and stromal tissue in the lesion. Glandular hyperplasia shows heterogeneous nodular lesion in the inner gland and surgical capsule on T2-weighted image. Stromal hyperplasia shows homogeneous low signal intensity on T2-weighted image.

PROSTATITIS

Acute prostatitis

Acute prostatitis presents with fever, pain, tenderness on digital rectal examination, dysuria, urgency, and pyuria. The prostate is enlarged with decreased echogenicity on transrectal US. The flow signals are diffusely increased on color or power Doppler US. Acute bacterial prostatitis generally responds well to antibiotic treatment. In some instances, however, acute prostatitis progresses to form a prostate abscess, and then transrectal US shows a hypoechoic or anechoic mass within the prostate. Transrectal US-guided aspiration or drainage may be useful in the diagnosis and treatment of a prostate abscess.

Chronic prostatitis

Chronic prostatitis presents with frequency, urgency, nocturia, dysuria, and hemospermia. The prostate may be tender and hard on digital rectal examination. On transrectal US, the prostate is usually not enlarged and has heterogeneous increased echogenicity. Inflammation of the seminal vesicle and vas deferens is often accompanied by chronic prostatitis. The wall of the seminal vesicle and vas deferens is thickened and the internal echogenicity is increased. Focal atrophy and infarction, which are indistinguishable from prostate cancer on transrectal US or MR imaging, may occur as sequelae of chronic prostatitis. In addition to the increased prostatic echogenicity, transrectal US often shows a thin, hypoechoic rim along the periphery of the prostate. This hypoechoic rim represents spared area of the inflammatory cell infiltration. The presence of peripheral hypoechoic rim in the prostate may be helpful in transrectal US diagnosis of chronic prostatitis.

Malacoplakia

Malacoplakia is a rare granulomatous inflammation that most commonly affects the bladder, followed in frequency by the kidney, ureter, testis, and prostate. Malacoplakia may appear as a hypoechoic lesion on transrectal US, which is indistinguishable from prostate cancer.

References

1. Lee HJ, Choe GY, Seong CG, et al: Hypoechoic rim of the chronic prostatic inflammation: Histopathologic findings. Korean J Radiol 2001; 2:159–163.
2. Cho JY, Kim SH, Lee SE: Peripheral hypoechoic lesions of the prostate: Evaluation with color and power Doppler US. Eur Urol 2000; 37:443–448.
3. Coakley FV, Hricak H: Radiologic anatomy of the prostate gland: A clinical approach. Radiol Clin North Am 2000; 38:15–30.
4. Lim JW, Ko YT, Lee DH, et al: Treatment of prostatic abscess: Value of transrectal ultrasonographically guided needle aspiration. J Ultrasound Med 2000; 19:609–617.
5. Grossfeld GD, Coakley FV: Benign prostatic hyperplasia: Clinical overview and value of diagnostic imaging. Radiol Clin North Am 2000; 38:31–47.
6. Varghese SL, Grossfeld GD: The prostate gland: Malignancies other than adenocarcinomas. Radiol Clin North Am 2000; 38:179–202.
7. Wasserman NF: Prostatitis: Clinical presentations and transrectal ultrasound findings. Semin Roentgenol 1999; 4:325–337.
8. Cho JY, Lee SE, Kim SH: Diffuse prostatic lesions: The role of color and power Doppler US. J Ultrasound Med 1998; 17:283–287.
9. Agrons GA, Wagner BJ, Lonergan GJ, et al: From the archives of the AFIP. Genitourinary rhabdomyosarcoma in children: Radiologic-pathologic correlation. Radiographics 1997; 17:919–937.
10. Yu KK, Hricak H, Alagappan R, et al: Detection of extracapsular extension of prostate carcinoma with endorectal and phased-array coil MR imaging: Multivariate feature analysis. Radiology 1997; 202:697–702.
11. Cheng SS, Rifkin MD, Bajas MA, et al: Does color Doppler increase the ability to identify prostate cancer? Radiology 1996; 201:338.
12. Collins GN, Raab GM, Hehir M, et al: Reproducibility and observer variability of the transrectal ultrasound measurements of prostatic volume. Ultrasound Med Biol 1995; 21:1101–1105.
13. Newman JS, Bree RL, Rubin JM: Prostate cancer: Diagnosis with color Doppler sonography with histologic correlation of each biopsy site. Radiology 1995; 195:86–90.
14. White S, Hricak H, Forstner R, et al: Prostate cancer: Effect of postbiopsy hemorrhage on interpretation of MR images. Radiology 1995; 195:385–390.
15. Hricak H, White S, Vignerone D, et al: Carcinoma of the prostate gland: MR imaging with pelvic phased-array coils versus integrated endorectal-pelvic phased-array coils. Radiology 1994; 193:703–709.
16. Ishida J, Sugimura K, Okizuka H, et al: Benign prostatic hyperplasia: Value of MR imaging for determining histologic type. Radiology 1994; 190:329–331.
17. Outwater EK, Petersen RO, Siegelman ES, et al: Prostate carcinoma: Assessment of diagnostic criteria for capsular penetration on endorectal coil MR images. Radiology 1994; 193:333–339.
18. Rifkin MD: Prostate imaging 1994. RSNA Categorical Course in Genitourinary Radiology. Oak Brook, IL, Radiological Society of North America, 1994, pp 175–182.
19. Kelly IM, Lees WR, Rickards D: Prostate cancer and the role of color Doppler US. Radiology 1993; 189:153–156.
20. Rifkin MD, Sudakoff GS, Alexander AA: Prostate: Techniques, results, and potential application of color Doppler US scanning. Radiology 1993; 186:509–513.
21. Schieber ML, Schnall MD, Pollack HM, et al: Current role of MR imaging in the staging of adenocarcinoma of the prostate. Radiology 1993; 189:339–352.
22. Kane RA, Littrup PJ, Babaian R, et al: Prostate-specific antigen levels in 1695 men without evidence of prostate cancer. Cancer 1992; 69:1201–1207.
23. Kirby RS: The clinical assessment of benign prostatic hyperplasia. Cancer 1992; 70:284–290.
24. Thrasher JB, Sutherland RS, Limoge JP, et al: Transrectal ultrasound and biopsy in diagnosis of malakoplakia of prostate. Urology 1992; 39:262–265.
25. Pollack HM: Imaging of the prostate. Eur Urol 1991; 20:50–58.
26. Schnall MD, Imai Y, Tomaszewski JE, et al: Prostate carcinoma: Local staging with endorectal surface coil MR imaging. Radiology 1991; 178:797–802.
27. Cooner WH, Mosley BR, Rutherford CL, et al: Prostate cancer detection in a clinical urological practice by ultrasonography, digital rectal examination, and prostatic-specific antigen. J Urol 1990; 143:1146–1154.
28. Rifkin MD, Dahnert W, Kurtz AB: State of the art: Endorectal sonography of the prostate gland. AJR Am J Roentgenol 1990; 154:691–700.
29. Rifkin MD, Zerhouni EA, Gatsonis CA, et al: Comparison of magnetic resonance imaging and ultrasonography in staging early prostate cancer: Results of multi-institutional cooperative trial. N Engl J Med 1990; 323:621–626.
30. Schnall MD, Pollack HM: Magnetic resonance imaging of the prostate gland. Urol Radiol 1990; 12:109–114.
31. Kahn T, Burrig K, Schmitz-Drager B, et al: Prostatic carcinoma and benign prostatic hyperplasia: MR imaging with histopathologic correlation. Radiology 1989; 173:847–851.
32. Schiebler ML, Tomaszewski JE, Bezzi M, et al: Prostatic carcinoma and benign prostatic hyperplasia: Correlation of high-resolution MR and histopathologic findings. Radiology 1989; 172:131–137.
33. Rifkin MD: Prostate ultrasound. Semin Ultrasound CT MR 1988; 9:352–369.
34. Rifkin MD: Endorectal sonography of the prostate: Clinical implications. AJR Am J Roentgenol 1987; 148:1137–1142.

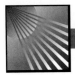

Illustrations • Prostate

1 • Normal prostate

2 • Prostate cancer: focal lesion

3 • Prostate cancer: diffuse lesion

4 • Prostate cancer: extraprostatic extension

5 • Prostate cancer: mucinous adenocarcinoma

6 • Prostate cancer: changes after treatment

7 • Other tumors of the prostate

8 • Focal prostatic lesions mimicking prostate cancer

9 • Benign prostatic hyperplasia

10 • Acute prostatitis

11 • Prostatic abscess

12 • Chronic prostatitis

13 • Other chronic inflammations of the prostate

14 • Prostatic calcifications

15 • Prostate biopsy and postbiopsy hemorrhage

1. Normal Prostate

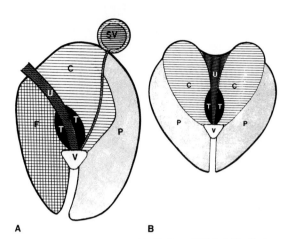

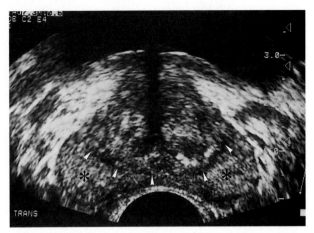

Fig. 1. Normal prostatic anatomy. (**A, B,** From Rifkin MD: Endorectal sonography of the prostate: Clinical implications. AJR Am J Roentgenol 1987; 148:1137–1142.)
A, B. Schematic drawing of the prostate in sagittal (**A**) and coronal (**B**) planes shows peripheral zone (P), central zone (C), transition zone (T), periurethral glandular tissue, and anterior fibromuscular stroma (F). V, verumontanum; U, urethra; SV, seminal vesicle.

Fig. 2. Transrectal US findings of normal prostate in a 50-year-old man. Transrectal US in axial plane demonstrates normal zonal anatomy of the prostate. The central gland shows slightly heterogeneous echogenicity, and there is mild benign hyperplasia *(arrowheads)*. The peripheral zone *(asterisks)* shows homogeneous echogenicity.

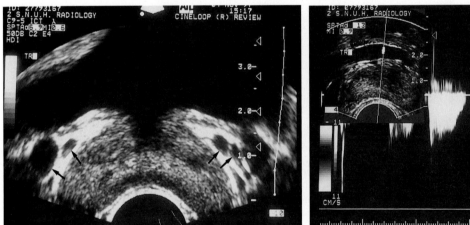

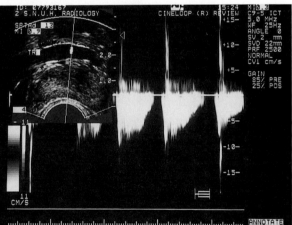

Fig. 3. Prominent Santorini's venous plexus on transrectal US in a 30-year-old man.
A. Transrectal US in axial plane shows a normal prostate and prominent anechoic structures *(arrows)* in the periprostatic fat, anterolateral to the prostate. **B.** Spectral Doppler US obtained at the anechoic structure with the patient performing repeated Valsalva maneuver demonstrates venous flow signals.

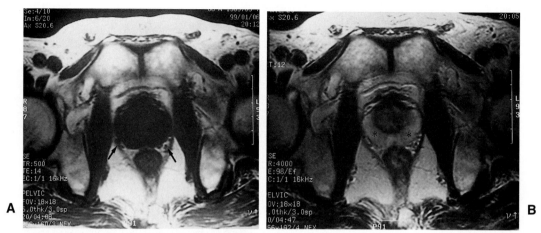

A   B

Fig. 4. MR imaging findings of a normal prostate in a 67-year-old man.
A. T1-weighted axial MR image shows homogeneous, low signal intensity of normal prostate. Note normal neurovascular bundles in posterolateral aspects of the prostate *(arrows)*. **B.** On T2-weighted MR image, the peripheral zone has homogeneous, high signal intensity *(asterisks)* and the central gland has heterogeneous signal intensity.

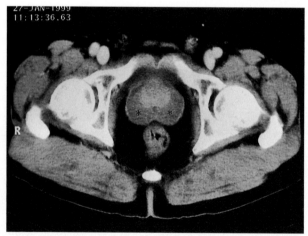

Fig. 5. CT findings of normal prostate in a 70-year-old man. Contrast-enhanced CT shows a normal prostate with a slightly low-attenuated peripheral zone *(asterisks)*. The enhancement pattern of the prostate on CT is variable.

2. Prostate Cancer: Focal Lesion

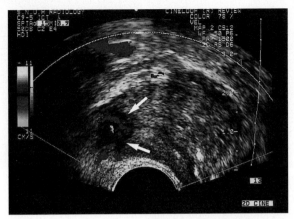

Fig. 1. Prostate cancer in a 68-year-old man. Color Doppler US shows a well-defined, hypoechoic lesion *(arrows)* in the right peripheral zone of the prostate. Note that the vascularity of the lesion is higher than that of the rest of the prostate. (See also Color Section.)

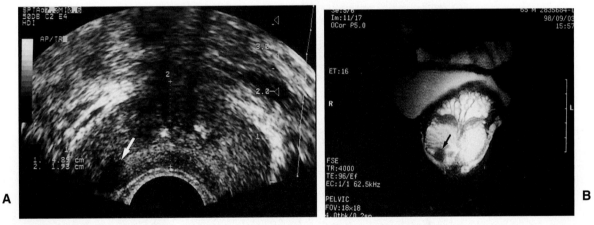

A   B

Fig. 2. Prostate cancer in a 65-year-old man.
A. Transrectal US in axial plane shows a well-defined, hypoechoic lesion *(arrow)* in the right peripheral zone of the prostate. **B.** T2-weighted coronal MR image well demonstrates a focal low-intensity lesion *(arrow)* in the right prostate.

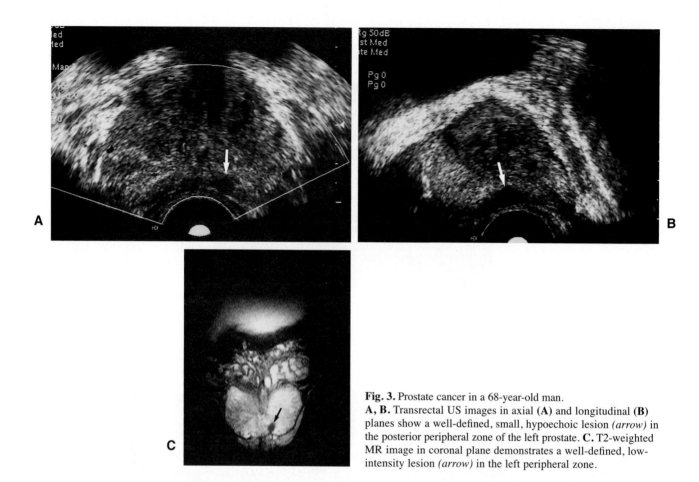

Fig. 3. Prostate cancer in a 68-year-old man.
A, B. Transrectal US images in axial (**A**) and longitudinal (**B**) planes show a well-defined, small, hypoechoic lesion *(arrow)* in the posterior peripheral zone of the left prostate. **C.** T2-weighted MR image in coronal plane demonstrates a well-defined, low-intensity lesion *(arrow)* in the left peripheral zone.

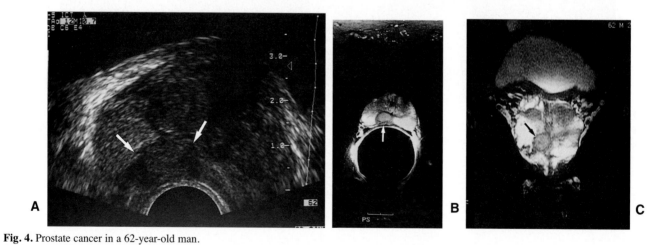

Fig. 4. Prostate cancer in a 62-year-old man.
A. Transrectal US of the prostate in axial plane shows a focal, hypoechoic lesion in the posterior peripheral zone of the right prostate *(arrows)*.
B, C. T2-weighted MR images in axial (**B**) and coronal (**C**) planes demonstrate a well-defined, low-intensity lesion *(arrow)*.

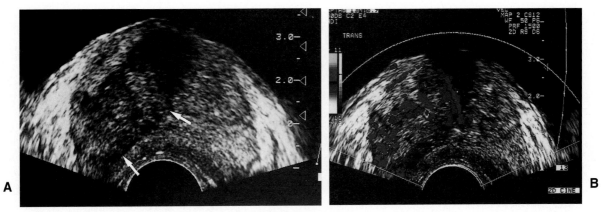

Fig. 5. Prostate cancer involving peripheral and central glands in a 59-year-old man.
A. Transrectal US in axial plane shows a large, well-defined, hypoechoic lesion *(arrows)* in the right aspect of the prostate. **B.** Color Doppler US well demonstrates that the lesion has marked hypervascularity. Note that the lesion involves not only the peripheral zone but also the central glands. **(B,** See also Color Section.)

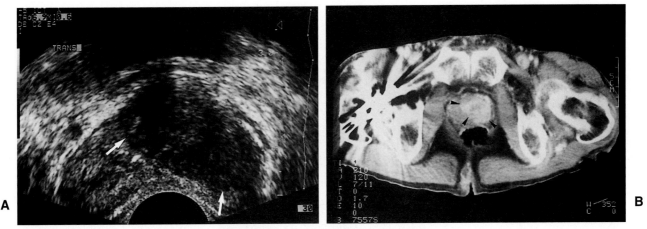

Fig. 6. Prostate cancer involving peripheral and central glands in a 60-year-old man.
A. Transrectal US in axial plane shows a large, hypoechoic lesion *(arrows)* in the left prostate involving both peripheral and central glands. **B.** Contrast-enhanced CT in early arterial phase demonstrates an enhancing lesion *(arrowheads)* in the left prostate.

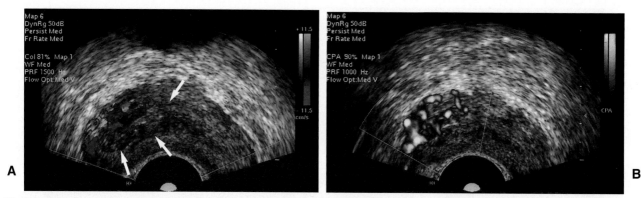

Fig. 7. Prostate cancer involving both peripheral and central glands in a 57-year-old man. (**A, B,** See also Color Section.)
A, B. Color Doppler (**A**) and power Doppler (**B**) US images of the prostate in axial plane show an ill-defined, hypoechoic lesion *(arrows)* in the central gland of the right prostate. Note that the vascularity is increased in the lesion.

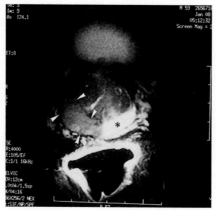

Fig. 8. Prostate cancer in a 59-year-old man. T2-weighted MR image shows a low-intensity lesion involving the right peripheral zone *(arrowheads)*. Note normal high signal intensity of the left peripheral zone *(asterisk)*.

3. Prostate Cancer: Diffuse Lesion

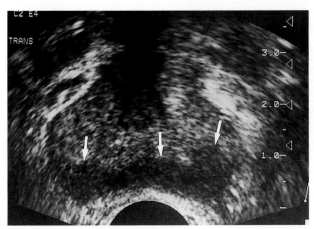

Fig. 1. Prostate cancer diffusely involving peripheral zone in a 62-year-old man. Transrectal US in axial plane shows hypoechoic lesions *(arrows)* involving the peripheral zone diffusely.

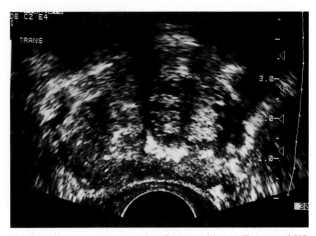

Fig. 2. Diffuse prostate cancer in a 74-year-old man. Transrectal US in axial plane shows a diffuse enlargement of the prostate with heterogeneous echogenicity and calcifications.

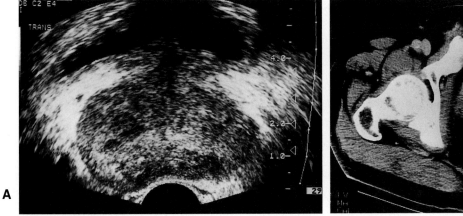

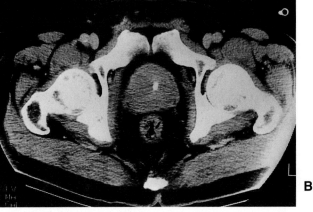

Fig. 3. Diffuse prostate cancer in a 78-year-old man.
A. Transrectal US of the prostate in axial plane shows enlarged prostate with heterogeneous echogenicity. Note scattered, ill-defined, hypoechoic lesions in the whole prostate and contour bulging of the right prostate. **B.** Contrast-enhanced CT shows large prostate with contour bulging on the right side.

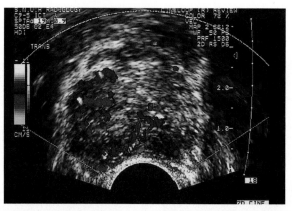

Fig. 4. Diffuse prostate cancer in a 68-year-old man. Color Doppler US shows ill-defined, diffuse, hypoechoic lesions with hypervascularity in the right and posterior peripheral zones of the prostate. (See also Color Section.)

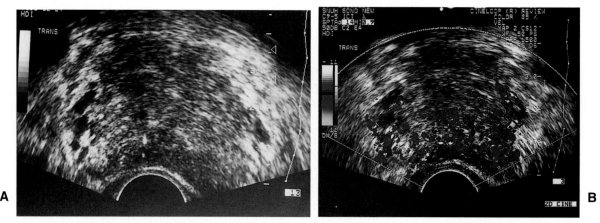

Fig. 5. Diffuse prostate cancer in a 65-year-old man.
A. Transrectal US in axial plane shows large prostate with diffusely heterogeneous echogenicity. **B.** On color Doppler US, vascularity is diffusely increased in the prostate. US-guided biopsy revealed diffuse prostate cancer with a Gleason's score of 8(4 + 4)/10. (**B,** See also Color Section.)

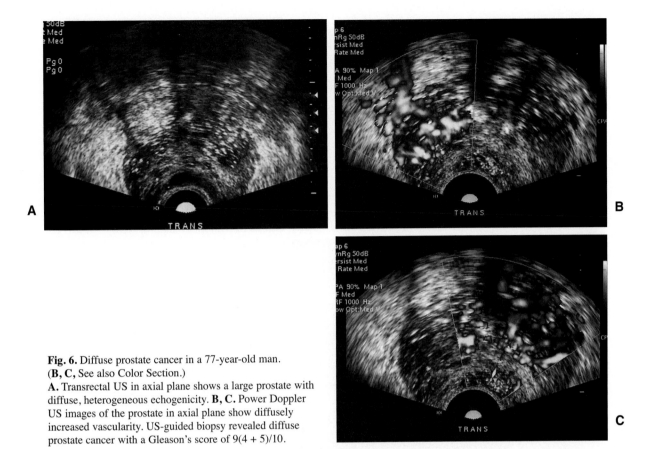

Fig. 6. Diffuse prostate cancer in a 77-year-old man.
(**B, C,** See also Color Section.)
A. Transrectal US in axial plane shows a large prostate with diffuse, heterogeneous echogenicity. **B, C.** Power Doppler US images of the prostate in axial plane show diffusely increased vascularity. US-guided biopsy revealed diffuse prostate cancer with a Gleason's score of 9(4 + 5)/10.

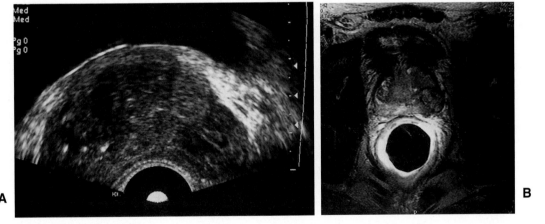

Fig. 7. Diffuse prostate cancer in a 66-year-old man.
A. Transrectal US in axial plane shows diffuse enlargement of the prostate with heterogeneous hypoechogenicity. **B.** T2-weighted MR image shows diffuse involvement of the peripheral zone with low-intensity lesions.

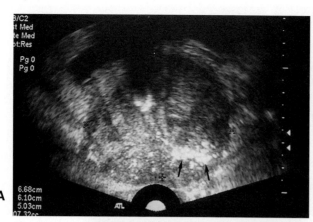

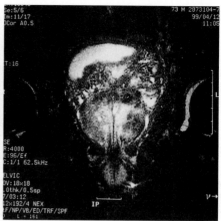

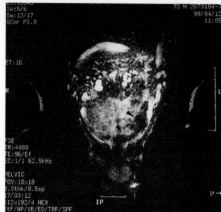

Fig. 8. Diffuse prostate cancer with calcifications in a 73-year-old man. **A.** Transrectal US in axial plane shows an enlarged prostate with heterogeneous echogenicity and dense calcifications *(arrows)* in the left prostate. **B, C.** T2-weighted MR images in coronal plane show diffuse low-intensity lesions in the peripheral zone. Note that the focal lesions of very low signal intensity in the left prostate *(arrowheads in* **C**) represent calcifications seen on transrectal US.

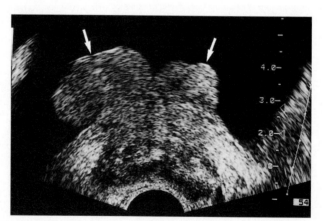

Fig. 9. Diffuse prostate cancer with severe benign prostatic hyperplasia in a 78-year-old man. Transrectal US in axial plane shows large benign hyperplastic nodules bulging into the bladder *(arrows)*. There are diffuse, ill-defined, hypoechoic lesions in the peripheral zone of the prostate.

4. Prostate Cancer: Extraprostatic Extension

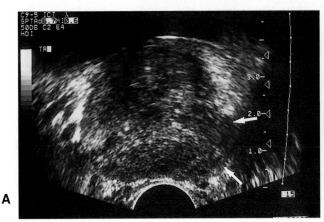

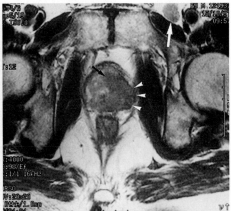

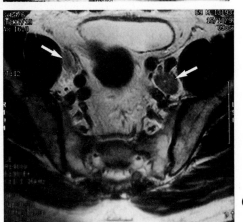

Fig. 1. Prostate cancer with periprostatic tumor extension in a
69-year-old man.
A. Transrectal US in axial plane shows ill-defined, hypoechoic
lesions in posterior and left lateral peripheral zones. Note bulging
of the prostatic contour at left lateral prostate *(arrow)*. **B.** T2-
weighted MR image in axial plane shows diffuse, low-intensity
lesions in the left and posterior peripheral zones. Note involvement
of the left central gland *(black arrow)*. Also note the contour
bulging in the left lateral aspect of the prostate *(arrowheads)*,
suggesting periprostatic tumor extension. There is an enlarged left
inguinal lymph node *(white arrow)*. **C.** T2-weighted MR image at a
higher level shows multiple metastatic pelvic lymph nodes
(arrows).

Fig. 2. Prostate cancer with periprostatic
tumor extension in a 65-year-old man.
A. T1-weighted MR image shows
bulging of the prostate contour at left
posterior aspect *(arrow)*. Note
obliteration of neurovascular bundle by
the tumor. **B.** T2-weighted MR image
shows diffuse obliteration of normal high
intensity of the peripheral zone. There is
a high-intensity, bulging mass in the left
posterior aspect of the prostate *(arrow)*.

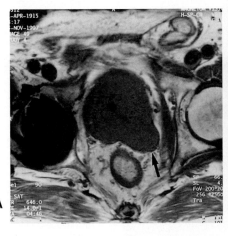

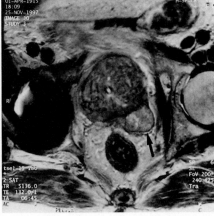

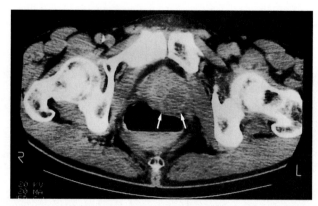

Fig. 3. Prostate cancer with periprostatic tumor extension in a 69-year-old man. Contrast-enhanced CT shows a low-attenuated lesion in the left prostate with contour bulging *(arrows)*.

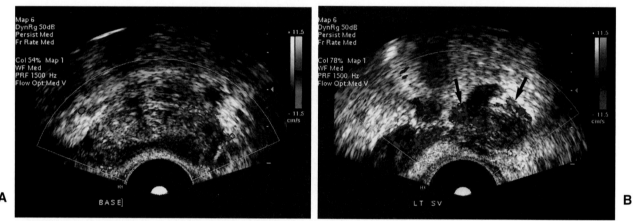

Fig. 4. Prostate cancer with involvement of the seminal vesicle in a 78-year-old man. (**A, B,** See also Color Section.)
A. Color Doppler US of the prostate in axial plane shows an ill-defined, hypoechoic lesion in the left posterolateral peripheral zone that has slight hypervascularity. **B.** Color Doppler US of the seminal vesicles in axial plane shows slightly enlarged left seminal vesicle that has slight hypervascularity *(arrows)*. US-guided biopsy revealed prostate cancer with involvement of the left seminal vesicle.

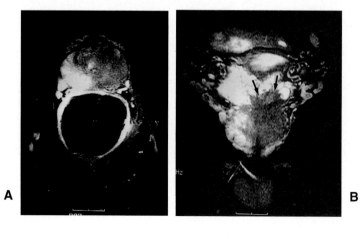

Fig. 5. Prostate cancer with involvement of the seminal vesicle in a 74-year-old man.
A. T2-weighted MR image in axial plane shows an ill-defined, low-intensity lesion in the left prostate. **B.** T2-weighted coronal MR image well demonstrates the involvement of the left prostate with a low-intensity lesion. Note invasion of the left seminal vesicle by the tumor *(arrows)*.

4. Prostate Cancer: Extraprostatic Extension

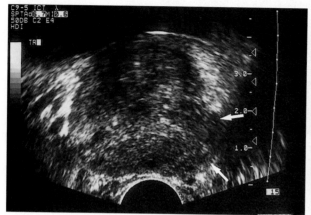

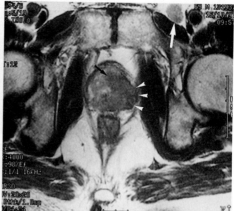

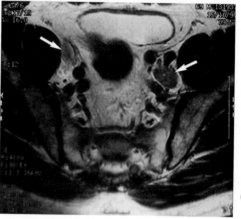

Fig. 1. Prostate cancer with periprostatic tumor extension in a 69-year-old man.
A. Transrectal US in axial plane shows ill-defined, hypoechoic lesions in posterior and left lateral peripheral zones. Note bulging of the prostatic contour at left lateral prostate *(arrow)*. **B.** T2-weighted MR image in axial plane shows diffuse, low-intensity lesions in the left and posterior peripheral zones. Note involvement of the left central gland *(black arrow)*. Also note the contour bulging in the left lateral aspect of the prostate *(arrowheads)*, suggesting periprostatic tumor extension. There is an enlarged left inguinal lymph node *(white arrow)*. **C.** T2-weighted MR image at a higher level shows multiple metastatic pelvic lymph nodes *(arrows)*.

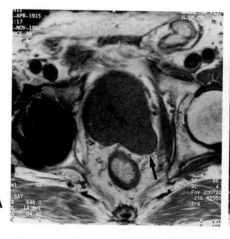

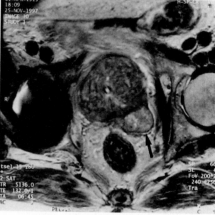

Fig. 2. Prostate cancer with periprostatic tumor extension in a 65-year-old man.
A. T1-weighted MR image shows bulging of the prostate contour at left posterior aspect *(arrow)*. Note obliteration of neurovascular bundle by the tumor. **B.** T2-weighted MR image shows diffuse obliteration of normal high intensity of the peripheral zone. There is a high-intensity, bulging mass in the left posterior aspect of the prostate *(arrow)*.

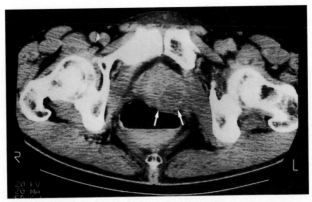

Fig. 3. Prostate cancer with periprostatic tumor extension in a 69-year-old man. Contrast-enhanced CT shows a low-attenuated lesion in the left prostate with contour bulging *(arrows)*.

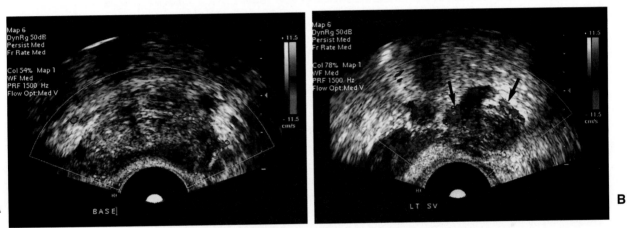

A

B

Fig. 4. Prostate cancer with involvement of the seminal vesicle in a 78-year-old man. (**A, B,** See also Color Section.)
A. Color Doppler US of the prostate in axial plane shows an ill-defined, hypoechoic lesion in the left posterolateral peripheral zone that has slight hypervascularity. **B.** Color Doppler US of the seminal vesicles in axial plane shows slightly enlarged left seminal vesicle that has slight hypervascularity *(arrows)*. US-guided biopsy revealed prostate cancer with involvement of the left seminal vesicle.

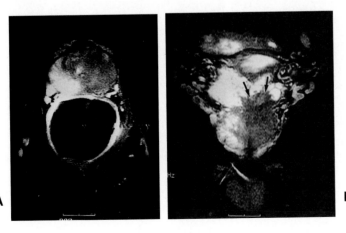

A

B

Fig. 5. Prostate cancer with involvement of the seminal vesicle in a 74-year-old man.
A. T2-weighted MR image in axial plane shows an ill-defined, low-intensity lesion in the left prostate. **B.** T2-weighted coronal MR image well demonstrates the involvement of the left prostate with a low-intensity lesion. Note invasion of the left seminal vesicle by the tumor *(arrows)*.

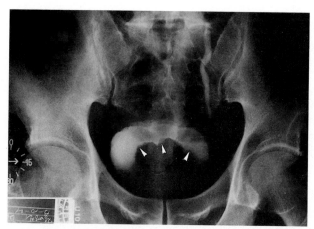

Fig. 6. Prostate cancer with bladder invasion in a 68-year-old man. IVU shows elevation of the bladder base with marginal nodularity and irregularity *(arrowheads)* due to invasion of the bladder by prostate cancer.

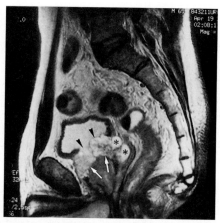

Fig. 7. Prostatic ductal adenocarcinoma of endometrioid type in a 65-year-old man with invasion of the bladder and seminal vesicles. T2-weighted sagittal MR image shows large, high-intensity mass in the base of the prostate *(arrows)* with involvement of the bladder base *(arrowheads)* and seminal vesicles *(asterisks)*.

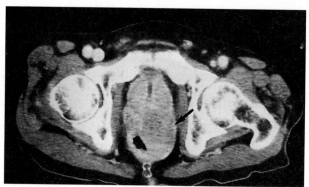

Fig. 8. Prostate cancer with rectal invasion in a 77-year-old man. Contrast-enhanced CT shows a large, low-attenuated mass *(arrow)* in the posterior aspect of the prostate with direct invasion of the rectum.

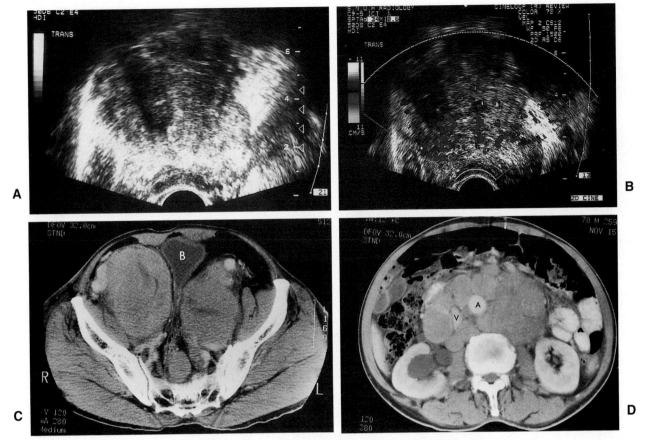

Fig. 9. Diffuse prostate cancer with extensive retroperitoneal nodal metastases in a 70-year-old man.
A. Transrectal US in axial plane shows an enlarged prostate with diffusely heterogeneous echogenicity. **B.** Color Doppler US shows diffusely increased vascularity of the prostate. (**B,** See also Color Section.) **C.** Contrast-enhanced CT of the pelvis shows multiple, large, metastatic lymph nodes in the pelvic cavity with compression of the bladder (B). **D.** Contrast-enhanced CT scan in the higher level shows extensive metastases to the retroperitoneal lymph nodes with encasement of the abdominal aorta (A) and inferior vena cava (V). Note that the nodal metastases extend behind the great vessels. Also note hydronephrosis of the right kidney.

5. Prostate Cancer: Mucinous Adenocarcinoma

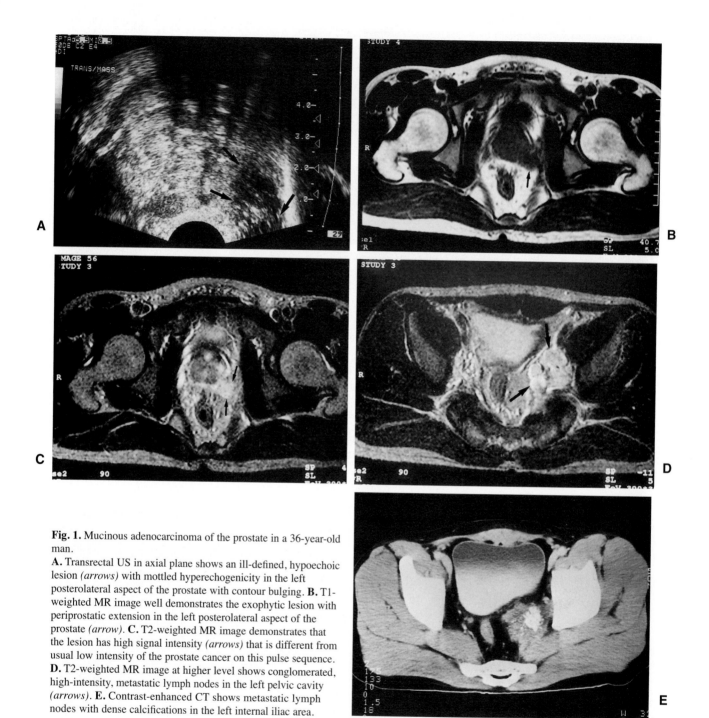

Fig. 1. Mucinous adenocarcinoma of the prostate in a 36-year-old man.
A. Transrectal US in axial plane shows an ill-defined, hypoechoic lesion *(arrows)* with mottled hyperechogenicity in the left posterolateral aspect of the prostate with contour bulging. **B.** T1-weighted MR image well demonstrates the exophytic lesion with periprostatic extension in the left posterolateral aspect of the prostate *(arrow)*. **C.** T2-weighted MR image demonstrates that the lesion has high signal intensity *(arrows)* that is different from usual low intensity of the prostate cancer on this pulse sequence. **D.** T2-weighted MR image at higher level shows conglomerated, high-intensity, metastatic lymph nodes in the left pelvic cavity *(arrows)*. **E.** Contrast-enhanced CT shows metastatic lymph nodes with dense calcifications in the left internal iliac area.

6. Prostate Cancer: Changes after Treatment

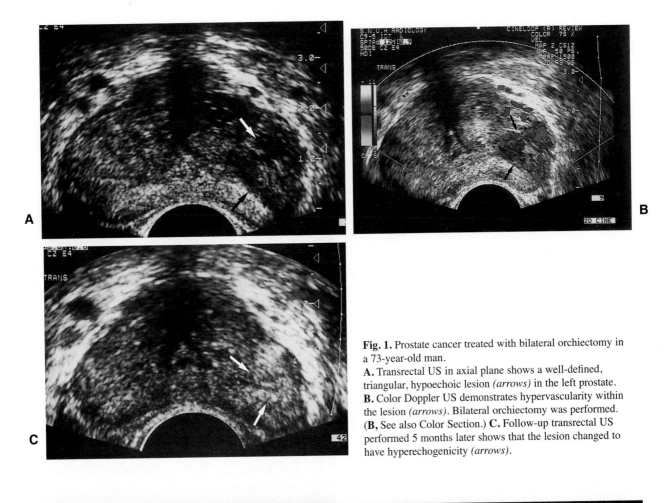

Fig. 1. Prostate cancer treated with bilateral orchiectomy in a 73-year-old man.
A. Transrectal US in axial plane shows a well-defined, triangular, hypoechoic lesion *(arrows)* in the left prostate.
B. Color Doppler US demonstrates hypervascularity within the lesion *(arrows)*. Bilateral orchiectomy was performed. **(B,** See also Color Section.) **C.** Follow-up transrectal US performed 5 months later shows that the lesion changed to have hyperechogenicity *(arrows)*.

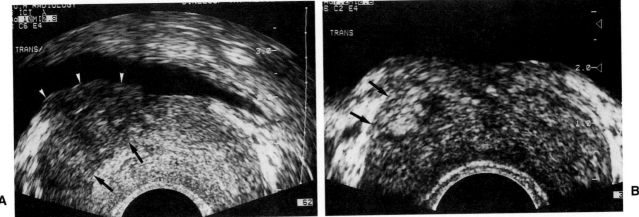

Fig. 2. Prostate cancer that was treated with radiation therapy in a 63-year-old man.
A. Transrectal US in axial plane shows a large, hypoechoic lesion in the right prostate *(arrows)* with invasion of the bladder wall *(arrowheads)*.
B. Follow-up transrectal US taken 9 months after radiation therapy shows that the prostatic mass is decreased in size and the echogenicity of the lesion is markedly increased *(arrows)*.

7. Other Tumors of the Prostate

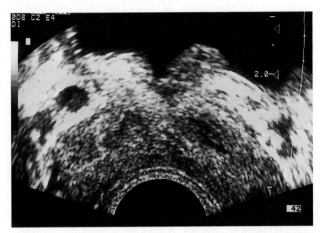

Fig. 1. Prostate lymphoma in a 16-year-old boy. Transrectal US in axial plane shows diffuse hypoechogenicity of the prostate without prostatic enlargement. US-guided biopsy revealed malignant lymphoma of diffuse large B-cell type.

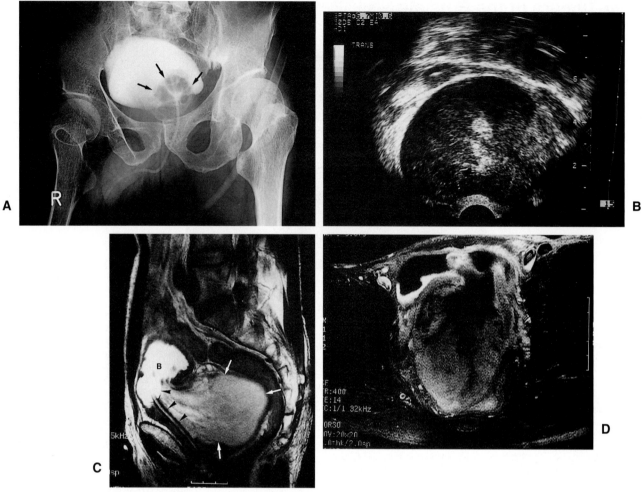

Fig. 2. Rhabdomyosarcoma of the prostate in a 17-year-old boy.
A. Bladder image of IVU shows a large, lobulated, prostatic mass bulging into the bladder *(arrows)*. Note the Foley catheter balloon filled with air. **B.** Transrectal US in axial plane shows markedly enlarged prostate with heterogeneous echogenicity. **C.** T2-weighted sagittal MR image shows a large prostatic mass *(arrows)* that bulges into the urinary bladder (B). The prostatic mass has homogeneous high signal intensity. Note Foley catheter in the bladder and elongated urethra *(arrowheads)*. **D.** Contrast-enhanced T1-weighted axial MR image shows poor enhancement of the prostatic mass.

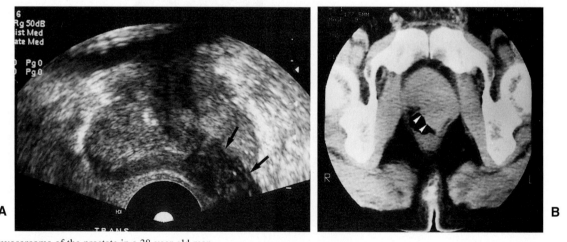

Fig. 3. Leiomyosarcoma of the prostate in a 38-year-old man.
A. Transrectal US in axial plane shows a large, exophytic, hypoechoic mass *(arrows)* in the posterolateral aspect of the left prostate. **B.** Contrast-enhanced CT shows a bulging mass in the left posterior aspect of the prostate with invasion of the rectal wall *(arrowheads)*.

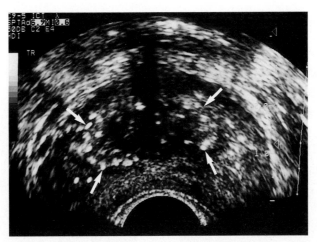

Fig. 4. Transitional cell carcinoma of the prostate involving central gland in a 73-year-old man. Transrectal US in axial plane shows an ill-defined, hypoechoic lesion with mottled hyperechoic spots suggesting calcifications in the central gland *(arrows)*. US-guided biopsy revealed primary transitional cell carcinoma of the prostate.

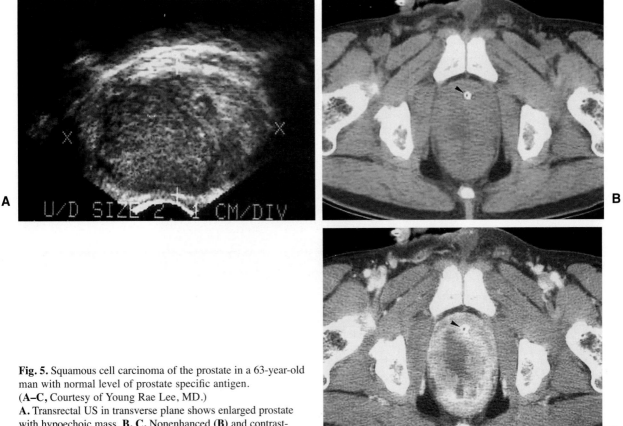

Fig. 5. Squamous cell carcinoma of the prostate in a 63-year-old man with normal level of prostate specific antigen. (**A–C,** Courtesy of Young Rae Lee, MD.)
A. Transrectal US in transverse plane shows enlarged prostate with hypoechoic mass. **B, C.** Nonenhanced (**B**) and contrast-enhanced (**C**) CT scans show large prostate with heterogeneous attenuation. Note a Foley catheter in the urethra *(arrowhead)*.

8. Focal Prostatic Lesions Mimicking Prostate Cancer

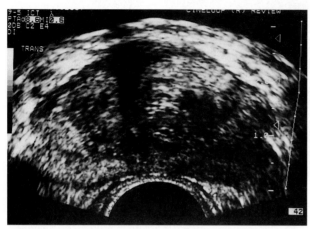

Fig. 1. Benign prostatic hyperplasia mimicking a prostate cancer in a 56-year-old man. Transrectal US in axial plane shows a large prostate and geographic hypoechoic lesions in the left prostate. US-guided biopsy revealed benign prostatic hyperplasia without evidence of prostate cancer.

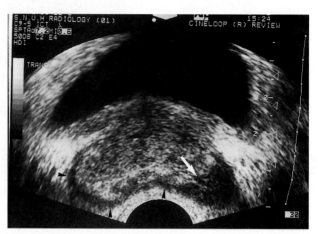

Fig. 2. Chronic prostatitis mimicking a prostate cancer in a 65-year-old man. Transrectal US in axial plane shows a focal hypoechoic lesion *(arrow)* in the left lateral peripheral zone. Also note diffusely increased echogenicity of the prostate and a thin, hypoechoic rim in the periphery of the prostate *(arrowheads)* suggesting chronic prostatitis. US-guided biopsy revealed chronic prostatitis and no evidence of prostate cancer.

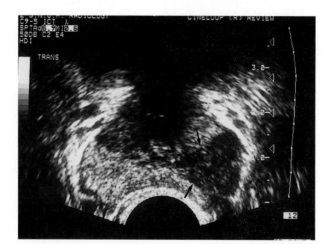

Fig. 3. Focal chronic inflammation of the prostate mimicking a prostate cancer in a 30-year-old man. Transrectal US in axial plane shows a well-defined, wedge-shaped, hypoechoic lesion in the left aspect of the prostate *(arrows)*. US-guided biopsy revealed chronic prostatitis.

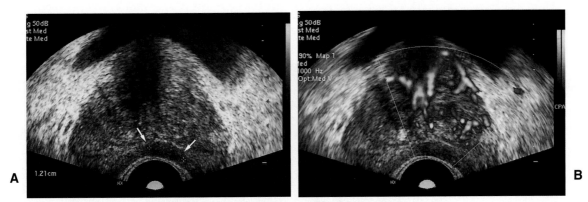

Fig. 4. Focal chronic inflammation of the prostate mimicking a prostate cancer in a 70-year-old man.
A. Transrectal US in axial plane shows a well-defined, hypoechoic lesion *(arrows)* in posterior peripheral zone. **B.** Power Doppler US shows that the vascularity of the lesion is lower than that of the rest of the prostate. (**B,** See also Color Section.)

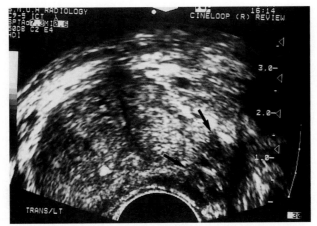

Fig. 5. Focal prostatic infarct mimicking a prostate cancer in a 65-year-old man. Transrectal US in axial plane shows an ill-defined, focal, hypoechoic lesion in the left posterolateral peripheral zone *(arrows)*. US-guided biopsy revealed prostatic infarct.

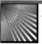

9. Benign Prostatic Hyperplasia

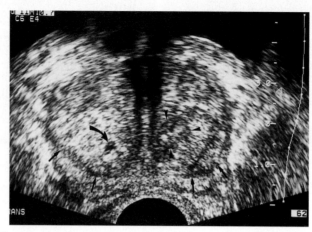

Fig. 1. Benign prostatic hyperplasia in a 71-year-old man. Transrectal US
in axial plane shows a large, well-demarcated, nodular mass in the
central gland surrounded by a thin hypoechoic rim *(arrows)* representing
a pseudocapsule. The mass has echogenicity similar to that of the rest of
the prostate. Note a small cyst *(curved arrow)* and a hypoechoic nodule
(arrowheads) within the mass.

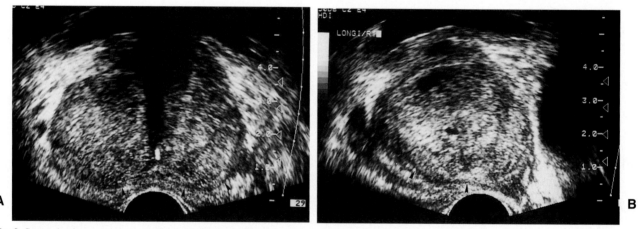

Fig. 2. Severe benign prostatic hyperplasia in a 66-year-old man.
A, B. Transrectal US images in axial (**A**) and midsagittal (**B**) planes show a large, heterogeneous, slightly hypoechoic, nodular mass in the central
gland with a peripheral hypoechoic rim *(arrowheads)*.

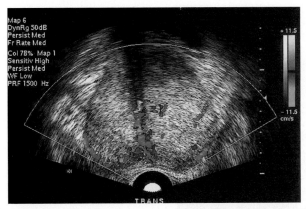

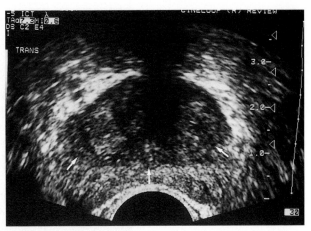

Fig. 3. Benign prostatic hyperplasia in a 56-year-old man. Color Doppler US shows large nodular masses in the central gland of the prostate and flow signals along the margin of the masses. (See also Color Section.)

Fig. 4. Benign prostatic hyperplasia in a 77-year-old man. Transrectal US in axial plane shows a well-defined, hypoechoic mass *(arrows)* in the central gland of the prostate.

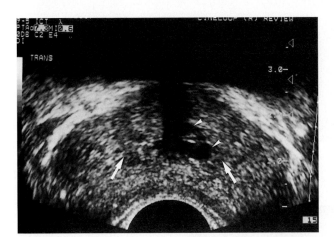

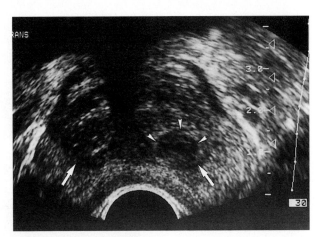

Fig. 5. Benign prostatic hyperplasia in a 67-year-old man. Transrectal US of the prostate in axial plane shows a slightly enlarged central gland without a distinct margin *(arrows)*. The lesion is heterogeneously hypoechoic. Note small cysts *(arrowheads)* within the lesion.

Fig. 6. Benign prostatic hyperplasia in a 59-year-old man. Transrectal US in axial plane shows large, nodular, hypoechoic masses in the central gland of the prostate *(arrows)*. Note a well-defined nodule *(arrowheads)* within the mass.

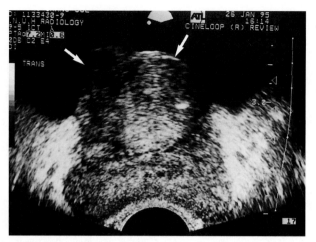

Fig. 7. Benign prostatic hyperplasia in a 73-year-old man. Transrectal US in axial plane shows a large nodular mass in the anterior part of the prostate bulging into the urinary bladder *(arrows)*. The mass is well demarcated and has heterogeneous echogenicity.

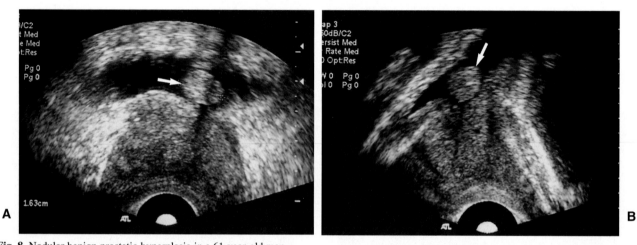

Fig. 8. Nodular benign prostatic hyperplasia in a 61-year-old man.
A, B. Transrectal US images in axial **(A)** and sagittal **(B)** planes show a round, nodular lesion *(arrow)* arising in the prostate and bulging into the bladder.

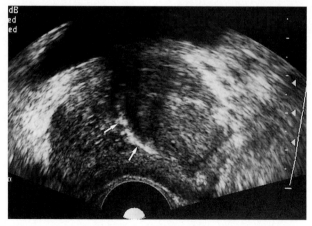

Fig. 9. Asymmetrical benign prostatic hyperplasia with marginal calcification in a 70-year-old man. Transrectal US in axial plane shows a large nodular mass in the left aspect of the prostate with dense marginal calcifications *(arrows)*.

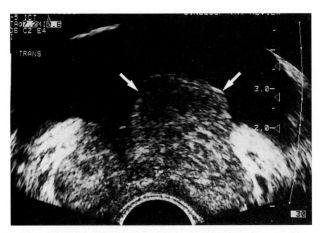

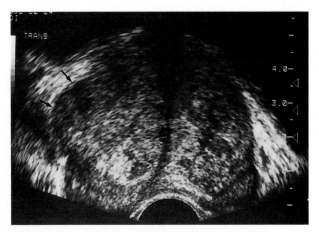

Fig. 10. Asymmetrical benign prostatic hyperplasia in a 60-year-old man. Transrectal US shows a large mass *(arrows)* in the central gland of the left prostate bulging into the urinary bladder. The mass has heterogeneous echogenicity.

Fig. 11. Benign prostatic hyperplasia in a 64-year-old man. Transrectal US in axial plane shows nodular enlargement of the central gland. Note focal bulging of the right lateral contour of the prostate *(arrows)*.

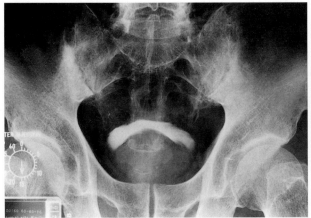

A

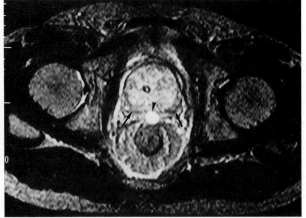

B

Fig. 12. MR imaging findings of benign prostatic hyperplasia in a 72-year-old man.
A. IVU shows marked elevation of the bladder base with smooth margin due to a large prostate. **B.** T2-weighted MR image shows a large, nodular mass in the central gland with marginal low signal intensity *(arrows)* representing a pseudocapsule. The peripheral zone is compressed by the central gland mass. Also note a small midline cyst *(arrowhead)*. **C.** T1-weighted contrast-enhanced MR image shows heterogeneous enhancement of the central gland mass.

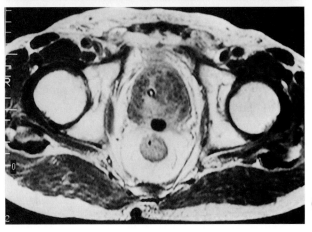

C

10. Acute Prostatitis

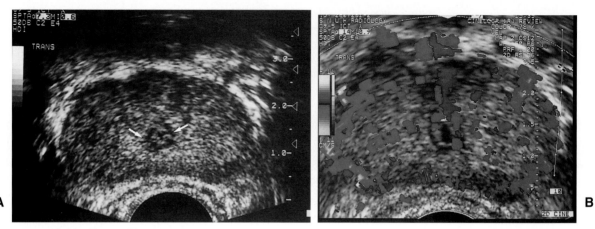

Fig. 1. Acute prostatitis in a 45-year-old man.
A. Transrectal US in axial plane shows a swollen prostate with diffuse peripheral hypoechogenicity. Note that prostatic echogenicity is increased in the central part, and the urethra is prominent with hypoechoic, edematous wall *(arrows)*. **B.** Color Doppler US of the prostate demonstrates diffusely increased vascularity of the prostate, especially in the peripheral portion. (**B,** See also Color Section.)

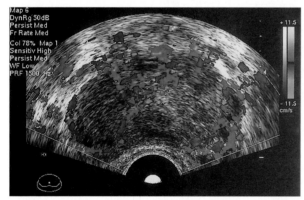

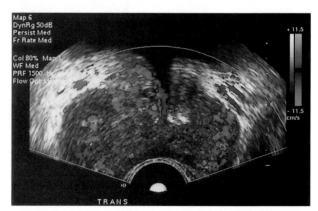

Fig. 2. Acute prostatitis in a 56-year-old man with diabetes. Color Doppler US of the prostate in axial plane shows enlarged prostate with diffuse, heterogeneous hypoechogenicity. Note that the vascularity of the prostate is diffusely increased. (See also Color Section.)

Fig. 3. Acute prostatitis in a 65-year-old man. Color Doppler US of the prostate in axial plane shows enlarged prostate with diffuse hypoechogenicity. The prostate has diffuse hypervascularity. (See also Color Section.)

11. Prostatic Abscess

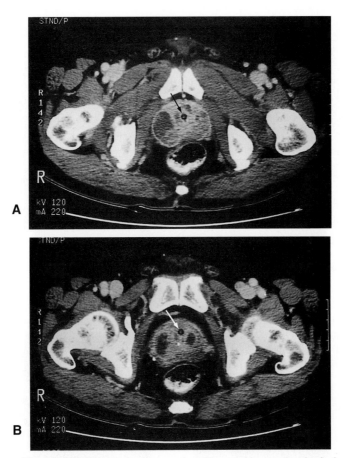

Fig. 1. Multiple prostatic abscesses in a 65-year-old man who also had abscesses in the brain and kidneys.

A, B. Contrast-enhanced CT scans show an enlarged prostate with multiple, low-attenuated abscess cavities in the prostate. Note a Foley catheter in the urethra *(arrow)*. Prostate-specific antigen was markedly elevated in this patient.

12. Chronic Prostatitis

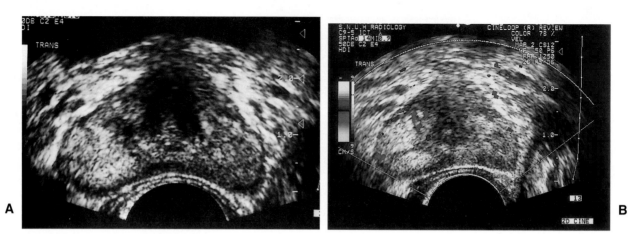

Fig. 1. Chronic prostatitis in a 47-year-old man.
A. Transrectal US of the prostate in axial plane shows markedly increased echogenicity of the prostate and hypoechoic rim in the periphery of the prostate. **B.** Color Doppler US of the prostate does not show increased vascularity of the prostate. (**B,** See also Color Section.)

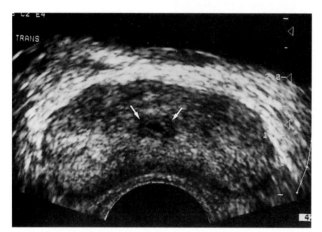

Fig. 2. Chronic prostatitis in a 55-year-old man. Transrectal US in axial plane shows diffusely increased echogenicity of the prostate and hypoechoic periphery. Note thickened wall of the urethra *(arrows).*

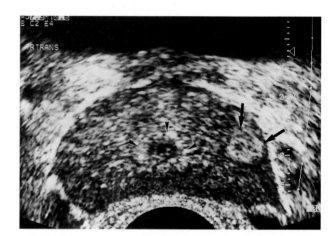

Fig. 3. Chronic prostatitis in a 41-year-old man. Transrectal US in axial plane shows diffusely increased prostatic echogenicity and a focal hyperechoic lesion *(arrows)* in the left aspect of the prostate. Note markedly increased echogenicity around the urethra *(arrowheads)* with a thickened urethral wall.

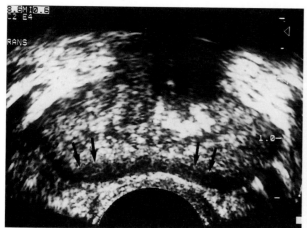

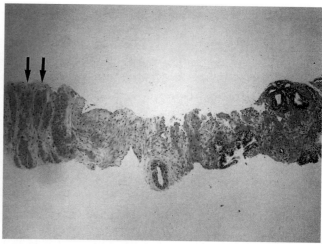

A

B

Fig. 4. A 64-year-old man with chronic prostatitis. (**A, B,** From Lee HJ, Choe GY, Seong CG, et al: Hypoechoic rim of the chronic prostatic inflammation: Histopathologic findings. Korean J Radiol 2001; 2:159–163.)

A. Transrectal US in axial plane shows heterogeneously increased prostatic echogenicity and a prominent hypoechoic rim in the periphery of the prostate *(arrows)*. **B.** Transrectal US–guided biopsy was performed and a photomicrograph of the biopsy specimen at lower-power field (×40) reveals that the peripheral portion, seen at transrectal US as a hypoechoic rim, is composed of loose connective tissue with few prostatic glands and sparse infiltration of inflammatory cells *(arrows)*. (**B,** See also Color Section.)

13. Other Chronic Inflammations of the Prostate

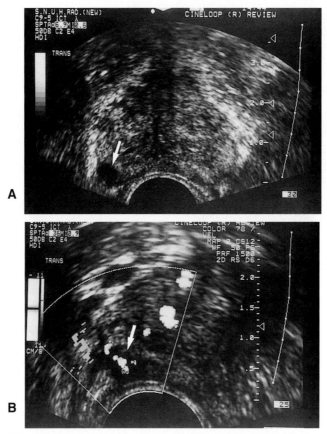

Fig. 1. Malacoplakia of the prostate in a 57-year-old man.
A. Transrectal US in axial plane shows a well-defined, hypoechoic nodule in the posterolateral aspect of the right peripheral zone *(arrow)*.
B. Doppler US shows flow signals within the lesion *(arrow)*. US-guided biopsy revealed prostatic malacoplakia.

14. Prostatic Calcifications

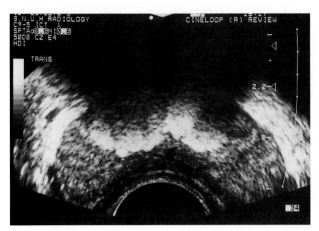

Fig. 1. Dense prostatic calcifications in a 57-year-old man with chronic prostatitis. Transrectal US in axial plane shows large calcifications with posterior sonic shadowing. US-guided biopsy revealed chronic prostatitis with calcifications.

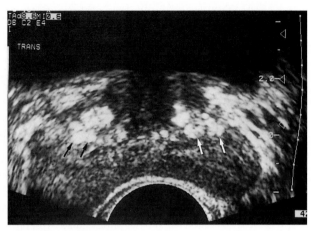

Fig. 2. Prostatic calcifications in a 40-year-old man with chronic prostatitis. Transrectal US in axial plane shows diffusely increased prostatic echogenicity and dense calcifications *(arrows)*.

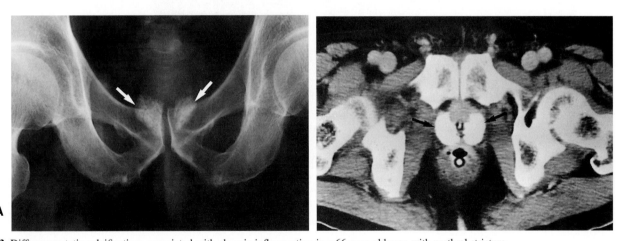

A   B

Fig. 3. Diffuse prostatic calcifications associated with chronic inflammation in a 66-year-old man with urethral stricture.
A. Plain radiograph shows diffuse calcifications in the prostatic regions *(arrows)*. **B.** CT scan shows dense calcifications in the peripheral glands of the prostate *(arrows)*.

15. Prostate Biopsy and Postbiopsy Hemorrhage

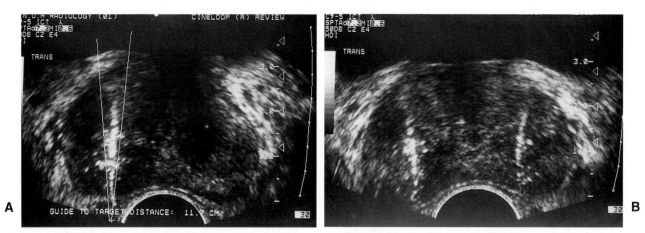

Fig. 1. Transrectal US–guided biopsy of the prostate in a 57-year-old man with chronic prostatitis.
A. Transrectal US during biopsy shows a needle in the right prostate. **B.** After biopsy, needle tracks appear as echogenic lines.

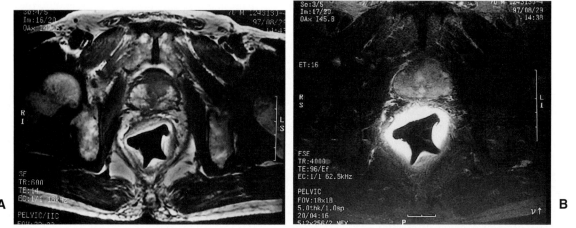

Fig. 2. MR imaging findings of postbiopsy hemorrhage of the prostate in a 70-year-old man with diffuse prostate cancer. MR imaging was performed 2 weeks after biopsy.
A. T1-weighted MR image shows diffuse, high signal intensity of the peripheral zone of the prostate due to postbiopsy hemorrhage. **B.** T2-weighted MR image shows diffusely decreased signal intensity of the prostate. With postbiopsy hemorrhage, it is difficult to define the prostatic cancerous lesion on MR imaging.

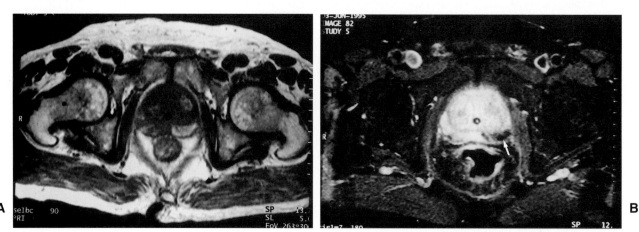

Fig. 3. Postbiopsy hemorrhage of the prostate in a 76-year-old man with prostate cancer. MR imaging was performed 7 days after biopsy.
A. T1-weighted MR image shows multifocal high-intensity lesions in the prostate due to postbiopsy hemorrhage. **B.** T2-weighted MR image demonstrates low-intensity of the hemorrhagic lesions *(arrow)*.

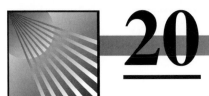

20

Imaging for Seminal Tracts

SEUNG HYUP KIM

ANATOMY

The seminal vesicles are paired accessory sex glands composed of convoluted tubes, located posterior and superior to the prostate. Their mucoid secretion helps activate spermatozoa. Normal seminal vesicles are usually symmetrical and are considered as dilated when an axial diameter exceeds 1.5 cm on imaging. The vas deferens is a continuation of the tail of the epididymis, and it courses through the inguinal ring as a part of the spermatic cord and along the superomedial aspect of the seminal vesicle, where it dilates to form the ampulla. The ampulla of the vas deferens joins the seminal vesicle to form the ejaculatory duct, which traverses the central zone of the prostate to open into the prostatic urethra on either side of the verumontanum. The utricle is a male counterpart of the uterus, which is usually a small dimple on the surface of the verumontanum. In as many as 10% of normal men, the utricle is larger and forms a slitlike aperture lying between the openings of the ejaculatory ducts and extending in a cephalad direction. Large persistent utricles are often associated with proximal hypospadias.

IMAGING STUDIES

Various imaging techniques including vasoseminal vesiculography, transrectal ultrasonography (US), and magnetic resonance (MR) imaging have been used to demonstrate the seminal tracts. Although conventional vasoseminal vesiculography remains as the most definite imaging modality for evaluation of the seminal tracts, the technique is invasive and is being replaced by noninvasive transrectal US or MR imaging.

Vasoseminal vesiculography

Vasoseminal vesiculography is an invasive technique to opacify seminal tracts by means of cannulation of a fine needle into the vas deferens. Although the technique of cannulation without scrotal incision has been reported, it is usually done by open exposure of the vas deferens in the scrotum. Injection of a small amount of water-soluble contrast material sequentially opacifies the vas deferens, ampulla of the vas, seminal vesicle, and ejaculatory duct, and then contrast material flows into the posterior urethra and the bladder. Epididymal obstruction can be evaluated with vasoepididymography by injecting contrast material with the needle directed distally. Vasoseminal vesiculography is usually performed to define the level of obstruc-

tion of the seminal tracts in men with azoospermia or severe oligospermia.

Transrectal ultrasonography

Transrectal US is being used as the first-line imaging modality for the evaluation of the seminal tracts. Transrectal US can demonstrate the abnormalities of the seminal tracts responsible for infertility or bloody ejaculation. Transrectal US can also be used to guide a needle for aspiration of the dilated seminal tracts and instillation of contrast material to obtain radiographs. On transrectal US, normal seminal vesicles appear as symmetrical, thin-walled, hypoechoic structures and have fine internal echoes. They may appear septated due to their convolutions. Vas deferens appears as a tubular structure, and its wall is thicker than that of the seminal vesicle. Normal ejaculatory ducts can be defined as a paired, thin echogenic line coursing through the central zone of the prostate to the verumontanum. The actual lumina of the ejaculatory ducts are normally not visible on transrectal US.

Computed tomography

Normal seminal vesicles are easily identified on computed tomographic (CT) scan as symmetrical soft tissue structures of a bow-tie shape posterior to the urinary bladder and cephalad to the prostate. Normal seminal vesicles should be separated from the bladder by a triangular fat plane, which is called the *seminal vesicle–bladder angle*.

MR imaging

The superb soft tissue contrast and multiplanar capability of MR imaging enabled detailed evaluation of internal architecture of the seminal tracts. The resolution has been enhanced further with endorectal MR imaging. On T1-weighted images, the seminal vesicles show homogeneous low to intermediate signal intensity, and T2-weighted images well exhibit convolutions with high-intensity fluid and low-intensity walls. The vas deferens appears as a low-intensity tubular structure due to its thicker walls.

CONGENITAL ANOMALIES

The common derivation of the seminal vesicles, vas deferens, and ureteric bud from the primitive mesonephric or wolffian

duct explains the frequent association of seminal tract and urinary tract anomalies.

Agenesis

Failure of development of a mesonephric duct results in agenesis of the ipsilateral kidney, ureter, bladder hemitrigone, seminal vesicle, vas deferens, and ejaculatory duct, singly or in combination. The vas deferens may be absent totally or partially, and part of the epididymis also may be missing. Although patients with vas agenesis may have a normal ipsilateral seminal vesicle, a combination of a sonographically absent seminal vesicle in a patient with no palpable ipsilateral vas is diagnostic of vas agenesis. The pudendal venous plexus may simulate small seminal vesicles on imaging studies.

Midline cyst

The classification of cysts involving the prostate and seminal tracts is based on their position and embryologic origin. The utricular cyst, müllerian duct cyst, and ejaculatory duct cyst all are located at or near the midline, and therefore they are collectively called *midline cyst*. Utricular cysts are of endodermal origin, usually smaller than müllerian duct cysts, communicate with the prostatic urethra, and are often associated with hypospadias. Müllerian duct cysts are of mesodermal origin, often extend well above the prostate, do not communicate with the prostatic urethra, and are not associated with genital anomalies. Ejaculatory duct cysts or wolffian duct cysts have connection with vas or seminal vesicles and thus could be differentiated from utricular cysts or müllerian duct cysts by the presence of sperm in their content. The differentiation among these cysts is theoretically clear but often difficult on imaging studies. Midline cysts may compress the ejaculatory duct, resulting in partial obstruction of the duct.

Seminal vesicle cyst

Seminal vesicle cysts are usually congenital in origin but can be acquired as a result of inflammation or hyperplasia of the prostate. Abnormal development of the distal mesonephric duct causes atresia of the ejaculatory duct and formation of a seminal vesicle cyst as well as failure of development of the ureteric bud, which results in renal agenesis or dysgenesis. The ipsilateral ureter may have an ectopic insertion into the mesonephric duct derivatives such as the bladder neck, prostatic urethra, ejaculatory duct, or seminal vesicle. Seminal vesicle cysts also can be associated with autosomal dominant polycystic kidney disease probably due to common structural defects in the basement membrane.

Seminal vesicle cyst appears as a unilocular cystic structure posterolateral to the bladder and may be complicated by infection or hemorrhage. Often imaging studies can demonstrate the dilated ipsilateral ureter inserting into the cyst. Occasionally the cyst wall is calcified. A small dysplastic ipsilateral kidney is often difficult to demonstrate.

Seminal vesicle cysts can be punctured under transrectal US guidance, and the aspirate usually reveals a viscous, brownish fluid that contains dead sperm. Instillation of contrast material following aspiration may demonstrate the relation of the cyst to the seminal and urinary tracts.

INFLAMMATION
Seminal vesiculitis

Seminal vesiculitis and abscess are usually found in association with inflammation of the prostate and vas deferens. Predisposing factors of seminal vesiculitis include urinary tract infection, instrumentation, indwelling catheters, diabetes, status postvasectomy, and anatomic abnormalities. The seminal vesicle is usually enlarged in acute inflammation but is shrunken in the chronic stage. US echogenicity and signal intensity on MR imaging are variable according to the stage of inflammation and association with hemorrhage. On vasoseminal vesiculography, the inflamed vas deferens may show a feathery appearance due to multiple small vasal diverticula. In chronic inflammation, vas deferens may show a beaded appearance due to strictures and dilation.

Tuberculosis

Seminal vesicle tuberculosis results from either upper urinary tract tuberculosis or primary genital tuberculosis. Tuberculosis of the seminal vesicle is usually associated with tuberculosis of the prostate and vas deferens. The seminal vesicles and vas deferens involved with tuberculosis demonstrate internal debris, wall thickening, contraction, or calcification.

EJACULATORY DUCT OBSTRUCTION

Ejaculatory duct obstruction (EDO) is one of the important causes of male infertility, and the condition is receiving increasing attention, since those lesions are potentially curable with endoscopic surgery. The condition, which is not as rare as previously thought, may be either congenital or acquired. Two thirds of EDO is considered congenital in origin and the remainder as caused by inflammation or trauma. Chronic infection or inflammation of the prostate resulting in calcifications along the ejaculatory duct has been proposed as a cause of partial EDO. Compression of the ejaculatory duct by a müllerian duct cyst or utricular cyst may also cause partial EDO. Transrectal US can easily differentiate patients with low ejaculatory volumes secondary to impaired seminal vesicle secretion from those with large vesicles due to EDO.

TUMORS

A variety of primary tumors, either benign or malignant, can occur in the seminal vesicles from either epithelial or mesenchymal elements. Among them, malignant tumors include adenocarcinoma, sarcoma, and seminoma, whereas benign tumors include leiomyoma, fibroma, cystadenoma, and dermoid cyst. Secondary involvement of the seminal vesicle by tumors of the urinary bladder, prostate, or rectum occurs more often than primary tumors of the seminal vesicle.

Usually the imaging findings of seminal vesicle tumors are nonspecific, but cystadenoma appears as a multicystic lesion. Endorectal MR imaging can detect invasion of the seminal vesicle by tumors of the adjacent organs before the development of contour changes. The high signal intensity of the normal seminal vesicle is replaced by low-intensity tumors on T2-weighted images. Care should be taken not to interpret

normal ampulla of the vas deferens as a sign of secondary invasion because it normally has thick, low-intensity walls.

MISCELLANEOUS CONDITIONS
Hematospermia

The most common cause of hematospermia is inflammation of the seminal tracts. In men older than 40 years of age, 5% to 10% of the cases of hematospermia are caused by carcinoma of the prostate. MR imaging well demonstrates the hemorrhagic fluid in the seminal vesicle by high signal intensity on T1-weighted image and low signal intensity on T2-weighted image.

Calcification of the seminal tract

Calcification of the seminal vesicle and vas deferens may be seen with diabetes, tuberculosis, schistosomiasis, chronic renal failure, and advanced age. Calculi may also develop in dilated seminal vesicles due to EDO.

References

1. Killi RM, Pourbagher A, Semerci B: Transrectal ultrasonography-guided echo-enhanced seminal vesiculography. BJU Int 1999; 84:521–523.
2. Kim SH, Paick JS, Lee IH, et al: Ejaculatory duct obstruction: TRUS-guided opacification of seminal tracts. Eur Urol 1998; 34:57–62.
3. Cornud F, Belin X, Delafontaine D, et al: Imaging of obstructive azoospermia. Eur Radiol 1997; 7:1079–1085.
4. Jones TR, Zagoria RJ, Jarow JP: Transrectal US–guided seminal vesiculography. Radiology 1997; 205:276–278.
5. McDermott VG, Meakem TJ III, Stolpen AH, et al: Prostatic and periprostatic cysts: Findings on MR imaging. AJR Am J Roentgenol 1995; 164:123–127.
6. Meacham RB, Townsend RR, Drose JA: Ejaculatory duct obstruction: Diagnosis and treatment with transrectal sonography. AJR Am J Roentgenol 1995; 165:1463–1466.
7. Lagalla R, Zappasodi F, Casto AL, et al: Cystadenoma of the seminal vesicle: US and CT findings. Abdom Imaging 1993; 18:298–300.
8. Pereira JK, Chait PG, Daneman A: Bilateral persisting mesonephric ducts. AJR Am J Roentgenol 1993; 160:367–369.
9. Ramchandani P, Banner MP, Pollack HM: Imaging of the seminal vesicles. Semin Roentgenol 1993; 28:83–91.
10. Kuligowska E, Baker CE, Oates RD: Male infertility: Role of transrectal US in diagnosis and management. Radiology 1992; 185:353–360.
11. Schnall MD, Pollack HM, Van Arsdalen K, et al: The seminal tract in patients with ejaculatory dysfunction: MR imaging with an endorectal surface coil. AJR Am J Roentgenol 1992; 159:337–341.
12. Abbitt PL, Watson L, Howards S: Abnormalities of the seminal tract causing infertility: Diagnosis with endorectal sonography. AJR Am J Roentgenol 1991; 157:337–339.
13. Alpern MB, Dorfman RE, Gross BH, et al: Seminal vesicle cysts: Association with adult polycystic kidney disease. Radiology 1991; 180:79–80.
14. Asch MR, Toi A: Seminal vesicles: Imaging and intervention using transrectal ultrasound. J Ultrasound Med 1991; 10:19–23.
15. King BF, Hattery RR, Lieber MM, et al: Congenital cystic disease of the seminal vesicle. Radiology 1991; 178:207–211.
16. Nghiem HT, Kellman GM, Sandberg SA, et al: Cystic lesions of the prostate. Radiographics 1990; 10:635–650.
17. Littrup PJ, Lee F, McLeary RD, et al: Transrectal US of the seminal vesicles and ejaculatory ducts: Clinical correlation. Radiology 1988; 168:625–628.
18. Thurnher S, Hricak H, Tanagho EA: Müllerian duct cyst: Diagnosis with MR imaging. Radiology 1988; 168:25–28.
19. Kenny PJ, Leeson MD: Congenital anomalies of the seminal vesicles: Spectrum of computed tomographic findings. Radiology 1983; 149:247–251.
20. Zagoria RJ, Papanicolaou N, Pfister RC, et al: Seminal vesicle abscess after vasectomy: Evaluation by transrectal sonography and CT. AJR Am J Roentgenol 1987; 149:137–138.
21. Dunnick NR, Ford K, Osborne D, et al: Seminal vesiculography: Limited value in vesiculitis. Urology 1982; 20:454–457.
22. Banner MP, Hassler R: The normal seminal vesiculogram. Radiology 1978; 128:339–344.

Illustrations • Imaging for Seminal Tracts

1 • Seminal tracts: normal findings

2 • Inflammatory diseases of the seminal tracts

3 • Calcifications in the seminal tracts

4 • Midline cysts

5 • Seminal vesicle cysts

6 • Ejaculatory duct obstruction

7 • Transrectal US–guided procedures for seminal tracts

8 • Tumors of the seminal tracts

1. Seminal Tracts: Normal Findings

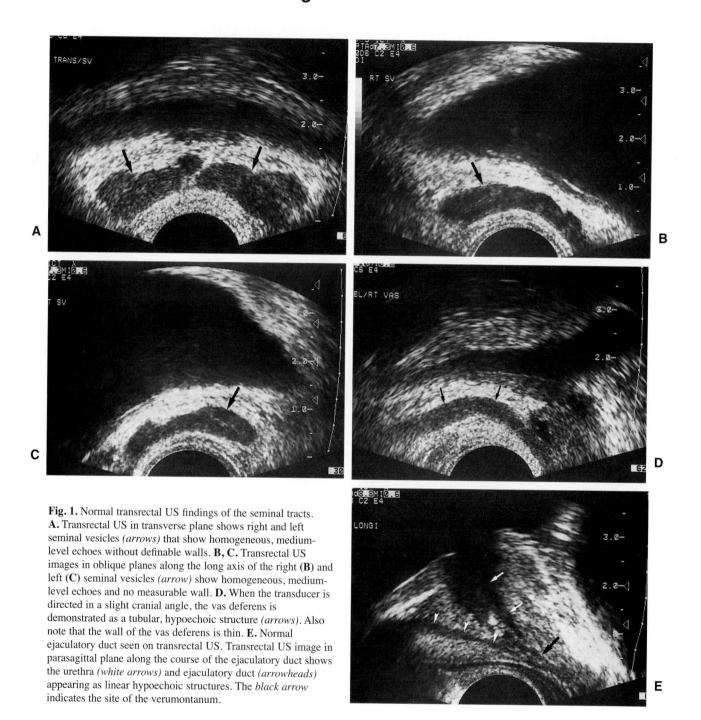

Fig. 1. Normal transrectal US findings of the seminal tracts. **A.** Transrectal US in transverse plane shows right and left seminal vesicles *(arrows)* that show homogeneous, medium-level echoes without definable walls. **B, C.** Transrectal US images in oblique planes along the long axis of the right **(B)** and left **(C)** seminal vesicles *(arrow)* show homogeneous, medium-level echoes and no measurable wall. **D.** When the transducer is directed in a slight cranial angle, the vas deferens is demonstrated as a tubular, hypoechoic structure *(arrows)*. Also note that the wall of the vas deferens is thin. **E.** Normal ejaculatory duct seen on transrectal US. Transrectal US image in parasagittal plane along the course of the ejaculatory duct shows the urethra *(white arrows)* and ejaculatory duct *(arrowheads)* appearing as linear hypoechoic structures. The *black arrow* indicates the site of the verumontanum.

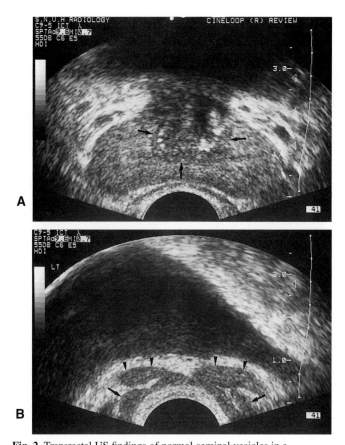

Fig. 2. Transrectal US findings of normal seminal vesicles in a 51-year-old man with mild prostatic hyperplasia.
A. Transrectal US in transverse plane shows a nodule of benign prostatic hyperplasia *(arrows)* containing mottled calcifications. The echogenicity of the prostate is homogeneous. **B.** The seminal vesicle *(arrows)* and vas deferens *(arrowheads)* are seen on the same image due to elevation of these structures by the enlarged prostate.

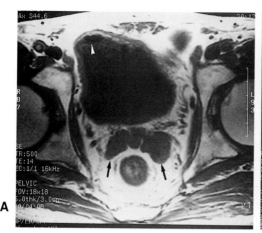

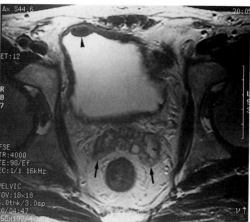

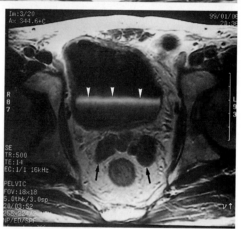

Fig. 3. Normal MR imaging findings of the seminal vesicles in a 67-year-old man.
A. T1-weighted MR image shows symmetrical, bow tie–shaped, low-intensity seminal vesicles *(arrows)* between the urinary bladder and rectum. **B.** T2-weighted MR image shows homogeneous, high-intensity content and low-intensity wall of the seminal vesicles *(arrows)*. A low-intensity lesion floating in the urinary bladder in **A** and **B** *(arrowhead)* is an air bubble in the urinary bladder that was introduced during cystoscopy.
C. Contrast-enhanced T1-weighted MR image reveals slight enhancement of the wall of the seminal vesicles *(arrows)*. A horizontal, high-intensity layer in the bladder *(arrowheads)* represents a layer of excreted contrast material in low concentration.

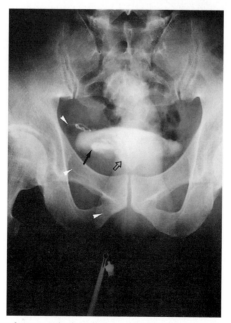

Fig. 4. Normal vasoseminal vesiculography in a 37-year-old man. The right vas deferens is cannulated with a needle at the scrotal level, and injection of contrast material demonstrates the right vas deferens *(arrowheads)*, seminal vesicle *(arrow)*, and ejaculatory duct *(open arrow)*. Note that the contrast material opacifies the urinary bladder, indicating a patent ejaculatory duct.

2. Inflammatory Diseases of the Seminal Tracts

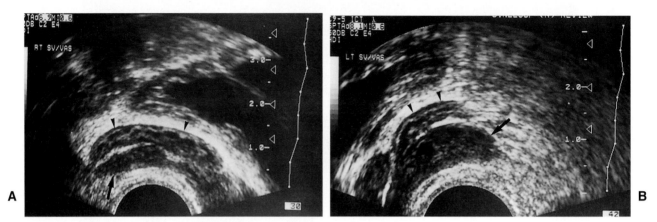

Fig. 1. Chronic inflammation of the seminal vesicle and vas deferens in a 44-year-old man.
A, B. Transrectal US images of the right **(A)** and left **(B)** seminal vesicles *(arrow)* and vasa deferens *(arrowheads)* show a thickened wall and increased internal echogenicity due to chronic inflammation of those structures.

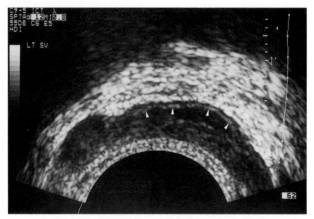

Fig. 2. Diffuse inflammation of the seminal vesicles in a 39-year-old man. Transrectal US in oblique plane along the left seminal vesicle shows diffusely increased echogenicity and a thickened wall *(arrowheads)*.

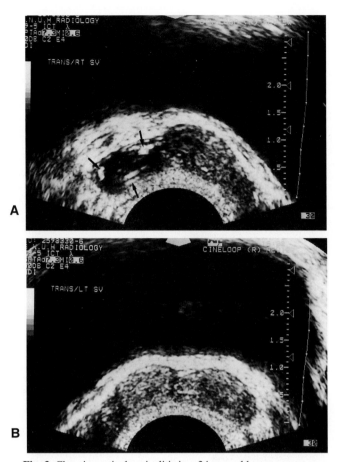

Fig. 3. Chronic seminal vesiculitis in a 34-year-old man.
A, B. Transrectal US images of the right (**A**) and left (**B**) seminal vesicles show increased echogenicity and wall thickening. Note small calcifications (*arrows* in **A**) attached to the thickened wall of the right seminal vesicle.

3. Calcifications in the Seminal Tracts

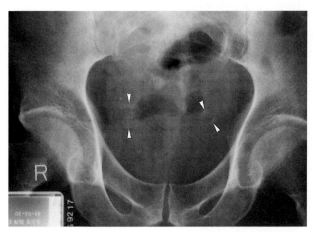

Fig. 1. Calcification of the vas deferens in a 55-year-old man with diabetes mellitus and chronic renal failure. Plain radiograph shows tortuous, tubular, tramline calcifications in vas deferens *(arrowheads)*.

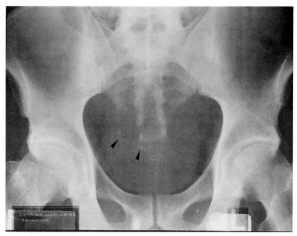

Fig. 2. Calcification of the vas deferens in a 46-year-old man with diabetes. Plain radiograph shows tubular calcification of the right vas deferens *(arrowheads)*.

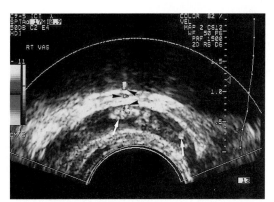

Fig. 3. Calcification of the vas deferens in a 69-year-old man. Color Doppler US of the right vas deferens shows echogenic lesions *(arrows)* that accompany color-twinkling artifacts *(arrowheads)*, suggesting calcifications. (See also Color Section.)

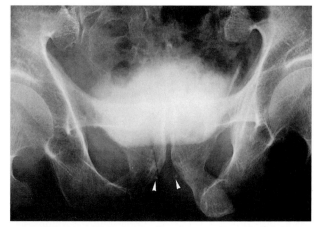

Fig. 4. Calcifications of the Cowper's gland in a 78-year-old man. IVU image of the urinary bladder shows small, symmetrical calcifications *(arrowheads)* just below the symphysis pubis, indicating calcifications of the Cowper's glands.

4. Midline Cysts

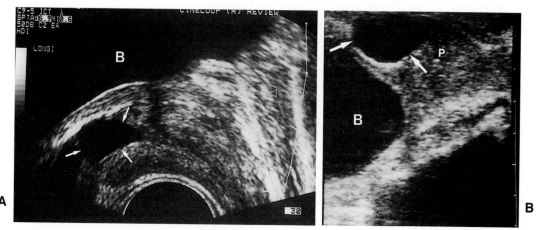

Fig. 1. Midline cysts.
A. A 57-year-old man with a midline cyst. Transrectal US with an end-firing transducer in longitudinal plane shows an ovoid midline cyst *(arrows)*. The cyst has a thin wall and anechoic content. B, urinary bladder. **B.** A 63-year-old man with a midline cyst. Transrectal US with a linear transducer shows a midline cyst *(arrows)* within the prostate (P). B, urinary bladder.

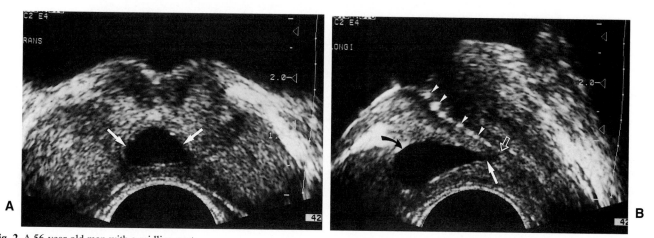

Fig. 2. A 56-year-old man with a midline cyst.
A. Transrectal US in transverse plane shows a midline cyst *(arrows)* in the base of the prostate. **B.** Longitudinal US shows a teardrop-shaped midline cyst *(curved arrow)*. Note that the neck *(arrow)* of the midline cyst is close to the verumontanum *(open arrow)*. Also note calcifications along the prostatic urethra *(arrowheads)*.

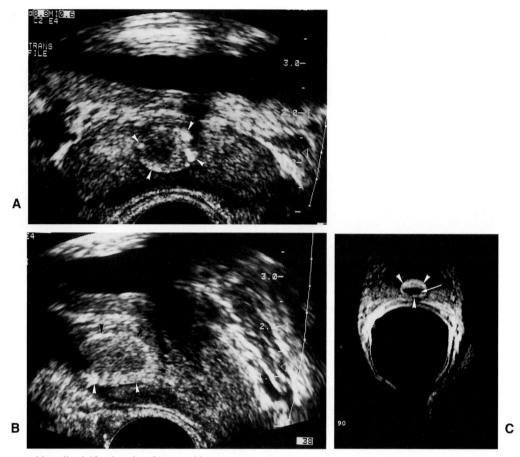

Fig. 3. A midline cyst with wall calcifications in a 31-year-old man.
A, B. Transrectal US images in transverse (**A**) and longitudinal (**B**) planes show a round midline cyst with calcified wall *(arrowheads)* in the base of the prostate. **C.** T2-weighted MR image in axial plane shows that the cyst *(arrowheads)* has a fluid-fluid level. The low signal intensity in the dependent portion of the cyst represents hemorrhagic content *(arrow)*.

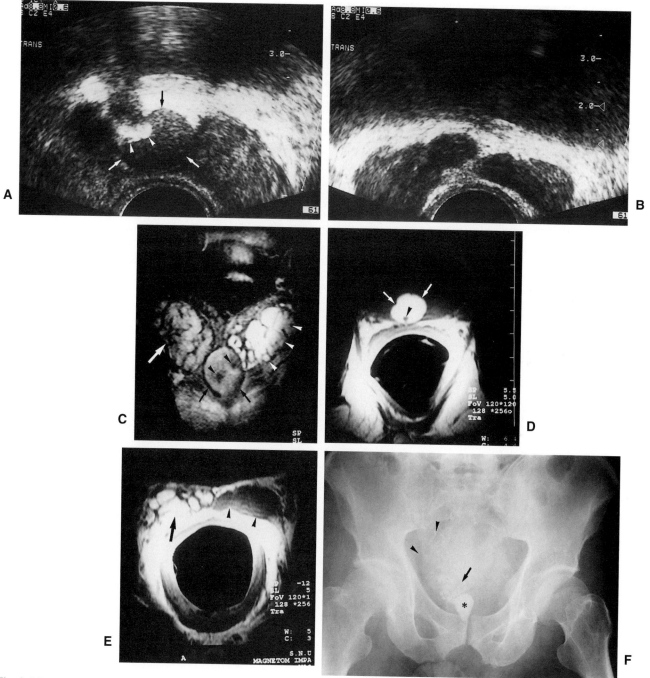

Fig. 4. A hemorrhagic ejaculatory duct cyst with calcification in a 40-year-old man.

A. Transrectal US in transverse plane shows a round midline cyst in the prostatic base *(arrows)* with calcifications *(arrowheads)*. **B.** Transrectal US in transverse plane at the level of the seminal vesicles shows prominent bilateral seminal vesicles. **C.** T2-weighted MR image in coronal plane shows the midline cyst *(black arrows)* that contains low-intensity calcifications *(black arrowheads)*. Note that the signal intensity of the cyst and right seminal vesicle *(white arrow)* is lower than the normal high signal intensity of the left seminal vesicle *(white arrowheads)*. **D.** T1-weighted MR image in axial plane at the level of the cyst shows that the cyst has high signal intensity, indicating hemorrhagic content *(arrows)*. Note a small low-intensity lesion indicating calcification *(arrowhead)*. **E.** T1-weighted MR image at the level of the seminal vesicles shows high-intensity, hemorrhagic content of the right seminal vesicle *(arrow)* and normal low signal intensity of the left seminal vesicle *(arrowheads)*. **F.** Transrectal US–guided aspiration and injection of contrast material reveal a cyst *(asterisk)* that communicates with the right seminal vesicle *(arrow)* and vas deferens *(arrowheads)*.

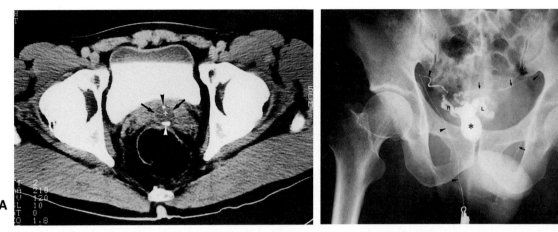

Fig. 5. A calcified midline cyst in a 44-year-old man with hematospermia.
A. Contrast-enhanced CT shows a round midline cyst *(arrows)* that contains calcifications *(arrowheads)*. **B.** Vasoseminal vesiculography with injection of contrast material into the right vas deferens opacifies the right vas deferens *(arrowheads)*, right seminal vesicle (R), and a large midline cyst *(asterisk)*. Left seminal vesicle (L) and vas deferens *(arrows)* were opacified by previous injection on the left side.

5. Seminal Vesicle Cysts

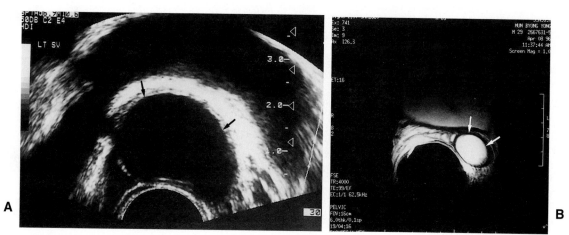

Fig. 1. A large seminal vesicle cyst in a 28-year-old man with a normal urinary tract.
A. Transrectal US of the left seminal vesicle shows a large cyst *(arrows)* with a thin wall and anechoic content. **B.** T2-weighted MR image in axial plane shows a cyst *(arrows)* with homogeneous high signal intensity in the left seminal vesicle.

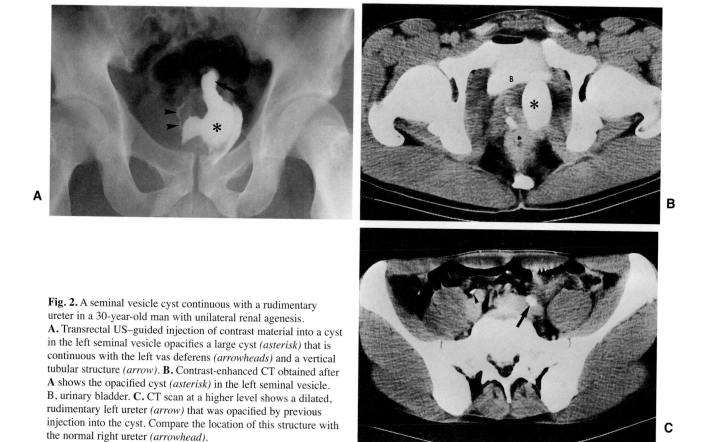

Fig. 2. A seminal vesicle cyst continuous with a rudimentary ureter in a 30-year-old man with unilateral renal agenesis.
A. Transrectal US–guided injection of contrast material into a cyst in the left seminal vesicle opacifies a large cyst *(asterisk)* that is continuous with the left vas deferens *(arrowheads)* and a vertical tubular structure *(arrow)*. **B.** Contrast-enhanced CT obtained after **A** shows the opacified cyst *(asterisk)* in the left seminal vesicle. B, urinary bladder. **C.** CT scan at a higher level shows a dilated, rudimentary left ureter *(arrow)* that was opacified by previous injection into the cyst. Compare the location of this structure with the normal right ureter *(arrowhead)*.

6. Ejaculatory Duct Obstruction

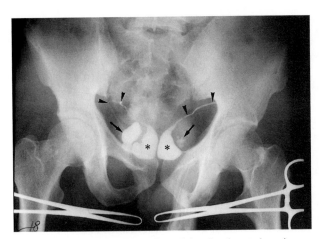

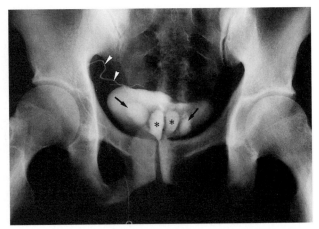

Fig. 1. Bilateral complete obstruction of the ejaculatory ducts in a 30-year-old infertile man. Bilateral vasoseminal vesiculography demonstrates complete obstruction of dilated ejaculatory ducts *(asterisks)*. Note opacified seminal vesicles *(arrows)* and vasa deferens *(arrowheads)*. Also note the nonopacified urinary bladder, indicating complete obstruction of the ejaculatory duct.

Fig. 2. Partial obstruction of the ejaculatory ducts in a 33-year-old man. Right vasoseminal vesiculography opacifies the right vas deferens *(arrowheads)*, dilated ampulla of vasa *(asterisks)*, and seminal vesicles *(arrows)*. Contrast material in the left seminal tract is due to a previous injection of contrast material into the left vas deferens. Note that the urinary bladder is opacified with contrast material, indicating that the ejaculatory duct obstruction is not complete.

7. Transrectal US–Guided Procedures for Seminal Tracts

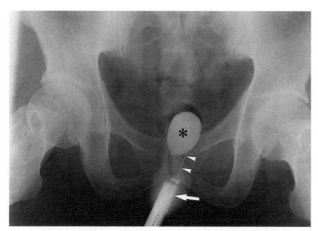

Fig. 1. A 36-year-old man who underwent transrectal US–guided aspiration and injection of contrast material. Plain radiograph shows an ovoid cyst *(asterisk)* that does not communicate with the seminal tracts. Note a needle *(arrowheads)* and the transducer of the transrectal US *(arrow)*.

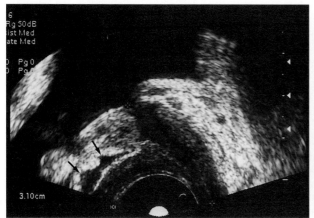

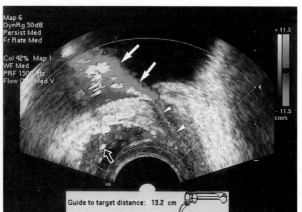

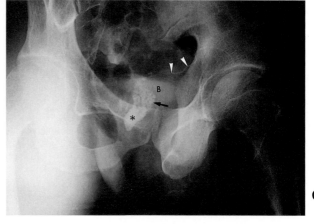

Fig. 2. Partial obstruction of the ejaculatory duct evaluated with transrectal US–guided aspiration in a 25-year-old man.
A. Transrectal US in longitudinal plane shows a dilated ejaculatory duct that has an echogenic margin *(arrows)* suggesting wall calcification. **B.** Transrectal US–guided aspiration was done, and contrast material was injected into the dilated ejaculatory duct. Color Doppler US in longitudinal plane, which was performed during the procedure, demonstrates flow of the fluid into the urethra *(arrowheads)* and bladder *(arrows)*. The *open arrow* indicates the tip of the needle in the dilated ejaculatory duct. (**B,** See also Color Section.) **C.** Plain radiograph in oblique projection that was obtained immediately after the procedure demonstrates the dilated ejaculatory duct *(asterisk)*, left seminal vesicle *(arrow)*, and left vas deferens *(arrowheads)*. Note that the urinary bladder (B) is faintly opacified, indicating partial obstruction of the ejaculatory duct.

8. Tumors of the Seminal Tracts

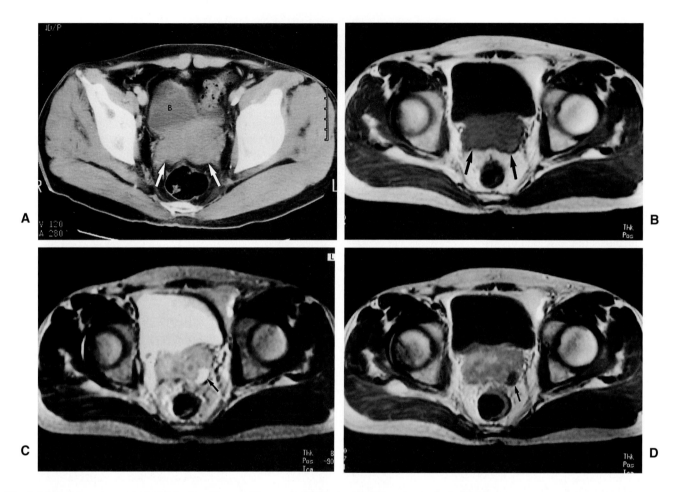

Fig. 1. Metastasis to the seminal vesicles in a 33-year-old man who had had testicular seminoma 2 years earlier.
A. Contrast-enhanced CT shows enlarged bilateral seminal vesicles with homogeneous attenuation *(arrows)*. B, urinary bladder. **B.** T1-weighted MR image shows homogeneous, intermediate signal intensity of the enlarged seminal vesicles *(arrows)*. **C.** T2-weighted MR image shows homogeneous, high attenuation of the enlarged seminal vesicles except for a small, high-attenuated cystic lesion *(arrow)* in the left seminal vesicle. **D.** Contrast-enhanced T1-weighted MR image demonstrates slightly heterogeneous enhancement of the masses in the seminal vesicles and a small, nonenhancing cystic lesion *(arrow)* in the left seminal vesicle.

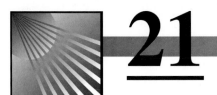

21

Scrotum

BOHYUN KIM

Clinical presentations often overlap among the different scrotal diseases, and misdiagnoses are quite common among testicular tumor, testicular torsion, and epididymitis, especially in young men. Physical examination is often limited due to swelling and pain. Therefore, imaging is essential in the differential diagnosis of the scrotal diseases.

ANATOMY OF THE TESTIS AND EPIDIDYMIS

The scrotal coverings consist of skin, the dartos tunic, external spermatic fascia, cremasteric muscle, internal spermatic fascia, and tunica vaginalis. The visceral layer of the tunica vaginalis surrounds the testis and epididymis and, along with the parietal layer, contains a small amount of serous fluid. The testis is covered with inelastic tunica albuginea. The testis consists of 200 to 250 lobuli *testis*, which are divided by fibrous septa called the *septula testis*. In each lobule, up to four seminiferous tubules exist. The seminiferous tubules drain into the rete testis, a meshwork of anastomosing tubules situated in the area of the testicular hilum (mediastinum testis), via straight tubules.

The epididymis consists of highly convoluted epididymal ducts and is subdivided into the head, body, and tail. Four types of appendages exist in the testis and epididymis: the appendix testis, appendix epididymis, paradidymis, and vas aberrans. Of these, the appendix testis in the upper pole of the testis and the appendix epididymis in the head of the epididymis are the most common.

Blood is supplied to the testis and adjacent structures by three arteries: the testicular, deferential, and cremasteric. Both the right and left testicular arteries arise directly from the aorta. Venous blood from the testis and a part of the epididymis drains into the pampiniform plexus, a venous plexus above the testis extending into the distal spermatic cord and becoming the testicular vein. The right testicular vein drains directly into the inferior vena cava, and the left vein drains into the left renal vein.

RADIOLOGIC MODALITIES

For imaging of the scrotum, ultrasonography (US) is usually the first-line imaging modality. Major indications include evaluation of a scrotal mass or pain, scrotal inflammation, scrotal fluid collection, varicocele, and impalpable testis. With the advent of color Doppler US, US became the most useful tool in the evaluation of scrotal diseases. It has largely replaced radioisotope scintigraphy in evaluating patients with acute scrotum.

Magnetic resonance (MR) imaging can be used as a problem-solving modality. It is indicated when US is equivocal or suboptimal or when there is a discrepancy between the clinical and US findings. MR imaging is particularly useful in localization of undescended testis, staging and follow-up of testicular cancer especially in patients with previous lymph node dissection in whom clip artifacts degrade CT images, and evaluation of scrotal trauma.

Other rather infrequently used imaging modalities include computed tomography (CT), radioisotope scintigraphy, and angiography. Because of limited spatial resolution and risk of radiation damage to the testis, CT is not as commonly used for imaging of the scrotum. However, it is useful in localization of undescended abdominal testis and is most commonly used for staging of testicular cancer. Radioisotope scan can be used for the differential diagnosis of acute scrotum. Because of the availability and shorter imaging time, color Doppler US is more frequently used in this circumstance. Angiography is rarely used in the imaging of the scrotum except for the diagnosis and treatment of varicoceles and evaluation of impalpable testis.

US AND MR IMAGING ANATOMY

On US, the normal testis has a homogeneous echo texture of medium echogenicity. The mediastinum testis is seen as a hyperechoic line extending caudally from the testicular hilum. The rete testis, a major constituent of the mediastinum testis, is usually not seen on US. Infrequently, however, it can be seen as a low-echoic area or a discrete cystic mass in which numerous tiny cysts are seen in the testicular parenchyma. The latter condition is called *tubular ectasia* of the seminiferous tubules and is often associated with distal obstruction and spermatocele. The tunica albuginea is usually not seen on US. The epididymis is seen as an elongated structure that surrounds the testis. The head, body, and tail of the epididymis vary in size, shape, and echogenicity. The echogenicity of the epididymis is similar to or lower than that of the testis. However, sometimes it is more echogenic. The head of the epididymis is usually more echogenic than the body or tail due to more interfaces among the tubules. The appendix of the testis and the appendix of the epididymis are rarely seen on US. In patients with hydrocele, these appendages can be seen as small stalked structures in the upper testis or epididymal head.

On MR images, the normal testis is seen as a sharply demarcated oval structure with homogeneous signal intensity. It demonstrates intermediate signal intensity on T1-weighted images and high signal intensity on T2-weighted images. The tunica albuginea is seen as a thin stripe of low signal intensity on both T1- and T2-weighted images. The mediastinum testis appears as a characteristic low-intensity stripe on T2-weighted images. The signal intensity of the epididymis is similar to that of the testis on T1-weighted images and much lower than that of the testis on T2-weighted images.

RADIOLOGIC FINDINGS

Undescended testis

When the testis is not palpated in the scrotum, it may be due to agenesis (3% to 5%), ectopia (1%), retractile testis (up to 70%), and true undescended testis (30%). *Undescended testis* refers to a testis that has been arrested during its descent to the scrotum. The incidence at birth has been reported to be 3.4% for full-term infants and 30.3% for premature infants. Bilaterality has been reported to be about 10% of cases. Undescended testis can be divided into three types by location: high scrotal, intracanalicular, and intra-abdominal. The high-scrotal type is most common, and the intra-abdominal testis is least common. The relative incidence has been reported to be 66% for high-scrotal, 16% for intracanalicular, and 10% for intra-abdominal testis in a large study. The undescended testis is nonpalpable in about 20% of cases. Approximately 80% of nonpalpable testes are intracanalicular, and the remaining 20% are intra-abdominal in location.

For the diagnostic evaluation of undescended testis, US, MR imaging, CT, angiography, and laparoscopy can be used. Owing to low cost and availability, US is often used as the primary imaging modality. Although US is the most practical approach, it has a small field of view and lacks tissue contrast and specificity. In contrast, owing to excellent tissue contrast, a large field of view, and multiplanar capability, MR imaging is more accurate than US in locating undescended testis. CT is reserved for the search for intra-abdominal testis.

On US, the undescended testis is oval in shape and has homogeneous echotexture. It is often small and hypoechoic due to incomplete development of the germinal epithelium. US is relatively accurate in detecting high-scrotal or intracanalicular testis but not as effective in depicting intra-abdominal testis as is CT or MR imaging.

MR imaging is an excellent modality for demonstrating high-scrotal and intracanalicular testis. The characteristic signal intensities of the testis, epididymis, and inner structures such as the mediastinum testis facilitate accurate localization of undescended testis and differentiation from inguinal nodes, regressed testis, or the pars infravaginalis gubernaculi.

Testicular venography was used for many years to localize undescended testis but now is less often used. The venographic findings of undescended testis include demonstration of a pampiniform plexus, testicular parenchyma, or a blind-ending testicular vein.

Testicular tumors

Testicular cancer is the most common malignancy among 15- to 34-year-old men and accounts for 1% of all cancers in men. About 95% of testicular tumors are of germ cell origin. Common histologic types include seminoma (35%), embryonal carcinoma (20%), teratoma (5%), teratocarcinoma (25%), and choriocarcinoma (1%). Non–germ cell tumors include gonadal stromal tumors, lymphoma, leukemia, and metastasis. Benign testicular tumors constitute only 3% to 4% of all testicular tumors, which include Leydig cell tumor, Sertoli cell tumor, gonadoblastoma, epidermoid cyst, and adrenal rest tumor.

Patients with testicular cancer often present with a lump or painless swelling of the testis. Approximately 30% of patients have scrotal pain, which may mimic epididymo-orchitis or testicular torsion. Reactive hydrocele is associated in 10% of patients. Gynecomastia occurs in 5% of patients with germ cell tumors and in 30% to 50% of patients with Leydig and Sertoli cell tumors.

Germ cell tumors can be classified into seminomas and non-seminomatous germ cell tumors (NSGCTs) because of the differences in treatment and prognosis. Seminomas are often treated by retroperitoneal radiotherapy following orchiectomy, whereas NSGCTs are treated by retroperitoneal lymph node dissection and/or chemotherapy following initial orchiectomy.

US serves as the primary imaging modality for detection of testicular tumors. US is highly sensitive in detecting intratesticular lesions and differentiating intratesticular and extratesticular masses. CT is most commonly used for staging. MR imaging can be used as a problem-solving modality when there is a discrepancy between clinical and US findings.

On US, most testicular tumors are hypoechoic. However, they are sometimes hyperechoic or mixed echogenic. Whereas seminomas often show homogeneous echotexture, NSGCTs tend to demonstrate heterogeneous echotexture most commonly due to hemorrhage and necrosis. Cystic spaces are often seen in teratomas and dense echogenic foci are present in about 35% of NSGCTs.

At the time of presentation, metastasis occurs in 20% to 25% of seminomas and in more than 40% of NSGCTs. Most germ cell tumors spread through the lymphatics. The primary draining site (sentinel nodes) is the aortocaval area from the right testis and the left para-aortic area from the left testis just below the level of renal hilum. Subsequent spread into the retroperitoneal and iliac lymph nodes occurs.

Tumor markers such as alpha fetoprotein, human chorionic gonadotropin, and lactic acid dehydrogenase and CT are commonly used for the staging and follow-up of cancer patients. The accuracy of CT, when used with tumor marker, is reported to be 80% to 90%. MR imaging is as accurate as CT and can be used as a problem-solving modality. It has been reported that MR imaging is better than CT in evaluating small retrocrural lymph nodes and for follow-up of patients with previous lymph node dissection in whom the artifacts may cause severe image degradation on CT.

On MR imaging, testicular tumors demonstrate a signal intensity similar to the normal testis on T1-weighted image and lower signal intensity than the testis on T2-weighted image. Seminomas are commonly homogeneously hypointense on T2-weighted image, whereas NSGCTs often show heterogeneous and higher signal intensity. Although MR imaging has a higher specificity than US in the differentiation of orchitis or hematoma from a testicular tumor, it cannot differentiate benign from malignant testicular tumors, and it is sometimes difficult to differentiate focal orchitis from tumors.

Epididymal and spermatic cord tumors

Tumors of the epididymis and spermatic cord are rare and occur about one tenth as frequently as testicular tumors. Although most testicular tumors are malignant, most extratesticular tumors are benign. The most common benign tumor of the epididymis is adenomatoid tumor, followed by papillary cystadenoma, which is often associated with von Hippel-Lindau disease.

On US, adenomatous tumors are commonly seen as a well-marginated, slightly echogenic mass in the epididymal tail or, less commonly, in the head. It is often difficult to differentiate the tumor from sperm granuloma. Papillary cystadenomas are seen as a unilocular or multiseptated cystic mass in the head of the epididymis.

In the spermatic cord, rhabdomyosarcoma is most common. Lipoma is the second most common tumor in the spermatic cord. Other mesenchymal sarcomas including leiomyosarcoma, liposarcoma, fibrosarcoma, and malignant fibrous histiocytoma are more common than their benign counterparts. Mesothelioma, originating from the tunica vaginalis, can occur in the scrotal wall. About 15% of the tumors are malignant.

The tumors of the spermatic cord or scrotal wall may demonstrate a soft tissue mass on US. However, US is often limited due to a small field of view and nonspecific findings. MR imaging can be useful in differentiating these tumors from other pathology such as inguinal hernia and in evaluating the tumor extent.

Testicular microlithiasis

Histologically, testicular microlithiasis represents calcified concretions within the lumen of the seminiferous tubules. It is often associated with cryptorchidism, testicular tumor, Klinefelter's syndrome, male pseudohermaphroditism, and infertility. Although it is not known whether testicular microlithiasis is directly related to development of testicular cancer, a high association between microlithiasis and tumor has been reported. In a recent report, a testis with less than five microliths was reported to have a lower prevalence of associated malignancy.

The microliths are seen on US as multiple tiny (1–2 mm in diameter), disseminated, echogenic foci throughout the testis. They commonly involve both testes and usually do not accompany acoustic shadowing.

Testicular torsion

Testicular torsion is defined as "rotation of the testis on the longitudinal axis of the spermatic cord." As any delay in the diagnosis of testicular torsion may result in irreversible loss of testicular function, prompt and accurate diagnosis is essential.

Testicular torsion can be classified as extravaginal, intravaginal, and mesorchial types, based on the site of twisting. Extravaginal type is a rare type that occurs in utero and is found exclusively in newborns. Intravaginal torsion is the most common form, in which the torsion occurs within the tunica vaginalis. The bell-clapper deformity, in which the testis is almost completely covered by the tunica vaginalis, often predisposes to intravaginal testicular torsion.

Approximately two thirds of cases with testicular torsion occur between 12 and 18 years of age. It is the most common cause of acute scrotal pain in this age. The typical symptoms include sudden scrotal pain and swelling. The patients usually have normal body temperature and clear urinalysis. Typically the pain radiates to the ipsilateral inguinal region or lower abdomen. Differentiation of torsion from epididymitis is often difficult.

Gray-scale US findings are nonspecific. Torsed testis may be enlarged with normal or decreased echogenicity. The epididymis may be enlarged with decreased echogenicity as well. Edema of scrotal skin and reactive hydrocele are often associated. Color Doppler US is an excellent modality for the diagnosis of testicular torsion, with reported sensitivities of 82% to 90% and a specificity of almost 100%. Lack of testicular perfusion can be easily depicted on color Doppler US. Although decreased testicular perfusion can also be assessed on radioisotope scintigraphy, color Doppler US is now more often used than scintigraphy.

MR imaging can be used as a problem-solving modality when color Doppler US findings are inconclusive. It is advocated particularly in the subacute phase of torsion. On MR imaging, the testis may be normal or enlarged and may demonstrate heterogeneous low signal intensity on T2-weighted images. The epididymis is often displaced anteroinferiorly. A twisted cord can be seen as multiple, low-intensity radiating structures in a "whirlpool pattern," and the point of the twist may be seen as an area of signal void ("torsion knot"). If present, these findings are specific for testicular torsion.

Appendiceal torsion

In children, appendiceal torsion occurs as commonly as testicular torsion, accounting for 20% to 40% of cases of acute scrotum in the pediatric age group. Out of four appendages of the testis and epididymis, 91% to 95% of appendiceal torsions occur in the appendix testis, and most of the rest involve the appendix epididymis.

Although torsion of an appendage may be asymptomatic, affected patients commonly present with the signs of acute scrotum. The onset of symptoms is less sudden, and initially the pain may be localized to the upper part of the hemiscrotum. In the early stage, the torsed appendix may show a characteristic "blue dot" through the scrotal skin.

US is the primary imaging modality for the diagnosis of appendiceal torsion. A torsed appendix may be seen as a swollen nodular structure floating in hydrocele on US. The testis and epididymis are normal in shape and echogenicity. The adjacent epididymal head may be enlarged. On color Doppler US, preservation of normal blood flow in the testis and epididymis can be helpful in the differentiation from testicular torsion.

Epididymitis and orchitis

Epididymitis is the most common cause of acute scrotum in adult men. The patients with acute epididymitis present with scrotal pain, fever, and swelling. On physical examination the epididymis and spermatic cord are tender and swollen. The scrotal pain is usually relieved by elevation of the scrotum (Prehn's sign). The presence of urethritis and localized swelling in distal epididymis may help the diagnosis of epididymitis. Reactive hydrocele and skin thickening are often associated.

US is the primary modality for evaluation of acute epididymitis and epididymo-orchitis. Color Doppler US is useful in

differentiating epididymitis from torsion. In acute stage the epididymis is markedly enlarged with heterogeneous echotexture. The echogenicity of the epididymis is often reduced. Epididymal abscess can be diagnosed when a well-circumscribed hypoechoic lesion is seen within the enlarged epididymis. In the chronic stage, US findings are often nonspecific. Only moderate enlargement of the epididymis may be seen. The diagnosis of epididymo-orchitis can be made when the echogenicity in the testis is focally or diffusely decreased. The diagnosis can be more confidently made if color Doppler US demonstrates increased vascularity in the epididymis and/or testis.

On MR imaging the epididymis is enlarged and demonstrates heterogeneous high signal intensity on T2-weighted images. The spermatic cord is often thickened and may show multiple, engorged vessels with signal void. In chronic epididymitis, the epididymis is enlarged and demonstrates low signal intensity. Associated orchitis may demonstrate a hypointense lesion within the testis.

Scrotal trauma

Scrotal trauma often results from direct or straddle injury. Direct injury may result in infarction of the testis and epididymis, testicular torsion, or rupture of the tunica albuginea. As surgical intervention is indicated for testicular rupture and massive intratesticular hematoma, assessment of the tunica integrity and the extent of scrotal hematoma is essential.

US is the primary imaging modality for the evaluation of scrotal injury. Gross rupture of the testis and intratesticular hematoma and hematocele can be accurately assessed with US. Characteristic US findings include irregular testicular contour with heterogeneous, hypoechoic or hyperechoic lesions. However, fracture lines are rarely seen, and a minor tear in the tunica albuginea without intratesticular hematoma or hematocele can be missed on US. Color Doppler US can be helpful in assessing testicular perfusion. Owing to high tissue contrast and multiplanar capability, MR imaging can be helpful in assessing the integrity of the tunica albuginea.

References

1. Bennett HF, Middleton WD, Bullock AD, et al: Testicular microlithiasis: US follow-up. Radiology 2001; 218:359–363.
2. Kim TJ, Kim SH, Sim JS, et al: Ultrasonographic findings of an intratesticular adenomatoid tumor. J Ultrasound Med 2000; 19:227–229.
3. Hricak H, Hamm B, Kim B: Anatomy and embryology. In Hricak H, Hamm B, Kim B (eds): Imaging of the Scrotum. New York, Raven Press, 1995, pp 1–5.
4. Hricak H, Hamm B, Kim B: Imaging techniques, anatomy, artifacts, and bioeffects. In Hricak H, Hamm B, Kim B (eds): Imaging of the Scrotum. New York, Raven Press, 1995, pp 11–36.
5. Hricak H, Hamm B, Kim B: Congenital anomalies of the testis. In Hricak H, Hamm B, Kim B (eds): Imaging of the Scrotum. New York, Raven Press, 1995, pp 37–48.
6. Hricak H, Hamm B, Kim B: Testicular tumors and tumorlike lesions. In Hricak H, Hamm B, Kim B (eds): Imaging of the Scrotum. New York, Raven Press, 1995, pp 49–91.
7. Caesar RE, Kaplan GW: Incidence of the bell-clapper deformity in an autopsy series. Urology 1994; 44:114–116.
8. Erden MI, Ozbek SS, Aytac SK, et al: Color Doppler imaging in acute scrotal disorders. Urol Int 1993; 50:39–42.
9. Patel MD, Olcott EW, Kerschmann RL, et al: Sonographically detected testicular microlithiasis and testicular carcinoma. J Clin Ultrasound 1993; 21:447–452.
10. Tartar VM, Trambert MA, Balsara ZN, et al: Tubular ectasia of the testicle: Sonographic and MR imaging appearance. AJR Am J Roentgenol 1993; 160:539–542.
11. Thomas RD, Dewbury KC: Ultrasound appearances of the rete testis. Clin Radiol 1993; 47:121–124.
12. Wilbert DM, Schaerfe CW, Stern WD, et al: Evaluation of the acute scrotum by color-coded Doppler ultrasonography. J Urol 1993; 149:1475–1477.
13. Fitzgerald SW, Erickson S, DeWire DM, et al: Color Doppler sonography in the evaluation of the adult acute scrotum. J Ultrasound Med 1992; 11:543–548.
14. Fritzsche PJ, Rifkin M, Hopkins CR, et al: Scrotum and testes. In Stark DD, Bradley WG (eds): Magnetic Resonance Imaging, 2nd ed, vol 2. St Louis, Mosby–Year Book, 1992, pp 2058–2077.
15. Höbarth K, Susani M, Szabo N, et al: Incidence of testicular microlithiasis. Urology 1992; 40:464–467.
16. Weingarten BJ, Kellman GM, Middleton WD, et al: Tubular ectasia within the mediastinum testis. J Ultrasound Med 1992; 11:349–353.
17. Zanzen DL, Mathieson JR, Marsh JI, et al: Testicular microlithiasis: Sonographic and clinical features. AJR Am J Roentgenol 1992; 157:1057–1060.
18. Johnson JO, Mattrey RF, Phillipson J: Differentiation of seminomatous from nonseminomatous testicular tumors with MR imaging. AJR Am J Roentgenol 1990; 154:539–543.
19. Mattery RF, Trambert M: MR imaging of the scrotum and testis. In Edelman RR, Hesselink JR (eds): Clinical Magnetic Resonance Imaging. Philadelphia, WB Saunders, 1990, pp 952–979.
20. Trambert MA, Mattrey RF, Levine D, et al: Subacute scrotal pain: Evaluation versus epididymitis with MR imaging. Radiology 1990; 175:53–56.
21. Ugarte R, Spaedy M, Cass AS: Accuracy of ultrasound in diagnosis of rupture after blunt testicular trauma. Urology 1990; 36:253–254.
22. Rosenfield AT, Blair DN, McCarthy S, et al: The pars infravaginalis gubernaculi: Importance in the identification of the undescended testis. AJR Am J Roentgenol 1989; 153:775–778.
23. Moul JW, Belman B: A review of surgical treatment of undescended testis with emphasis on anatomical position. J Urol 1988; 140:125–128.
24. Schwerk WB, Schwerk WN, Rodeck G: Testicular tumors: Prospective analysis of real-time US patterns and abdominal staging. Radiology 1987; 164:369–374.
25. Anderson PA, Giacomantonio JM: The acutely painful scrotum in children: Review of 113 consecutive cases. Can Med Assoc J 1985; 132:1153–1155.
26. Grantham JG, Charboneau JW, James EM, et al: Testicular neoplasms: Twenty-nine tumors studied by high-resolution US. Radiology 1985; 157:775–780.
27. Rifkin MD, Kurtz AB, Pasto ME, et al: Diagnostic capabilities of high-resolution scrotal ultrasonography: Prospective evaluation. J Ultrasound Med 1985; 4:13–19.
28. Tesoro-Tess JD, Pizzocaro G, Zanoni F, et al: Lymphangiography and computed tomography in testicular carcinoma—how accurate in early-stage disease? J Urol 1985; 133:967–970.
29. Ellis JH, Bies JR, Kopecky KK, et al: Comparison of NMR and CT imaging in the evaluation of metastatic retroperitoneal lymphadenopathy from testicular carcinoma. J Comput Assist Tomogr 1984; 8:709–719.
30. Anderson KA, McAninch JW, Jeffrey RB, et al: Ultrasonography for the diagnosis and staging of blunt scrotal trauma. J Urol 1983; 130:933–935.
31. Jeffrey RB, Laing FC, Hricak H, et al: Sonography of testicular trauma. AJR Am J Roentgenol 1983; 141:993–995.

Illustrations • Scrotum

1 • Normal US findings of the scrotum

2 • Spermatocele and dilated seminiferous tubules and ductules

3 • Undescended testis

4 • Testicular tumors: seminoma

5 • Testicular tumors: nonseminomatous germ cell tumors

6 • Testicular tumors: lymphoma

7 • Other testicular tumors

8 • Testicular tumors in undescended testis

9 • Tumors of the epididymis and scrotal wall

10 • Retroperitoneal nodal metastases in testicular tumors

11 • Testicular microlithiasis

12 • Testicular torsion

13 • Epididymitis

14 • Orchitis and epididymo-orchitis

15 • Scrotal trauma

16 • Miscellaneous conditions of the scrotum

1. Normal US Findings of the Scrotum

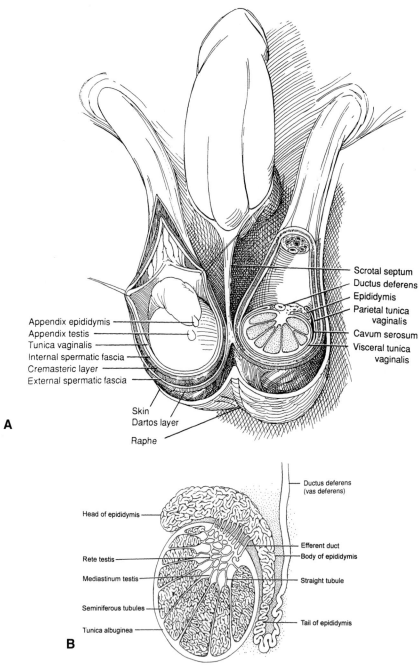

Fig. 1. Anatomy of the scrotum and its contents. (**A, B,** From Hricak H, Hamm B, Kim B: Anatomy and embryology. In Hricak H, Hamm B, Kim B [eds]: Imaging of the Scrotum. New York, Raven Press, 1995, pp 1–5.)
A. Schematic drawing of the scrotum. **B.** Schematic drawing of the testis and epididymis.

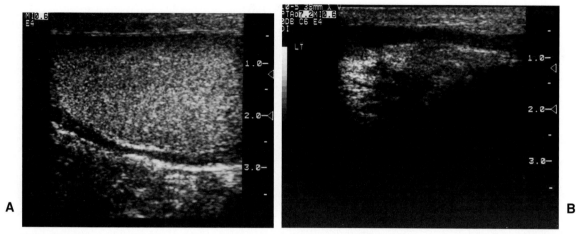

A B

Fig. 2. Normal US of the testis and epididymis in a 46-year-old man.
A. Longitudinal US of the right testis shows homogeneous, intermediate echoes of the testis. **B.** Longitudinal US along the course of the epididymal body shows homogeneous echoes of the epididymis. Note that the echogenicity of the epididymis is slightly lower than that of the testis.

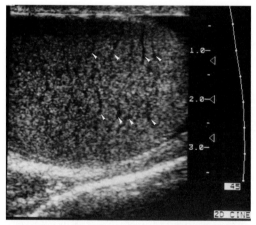

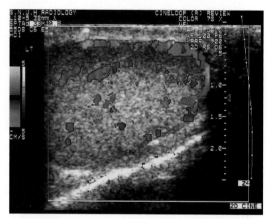

Fig. 3. Normal US of the testis showing prominent seminiferous tubules in a 53-year-old man. Longitudinal US of the left testis shows prominent, linear, hypoechoic structures throughout the testis representing prominent seminiferous tubules *(arrowheads)*.

Fig. 4. Normal color Doppler US of the testis in a 51-year-old man. Longitudinal color Doppler US of the left testis shows normal capsular vessels and branching intratesticular vessels. (See also Color Section.)

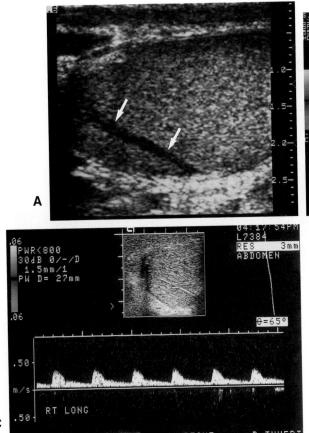

A

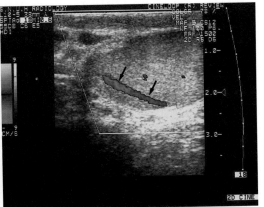

B

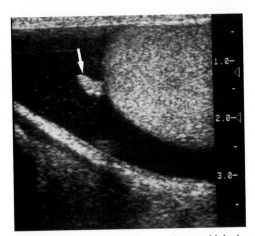

C

Fig. 5. Normal US of the testis showing prominent, linear, intratesticular vessels appearing as a hypoechoic band. (**B, C,** See also Color Section.) **A.** Longitudinal US shows a linear, hypoechoic band *(arrows)* obliquely traversing the testis. **B.** Color Doppler US demonstrates blood flow within the hypoechoic band *(arrows)*. **C.** Spectral Doppler US from the hypoechoic band shows arterial flow.

Fig. 6. Normal appendix testis in a 46-year-old man with hydrocele. Longitudinal US shows a small, stalked appendage *(arrow)* attached to the testis, which is well demonstrated against surrounding hydrocele.

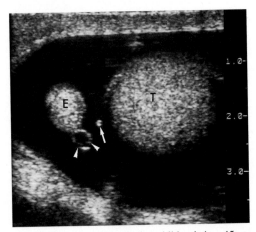

Fig. 7. The appendix testis and appendix epididymis in a 45-year-old man with hydrocele. Longitudinal US demonstrates an echogenic dot attached to the cranial portion of the testis (T) representing the appendix testis *(arrow)* and a small cystic lesion attached to the head of the epididymis (E) representing the appendix epididymis *(arrowheads)*. These structures are well visualized against surrounding hydrocele.

2. Spermatocele and Dilated Seminiferous Tubules and Ductules

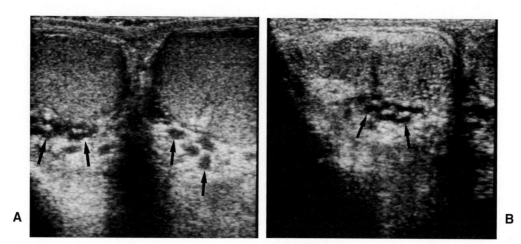

Fig. 1. Tubular ectasia of the rete testis in a 32-year-old man who had undergone vasectomy 6 years earlier.
A. Transverse US of the scrotum shows dilated, tubular structures in the region of mediastinum testis, bilaterally *(arrows)*. **B.** Longitudinal US of the right scrotum well demonstrates dilated, tubular structures in the mediastinum testis *(arrows)*.

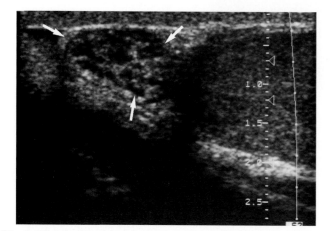

Fig. 2. Dilated efferent ductules in the epididymal head in a 22-year-old man with agenesis of the right vas deferens. Longitudinal US of the right scrotum demonstrates dilated efferent ductules in the right epididymal head *(arrows)*.

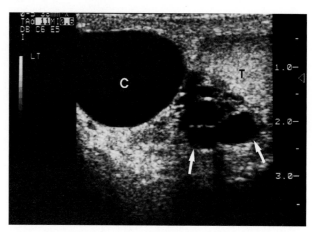

Fig. 3. A large spermatocele and dilated efferent ductules in a 23-year-old man. Longitudinal US demonstrates a large cystic lesion (C) in the superior aspect of the right testis (T). The tortuous cystic lesions in the posterior aspect of the right testis represent dilated rete testes and efferent ductules *(arrows)*.

3. Undescended Testis

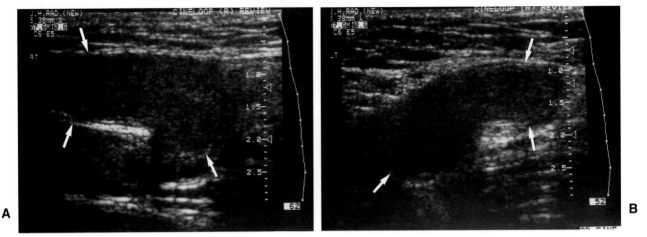

A   B

Fig. 1. Bilateral undescended testes in a 44-year-old man.
A, B. US images of both inguinal regions show elongated, hypoechoic, undescended testes *(arrows)*, partly within the inguinal canal and partly in the superficial inguinal pouch.

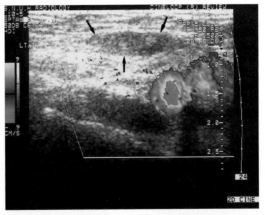

Fig. 2. Undescended testis in the superficial inguinal pouch in a 24-year-old man. Color Doppler US demonstrates a small, atrophic, undescended testis *(arrows)* anteromedial to the femoral vessels. (See also Color Section.)

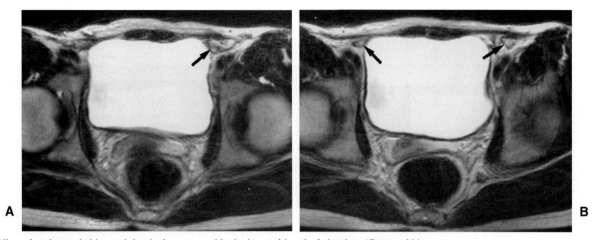

Fig. 3. Bilateral undescended intra-abdominal testes outside the internal inguinal ring in a 17-year-old boy.
A, B. T2-weighted axial MR images of the lower pelvis demonstrate bilateral intra-abdominal testes *(arrows)* outside the internal inguinal ring.

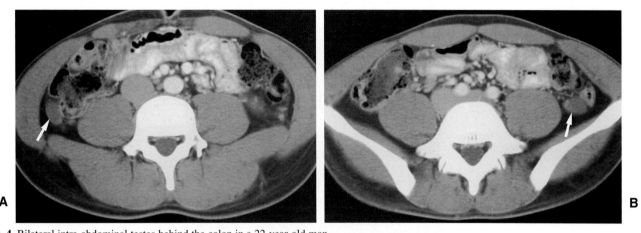

Fig. 4. Bilateral intra-abdominal testes behind the colon in a 22-year-old man.
A, B. Contrast-enhanced CT scans show bilateral intra-abdominal testes *(arrow)* behind the ascending and descending colons.

4. Testicular Tumors: Seminoma

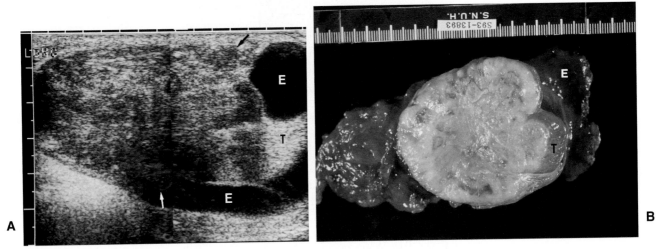

Fig. 1. Seminoma in a 32-year-old man.
A. Longitudinal US of the right testis shows diffusely enlarged testis replaced by tumor of heterogeneous echogenicity. The tumor has a lobulated margin *(arrows),* suggesting extratesticular extension, which was confirmed at surgery. Note the remnant normal testis at caudal portion (T) and cystic dilation of the epididymis (E). **B.** Gross specimen of the removed testis and epididymis correlates well with the US findings. Note the large tumor, remnant testis (T), and dilated epididymis (E). (**B,** See also Color Section.)

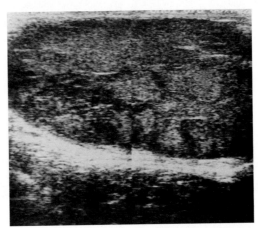

Fig. 2. Seminoma in a 45-year-old man. Longitudinal US of the right testis shows a heterogeneous, hypoechoic mass replacing the whole testis.

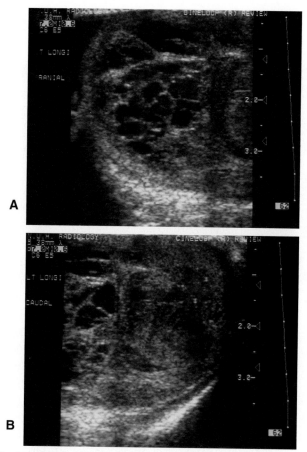

Fig. 3. Anaplastic seminoma in a 46-year-old man.
A, B. Longitudinal US images of the cranial (**A**) and caudal (**B**) parts of
the enlarged left testis show a solid and cystic, heterogeneously
hypoechoic mass replacing nearly the whole testis.

5. Testicular Tumors: Nonseminomatous Germ Cell Tumors

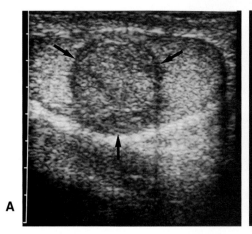
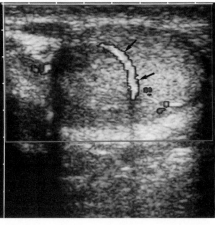

Fig. 1. Teratocarcinoma of the right testis in a 39-year-old man who had undergone left orchiectomy for seminoma 10 years earlier.
A. Longitudinal US of the right testis shows a well-demarcated, round, intratesticular mass *(arrows)* with homogeneous echogenicity.
B. Doppler US shows prominent vessels in the periphery of the tumor *(arrows)*.

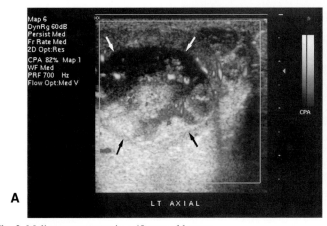
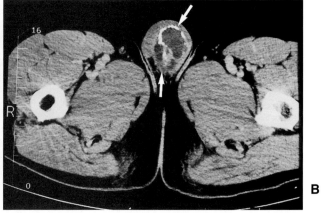

Fig. 2. Malignant teratoma in a 48-year-old man.
A. Color Doppler US of the left testis in transverse plane shows a solid and cystic mass with heterogeneous echogenicity *(arrows)*. The vascularity is slightly increased in the mass. (**A,** See also Color Section.) **B.** Contrast-enhanced CT shows left testicular mass *(arrows)* with dense calcifications and necrosis.

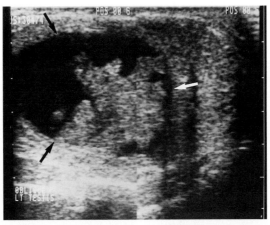

Fig. 3. Mixed germ cell tumor (embryonal cell carcinoma mixed with teratocarcinoma) in a 57-year-old man. US of the left testis shows an enlarged testis with a large cystic and solid mass *(arrows).*

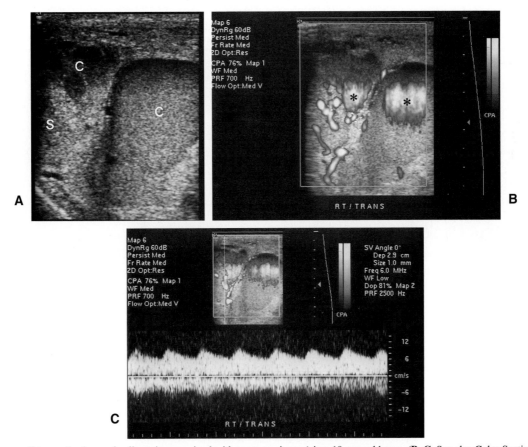

Fig. 4. Mixed germ cell tumor (embryonal cell carcinoma mixed with teratocarcinoma) in a 19-year-old man. (**B, C,** See also Color Section.)
A. Transverse US of the right scrotum shows a markedly enlarged testis totally replaced by mixed cystic (C) and solid (S) tumors. **B.** Color Doppler US shows increased vascularity in the solid component of the tumor. Color signals in the cystic components *(asterisks)* are due to blooming artifacts of the color Doppler US. **C.** Spectral Doppler US obtained from the solid component shows low-resistance arterial flow.

6. Testicular Tumors: Lymphoma

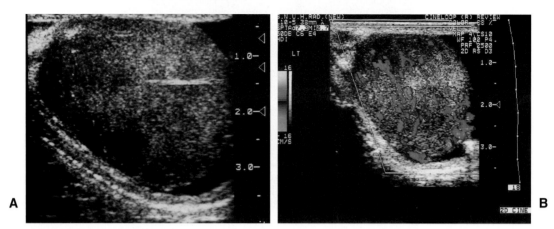

A

B

Fig. 1. Malignant testicular lymphoma in a 66-year-old man.
A. Longitudinal US of the left testis shows an enlarged testis and poorly defined, hypoechoic areas in the testis. **B.** Color Doppler US of the left testis shows diffusely increased vascularity in the tumor. (**B,** See also Color Section.)

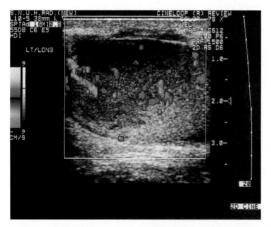

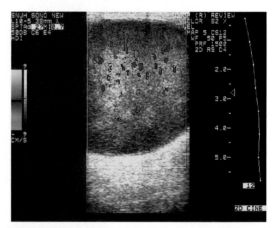

Fig. 2. Malignant lymphoma of the testis in a 60-year-old man. Color Doppler US of the left testis in longitudinal plane shows an enlarged testis with a poorly defined, hypoechoic lesion. Note increased vascularity in the mass. (See also Color Section.)

Fig. 3. Malignant lymphoma involving both testes in a 55-year-old man. Color Doppler US of the right testis in transverse plane shows an enlarged testis with poorly defined, hypoechoic areas and diffusely increased vascularity. The patient also had lymphomatous involvement of the nasal cavity and both adrenal glands. (See also Color Section.)

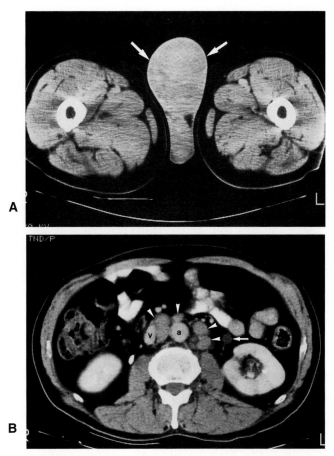

Fig. 4. Malignant lymphoma of the testis in a 75-year-old man.
A. Contrast-enhanced CT shows diffusely an enlarged left testis *(arrows)*
with slightly heterogeneous enhancement. **B.** CT scan of the abdomen
shows multiple, enlarged, retroperitoneal lymph nodes *(arrowheads)* due
to lymphomatous involvement. Note hydronephrosis and hydroureter
(arrow) on the left side. a, abdominal aorta; v, inferior vena cava.

7. Other Testicular Tumors

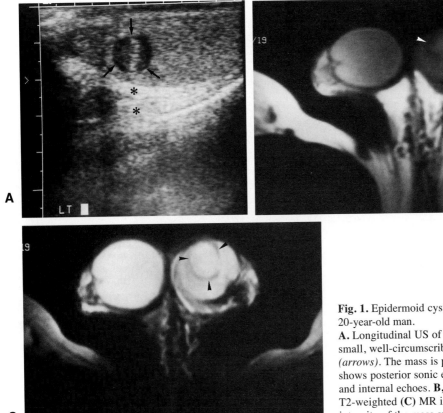

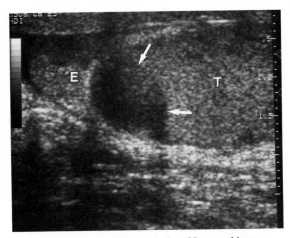

Fig. 1. Epidermoid cyst of the testis in a 20-year-old man. **A.** Longitudinal US of the left testis shows a small, well-circumscribed, round mass *(arrows)*. The mass is primarily cystic and shows posterior sonic enhancement *(asterisks)* and internal echoes. **B, C.** T1-weighted **(B)** and T2-weighted **(C)** MR images show high signal intensity of the mass surrounded by a low-intensity rim *(arrowheads)*.

Fig. 2. Adenomatoid tumor of the testis in a 29-year-old man. Longitudinal US of the right testis shows a normal-contoured testis with a well-defined, homogeneously hypoechoic lesion *(arrows)* in the cranial part of the testis (T). E, epididymis. (From Kim TJ, Kim SH, Sim JS, et al: Ultrasonographic findings of an intratesticular adenomatoid tumor. J Ultrasound Med 2000; 19:227–229.)

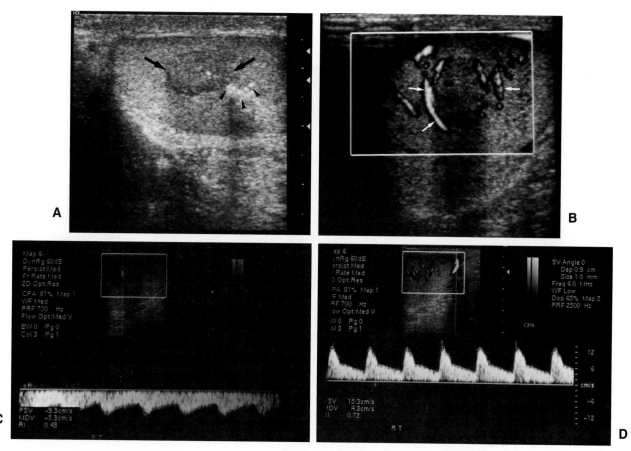

Fig. 3. A 30-year-old man with Sertoli cell tumor.
A. Longitudinal US of the right testis shows a well-circumscribed, homogeneously hypoechoic lesion *(arrows)* in the normal contoured testis. Note that the lesion accompanies posterior sonic attenuation. Also note the localized testicular microlithiasis *(arrowheads)* adjacent to the mass. **B.** Power Doppler US shows slightly increased vascularity along the tumor margin *(arrows).* **C.** Spectral Doppler US obtained from peripheral tumor vessel shows low-resistance pattern with a resistive index of 0.43. **D.** Spectral Doppler US obtained from uninvolved portion of the right testis shows higher-resistance pattern with a resistive index of 0.72.

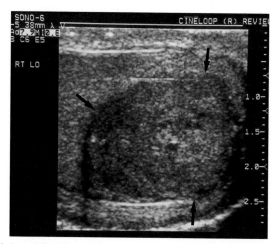

Fig. 4. Sertoli-Leydig cell tumor in a 38-year-old man. Longitudinal US of the right testis shows a well-circumscribed, hypoechoic mass *(arrows).*

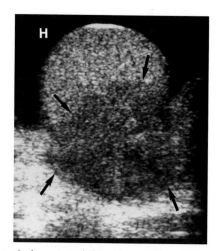

Fig. 5. Intratesticular metastasis in a 49-year-old man who underwent right hemicolectomy for ascending colon cancer. Transverse US of the right testis shows a heterogeneous, hypoechoic mass *(arrows)* involving the testicular mediastinum and paratesticular soft tissue. Note the large amount of hydrocele (H).

8. Testicular Tumors in Undescended Testis

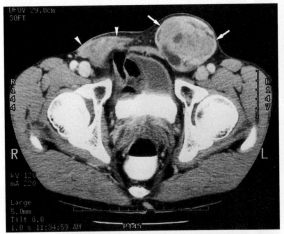
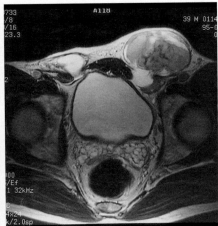

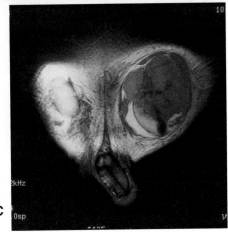

Fig. 1. Bilateral undescended testis with seminoma arising from the left testis in a 39-year-old man.
A. Contrast-enhanced CT of the inguinal area shows a well-demarcated, heterogeneously enhancing mass *(arrows)* in the left inguinal canal. Also note the undescended testis in the right inguinal region *(arrowheads).*
B, C. T2-weighted axial **(B)** and coronal **(C)** MR images show that the mass has heterogeneous signal intensity.

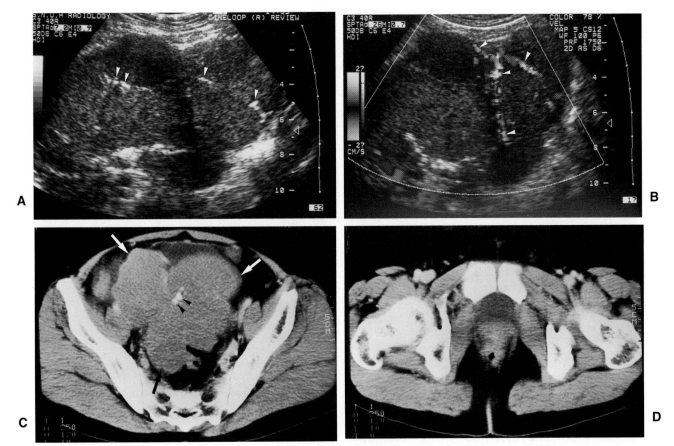

Fig. 2. Bilateral undescended testes with seminoma arising in the undescended right testis in a 28-year-old man.
A. US of the pelvis shows a large mass with a lobulated contour and foci of increased echogenicity *(arrowheads)* representing calcifications.
B. Doppler US of the mass demonstrates prominent linear vessels *(arrowheads)* in the mass. **C.** Contrast-enhanced CT of the pelvic area shows a huge, lobulated, well-enhancing mass *(arrows)* in the right pelvic cavity. Note small calcifications *(arrowheads)* in the mass. **D.** CT scan of the inguinal area shows absence of the spermatic cord in both inguinal regions.

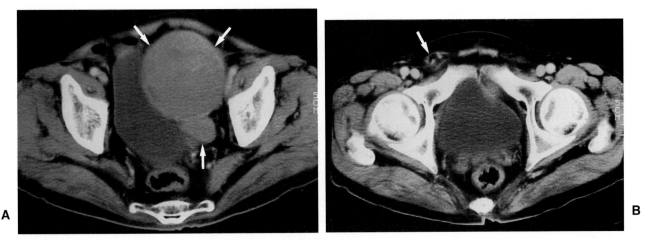

Fig. 3. Undescended left testis with anaplastic seminoma in a 58-year-old man.
A. Contrast-enhanced CT scan of the pelvic cavity shows a large, lobulated, solid mass *(arrows)* in the left suprapubic area. Note that the mass enhances homogeneously. **B.** CT scan of the inguinal area shows an absence of the left spermatic cord in the inguinal canal. The *arrow* indicates the right spermatic cord.

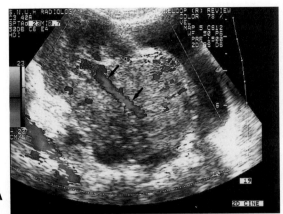

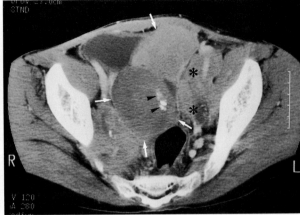

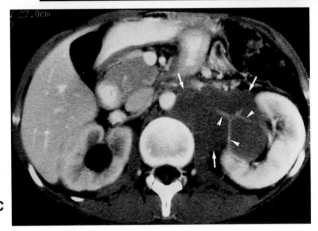

A

B

C

Fig. 4. Undescended left testis with seminoma in an
18-year-old man.
A. Color Doppler US shows a lobulated pelvic mass with a linear,
intratumoral vessel *(arrows).* (**A,** See also Color Section.)
B. Contrast-enhanced CT scan of the pelvic area shows a large,
lobulated mass *(arrows)* with focal calcifications *(arrowheads).*
Note the extensive metastatic lymphadenopathy in the bilateral
pelvic node chain *(asterisks).* **C.** CT scan of the abdomen shows
multiple, enlarged, retroperitoneal lymph nodes *(arrows)* encasing
the left renal vessels *(arrowheads).* Note hydronephrosis of the
right kidney due to ureteral invasion by the pelvic mass.

9. Tumors of the Epididymis and Scrotal Wall

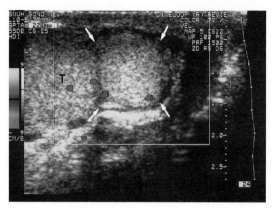

Fig. 1. Adenomatoid tumor of the epididymis in a 30-year-old man. Longitudinal color Doppler US of the left scrotum shows a round, solid mass *(arrows)* in the tail of the epididymis. Note that the echogenicity and vascularity of the mass are similar to those of the testis (T). (See also Color Section.)

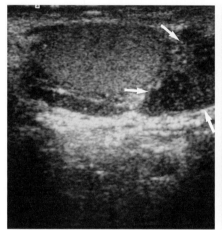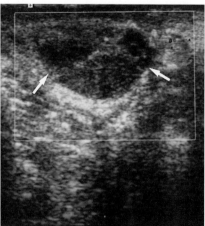

Fig. 2. Sperm granuloma in a 42-year-old man with scrotal mass.
A, B. US of the left scrotum in longitudinal **(A)** and transverse **(B)** planes shows a well-demarcated mass *(arrows)* in the tail of the epididymis. The mass is hypoechoic and has fine, internal echoes and septa.

A

B

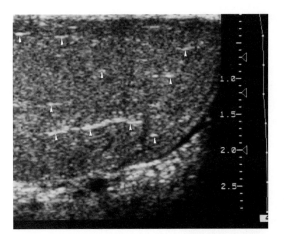

Fig. 3. Epidermoid cyst in scrotal wall in a 29-year-old man. US of the mass shows a well-circumscribed mass of homogeneous echogenicity with scattered echogenic foci *(arrowheads)*. The testis and epididymis were normal (not shown). At surgery, the mass was located in the subdartos layer of the scrotal wall, and the mass was filled with greasy material.

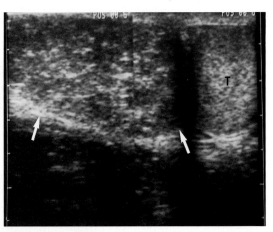

Fig. 4. Epidermal inclusion cyst of the scrotal wall in a 37-year-old man. Longitudinal US of the right scrotum shows a large mass *(arrows)* filled with speckled, echogenic materials cranial to the right testis (T). At surgery, this mass was located in the subcutaneous layer of the scrotal wall, and pathologic examination revealed an epidermal inclusion cyst.

10. Retroperitoneal Nodal Metastases in Testicular Tumors

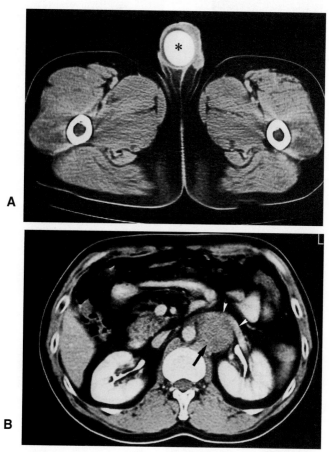

Fig. 1. Retroperitoneal nodal metastasis from a testicular tumor in a 34-year-old man who underwent right orchiectomy and prosthesis insertion.
A. Contrast-enhanced CT scan shows a round testicular prosthesis *(asterisk)* in the right scrotum. **B.** CT scan of the abdomen at renal hilar level shows a large, metastatic lymph node *(arrow)* in the left para-aortic region with anterior displacement of the left renal vein *(arrowheads).*

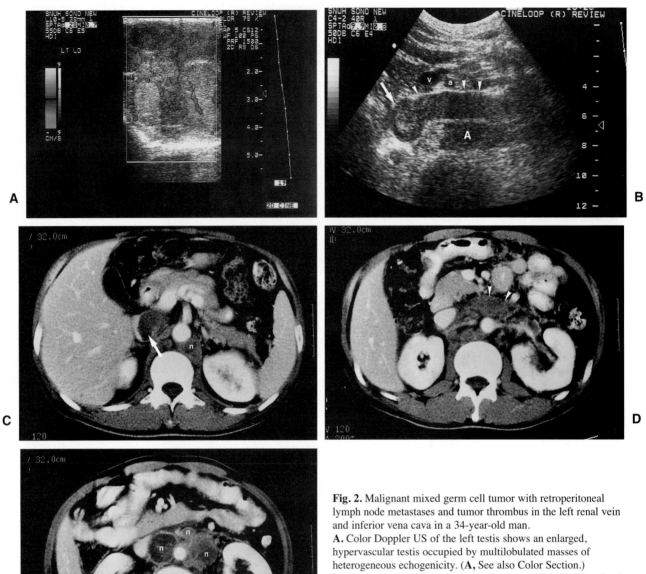

Fig. 2. Malignant mixed germ cell tumor with retroperitoneal lymph node metastases and tumor thrombus in the left renal vein and inferior vena cava in a 34-year-old man.
A. Color Doppler US of the left testis shows an enlarged, hypervascular testis occupied by multilobulated masses of heterogeneous echogenicity. (**A,** See also Color Section.)
B. Transverse US of the abdomen shows the dilated left renal vein *(arrowheads)* and inferior vena cava *(arrow)* filled with echogenic thrombi. A, abdominal aorta; a, superior mesenteric artery; v, superior mesenteric vein. **C–E.** Contrast-enhanced CT scans from cranial to caudal show thrombi in the inferior vena cava *(arrow* in **C**) and left renal vein *(arrowheads* in **D**). Also note the multiple necrotic metastatic lymph nodes (n).

10. Retroperitoneal Nodal Metastases in Testicular Tumors

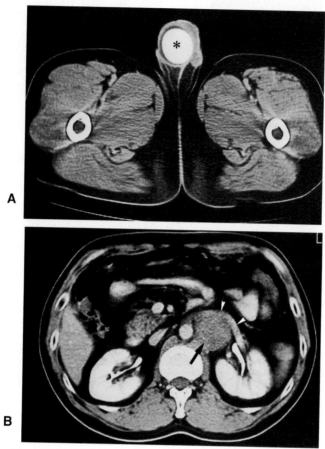

Fig. 1. Retroperitoneal nodal metastasis from a testicular tumor in a
34-year-old man who underwent right orchiectomy and prosthesis
insertion.
A. Contrast-enhanced CT scan shows a round testicular prosthesis
(asterisk) in the right scrotum. **B.** CT scan of the abdomen at renal hilar
level shows a large, metastatic lymph node *(arrow)* in the left para-aortic
region with anterior displacement of the left renal vein *(arrowheads)*.

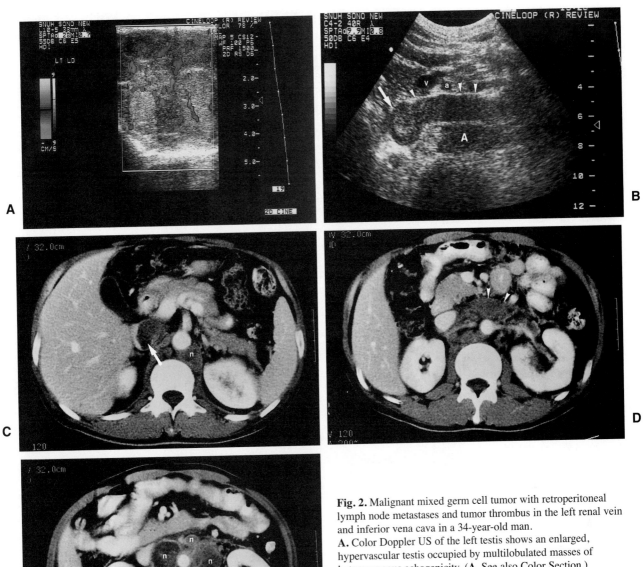

Fig. 2. Malignant mixed germ cell tumor with retroperitoneal lymph node metastases and tumor thrombus in the left renal vein and inferior vena cava in a 34-year-old man.
A. Color Doppler US of the left testis shows an enlarged, hypervascular testis occupied by multilobulated masses of heterogeneous echogenicity. (**A,** See also Color Section.)
B. Transverse US of the abdomen shows the dilated left renal vein *(arrowheads)* and inferior vena cava *(arrow)* filled with echogenic thrombi. A, abdominal aorta; a, superior mesenteric artery; v, superior mesenteric vein. **C–E.** Contrast-enhanced CT scans from cranial to caudal show thrombi in the inferior vena cava *(arrow* in **C**) and left renal vein *(arrowheads* in **D**). Also note the multiple necrotic metastatic lymph nodes (n).

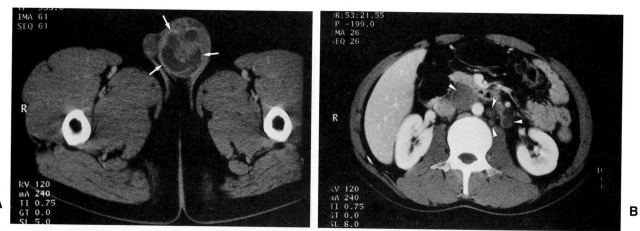

Fig. 3. Malignant mixed germ cell tumor of the left testis and retroperitoneal lymph node metastases in a 27-year-old man.
A. Contrast-enhanced CT shows a large tumor in the left testis with extensive necrosis and peripheral enhancement *(arrows)*. **B.** CT scan of the abdomen shows multiple, metastatic lymph nodes in the retroperitoneum *(arrowheads)*. Note that some of the metastatic nodes are low attenuated due to necrosis.

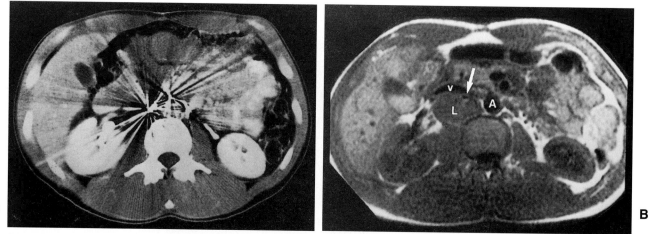

Fig. 4. Recurrent retroperitoneal nodal metastasis from a testicular tumor in a 35-year-old man who underwent radical orchiectomy and retroperitoneal lymph node dissection. (**A, B,** From Hricak H, Hamm B, Kim B: Imaging techniques, anatomy, artifacts, and bioeffects. In Hricak H, Hamm B, Kim B [eds]: Imaging of the Scrotum. New York, Raven Press, 1995, pp 11–36.)
A. On contrast-enhanced CT, evaluation of the retroperitoneum is difficult due to severe artifacts from surgical clips that were used in the retroperitoneal lymph node dissection. **B.** T1-weighted MR image demonstrates a large, retrocaval, metastatic lymph node (L). Note that a small, signal-void focus in the mass *(arrow)* represents a surgical clip. A, abdominal aorta; v, inferior vena cava.

11. Testicular Microlithiasis

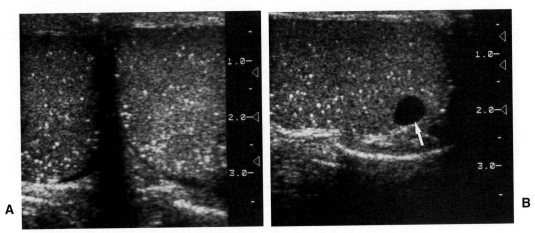

Fig. 1. Testicular microlithiasis in a 15-year-old boy with left-sided varicocele.
A. Transverse US of the scrotum demonstrates multiple echogenic foci scattered throughout both testes. **B.** Longitudinal US of the left testis shows microlithiasis and a small testicular cyst *(arrow)*.

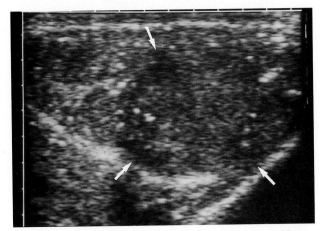

Fig. 2. Testicular microlithiasis associated with seminoma in a 37-year-old man. Longitudinal US of the left testis demonstrates scattered echogenic foci throughout the testis. Note a large, ill-defined, hypoechoic mass *(arrows)* in the testis, which was confirmed as seminoma.

12. Testicular Torsion

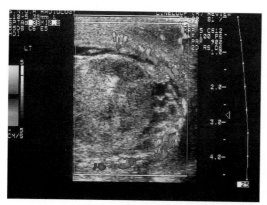

Fig. 1. Testicular torsion in a 16-year-old boy. Color Doppler US of the left scrotum shows a swollen, heterogeneously hypoechoic testis. Note the lack of blood flow in the testis and the hypervascular rim in the scrotal wall. (See also Color Section.)

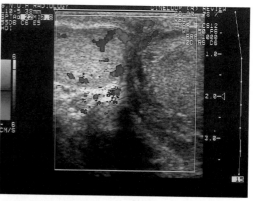

Fig. 2. Testicular torsion in a 30-year-old man. Color Doppler US of the scrotum in transverse plane shows a markedly enlarged left testis with decreased echogenicity. Note the normal blood flow in the right testis but no demonstrable flow in the left testis. (See also Color Section.)

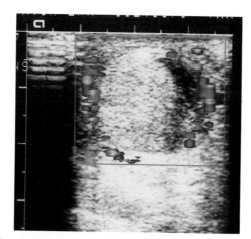

Fig. 3. Extravaginal torsion of the left testis in an infant. Transverse color Doppler US reveals an enlarged, echogenic left testis. The blood flow is decreased in the testis but increased in the scrotal wall. (See also Color Section.)

Fig. 4. Left testicular atrophy in a 33-year-old man with a history of testicular torsion.
A. Transverse US of the scrotum demonstrates markedly shrunken, hypoechoic left testis (L). R, right testis. **B.** Longitudinal US of the left testis demonstrates a small testis with heterogeneous, low echogenicity.

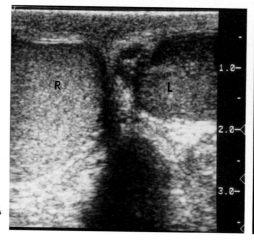

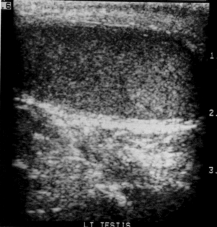

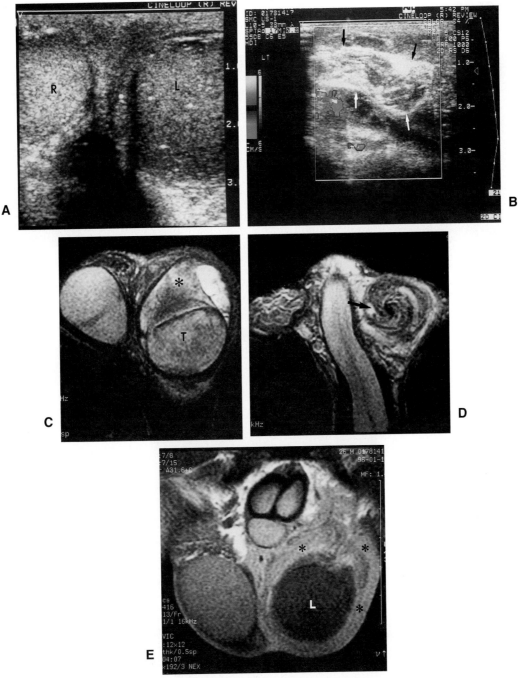

Fig. 5. Chronic testicular torsion in a 26-year-old man.
A. Transverse US of the scrotum shows enlarged, hypoechoic left testis (L). R, right testis. **B.** Longitudinal color Doppler US of the cranial portion of the left scrotum shows the twisted spermatic cord appearing as an echogenic mass *(arrows).* (**B,** See also Color Section.) **C.** Transverse T2-weighted MR image of the scrotum shows a posteriorly displaced left testis and a large amount of hematocele *(asterisk).* The left testis (T) is slightly enlarged and shows heterogeneous signal intensity. **D.** Transverse T2-weighted MR image through the high-scrotal area shows a "torsion knot" and "whirlpool sign" of the left spermatic cord *(arrow).* **E.** Contrast-enhanced T1-weighted MR image in coronal plane shows lack of enhancement in the left testis (L). Note that the left scrotal wall is thickened and shows diffuse enhancement *(asterisks).*

13. Epididymitis

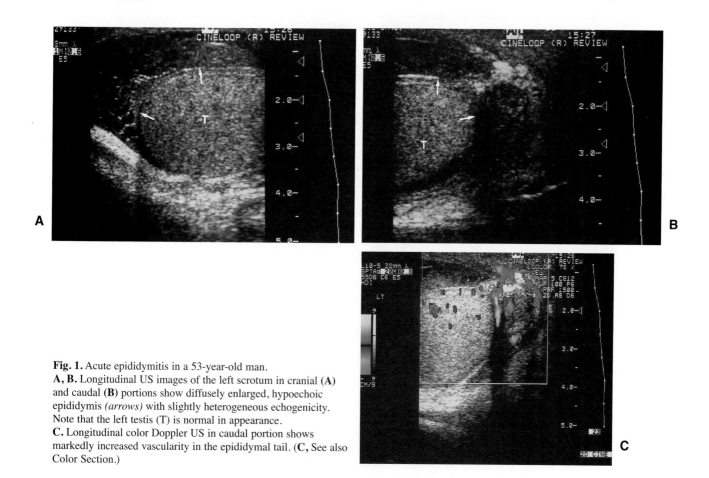

Fig. 1. Acute epididymitis in a 53-year-old man.
A, B. Longitudinal US images of the left scrotum in cranial (**A**) and caudal (**B**) portions show diffusely enlarged, hypoechoic epididymis *(arrows)* with slightly heterogeneous echogenicity. Note that the left testis (T) is normal in appearance.
C. Longitudinal color Doppler US in caudal portion shows markedly increased vascularity in the epididymal tail. (**C,** See also Color Section.)

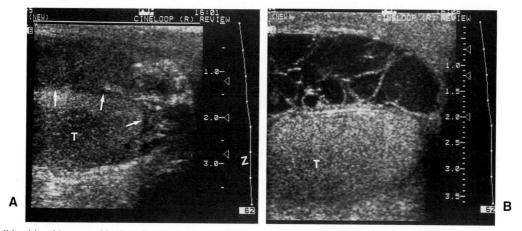

Fig. 2. Acute epididymitis with septated hydrocele in a 45-year-old man.
A. Longitudinal US of the left scrotum shows a diffusely enlarged epididymis *(arrows)* with slightly heterogeneous echogenicity. T, testis.
B. Longitudinal US in other plane shows hydrocele with abundant septations. T, testis.

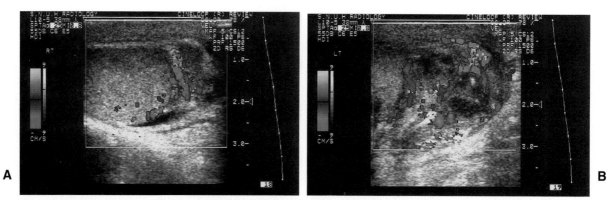

A   B

Fig. 3. Bilateral epididymitis in a 63-year-old man with acute scrotal pain. (**A, B,** See also Color Section.)
A, B. Longitudinal color Doppler US images of the right (**A**) and left (**B**) testes show swelling and increased vascularity in the enlarged epididymis at the tail portion. Note diffuse thickening of the scrotal wall.

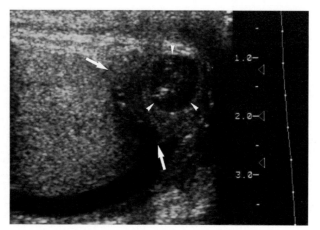

Fig. 4. Acute epididymitis in a 58-year-old man. Longitudinal US of the right scrotum shows a well-circumscribed, hypoechoic lesion *(arrowheads)* in the enlarged epididymal tail *(arrows)*. These findings suggest acute epididymitis with abscess formation. The patient was treated with antibiotics and improved.

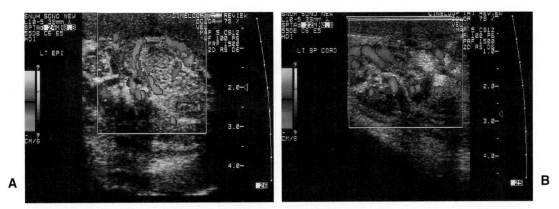

Fig. 5. Acute epididymitis in a 28-year-old man. (**A, B,** See also Color Section.)
A. Color Doppler US shows a diffusely enlarged epididymis with increased vascularity. Note the thickened scrotal wall. **B.** Color Doppler US along the left spermatic cord shows a thickened spermatic cord with increased vascularity.

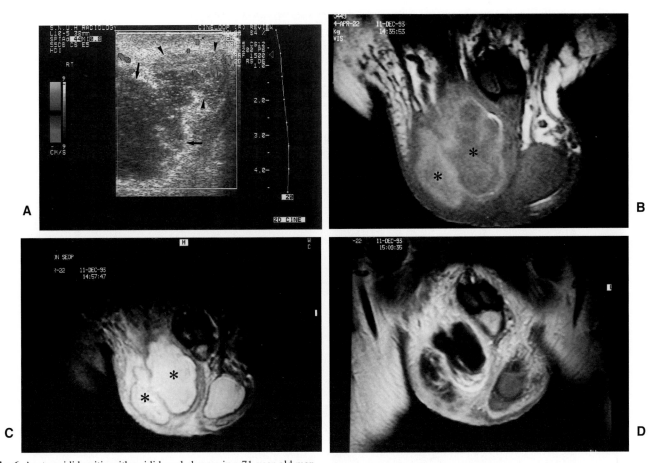

Fig. 6. Acute epididymitis with epididymal abscess in a 71-year-old man.
A. Color Doppler US of the right scrotum shows an enlarged epididymis with increased vascularity *(arrowheads)* and a large hypoechoic lesion suggesting an abscess cavity *(arrows)*. (**A,** See also Color Section.) **B, C.** T1-weighted (**B**) and T2-weighted (**C**) MR images in coronal plane show right scrotal swelling and irregular abscess cavities *(asterisks)*. **D.** Contrast-enhanced T1-weighted MR image in coronal plane shows an absence of enhancement of the abscess cavities and strong enhancement of the thickened scrotal wall.

14. Orchitis and Epididymo-orchitis

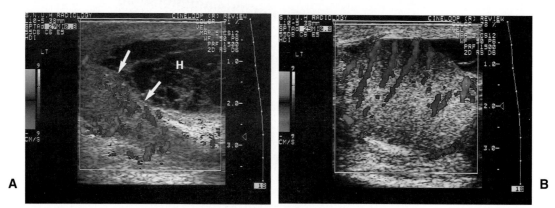

Fig. 1. Acute epididymo-orchitis in a 21-year-old man. (**A, B,** See also Color Section.)
A. Color Doppler US along the left epididymis shows a diffusely enlarged epididymis with decreased echogenicity and increased vascularity *(arrows).* Note the septated hydrocele (H). **B.** Color Doppler US of the left testis shows markedly increased vascularity and slightly decreased echogenicity, suggesting associated orchitis.

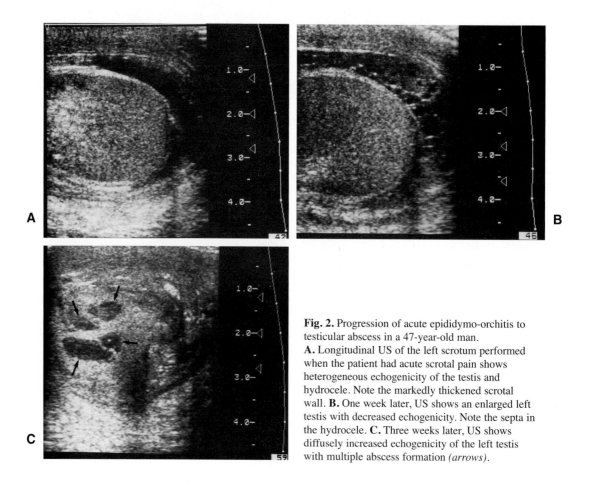

Fig. 2. Progression of acute epididymo-orchitis to testicular abscess in a 47-year-old man.
A. Longitudinal US of the left scrotum performed when the patient had acute scrotal pain shows heterogeneous echogenicity of the testis and hydrocele. Note the markedly thickened scrotal wall. **B.** One week later, US shows an enlarged left testis with decreased echogenicity. Note the septa in the hydrocele. **C.** Three weeks later, US shows diffusely increased echogenicity of the left testis with multiple abscess formation *(arrows).*

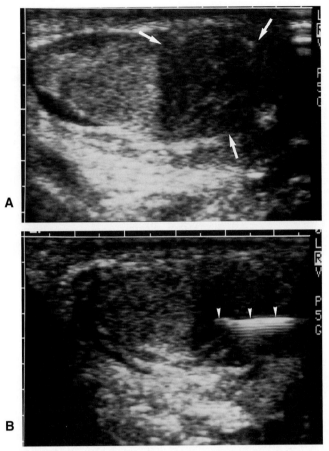

Fig. 3. Malacoplakia of the testis in a 54-year-old man who had undergone partial cystectomy for bladder cancer 1 year earlier. **A.** Longitudinal US of the right scrotum shows a large hypoechoic mass *(arrows)* occupying the caudal half of the right testis. **B.** US-guided biopsy was performed, and pathologic examination revealed testicular malacoplakia. Note a biopsy needle *(arrowheads)* within the lesion.

15. Scrotal Trauma

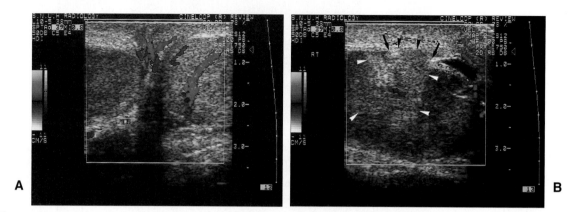

Fig. 1. A 20-year-old man with testicular rupture due to blunt scrotal trauma received 4 days earlier. (**A, B,** See also Color Section.)
A. Transverse color Doppler US of the scrotum shows decreased echogenicity of the right testis with decreased vascularity. **B.** Color Doppler US of the right testis in longitudinal plane shows discontinuity of the tunica albuginea in the anterior aspect *(arrows)*. Note the decreased echogenicity and decreased vascularity of the right testis. Also note the ill-defined, increased echogenicity *(arrowheads)* across the tunical defect, suggesting intratesticular and extratesticular hematoma.

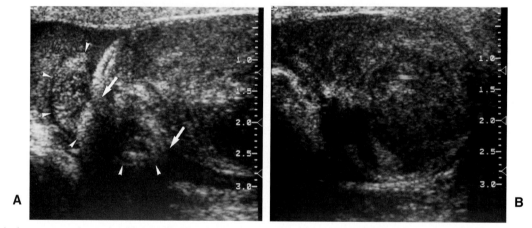

Fig. 2. Left testicular rupture and associated intratesticular and extratesticular hematomas in a 24-year-old man who had received blunt trauma to the scrotum 4 days earlier.
A. Longitudinal US demonstrates a heterogeneous echogenic mass *(arrowheads)* across the defect in the tunica albuginea *(arrows)* in the superior aspect of the left testis. **B.** Transverse US shows an enlarged, hypoechoic, left testis with extensive intratesticular hematoma.

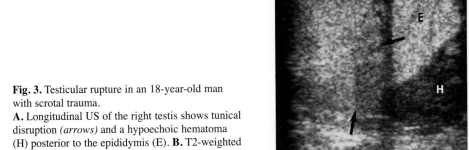

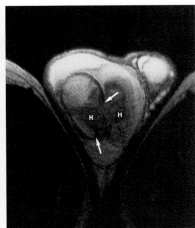

Fig. 3. Testicular rupture in an 18-year-old man with scrotal trauma.
A. Longitudinal US of the right testis shows tunical disruption *(arrows)* and a hypoechoic hematoma (H) posterior to the epididymis (E). **B.** T2-weighted MR image well demonstrates disruption of the tunica albuginea *(arrows)* and intratesticular and extratesticular hematoma (H).

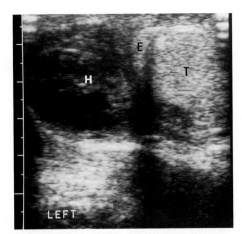

Fig. 4. A 43-year-old man with postvasectomy scrotal hematoma. Longitudinal US of the left scrotum shows a large, hypoechoic hematoma (H) superior to the testis (T) and epididymis (E).

16. Miscellaneous Conditions of the Scrotum

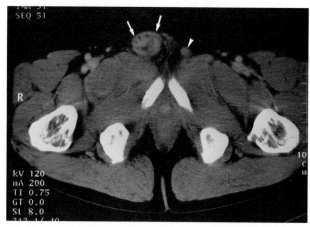

Fig. 1. Metastasis to the spermatic cord in a 64-year-old man with pancreatic cancer. Contrast-enhanced CT of the inguinal area shows a mass of heterogeneous attenuation involving the right spermatic cord *(arrows)*. Note the normal left spermatic cord *(arrowhead)*.

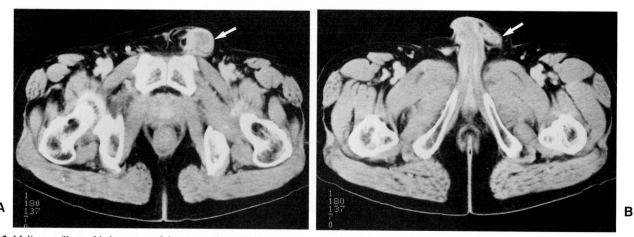

Fig. 2. Malignant fibrous histiocytoma of the spermatic cord in a 71-year-old man.
A, B. Contrast-enhanced CT scans of the inguinal region show a soft tissue mass that involves the left spermatic cord *(arrow)*. The mass has slightly heterogeneous attenuation and infiltrates into the surrounding tissue.

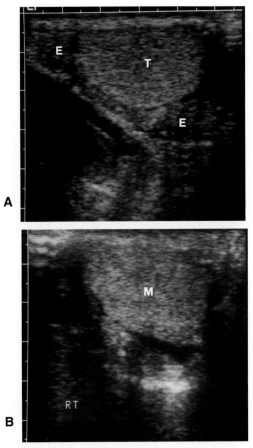

Fig. 3. Fibrous pseudotumor of the periependymal region in a
33-year-old man who presented with a supratesticular mass for 3 years.
A. Longitudinal US of the right scrotum shows normal testis (T) and
epididymis (E). **B.** Longitudinal US of the right supratesticular region
shows a solid mass (M) of homogeneous echogenicity in the right
scrotum. The echogenicity of the mass is slightly higher than that of the
testis. At surgery, this mass was separate from the testis or epididymis,
and the pathologic examination revealed a fibrous pseudotumor.

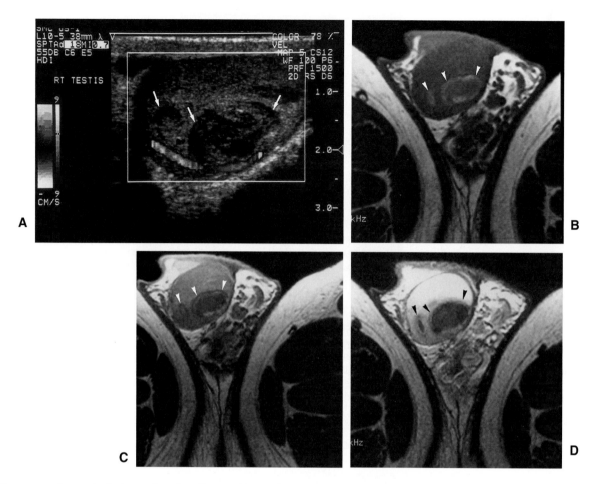

Fig. 4. Spontaneous intratesticular hemorrhage in a 42-year-old man with Henoch-Schönlein purpura.
A. Longitudinal Doppler US of the right scrotum demonstrates intratesticular masses of heterogeneous hypoechogenicity *(arrows)*. **B, C.** On T1-weighted **(B)** and T2-weighted **(C)** MR images, the intratesticular lesions are demarcated by rims of variable signal intensities *(arrowheads)*.
D. Contrast-enhanced T1-weighted MR image shows no enhancement of the intratesticular lesions *(arrowheads)*.

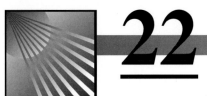

22

Varicocele

SEUNG HYUP KIM

DEFINITION, INCIDENCE, AND PATHOPHYSIOLOGY

A varicocele consists of a group of dilated veins in the spermatic cord and pampiniform plexus, almost exclusively on the left side. Most varicoceles are caused by incompetent valves of the internal spermatic vein or collateral bypass of competent valves with resultant free reflux of venous blood into the pampiniform plexus. Although the mechanism of action is not well known, it is certain that a varicocele influences spermatogenesis, causing decreased sperm count and abnormal sperm motility and morphology. Varicoceles can be associated with testicular atrophy and abnormal testis histology. Varicoceles occur more commonly in infertile men than in the rest of the population, and repair of varicoceles can improve semen parameters and fertility rates.

Primary varicoceles are present in 10% to 20% of men and almost all involve the left side. The left-sided predominance is possibly related to the left spermatic venous drainage into the left renal vein, which may be compressed by a nutcracker phenomenon between the aorta and superior mesenteric artery. Solitary right-sided varicocele is rare, accounting for less than 2% of all cases of varicocele. When one encounters unilateral right-sided varicoceles, the possibility of a retroperitoneal mass obstructing the right spermatic vein should be considered. Total situs inversus is another cause of solitary right-sided varicocele. Bilateral varicoceles occur in approximately 9% to 15% of patients with varicoceles.

Primary varicoceles distend when the patient is standing or performs a Valsalva maneuver. However, secondary varicoceles, caused by obstruction or increased pressure on the spermatic vein by a retroperitoneal mass, renal vein thrombosis, or a hydronephrotic kidney, usually occur in older patients and do not decompress when the patient changes positions.

CLINICAL ASPECT

On physical examination, large varicoceles are easily palpated as multiple tubular structures within the scrotum. Small varicoceles require palpation during a Valsalva maneuver while the patient is standing. Varicoceles have been classified into three grades: grade 1 indicates dilated veins palpable only during a Valsalva maneuver; grade 2, dilated veins palpable without a Valsalva maneuver; and grade 3, dilated veins palpable and visible without a Valsalva maneuver. Subclinical varicocele is a varicocele that is not palpable even with a Valsalva maneuver. The incidence of subclinical varicocele is not known, but its importance in male infertility may be significant.

DIAGNOSIS

On ultrasound (US), varicoceles appear as tubular, serpiginous structures larger than 2 to 3 mm in diameter along the course of the spermatic cord or in the peritesticular region, typically above and posterior to the testis. Color Doppler US is helpful in confirming the presence of a varicocele and detecting a subclinical varicocele. Color and spectral Doppler US can demonstrate the direction of venous flow in the internal spermatic vein. A Valsalva maneuver or an upright position enhances visualization of small clinical or subclinical varicoceles by demonstrating flow reversal. Spectral Doppler US is sometimes difficult because the cremasteric muscle contracts and the veins leave the Doppler sample volume. The use of a wide sample volume can overcome this problem.

Varicoceles may be classified into stop type and shunt type on the basis of Doppler US findings. The stop-type varicocele reveals a retrograde flow at the beginning of a Valsalva maneuver. A varicocele is considered shunt type when a continuous retrograde flow is detected that is intensified by a Valsalva maneuver. Varicocele may extend into the testicle resulting in intratesticular varicocele, which can be depicted by color Doppler US.

Internal spermatic venography seems to be the most sensitive test to detect reflux, and transcatheter treatment can be performed in the same session. The major venographic finding of varicocele is free retrograde flow of contrast material into the dilated pampiniform plexus. Varicocele may be caused by retrograde flow into the internal spermatic vein despite competent valves through bypassing anastomoses with other retroperitoneal veins. Sometimes retrograde flow into the internal spermatic vein drains through the external spermatic vein to the common iliac vein. Varicocele may also be caused by obstruction at the level of the common iliac vein.

TREATMENT

If a varicocele is large and symptomatic, it may be treated. Treatment is also indicated in subfertile men with clinical or subclinical varicoceles who have been infertile for at least 2 years and who have oligoasthenospermia without an apparent cause of infertility. Treatment of varicocele is either by surgical ligation or by transcatheter occlusion of the internal spermatic vein. Either form of treatment has a high recurrence rate, reportedly up to 50%. The significant pressure gradient, more than 3 mm Hg gradient between the left renal vein and inferior

vena cava, represents a poor prognostic sign for recurrence of varicocele after treatment.

Using the Seldinger technique, a gently curved 5- to 7-French torque control catheter with side holes is introduced deep into the left renal vein, and the venography is performed during a Valsalva maneuver. Some recommend using the transjugular approach to facilitate catheterization and to obtain a venogram with the patient in upright position. If reflux into the internal spermatic vein is noted on the left renal venogram, selective internal spermatic venography is performed to demonstrate detailed anatomy of the vein and its collaterals. In most cases, the left internal spermatic vein originates from the inferior surface of the left renal vein, usually 2 or 3 cm away from the junction of the renal vein and the inferior vena cava.

For interventional radiologic treatment, a catheter should be located deep into the internal spermatic vein. Sometimes, it is difficult to advance the catheter into the internal spermatic vein since it tends to buckle at the orifice of the left renal vein. In those cases, use of a guiding catheter may be helpful. An 8-French curved guiding catheter is located at the orifice of the internal spermatic vein and a 5-French straight catheter is introduced through the guiding catheter using a coaxial technique. The right internal spermatic vein is more difficult to catheterize than the left one. A sidewinder catheter is used, and the orifice of the vein is searched for at the anterolateral surface of the inferior vena cava, just caudal to the orifice of the right renal vein.

There are many kinds of embolic materials used for transcatheter occlusion of the varicocele. They include coils, detachable balloons, spiders, compressed Ivalon (Spiderlon) plugs, spider combined with Ivalon, brushes, plastics, and Gelfoam. Among these embolic materials, coils have been most commonly used. The diameter of the coils should be slightly larger than that of the internal spermatic veins. The ends of the coil may be modified to prevent dislodgment. Because of multiple internal spermatic veins and their collateral vessels, embolic devices are usually placed caudally at the level of the inguinal canal and cranially near to the orifice. Between them, the locations of embolic devices are decided according to the anatomy of the vessels.

Various sclerosing agents also have been used for transcatheter treatment of varicoceles. They include hypertonic glucose with monoethanolamine, Varicocid (the salt of a fatty acid of cod liver oil), aethoxysclerol, sodium tetradecyl sulfate (Sotradecol), and heated contrast material. An occlusion balloon catheter may be used to reduce the risk of spill of sclerosing agents into the renal vein. The advantages of sclerosing agents or tissue adhesives in the management of varicocele include ease of delivery, minimal patient discomfort, a higher success rate, and the ability to occlude all collateral vessels that may be the cause of persistent or recurrent varicocele after treatment. The disadvantages of those materials include the risk of reflux of the agents into the renal vein or pampiniform plexus, which may cause renal vein thrombosis and testicular thrombophlebitis, respectively.

References

1. Cornud F, Belin X, Amar E, et al: Varicocele: Strategies in diagnosis and treatment. Eur Radiol 1999; 9:536–545.
2. Kim SH: Embolotherapy of varicocele. In Han MC, Park JH (eds): Interventional Radiology. Seoul, Ilchokak, 1999, pp 53–59.
3. Marsman JWP: The aberrantly fed varicocele: Frequency, venographic appearance, and results of transcatheter embolization. AJR Am J Roentgenol 1995; 164:649–657.
4. Kim SH, Park JH, Han MC, et al: Embolization of the internal spermatic vein in varicocele: Significance of venous pressure. Cardiovasc Intervent Radiol 1992; 15:102–107.
5. Weiss AJ, Kellman CM, Middleton WD, et al: Intratesticular varicocele: Sonographic findings in two patients. AJR Am J Roentgenol 1992; 158:1061–1063.
6. Demas BE, Hricak H, McClure D: Varicoceles: Radiologic diagnosis and treatment. Radiol Clin North Am 1991; 29:619–627.
7. Gonda RL Jr, Karo JJ, Forte RA, et al: Diagnosis of subclinical varicocele in infertility. AJR Am J Roentgenol 1987; 148:71–75.
8. Sigmund G, Gall H, Baehren W: Stop-type and shunt-type varicoceles: Venographic findings. Radiology 1987; 163:105–110.
9. Marsman JWP: Clinical versus subclinical varicocele: Venographic findings and improvement of fertility after embolization. Radiology 1985; 155:635–638.

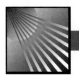

Illustrations • Varicocele

1. Demonstration of Varicocele with Color Doppler US

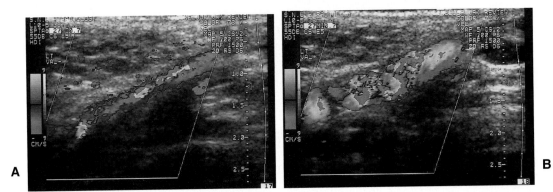

Fig. 1. Left varicocele in a 29-year-old man. (**A, B,** See also Color Section.)
A. Color Doppler US in left inguinal region with the patient at rest shows prominent left internal spermatic vein with the flow in the cranial direction.
B. Color Doppler US with Valsalva maneuver shows markedly dilated internal spermatic vein with turbulent, reversed flow in the caudal direction.

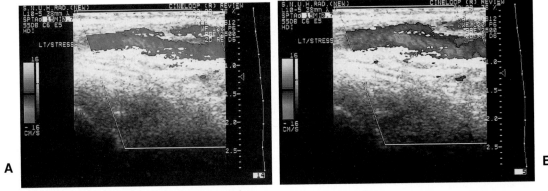

Fig. 2. Left varicocele in a 27-year-old man. (**A, B,** See also Color Section.)
A, B. Color Doppler US of the left inguinal region shows changing direction of blood flow with Valsalva maneuver. Without Valsalva maneuver (**A**), the vein is filled with red, representing the cranial direction of flow. With Valsalva maneuver (**B**), the color signal changed to blue, representing the caudal direction of the flow.

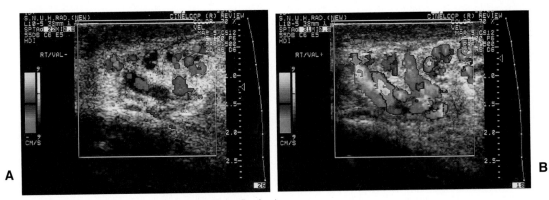

Fig. 3. Left varicocele in a 20-year-old man. (**A, B,** See also Color Section.)
A, B. Color Doppler US of the left scrotum in the region of pampiniform plexus in rest (**A**) and with Valsalva maneuver (**B**). Without Valsalva maneuver, the vessels are dilated in pampiniform plexus and some of them show color flow signals. With Valsalva maneuver, the venous channels are dilated and totally filled with prominent flow signals.

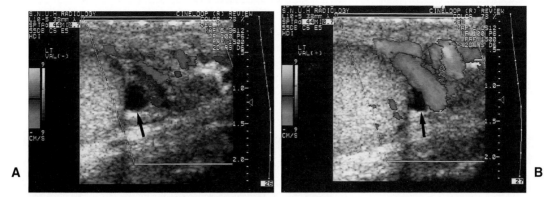

Fig. 4. Left varicocele in a 37-year-old man. (**A, B,** See also Color Section.)
A. Color Doppler US in the caudal portion of the left scrotum shows slightly dilated vessels with scanty flow signals in them. Note a small cyst in the tail of the epididymis *(arrow).* **B.** Color Doppler US with Valsalva maneuver shows dilation of the vessels with prominent flow signals. Note a small cyst in the tail of the epididymis *(arrow).*

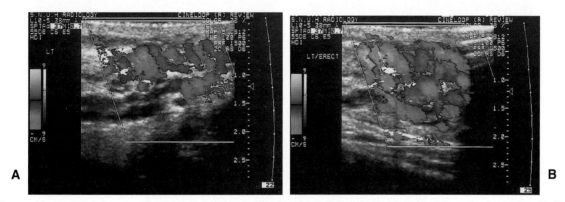

Fig. 5. A 22-year-old man with left varicocele showing changes of color Doppler findings with the changes of the patient's position. (**A, B,** See also Color Section.)
A. Color Doppler US with the patient in supine position shows tortuous, dilated vessels with flow signals in some of them. **B.** With the patient in erect position, the vessels are more dilated and all vessels are filled with flow signals of higher velocity.

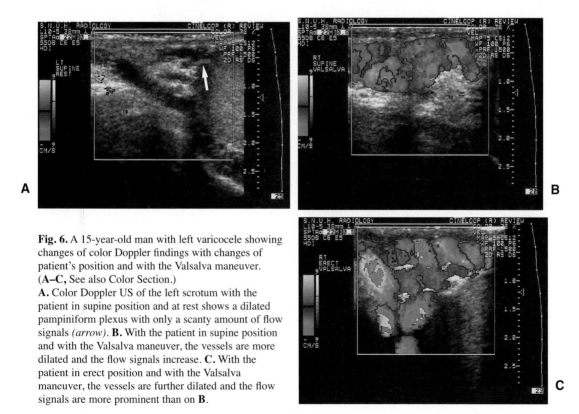

Fig. 6. A 15-year-old man with left varicocele showing changes of color Doppler findings with changes of patient's position and with the Valsalva maneuver. (**A–C,** See also Color Section.)
A. Color Doppler US of the left scrotum with the patient in supine position and at rest shows a dilated pampiniform plexus with only a scanty amount of flow signals *(arrow).* **B.** With the patient in supine position and with the Valsalva maneuver, the vessels are more dilated and the flow signals increase. **C.** With the patient in erect position and with the Valsalva maneuver, the vessels are further dilated and the flow signals are more prominent than on **B**.

669

2. Spectral Doppler US of Varicocele

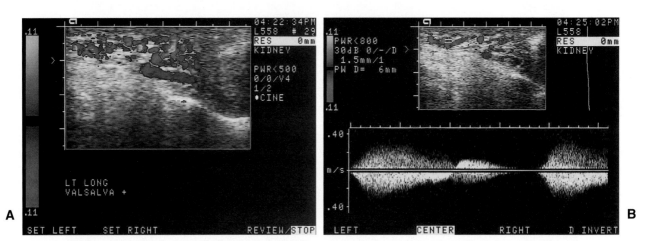

Fig. 1. Left varicocele in a 22-year-old man. (**A, B,** See also Color Section.)
A. Color Doppler US of the left scrotum with the Valsalva maneuver shows a dilated pampiniform plexus with flow signals. **B.** Spectral Doppler US obtained from the dilated plexus shows venous flow that changes its direction with Valsalva maneuvers.

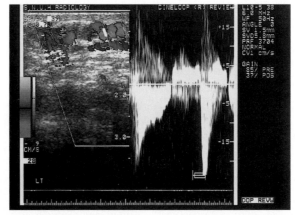

Fig. 2. Left varicocele in a 23-year-old man. Spectral Doppler US obtained from the dilated pampiniform plexus shows venous flow that changes its direction with Valsalva maneuvers. (See also Color Section.)

3. Intratesticular Varicocele

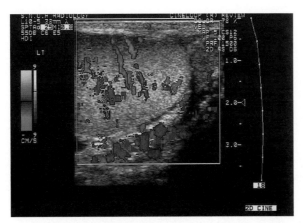

Fig. 1. Intratesticular varicocele in a 74-year-old man. Color Doppler US of the left scrotum shows dilated veins around the testis. Also note dilated vessels in the testis. (See also Color Section.)

4. Internal Spermatic Venography of Varicocele

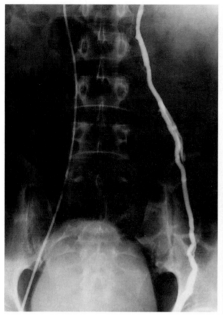

A

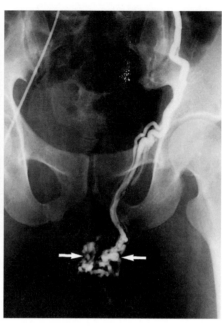

B

Fig. 1. Left varicocele in a 50-year-old man.
A, B. Left gonadal venography opacifies the dilated internal spermatic vein down to the pampiniform plexus (*arrows* in **B**).

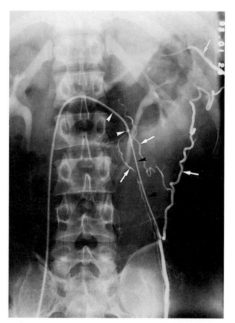

Fig. 2. Left varicocele in a 27-year-old man. Selective left gonadal venography using a coaxial catheter technique opacifies the internal spermatic vein that communicates with the renal capsular veins (*arrows*). Note an 8-French guiding catheter (*white arrowheads*) and an inner 5-French catheter (*black arrowheads*) that was inserted into the gonadal vein.

5. Embolotherapy for Varicocele

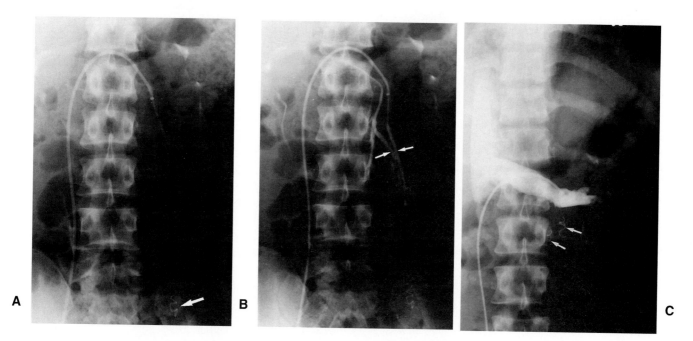

Fig. 1. Embolotherapy of left varicocele with coaxial catheter technique in a 19-year-old man.
A. Caudal portion of the left internal spermatic vein was embolized with a 5-mm spring coil *(arrow).* **B.** Injection of contrast material into the left internal spermatic vein opacifies two parallel channels *(arrows).* **C.** Each venous channel was embolized with a 5-mm spring coil *(arrows).* Note that the left internal spermatic vein is no more opacified at left renal venogram.

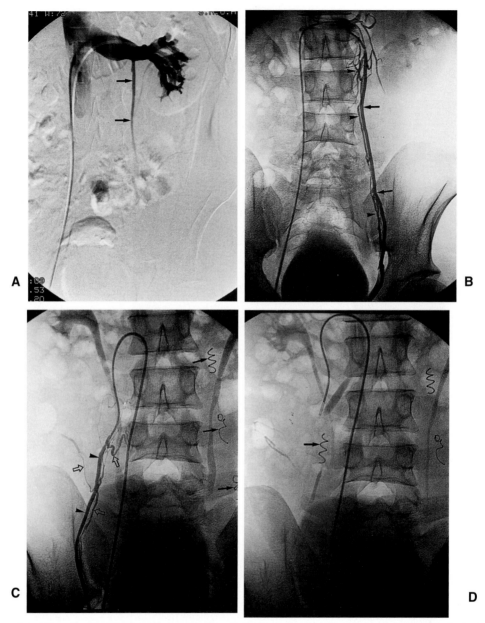

Fig. 2. Embolotherapy of the bilateral varicoceles in a 27-year-old man. (**A–D**, From Kim SH: Embolotherapy of varicocele. In Han MC, Park JH [eds]: Interventional Radiology. Seoul, Ilchokak, 1999, pp 53–59.)
A. Left renal venogram taken with the Valsalva maneuver shows reflux of contrast material into the left internal spermatic vein, which is deficient of valves *(arrows)*. **B.** Selective venogram of the left internal spermatic vein opacifies the whole length of the left internal spermatic vein *(arrows)* and multiple parallel channels *(arrowheads)*. **C.** The left internal spermatic vein was embolized with three 6-mm Gianturco coils *(arrows)*. Then, selective venogram for the right internal spermatic vein was performed, which opacified the right internal spermatic vein *(arrowheads)* and parallel channels *(open arrows)*. **D.** The right internal spermatic vein was embolized with a 6-mm Gianturco coil *(arrow)*.

6. Recurrent Varicocele and the Significance of a Nutcracker Phenomenon

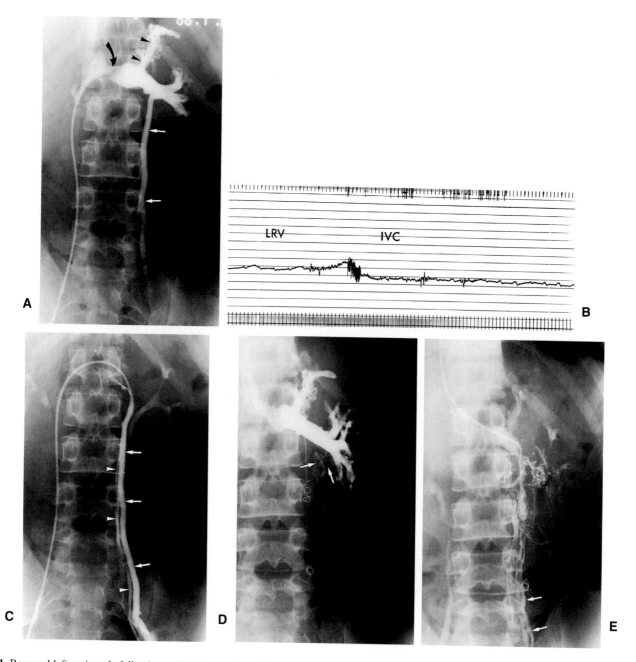

Fig. 1. Recurred left varicocele following embolotherapy in an 18-year-old man. (**A–E,** From Kim SH, Park JH, Han MC, et al: Embolization of the internal spermatic vein in varicocele: Significance of venous pressure. Cardiovasc Intervent Radiol 1992; 15:102–107.)
A. The left renal venogram shows reflux of contrast material into the dilated left internal spermatic vein *(arrows)* and prominent left adrenal vein *(arrowheads)*. Note the compression effect on the left renal vein *(curved arrow)* at the site where the vein locates itself between the superior mesenteric artery and the aorta. **B.** The pressure gradient between the left renal vein (LRV) and the inferior vena cava (IVC) was 5 mm Hg.
C. Selective left internal spermatic venogram opacifies the internal spermatic vein *(arrows)* and small parallel anastomotic veins *(arrowheads)*. **D.** The left internal spermatic vein was embolized with two 5-mm Gianturco coils. Left renal venogram obtained 10 minutes after the embolization shows no evidence of contrast material refluxing distal to the coils, but fine periureteral collateral veins are opacified *(arrows)*. **E.** This selective left internal spermatic venogram was obtained through transjugular approach 3 months after the embolization. It shows abundant, fine, collateral channels reconstructing the pelvic portion of the left internal spermatic vein *(arrows)*, which is the cause of the recurrence of varicocele.

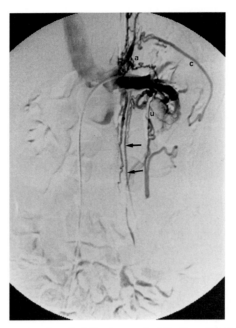

Fig. 2. Recurrent varicocele following surgical ligation of the internal spermatic vein in a 20-year-old man. Left renal venogram shows reflux of contrast material into a thin internal spermatic vein *(arrows)* and multiple collateral channels, including adrenal veins (a), renal capsular veins (c), and periureteral veins (u). The patient showed a nutcracker phenomenon, and the pressure gradient between the left renal vein and the inferior vena cava was 8 mm Hg. (From Kim SH: Embolotherapy of varicocele. In Han MC, Park JH [eds]: Interventional Radiology. Seoul, Ilchokak, 1999, pp 53–59.)

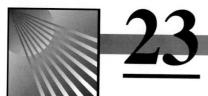

23

Erectile Dysfunction and Penile Diseases

SEUNG HYUP KIM

Penile erection is a complex phenomenon comprising coordinated interaction among the nervous, arterial, venous, and sinusoidal systems. A defect in any of these systems can result in erectile dysfunction. *Erectile dysfunction* is defined as the consistent inability to generate or maintain an erection of sufficient rigidity for sexual intercourse. Although the introduction of sildenafil citrate (Viagra) made the information obtained from imaging studies less critical in the management of patients with erectile dysfunction, the imaging studies such as Doppler ultrasonography (US), penile arteriography, and cavernosography with cavernosometry remain the major modalities in the evaluation of erectile dysfunction.

PHYSIOLOGY OF ERECTION

The normal chain of events leading to penile erection begins with psychological factors that cause transmission of parasympathetic impulses to the penis. The walls of the arterioles and sinusoids of the corpora cavernosa relax, leading to increased inflow of blood through the cavernosal artery. With filling of the sinusoidal spaces, the corporal veno-occlusive mechanism works. The emissary veins leaving the corpora are compressed passively against the fibrous tunica albuginea, and rigid penile erection is achieved and maintained. Detumescence occurs after ejaculation by neurologically stimulated contraction of trabecular smooth muscle in the corpora cavernosa.

Erectile dysfunction is caused by interruptions in the chain of erection, including psychogenic, neurogenic, arteriogenic, and venogenic causes. Often multiple causes are involved. Establishing a specific cause is important particularly in young men because of the high frequency of correctable vascular abnormalities in these patients. Organic causes are found in 50% to 90%, and organic impotence in the presence of normal endocrine balance and an intact nervous system is vascular in origin (either arterial insufficiency or venous incompetence) in about 50% to 70%. Pure arteriogenic impotence accounts for about 30% of cases, and isolated venogenic impotence is found in about 15%. Often erectile dysfunction is caused by combined arteriogenic and venogenic causes. Occasionally, organic impotence is caused by morphologic abnormalities of the penis such as Peyronie's disease.

PENILE ANATOMY

The penis is made up of three corporal bodies: two corpora cavernosa and one corpus spongiosum. The corpora cavernosa are the main erectile bodies and the corpus spongiosum contains the urethra. A septum divides the two corpora cavernosa but contains fenestrations that provide communications between both corpora.

The blood supply of the penis comes primarily from the internal pudendal arteries that originate from the anterior division of the internal iliac arteries. Each internal pudendal artery gives off a scrotal branch, a bulbar artery, and a very small urethral artery before continuing as the penile artery proper, which branches into a cavernosal artery and a dorsal artery at the base of the penis. The cavernosal arteries are the primary source of blood flow to the corpora cavernosa, whereas dorsal arteries, which lie outside the tunica albuginea, supply blood to the skin and glans of the penis. However, multiple anastomotic channels connect the cavernosal arteries with the dorsal arteries. Each cavernosal artery travels near the center of each corpus cavernosum as it sends small helicine arteries, which communicate directly with the sinusoidal spaces. Venous drainage from the corpora cavernosa occurs through small emissary veins, which then drain into the dorsal and cavernosal (crural) veins.

PENILE DOPPLER ULTRASONOGRAPHY

During the past several years, important changes have occurred in the understanding, diagnosis, and treatment of erectile dysfunction. Although there are controversies concerning the value of imaging studies in the evaluation of erectile dysfunction, Doppler US of penile vessels remains a first-line test to discriminate between hemodynamic abnormalities in the penile inflow and outflow vessels. The diagnosis of an arteriogenic or venogenic impotence, however, should be confirmed by penile arteriography or cavernosometry with cavernosography, respectively.

The hemodynamic function of the penis can be evaluated noninvasively by performing color or power Doppler US with spectral analysis after injection of a vasoactive pharmacologic agent such as papaverine, phentolamine, or prostaglandin E_1 as a single agent or in combination to induce an erection. Compared with papaverine, prostaglandin E_1 has advantages of slower onset, longer maintenance, and less chance of priapism and is at least as effective as papaverine in increasing penile blood flow.

Doppler US is performed in a longitudinal, parasagittal plane from a ventral approach, with the patient supine and the penis in an anatomic position on the anterior abdominal wall. High-resolution US scanners with frequencies of 5 to 10 MHz

are used. Color or power Doppler US improves the localization of the penile vessels and thus permits more rapid acquisition of Doppler waveforms. Power Doppler US is superior to conventional color Doppler US in visualizing cavernosal microcirculation. The value of spectral Doppler ultrasound in the flaccid penis is questionable. Audiovisual stimulation can be used to accelerate the erectile response. There are controversies with regard to the value of a second injection of vasoactive agents when the results are inconclusive.

The following is our protocol of penile Doppler US. In the flaccid state, the inner diameter of the cavernosal artery is measured. Three to five minutes after an intracavernosal injection of 10 to 15 μg of prostaglandin E_1, the inner diameter of the cavernosal artery is measured again and Doppler spectra are obtained from the proximal cavernosal arteries at the base of the penis. Some recommend using a tourniquet when a vasoactive agent is being injected, but we do not use it. Because the time after intracavernosal injection at which the highest peak systolic velocity is achieved varies among individuals, it is important to obtain multiple measurements, especially when the velocity is subnormal. The dorsal penile arteries and deep dorsal vein are also evaluated. Doppler angle is kept between 30 and 60 degrees. The sample volume and wall filter are set at minimum to maximize the Doppler signal. Patients should be informed that a prolonged erection for more than 2 hours after the examination may be hazardous and they should return to the hospital if the rigid erection lasts longer.

NORMAL PENILE DOPPLER ULTRASONOGRAPHY

Normally the corpora cavernosa are symmetrical and have homogeneous medium-level echoes. The tunica albuginea appears as a thin, echogenic line surrounding the corpora. The cavernosal arteries are located slightly medially in the center of the corpora. The inner diameters of cavernosal arteries are 0.3 to 0.5 mm in the flaccid state and 0.6 to 1.0 mm after an injection of a vasoactive agent.

The normal progression of cavernosal arterial flow during penile erection is well known. In the flaccid state, monophasic flow is present with minimal diastolic flow. With the onset of erection, there is an increase in both systolic and diastolic flows. As intracavernosal pressure increases, a dicrotic notch appears and a decrease in diastolic flow occurs. With continuously increasing intracavernosal pressure, end-diastolic flow declines to zero and then undergoes diastolic flow reversal. Then the systolic envelope is narrowed, and diastolic flow disappears completely with firm erection.

PARAMETERS FOR PENILE DOPPLER ULTRASONOGRAPHY

Several parameters have been used to quantify penile arterial blood flow, including peak systolic velocity (PSV), end-diastolic velocity (EDV), and resistive index. Among these indexes, PSV is the most commonly used. The reported criteria of PSV used to distinguish normal from impaired arterial function vary from 25 to 40 cm/sec. However, it is generally agreed that a PSV lower than 25 cm/sec indicates arterial insufficiency, higher than 30 cm/sec is normal, and 25 to 30 cm/sec is equivocal.

It has been reported that PSV varies significantly according to the sampling location along the course of a cavernosal artery. The proximal cavernosal artery, where it angles posteriorly toward the crus, should be the standard sampling location for Doppler US of the cavernosal arteries. Doppler spectral pattern and PSV of the dorsal penile arteries are quite variable and are usually different from those of the cavernosal arteries.

Arterial compliance reflecting an ability of the vessel to dilate is another important parameter. A 60% to 75% increase in diameter of the cavernosal arteries after an intracavernosal injection of vasoactive agents with evident pulsation is considered adequate compliance of the arteries.

ARTERIOGENIC AND VENOGENIC IMPOTENCE

The parameters indicating arterial disease are a subnormal clinical response to vasoactive agents, a less than 60% increase in the diameter of the cavernosal artery, and a PSV of the cavernosal arteries lower than 30 cm/sec. If a significant discrepancy exists between the velocities of the two cavernosal arteries (>10 cm/sec difference), unilateral arterial disease should be suspected.

In the presence of normal arterial function, Doppler findings suggestive of an abnormal venous leak are persistent EDV of the cavernosal artery above 5 cm/sec and demonstration of flow in the deep dorsal vein. However, venous leak through the crural veins could not be demonstrated with Doppler US. The development of reversal of the diastolic flow of the cavernosal artery after intracavernosal injection of vasoactive agents is regarded as a reliable indicator of venous competence. Patients with arterial insufficiency and competent veins who do not achieve adequate rigidity might show persistent end-diastolic flow in cavernosal arteries and prominent flow in the dorsal veins. Therefore, it is difficult to distinguish the patients with isolated arteriogenic impotence from those with combined arteriogenic and venogenic impotence with Doppler US alone.

MISCELLANEOUS CONDITIONS

Other conditions of the penis causing erectile dysfunction that may be evaluated with US and Doppler US are congenital anomalies, masses, priapism, Peyronie's disease, and trauma-related abnormalities. Priapism is defined as prolonged, usually painful, penile erection not initiated by sexual stimuli. It is important to distinguish between the two types of priapism, high (arterial) and low (venous) flow, because their treatment and prognosis differ. In addition to the gray-scale US findings of Peyronie's disease such as fibrous thickening and calcification of tunica albuginea, Doppler US after an intracavernosal injection of vasoactive agents may confirm the correlation of the plaques and the penile vessels. Arteriosinusoidal or arteriovenous fistulas within the corporal tissue may cause priapism, and color Doppler US can identify the location of the fistula.

PENILE ARTERIOGRAPHY

Initial flush arteriography, with catheter located just above the iliac bifurcation, is performed to delineate the anatomy of the aortic bifurcation and pelvic arteries. Prostaglandin E_1 (20 μg) is then injected into a corpus cavernosum. Each internal pudendal artery is selectively catheterized, and an arteri-

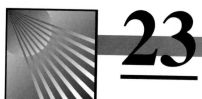

23

Erectile Dysfunction and Penile Diseases

SEUNG HYUP KIM

Penile erection is a complex phenomenon comprising coordinated interaction among the nervous, arterial, venous, and sinusoidal systems. A defect in any of these systems can result in erectile dysfunction. *Erectile dysfunction* is defined as the consistent inability to generate or maintain an erection of sufficient rigidity for sexual intercourse. Although the introduction of sildenafil citrate (Viagra) made the information obtained from imaging studies less critical in the management of patients with erectile dysfunction, the imaging studies such as Doppler ultrasonography (US), penile arteriography, and cavernosography with cavernosometry remain the major modalities in the evaluation of erectile dysfunction.

PHYSIOLOGY OF ERECTION

The normal chain of events leading to penile erection begins with psychological factors that cause transmission of parasympathetic impulses to the penis. The walls of the arterioles and sinusoids of the corpora cavernosa relax, leading to increased inflow of blood through the cavernosal artery. With filling of the sinusoidal spaces, the corporal veno-occlusive mechanism works. The emissary veins leaving the corpora are compressed passively against the fibrous tunica albuginea, and rigid penile erection is achieved and maintained. Detumescence occurs after ejaculation by neurologically stimulated contraction of trabecular smooth muscle in the corpora cavernosa.

Erectile dysfunction is caused by interruptions in the chain of erection, including psychogenic, neurogenic, arteriogenic, and venogenic causes. Often multiple causes are involved. Establishing a specific cause is important particularly in young men because of the high frequency of correctable vascular abnormalities in these patients. Organic causes are found in 50% to 90%, and organic impotence in the presence of normal endocrine balance and an intact nervous system is vascular in origin (either arterial insufficiency or venous incompetence) in about 50% to 70%. Pure arteriogenic impotence accounts for about 30% of cases, and isolated venogenic impotence is found in about 15%. Often erectile dysfunction is caused by combined arteriogenic and venogenic causes. Occasionally, organic impotence is caused by morphologic abnormalities of the penis such as Peyronie's disease.

PENILE ANATOMY

The penis is made up of three corporal bodies: two corpora cavernosa and one corpus spongiosum. The corpora cavernosa

are the main erectile bodies and the corpus spongiosum contains the urethra. A septum divides the two corpora cavernosa but contains fenestrations that provide communications between both corpora.

The blood supply of the penis comes primarily from the internal pudendal arteries that originate from the anterior division of the internal iliac arteries. Each internal pudendal artery gives off a scrotal branch, a bulbar artery, and a very small urethral artery before continuing as the penile artery proper, which branches into a cavernosal artery and a dorsal artery at the base of the penis. The cavernosal arteries are the primary source of blood flow to the corpora cavernosa, whereas dorsal arteries, which lie outside the tunica albuginea, supply blood to the skin and glans of the penis. However, multiple anastomotic channels connect the cavernosal arteries with the dorsal arteries. Each cavernosal artery travels near the center of each corpus cavernosum as it sends small helicine arteries, which communicate directly with the sinusoidal spaces. Venous drainage from the corpora cavernosa occurs through small emissary veins, which then drain into the dorsal and cavernosal (crural) veins.

PENILE DOPPLER ULTRASONOGRAPHY

During the past several years, important changes have occurred in the understanding, diagnosis, and treatment of erectile dysfunction. Although there are controversies concerning the value of imaging studies in the evaluation of erectile dysfunction, Doppler US of penile vessels remains a first-line test to discriminate between hemodynamic abnormalities in the penile inflow and outflow vessels. The diagnosis of an arteriogenic or venogenic impotence, however, should be confirmed by penile arteriography or cavernosometry with cavernosography, respectively.

The hemodynamic function of the penis can be evaluated noninvasively by performing color or power Doppler US with spectral analysis after injection of a vasoactive pharmacologic agent such as papaverine, phentolamine, or prostaglandin E_1 as a single agent or in combination to induce an erection. Compared with papaverine, prostaglandin E_1 has advantages of slower onset, longer maintenance, and less chance of priapism and is at least as effective as papaverine in increasing penile blood flow.

Doppler US is performed in a longitudinal, parasagittal plane from a ventral approach, with the patient supine and the penis in an anatomic position on the anterior abdominal wall. High-resolution US scanners with frequencies of 5 to 10 MHz

are used. Color or power Doppler US improves the localization of the penile vessels and thus permits more rapid acquisition of Doppler waveforms. Power Doppler US is superior to conventional color Doppler US in visualizing cavernosal microcirculation. The value of spectral Doppler ultrasound in the flaccid penis is questionable. Audiovisual stimulation can be used to accelerate the erectile response. There are controversies with regard to the value of a second injection of vasoactive agents when the results are inconclusive.

The following is our protocol of penile Doppler US. In the flaccid state, the inner diameter of the cavernosal artery is measured. Three to five minutes after an intracavernosal injection of 10 to 15 μg of prostaglandin E_1, the inner diameter of the cavernosal artery is measured again and Doppler spectra are obtained from the proximal cavernosal arteries at the base of the penis. Some recommend using a tourniquet when a vasoactive agent is being injected, but we do not use it. Because the time after intracavernosal injection at which the highest peak systolic velocity is achieved varies among individuals, it is important to obtain multiple measurements, especially when the velocity is subnormal. The dorsal penile arteries and deep dorsal vein are also evaluated. Doppler angle is kept between 30 and 60 degrees. The sample volume and wall filter are set at minimum to maximize the Doppler signal. Patients should be informed that a prolonged erection for more than 2 hours after the examination may be hazardous and they should return to the hospital if the rigid erection lasts longer.

NORMAL PENILE DOPPLER ULTRASONOGRAPHY

Normally the corpora cavernosa are symmetrical and have homogeneous medium-level echoes. The tunica albuginea appears as a thin, echogenic line surrounding the corpora. The cavernosal arteries are located slightly medially in the center of the corpora. The inner diameters of cavernosal arteries are 0.3 to 0.5 mm in the flaccid state and 0.6 to 1.0 mm after an injection of a vasoactive agent.

The normal progression of cavernosal arterial flow during penile erection is well known. In the flaccid state, monophasic flow is present with minimal diastolic flow. With the onset of erection, there is an increase in both systolic and diastolic flows. As intracavernosal pressure increases, a dicrotic notch appears and a decrease in diastolic flow occurs. With continuously increasing intracavernosal pressure, end-diastolic flow declines to zero and then undergoes diastolic flow reversal. Then the systolic envelope is narrowed, and diastolic flow disappears completely with firm erection.

PARAMETERS FOR PENILE DOPPLER ULTRASONOGRAPHY

Several parameters have been used to quantify penile arterial blood flow, including peak systolic velocity (PSV), end-diastolic velocity (EDV), and resistive index. Among these indexes, PSV is the most commonly used. The reported criteria of PSV used to distinguish normal from impaired arterial function vary from 25 to 40 cm/sec. However, it is generally agreed that a PSV lower than 25 cm/sec indicates arterial insufficiency, higher than 30 cm/sec is normal, and 25 to 30 cm/sec is equivocal.

It has been reported that PSV varies significantly according to the sampling location along the course of a cavernosal artery. The proximal cavernosal artery, where it angles posteriorly toward the crus, should be the standard sampling location for Doppler US of the cavernosal arteries. Doppler spectral pattern and PSV of the dorsal penile arteries are quite variable and are usually different from those of the cavernosal arteries.

Arterial compliance reflecting an ability of the vessel to dilate is another important parameter. A 60% to 75% increase in diameter of the cavernosal arteries after an intracavernosal injection of vasoactive agents with evident pulsation is considered adequate compliance of the arteries.

ARTERIOGENIC AND VENOGENIC IMPOTENCE

The parameters indicating arterial disease are a subnormal clinical response to vasoactive agents, a less than 60% increase in the diameter of the cavernosal artery, and a PSV of the cavernosal arteries lower than 30 cm/sec. If a significant discrepancy exists between the velocities of the two cavernosal arteries (>10 cm/sec difference), unilateral arterial disease should be suspected.

In the presence of normal arterial function, Doppler findings suggestive of an abnormal venous leak are persistent EDV of the cavernosal artery above 5 cm/sec and demonstration of flow in the deep dorsal vein. However, venous leak through the crural veins could not be demonstrated with Doppler US. The development of reversal of the diastolic flow of the cavernosal artery after intracavernosal injection of vasoactive agents is regarded as a reliable indicator of venous competence. Patients with arterial insufficiency and competent veins who do not achieve adequate rigidity might show persistent end-diastolic flow in cavernosal arteries and prominent flow in the dorsal veins. Therefore, it is difficult to distinguish the patients with isolated arteriogenic impotence from those with combined arteriogenic and venogenic impotence with Doppler US alone.

MISCELLANEOUS CONDITIONS

Other conditions of the penis causing erectile dysfunction that may be evaluated with US and Doppler US are congenital anomalies, masses, priapism, Peyronie's disease, and trauma-related abnormalities. Priapism is defined as prolonged, usually painful, penile erection not initiated by sexual stimuli. It is important to distinguish between the two types of priapism, high (arterial) and low (venous) flow, because their treatment and prognosis differ. In addition to the gray-scale US findings of Peyronie's disease such as fibrous thickening and calcification of tunica albuginea, Doppler US after an intracavernosal injection of vasoactive agents may confirm the correlation of the plaques and the penile vessels. Arteriosinusoidal or arteriovenous fistulas within the corporal tissue may cause priapism, and color Doppler US can identify the location of the fistula.

PENILE ARTERIOGRAPHY

Initial flush arteriography, with catheter located just above the iliac bifurcation, is performed to delineate the anatomy of the aortic bifurcation and pelvic arteries. Prostaglandin E_1 (20 μg) is then injected into a corpus cavernosum. Each internal pudendal artery is selectively catheterized, and an arteri-

ogram is obtained at a 30-degree ipsilateral anterior oblique projection with an injection of 10 to 15 mL of non-ionic contrast material. Deep selection of the internal pudendal artery should be avoided since it often causes vasospasm. Arteriography with catheter tip at internal iliac artery usually demonstrates penile arterial anatomy adequately.

The vascular patterns are highly variable and frequently different from classic descriptions. Common anatomic variations are dorsal penile–cavernosal perforators, accessory cavernosal arteries, and bilateral cavernosal arteries arising from one penile artery through transverse root communicators.

CAVERNOSOMETRY WITH CAVERNOSOGRAPHY

Although significantly different protocols exist, basically cavernosometry with cavernosography evaluates the veno-occlusive function of the corpora cavernosa. Since it is an invasive study, cavernosometry with cavernosography should be reserved for selected patients who are candidates for surgical or interventional management.

The following are the protocols of cavernosometry with cavernosography that were described by Krysiewicz and that we are using. Two 21-gauge butterfly needles are placed, one in each corpus cavernosum at the proximal shaft, one needle for infusion and the other for recording of intracavernosal pressure. Baseline intracavernosal pressure is recorded, and then 20 μg of prostaglandin E_1 is administered. The clinical response is noted and postinjection intracavernosal pressure is recorded 10 minutes after injection. In normal full erection this pressure should be somewhere between 80 and 100 mm Hg.

Then normal saline is infused with the use of an infusion pump to attain an intracavernosal pressure of 150 mm Hg. At this point the infusion is stopped and the rate of fall of intracavernosal pressure is recorded over a 30-second interval. After this, saline is infused again to attain an intracavernosal pressure of 100 mm Hg, and the flow rate needed to maintain this pressure is noted. From these cavernosometric measurements obtained, the presence or absence of a venous leak is determined.

Findings that indicate venous insufficiency are a subnormal clinical response to intracavernosal injection of prostaglandin E_1, a postinjection intracavernosal pressure of less than 80 mm Hg, a greater than 1 mm Hg/sec drop in intracavernosal pressure after stopping intracavernosal infusion of saline at an intracavernosal pressure of 150 mm Hg, and a flow rate greater than 10 mL/min to maintain an intracavernosal pressure of 100 mm Hg.

If venous leak is suspected at cavernosometry, cavernosography is performed to demonstrate abnormal draining veins by infusing diluted contrast material at the rate needed to maintain intracavernosal pressure of 100 mm Hg. Identification of the veins that are incompetent is important in those patients who will subsequently undergo surgical ligation or interventional occlusion of the veins.

References

1. Kim SH: Doppler US evaluation of erectile dysfunction. Abdom Imaging 2002; 27:578–587.
2. Kim SH: Imaging for evaluation of erectile dysfunction. J Korean Soc Med US 2001; 20:1–13.
3. Chen J, Greenstein A, Matzkin H: Is a second injection of vasoactive medication necessary during color duplex Doppler evaluation of young patients with veno-occlusive erectile dysfunction? Urology 2000; 55:927–930.
4. King BF Jr, McKusick CA, Nehra A: Diagnostic imaging of male sexual dysfunction. In Pollack HM, McClennan BL (eds): Clinical Urography, 2nd ed, vol 3. Philadelphia, WB Saunders, 2000, pp 2615–2629.
5. Klingler HC, Kratzik C, Pycha A, et al: Value of power Doppler sonography in the investigation of erectile dysfunction. Eur Urol 1999; 36:320–326.
6. Chiou RK, Pomeroy BD, Chen WS, et al: Hemodynamic patterns of pharmacologically induced erection: Evaluation by color Doppler sonography. J Urol 1998; 159:109–112.
7. Chung WS, Park YY, Kwon SW: The impact of aging on penile hemodynamics in normal responders to pharmacological injection: A Doppler sonographic study. J Urol 1997; 157:2129–2131.
8. Harmon WJ, Nehra A: Priapism: Diagnosis and management. Mayo Clin Proc 1997; 72:350–355.
9. Meuleman EJ, Diemont WL: Investigation of erectile dysfunction: Diagnostic testing for vascular factors in erectile dysfunction. Urol Clin North Am 1995; 22:803–819.
10. Kim SH, Paick JS, Lee SE, et al: Doppler sonography of deep cavernosal artery of the penis: Variation of peak systolic velocity according to sampling location. J Ultrasound Med 1994; 13:591–594.
11. Amin Z, Patel U, Friedman EP, Vale JA, et al: Colour Doppler and duplex ultrasound assessment of Peyronie's disease in impotent men. Br J Radiol 1993; 66:398–402.
12. Benson CB, Aruny JE, Vickers MA Jr: Correlation of duplex sonography with arteriography in patients with erectile dysfunction. AJR Am J Roentgenol 1993; 160:71–73.
13. Feldstein VA: Posttraumatic "high-flow" priapism: Evaluation with color flow Doppler sonography. J Ultrasound Med 1993; 12:589–593.
14. Jarow JP, Pugh VW, Routh WD, et al: Comparison of penile duplex ultrasonography: Variant penile arterial anatomy affects interpretation of duplex ultrasonography. Invest Radiol 1993; 28:806–810.
15. Valji K, Bookstein JJ: Diagnosis of arteriogenic impotence: Efficacy of duplex sonography as a screening tool. AJR Am J Roentgenol 1993; 160:65–69.
16. Fitzgerald SW, Erickson SJ, Foley WD, et al: Color Doppler sonography in the evaluation of erectile dysfunction. Radiographics 1992; 12:3–17.
17. Benson CB, Vickers MA, Aruny J: Evaluation of impotence. Semin Ultrasound CT MR 1991; 12:176–190.
18. Fitzgerald SW, Foley WD: Color Doppler imaging of the genitourinary system. In Foley WD (ed): Color Doppler Flow Imaging. Reading, MA, Andover, 1991, pp 153–170.
19. Hattery RR, King BF Jr, Lewis RW, et al: Vasculogenic impotence: Duplex and color Doppler imaging. Radiol Clin North Am 1991; 29:629–645.
20. Kim SH, Lee SE, Han MC: Penile hemangioma: US and MR imaging demonstration. Urol Radiol 1991; 13:126–128.
21. Rosen MP, Schwartz AN, Levine FJ, et al: Radiologic assessment of impotence: Angiography, sonography, cavernosography, and scintigraphy. AJR Am J Roentgenol 1991; 157:923–931.
22. Cohan RH, Dunnick NR, Carson CC: Radiology of penile prosthesis. AJR Am J Roentgenol 1989; 152:925–931.
23. Krysiewicz S, Mellinger BC: The role of imaging in the evaluation of impotence. AJR Am J Roentgenol 1989; 153:1133–1139.
24. Quam JP, King BF, James EM, et al: Duplex and color Doppler sonographic evaluation of vasculogenic impotence. AJR Am J Roentgenol 1989; 153:1141–1147.
25. Schwartz AN, Wang KY, Mack LA, et al: Evaluation of normal erectile function with color flow Doppler sonography. AJR Am J Roentgenol 1989; 153:1155–1160.
26. Bookstein JJ: Penile angiography: The last angiographic frontier. AJR Am J Roentgenol 1988; 150:47–54.
27. Schwartz AN, Freidenberg D, Harley JD: Nonselective angiography after intracorporal papaverine injection: An alternative technique for evaluating penile arterial integrity. Radiology 1988; 167:249–253.
28. Bookstein JJ: Cavernosal veno-occlusive insufficiency in male impotence: Evaluation of degree and location. Radiology 1987; 164:175–178.
29. Bookstein JJ, Lang EV: Penile magnification pharmacoarteriography: Details of intrapenile arterial anatomy. AJR Am J Roentgenol 1987; 148:883–888.
30. Lurie AL, Bookstein JJ, Kessler WO: Post-traumatic impotence: Angiographic evaluation. Radiology 1987; 165:115–119.
31. Lue T, Hricak H, Marich KW, et al: Vasculogenic impotence evaluated by high-resolution ultrasonography and pulsed Doppler spectrum analysis. Radiology 1985; 155:777–781.

Illustrations • Erectile Dysfunction and Penile Diseases

1. Penile Vascular Anatomy

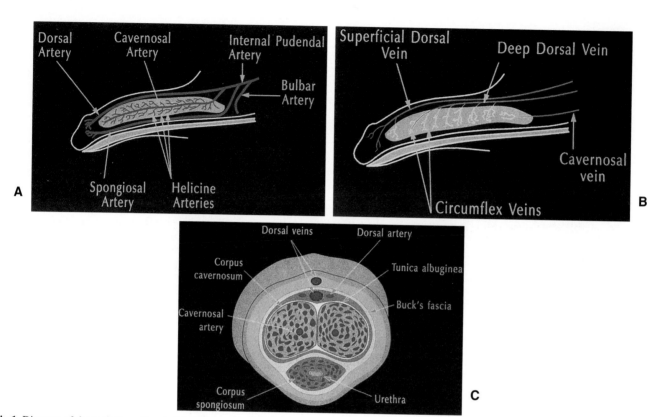

Fig 1. Diagram of the typical penile arterial anatomy. (**A–C,** From Fitzgerald SW, Erickson SJ, Foley WD, et al: Color Doppler sonography in the evaluation of erectile dysfunction. Radiographics 1992; 12:3–17.) (**A–C,** See also Color Section.)
A. Penile arterial anatomy. Penile arteries arise as branches of the internal pudendal artery. The cavernosal arteries and their helicine branches supply the sinusoidal spaces of the corpora cavernosa. **B.** Penile venous anatomy. Superficial dorsal vein drains the distal corporal spaces, while most of the corporal sinusoidal outflow occurs through the deep dorsal vein. Proximal corporal spaces are drained by the cavernosal (crural) veins directly into the periprostatic venous plexus. Venous flow in the cavernosal veins is usually not visualized at Doppler US. **C.** Cross-sectional diagram of the penile shaft. Corpora cavernosa are enclosed within the tunica albuginea and Buck's fascia. The cavernosal arteries are located slightly medially in the center of the corpora cavernosa.

2. Penile Doppler US: Technique and Normal Findings

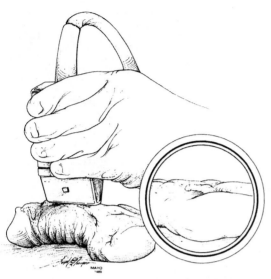

Fig. 1. Position of the penis during penile US. Doppler US is performed in a longitudinal plane from a ventral approach with the penis in the anatomic position lying on the anterior abdominal wall. (From Quam JP, King BF, James EM, et al: Duplex and color Doppler sonographic evaluation of vasculogenic impotence. AJR Am J Roentgenol 1989; 153:1141–1147.)

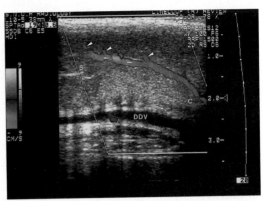

Fig. 2. Normal color Doppler US of the cavernosal artery. Longitudinal color Doppler US obtained through a plane including the right cavernosal artery and deep dorsal vein shows the right cavernosal artery running from the crus of the corpus cavernosum (C) to the penile shaft (S) and sending small helicine branches (*arrowheads*). Note the absence of flow in the deep dorsal vein (DDV). (See also Color Section.)

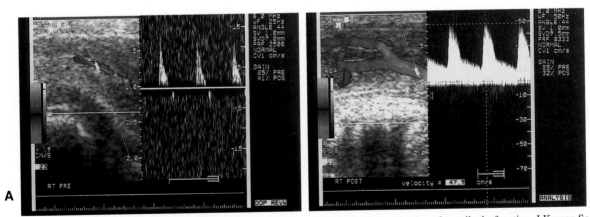

Fig. 3. Normal color Doppler US of the cavernosal artery. (**A, B,** From Kim SH: Imaging for evaluation of erectile dysfunction. J Korean Soc Med US 2001; 20:1–13.) (**A, B,** See also Color Section.)
A. Longitudinal color and spectral Doppler US of the right cavernosal artery in the flaccid state. Color Doppler US shows a very small right cavernosal artery, and spectral Doppler US shows very weak flow with a low peak systolic velocity of about 10 cm/sec. **B.** Color and spectral Doppler US of the same artery obtained 3 minutes after an injection of 10 µg of prostaglandin E$_1$ shows a dilated artery and increased systolic and diastolic flow with a peak systolic velocity of 48 cm/sec. The right dorsal artery is not included in this image.

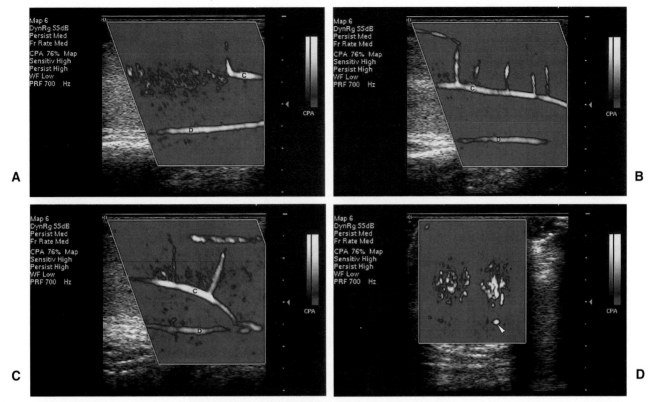

Fig. 4. Normal power Doppler US of the penis. (**A–D,** See also Color Section.)
A–C. Longitudinal power Doppler US images through distal (**A**), middle (**B**), and proximal (**C**) portions of the left corpus cavernosum well demonstrate the left cavernosal (C) and dorsal (D) arteries. Note small helicine branches that are demonstrated better here than on color Doppler US. **D.** Power Doppler US in transverse plane at the level of the distal penile shaft shows prominent flow signals in the helicine branches of the cavernosal arteries. Note a prominent flow signal from the left dorsal penile artery *(arrowhead)*, but the right dorsal artery is not well demonstrated. This asymmetry of the right and left dorsal arteries is a common variation.

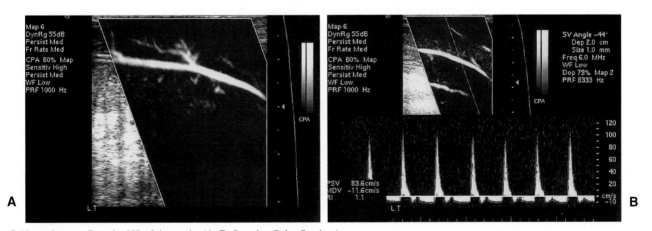

Fig. 5. Normal power Doppler US of the penis. (**A, B,** See also Color Section.)
A. Power Doppler US of the left cavernosal artery using a different color map clearly shows the left cavernosal artery and helicine branches. **B.** Power Doppler US with spectral Doppler shows a high-resistance pattern of the left cavernosal artery with a peak systolic velocity of 83 cm/sec. Note reversed end-diastolic flow (–11 cm/sec).

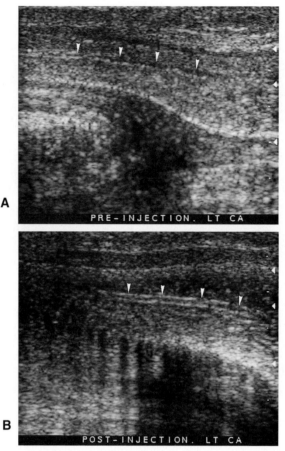

Fig. 6. Measurement of the inner diameter of the cavernosal artery.
(**A, B,** From Kim SH: Imaging for evaluation of erectile dysfunction.
J Korean Soc Med US 2001; 20:1–13.)
A, B. Gray-scale US of the left corpus cavernosum in a longitudinal
plane before (**A**) and after (**B**) intracavernosal injection of prostaglandin
E_1 shows the left cavernosal artery *(arrowheads)*. Note that the artery is
dilated and has a highly echogenic wall after injection on **B**. The inner
diameter of the artery is measured on gray-scale US images before and
after injection.

3. Penile Doppler US: Color and Power Doppler US

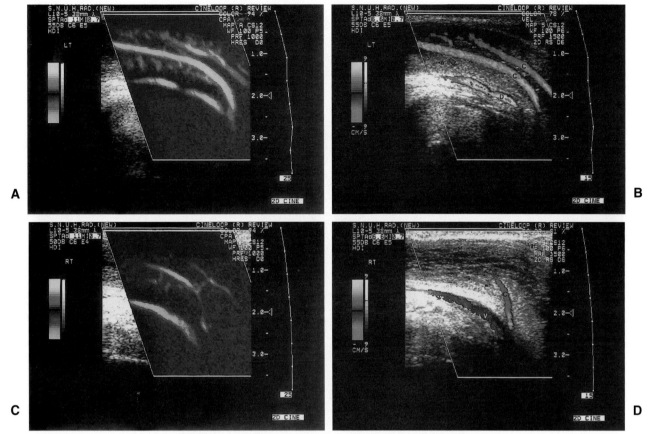

Fig. 1. Power Doppler US reveals slow blood flow more sensitively than color Doppler US does, but it does not provide directional information. Therefore, power Doppler US should be used in conjunction with color Doppler or spectral Doppler US. (**A–D,** See also Color Section.)
A. Power Doppler US of the left corpus cavernosum shows three vessels. **B.** Color Doppler US in the same patient as **A** shows two cavernosal arteries (C) and a dorsal artery (D). **C.** Power Doppler US of the right corpus cavernosum in another patient shows multiple vessels. **D.** Color Doppler US in the same patient as **C** shows a cavernosal artery (C) and venous flow in the deep dorsal vein (V).

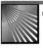

4. Temporal Changes of Doppler Spectra of the Cavernosal Artery

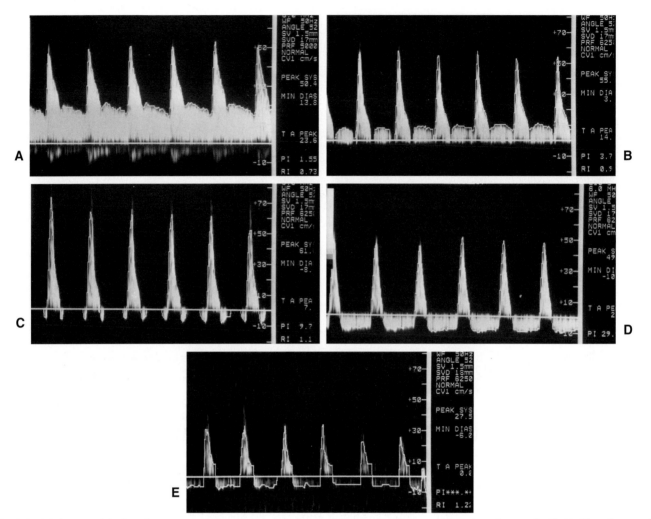

Fig. 1. Serial changes of the Doppler spectrum of the right cavernosal artery following intracavernosal injection of prostaglandin E₁. Note changes of peak systolic velocity (PSV) and end-diastolic velocity (EDV) and compare them with changes of curve in Fig. 2 (Illustration 4). (**A–E,** From Kim SH: Imaging for evaluation of erectile dysfunction. J Korean Soc Med US 2001; 20:1–13.)
A. Three minutes after injection. Note increased systolic and diastolic velocities (peak systolic velocity [PSV] 50.4 cm/sec, end-diastolic velocity [EDV] 13.8 cm/sec). **B.** Six minutes after the injection. Note more increased systolic velocity but decreased diastolic velocity (PSV 55.9 cm/sec, EDV 3.1 cm/sec). **C.** Slightly later, more increased systolic velocity and absent or slightly reversed diastolic flow (PSV 61 cm/sec, EDV –8 cm/sec). **D.** Seven minutes after the injection. Note decreased systolic velocity and markedly reversed diastolic flow (PSV 49.8 cm/sec, EDV –10.1 cm/sec). **E.** Full erection state at 9 minutes after the injection. Note weak Doppler signal due to markedly decreased flow (PSV 27.5 cm/sec, EDV –6 cm/sec).

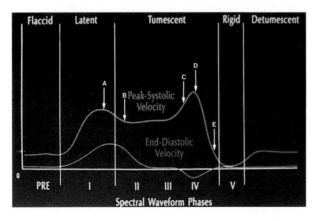

Fig. 2. Time-velocity curves showing the progression of cavernosal arterial blood flow during erection. No specific time frame is shown because of the wide variation in temporal response to intracavernosal injection of vasoactive agent. A–E correspond to the Doppler sampling time in **A–E** of Figure 1 (Illustration 4). (Modified from Fitzgerald SW, Erickson SJ, Foley WD, et al: Color Doppler sonography in the evaluation of erectile dysfunction. Radiographics 1992; 12:3–17.) (See also Color Section.)

5. Penile Doppler US: Technical Considerations

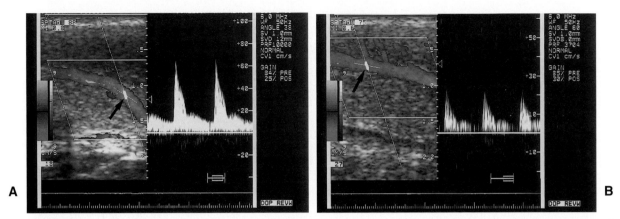

Fig. 1. The peak systolic velocity of the cavernosal artery varies significantly according to the sampling location. Doppler waveforms obtained at proximal and distal portions of a cavernosal artery in early tumescent stage of erection. (**A, B,** From Kim SH, Paick JS, Lee SE, et al: Doppler sonography of deep cavernosal artery of the penis: Variation of peak systolic velocity according to sampling location. J Ultrasound Med 1994; 13:591–594.) (**A, B,** See also Color Section.)
A. Doppler waveform obtained at the base of the penis, where the vessel angles posteriorly *(arrow)*. Peak systolic velocity at this sampling location is 63 cm/sec. **B.** Doppler waveform of the same artery obtained immediately after **A** at the distal portion of the shaft, where the artery's course is straight *(arrow)*. Peak systolic velocity at this sampling location is 23 cm/sec.

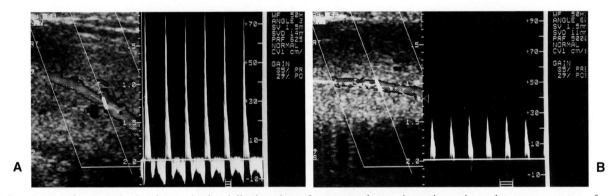

Fig. 2. Doppler waveforms obtained at the proximal and distal portions of a cavernosal artery in another patient at late tumescent stage of erection. (**A, B,** From Kim SH: Imaging for evaluation of erectile dysfunction. J Korean Soc Med US 2001; 20:1–13.)
A. Doppler waveform obtained at the base of the penis. Peak systolic velocity at this sampling location is 73 cm/sec. **B.** Doppler waveform of the same artery obtained immediately after **A** at the distal portion of the shaft. Peak systolic velocity at this sampling location is 29 cm/sec.

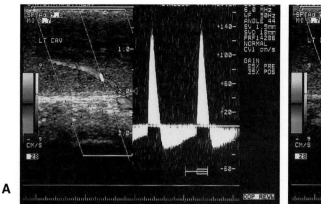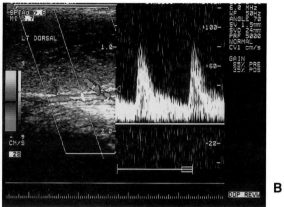

Fig. 3. Doppler waveforms are quite different between the cavernosal artery and the dorsal artery since the dorsal artery is located outside the tunica albuginea. (**A, B,** From Kim SH: Imaging for evaluation of erectile dysfunction. J Korean Soc Med US 2001; 20:1–13.) (**A, B,** See also Color Section.)
A. Doppler waveform obtained at the left cavernosal artery shows a high-resistance pattern with reversed diastolic flow. **B.** Doppler waveform obtained at the left dorsal artery of the same patient immediately after **A** shows low-resistance pattern with prominent, antegrade, diastolic flow.

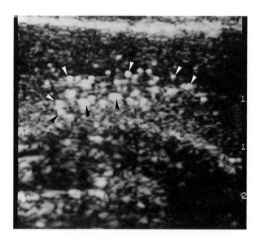

Fig. 4. Air bubbles introduced into the corpus cavernosum during injection of a vasoactive agent may hinder adequate Doppler examination of the penis. The cavernosal artery is not well demonstrated due to air bubbles appearing as multiple, echogenic dots *(arrowheads)* with posterior sonic shadowing.

6. Penile Arteriography: Normal and Variations

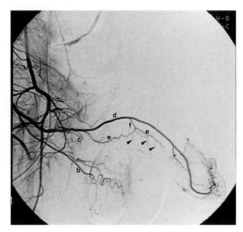

Fig. 1. Normal internal pudendal arteriogram. Right internal pudendal arteriogram in right anterior oblique projection performed following intracavernosal injection of 20 μg of prostaglandin E$_1$ well demonstrates the internal pudendal artery (a), scrotal branch (b), artery to the bulb of corpus spongiosum (c), dorsal penile artery (d), cavernosal arteries (e), and helicine branches *(arrowheads)*. Note a dorsal penile–cavernosal perforator (f). (From Kim SH: Imaging for evaluation of erectile dysfunction. J Korean Soc Med US 2001; 20:1–13.)

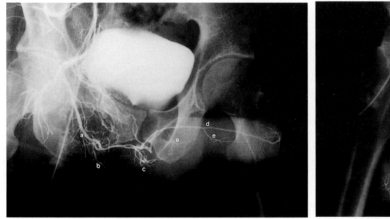
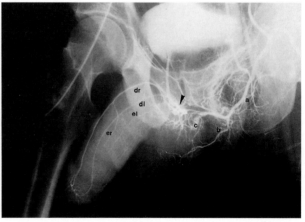

A **B**

Fig. 2. Normal internal pudendal arteriogram.
A. Right internal pudendal arteriogram shows the right internal pudendal artery (a), scrotal branch (b), artery to the bulb of corpus spongiosum (c), dorsal penile artery (d), and cavernosal arteries (e). **B.** Left internal pudendal arteriogram opacifies both left and right penile arteries through transverse root communicator *(arrowhead)*. a, left internal pudendal artery; b, left scrotal branch; c, left artery to the bulb of corpus spongiosum; dl, left dorsal artery; dr, right dorsal artery; el, left cavernosal artery; er, right cavernosal artery.

7. Arteriogenic Impotence

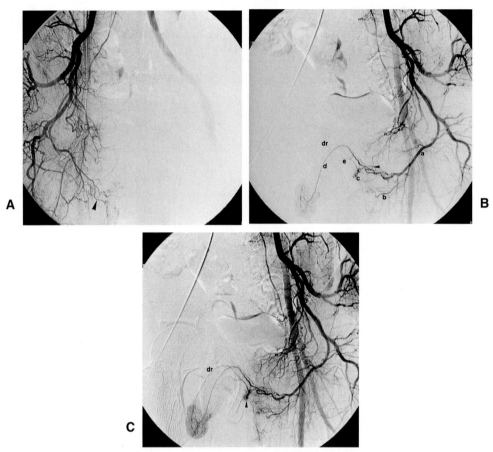

Fig. 1. A 30-year-old man who had received a pelvic bone fracture and urethral rupture during a traffic accident 2 years earlier. Penile Doppler US revealed significantly lower peak systolic velocity of the right cavernosal artery (14 cm/sec) than that of the left cavernosal artery (43 cm/sec). (**A–C,** From Kim SH: Imaging for evaluation of erectile dysfunction. J Korean Soc Med US 2001; 20:1–13.)
A. Right internal pudendal arteriogram shows occlusion of the right internal pudendal artery distal to the origin of the scrotal branch *(arrowhead)*. **B.** Left internal pudendal arteriogram in the early phase shows the left internal pudendal artery (a), scrotal branch (b), artery to the bulb of corpus spongiosum (c), left dorsal penile artery (d), and left cavernosal artery (e). Note faint opacification of the right dorsal penile artery (dr) through a root communicator *(arrowhead)*. **C.** Late phase of left internal pudendal arteriogram well demonstrates the right dorsal penile artery (dr), but the right cavernosal artery is not opacified. Note staining of the bulb of the corpus spongiosum *(arrowhead)*. A right dorsal artery to right inferior epigastric artery anastomosis was performed in this patient.

Fig. 2. A 32-year-old impotent man who had received a left femur fracture due to a traffic accident 3 years earlier. Penile Doppler US revealed subnormal peak systolic velocities of both cavernosal arteries (right, 14.9 cm/sec; left, 25.2 cm/sec). Peak systolic velocities of right and left dorsal penile arteries were asymmetrical (right, 71.3 cm/sec; left, 28 cm/sec). (**A, C, D,** See also Color Section.)
A, B. Power Doppler US image (**A**) and spectra (**B**) of the penis in axial plane show communication of the right dorsal penile artery *(arrow in* **A***)* with the left cavernosal artery *(arrowhead in* **A***)*. Doppler spectra have an upward direction, indicating that the flow direction is from the right dorsal artery to the left cavernosal artery. **C.** Power Doppler US image in axial plane slightly distal to the level of **A** and **B** shows communication between the left dorsal penile artery *(arrow)* and the right cavernosal artery *(arrowhead)*. **D.** Power Doppler US image in axial plane immediately distal to **C** shows communication between the right *(arrow)* and left *(arrowhead)* cavernosal arteries. **E.** Pelvic arteriogram in anteroposterior projection shows opacification of both right and left, internal and external iliac arteries. Also note both the right and left inferior epigastric arteries *(arrowheads)*, which are important when vascular reconstructive surgery is considered. **F, G.** Right internal pudendal arteriograms at early (**F**) and late (**G**) phases show right dorsal penile artery (dr) communicating with the left cavernosal artery that sends two cavernosal arteries distally *(arrowheads)*. There is a vessel connecting the cavernosal arteries and left dorsal penile artery *(asterisk)*. A, C, D represent the site where Doppler US revealed communications in **A, C, D,** respectively. Also note that the distal portion of the right dorsal penile artery *(open arrowheads)* is small, probably due to a steal phenomenon caused by communicating vessels. **H.** Left internal pudendal arteriogram shows nonopacification of the left penile arteries.

6. Penile Arteriography: Normal and Variations

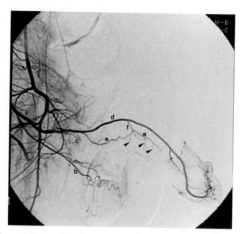

Fig. 1. Normal internal pudendal arteriogram. Right internal pudendal arteriogram in right anterior oblique projection performed following intracavernosal injection of 20 μg of prostaglandin E_1 well demonstrates the internal pudendal artery (a), scrotal branch (b), artery to the bulb of corpus spongiosum (c), dorsal penile artery (d), cavernosal arteries (e), and helicine branches *(arrowheads)*. Note a dorsal penile–cavernosal perforator (f). (From Kim SH: Imaging for evaluation of erectile dysfunction. J Korean Soc Med US 2001; 20:1–13.)

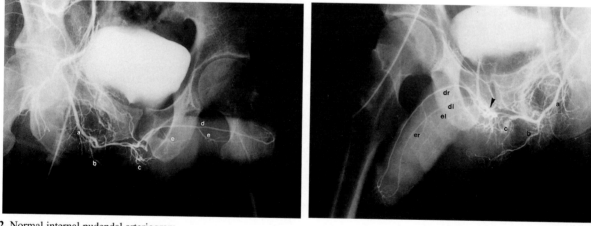

A **B**

Fig. 2. Normal internal pudendal arteriogram.
A. Right internal pudendal arteriogram shows the right internal pudendal artery (a), scrotal branch (b), artery to the bulb of corpus spongiosum (c), dorsal penile artery (d), and cavernosal arteries (e). **B.** Left internal pudendal arteriogram opacifies both left and right penile arteries through transverse root communicator *(arrowhead)*. a, left internal pudendal artery; b, left scrotal branch; c, left artery to the bulb of corpus spongiosum; dl, left dorsal artery; dr, right dorsal artery; el, left cavernosal artery; er, right cavernosal artery.

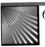

7. Arteriogenic Impotence

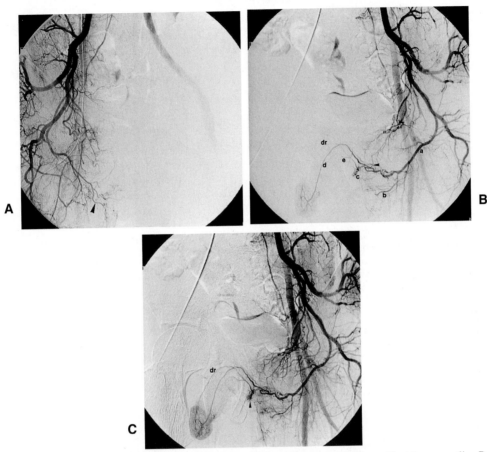

Fig. 1. A 30-year-old man who had received a pelvic bone fracture and urethral rupture during a traffic accident 2 years earlier. Penile Doppler US revealed significantly lower peak systolic velocity of the right cavernosal artery (14 cm/sec) than that of the left cavernosal artery (43 cm/sec). (**A–C,** From Kim SH: Imaging for evaluation of erectile dysfunction. J Korean Soc Med US 2001; 20:1–13.)
A. Right internal pudendal arteriogram shows occlusion of the right internal pudendal artery distal to the origin of the scrotal branch *(arrowhead)*. **B.** Left internal pudendal arteriogram in the early phase shows the left internal pudendal artery (a), scrotal branch (b), artery to the bulb of corpus spongiosum (c), left dorsal penile artery (d), and left cavernosal artery (e). Note faint opacification of the right dorsal penile artery (dr) through a root communicator *(arrowhead)*. **C.** Late phase of left internal pudendal arteriogram well demonstrates the right dorsal penile artery (dr), but the right cavernosal artery is not opacified. Note staining of the bulb of the corpus spongiosum *(arrowhead)*. A right dorsal artery to right inferior epigastric artery anastomosis was performed in this patient.

Fig. 2. A 32-year-old impotent man who had received a left femur fracture due to a traffic accident 3 years earlier. Penile Doppler US revealed subnormal peak systolic velocities of both cavernosal arteries (right, 14.9 cm/sec; left, 25.2 cm/sec). Peak systolic velocities of right and left dorsal penile arteries were asymmetrical (right, 71.3 cm/sec; left, 28 cm/sec). (**A, C, D,** See also Color Section.)
A, B. Power Doppler US image (**A**) and spectra (**B**) of the penis in axial plane show communication of the right dorsal penile artery *(arrow in **A**)* with the left cavernosal artery *(arrowhead in **A**)*. Doppler spectra have an upward direction, indicating that the flow direction is from the right dorsal artery to the left cavernosal artery. **C.** Power Doppler US image in axial plane slightly distal to the level of **A** and **B** shows communication between the left dorsal penile artery *(arrow)* and the right cavernosal artery *(arrowhead)*. **D.** Power Doppler US image in axial plane immediately distal to **C** shows communication between the right *(arrow)* and left *(arrowhead)* cavernosal arteries. **E.** Pelvic arteriogram in anteroposterior projection shows opacification of both right and left, internal and external iliac arteries. Also note both the right and left inferior epigastric arteries *(arrowheads)*, which are important when vascular reconstructive surgery is considered. **F, G.** Right internal pudendal arteriograms at early (**F**) and late (**G**) phases show right dorsal penile artery (dr) communicating with the left cavernosal artery that sends two cavernosal arteries distally *(arrowheads)*. There is a vessel connecting the cavernosal arteries and left dorsal penile artery *(asterisk)*. A, C, D represent the site where Doppler US revealed communications in **A, C, D,** respectively. Also note that the distal portion of the right dorsal penile artery *(open arrowheads)* is small, probably due to a steal phenomenon caused by communicating vessels. **H.** Left internal pudendal arteriogram shows nonopacification of the left penile arteries.

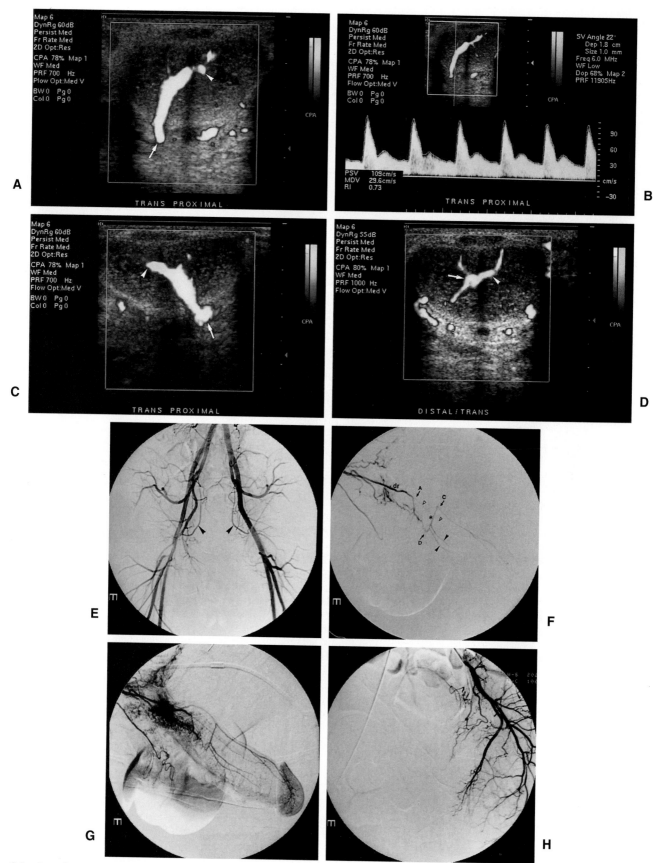

Fig. 2 *See legend on opposite page*

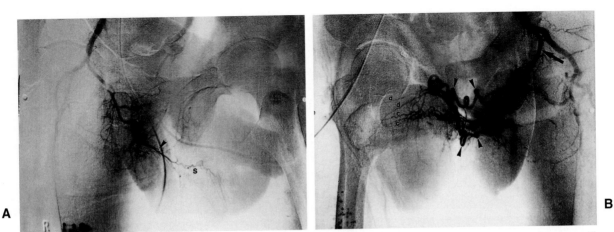

Fig. 3. A 45-year-old man who received urethral injury due to a traffic accident 14 years earlier. Doppler US revealed subnormal peak systolic velocity in both right and left cavernosal arteries.
A. Right internal pudendal arteriogram shows occlusion of the internal pudendal artery *(arrowhead)* immediately distal to the origin of the scrotal branch (s). **B.** Left internal pudendal arteriogram shows a dilated left internal pudendal artery *(arrow)* and tortuous collateral vessels *(arrowheads)* supplying both right and left dorsal penile arteries (d) and cavernosal arteries (c).

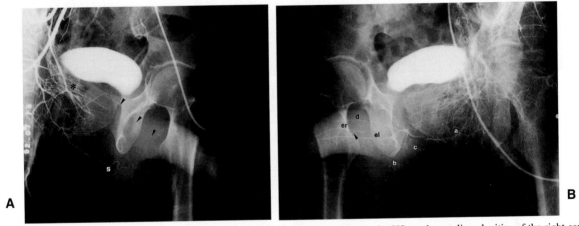

Fig. 4. A 52-year-old man with Buerger's disease complaining of erectile dysfunction. At Doppler US, peak systolic velocities of the right cavernosal artery were significantly lower (14 cm/sec) than those of the left cavernosal artery (41 cm/sec).
A. Right internal pudendal arteriogram shows occlusion of the internal pudendal artery distal to the origin of the scrotal branch (s). Note the fine collateral vessels *(asterisk)* from the branches of anterior trunk vessels of the right internal iliac artery and faint opacification of the right dorsal penile artery *(arrowheads)*. **B.** Late-phase image of left internal pudendal arteriogram faintly opacifies the left internal pudendal artery (a), scrotal branch (b), artery to the bulb of corpus spongiosum (c), left dorsal penile artery (d), and left cavernosal artery (el). Distal portion of the right cavernosal artery (er) is opacified through the communication *(arrowhead)* between the right and left cavernosal arteries.

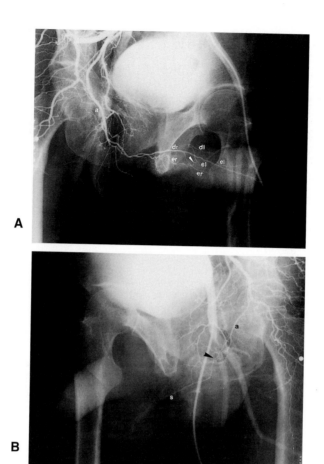

A

B

Fig. 5. A 52-year-old man with Buerger's disease who had undergone bilateral sympathectomy 10 years earlier. Peak systolic velocities at penile Doppler US were 24 cm/sec for the right cavernosal artery, 26 cm/sec for the left cavernosal artery, and 66 cm/sec for the right dorsal penile artery. Left dorsal penile arterial flow was not demonstrable at Doppler US. **A.** Right internal pudendal arteriogram opacifies the right internal pudendal artery (a) and right dorsal (dr) and right cavernosal (er) arteries. Distal portions of the left dorsal (dl) and left cavernosal (el) arteries are opacified through a communication between the right and left cavernosal arteries *(arrowhead)*. er, right cavernosal artery. **B.** Left internal pudendal arteriogram shows the small right internal pudendal artery (a), which is occluded *(arrowhead)* after the origin of the scrotal branch (s).

8. Cavernosometry/Cavernosography

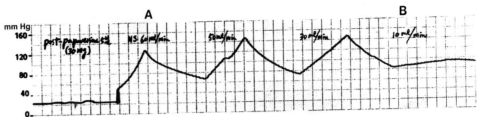

Fig. 1. Cavernosometric graph determining the flow rate to maintain intracavernosal pressure of 100 mm Hg. Flow rate was decreased from 60 mL/min (**A**) to 10 mL/min (**B**). In this patient maintenance flow rate is 10 mL/min. (From Kim SH: Imaging for evaluation of erectile dysfunction. J Korean Soc Med US 2001; 20:1–13.)

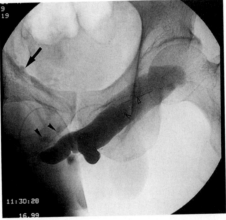

Fig. 2. Cavernosography. With infusion of diluted contrast material, penile erection is achieved and both right and left corpora cavernosa are opacified. Note that a small amount of venous leak occurs through the fine crural perforating veins (*arrowheads*) into the periprostatic venous plexus and right internal iliac vein (*arrow*). Also note two needle tips (*open arrowheads*) in the corpora cavernosa. (From Kim SH: Imaging for evaluation of erectile dysfunction. J Korean Soc Med US 2001; 20:1–13.)

9. Venogenic Impotence

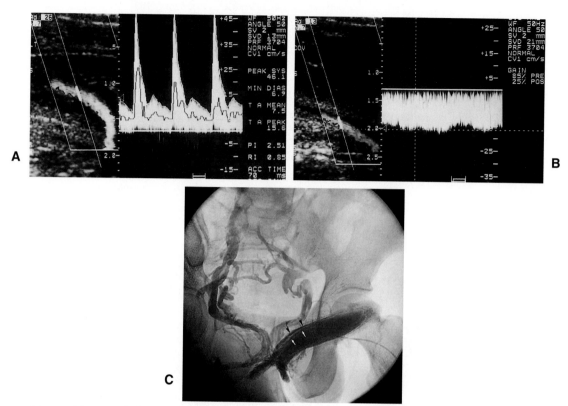

Fig. 1. A 44-year-old man with venogenic impotence. (**A–C,** From Kim SH: Imaging for evaluation of erectile dysfunction. J Korean Soc Med US 2001; 20:1–13.)
A. Doppler US of the left cavernosal artery in erection status shows normal peak systolic velocity (46 cm/sec) but slightly high end-diastolic velocity (6.9 cm/sec). **B.** Doppler US at the deep dorsal vein shows prominent venous leak with peak velocity of 16.7 cm/sec. **C.** Cavernosography shows corpora cavernosa and venous leak through the deep *(arrows)* and superficial *(arrowheads)* dorsal veins.

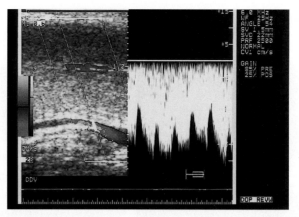

Fig. 2. Another patient with venogenic impotence. Color Doppler US shows prominent venous leak with pulsatile flow pattern. (See also Color Section.)

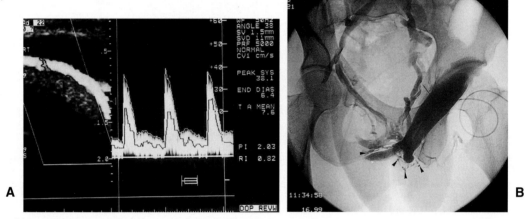

Fig. 3. A 25-year-old man with venogenic impotence. (**A, B,** From Kim SH: Imaging for evaluation of erectile dysfunction. J Korean Soc Med US 2001; 20:1–13.)
A. Doppler US of the right cavernosal artery in erection status shows normal peak systolic velocity (38 cm/sec) but slightly prominent end-diastolic velocity (6.4 cm/sec). Venous flow was not demonstrated in the dorsal veins. **B.** Cavernosography shows corpora cavernosa and prominent venous leak through the crural perforating veins *(arrowheads)* that drain into the periprostatic venous plexus and internal iliac veins. Note that the dorsal veins are not opacified.

10. Peyronie's Disease

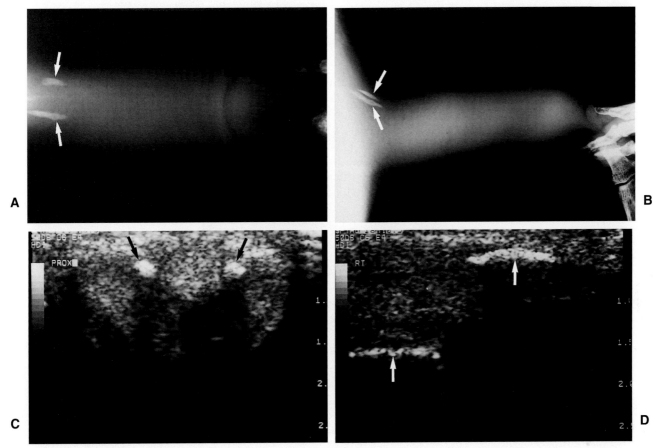

Fig. 1. A 70-year-old man with Peyronie's disease.
A, B. Plain radiographs in craniocaudal (**A**) and lateral (**B**) projections show two linear calcifications in the dorsal aspect of the penile root area *(arrows)*. **C, D.** US images in transverse (**C**) and coronal (**D**) planes show densely echogenic lesions with posterior sonic shadowing in both right and left corpora cavernosa *(arrows)*.

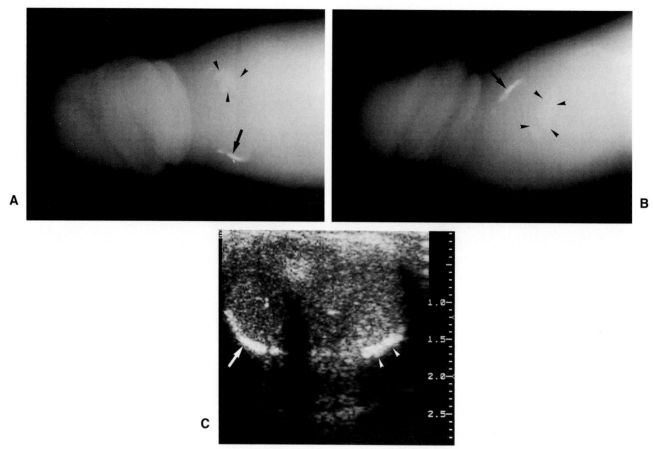

Fig. 2. A 46-year-old man with Peyronie's disease.
A, B. Plain radiographs in craniocaudal (**A**) and lateral (**B**) projections show dense *(arrow)* and faint *(arrowheads)* calcifications in the dorsal aspect of the penis in the distal shaft. Note that the left-sided calcification is dense *(arrow)* and the right-sided one is faint *(arrowheads)*. Also note that the penis is slightly curved upward in lateral projection (**B**). **C.** Transverse US shows curvilinear calcifications in the dorsal aspect of both right *(arrow)* and left *(arrowheads)* corpora cavernosa in the region of the tunica albuginea.

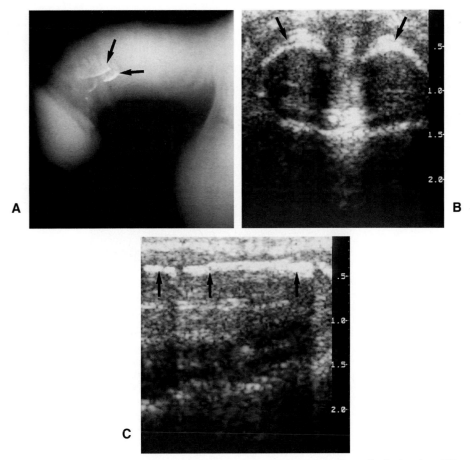

Fig. 3. A 50-year-old man with Peyronie's disease. (**A–C,** From Kim SH: Imaging for evaluation of erectile dysfunction. J Korean Soc Med US 2001; 20:1–13.)
A. Plain radiograph in lateral projection shows two calcifications *(arrows)* in the distal penile shaft. Note that the penis is angulated downward.
B. Transverse US shows curvilinear calcifications *(arrows)* in the ventral aspect of both right and left corpora cavernosa in the region of the tunica albuginea. **C.** Longitudinal US in left corpus cavernosum shows linear calcifications in the ventral aspect of the tunica albuginea *(arrows).*

11. Priapism

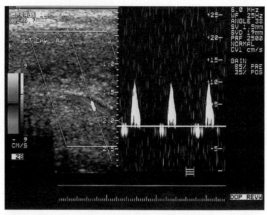

Fig. 1. A 49-year-old man with low-flow priapism. He complained of persistent painful erection for 4 days following an intracavernosal injection of a vasoactive agent. Doppler US of the left cavernosal artery without intracavernosal injection of vasoactive agent shows weak flow signal with low peak systolic velocity (10 cm/sec) and high-resistance pattern. Aspiration of the corpus cavernosum revealed anoxic blood. Priapism was relieved after repeated aspiration of cavernosal blood, and follow-up Doppler US revealed restored cavernosal blood flow. (From Kim SH: Imaging for evaluation of erectile dysfunction. J Korean Soc Med US 2001; 20:1–13.) (See also Color Section.)

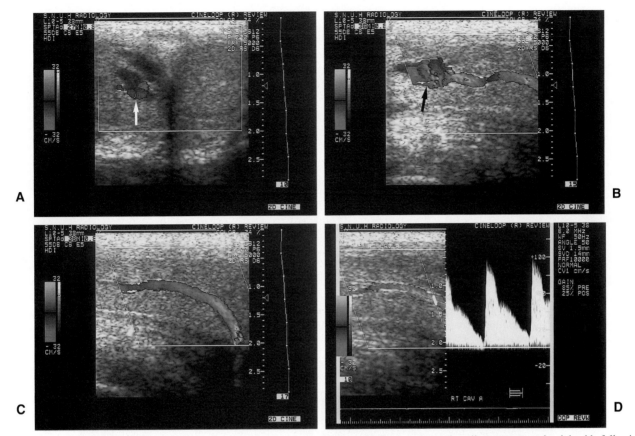

Fig. 2. A 30-year-old man with high-flow priapism. He complained of intermittent persistent erection and penile curvature to the right side following a blunt trauma to the penis that had occurred 3 years earlier. (**A–D,** From Kim SH: Imaging for evaluation of erectile dysfunction. J Korean Soc Med US 2001; 20:1–13.) (**A–D,** See also Color Section.)
A. Color Doppler US in transverse plane without intracavernosal injection of vasoactive agent shows prominent cavernosal vessels in the right corpus cavernosum *(arrow).* **B, C.** Color Doppler US images of the right corpus cavernosum in longitudinal plane at the region of the distal (**B**) and proximal (**C**) shaft show prominent blood flow in the cavernosal artery forming an entangled vascular mass *(arrow* in **B)** in the distal penile shaft. **D.** Spectral Doppler US obtained in the proximal portion of the right cavernosal artery shows prominent blood flow with very high peak systolic velocity (100 cm/sec).

12. Penile Prosthesis

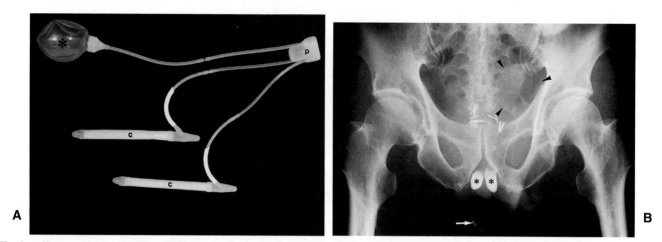

Fig. 1. A 60-year-old man who has an inflatable penile prosthesis (AMS 700 CXM [American Medical Systems, Minnetonka, Minn.]).
A. Photograph of an AMS 700 CXM prosthesis. The reservoir *(asterisk)* is filled with normal saline or isotonic contrast material and positioned in the lower pelvis. The pump (p) is inserted into the scrotum and corporal cylinders (c) into the corpora cavernosa. **B.** Plain radiograph of the pelvis shows the reservoir *(arrowheads)*, metallic part of pump *(arrow)*, and radiopaque cylinder tips *(asterisks)*.

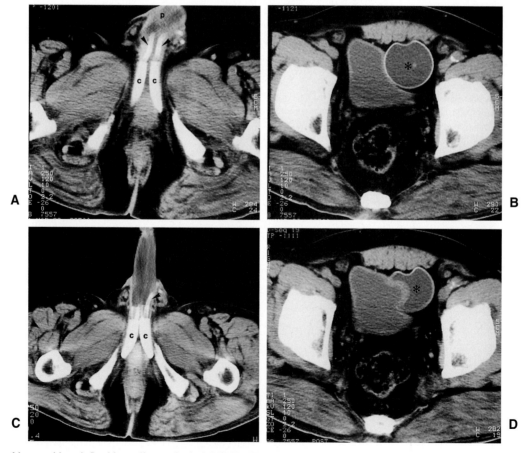

Fig. 2. A 71-year-old man with an inflatable penile prosthesis (AMS 700 CXM).
A–D. CT scans showing the penile prosthesis in the noninflated state **(A, B)** and inflated state **(C, D)**. Note that the reservoir is partially collapsed in the inflated state **(D)**. p, penis; c, radiopaque tips of cylinder; *arrowheads*, tubing; *asterisk*, reservoir.

13. Miscellaneous Conditions of the Penis

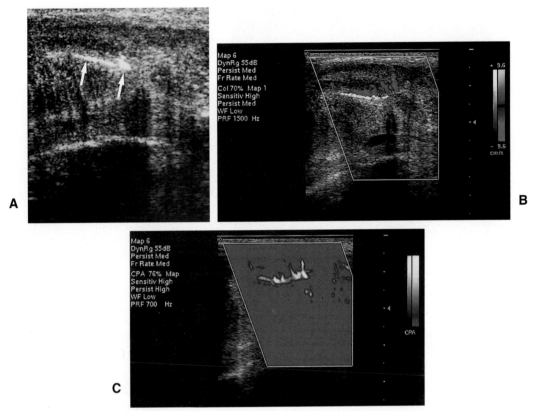

Fig. 1. Erectile dysfunction in a 60-year-old man with hypercholesterolemia. (**A, B,** From Kim SH: Imaging for evaluation of erectile dysfunction. J Korean Soc Med US 2001; 20:1–13.) (**B, C,** See also Color Section.)
A. Longitudinal US of the right corpus cavernosum shows a linear calcification in the distal shaft region *(arrows)*. **B, C.** Color (**B**) and power (**C**) Doppler US images of the same area reveal that the calcification is along the course of the cavernosal artery, indicating arterial wall calcification.

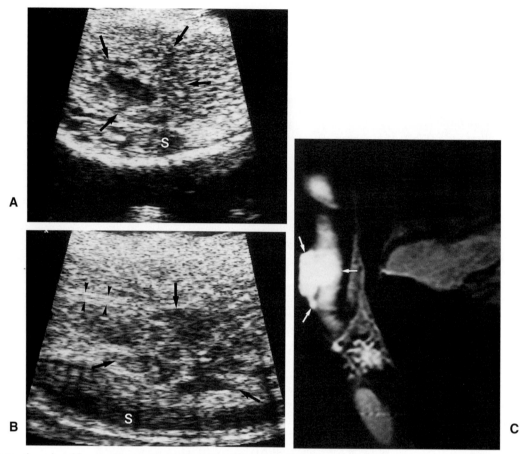

Fig. 2. Penile hemangioma in a 27-year-old man. (**A–C,** From Kim SH, Lee SE, Han MC: Penile hemangioma: US and MR imaging demonstration. Urol Radiol 1991; 13:126–128.)
A. US in axial plane taken from the dorsal surface of the midshaft of the penis shows an ill-defined, hypoechoic lesion in the right side of the penis with deep extension into the right corpus cavernosum *(arrows)*. S, corpus spongiosum. **B.** US in longitudinal plane shows a large hypoechoic mass *(arrows)* in the right corpus cavernosum. Note the right cavernosal artery *(arrowheads)* and corpus spongiosum (S). **C.** T2-weighted MR imaging in sagittal plane shows a high-intensity mass *(arrows)* in the ventral aspect of the penis with extension into the right corpus cavernosum.

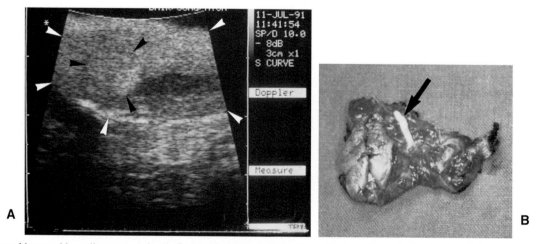

Fig. 3. A 51-year-old man with penile sparganosis. (**A, B,** From Kim SH: Imaging for evaluation of erectile dysfunction. J Korean Soc Med US 2001; 20:1–13.)
A. Penile US in longitudinal plane shows an ill-defined mass lesion *(white arrowheads)* in the dorsal subcutaneous tissue of the penis. There is a well-defined, round, hyperechoic lesion *(black arrowheads)* within the mass. Intermittent whirling movements were observed during the US examination.
B. Photograph of the removed mass. A white live worm *(arrow)* was found. (**B,** See also Color Section.)

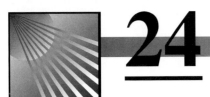

Retroperitoneal Diseases

SEUNG HYUP KIM

The retroperitoneal or extraperitoneal space is the region between the posterior parietal peritoneum and the transversalis fascia. It extends from the diaphragm cranially to the pelvis caudally. The retroperitoneal space at the abdomen level can be divided into three spaces: perirenal, anterior pararenal, and posterior pararenal. These spaces are bounded by the posterior parietal peritoneum, anterior renal fascia, posterior renal fascia, lateroconal fascia, and transversalis fascia. The perirenal space contains kidney and adrenal glands, whereas the anterior pararenal space includes pancreas, duodenum, and ascending and descending colon. The posterior pararenal space does not include visceral organs but contains only fatty tissue.

The diseases that may occur in the retroperitoneal spaces can be divided into primary retroperitoneal tumors, retroperitoneal fibrosis, retroperitoneal lymphadenopathy, and miscellaneous retroperitoneal fluid collections.

PRIMARY RETROPERITONEAL TUMORS

There is a wide range of histology for tumors that primarily occur in the retroperitoneum. Most of the primary retroperitoneal tumors arise from the mesenchymal tissues, neurogenic tissues, or embryonic rests and notochords (Table 24–1). The great majority of the retroperitoneal tumors are malignant. The three most common malignant tumors of the retroperitoneum are malignant fibrous histiocytoma, liposarcoma, and leiomyosarcoma.

Malignant fibrous histiocytoma is reported to be the most common primary malignant retroperitoneal tumor and occurs most commonly in middle to later adult life. Many tumors previously considered fibrosarcoma are now diagnosed as malignant fibrous histiocytoma. Retroperitoneal malignant fibrous histiocytoma appears as a nonspecific soft tissue mass. The lesion is either homogenous or heterogeneous with intratumoral necrosis. Areas of dystrophic calcification are seen in about 25%.

Liposarcoma is the second most common primary malignant retroperitoneal tumor. Liposarcomas have three histologic types. Well-differentiated liposarcoma is made up mostly of fat with only a small amount of solid, fibrotic strands running through it. This type must be differentiated from benign lipoma and from angiomyolipoma extending from the kidney. Myxoid liposarcoma contains no mature fat and shows a relatively low-attenuated mass of ground-glass opacity on CT. Pleomorphic liposarcoma appears as a muscle attenuation mass with regions of necrosis. This type of liposarcoma cannot be differentiated from malignant fibrous histiocytoma on imaging.

Leiomyosarcoma is the third most common primary malignant tumor of the retroperitoneum. The imaging characteristics of leiomyosarcoma are nonspecific, but the diagnosis can be suggested when a tumor is intimately associated with the renal veins or inferior vena cava, from which it often arises.

Various benign tumors can occur in the retroperitoneum. Benign neurogenic tumors such as neurilemmoma, neurofibroma, ganglioneuroma, and paraganglioma are the most common among them. Neurilemmoma and paraganglioma often show cystic degeneration. Neurofibroma has low attenuation on nonenhanced CT and often shows near-water attenuation. Teratoma is another common benign tumor of the retroperitoneum. Teratoma characteristically shows a mixture of various tissues including fat and calcifications. Although imaging findings are nonspecific in most retroperitoneal tumors, occasionally a specific diagnosis may be suggested on the basis of following clinical and imaging findings: mixed components including fat and calcifications in teratoma; homogenous fatty mass in lipoma; presence of fat

Table 24–1	Primary Retroperitoneal Tumors and Their Origins

Tissue of Origin	Tumors
Mesenchymal tissues	
Adipose tissue	Lipoma, liposarcoma
Smooth muscle	Leiomyoma, leiomyosarcoma
Striated muscle	Rhabdomyoma, rhabdomysarcoma
Connective tissue	Fibroma, fibrosarcoma
Lymph vessel	Lymphangioma, lymphangiosarcoma
Blood vessel	Hemangioendothelioma, hemangiopericytoma, angiosarcoma
Others	Myxoma, myxosarcoma
Nervous tissues	
Nerve sheath	Neurofibroma, neurilemmoma, malignant schwannoma
Sympathetic nervous system	Ganglioneuroma, ganglioneuroblastoma, neuroblastoma
Heterotopic adrenal tissue	Paraganglioma
Embryonic rests	
Embryonic rests	Benign and malignant teratoma
Notochord	Chordoma
Embryonic hindgut	Tailgut cyst (retrorectal cystic hamartoma)

in a mass of heterogeneous density in liposarcoma; large regions of necrosis in leiomyosarcoma; calcified tumor in a child in neuroblastoma; hypervascularity in hemangioma and hemangiopericytoma; catecholamine excess and para-aortic location in paraganglioma; homogeneous low attenuation in neurofibroma; and prominent cystic degeneration in neurilemmoma.

Retroperitoneal fibrosis

Retroperitoneal fibrosis is a disease process with a number of different causes. The process frequently involves the ureters and causes hydronephrosis and hydroureter either unilaterally or bilaterally. The process usually surrounds the abdominal aorta and inferior vena cava at the lower lumbar level but sometimes may involve smaller vessels. Retroperitoneal fibrosis may extend cranially or caudally, and the duodenum or sigmoid colon may be involved. The process can be extensive in the retroperitoneum or can be localized. Occasionally it is localized around the ureter.

The etiology of the process can be both benign and malignant. The malignant causes are usually metastatic neoplasms to the retroperitoneum that stimulate a fibrotic reaction leading to a fibrotic mass. The most common malignancies to metastasize to the retroperitoneum causing fibrosis are breast, stomach, pancreas, lung, and colon. Hodgkin's lymphoma also may cause malignant retroperitoneal fibrosis.

Benign retroperitoneal fibrosis may be caused by a number of conditions. The drug methysergide maleate has been known to cause this condition. Perianeurysmal fibrosis associated with aortic disease may cause similar soft tissue mantles around the aorta. The presence of an aneurysm with an intimately associated rind of fibrotic tissue is usually diagnostic of this condition. However, this change can be seen without an associated aneurysm. If none of these causes can be found, then the diagnosis of idiopathic retroperitoneal fibrosis can be made.

Obstruction and medial deviation of the ureter are common findings in retroperitoneal fibrosis. The ureteral lumen is usually narrowed but not occluded. Loss of peristalsis in the involved ureteral segment due to surrounding fibrosis causes severe passage disturbance of urine and may cause acute renal failure when both ureters are involved. The disease progresses slowly, but the symptoms often develop suddenly.

On CT and MR imaging, a fibrotic soft tissue mantle is seen around the retroperitoneal structures. In the acute phase of this disease, the fibrotic tissue is highly vascular and enhances greatly on contrast-enhanced CT or MR imaging. Steroid therapy may be effective in this phase of the disease. Chronic cases usually do not respond to steroid therapy, and urinary diversion is usually necessary if hydronephrosis is present.

RETROPERITONEAL LYMPHADENOPATHY

Retroperitoneal lymph nodes are evaluated most commonly with CT or MR imaging. Normal abdominal lymph nodes can measure 3 to 10 mm in diameter. They are seen mainly around the aorta and inferior vena cava. Lymph nodes larger than 10 mm are usually considered abnormal. A single slightly enlarged node is not necessarily abnormal, but a cluster of slightly enlarged nodes is almost always a sign of disease. In measuring the size of the lymph nodes, a minimal axial diameter should be measured instead of a maximal axial diameter.

Nodal enlargement must be distinguished from other structures such as diaphragmatic crura, prominent vessels, unopacified bowel loops, and psoas minor muscles. Adequate contrast enhancement, both oral and intravenous, is often necessary to differentiate enlarged lymph nodes from other normal structures.

Abnormal lymph nodes may have certain imaging findings that may suggest their specific causes. Calcified nodes are seen in patients with tuberculosis and those who have had previous chemotherapy or radiation therapy. Low-attenuated necrotic nodes may be seen in tuberculosis and occasionally in metastatic testicular tumor. High-attenuated nodes are seen in patients with Kaposi's sarcoma. Extensive retroperitoneal lymphadenopathy with calcification may occur in Castleman's disease.

MISCELLANEOUS RETROPERITONEAL FLUID COLLECTIONS

The retroperitoneal space is also the site for fluid collection, including hematomas, abscesses, urinomas, and lymphoceles. On the basis of clinical history and imaging findings, these collections can be readily differentiated from neoplastic processes. The majority of infectious processes involving the perirenal space originate from the kidney. Imaging findings in infection include interstitial inflammatory edema or collections of fluid in and around the perirenal space, diffuse or localized gas formation, enlargement of the adjacent kidney, and thickening of the renal fascia. Xanthogranulomatous pyelonephritis may extend into the perirenal space.

Urinomas are collections of urine that have leaked into the perirenal space or beyond. The release of urine causes rapid lipolysis, which produces a fibrous sac around the urine collection.

Perirenal hematoma may occur after trauma or spontaneously. The two most common causes of spontaneous perirenal hematoma are renal cell carcinoma and angiomyolipoma. Hemorrhage that originates from the kidney may be subcapsular or perirenal. Imaging findings of perirenal hematoma include irregular reticular or confluent collections in the perirenal space. The collection has high attenuation when subacute. Subcapsular hematoma may be differentiated from perirenal hematoma, although such differentiation is occasionally difficult. Subcapsular hematomas produce a lenticular or linear shape, whereas perirenal hematoma produces a crescentic shape. One potential pitfall that can obscure the difference between these two forms of retroperitoneal hematomas occurs when the posterior renorenal bridging septum confines a perirenal hematoma, simulating the appearance of a subcapsular hematoma.

References

1. Friedenberg RM, Harris RD: Excretory urography in adult. In Pollack HM, McClennan BL (eds): Clinical Urography, 2nd ed, vol 1. Philadelphia, WB Saunders, 2000, pp 180–185.
2. Lee JS, Seong CK, Sim JS, et al: Retroperitoneal fibrosis: Spectrum of imaging findings. J Korean Radiol Soc 1999; 41:1177–1182.
3. Chang YJ, Lee HK, Kim HH, et al: Radiologic findings of malignant retroperitoneal fibrosis. J Korean Radiol Soc 1997; 37:899–904.
4. Choi SH, Lim HK, Lee WJ: Idiopathic retroperitoneal fibrosis with rectosigmoid obstruction: Imaging findings. J Korean Radiol Soc 1997; 37:881–883.
5. Bechtold RE, Dyer RB, Zagoria RL, et al: The perirenal space: Relationship of pathologic processes to normal retroperitoneal anatomy. Radiographics 1996; 16:841–854.

6. Kottra JJ, Dunnick NR: Retroperitoneal fibrosis. Radiol Clin North Am 1996; 34:1259–1275.

7. Liessi G, Cesari S, Pavanello M, et al: Tailgut cyst: CT and MR findings. Abdom Imaging 1995; 20:256–258.

8. Bass JC, Koroblkin M, Francis IR, et al: Retroperitoneal plexiform neurofibromas: CT findings. AJR Am J Roentgenol 1994; 163:617–620.

9. Bosnak MA: Imaging of Retroperitoneal Disease. Syllabus for NICER Course. Oslo, Norway, Nycomed Amersham Intercontinental Continuing Education in Radiology, 1994, pp 234–242.

10. Johnson WK, Ross PR, Powers C, et al: Castleman disease mimicking an aggressive retroperitoneal neoplasm. Abdom Imaging 1994; 19:342–344.

11. Kim SH, Kim SC, Choi BI, et al: Uterine cervical carcinoma: Evaluation of pelvic lymph node metastasis with MR imaging. Radiology 1994; 190:807–811.

12. Yang DM, Song EH, Han H, et al: Castleman disease in the retroperitoneum: Report of 2 cases. J Korean Radiol Soc 1994; 31:355–357.

13. Hartman DS, Hayes WS, Choyke PL, et al: Leiomyosarcoma of the retroperitoneum and inferior vena cava: Radiologic-pathologic correlation. Radiographics 1992; 12:1203–1220.

14. Kim SH, Choi BI, Han MC, et al: Retroperitoneal neurilemoma: CT and MR findings. AJR Am J Roentgenol 1992; 159:1023–1026.

15. Davidson AJ, Hartman DS: Lymphangioma of the retroperitoneum: CT and sonographic characteristics. Radiology 1990; 175:507–510.

16. Hayes WS, Davidson AJ, Grimley PM, et al: Extra-adrenal retroperitoneal paraganglioma: Clinical, pathologic, and CT findings. AJR Am J Roentgenol 1990; 155:1247–1250.

17. Choi BI, Kim SH, Chang KH, et al: MR imaging of retroperitoneal teratoma: Correlation with CT and pathology. J Comput Assist Tomogr 1989; 13:1083–1086.

18. Davidson AJ, Hartman DS, Goldman SM: Mature teratoma of the retroperitoneum: Radiologic, pathologic, and clinical correlation. Radiology 1989; 172:421–425.

19. Koci TM, Worthen NJ, Phillips JJ, et al: Perirenal hemangioendothelioma in a newborn: Sonographic and MR findings. J Comput Assist Tomogr 1989; 13:145–147.

20. Lane RH, Stephens DH, Reman HM: Primary retroperitoneal neoplasms: CT findings in 90 cases with clinical and pathologic correlation. AJR Am J Roentgenol 1989; 152:83–89.

21. Cohan RH, Baker ME, Cooper C, et al: Computed tomography of primary retroperitoneal malignancies. J Comput Assist Tomogr 1988; 12:804–810.

22. Goldman SM, Davidson AJ, Neal J: Retroperitoneal and pelvic hemangiopericytomas: Clinical, radiologic, and pathologic correlation. Radiology 1988; 168:13–17.

23. Levine E, Huntrakoon M, Werzel LH: Malignant nerve-sheath neoplasms in neurofibromatosis: Distinction from benign tumors by using imaging techniques. AJR Am J Roentgenol 1987; 149:1059–1064.

24. Quint LE, Gluzer GM, Francis IR, et al: Pheochromocytoma and paraganglioma: Comparison of MR imaging with CT and I-131 MIBG scintigraphy. Radiology 1987; 165:89–93.

25. Alpern MB, Thorsen K, Kellman GM, et al: CT appearance of hemangiopericytoma. J Comput Assist Tomogr 1986; 10:264–267.

26. Johnson AR, Ros PR, Hjermstad BM: Tailgut cyst: Diagnosis with CT and sonography. AJR Am J Roentgenol 1986; 147:1309–1311.

27. Goodman K, Bain RS, Clair MR, et al: Angiomatous lymphoid hamartoma of the pelvis: Characteristic calcification and computed tomographic appearance. Radiology 1983; 146:728.

Illustrations • Retroperitoneal Diseases

1. Normal Anatomy and Variations

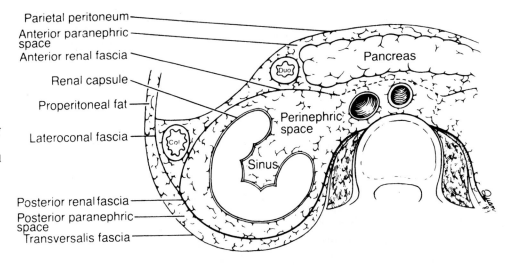

Parietal peritoneum
Anterior paranephric space
Anterior renal fascia
Renal capsule
Properitoneal fat
Lateroconal fascia
Pancreas
Duo
Perinephric space
Col
Sinus
Posterior renal fascia
Posterior paranephric space
Transversalis fascia

Fig. 1. Schematic drawing of cross-sectional anatomy of the right side of the retroperitoneum showing retroperitoneal compartments divided by renal fascial planes. (From Friedenberg RM, Harris RD: Excretory urography in adult. In Pollack HM, McClennan BL [eds]: Clinical Urography, 2nd ed, vol 1. Philadelphia, WB Saunders, 2000, pp 180–185.)

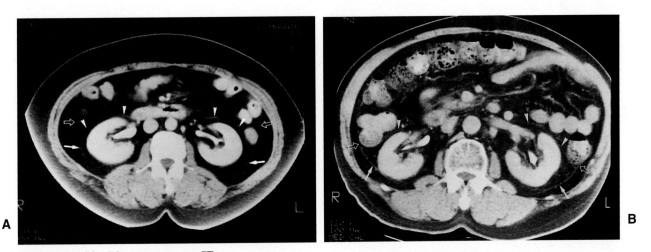

A **B**

Fig. 2. Retroperitoneal fascial anatomy seen on CT.
A. Contrast-enhanced CT in a 46-year-old woman well demonstrates anterior renal fascia *(arrowheads)*, posterior renal fascia *(arrows)*, and lateroconal fascia *(open arrows)*. **B.** Contrast-enhanced CT in an 88-year-old man shows normal kidneys, anterior renal fascia *(arrowheads)*, posterior renal fascia *(arrows)*, and lateroconal fascia *(open arrows)*.

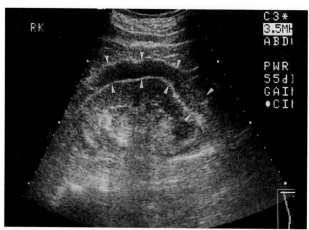

Fig. 3. Prominent, hypoechoic, perirenal fat in a 66-year-old man with diabetic nephropathy. US of the right kidney shows increased renal parenchymal echogenicity and prominent, hypoechoic, perirenal fat mimicking perirenal fluid collection *(arrowheads)*. The echogenicity of retroperitoneal fat is variable and sometimes may be quite hypoechoic.

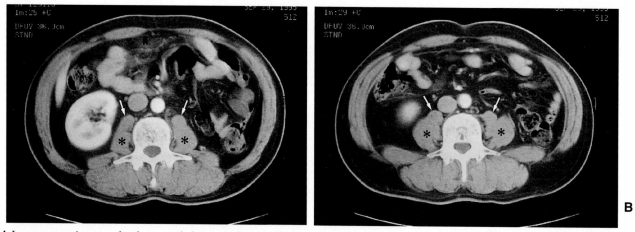

A **B**

Fig. 4. Large psoas minor muscles that can mimic retroperitoneal lymphadenopathy in a 49-year-old man who underwent left radical nephrectomy for renal cell carcinoma.
A, B. Contrast-enhanced CT scans show prominent psoas minor muscles *(arrows)* located anterior to the psoas major muscles *(asterisks)*. The prominent psoas minor muscles may be confused with retroperitoneal lymphadenopathy, especially in a patient with a history of malignancy.

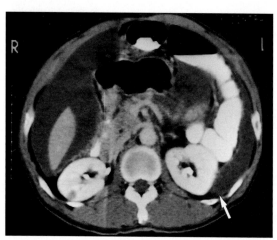

Fig. 5. Extension of ascites posterior to the kidney in a 58-year-old man with peritoneal carcinomatosis from an unknown primary tumor. Contrast-enhanced CT shows large amount of ascites in the peritoneal cavity. Note that the ascites *(arrow)* in the left paracolic gutter extends posterior to the left kidney by dissecting between two leaves of the posterior renal fascia.

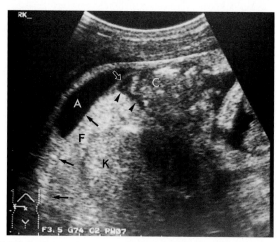

Fig. 6. US demonstration of retroperitoneal fascial anatomy in a 51-year-old man who was receiving peritoneal dialysis for chronic renal failure. Transverse US of the right abdomen demonstrates ascites (A), right kidney (K), perirenal fat (F), anterior renal fascia *(arrowheads)*, posterior renal fascia *(arrows)*, and lateroconal fascia *(open arrow)*. C, ascending colon.

2. Retroperitoneal Lipoma and Liposarcoma

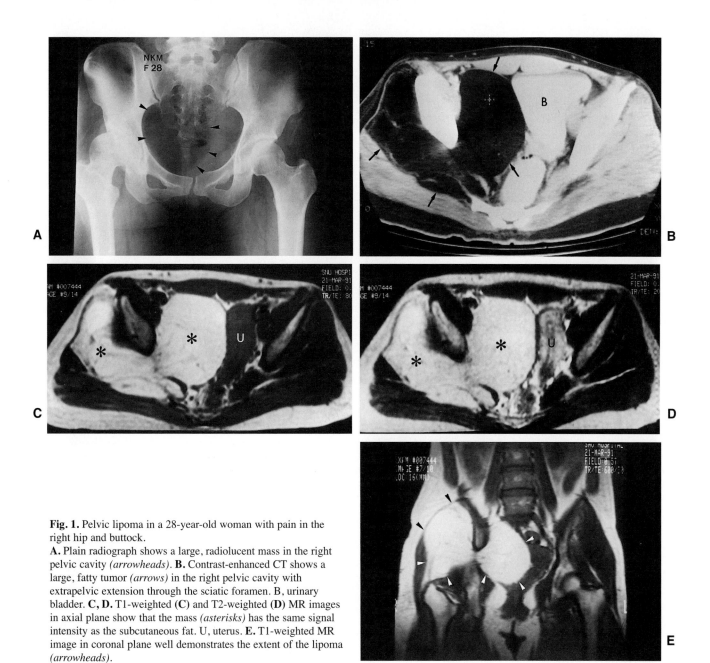

Fig. 1. Pelvic lipoma in a 28-year-old woman with pain in the right hip and buttock.
A. Plain radiograph shows a large, radiolucent mass in the right pelvic cavity *(arrowheads)*. **B.** Contrast-enhanced CT shows a large, fatty tumor *(arrows)* in the right pelvic cavity with extrapelvic extension through the sciatic foramen. B, urinary bladder. **C, D.** T1-weighted **(C)** and T2-weighted **(D)** MR images in axial plane show that the mass *(asterisks)* has the same signal intensity as the subcutaneous fat. U, uterus. **E.** T1-weighted MR image in coronal plane well demonstrates the extent of the lipoma *(arrowheads)*.

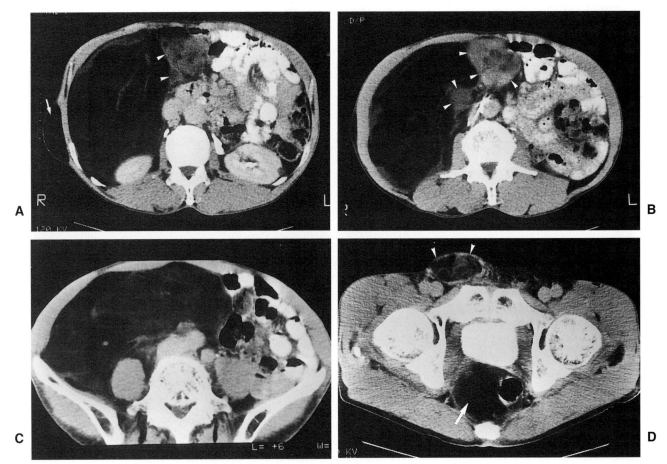

Fig. 2. Retroperitoneal liposarcoma of well-differentiated type in a 67-year-old man.
A–D. Contrast-enhanced CT scans show a large, retroperitoneal, fatty mass in the right abdomen extending down to the perirectal area (*arrow* in **D**). The mass has a nonfatty, soft tissue component in its medial aspect (*arrowheads* in **A** and **B**), suggesting liposarcoma. Also note a lipoma in the subcutaneous fat of the right lateral abdomen (*arrow* in **A**) and right inguinal hernia (*arrowheads* in **D**).

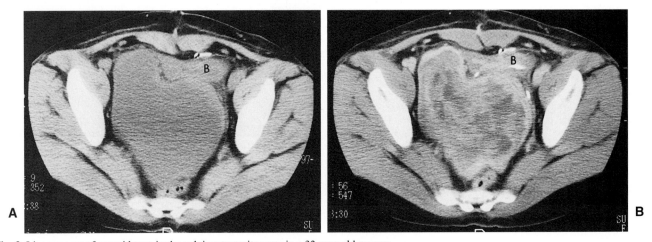

Fig. 3. Liposarcoma of myxoid type in the pelvic retroperitoneum in a 32-year-old woman.
A. Nonenhanced CT shows a large pelvic mass of slightly low attenuation posterior to the urinary bladder (B). **B.** Contrast-enhanced CT shows heterogeneous enhancement of the mass. B, urinary bladder.

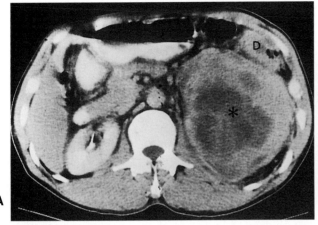

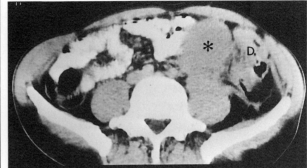

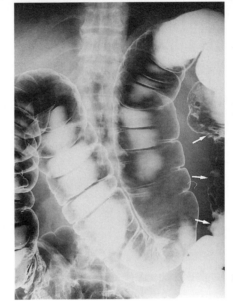

Fig. 4. Retroperitoneal liposarcoma of pleomorphic type in a 50-year-old man.
A, B. Contrast-enhanced CT scans show a large retroperitoneal mass of heterogeneous attenuation in the left abdomen *(asterisk)*. The descending colon is involved by the mass with thickening of the wall (D). **C.** Colon study shows irregularities and nodularities along the medial border of the descending colon *(arrows)*. At operation, the descending colon was found to be involved by the tumor.

3. Retroperitoneal Leiomyoma and Leiomyosarcoma

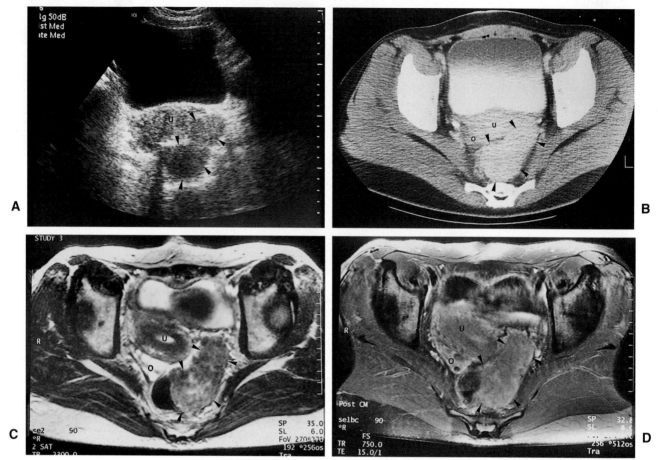

Fig. 1. Retroperitoneal leiomyoma in a 33-year-old woman. At surgery, the mass was located in the pelvic retroperitoneum.
A. US shows a pelvic mass *(arrowheads)* adjacent to the uterus (U). The mass has a lobulated margin and the echogenicity is similar to that of the uterus. **B.** Contrast-enhanced CT shows that the mass *(arrowheads)* enhances well and its attenuation is similar to that of the uterus (U). O, right ovary. **C.** T2-weighted MR image shows that the mass *(arrowheads)* has heterogeneous signal intensity and is not continuous with the uterus (U). O, right ovary. **D.** On contrast-enhanced T1-weighted MR image, the mass enhances similarly with the uterus (U). O, right ovary.

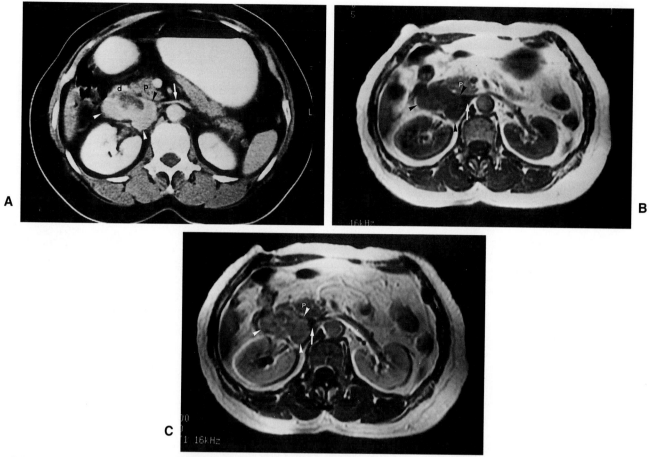

Fig. 2. Retroperitoneal leiomyosarcoma arising in the wall of the inferior vena cava in a 56-year-old woman.
A. Contrast-enhanced CT shows a soft tissue mass of heterogeneous attenuation *(arrowheads)* posterior to the head of the pancreas (p). The left renal vein *(arrow)* is well demonstrated, but the inferior vena cava cannot be identified from the mass. d, duodenum. **B, C.** T1-weighted **(B)** and contrast-enhanced T1-weighted **(C)** MR images well demonstrate the enhancing mass *(arrowheads)*. Also note that inferior vena cava, which was not identifiable on CT, is well defined as a signal-void structure *(arrow)*. p, pancreas head.

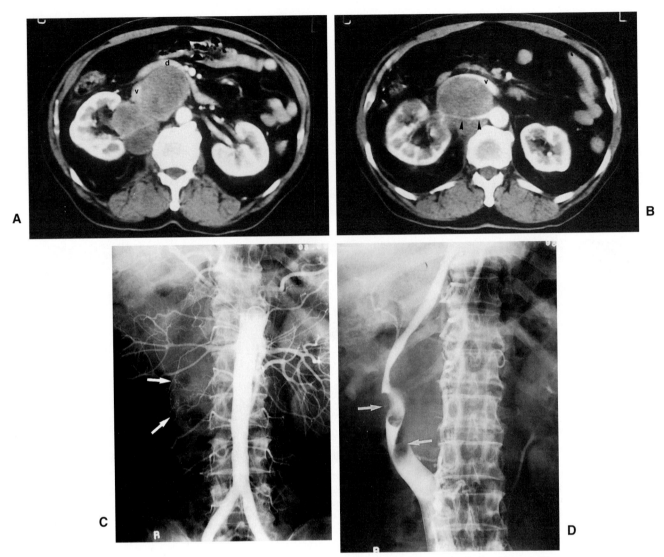

Fig. 3. Retroperitoneal leiomyosarcoma arising from the wall of the inferior vena cava and right renal vein in a 60-year-old man.
A, B. Contrast-enhanced CT scans show a large, lobulated, soft tissue mass in the region of the inferior vena cava and right renal vein. The inferior vena cava (v), duodenum (d), and right renal artery *(arrowheads* in **B)** are severely displaced by the mass. Note that the perfusion to the right kidney is well preserved. **C.** Abdominal aortogram shows tortuous tumor vessels *(arrows)* supplied by the lumbar arteries. **D.** Inferior venacavogram shows deviation of the inferior vena cava by the mass that protrudes into the vena cava *(arrows).*

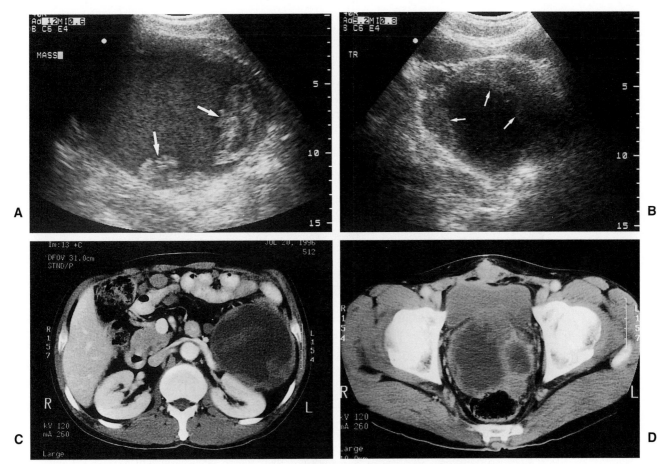

Fig. 4. Multiple retroperitoneal leiomyosarcomas in the left abdomen and pelvic cavity in a 57-year-old man.
A, B. US images of the left abdomen (**A**) and pelvic cavity (**B**) show large masses with extensive cystic degeneration. Some solid portions are seen in the periphery of the mass *(arrows)*. **C, D.** Contrast-enhanced CT scans in the left abdomen (**C**) and pelvic cavity (**D**) demonstrate the tumors with extensive central necrosis.

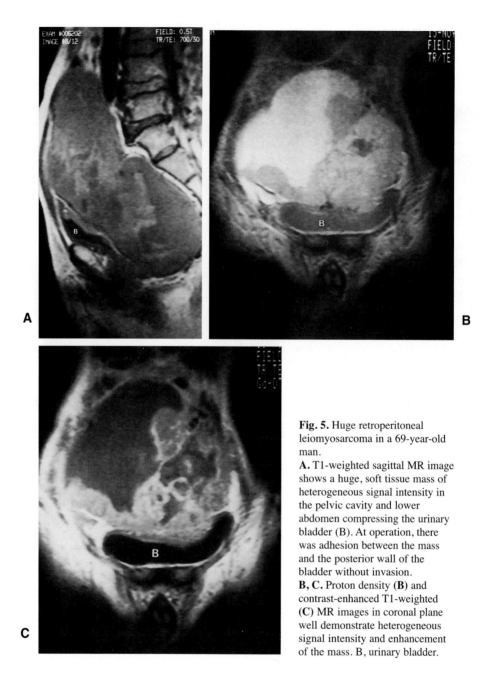

Fig. 5. Huge retroperitoneal leiomyosarcoma in a 69-year-old man.

A. T1-weighted sagittal MR image shows a huge, soft tissue mass of heterogeneous signal intensity in the pelvic cavity and lower abdomen compressing the urinary bladder (B). At operation, there was adhesion between the mass and the posterior wall of the bladder without invasion.

B, C. Proton density (**B**) and contrast-enhanced T1-weighted (**C**) MR images in coronal plane well demonstrate heterogeneous signal intensity and enhancement of the mass. B, urinary bladder.

4. Retroperitoneal Rhabdomyosarcoma

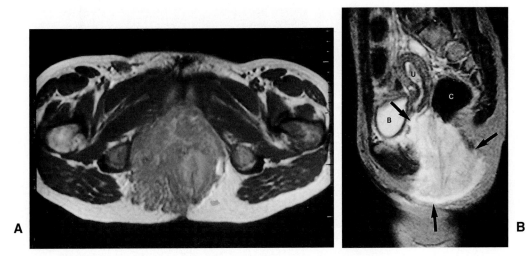

Fig. 1. Perineal rhabdomyosarcoma of alveolar cell type in a 15-year-old girl.
A. T1-weighted MR image in axial plane shows a large soft tissue mass with an infiltrating margin in the perineum. The signal intensity of the mass is higher than that of the muscles. **B.** T2-weighted sagittal MR image well demonstrates the extent of the mass *(arrows)*. The signal intensity of the mass is very high on this T2-weighted image. B, urinary bladder; C, rectosigmoid colon; U, uterus.

5. Retroperitoneal Malignant Fibrous Histiocytoma

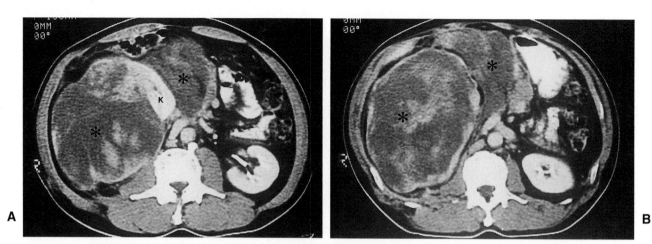

Fig. 1. Retroperitoneal malignant fibrous histiocytoma in a 55-year-old man. This mass also showed a feature of myxoid-type liposarcoma pathologically.
A, B. Contrast-enhanced CT scans show a large, lobulated, soft tissue mass *(asterisks)* of heterogeneous attenuation in the right abdomen with invasion of the right kidney (K).

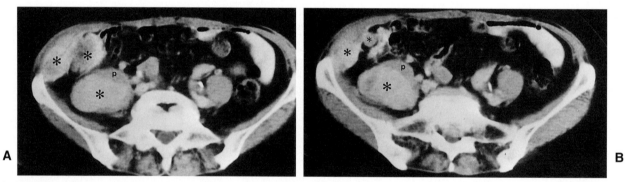

Fig. 2. Retroperitoneal malignant fibrous histiocytoma in a 58-year-old woman.
A, B. Contrast-enhanced CT scans show multiple, soft tissue masses *(asterisks)* behind the right psoas muscle (p) and in the right extraperitoneal fat layer beneath the anterior abdominal wall. Biopsy of the mass in the abdominal wall revealed malignant fibrous histiocytoma.

6. Retroperitoneal Lymphangioma

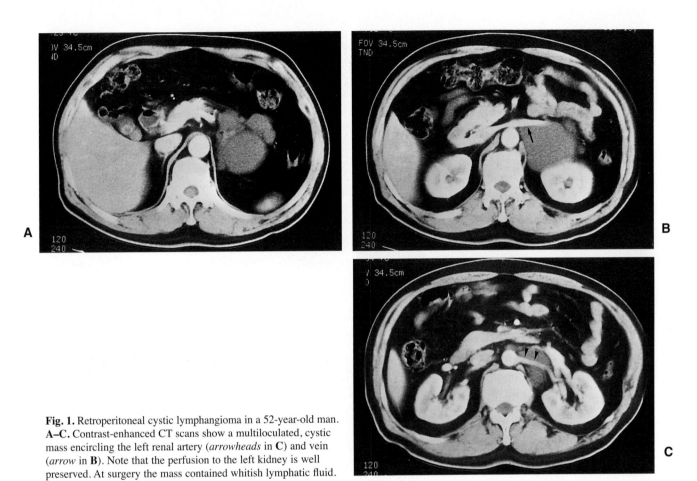

Fig. 1. Retroperitoneal cystic lymphangioma in a 52-year-old man. **A–C.** Contrast-enhanced CT scans show a multiloculated, cystic mass encircling the left renal artery (*arrowheads* in **C**) and vein (*arrow* in **B**). Note that the perfusion to the left kidney is well preserved. At surgery the mass contained whitish lymphatic fluid.

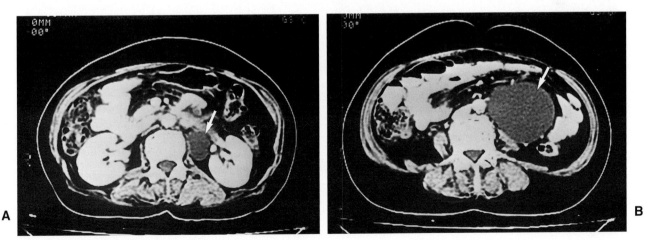

Fig. 2. Retroperitoneal cystic lymphangioma in a 63-year-old woman. **A, B.** Contrast-enhanced CT scans show a round, thin-walled, unilocular, cystic mass *(arrow)* in the left abdomen, medial and inferior to the left kidney.

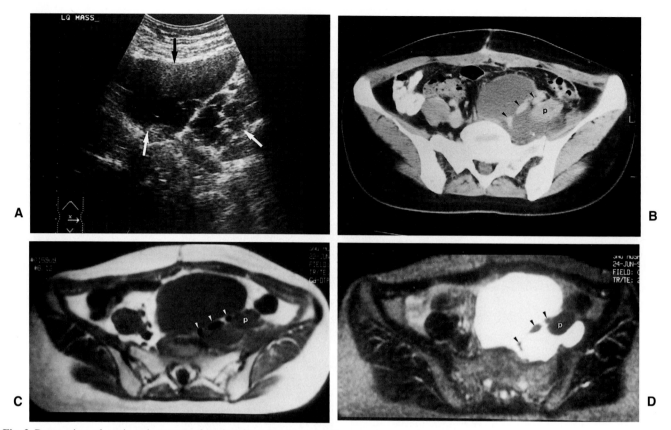

Fig. 3. Retroperitoneal cystic and cavernous lymphangioma in a 31-year-old woman.
A. US of the left lower abdomen in transverse plane shows a multiloculated cystic mass *(arrows)*. **B.** Contrast-enhanced CT scan shows the cystic mass encircling the left iliac vessels *(arrowheads)* and psoas muscle (p). **C, D.** T1-weighted **(C)** and T2-weighted **(D)** MR images show that the mass has the signal intensity of fluid and the feature of creeping between the iliac vessels *(arrowheads)* and psoas muscle (p).

7. Retroperitoneal Hemangiopericytoma

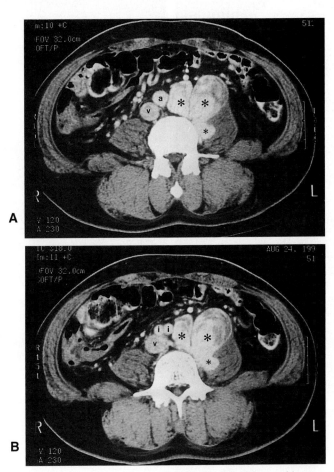

Fig. 1. Retroperitoneal hemangiopericytoma in a 46-year-old man.
A, B. Contrast-enhanced CT scans show a lobulated mass with very
strong enhancement *(asterisks)* in the region of iliac bifurcation (i),
anteromedial to the left psoas muscle. a, aorta; v, vena cava.

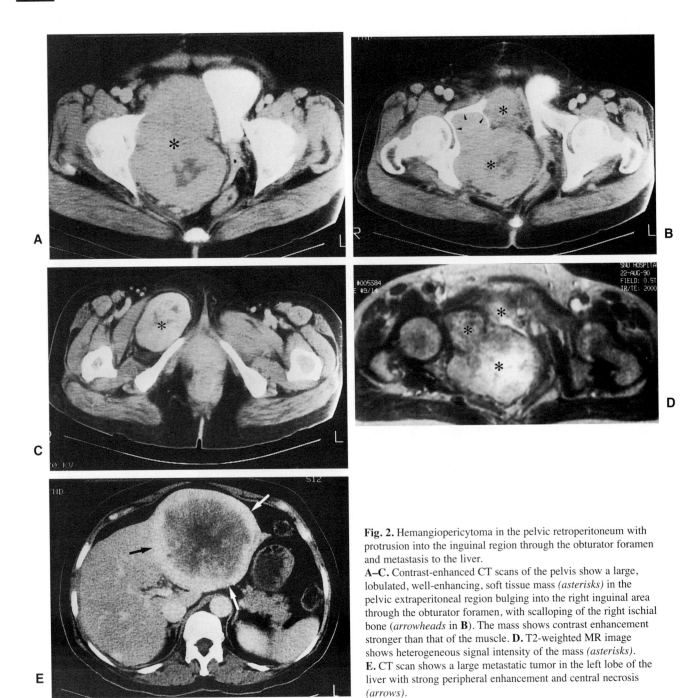

Fig. 2. Hemangiopericytoma in the pelvic retroperitoneum with protrusion into the inguinal region through the obturator foramen and metastasis to the liver.
A–C. Contrast-enhanced CT scans of the pelvis show a large, lobulated, well-enhancing, soft tissue mass *(asterisks)* in the pelvic extraperitoneal region bulging into the right inguinal area through the obturator foramen, with scalloping of the right ischial bone *(arrowheads* in **B**). The mass shows contrast enhancement stronger than that of the muscle. **D.** T2-weighted MR image shows heterogeneous signal intensity of the mass *(asterisks)*.
E. CT scan shows a large metastatic tumor in the left lobe of the liver with strong peripheral enhancement and central necrosis *(arrows)*.

8. Retroperitoneal Chondrosarcoma

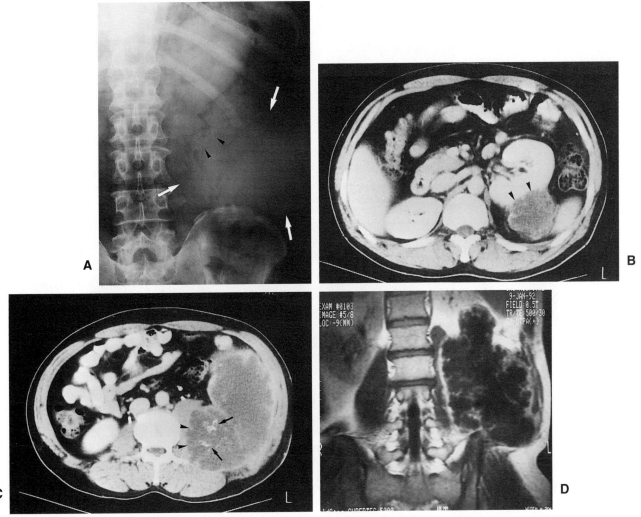

Fig. 1. Retroperitoneal chondrosarcoma in the left abdomen in a 43-year-old man.
A. Plain radiograph shows a large, soft tissue mass in the left abdomen *(arrows)* that contains mottled calcifications *(arrowheads)*. **B, C.** Contrast-enhanced CT scans show a large, low-attenuated mass in the left perirenal and posterior pararenal spaces with invasion of the left psoas muscle and left kidney *(arrowheads)*. Note mottled calcifications in the mass *(arrows* in **C**). **D.** Contrast-enhanced T1-weighted coronal MR image shows a large necrotic mass in the left abdomen.

9. Retroperitoneal Neurofibroma

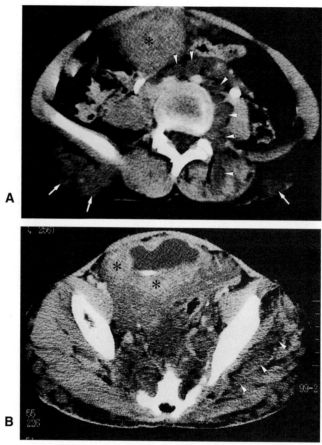

Fig. 1. Neurofibromatosis in a 9-year-old boy with diffuse involvement of the retroperitoneum, urinary bladder, and muscles and subcutaneous fat of the back and buttock.
A. Contrast-enhanced CT scan of the lower abdomen shows markedly thickened wall of the urinary bladder in the dome *(asterisk)*, and multiple, low-attenuated masses *(arrowheads)* in the left retroperitoneum and back muscle. Also note masses in the subcutaneous fat in the back *(arrows)*. **B.** CT scan at a lower level shows innumerable masses in the pelvic retroperitoneum and posterior subcutaneous fat. Note nodular thickening of the bladder wall *(asterisks)*. Also note similar masses in the left gluteus muscles *(arrowheads)*.

10. Retroperitoneal Neurilemmoma

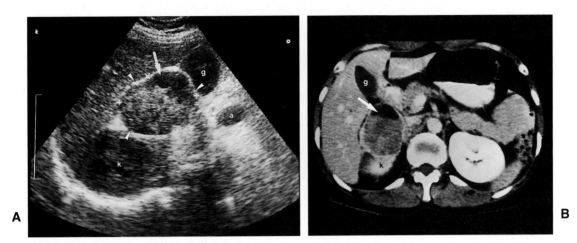

Fig. 1. Retroperitoneal neurilemmoma in a 41-year-old woman.
A. US of right upper abdomen in transverse plane shows a round mass *(arrowheads)* that has a focal cystic portion *(arrow)*. a, aorta; g, gallbladder; k, right kidney. **B.** Contrast-enhanced CT shows a low-attenuated mass with a cystic portion *(arrow)* above the right kidney (k). At surgery, the right adrenal gland was intact. g, gallbladder.

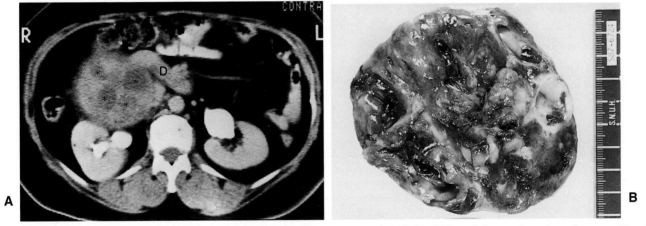

Fig. 2. Retroperitoneal neurilemmoma in a 48-year-old woman. (**A, B,** From Kim SH, Choi BI, Han MC, et al: Retroperitoneal neurilemoma: CT and MR findings. AJR Am J Roentgenol 1992; 159:1023–1026.)
A. Contrast-enhanced CT shows a round mass anterior to the right kidney containing multiple, round necrotic areas *(asterisks)*. D, duodenum. **B.** Cut surface of gross specimen shows multiple areas of cystic and hemorrhagic degeneration and intervening non-necrotic portions.

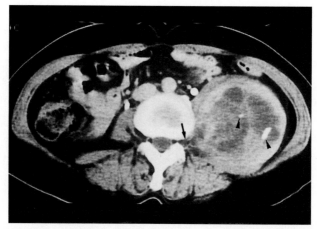

Fig. 3. Retroperitoneal neurilemmoma with calcification in a 52-year-old woman. Contrast-enhanced CT shows a large, round mass containing areas of cystic degeneration and calcifications *(arrowheads)*. Also note that the mass has a stalk in the neural foramen of the vertebra *(arrow)*.

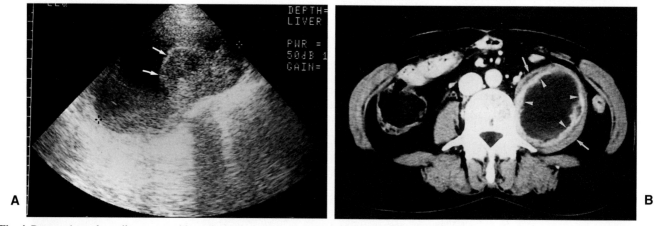

Fig. 4. Retroperitoneal neurilemmoma with cystic degeneration and calcification in a 55-year-old woman.
A. Longitudinal US shows a cystic mass with internal echogenic component *(arrows)* in the left abdomen. **B.** Contrast-enhanced CT shows a round mass in the left paraspinal region with extensive cystic degeneration and calcifications along the margin of the degenerated cystic cavity *(arrowheads)*. Note the thinned psoas muscle *(arrows)* around the mass.

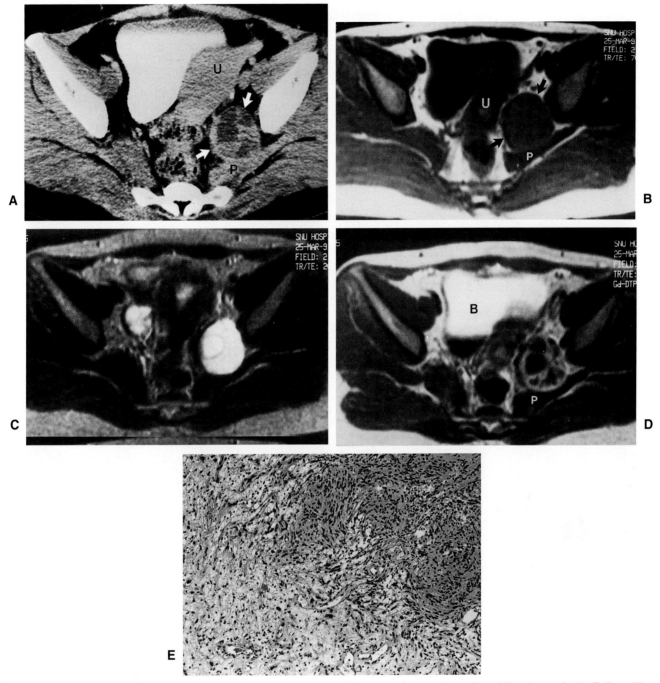

Fig. 5. A 35-year-old woman with pelvic extraperitoneal neurilemmoma in the left presacral area in front of the piriformis muscle. (**A–E,** From Kim SH, Choi BI, Han MC, et al: Retroperitoneal neurilemoma: CT and MR findings. AJR Am J Roentgenol 1992; 159:1023–1026.)
A. Contrast-enhanced CT shows a well-defined, round mass *(arrows)* containing multiple necrotic areas of low attenuation in the left pelvic retroperitoneum in front of the piriformis muscle (P). U, uterus. **B.** T1-weighted MR image shows a round mass of homogeneous, intermediate signal intensity *(arrows)* similar to that of the skeletal muscles. The mass is abutting and compressing the piriformis muscle (P). U, uterus. **C.** T2-weighted MR image shows markedly increased signal intensity of the mass with a relatively homogeneous appearance. **D.** Contrast-enhanced T1-weighted MR image shows the mass composed of radially distributed, nonenhancing, necrotic areas and highly enhancing, non-necrotic portions. P, piriformis muscle; B, urinary bladder. **E.** Photomicrograph of the non-necrotic portion of the tumor shows two components of the tumor: highly cellular Antoni A tissue *(upper right)* and loose hypocellular Antoni B tissue *(lower left)*. Areas of Antoni B tissue were more prominent than those of Antoni A tissue in this case.

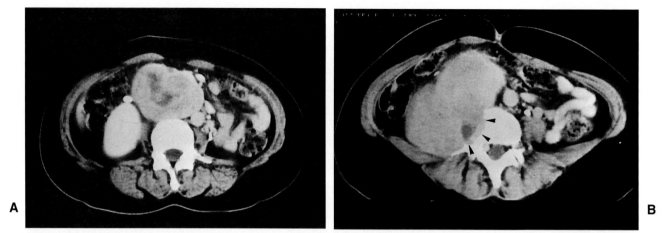

Fig. 6. Multilobulated retroperitoneal neurilemmoma with vertebral erosion in a 33-year-old woman.
A. Contrast-enhanced CT at the level of the lower pole of the right kidney shows a round, soft tissue mass with central degeneration in front of the vertebra. **B.** CT scan at a lower level shows a multilobulated mass with erosion of the vertebra *(arrowheads)*. In the neurogenic tumors, this finding of vertebral erosion is not a sign of malignancy.

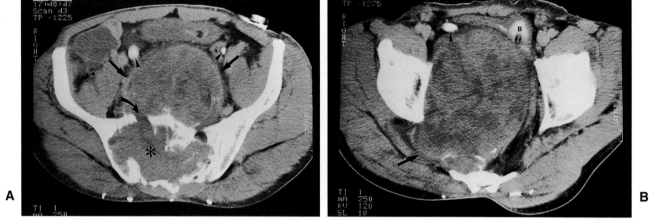

Fig. 7. Retroperitoneal neurilemmoma with extensive sacral bony destruction in a 56-year old man.
A. Contrast-enhanced CT scan at the pelvic inlet level shows a large presacral mass *(arrows)*. The sacral bone is severely destroyed by the mass *(asterisk)*, which is continuous with the presacral mass through the right sacral neural foramen *(curved arrow)*. Note the dilated right ureter and normal-sized left ureter displaced anteriorly *(arrowheads)*. **B.** CT scan at a lower level shows a huge mass of heterogeneous attenuation bulging into the right sciatic foramen *(arrow)*. Note the anteriorly displaced right ureter *(arrowhead)* and urinary bladder (B).

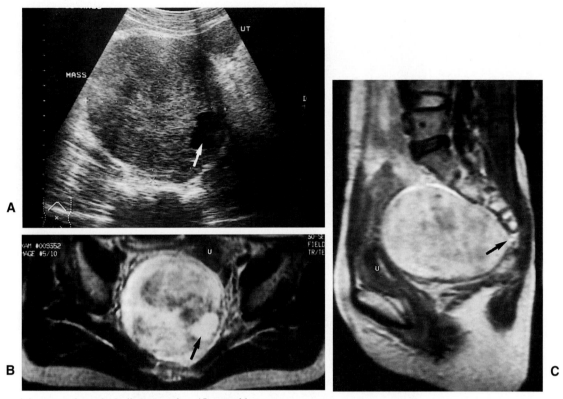

Fig. 8. Large pelvic retroperitoneal neurilemmoma in a 45-year-old woman.
A. Transverse US shows a large pelvic mass with a focal cystic component *(arrow)*. **B.** T2-weighted axial MR image shows heterogeneous signal intensity of the mass and a focal cystic component *(arrow)*. The uterus is displaced anteriorly (U). **C.** T2-weighted sagittal MR image shows that the mass is attached to the coccyx *(arrow)*. U, uterus.

11. Retroperitoneal Ganglioneuroma

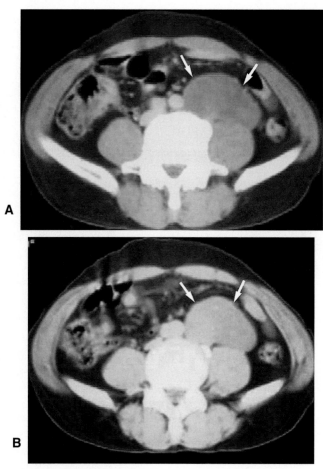

Fig. 1. Retroperitoneal ganglioneuroma in a 51-year-old man.
A, B. Contrast-enhanced CT scans in early arterial (**A**) and late
arteriovenous (**B**) phases show a smooth-marginated mass in the left
retroperitoneum *(arrows)*. The mass shows low attenuation on arterial-
phase CT with homogeneous enhancement on arteriovenous-phase CT,
suggesting slow enhancement and slow washout.

12. Retroperitoneal Malignant Schwannoma

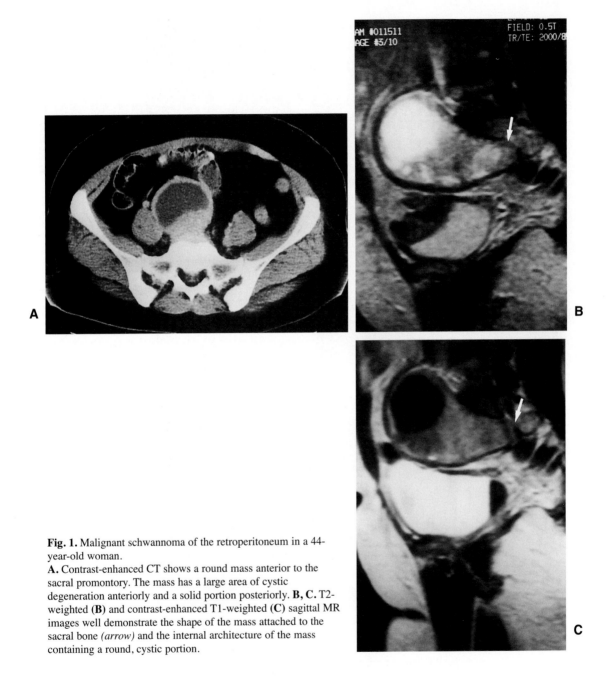

Fig. 1. Malignant schwannoma of the retroperitoneum in a 44-year-old woman.
A. Contrast-enhanced CT shows a round mass anterior to the sacral promontory. The mass has a large area of cystic degeneration anteriorly and a solid portion posteriorly. **B, C.** T2-weighted (**B**) and contrast-enhanced T1-weighted (**C**) sagittal MR images well demonstrate the shape of the mass attached to the sacral bone *(arrow)* and the internal architecture of the mass containing a round, cystic portion.

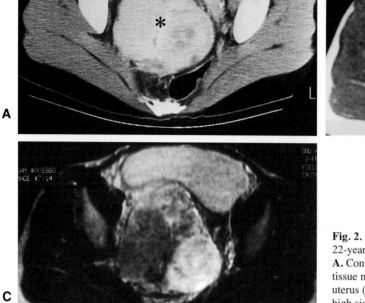

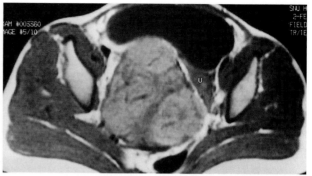

Fig. 2. Malignant schwannoma of the pelvic retroperitoneum in a 22-year-old woman.
A. Contrast-enhanced CT shows a large, well-enhancing, soft tissue mass *(asterisk)* in the pelvic cavity with displacement of the uterus (U). **B.** On T1-weighted MR image, the mass has relatively high signal intensity. U, uterus. **C.** T2-weighted MR image shows heterogeneous signal intensity of the mass.

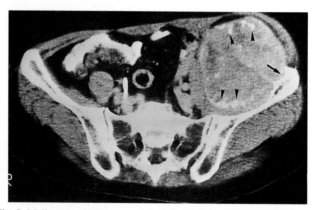

Fig. 3. Malignant schwannoma of the left pelvis in a 62-year-old woman. Contrast-enhanced CT shows a large, round, soft tissue mass with peripheral calcifications *(arrowheads)* in the left pelvis. Note scalloping of the iliac bone caused by the mass *(arrow)*.

13. Retroperitoneal Neuroblastoma

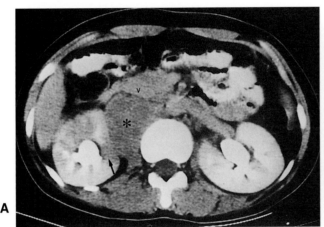

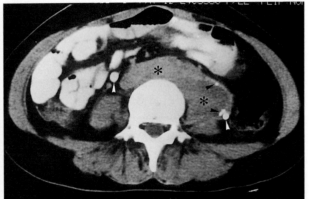

Fig. 1. Retroperitoneal neuroblastoma in a 22-year-old woman. **A.** Contrast-enhanced CT shows a low-attenuated mass in the right paravertebral region *(asterisk)* displacing the inferior vena cava (v) anteriorly. Note bilateral hydronephrosis and a focal low-attenuated lesion in the right kidney *(arrow)*, suggesting renal invasion. **B.** CT scan at the level of the lower abdomen shows other masses *(asterisks)* in the retroperitoneum crossing the midline and obliterating the great vessels. Note the small calcifications *(black arrowheads)* in the mass and dilated ureters *(white arrowheads)*. **C.** CT scan at a lower level shows another large mass *(asterisk)* in the right pelvic cavity displacing the uterus (U) and urinary bladder (B) to the left side. Note that both ureters *(arrowheads)* are also displaced.

14. Retroperitoneal Paraganglioma

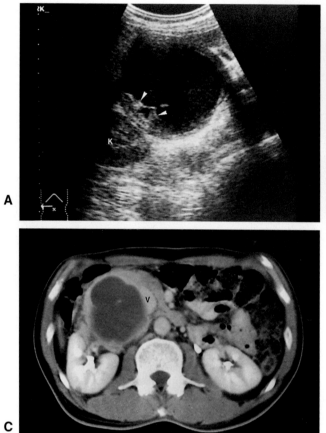

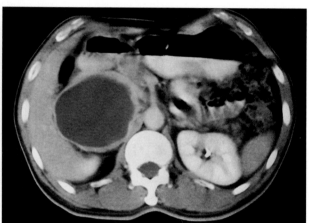

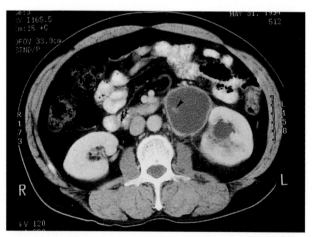

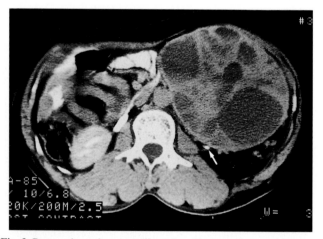

Fig. 1. Retroperitoneal paraganglioma (extra-adrenal pheochromocytoma) in a 56-year-old man.
A. US of the right abdomen in transverse plane shows a round, thick-walled, cystic mass with focal solid components *(arrowheads)*. K, right kidney. **B, C.** Contrast-enhanced CT scans show a thick-walled, cystic mass between the inferior vena cava (v) and right kidney.

Fig. 2. Retroperitoneal paraganglioma in a 47-year-old man. Contrast-enhanced CT shows a round, thick-walled, cystic mass in the left abdomen between the aorta and left kidney. Note the focal solid component in the mass *(arrowhead)* and hydronephrosis of the left kidney.

Fig. 3. Retroperitoneal paraganglioma in a 51-year-old man with severe hypertension and elevated vanillylmandelic acid level in a 24-hour urine specimen. Contrast-enhanced CT shows a large, soft tissue mass of heterogeneous attenuation in the left abdomen in front of the left ureter *(arrow)*. The mass contains multifocal areas of cystic degeneration.

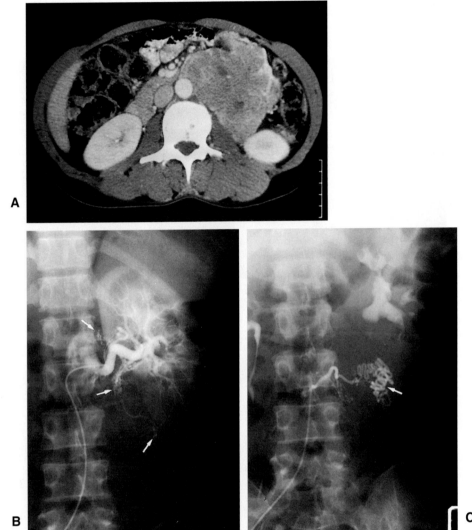

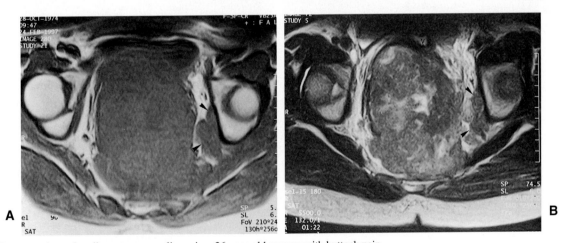

Fig. 4. Retroperitoneal paraganglioma in a 41-year-old woman.
A. Contrast-enhanced CT shows a large, solid mass with heterogeneous enhancement in the left para-aortic region.
B, C. Left renal arteriogram (**B**) and lumbar arteriogram (**C**) demonstrate tortuous tumor vessels *(arrows)* supplying the tumor.

Fig. 5. Pelvic retroperitoneal malignant paraganglioma in a 26-year-old woman with buttock pain.
A, B. T1-weighted (**A**) and T2-weighted (**B**) MR images show a huge mass in the pelvic cavity with displacement of the vagina (V) and urinary bladder anteriorly. The mass has homogeneous, intermediate signal intensity on T1-weighted image and heterogenous signal intensity on T2-weighted image. Note the multiple lymphadenopathy *(arrowheads)* in the left pelvic wall.

15. Retroperitoneal Primitive Neuroectodermal Tumor

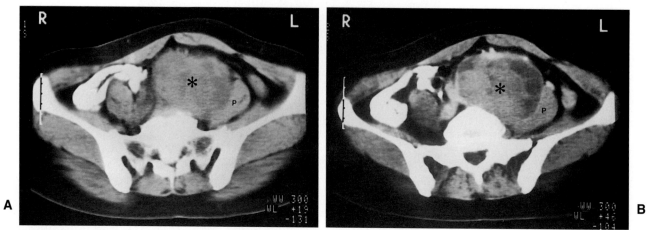

Fig. 1. Retroperitoneal primitive neuroectodermal tumor in a 53-year-old woman.
A, B. Nonenhanced **(A)** and contrast-enhanced **(B)** CT scans show a retroperitoneal mass *(asterisk)* of heterogeneous attenuation causing lateral displacement of the left psoas muscle (P).

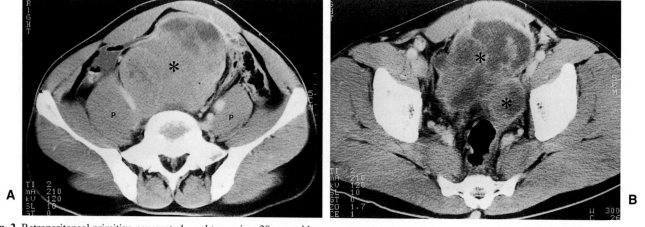

Fig. 2. Retroperitoneal primitive neuroectodermal tumor in a 30-year-old man.
A, B. Contrast-enhanced CT scans show multilobulated, soft tissue masses *(asterisks)* of heterogeneous attenuation in the lower abdomen and pelvic cavity. P, psoas muscles.

16. Retroperitoneal Teratoma

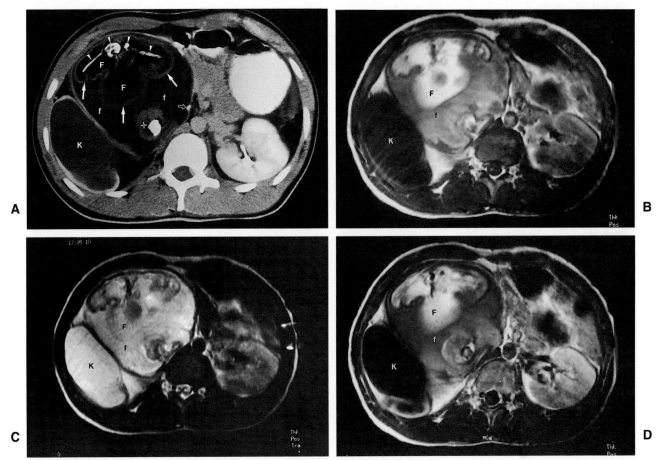

Fig. 1. Mature cystic teratoma of the retroperitoneum causing hydronephrosis in a 19-year-old man.
A. Contrast-enhanced CT shows a large mass containing solid fat (F), fluid fat (f), bone and calcifications, and skin. A fetus-like structure covered by skin *(arrows)* is seen, which contains solid fat and vertebra-like bony tissue *(arrowheads)*. Note a small calcification *(open arrow)* in the wall of the cystic mass. Also note that the right kidney shows severe hydronephrosis (K). **B–D.** T1-weighted **(B)**, T2-weighted **(C)**, and contrast-enhanced T1-weighted **(D)** MR images show various signal intensities in the mass. Note that the signal intensity of the solid fat (F) is different from that of the fluid fat (f) on T1-weighted images **(B, D)** but is similar on T2-weighted image **(C)**. K, hydronephrotic right kidney.

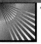
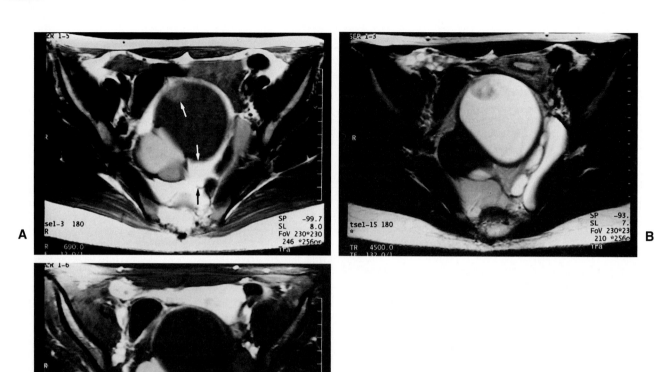

Fig. 2. Presacral teratoma in a 19-year-old woman.
A, B. T1-weighted (**A**) and T2-weighted (**B**) axial MR images of the pelvis show a large pelvic mass of variable signal intensity. Note high-intensity lesions on T1-weighted image (*arrows* in **A**), which show signal suppression on **C. C.** Contrast-enhanced, fat-suppressed, T1-weighted MR image well demonstrates suppression of signal intensity in some parts of the mass, indicating the presence of fat.

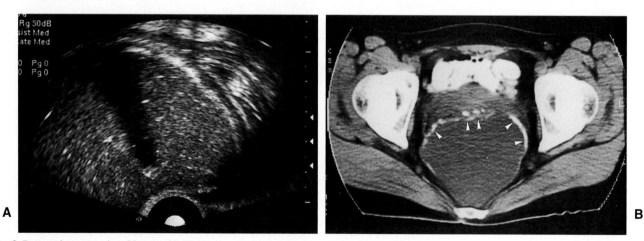

Fig. 3. Presacral teratoma in a 29-year-old woman.
A. Transvaginal US shows a cystic mass that contains echogenic debris and posterior sonic shadowing, suggesting the presence of calcification.
B. Contrast-enhanced CT shows a presacral cystic mass with peripheral calcifications (*arrowheads*). The attenuation of the mass is not suggestive of fat.

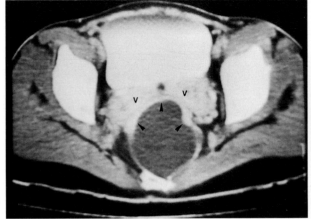

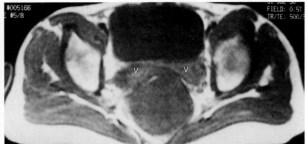

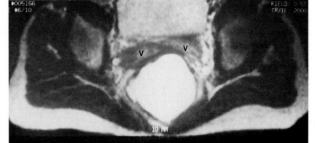

Fig. 4. Infected presacral dermoid cyst in a 30-year-old woman who complained of constipation.
A. Contrast-enhanced CT shows a round, cystic mass in the presacral region. The mass has a focally thick, enhancing anterior wall *(arrowheads)* and contains fluid of nonfatty attenuation. V, upper vagina. **B.** T1-weighted MR image shows that the mass has signal intensity higher than that of the urine in the bladder but similar to that of the skeletal muscle. V, upper vagina. **C.** On T2-weighted MR image, the mass has very high signal intensity, which is much higher than that of urine in the bladder. V, upper vagina.

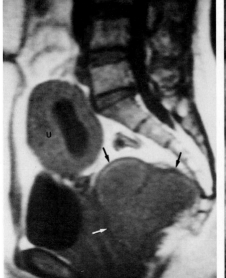

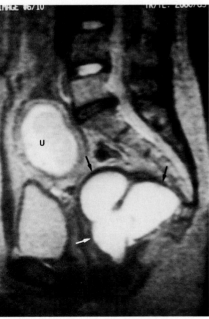

Fig. 5. Infected presacral dermoid cyst in a 26-year-old woman with a 9-week pregnancy.
A, B. T1-weighted **(A)** and T2-weighted **(B)** MR images show a lobulated mass in the presacral area *(arrows)* that contains the fluid of intermediate signal intensity on T1-weighted image and very high signal intensity on T2-weighted image. U, pregnant uterus with gestational sac.

17. Other Primary Retroperitoneal Tumors

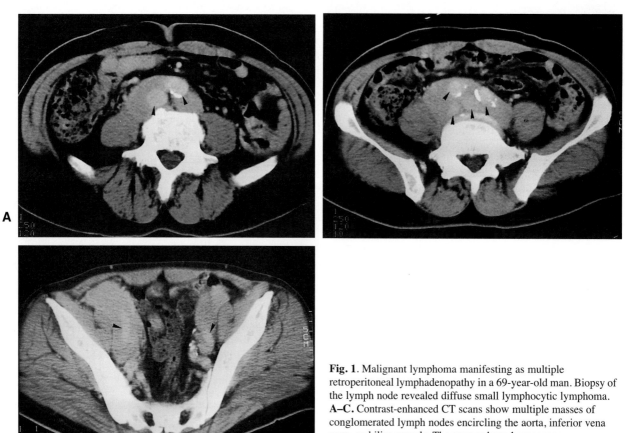

Fig. 1. Malignant lymphoma manifesting as multiple retroperitoneal lymphadenopathy in a 69-year-old man. Biopsy of the lymph node revealed diffuse small lymphocytic lymphoma. **A–C.** Contrast-enhanced CT scans show multiple masses of conglomerated lymph nodes encircling the aorta, inferior vena cava, and iliac vessels. The masses have homogeneous attenuation similar to that of the muscles. Note encased vessels *(arrowheads)* within the masses.

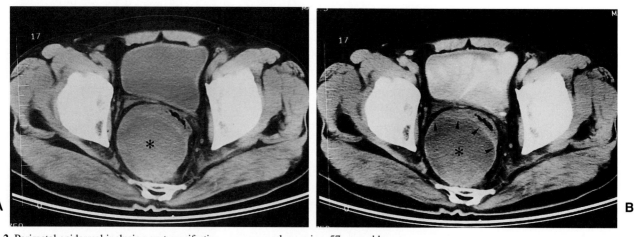

Fig. 2. Perirectal epidermal inclusion cyst manifesting as a presacral mass in a 57-year-old man.
A, B. Nonenhanced (**A**) and contrast-enhanced (**B**) CT scans of the pelvis show a round, cystic mass *(asterisk)* in the presacral region. The mass has homogeneous attenuation and does not enhance after injection of contrast material. The rectum is stretched by the mass *(arrowheads)*.

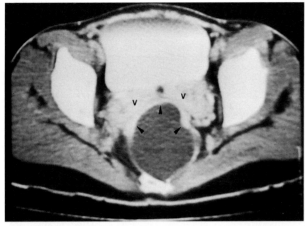

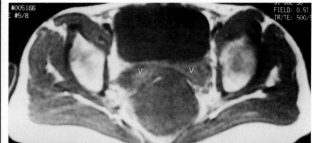

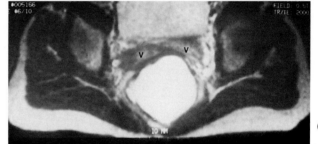

Fig. 4. Infected presacral dermoid cyst in a 30-year-old woman who complained of constipation.
A. Contrast-enhanced CT shows a round, cystic mass in the presacral region. The mass has a focally thick, enhancing anterior wall *(arrowheads)* and contains fluid of nonfatty attenuation. V, upper vagina. **B.** T1-weighted MR image shows that the mass has signal intensity higher than that of the urine in the bladder but similar to that of the skeletal muscle. V, upper vagina. **C.** On T2-weighted MR image, the mass has very high signal intensity, which is much higher than that of urine in the bladder. V, upper vagina.

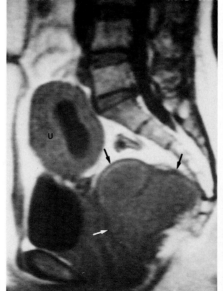

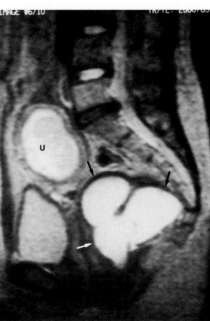

Fig. 5. Infected presacral dermoid cyst in a 26-year-old woman with a 9-week pregnancy.
A, B. T1-weighted **(A)** and T2-weighted **(B)** MR images show a lobulated mass in the presacral area *(arrows)* that contains the fluid of intermediate signal intensity on T1-weighted image and very high signal intensity on T2-weighted image. U, pregnant uterus with gestational sac.

17. Other Primary Retroperitoneal Tumors

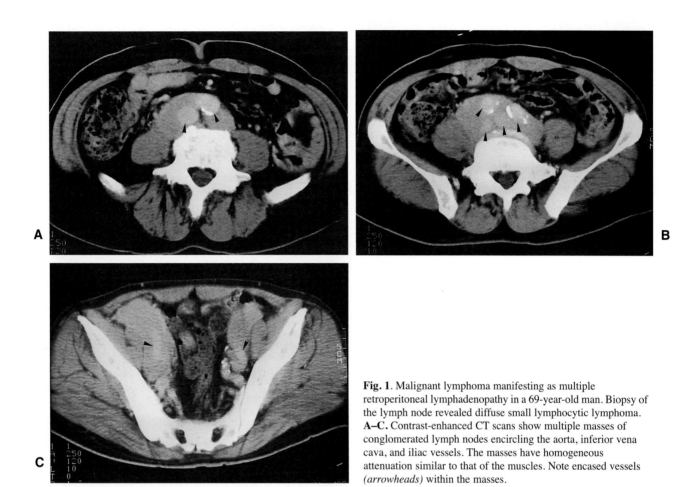

Fig. 1. Malignant lymphoma manifesting as multiple retroperitoneal lymphadenopathy in a 69-year-old man. Biopsy of the lymph node revealed diffuse small lymphocytic lymphoma. **A–C.** Contrast-enhanced CT scans show multiple masses of conglomerated lymph nodes encircling the aorta, inferior vena cava, and iliac vessels. The masses have homogeneous attenuation similar to that of the muscles. Note encased vessels *(arrowheads)* within the masses.

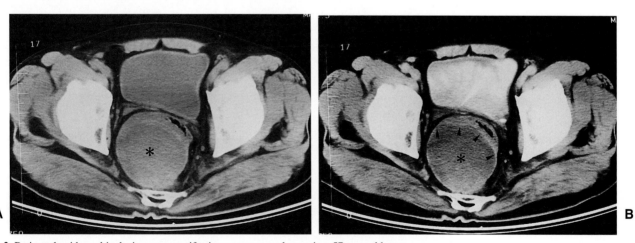

Fig. 2. Perirectal epidermal inclusion cyst manifesting as a presacral mass in a 57-year-old man.
A, B. Nonenhanced **(A)** and contrast-enhanced **(B)** CT scans of the pelvis show a round, cystic mass *(asterisk)* in the presacral region. The mass has homogeneous attenuation and does not enhance after injection of contrast material. The rectum is stretched by the mass *(arrowheads)*.

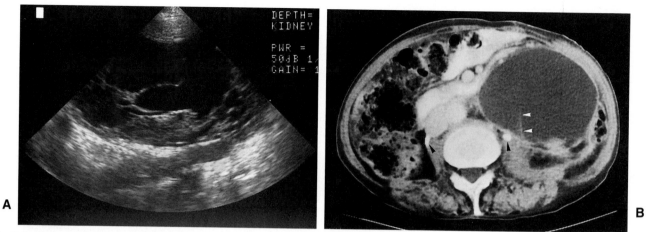

Fig. 3. Enteric cyst in a 61-year-old woman.
A. US shows a large cystic mass with abundant septa and some solid-appearing lesions. **B.** Contrast-enhanced CT shows a large cystic mass with a slightly thick wall in the left abdomen. The mass has a septum *(white arrowheads)*, but this finding is not so prominent as on US. The *black arrowheads* indicate ureters.

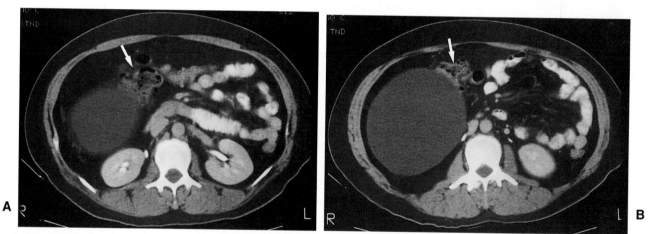

Fig. 4. Retroperitoneal mucinous cystadenoma in a 45-year-old man.
A, B. Contrast-enhanced CT scans of the abdomen show a large, thin-walled, unilocular cystic mass in the right abdomen with displacement of the ascending colon *(arrow)* to the anteromedial side, indicating a retroperitoneal location of the mass. Mucinous cystadenoma can be found in the retroperitoneum from either heterotopic ovarian tissue or invagination of peritoneal mesothelial layer with metaplasia.

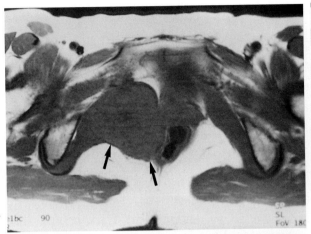

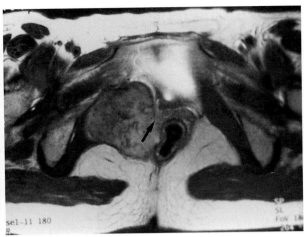

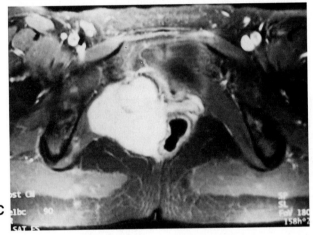

Fig. 5. Pelvic fibromatosis in a 29-year-old woman.
A. T1-weighted MR image shows a soft tissue mass in the right ischiorectal fossa *(arrows)*. The mass has homogeneous signal intensity, which is same as that of the pelvic muscles. **B.** T2-weighted MR image well demonstrates the mass. The mass is continuous with the vaginal wall *(arrow)*, suggesting the origin of the mass. **C.** Contrast-enhanced T1-weighted MR image shows homogeneous, strong enhancement of the mass.

18. Metastatic Tumors of the Retroperitoneum

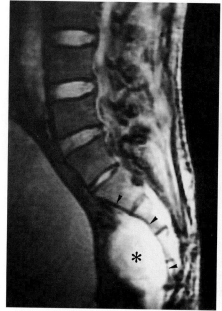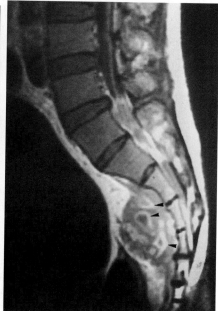

Fig. 1. Presacral chloroma in a 34-year-old man with acute myelocytic leukemia.
A. T2-weighted sagittal MR image shows a high-intensity presacral mass *(asterisk)* with broad-based attachment to the sacral bone *(arrowheads)*. Note the very large bladder due to a neurogenic bladder.
B. Contrast-enhanced T1-weighted MR image shows multifocal, necrotic areas with strong enhancement along their margins *(arrowheads)*.

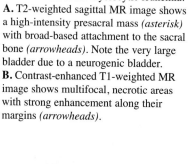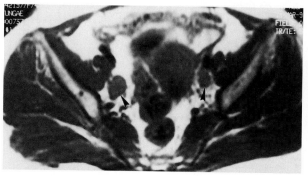

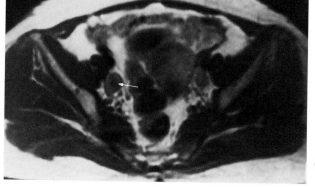

Fig. 2. Metastatic pelvic lymph nodes in a patient with uterine cervical carcinoma. (**A–C,** From Kim SH, Kim SC, Choi BI, et al: Uterine cervical carcinoma: Evaluation of pelvic lymph node metastasis with MR imaging. Radiology 1994; 190:807–811.)
A, B. T1-weighted (**A**) and T2-weighted (**B**) MR images show bilaterally enlarged pelvic lymph nodes *(arrowheads)*.
C. Contrast-enhanced MR image shows enhancement of the nodes. Note absent enhancement of the center of the right pelvic node, suggesting central necrosis *(arrow)*. At pathologic examination, this node had central necrosis and fibrosis.

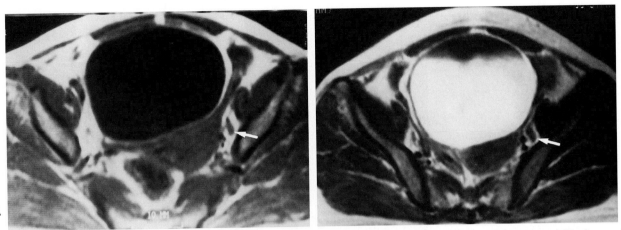

Fig. 3. Ovoid nonmetastatic lymph node in a patient with uterine cervical carcinoma. (**A, B,** From Kim SH, Kim SC, Choi BI, et al: Uterine cervical carcinoma: Evaluation of pelvic lymph node metastasis with MR imaging. Radiology 1994; 190:807–811.)
A, B. T1-weighted (**A**) and contrast-enhanced T1-weighted (**B**) MR images show an ovoid node in the left pelvic cavity *(arrow)* that enhances slightly after injection of contrast material. At pathologic examination, there was no metastasis in any of the 39 pelvic nodes sampled.

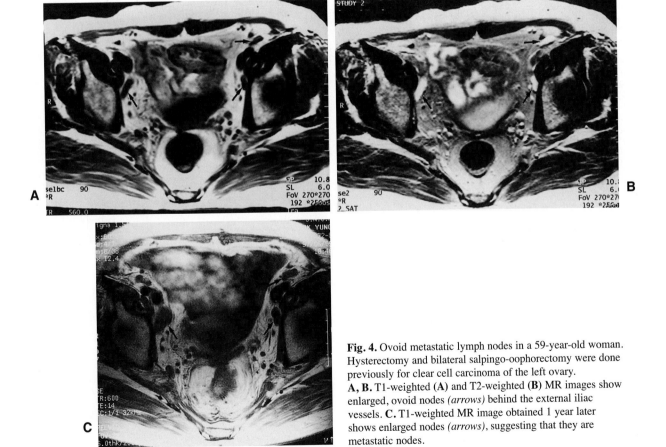

Fig. 4. Ovoid metastatic lymph nodes in a 59-year-old woman. Hysterectomy and bilateral salpingo-oophorectomy were done previously for clear cell carcinoma of the left ovary.
A, B. T1-weighted (**A**) and T2-weighted (**B**) MR images show enlarged, ovoid nodes *(arrows)* behind the external iliac vessels. **C.** T1-weighted MR image obtained 1 year later shows enlarged nodes *(arrows)*, suggesting that they are metastatic nodes.

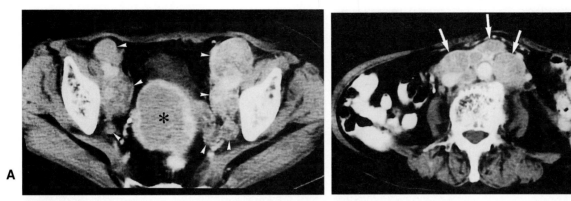

Fig. 5. Extensive metastatic lymphadenopathy in a 70-year-old woman with uterine cervical carcinoma.
A. Contrast-enhanced CT of the pelvic cavity shows a large mass in the uterine cervix *(asterisk)* and bilateral pelvic node metastases *(arrowheads)*.
B. CT scan at the level of lower abdomen shows extensive node metastases *(arrows)* around the aorta and inferior vena cava.

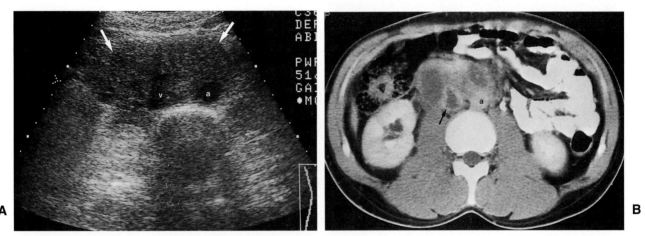

Fig. 6. Retroperitoneal metastatic lymphadenopathy in a 26-year-old man with testis tumor.
A. US of the lower abdomen in transverse plane shows a large mass *(arrows)* around the aorta (a) and inferior vena cava (v). Note that the echogenicity of the inferior vena cava is higher than that of the aorta, suggesting thrombosis. **B.** Contrast-enhanced CT shows the masses of heterogeneous attenuation caused by conglomerated metastatic lymph nodes. Note the thrombosis of the inferior vena cava *(arrow)*. a, aorta.

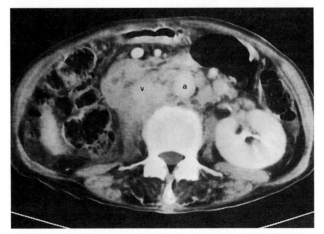

Fig. 7. Retroperitoneal metastatic lymphadenopathy in a 68-year-old woman who underwent right nephroureterectomy 2 years earlier for transitional cell carcinoma of the renal pelvis. Contrast-enhanced CT shows extensive retroperitoneal node metastases. a, aorta; v, inferior vena cava.

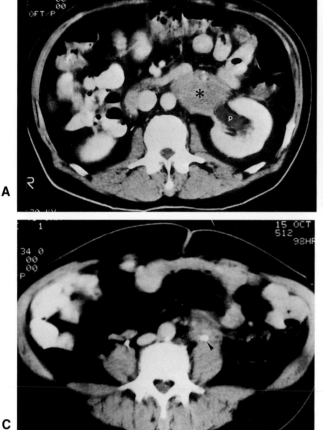

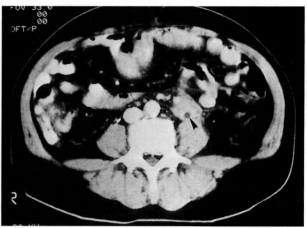

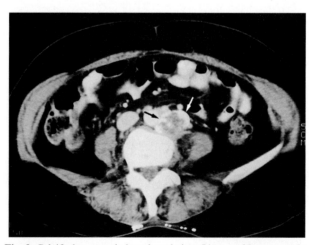

Fig. 8. Retroperitoneal metastasis along the course of the left ureter in a 55-year-old man who underwent left orchiectomy for malignant lymphoma of diffuse large cell type.
A. Contrast-enhanced CT shows a mass of homogeneous attenuation in the left renal hilar region *(asterisk)* with dilation of the left renal pelvis (p). **B.** CT scan at a lower level shows a mass encasing the left ureter *(arrowhead)*. **C.** Delayed CT scan confirms that the low-attenuated structure in the mass is the ureter *(arrowhead)*.

Fig. 9. Calcified metastatic lymph node in a 54-year-old woman who received chemotherapy for recurrent uterine cervical carcinoma. Contrast-enhanced CT shows a para-aortic lymph node with dense calcification *(arrows)*.

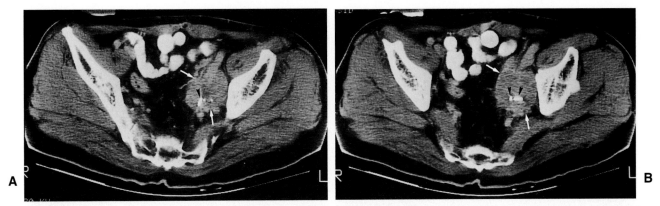

Fig. 10. Metastatic pelvic lymphadenopathy engulfing surgical clips that were used in a radical cystectomy for transitional cell carcinoma of the urinary bladder in a 74-year-old man.
A, B. Contrast-enhanced CT scans show large lymph nodes *(arrows)* engulfing surgical clips *(arrowheads)* in the left pelvic cavity.

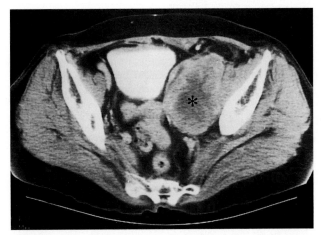

Fig. 11. Large metastatic pelvic lymph node in a 66-year-old woman with malignant melanoma. Contrast-enhanced CT shows a large metastatic node *(asterisk)* in the left pelvic cavity adjacent to the iliopsoas muscle.

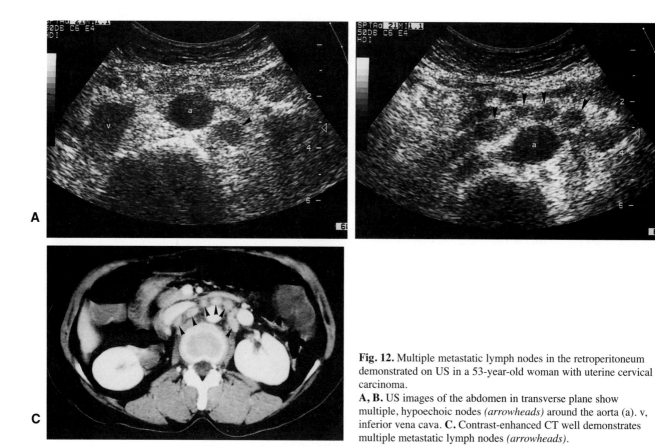

Fig. 12. Multiple metastatic lymph nodes in the retroperitoneum demonstrated on US in a 53-year-old woman with uterine cervical carcinoma.
A, B. US images of the abdomen in transverse plane show multiple, hypoechoic nodes *(arrowheads)* around the aorta (a). v, inferior vena cava. **C.** Contrast-enhanced CT well demonstrates multiple metastatic lymph nodes *(arrowheads)*.

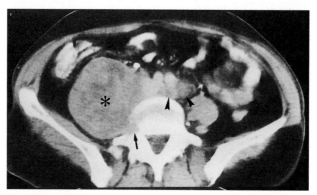

Fig. 13. Retroperitoneal metastatic lymphadenopathy mimicking a primary retroperitoneal tumor in a 39-year-old woman with uterine cervical carcinoma. Contrast-enhanced CT shows a round retroperitoneal mass *(asterisk)* mimicking a primary retroperitoneal tumor such as neurogenic tumor. Note destruction of the vertebra by the mass *(arrow)*. There are other small lymph nodes *(arrowheads)* behind the common iliac arteries, suggesting metastatic lymphadenopathy.

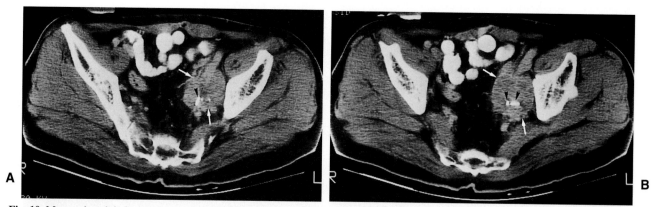

Fig. 10. Metastatic pelvic lymphadenopathy engulfing surgical clips that were used in a radical cystectomy for transitional cell carcinoma of the urinary bladder in a 74-year-old man.
A, B. Contrast-enhanced CT scans show large lymph nodes *(arrows)* engulfing surgical clips *(arrowheads)* in the left pelvic cavity.

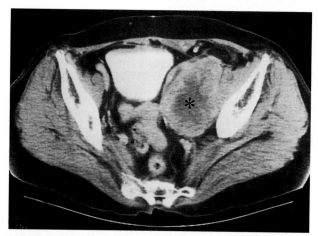

Fig. 11. Large metastatic pelvic lymph node in a 66-year-old woman with malignant melanoma. Contrast-enhanced CT shows a large metastatic node *(asterisk)* in the left pelvic cavity adjacent to the iliopsoas muscle.

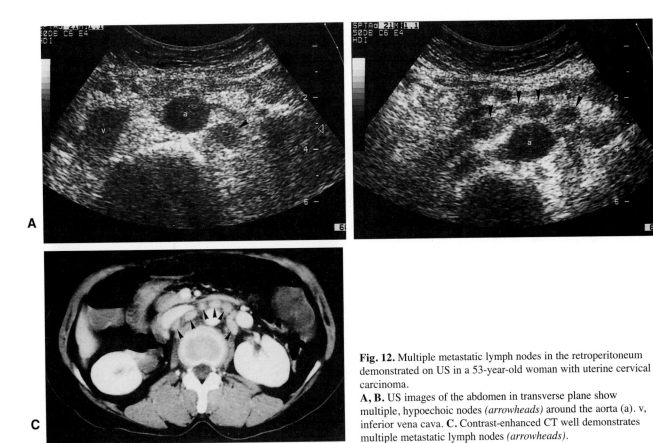

Fig. 12. Multiple metastatic lymph nodes in the retroperitoneum demonstrated on US in a 53-year-old woman with uterine cervical carcinoma.

A, B. US images of the abdomen in transverse plane show multiple, hypoechoic nodes *(arrowheads)* around the aorta (a). v, inferior vena cava. **C.** Contrast-enhanced CT well demonstrates multiple metastatic lymph nodes *(arrowheads)*.

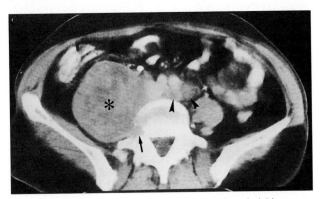

Fig. 13. Retroperitoneal metastatic lymphadenopathy mimicking a primary retroperitoneal tumor in a 39-year-old woman with uterine cervical carcinoma. Contrast-enhanced CT shows a round retroperitoneal mass *(asterisk)* mimicking a primary retroperitoneal tumor such as neurogenic tumor. Note destruction of the vertebra by the mass *(arrow)*. There are other small lymph nodes *(arrowheads)* behind the common iliac arteries, suggesting metastatic lymphadenopathy.

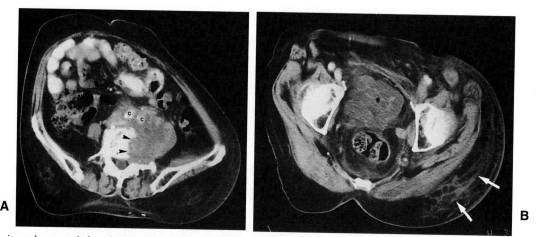

Fig. 14. Retroperitoneal metastatic lymphadenopathy with ipsilateral lymphedema.
A. Contrast-enhanced CT shows a large mass composed of conglomerated metastatic lymph nodes in the left retroperitoneum. Note that the mass extends behind the common iliac arteries (c) and destroys the vertebra *(arrowheads)*. **B.** CT scan at the pelvis level shows increased soft tissue streaks in the subcutaneous tissue *(arrows)* on the left side due to lymphedema.

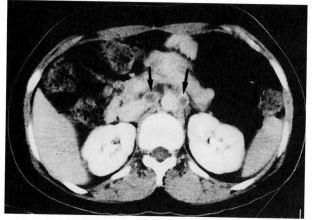

Fig. 15. Necrotic nodes in tuberculous lymphadenopathy. Contrast-enhanced CT shows multiple, enlarged lymph nodes, which have low attenuation due to caseation necrosis *(arrows)*.

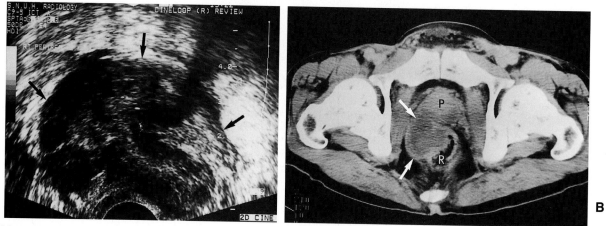

Fig. 16. Metastatic melanoma in the perirectal region in a 63-year-old man who underwent surgery for malignant melanoma in the left inguinal region 2 years earlier.
A. Transrectal US shows a large mass of heterogeneous echogenicity *(arrows)* adjacent to the prostate. **B.** Contrast-enhanced CT shows a mass of heterogeneous attenuation *(arrows)* between the prostate (P) and rectum (R), with invasion of those organs. Note the fibrotic scar in the left inguinal region due to previous surgery for the primary tumor in this region.

19. Retroperitoneal Fibrosis

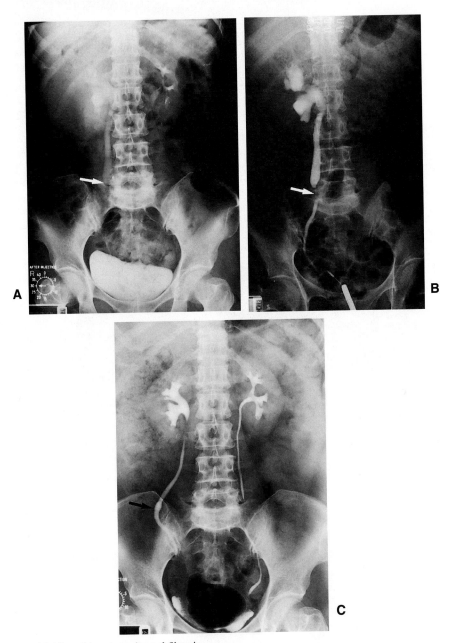

Fig. 1. A 55-year-old woman with idiopathic retroperitoneal fibrosis.
A. IVU taken 30 minutes after injection of contrast material shows hydronephrosis and hydroureter on the right side due to ureteral obstruction *(arrow)*. **B.** RGP shows severe focal stenosis of the right distal ureter *(arrow)* with smooth margin. (**B,** From Lee JS, Seong CK, Sim JS, et al: Retroperitoneal fibrosis: Spectrum of imaging findings. J Korean Radiol Soc 1999; 41:1177–1182.) **C.** Surgery disclosed severe retroperitoneal fibrosis. Adhesiolysis, ureteroureterostomy, and intraperitonealization of the ureter were performed on the right side. Follow-up IVU shows relieved ureteral obstruction and lateral deviation of the right ureter due to previous intraperitonealization *(arrow)*.

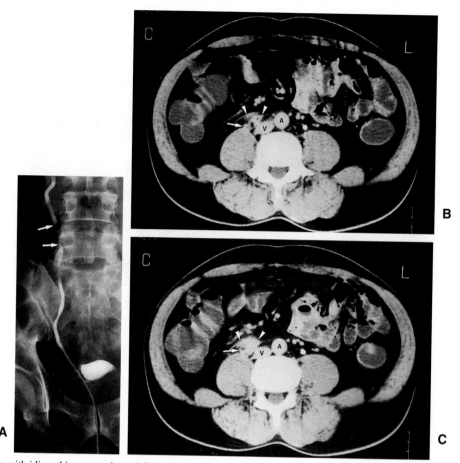

Fig. 2. A 58-year-old man with idiopathic retroperitoneal fibrosis.
A. RGP shows smooth stricture of the right distal ureter *(arrows)*. **B, C.** Contrast-enhanced CT scans show a soft tissue mass *(arrowheads)* involving right ureter *(arrow)*. V, inferior vena cava; A, aorta.

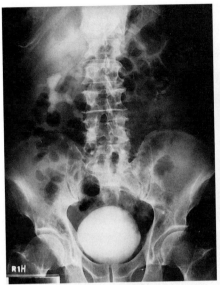

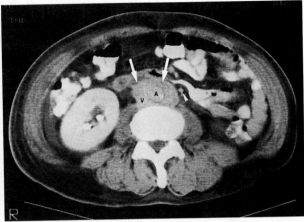

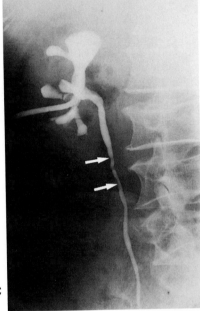

Fig. 3. A 67-year-old man with idiopathic retroperitoneal fibrosis.
A. IVU shows dilated pelvocalyces and proximal ureter on the right side.
B. Contrast-enhanced CT shows a soft tissue mantle *(arrows)* around the abdominal aorta (A) and inferior vena cava (V). Note that the right ureter is encased by the soft tissue mantle and therefore is not identified, but the left ureter is not involved and is well demonstrated *(arrowhead)*. (**B,** From Lee JS, Seong CK, Sim JS, et al: Retroperitoneal fibrosis: Spectrum of imaging findings. J Korean Radiol Soc 1999; 41:1177–1182.)
C. Percutaneous nephrostomy was performed and the nephrostogram shows smooth narrowing of the right midureter *(arrows)*.

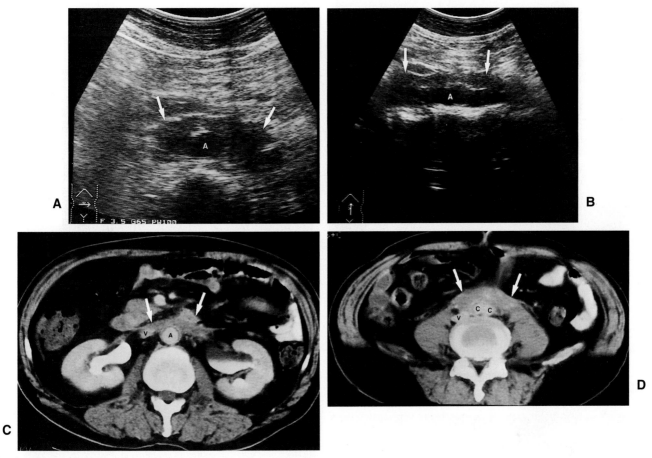

Fig. 4. A 67-year-old man with retroperitoneal fibrosis.
A, B. Abdominal US images in transverse (**A**) and longitudinal (**B**) planes show a hypoechoic soft tissue mantle *(arrows)* anterior and lateral to the aorta (A). **C, D.** Contrast-enhanced CT scans show bilateral hydronephrosis and a soft tissue mantle *(arrows)* adjacent to the distal abdominal aorta (A), inferior vena cava (V), and proximal common iliac arteries (C). Note that both ureters are encased by the mass and are not identified.

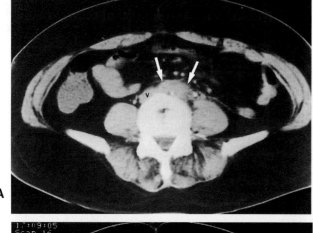

A

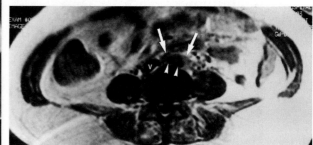

B

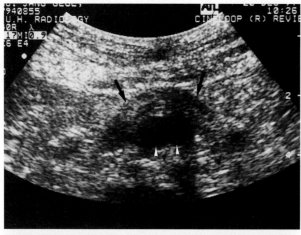

C

Fig. 5. A 58-year-old woman with retroperitoneal fibrosis treated with steroid therapy.
A. Contrast-enhanced CT shows a soft tissue mantle *(arrows)* obliterating the proximal common iliac arteries and left ureter. V, inferior vena cava. **B.** Contrast-enhanced T1-weighted MR image shows enhancing soft tissue mass *(arrows)* with encasement of the proximal common iliac arteries *(arrowheads)*. V, inferior vena cava. **C.** Follow-up, contrast-enhanced CT obtained 4 months later shows disappeared soft tissue mantle around the proximal common iliac arteries *(arrowheads)*. Also note that the left ureter is well identified and opacified with contrast material *(arrow)*. V, inferior vena cava.

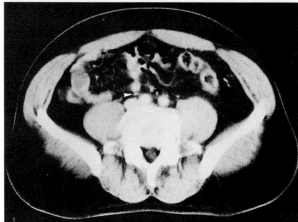

A

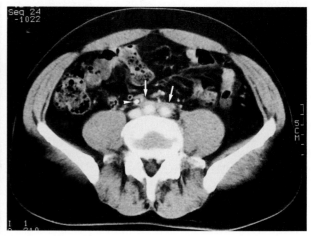

B

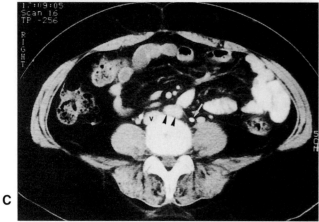

C

Fig. 6. A 42-year-old man with retroperitoneal fibrosis treated with steroid.
A. US of the abdomen in transverse plane shows a soft tissue mantle *(arrows)* anterior and lateral to the common iliac arteries *(arrowheads)*. **B.** Contrast-enhanced CT shows enhancing soft tissue mantle *(arrows)* around the common iliac arteries. Note that the right ureter *(arrowhead)* is dilated and encased by the lesion. **C.** Follow-up CT scan obtained 4 months later after steroid therapy shows disappeared soft tissue mantle and improved ureteral obstruction. The *arrowhead* indicates the normalized right ureter.

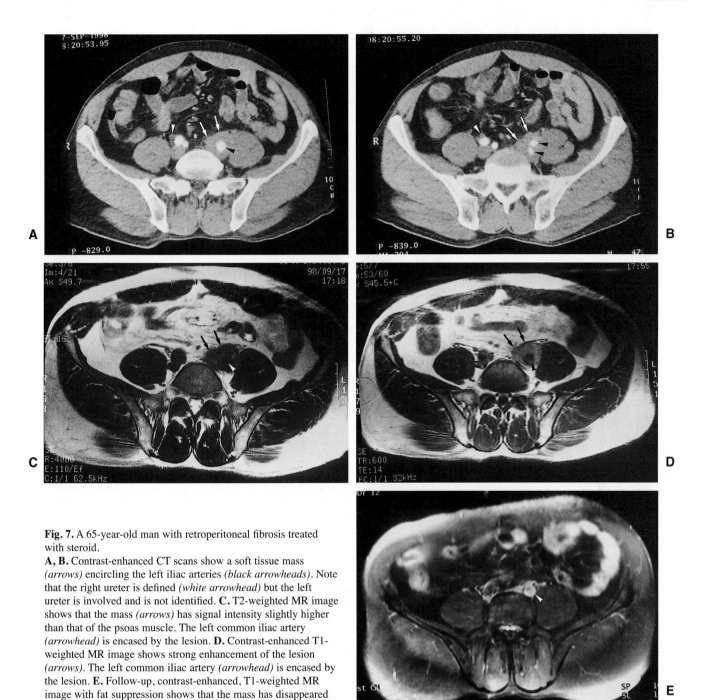

Fig. 7. A 65-year-old man with retroperitoneal fibrosis treated with steroid.
A, B. Contrast-enhanced CT scans show a soft tissue mass *(arrows)* encircling the left iliac arteries *(black arrowheads)*. Note that the right ureter is defined *(white arrowhead)* but the left ureter is involved and is not identified. **C.** T2-weighted MR image shows that the mass *(arrows)* has signal intensity slightly higher than that of the psoas muscle. The left common iliac artery *(arrowhead)* is encased by the lesion. **D.** Contrast-enhanced T1-weighted MR image shows strong enhancement of the lesion *(arrows)*. The left common iliac artery *(arrowhead)* is encased by the lesion. **E.** Follow-up, contrast-enhanced, T1-weighted MR image with fat suppression shows that the mass has disappeared and the left common iliac artery is well identified *(arrowhead)*.

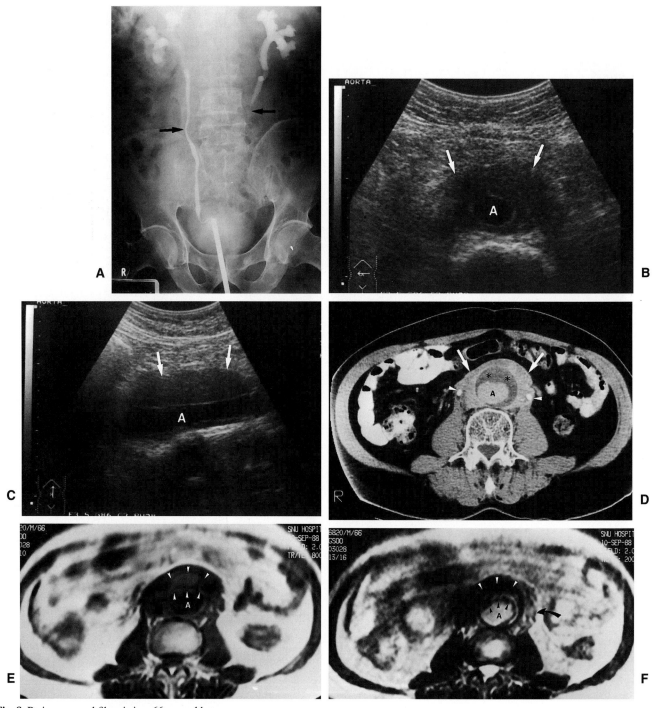

Fig. 8. Perianeurysmal fibrosis in a 66-year-old man.
A. RGP shows smooth stenosis on both midureters *(arrows)*. **B, C.** Abdominal US images in transverse **(B)** and longitudinal **(C)** planes show a large, hypoechoic, soft tissue mantle *(arrows)* around the dilated aorta (A). **D.** Contrast-enhanced CT shows the soft tissue mantle *(arrows)* around the dilated abdominal aorta (A). Note that the aorta has thick mural thrombi *(asterisks)*. Both ureters *(arrowheads)* are adherent to the periphery of the soft tissue mantle. **E, F.** T1-weighted **(E)** and T2-weighted **(F)** MR images show low signal intensity of the mass on both pulse sequences. Note that the signal intensity is higher in the left aspect of the mass *(curved arrow)*. Also note that the signal intensity of the mural thrombi *(arrowheads)* in the aorta (A) is heterogeneous.

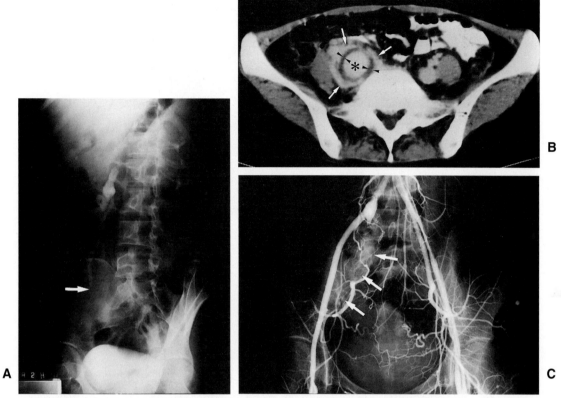

Fig. 9. A 29-year-old woman with perianeurysmal fibrosis with ureteral obstruction caused by mycotic aneurysm of the iliac artery.
A. Two-hour-delayed IVU in oblique projection shows obstruction of the right distal ureter *(arrow)* with hydronephrosis and hydroureter. Contrast material already has been excreted from the left urinary tract. **B.** Contrast-enhanced CT shows an aneurysm of the right iliac artery *(asterisk)* with low-attenuated mural thrombi *(arrowheads)* and enhancing soft tissue mantle *(arrows)* around the aneurysm. (**B,** From Lee JS, Seong CK, Sim JS, et al: Retroperitoneal fibrosis: Spectrum of imaging findings. J Korean Radiol Soc 1999; 41:1177–1182.) **C.** Arteriography shows faintly opacified, large aneurysms *(arrows)* in the right internal iliac artery.

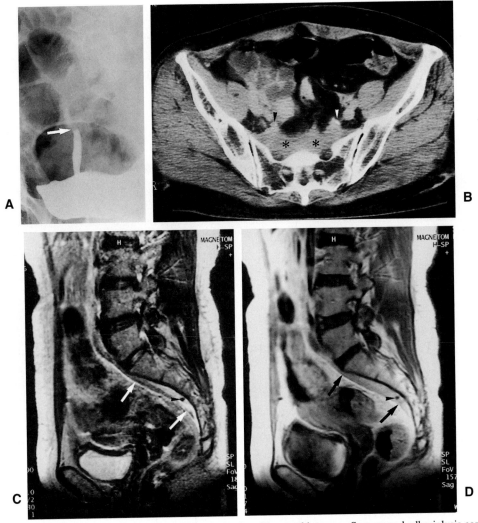

Fig. 10. Presacral retroperitoneal fibrosis causing right ureteral obstruction in a 55-year-old woman. Surgery and adhesiolysis confirmed the diagnosis of idiopathic retroperitoneal fibrosis. (**B, D**, From Lee JS, Seong CK, Sim JS, et al: Retroperitoneal fibrosis: Spectrum of imaging findings. J Korean Radiol Soc 1999; 41:1177–1182.)
A. RGP shows obstruction of the right distal ureter *(arrow).* **B.** Contrast-enhanced CT shows thick, soft tissue mantle in the presacral area *(asterisks).* Note that both ureters are adherent to the presacral lesion. The left ureter is opacified with contrast material *(white arrowhead),* but the right ureter *(black arrowhead)* is not opacified due to obstruction. **C.** T2-weighted sagittal MR image shows heterogeneous signal intensity of the presacral lesion *(arrows).* Note that the lesion encases a vessel that appears as a signal-void structure *(arrowhead).* **D.** Contrast-enhanced T1-weighted sagittal MR image shows that the lesion enhances well *(arrows).* The encased vessel is also seen as a signal-void structure on this image *(arrowhead).*

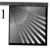

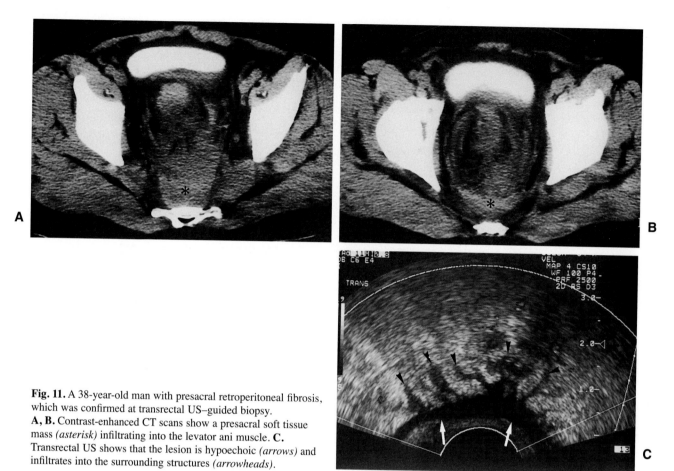

Fig. 11. A 38-year-old man with presacral retroperitoneal fibrosis, which was confirmed at transrectal US–guided biopsy.
A, B. Contrast-enhanced CT scans show a presacral soft tissue mass *(asterisk)* infiltrating into the levator ani muscle. **C.** Transrectal US shows that the lesion is hypoechoic *(arrows)* and infiltrates into the surrounding structures *(arrowheads)*.

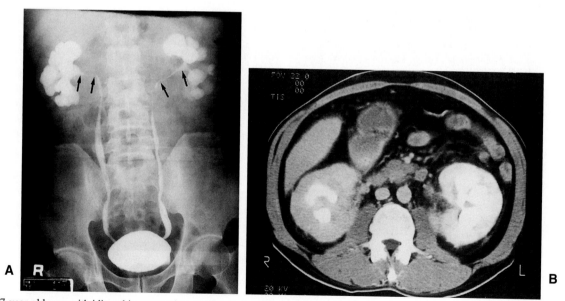

Fig. 12. A 47-year-old man with idiopathic retroperitoneal fibrosis involving the renal sinus.
A. IVU shows bilateral hydronephrosis caused by smooth narrowing of the renal pelvis *(arrows)*. **B.** Contrast-enhanced CT shows dilated calyces. Renal sinus fat is not demonstrable due to infiltration of soft tissue lesion in the renal sinus with narrowing of the renal pelvis and calyceal infundibula.

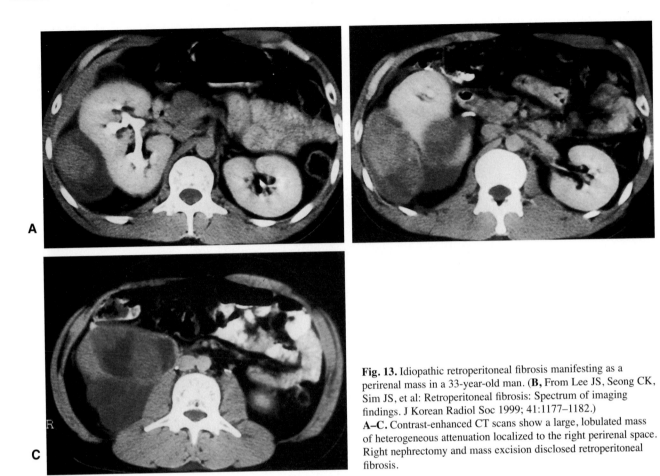

Fig. 13. Idiopathic retroperitoneal fibrosis manifesting as a perirenal mass in a 33-year-old man. (**B,** From Lee JS, Seong CK, Sim JS, et al: Retroperitoneal fibrosis: Spectrum of imaging findings. J Korean Radiol Soc 1999; 41:1177–1182.)
A–C. Contrast-enhanced CT scans show a large, lobulated mass of heterogeneous attenuation localized to the right perirenal space. Right nephrectomy and mass excision disclosed retroperitoneal fibrosis.

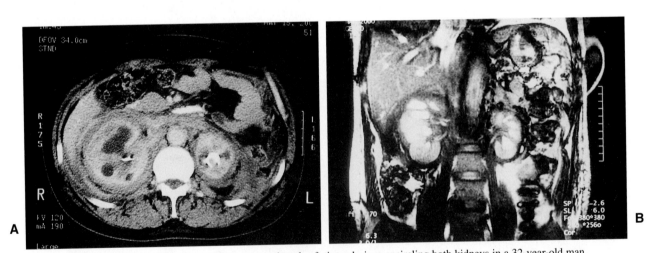

Fig. 14. Idiopathic retroperitoneal fibrosis manifesting as perirenal soft tissue lesions encircling both kidneys in a 32-year-old man.
A. Contrast-enhanced CT shows a soft tissue mantle in the perirenal spaces encircling both kidneys. Note the ureteral stents in both kidneys.
B. T2-weighted coronal MR image shows dark signal of the perirenal lesions, indicating that the lesions are composed of mature fibrotic tissue.

20. Retroperitoneal Abscess

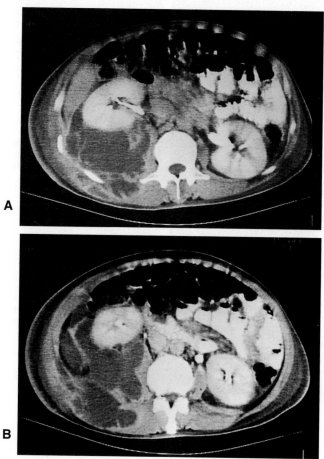

Fig. 1. A 50-year-old diabetic man with retroperitoneal abscess.
A, B. Contrast-enhanced CT scans show a large retroperitoneal abscess involving the right perirenal and posterior pararenal spaces and back muscles. The right kidney is displaced anteriorly by the abscess. Incision and drainage were performed, and the causative organism was determined to be *Staphylococcus aureus*.

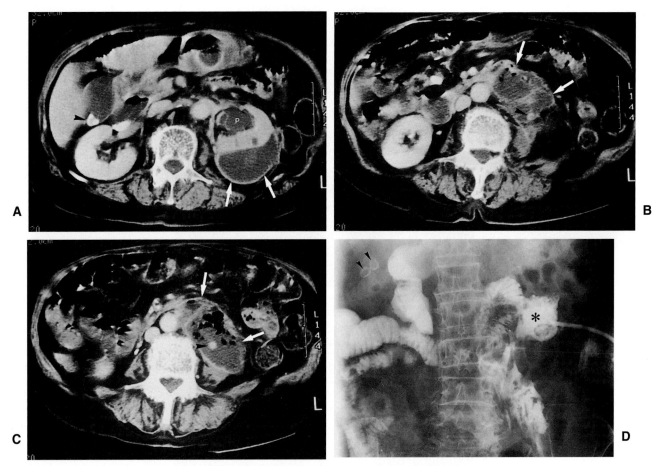

Fig. 2. Subcapsular and perirenal abscesses communicating with the small intestine in a 82-year-old woman with longstanding diabetes mellitus.
A. Contrast-enhanced CT shows subcapsular fluid collection *(arrows)* posterior to the left kidney. Also note the dilated left renal pelvis (P) and a stone in the gallbladder *(arrowhead)*. **B, C.** CT scans at lower level show that the abscess *(arrows)* extends to the lower perirenal space encircling the proximal ureter *(arrowhead)*. Note gas bubbles in the abscess cavity, suggesting either gas-forming bacterial infection or communication with the bowel. **D.** Percutaneous catheter drainage was done, and injection of contrast material through the catheter demonstrates abscess cavity *(asterisk)* communicating with the small bowels. Also note stones in the gallbladder *(arrowheads)*.

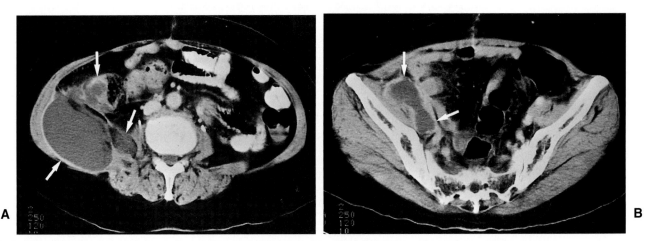

Fig. 3. A 60-year-old woman with retroperitoneal abscess that occurred after radical hysterectomy for uterine cervical carcinoma.
A, B. Contrast-enhanced CT scans show multiloculated abscesses *(arrows)* with a thick, enhancing rim in the left pelvic wall, which were managed with percutaneous catheter drainage.

21. Retroperitoneal Urinoma

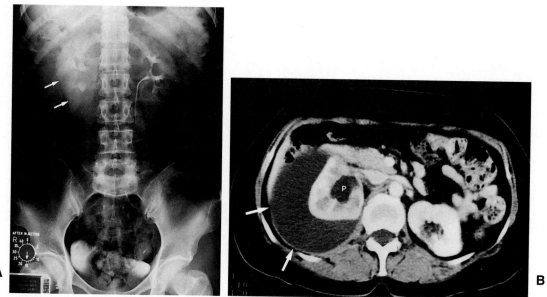

A **B**

Fig. 1. A 55-year-old woman with a large urinoma in the right perirenal space. The patient had right ureteral obstruction due to retroperitoneal fibrosis. **A.** IVU shows obstruction of the right urinary tract and indentation on the right renal contour at the lower lateral aspect *(arrows)*. **B.** Contrast-enhanced CT shows a large amount of fluid collection in the right perirenal space *(arrows)* due to urinoma. Also note the dilated renal pelvis (P) and delayed excretion in the right kidney. (**B,** From Lee JS, Seong CK, Sim JS, et al: Retroperitoneal fibrosis: Spectrum of imaging findings. J Korean Radiol Soc 1999; 41:1177–1182.)

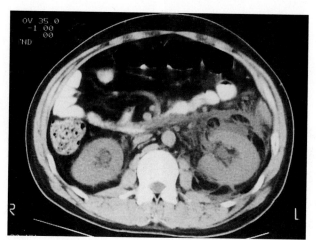

Fig. 2. Urine leak into the perirenal space in a 40-year-old man who had bilateral hydronephrosis following Miles operation for rectal cancer. Nonenhanced CT shows bilateral hydronephrosis and urine leak in the left perirenal space. Note accentuated bridging septa due to leak of urine.

22. Retroperitoneal Hematoma

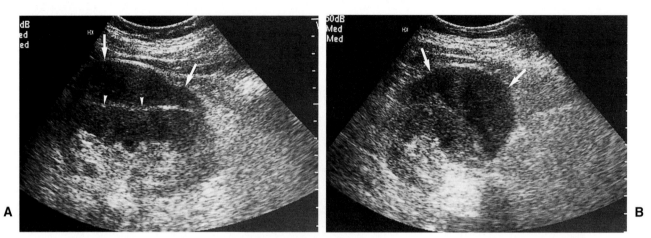

Fig. 1. Subcapsular hematoma that occurred following extracorporeal shock-wave lithotripsy.
A, B. US images in longitudinal (**A**) and transverse (**B**) planes show a crescent-shaped fluid collection *(arrows)* lateral to the left kidney. Note that the left renal contour is slightly deformed *(arrowheads* in **A**) due to compression by the fluid collection. Note that the lesion has fine internal echoes. The subcapsular hematoma resorbed spontaneously on follow-up.

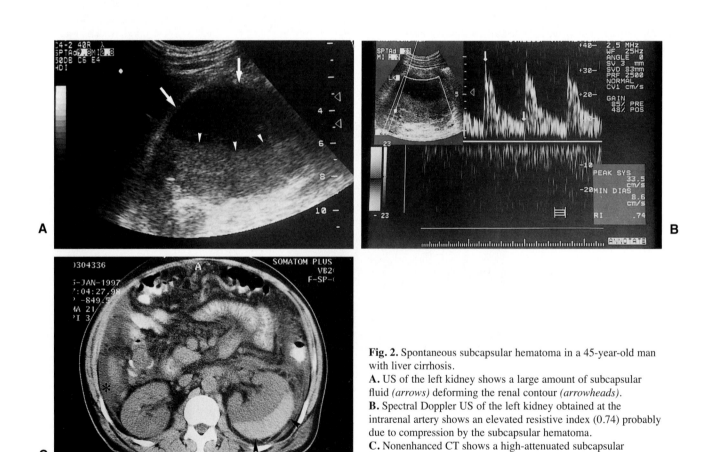

Fig. 2. Spontaneous subcapsular hematoma in a 45-year-old man with liver cirrhosis.
A. US of the left kidney shows a large amount of subcapsular fluid *(arrows)* deforming the renal contour *(arrowheads)*.
B. Spectral Doppler US of the left kidney obtained at the intrarenal artery shows an elevated resistive index (0.74) probably due to compression by the subcapsular hematoma.
C. Nonenhanced CT shows a high-attenuated subcapsular hematoma *(arrowheads)* posterior to the left kidney. Also note ascites in the peritoneal cavity *(asterisk)*.

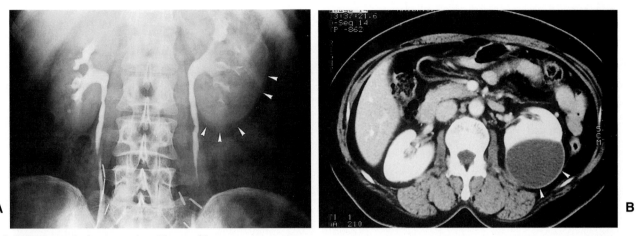

Fig. 3. Old subcapsular hematoma in a 46-year-old woman.
A. A 15-minute IVU shows a large left kidney and compressed calyces. Note the double contour of the kidney in the lower polar region *(arrowheads)*.
B. Contrast-enhanced CT shows a large subcapsular mass with a thick wall *(arrowheads)* that suggests an old subcapsular hematoma.

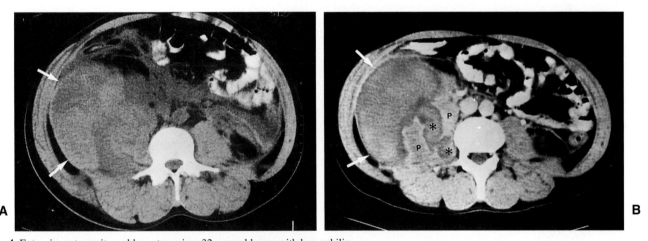

Fig. 4. Extensive retroperitoneal hematoma in a 32-year-old man with hemophilia.
A, B. Nonenhanced **(A)** and contrast-enhanced **(B)** CT scans of the abdomen show extensive hematoma in the right retroperitoneum *(arrows)*. Note that the hematoma has heterogeneous high attenuation on nonenhanced CT and the extent of the hematoma is well delineated on contrast-enhanced CT. Note that the hematoma *(asterisks)* extends into the psoas muscle (P).

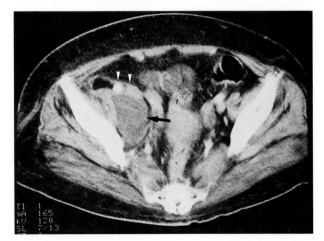

Fig. 5. Retroperitoneal hematoma that occurred following traumatic catheterization of the femoral artery for coronary arteriography in a 56-year-old woman. Contrast-enhanced CT shows a hematoma *(arrow)* posterior to the right external iliac vessels *(arrowheads)*.

23. Other Fluid Collections of the Retroperitoneum

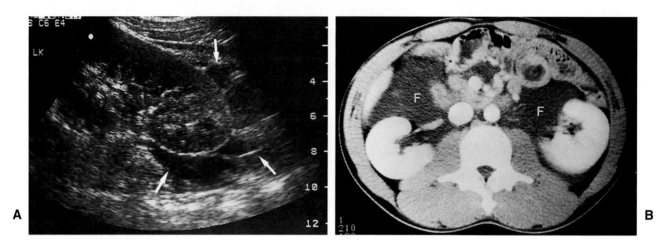

Fig. 1. Perirenal lymphangiectasia in a 30-year-old man with mediastinal lymphoma.
A. US of the left kidney in longitudinal plane shows perirenal fluid collection with septations *(arrows)* below the left kidney. **B.** Contrast-enhanced CT shows fluid collection in the perirenal and anterior pararenal spaces bilaterally (F).

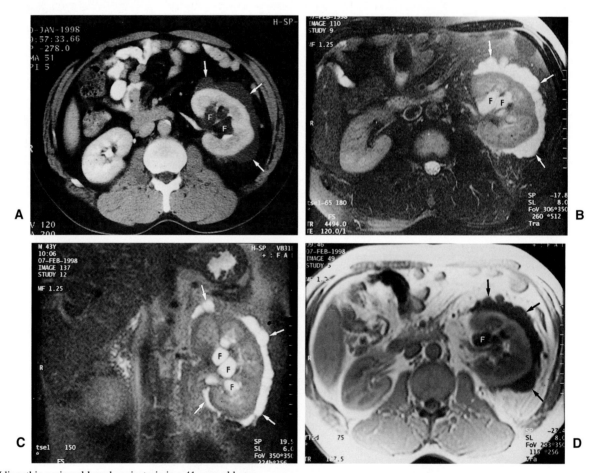

Fig. 2. Idiopathic perirenal lymphangiectasia in a 41-year-old man.
A. Contrast-enhanced CT shows fluid collection around the left kidney, probably in the perirenal space and marginated by the bridging septa *(arrows)*. Also note the parapelvic cysts in the renal sinus (F). **B, C.** T2-weighted MR images in axial **(B)** and coronal **(C)** planes show that the lesions in the perirenal space *(arrows)* and renal sinus (F) have homogeneous high intensity. **D.** Contrast-enhanced T1-weighted MR image in axial plane shows that the lesions *(arrows* and F) do not enhance.

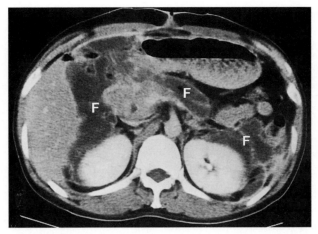

Fig. 3. Retroperitoneal fluid collection in traumatic pancreas avulsion of the pancreatic head in a 50-year-old man. Contrast-enhanced CT scan shows extensive fluid collection (F) in the perirenal and anterior pararenal spaces.

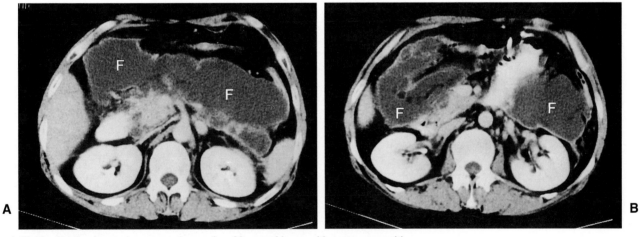

Fig. 4. Fluid collection in anterior pararenal space in a 39-year-old man with acute pancreatitis.
A, B. Contrast-enhanced CT scans show a large amount of fluid collection in the anterior pararenal space (F).

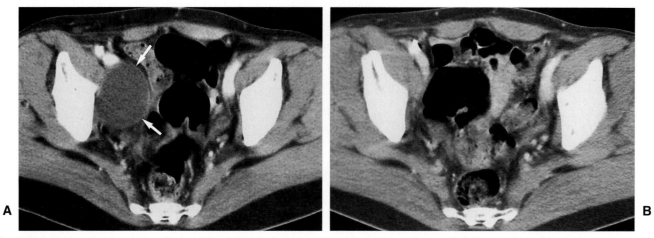

Fig. 5. Postoperative lymphocele in a 53-year-old woman who had undergone radical hysterectomy and pelvic node dissection for uterine cervical carcinoma 2 years earlier.
A. Contrast-enhanced CT shows a round, thin-walled, cystic lesion *(arrows)* in the right pelvic wall. Transvaginal US–guided aspiration revealed clear serous fluid. **B.** Follow-up CT scan obtained 1 year later shows disappeared cystic lesion.

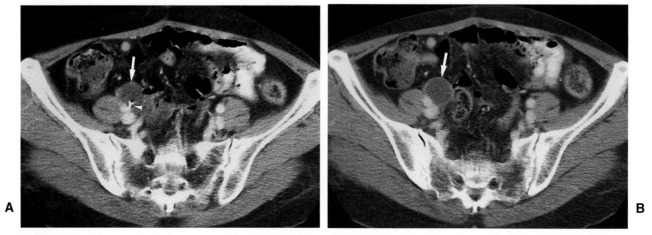

Fig. 6. Small postoperative lymphocele in a 54-year-old woman who underwent hysterectomy and bilateral salpingo-oophorectomy and pelvic node biopsy 1 year earlier.
A, B. Contrast-enhanced CT scans show a small, round, thin-walled, cystic lesion *(arrow)* in the right pelvic wall. Note a surgical clip *(arrowhead in* **A***)* adjacent to the cystic lesion.

24. Miscellaneous Retroperitoneal Diseases and Calcifications

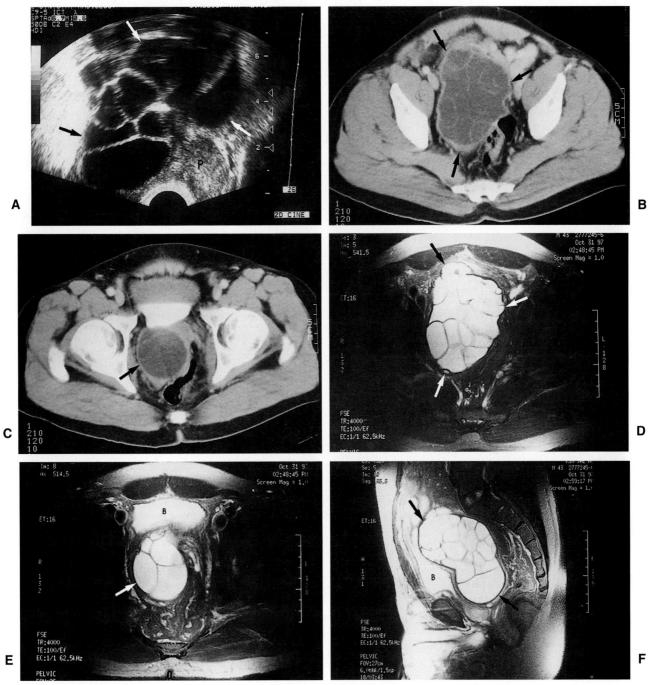

Fig. 1. Echinococcal cysts in a 43-year-old man who had visited Saudi Arabia 10 years earlier.
A. Transrectal US in transverse plane shows a large, septated, cystic mass *(arrows)* in the right pelvic cavity above the prostate (P). **B, C.** Contrast-enhanced CT scans show a thick-walled, cystic mass with abundant septa in the right pelvic cavity *(arrows)*. **D–F.** T2-weighted axial **(D, E)** and sagittal **(F)** MR images well demonstrate the septated cystic mass *(arrows)*. B, urinary bladder.

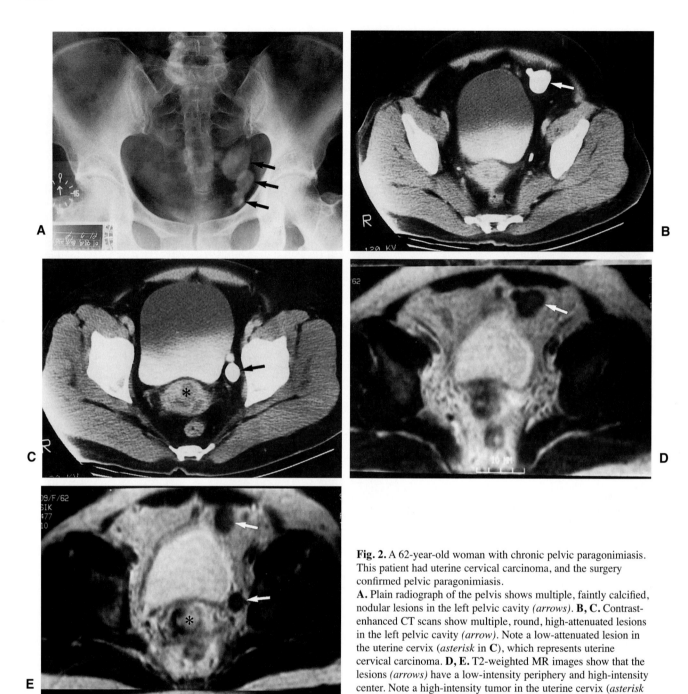

Fig. 2. A 62-year-old woman with chronic pelvic paragonimiasis. This patient had uterine cervical carcinoma, and the surgery confirmed pelvic paragonimiasis.
A. Plain radiograph of the pelvis shows multiple, faintly calcified, nodular lesions in the left pelvic cavity *(arrows)*. **B, C.** Contrast-enhanced CT scans show multiple, round, high-attenuated lesions in the left pelvic cavity *(arrow)*. Note a low-attenuated lesion in the uterine cervix *(asterisk in* **C**), which represents uterine cervical carcinoma. **D, E.** T2-weighted MR images show that the lesions *(arrows)* have a low-intensity periphery and high-intensity center. Note a high-intensity tumor in the uterine cervix *(asterisk in* **E**).

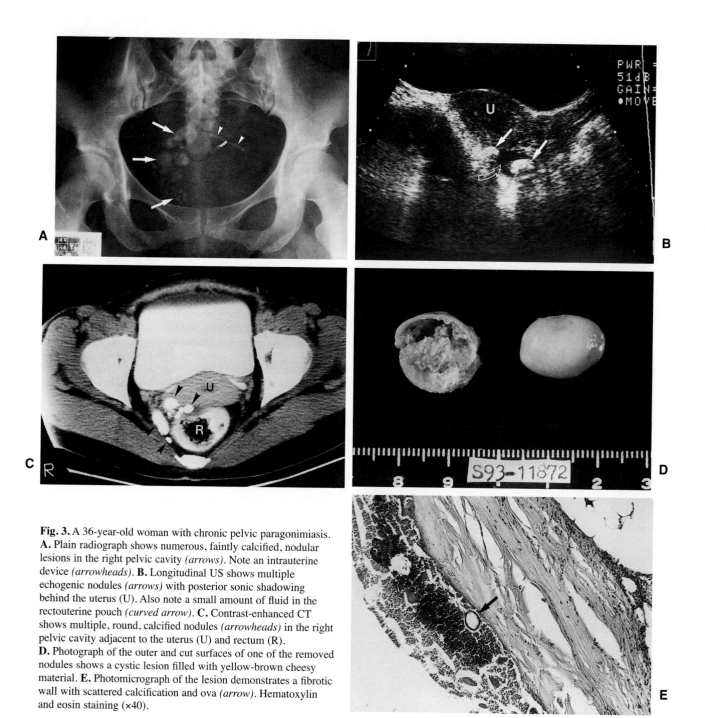

Fig. 3. A 36-year-old woman with chronic pelvic paragonimiasis. **A.** Plain radiograph shows numerous, faintly calcified, nodular lesions in the right pelvic cavity *(arrows)*. Note an intrauterine device *(arrowheads)*. **B.** Longitudinal US shows multiple echogenic nodules *(arrows)* with posterior sonic shadowing behind the uterus (U). Also note a small amount of fluid in the rectouterine pouch *(curved arrow)*. **C.** Contrast-enhanced CT shows multiple, round, calcified nodules *(arrowheads)* in the right pelvic cavity adjacent to the uterus (U) and rectum (R). **D.** Photograph of the outer and cut surfaces of one of the removed nodules shows a cystic lesion filled with yellow-brown cheesy material. **E.** Photomicrograph of the lesion demonstrates a fibrotic wall with scattered calcification and ova *(arrow)*. Hematoxylin and eosin staining (×40).

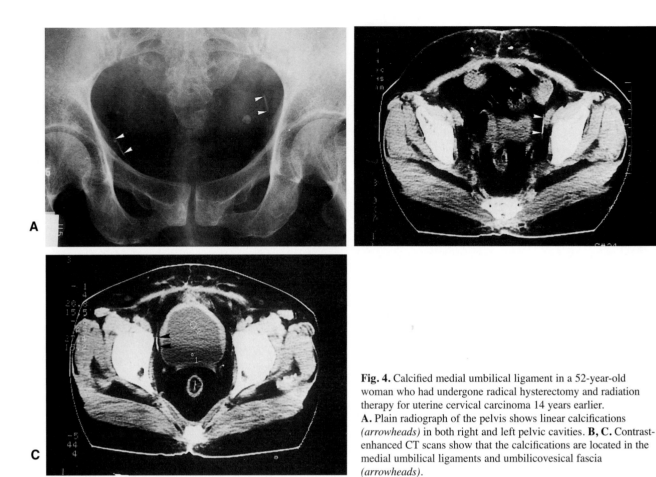

Fig. 4. Calcified medial umbilical ligament in a 52-year-old woman who had undergone radical hysterectomy and radiation therapy for uterine cervical carcinoma 14 years earlier.
A. Plain radiograph of the pelvis shows linear calcifications *(arrowheads)* in both right and left pelvic cavities. **B, C.** Contrast-enhanced CT scans show that the calcifications are located in the medial umbilical ligaments and umbilicovesical fascia *(arrowheads)*.

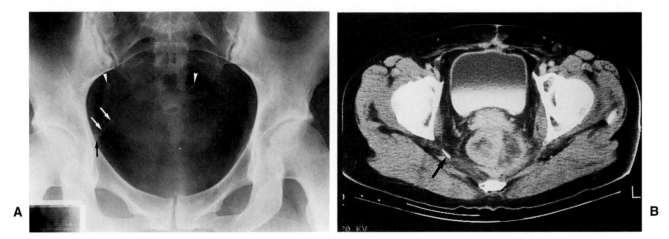

Fig. 5. Sacrospinous ligament calcification in a 42-year-old woman with rectal cancer.
A. Plain radiograph shows a linear calcification *(white arrows)* continuous with the right ischial spine *(black arrow)*. Also note radiopacities of rings for tubal ligation *(arrowheads)*. **B.** Contrast-enhanced CT confirms that the calcification *(arrow)* is located in the course of the sacrospinous ligament.

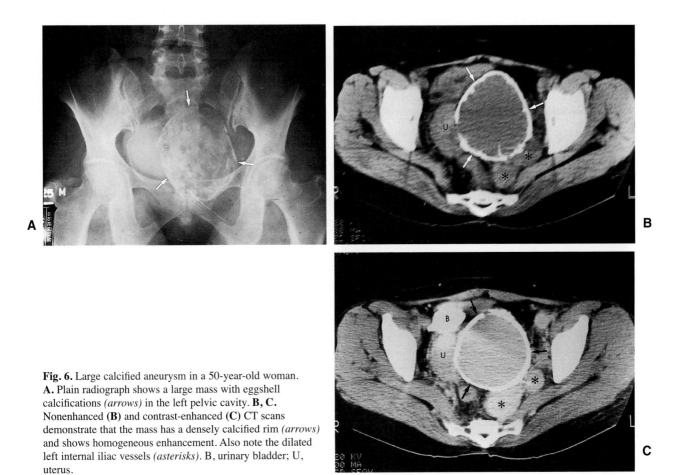

Fig. 6. Large calcified aneurysm in a 50-year-old woman.
A. Plain radiograph shows a large mass with eggshell
calcifications *(arrows)* in the left pelvic cavity. **B, C.**
Nonenhanced **(B)** and contrast-enhanced **(C)** CT scans
demonstrate that the mass has a densely calcified rim *(arrows)*
and shows homogeneous enhancement. Also note the dilated
left internal iliac vessels *(asterisks)*. B, urinary bladder; U,
uterus.

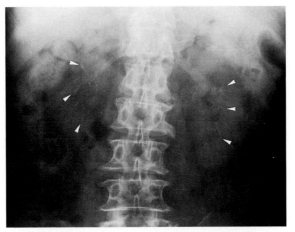

Fig. 7. Calcified renal arterial branches in a 62-year-old woman who
suffered from diabetes mellitus for 15 years. Plain radiograph shows
linear, branching calcifications in both kidneys *(arrowheads)*.

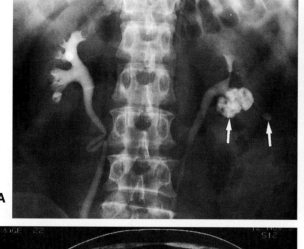

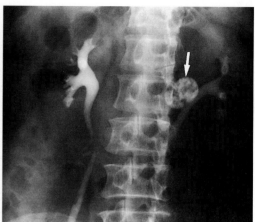

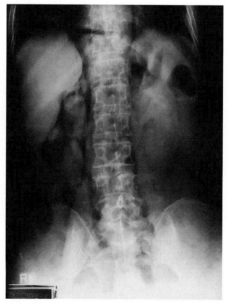

Fig. 8. Calcified mesenteric lymph nodes in a 58-year-old man with a history of pulmonary tuberculosis.

A, B. IVU images in anteroposterior **(A)** and oblique **(B)** projections show calcifications *(arrows)* anterior to the left kidney. **C.** Contrast-enhanced CT scans show that the lesions are calcified mesenteric lymph nodes *(arrows).*

Fig. 9. Pneumoretroperitoneum due to perforation of the sigmoid colon during colonoscopy in a 57-year-old woman. Plain radiograph shows air collections in the retroperitoneal spaces.

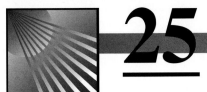

25

Adrenal Gland

JUNG SUK SIM AND WILLIAM H. BUSH, JR.

The adrenal gland, when functionally abnormal, is closely related to systemic diseases. Its abnormal production of hormones can give rise to endocrinologic diseases, and some endocrinologic diseases influence the adrenal glands. Various primary and metastatic tumors occur in the adrenal glands. Invasive methods such as venous sampling or biopsy have been used to evaluate the adrenal gland, but they have been largely replaced by computed tomography (CT) or magnetic resonance (MR) imaging.

The adrenal gland is a small organ, composed of the cortex and medulla. The adrenal cortex has three layers: zona glomerularis, zona fasciculata, and zona reticularis. These zones produce the hormones aldosterone, cortisol, and androgen, respectively. The adrenal medulla is made up of paraganglionic chromaffin cells originated from neuroectoderm. Catecholamine is released from the adrenal medulla.

CUSHING'S SYNDROME

Cushing's syndrome is caused by any condition in which the plasma cortisol level is elevated. The two major mechanisms that cause Cushing's syndrome are overstimulation of the adrenal glands by adrenocorticotropic hormone (ACTH) and autonomous overproduction of cortisol from the adrenal glands. About 80% of Cushing's syndrome is caused by a pituitary adenoma inducing excess ACTH. The remaining 20% of Cushing's syndrome is caused by an adrenal adenoma, an adrenal cortical carcinoma, or ectopic ACTH production by nonadrenal tumors. Differentiation among these causes relies basically on biochemical studies, such as the dexamethasone suppression test with 24-hour urine collection. If dexamethasone can suppress cortisol production, the work-up can be focused on searching for a pituitary adenoma, best done first by MR imaging of the sella.

In unsuppressed cases on dexamethasone suppression test, CT should be done in search of adrenal masses. Characteristic findings of functioning adrenal adenoma are 2- to 4-cm, round, well-marginated masses of homogeneous attenuation. The Hounsfield unit (HU) of an adrenal adenoma is usually less than 10 due to the rich content of cholesterol.

In addition to adrenal adenoma, several diseases can produce cortisol autonomously. Longstanding stimulation by the pituitary gland can cause a condition called *multinodular hyperplasia* that is dependent on ACTH. However, sometimes these nodules can become larger and function autonomously.

This condition is called *massive macronodular hyperplasia*. Primary pigmented nodular adrenal disease is another entity that shows autonomy; the adrenals are composed of multiple, small, yellow nodules made up of lipofuscin pigment. An adrenal mass in a cushingoid patient always has the possibility of being a cortical carcinoma, especially when the mass is larger than 5 cm. Adrenal cortical carcinoma often infiltrates into the adjacent structures, including the liver, kidney, and inferior vena cava.

An ectopic ACTH-producing tumor is another condition that may cause Cushing's syndrome. Small cell cancer of the lung and bronchial or thymic carcinoid are common ones. Because carcinoids are usually small and grow very slowly, one can miss the diagnosis even when the signs of Cushing's syndrome are obvious.

CONN'S SYNDROME

Conn's syndrome represents excess production of aldosterone resulting in hypertension and hypokalemia. More than 80% of Conn's syndrome is due to a benign adrenal adenoma, an aldosteronoma. Aldosteronoma is a small nodular tumor, usually less than 1 cm. Therefore, it is difficult to detect the aldosteronoma or differentiate it from multinodular adrenal hyperplasia, even in patients who have hyperaldosteronism. The diagnosis of hyperaldosteronism is made by laboratory test. The goal of imaging is to detect a dominant adenoma that would allow for surgical excision and cure, thereby avoiding the need for medical suppressive therapy with attendant side effects. CT is the most suitable radiologic method to detect aldosteronoma. However, CT can miss small aldosteronomas if careful technique with thin slices is not used.

VIRILIZATION

Virilization means an expression of masculine features in prepubertal boys and in women of any age. Adrenal hyperplasia that is due to congenital deficiency of 21-hydroxylase is a main cause of virilization. Deficiency of that enzyme blocks the synthesis of adrenocortical steroids, which induces chronic overproduction of ACTH in the pituitary gland and then the steroid precursor, pregnanetriol, in the adrenal gland, causing virilization.

Adrenal glands of congenital adrenal hyperplasia are enlarged but have a smooth contour. An adrenal limb thicker

than 1 cm or thicker than the adjacent diaphragm is considered hyperplastic. The rarer causes of virilization are tumors of adrenal glands or ovaries. Among adrenal tumors, malignancy is a much more common cause of virilization than are benign lesions. CT usually demonstrates the causative tumors.

PHEOCHROMOCYTOMA

Pheochromocytoma is a tumor of paraganglionic chromaffin cells in the adrenal medulla that secretes epinephrine and norepinephrine. The name *pheochromocytoma* is applied when the tumor is in the adrenal gland. If the tumor is found in an extra-adrenal site, it is called *paraganglioma*, although it has the same histology. Pheochromocytomas associated with von Hippel-Lindau disease or multiple endocrine neoplasia type 2 or 3 are frequently bilateral, and some of them have normal levels of catecholamine. Diagnosis is based on laboratory tests and can be made on the basis of 24-hour urine vanillylmandelic acid and plasma catecholamine levels.

CT findings of pheochromocytoma are variable. Small tumors are well defined and show homogeneous attenuation, whereas larger tumors usually have areas of necrosis and cystic changes. Calcification is rare in pheochromocytoma. Pheochromocytoma often appears as a well-marginated, high signal intensity mass on T2-weighted MR imaging. However, about one third have low signal areas due to old hemorrhage. Needle biopsy or aspiration should never be tried because mechanical stimulation of a pheochromocytoma can lead to hypertensive crisis.

About 10% of pheochromocytomas are bilateral, although these are more often associated with a syndrome. The incidence of malignancy is also about 10%, though more often with a solitary pheochromocytoma. Common metastatic sites are bones, lymph nodes, lungs, and liver. Meta-iodobenzylguanidine (MIBG) scan is the most suitable method to look for metastatic lesions.

ADDISON'S DISEASE

Addison's disease is a consequence of adrenal insufficiency. Infection, metastasis, shock, and hemorrhage are the major causes. Histoplasmosis and tuberculosis are the most common infections that lead to calcification. Not all bilateral adrenal calcification means adrenal insufficiency.

ADRENAL ADENOMA VERSUS METASTASIS

Both adenoma and metastasis are relatively common tumors in the adrenal glands. Incidentally found adenomas are small and usually contain much lipid. They grow slowly and may have a subclinical level of endocrine activity. Adrenal metastasis is rare in patients who do not have a known primary site. Metastases may be small, but more than 80% of them are larger than 3 cm when discovered. They never have fat unless they are from liposarcoma.

Once an unexpected adrenal mass is found on nonenhanced CT, a mass with attenuation of less than 10 HU is most likely an adenoma, and when the attenuation is 0 HU or less, the specificity approaches 100%. This is a very specific finding, but many benign adenomas have attenuation numbers greater than 10 HU. An adrenal mass in a patient who has known malignancy of another organ is more likely a metastasis, especially when the patient has metastasis at other sites.

Identification of lipid in the mass is the key for differentiation between adrenal adenoma and metastasis. Among MR sequences, chemical shift imaging shows the most sensitive results. Significant difference of signal intensity between in-phase and out-of-phase MR images means the presence of a considerable amount of lipid in the mass and confirms an adenoma. Fat saturation images have proved not to be sensitive enough. In some cases needle biopsy may be necessary. In the differentiation of incidentally found adrenal mass in a patient who does not have known malignancy, size plays an important role. If the mass is larger than 3 cm, MR imaging or biopsy should be performed to exclude the possibility of malignancy, such as metastasis or adrenal carcinoma.

Chemical shift MR imaging has the same sensitivity as nonenhanced CT for detecting characteristic lipid content. Neither can confirm a lipid-poor adenoma as being benign. "Contrast-washout" series CT imaging can identify the lipid-poor adenoma, because washout is more rapid from adenomas than from metastases.

OTHER TUMORS OF THE ADRENAL GLAND

Lymphoma

Reportedly 25% of patients who die of lymphoma have adrenal involvement. Non-Hodgkin's lymphoma involves adrenal glands more frequently than does Hodgkin's disease. Adrenal involvement is common when the kidney and retroperitoneum are also involved. Diffuse adrenal enlargement is the most common manifestation, and adrenal function is usually preserved.

Myelolipoma

Adrenal myelolipoma is a hamartoma of the adrenal gland composed of fat and myeloid tissue. It is usually bilateral and frequently hemorrhagic. Depending on the amount of fat, myelolipoma presents as a fatty mass or a nonfatty, soft tissue mass. Calcification is present in 25% of adrenal myelolipomas.

Leiomyoma

Several cases of adrenal leiomyoma have been reported, mainly in patients with acquired immunodeficiency syndrome. They are small and round with peripheral enhancement. Differential diagnosis should include Kaposi's sarcoma, lymphoma, tuberculosis, and hemorrhage.

Hemangioma

Adrenal hemangioma is a vascular mass, frequently with calcifications. Enhancement pattern is similar to hemangioma of other organs. Since it is not clearly differentiated from carcinoma on imaging studies, most of them are surgically removed.

ADRENAL CYSTS

Adrenal cysts may be congenital, but more often they are formed from previous hemorrhage or trauma. Cysts can grow and cause pain, especially when hemorrhage is associated. Calcification may be found in the cyst wall, and infection may be a complication.

ADRENAL HEMORRHAGE

The appearance of adrenal hemorrhage depends on the patient's age and timing of hemorrhage. Neonatal adrenal hemorrhage is initially found as a cystic mass and changes into a small, solid mass and then eventually disappears. Neonatal adrenal hemorrhage is more frequent on the right side. The explanation for higher susceptibility of the right adrenal is the greater likelihood of compression between the liver and the spine, and because the right adrenal vein usually drains directly into the inferior vena cava. Differentiation from neuroblastoma is always problematic. In adults, adrenal hematoma is caused by stress, burns, sepsis, renal vein thrombosis, liver transplantation, or trauma. Hemorrhage may also occur during the first 3 weeks of initiation of anticoagulation therapy.

ADRENAL CALCIFICATION

Adrenal calcification is caused by tuberculosis, histoplasmosis, and hemorrhage. Calcification is often seen in adrenal neuroblastoma. Wolman's disease, which is a familial xanthomatosis due to accumulation of triglyceride and cholesterol ester, also can cause splenomegaly and adrenal calcification.

Benign cysts often have calcification in the wall, and at times it may be quite thick. Adrenal carcinoma frequently has heterogeneous calcifications.

References

1. Caoli EM, Korobkin M, Francis IR, et al: Delayed enhanced CT of lipid-poor adrenal adenomas. AJR Am J Roentgenol 2000; 175:1411–1415.
2. Pena CS, Boland GWL, Hahn PF, et al: Characterization of indeterminate (lipid-poor) adrenal masses: Use of washout characteristics at contrast-enhanced CT. Radiology 2000; 217:798–802.
3. Korobkin M, Brodeur FJ, Francis IR, et al: CT time-attenuation washout curves of adrenal adenomas and nonadenomas. AJR Am J Roentgenol 1998; 170:747–752.
4. Marotti M, Sucic Z, Krolo I, et al: Adrenal cavernous hemangioma: MRI, CT, and US appearance. Eur Radiol 1997; 7:691–694.
5. Cyran KM, Kenney PJ, Memel DS, et al: Adrenal myelolipoma. AJR Am J Roentgenol 1996; 166:395–400.
6. Dunnick NR, Korobkin M, Francis I: Adrenal radiology: Distinguishing benign from malignant adrenal masses. AJR Am J Roentgenol 1996; 167:861–867.
7. Korobkin M, Giordano TJ, Brodeur FJ, et al: Adrenal adenomas: Relationship between histologic lipid and CT and MR findings. Radiology 1996; 200:743–747.
8. Parola P, Petit N, Azzedine A, et al: Symptomatic leiomyoma of the adrenal gland in a woman with AIDS. Aids 1996; 10:340–341.
9. Rozenblit A, Morehouse HT, Amis ES Jr: Cystic adrenal lesions: CT features. Radiology 1996; 201:541–548.
10. Boraschi P, Campatelli A, Di Vito A, et al: Hemorrhage in cavernous hemangioma of the adrenal gland: US, CT, and MRI appearances with pathologic correlation. Eur J Radiol 1995; 21:41–43.
11. Korobkin M, Dunnick NR: Characterization of adrenal masses. AJR Am J Roentgenol 1995; 164:643–644.
12. Korobkin M, Francis IR: Adrenal imaging. Semin Ultrasound CT MR 1995; 16:317–330.
13. Dahan H, Beges C, Weiss L, et al: Leiomyoma of the adrenal gland in a patient with AIDS. Abdom Imaging 1994; 19:259–261.
14. Lee MJ, Mayo-Smith WW, Hahn PF, et al: State-of-the-art MR imaging of the adrenal gland. Radiographics 1994; 14:1015–1029.
15. Loughlin RF, Bilbey JH: Tumors of the adrenal gland: Findings on CT and MR imaging. AJR Am J Roentgenol 1994; 163:1413–1418.
16. Doppman JL: The dilemma of bilateral adrenocortical nodularity in Conn's and Cushing's syndromes. Radiol Clin North Am 1993; 31:1039–1050.
17. Dunnick NR, Leight GS Jr, Roubidoux MA, et al: CT in the diagnosis of primary aldosteronism: Sensitivity in 29 patients. AJR Am J Roentgenol 1993; 160:321–324.
18. Doppman JL, Gill JR Jr, Miller DL, et al: Distinction between hyperaldosteronism due to bilateral hyperplasia and unilateral aldosteronoma: Reliability of CT. Radiology 1992; 184:677–682.
19. Radin DR, Manoogian C, Nadler JL: Diagnosis of primary hyperaldosteronism: Importance of correlating CT findings with endocrinologic studies. AJR Am J Roentgenol 1992; 158:553–557.
20. Sivit CJ, Hung W, Taylor GA, et al: Sonography in neonatal congenital adrenal hyperplasia. AJR Am J Roentgenol 1991; 156:141–143.
21. Doppman JL, Miller DL, Dwyer AJ, et al: Macronodular adrenal hyperplasia in Cushing disease. Radiology 1988; 166:347–352.
22. Wilson DA, Muchmore HG, Tisdal RG, et al: Histoplasmosis of the adrenal glands studied by CT. Radiology 1984; 150:779–783.

Illustrations • Adrenal Gland

1 • Adrenal hyperplasia

2 • Adrenal adenoma

3 • Adrenal myelolipoma

4 • Adrenal ganglioneuroma

5 • Adrenal carcinoma

6 • Pheochromocytoma

7 • Adrenal metastasis

8 • Other tumors of the adrenal gland

9 • Adrenal hemorrhage

10 • Adrenal tuberculosis

11 • Adrenal calcification

1. Adrenal Hyperplasia

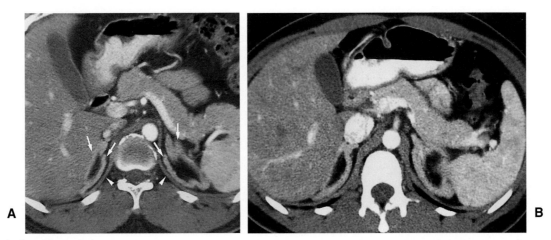

Fig. 1. Bilateral adrenal hyperplasia.
A. Bilateral adrenal hyperplasia in a 25-year-old woman. Contrast-enhanced CT shows diffuse enlargement of the adrenal glands *(arrows)*. Note that the adrenal glands are thicker than the diaphragm *(arrowheads)*. **B.** A 24-year-old woman with bilateral adrenal hyperplasia. Contrast-enhanced CT shows diffuse enlargement of the adrenal glands.

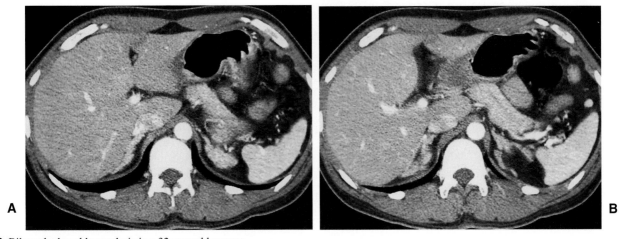

Fig. 2. Bilateral adrenal hyperplasia in a 32-year-old woman.
A, B. Contrast-enhanced CT scans show diffuse enlargement and nodular thickening of both adrenal glands.

2. Adrenal Adenoma

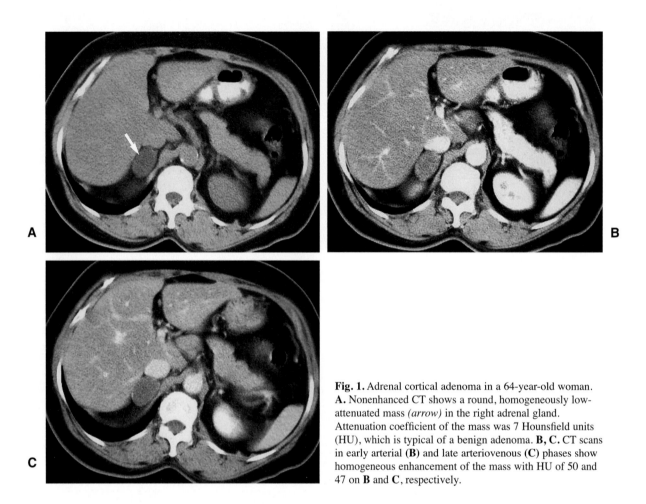

A

B

C

Fig. 1. Adrenal cortical adenoma in a 64-year-old woman.
A. Nonenhanced CT shows a round, homogeneously low-attenuated mass *(arrow)* in the right adrenal gland.
Attenuation coefficient of the mass was 7 Hounsfield units (HU), which is typical of a benign adenoma. B, C. CT scans in early arterial (B) and late arteriovenous (C) phases show homogeneous enhancement of the mass with HU of 50 and 47 on B and C, respectively.

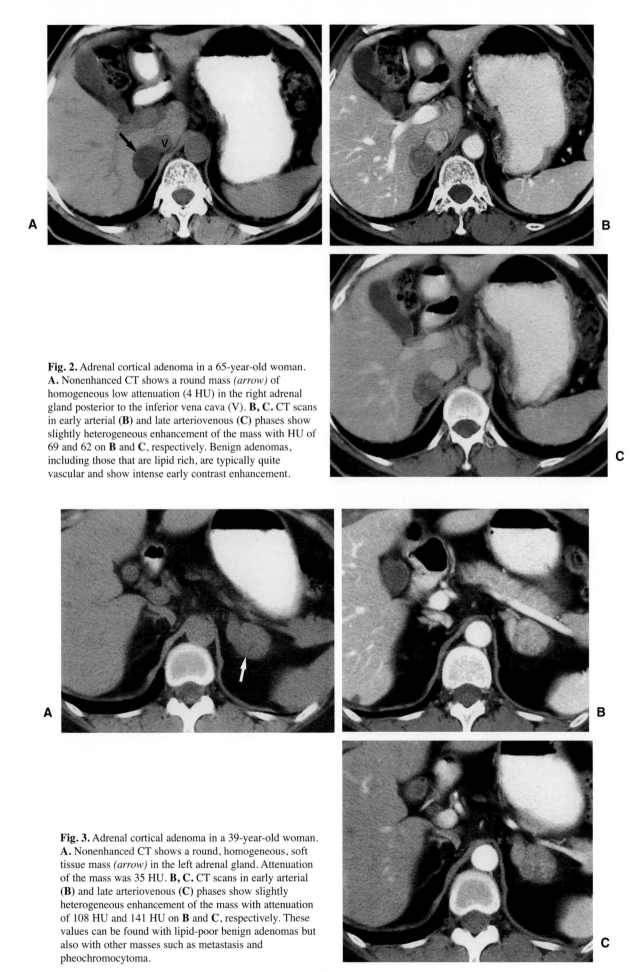

Fig. 2. Adrenal cortical adenoma in a 65-year-old woman.
A. Nonenhanced CT shows a round mass *(arrow)* of
homogeneous low attenuation (4 HU) in the right adrenal
gland posterior to the inferior vena cava (V). **B, C.** CT scans
in early arterial **(B)** and late arteriovenous **(C)** phases show
slightly heterogeneous enhancement of the mass with HU of
69 and 62 on **B** and **C**, respectively. Benign adenomas,
including those that are lipid rich, are typically quite
vascular and show intense early contrast enhancement.

Fig. 3. Adrenal cortical adenoma in a 39-year-old woman.
A. Nonenhanced CT shows a round, homogeneous, soft
tissue mass *(arrow)* in the left adrenal gland. Attenuation
of the mass was 35 HU. **B, C.** CT scans in early arterial
(B) and late arteriovenous **(C)** phases show slightly
heterogeneous enhancement of the mass with attenuation
of 108 HU and 141 HU on **B** and **C**, respectively. These
values can be found with lipid-poor benign adenomas but
also with other masses such as metastasis and
pheochromocytoma.

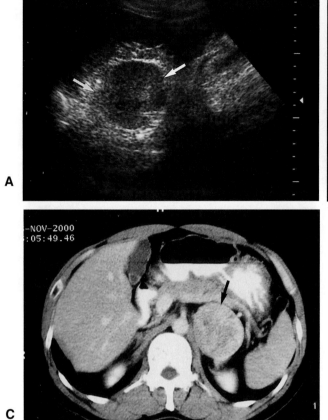

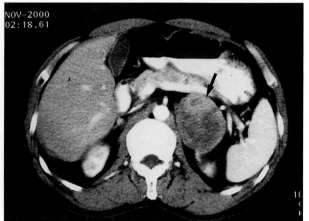

A

B

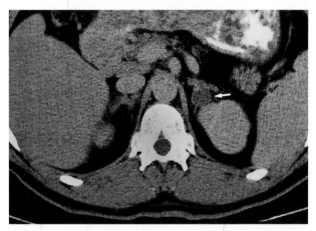

C

Fig. 4. Large adrenal cortical adenoma in a 39-year-old man.
A. US of the left flank shows a well-marginated, hypoechoic mass
(arrows) in the left adrenal gland. **B, C.** Contrast-enhanced CT
scans in early arterial **(B)** and late arteriovenous **(C)** phases show
a round, well-marginated, heterogeneously enhancing mass in the
left adrenal gland *(arrow)*.

Fig. 5. Adrenal adenoma in a 43-year-old man with hypertension and
prior cerebral hemorrhage. Laboratory evaluation revealed hypokalemia.
Nonenhanced CT shows a round, 1.8 cm, low-attenuating mass in the left
adrenal gland *(arrow)* representing a dominant aldosteronoma. In
addition, there is mild bilateral micronodular hyperplasia without any
other major nodule. The dominant adenoma in the left adrenal gland was
surgically removed, and this improved medical control of the patient's
symptoms resulting from Conn's syndrome.

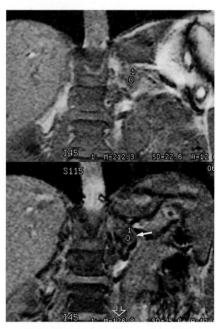

Fig. 6. Adrenocortical adenoma in a 58-year-old woman who was being
evaluated (staged) for malignant melanoma. Prior contrast-enhanced CT
(not shown) had revealed a 2-cm left adrenal mass. MR chemical shift
imaging in the coronal plane shows drop in signal intensity *(open arrow)*
of the 2-cm mass in the left adrenal gland *(arrow)* on the out-of-phase
sequence *(lower panel)*. This is indicative of a benign, lipid-rich adrenal
adenoma.

3. Adrenal Myelolipoma

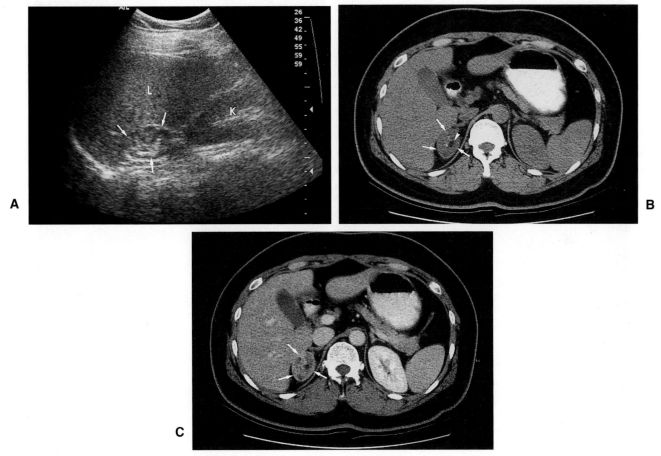

Fig. 1. Adrenal myelolipoma in a 50-year-old man. (**A–C,** Courtesy of Bohyun Kim, MD.)
A. Longitudinal US shows a mass of heterogeneous echogenicity in the right adrenal gland *(arrows)*. L, liver; K, right kidney. **B.** Nonenhanced CT scan shows heterogeneous attenuation of the mass *(arrows)* with small calcifications and low-attenuated fat *(arrowhead)*. **C.** Contrast-enhanced CT shows heterogeneous enhancement of the mass *(arrows)*.

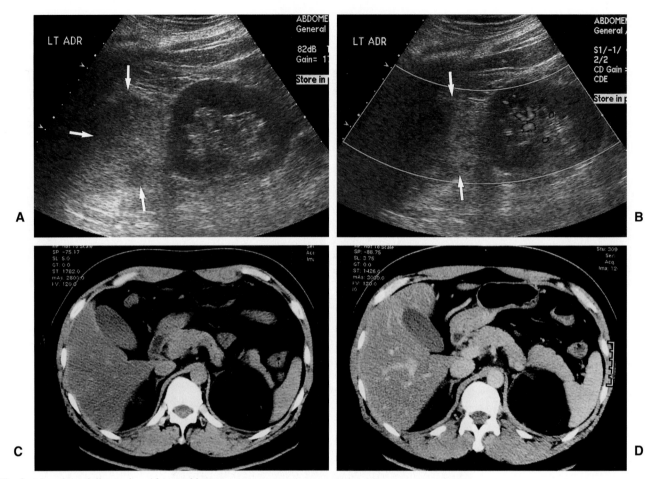

Fig. 2. Adrenal myelolipoma in a 46-year-old man.
A. Longitudinal US shows an ill-defined, large, echogenic mass *(arrows)* in the left adrenal region above the kidney. **B.** Color Doppler US shows the hypovascular nature of the mass *(arrows)*. (**B,** See also Color Section.) **C, D.** Nonenhanced (**C**) and contrast-enhanced (**D**) CT scans show a large, fatty mass in the left adrenal gland. Note subtle enhancement following the injection of contrast material.

4. Adrenal Ganglioneuroma

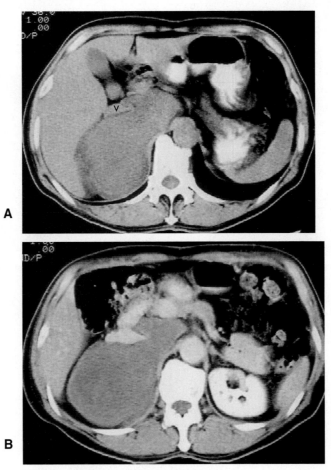

Fig. 1. Adrenal ganglioneuroma in a 58-year-old man.
A. Nonenhanced CT shows a large, homogeneous, soft tissue mass in the right adrenal region. The mass grows anteriorly and displaces the inferior vena cava (V) laterally. **B.** Contrast-enhanced CT shows poor enhancement of the mass.

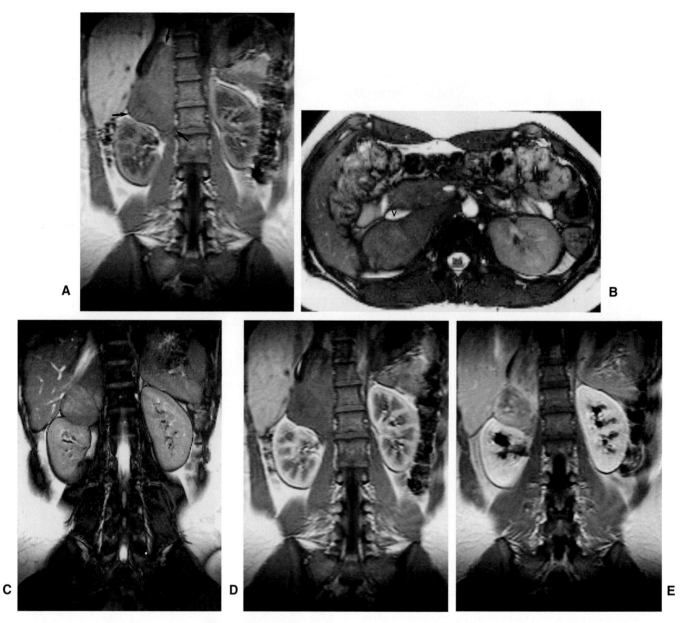

Fig. 2. Adrenal ganglioneuroma in a 25-year-old woman.
A. T1-weighted coronal MR image shows a triangular-shaped mass *(arrows)* in the right adrenal gland with displacement of the right kidney inferolaterally. The mass has homogeneous, intermediate signal intensity. **B, C.** T2-weighted axial (**B**) and coronal (**C**) MR images show heterogeneous, intermediate signal intensity of the mass, which is slightly lower than that of the kidney. Also note that the mass grows anteriorly and displaces the inferior vena cava (V) laterally. **D, E.** Contrast-enhanced T1-weighted MR images in early cortical (**D**) and late excretory (**E**) phases reveal delayed enhancement of the mass.

5. Adrenal Carcinoma

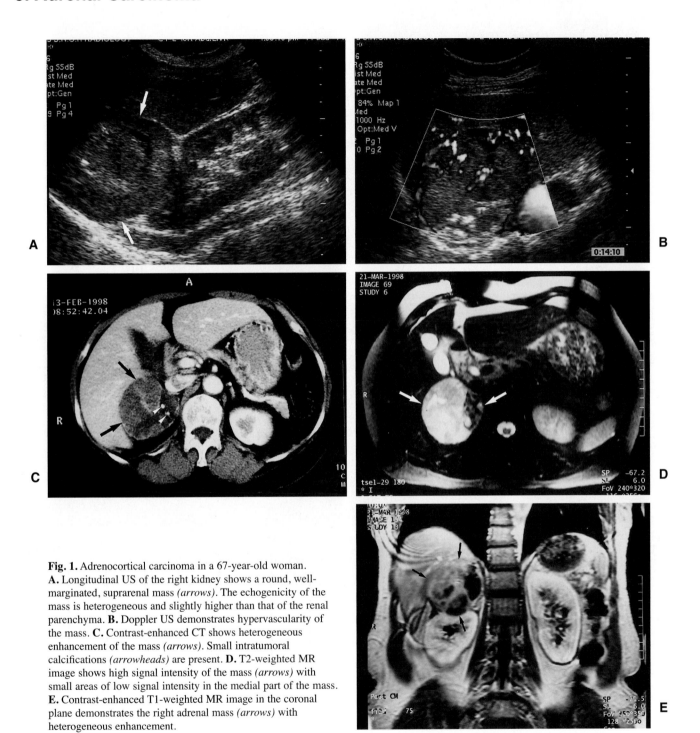

Fig. 1. Adrenocortical carcinoma in a 67-year-old woman.
A. Longitudinal US of the right kidney shows a round, well-marginated, suprarenal mass *(arrows)*. The echogenicity of the mass is heterogeneous and slightly higher than that of the renal parenchyma. **B.** Doppler US demonstrates hypervascularity of the mass. **C.** Contrast-enhanced CT shows heterogeneous enhancement of the mass *(arrows)*. Small intratumoral calcifications *(arrowheads)* are present. **D.** T2-weighted MR image shows high signal intensity of the mass *(arrows)* with small areas of low signal intensity in the medial part of the mass. **E.** Contrast-enhanced T1-weighted MR image in the coronal plane demonstrates the right adrenal mass *(arrows)* with heterogeneous enhancement.

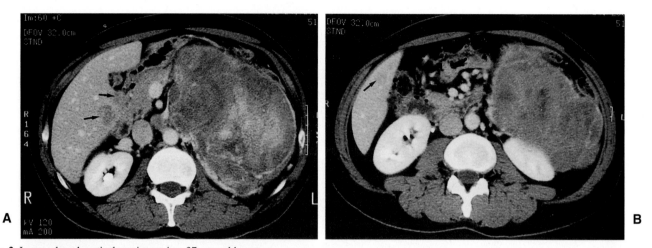

Fig. 2. Large adrenal cortical carcinoma in a 37-year-old man.
A, B. Contrast-enhanced CT scans show a huge soft tissue mass arising in the left adrenal gland. The mass is slightly heterogeneous in enhancement, but there is no prominent necrosis in the tumor. Metastatic lesions *(arrows)* are present in the liver.

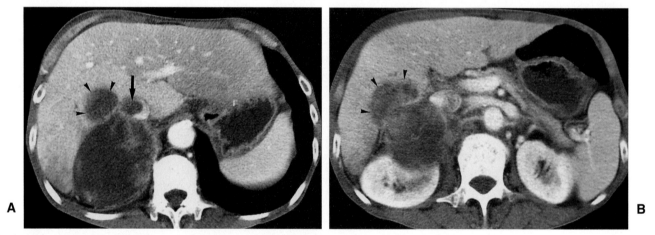

Fig. 3. Adrenocortical carcinoma with invasion into the liver and inferior vena cava in a 71-year-old man.
A, B. Contrast-enhanced CT scans show a large, low-attenuation mass with lobulated contour in the right adrenal gland. Note involvement of the liver by the tumor *(arrowheads)* and tumor thrombosis in the inferior vena cava *(arrow in **A**)*.

6. Pheochromocytoma

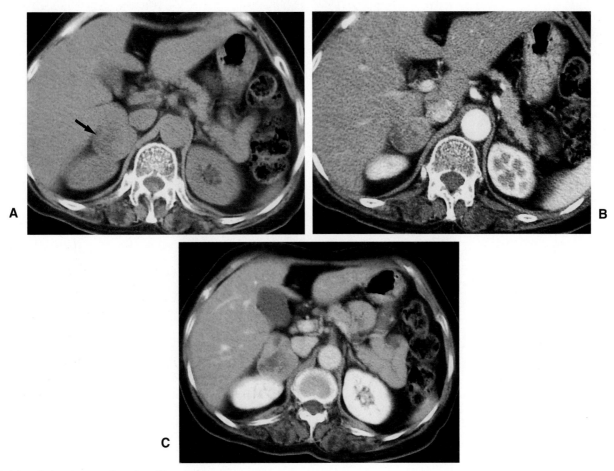

Fig. 1. Adrenal pheochromocytoma in a 58-year-old woman.
A. Nonenhanced CT shows a round, soft tissue density mass in the right adrenal gland *(arrow)*. **B, C.** Contrast-enhanced CT scans in cortical **(B)** and nephrographic **(C)** phases show heterogeneous enhancement of the mass.

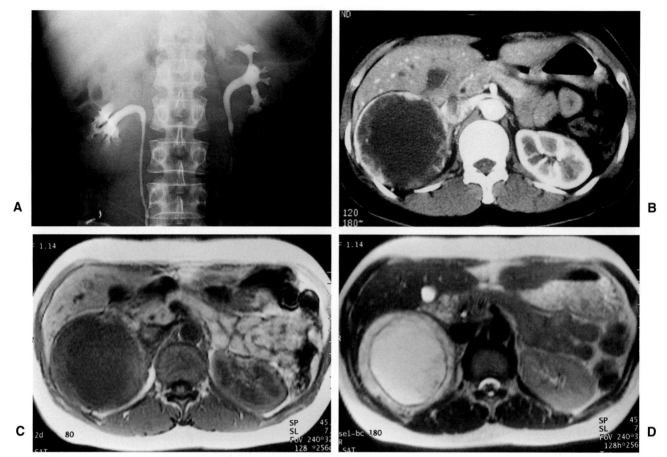

Fig. 2. Adrenal pheochromocytoma in a 40-year-old woman.
A. IVU shows downward displacement of the right kidney suggesting a suprarenal mass. **B.** Contrast-enhanced CT in cortical phase shows a large, round, well-marginated, peripherally enhancing mass with extensive central necrosis. **C.** T1-weighted MR image shows intermediate-intensity periphery and low-intensity center. **D.** T2-weighted MR image shows high signal intensity of the mass. A low-intensity rim is seen between the central necrotic area and peripheral solid portion.

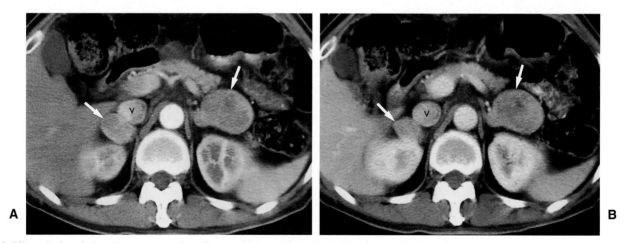

Fig. 3. Bilateral adrenal pheochromocytomas in a 47-year-old man with multiple endocrine neoplasia syndrome.
A, B. Contrast-enhanced CT scans in cortical (**A**) and nephrographic (**B**) phases show bilateral adrenal masses with heterogeneous enhancement *(arrows)*. V, inferior vena cava.

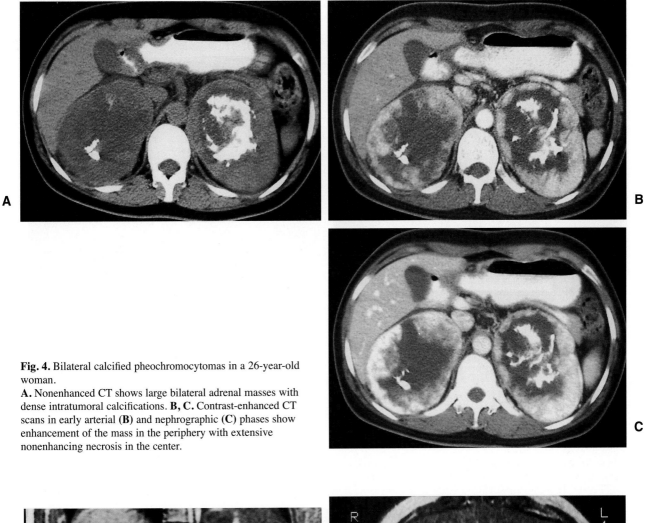

Fig. 4. Bilateral calcified pheochromocytomas in a 26-year-old woman.
A. Nonenhanced CT shows large bilateral adrenal masses with dense intratumoral calcifications. **B, C.** Contrast-enhanced CT scans in early arterial (**B**) and nephrographic (**C**) phases show enhancement of the mass in the periphery with extensive nonenhancing necrosis in the center.

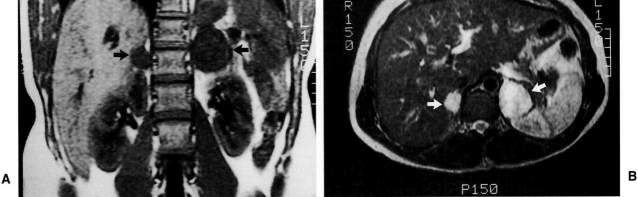

Fig. 5. Bilateral pheochromocytomas in a 22-year-old woman with persistent hypertension. There was family history of pheochromocytoma in her father. Laboratory studies revealed elevated catecholamine levels.
A. T1-weighted coronal MR image shows bilateral, intermediate-signal-intensity adrenal masses *(arrows)*. **B.** T2-weighted axial MR image shows that both of the adrenal masses *(arrows)* have relatively uniform high signal intensity. Both of the pheochromocytomas were removed surgically.

7. Adrenal Metastasis

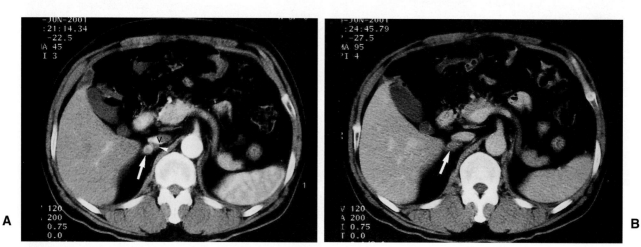

A   B

Fig. 1. Small metastatic lesion in the right adrenal gland in a 48-year-old man who underwent left nephrectomy for renal cell carcinoma 1 year earlier. **A.** Contrast-enhanced CT in early arterial phase shows a small nodular mass *(arrow)* in the right adrenal gland. The mass shows enhancement much stronger than the rest of the adrenal gland *(arrowhead)*. V, inferior vena cava. **B.** Late arterial-phase CT shows attenuation of the mass *(arrow)* that is similar to that of the remnant adrenal gland in this image.

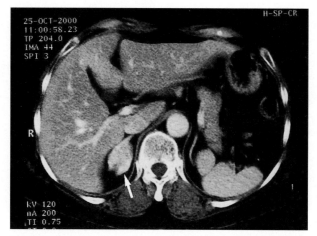

Fig. 2. Right adrenal metastasis in a 56-year-old woman who had undergone left nephrectomy for renal cell carcinoma 2 years earlier. Contrast-enhanced CT shows a round, enhancing mass in the right adrenal gland *(arrow)*.

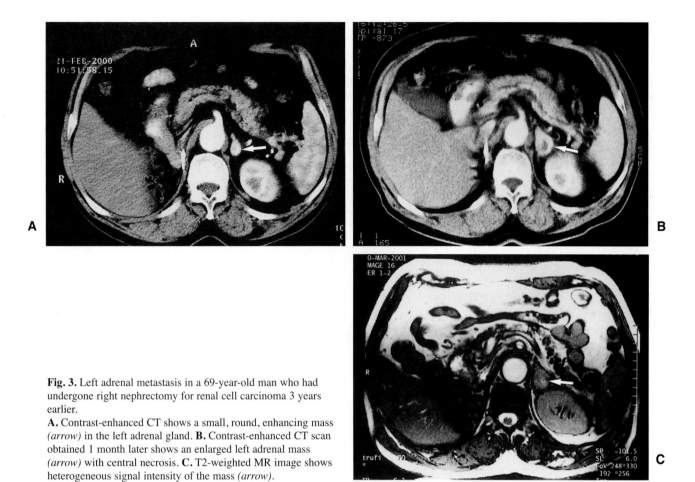

Fig. 3. Left adrenal metastasis in a 69-year-old man who had undergone right nephrectomy for renal cell carcinoma 3 years earlier.
A. Contrast-enhanced CT shows a small, round, enhancing mass *(arrow)* in the left adrenal gland. **B.** Contrast-enhanced CT scan obtained 1 month later shows an enlarged left adrenal mass *(arrow)* with central necrosis. **C.** T2-weighted MR image shows heterogeneous signal intensity of the mass *(arrow)*.

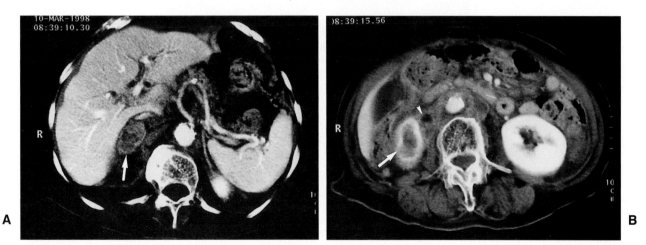

Fig. 4. Right adrenal metastasis in a 78-year-old woman with gastric carcinoma.
A. Contrast-enhanced CT scan in the early arterial phase shows a mass in the right adrenal gland with heterogeneous attenuation *(arrow)*. **B.** CT scan at a lower level shows diffuse metastases in the retroperitoneum and mesentery. Note the lower pole of the hydronephrotic right kidney *(arrow)* and the dilated right ureter *(arrowhead)*.

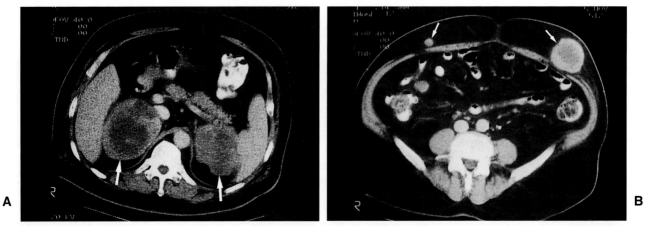

Fig. 5. Bilateral adrenal metastases from prostate cancer in a 66-year-old man.
A. Contrast-enhanced CT shows bilateral, large, adrenal masses with heterogeneous attenuation *(arrows)*. **B.** CT scan at a lower level shows multiple metastatic lesions *(arrows)* in the subcutaneous fat of the anterior abdomen.

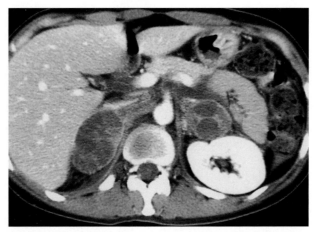

Fig. 6. Bilateral adrenal metastases from lung cancer in a 40-year-old woman. Contrast-enhanced CT shows bilateral adrenal masses with heterogeneous attenuation.

8. Other Tumors of the Adrenal Gland

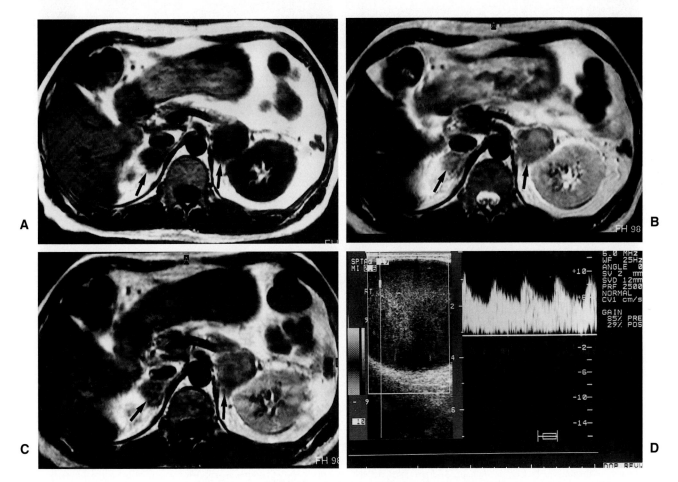

Fig. 1. Bilateral adrenal lymphoma in a 51-year-old man. This patient also had lymphomatous involvement of the paranasal sinuses and testes. **A.** T1-weighted MR image shows bilateral adrenal masses of homogeneous, low signal intensity *(arrows)*. **B.** T2-weighted MR image shows slightly heterogeneous low intensity of the masses *(arrows)*. **C.** Contrast-enhanced T1-weighted MR image shows homogeneous enhancement of the masses *(arrows)*. **D.** Doppler US of the right testis shows globular enlargement of the testis with heterogeneous hypoechogenicity. Spectral Doppler US reveals a low-resistance pattern of intratesticular arterial blood flow.

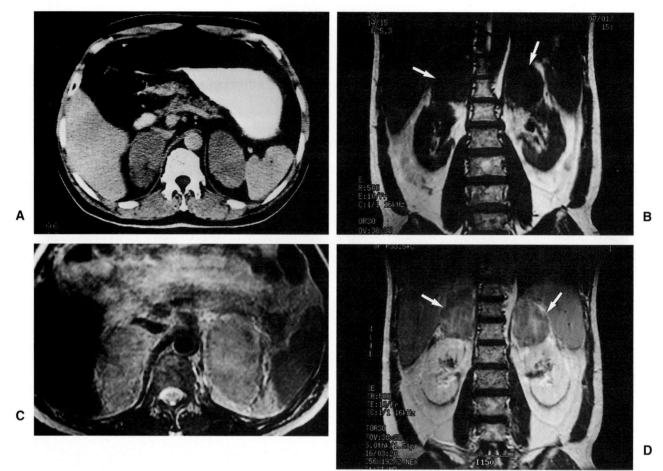

Fig. 2. Bilateral adrenal lymphoma in a 60-year-old man.
A. Contrast-enhanced CT scan shows bilateral adrenal masses of homogeneous, intermediate attenuation. **B.** T1-weighted coronal MR image shows homogeneous, intermediate signal intensity, bilateral adrenal masses *(arrows)*. **C.** T2-weighted axial MR image shows relatively homogeneous high signal intensity of the masses. **D.** Contrast-enhanced T1-weighted coronal MR image shows heterogeneous enhancement of the adrenal masses *(arrows)*.

8. Other Tumors of the Adrenal Gland

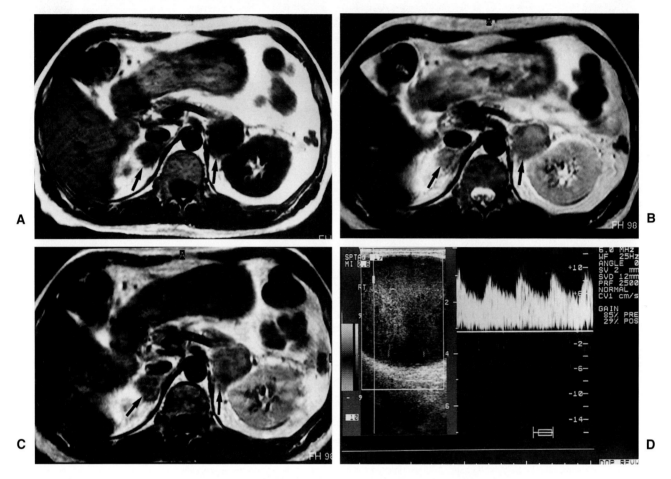

Fig. 1. Bilateral adrenal lymphoma in a 51-year-old man. This patient also had lymphomatous involvement of the paranasal sinuses and testes. **A.** T1-weighted MR image shows bilateral adrenal masses of homogeneous, low signal intensity *(arrows)*. **B.** T2-weighted MR image shows slightly heterogeneous low intensity of the masses *(arrows)*. **C.** Contrast-enhanced T1-weighted MR image shows homogeneous enhancement of the masses *(arrows)*. **D.** Doppler US of the right testis shows globular enlargement of the testis with heterogeneous hypoechogenicity. Spectral Doppler US reveals a low-resistance pattern of intratesticular arterial blood flow.

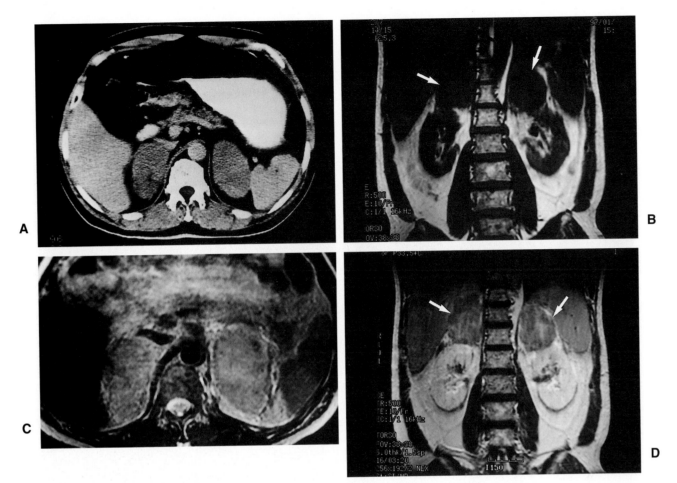

Fig. 2. Bilateral adrenal lymphoma in a 60-year-old man.
A. Contrast-enhanced CT scan shows bilateral adrenal masses of homogeneous, intermediate attenuation. **B.** T1-weighted coronal MR image shows homogeneous, intermediate signal intensity, bilateral adrenal masses *(arrows)*. **C.** T2-weighted axial MR image shows relatively homogeneous high signal intensity of the masses. **D.** Contrast-enhanced T1-weighted coronal MR image shows heterogeneous enhancement of the adrenal masses *(arrows)*.

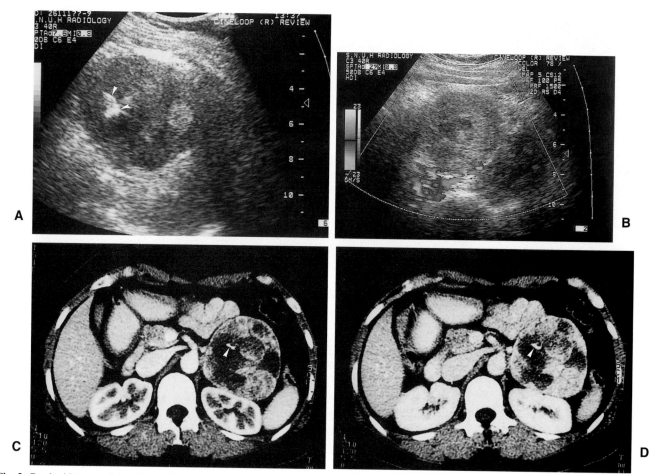

Fig. 3. Carcinoid tumor of the adrenal gland in a 41-year-old woman.
A. US shows a well-marginated mass with heterogeneous echogenicity in the left suprarenal area. There is a strong hyperechogenicity within the mass suggesting calcification *(arrowheads)*. **B.** Color Doppler US shows the hypovascular nature of the tumor. (**B,** See also Color Section.) **C, D.** Contrast-enhanced CT scans in cortical (**C**) and nephrographic (**D**) phases show heterogeneous enhancement of the left adrenal mass. Note that the mass has a small calcification *(arrowhead)*.

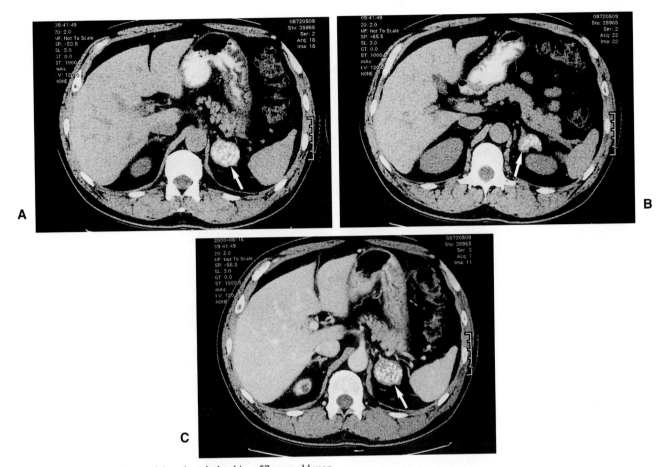

Fig. 4. Cavernous hemangioma of the adrenal gland in a 57-year-old man.
A, B. Nonenhanced CT scans show a well-defined mass in the left adrenal gland *(arrow)*. Note mottled, dense calcifications in the mass. **C.** Contrast-enhanced CT shows only mild enhancement of the mass *(arrow)*.

9. Adrenal Hemorrhage

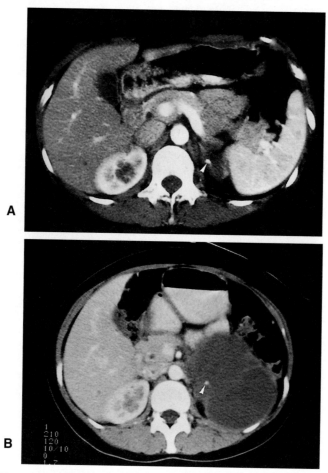

Fig. 1. Cyst formation after postpartum adrenal hemorrhage in a 29-year-old woman with history of delivery 4 weeks earlier.
A, B. Contrast-enhanced CT scans show a large, lobulated, cystic mass in the left adrenal gland. Note small calcifications *(arrowhead)* in the wall and septum of the cyst.

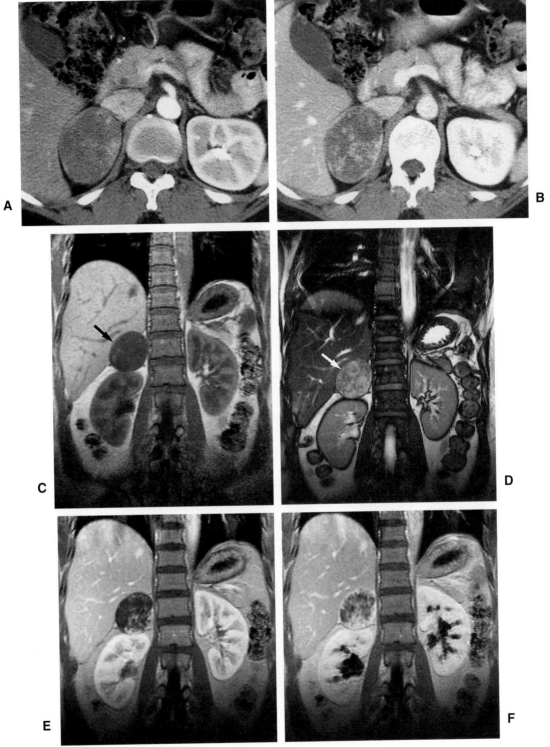

Fig. 2. Organizing hematoma of the adrenal gland mimicking a tumor in a 41-year-old woman.
A. Contrast-enhanced CT in early cortical phase shows a large, low-attenuated mass in the right adrenal gland. The mass shows faint peripheral enhancement. **B.** Contrast-enhanced CT in nephrographic phase shows mottled enhancement in the center of the tumor in addition to the peripheral enhancement. **C.** T1-weighted gradient-echo MR image in coronal plane shows a round mass in the right adrenal gland *(arrow)*. The mass has low signal intensity with mottled high intensities. **D.** T2-weighted gradient-echo MR image shows high signal intensity of the mass *(arrow)* with low-intensity mottling. **E, F.** Contrast-enhanced MR images in cortical **(E)** and nephrographic **(F)** phases show progressive mottled enhancement of the mass.

10. Adrenal Tuberculosis

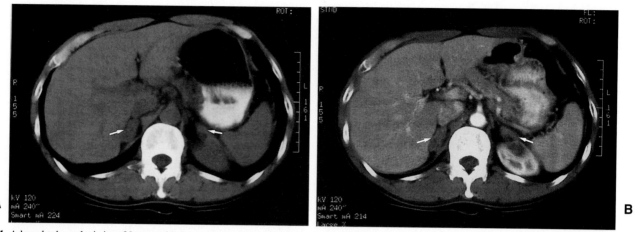

Fig. 1. Adrenal tuberculosis in a 30-year-old man.
A. Nonenhanced CT shows diffuse enlargement of both right and left adrenal glands *(arrows)*. **B.** Contrast-enhanced CT shows weak enhancement of the lesions *(arrows)*.

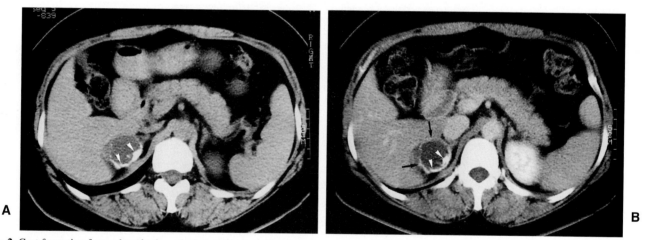

Fig. 2. Cyst formation from adrenal tuberculosis in a 41-year-old woman.
A. Nonenhanced CT shows a round, low-attenuated mass in the right adrenal gland with dense peripheral calcifications *(arrowheads)*. **B.** Contrast-enhanced CT shows peripheral enhancement of the cyst wall *(arrows)*. Note dense calcifications in the wall *(arrowheads)*.

11. Adrenal Calcification

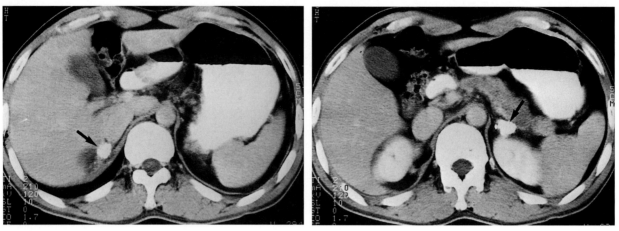

A   B

Fig. 1. Calcified adrenal glands in a 42-year-old man with Addison's disease.
A, B. Contrast-enhanced CT scans show densely calcified right and left adrenal glands *(arrow)*.

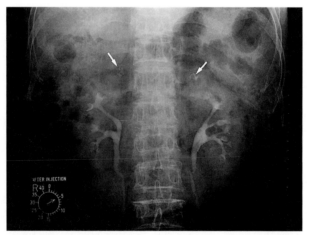

Fig. 2. Bilateral adrenal calcifications in a 66-year-old asymptomatic
woman. On IVU, there are small calcifications in both adrenal glands
(arrows). The likely causes are remote hemorrhage or remote infection,
such as tuberculosis.

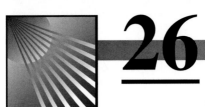

26

Renal Trauma

JUNG SUK SIM AND LEE B. TALNER

The kidneys are injured in approximately 10% of all abdominal trauma cases. Blunt trauma is responsible for 80% of renal injuries, and penetrating trauma causes about half of major renal injuries. Since conservative, nonoperative management is preferred even in major renal injuries, accurate assessment with imaging, especially computed tomography (CT), becomes central for guiding patient management.

GRADING OF RENAL TRAUMA

Various classification systems have been proposed, but now the American Association for the Surgery of Trauma (AAST) scheme is widely accepted (Table 26–1). This grading system is based on CT findings.

The only absolute indication for intervention (surgery or embolization) is persistent bleeding. The other conditions, such as devitalization of renal tissue, urinary extravasation, and vascular injury, are relative indications that depend on the patient's condition, evolution of findings on serial examination, and the strategy of clinicians.

Table 26–1	American Association for the Surgery of Trauma (AAST) Grading System for Renal Injury

Grade	Type of Injury	Definition
Minor		
I	Contusion	Microscopic or gross hematuria, urologic studies normal
	Hematoma	Subcapsular, nonexpanding without parenchymal laceration
II	Hematoma	Nonexpanding perirenal hematoma
	Laceration	< 1 cm depth of renal cortex without urinary extravasation
Major		
III	Laceration	> 1 cm depth of renal cortex, without collecting system rupture or urinary extravasation
IV	Laceration	Parenchymal laceration extending through the renal cortex, medulla, and collecting system, with urine extravasation
	Vascular	Main renal artery or vein injury with contained hemorrhage
V	Laceration	Shattered kidney
	Vascular	Avulsion of renal hilum which devascularizes kidney

CLINICAL CONSIDERATIONS

Most blunt renal injuries can be managed conservatively. Certain features, such as persistent gross hematuria, hemodynamic instability, and penetrating injuries, or rapid deceleration trauma is more often associated with major renal injuries.

Gross hematuria from blunt trauma is often a sign of severe urologic injury, but the amount of hematuria does not correlate with the grade of renal injury. Penetrating trauma to the back or flank should be evaluated with triple-contrast CT. Most patients with penetrating injuries of the kidneys have damage to other organs as well. Before the era of CT, these patients usually underwent surgical exploration. In recent years, CT images in conjunction with clinical findings can determine whether exploration is needed. Motor vehicle crashes, direct blows to the flank, or falls from a height can produce rapid-deceleration injury. Rapid deceleration stretches the renal pedicle and may result in avulsion or occlusion of renal vessels, or avulsion of the ureter, which are examples of grade IV or V injury.

ROLE OF IMAGING

Computed tomography

CT is the imaging modality of choice in evaluating renal trauma. It accurately demonstrates all degrees of renal injuries, including intrarenal minor injuries, parenchymal and collecting system lacerations, extent of hematomas and urinomas, and associated abdominal and retroperitoneal injuries. In all renal injuries of grade III or higher, delayed CT scans (e.g., at 10 minutes) should be added to avoid missing a laceration of the collecting system or ureter.

Intravenous urography

Until the 1980s, most patients with abdominal trauma and hematuria were evaluated with intravenous urography (IVU). However, it has been largely replaced by CT. IVU is neither sensitive in detecting renal injuries nor accurate in grading them. One-shot IVU, taken 10 minutes after administration of high-dose intravenous contrast material, may be used for emergency evaluation of renal trauma in hemodynamically unstable patients, especially those with penetrating injuries. The purpose of one-shot IVU is not to evaluate the injured kidney but to determine urinary extravasation and the presence of a functioning contralateral kidney.

Angiography

The use of angiography for diagnosis of renal injury has diminished, but angiography can provide the opportunity for embolization. In major trauma centers, angioembolization is the procedure of choice for persistent bleeding.

Ultrasonography

Ultrasonography (US) can delineate renal injuries, including hematoma and laceration. US is also sensitive in demonstrating hemoperitoneum. Color or power Doppler US easily demonstrates the abnormalities of renal perfusion caused by trauma. However, US is usually inadequate for determining the grade of renal trauma. US for renal trauma is more popular in Asia and Europe than in the United States, where CT is used almost exclusively.

IMAGING FINDINGS OF RENAL TRAUMA

Increasing use of conservative management and advances in CT technology make CT the cornerstone of evaluation and management of patients with renal trauma. The following sections discuss the frequent findings of renal trauma. Among them, renal shattering, vascular avulsion, and urinary retention are particularly important, because they indicate the need for surgical exploration.

Renal contusion

Contusion consists of focal interstitial edema, intraparenchymal extravasation of small amounts of bloody urine. The contused renal parenchyma shows slightly higher attenuation on nonenhanced CT due to hemorrhage, decreased nephrogram, and delayed excretion due to increased tubular pressure on contrast-enhanced CT. Delayed images often show contrast staining of the contused parenchyma.

Subcapsular hematoma

A subcapsular hematoma is diagnosed when hemorrhage is between the renal parenchyma and capsule. Typically it shows a lenticular or semicircular shape, but often differentiation from perirenal hematoma is difficult, and the two types often coexist.

Perirenal hematoma

Perirenal hematoma spreads around the kidney and can be quite large. The kidney is displaced from the site of bleeding, and anterior displacement is most common. A large perirenal hematoma may cross the midline.

Renal laceration

Renal laceration causes irregular, moderately well-defined, linear or wedge-shaped defects in the enhanced renal parenchyma. Various terms have been used to describe renal laceration: *Complete laceration* means a laceration involving the collecting system with urine leakage; *renal fracture* means complete discontinuity between the poles of the kidney; and *shattered kidney* means fragmentation of the renal parenchyma into several pieces.

Vascular occlusion

Vascular occlusion is an important complication of deceleration injury. On contrast-enhanced CT, the kidney does not enhance at all except for a thin rim of subcapsular cortex that is supplied from capsular arteries (cortical rim sign). Angiographic confirmation is not needed.

Vascular avulsion

Avulsion of the main renal artery or vein from blunt trauma results in massive hemorrhage, often extending through multiple retroperitoneal compartments. Renal enhancement is absent in renal arterial avulsion but not in venous avulsion. A stab wound is most likely to lacerate a branch of the renal artery, which also can cause massive hemorrhage. Renal pseudoaneurysm, with delayed rebleeding, is an important complication of stab wounds to the kidney.

TRAUMA TO THE ABNORMAL KIDNEYS

Kidneys with congenital renal anomalies are more vulnerable to trauma. Horseshoe kidney, in which bridging renal parenchyma is located in front of unyielding lumbar vertebrae, is frequently injured. Hydronephrotic kidney, most commonly from ureteropelvic junction obstruction, is easily ruptured to form urinoma.

References

1. Federle MP: Renal trauma. In Pollack HM, McClennan BL (eds): Clinical Urography, 2nd ed, vol 2. Philadelphia, WB Saunders, 2000, pp 1772–1784.
2. Lentz KA, McKenney MG, Nunez DB Jr, et al: Evaluating blunt abdominal trauma: Role for ultrasonography. J Ultrasound Med 1996; 15:447–451.
3. McKenney MG, Martin L, Lentz K, et al: One thousand consecutive ultrasounds for blunt abdominal trauma. J Trauma 1996; 40:607–610.
4. Miller KS, McAninch JW: Radiographic assessment of renal trauma: Our 15-year experience. J Urol 1995; 154:352–355.
5. Stevenson J, Battistella FD: The "one-shot" intravenous pyelogram: Is it indicated in unstable trauma patients before celiotomy? J Trauma 1994; 36:828–833.
6. Fanney DR, Casillas J, Murphy BJ: CT in the diagnosis of renal trauma. Radiographics 1990; 10:29–40.
7. Fletcher TB, Setiawan H, Harrell RS, et al: Posterior abdominal stab wounds: Role of CT evaluation. Radiology 1989; 173:621–625.
8. Pollack HM, Wein AJ: Imaging of renal trauma. Radiology 1989; 172:297–308.
9. Nicolaisen GS, McAninch JW, Marshall GA, et al: Renal trauma: Reevaluation of the indications for radiographic assessment. J Urol 1985; 133:183–187.
10. Rhyner P, Federle MP, Jeffrey RB: CT of trauma to the abnormal kidney. AJR Am J Roentgenol 1984; 142:747–750

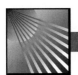

Illustrations • Renal Trauma

1 • Superficial cortical laceration

2 • Deep parenchymal laceration

3 • Shattered kidney

4 • Main vascular injury

5 • Iatrogenic renal trauma

6 • Trauma to the kidney with underlying abnormality

1. Superficial Cortical Laceration

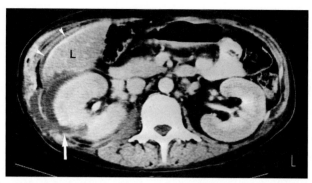

Fig. 1. Superficial cortical laceration in a 37-year-old woman who received a penetrating injury to her right flank. Contrast-enhanced CT shows cortical laceration *(arrow)* of the right kidney with a hematoma in the perirenal and posterior pararenal spaces, and abdominal wall. Note a small amount of ascites *(arrowheads)* around the liver (L).

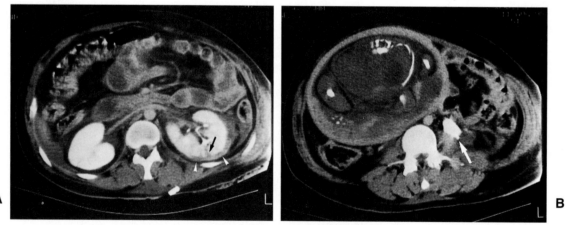

Fig. 2. Superficial cortical laceration and ureteral transection in a 33-year-old pregnant woman after she was in a traffic accident. She also had a splenic laceration, and the fetus was dead.
A. Contrast-enhanced CT shows a superficial cortical laceration *(arrow)* in the left kidney with perirenal hematoma *(arrowheads)*. **B.** CT scan at a lower level shows leak of contrast material from the left ureter due to ureteral transection *(arrow)*. Note the pregnant uterus in the right abdomen.

2. Deep Parenchymal Laceration

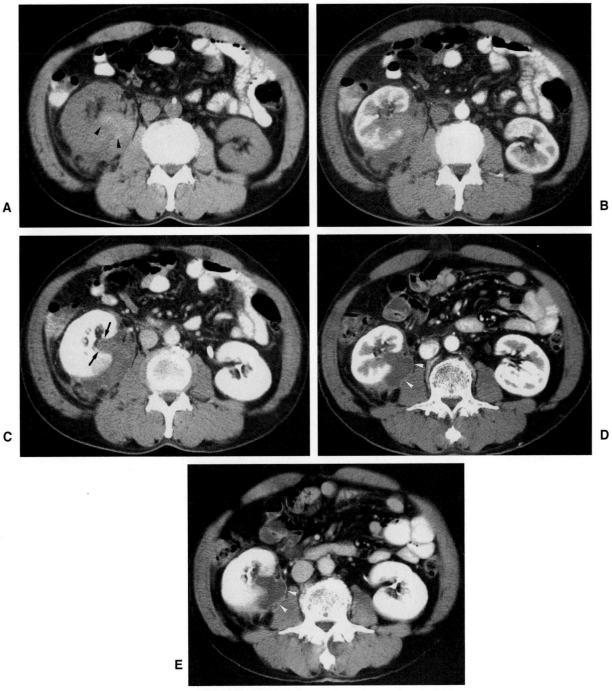

Fig. 1. Deep parenchymal laceration in a 64-year-old man who was in a traffic accident.
A. Nonenhanced CT shows right perirenal hematoma, which has focal high-attenuated foci *(arrowheads)*. **B.** Contrast-enhanced CT scan in cortical phase shows discontinuity of medial renal cortex and perirenal hematoma. **C.** Contrast-enhanced CT in excretory phase well demonstrates the deep parenchymal laceration *(arrows)*. **D, E.** Follow-up contrast-enhanced CT scans obtained 6 weeks later show a decreased amount of perirenal hematoma with thickened enhancing rim *(arrowheads)*.

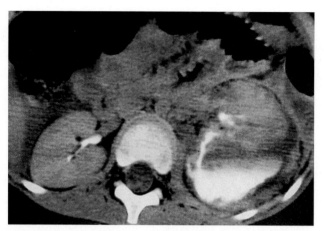

Fig. 2. Grade IV renal laceration. CT scan obtained 10 minutes after injection of contrast material shows extravasation of opacified urine from laceration that involves the pelvocalyceal system.

3. Shattered Kidney

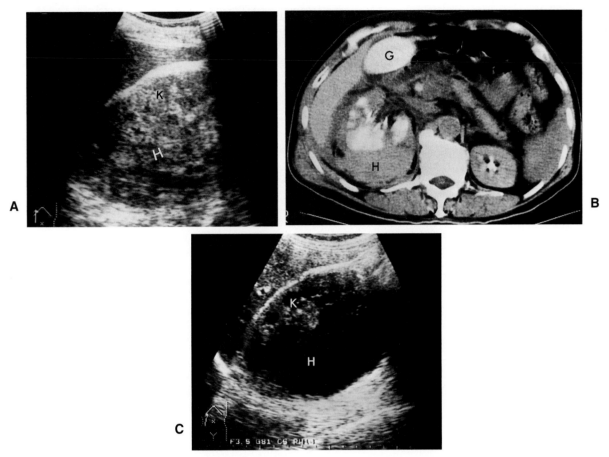

Fig. 1. Shattered kidney in a 73-year-old man who received a blunt trauma when he was drunk.
A. Longitudinal US of the right flank shows an indistinct outline of the right kidney (K) and large amount of perirenal hematoma (H), which has heterogeneous echogenicity posterior to the kidney. **B.** Contrast-enhanced CT shows fragmented renal parenchyma due to multiple fractures of the right kidney. There is a large amount of perirenal hematoma (H). Note that gallbladder (G) is opacified due to vicarious excretion of contrast material from an earlier CT. **C.** On follow-up US taken 1 month later, perirenal hematoma (H) became hypoechoic due to liquefaction. K, right kidney.

4. Main Vascular Injury

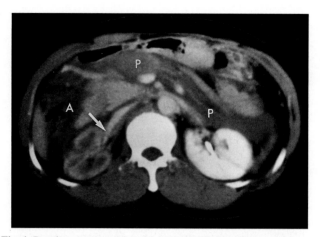

Fig. 1. Renal artery trauma in a 37-year-old woman who received a seat-belt injury 1 month earlier. Contrast-enhanced CT shows a small right kidney with diminished and delayed perfusion. Note that the right renal vein is well opacified probably due to retrograde filling *(arrow)*. Also note peripancreatic fluid collection (P) and ascites (A) due to transection of the pancreas head.

5. Iatrogenic Renal Trauma

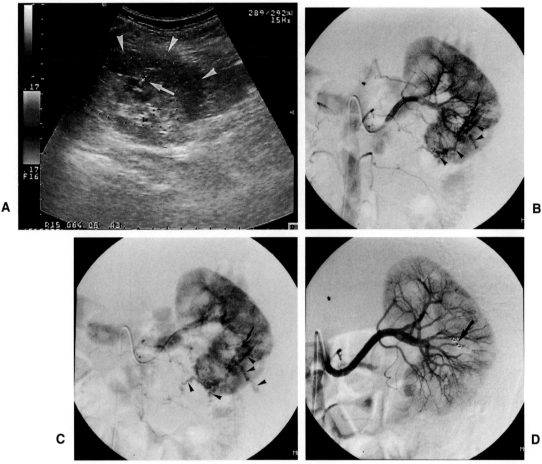

Fig. 1. Postbiopsy active bleeding in a 42-year-old woman with chronic renal parenchymal disease.
A. Color Doppler US performed immediately after US-guided biopsy of the left kidney shows a developing perirenal hematoma *(arrowheads)*. There were flow signals *(arrow)* crossing the renal capsule into the perirenal hematoma. (**A,** See also Color Section.) **B, C.** Left renal arteriograms demonstrate a leak of contrast material *(arrow)* from the kidney, which spreads in the perirenal space *(arrowheads)*. **D.** Transcatheter embolization was performed by using microcoils *(arrow)*.

6. Trauma to the Kidney with Underlying Abnormality

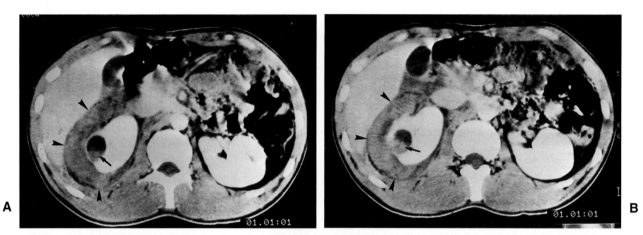

Fig. 1. Trauma to the right kidney, which has a renal cyst, in a 23-year-old man who had had a traffic accident 1 week earlier.
A, B. Contrast-enhanced CT scans show a right perirenal hematoma *(arrowheads)* and hemorrhage into the right renal cyst resulting in a fluid-blood level *(arrow)*.

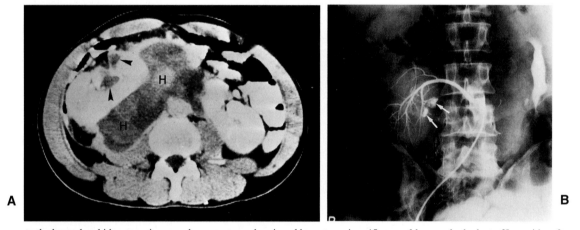

Fig. 2. Trauma to the horseshoe kidney causing pseudoaneurysm and perirenal hematoma in a 45-year-old man who had a traffic accident 3 weeks earlier.
A. Contrast-enhanced CT shows large amount of perirenal hematoma (H) on the right side. Also note low-attenuated intrarenal hematomas *(arrowheads)* in the right kidney. **B.** Selective arteriography of the right kidney shows two pseudoaneurysms *(arrows)*, which were treated with transcatheter embolization.

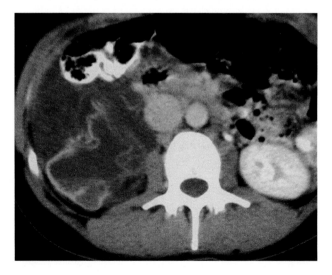

Fig. 3. Rupture of the renal pelvis and large retroperitoneal urine extravasation caused by blunt trauma to the kidney with preexisting ureteropelvic junction obstruction. Contrast-enhanced CT shows partially collapsed wall of the renal pelvis and marked thinning of the renal parenchyma from obstructive atrophy.

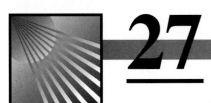

27

Transplanted Kidneys

BOHYUN KIM

Various complications may develop at any time following renal transplantation, but most of the severe complications occur during the first postoperative month. The complications can be divided into four categories: renal, vascular, and urologic complications, and fluid collections. The major role of imaging studies is to differentiate vascular and urologic complications that do not require renal biopsy from renal complications that do need renal biopsy. Because of its high sensitivity and wide availability, color Doppler ultrasonography (US) is most commonly used. Other frequently used imaging modalities include intravenous urography (IVU), computed tomography (CT), magnetic resonance (MR) imaging, angiography, and renal scintigraphy.

RENAL COMPLICATIONS

Imaging findings of renal complications are often nonspecific, and the specific diagnosis can be made only by renal biopsy. However, the occurrence time of renal complications after transplantation, along with the clinical and radiologic findings, may help differentiate among renal complications. Acute tubular necrosis commonly occurs during or immediately after transplantation, and cyclosporin toxicity often occurs in the first to third postoperative months. Allograft rejection may vary in onset time according to the type of rejection. Acute rejection most commonly occurs 1 to 4 weeks after surgery, and chronic rejection occurs months to years after transplantation.

Acute tubular necrosis

Acute tubular necrosis usually occurs immediately after transplantation, most often within the first 48 hours, and is caused by ischemia of the transplanted kidney. It most commonly occurs in cadaveric allografts but may also occur in the living donor due to the delay between the donor nephrectomy and vascular anastomosis in the recipient. The affected patient may present with anuria, azotemia, and graft swelling. It usually resolves within 7 to 10 days following transplantation but may persist for several weeks.

Graft rejection

Graft rejection is often classified into five categories according to the onset of the disease: hyperacute, accelerated acute, acute, chronic, and acute superimposed on chronic. Because of

difference in treatment, it is essential to differentiate graft rejection from other causes of graft dysfunction.

Hyperacute rejection is mediated by humoral antibodies and frequently occurs during surgery or a few hours following transplantation. The vascular endothelium of small vessels is damaged by complement-mediated reaction resulting in thrombosis and extensive cortical necrosis. The affected graft is usually unsalvageable and should be removed immediately by transplant nephrectomy.

Accelerated acute rejection occurs within the first few days after surgery. Diagnosis can be made when rejection occurs in the first week of transplantation.

Acute rejection most commonly occurs during the first week after transplantation but may occur at any time following surgery. It presents with oliguria, azotemia, graft swelling and tenderness, and fever. Acute rejection can be divided into interstitial and vascular rejection. Interstitial rejection is a cell-mediated process, and vascular rejection is mediated by humoral and cellular immune reaction. Histologically, in interstitial rejection the major changes occur in the interstitium, sparing the glomeruli, arterioles, and arteries, whereas arterioles and arteries are mainly affected in vascular rejection. Pure vascular rejection shows a poorer prognosis but is rare.

Chronic rejection is mediated by both humoral and cellular mechanisms. It usually occurs months to years after surgery. The affected patients may present with progressive azotemia and hypertension. Histologically it often results in interstitial fibrosis. The changes are usually irreversible.

Cyclosporin nephrotoxicity

Cyclosporin is toxic to both the liver and kidneys. Renal dysfunction commonly occurs during the first month of transplantation. The diagnosis can be made by exclusion of other causes of renal dysfunction. Measurement of blood cyclosporin levels may be helpful but does not always correlate with the severity of nephrotoxicity. Imaging studies can be beneficial in these circumstances, but renal biopsy is often needed. Treatment mainly includes reducing the cyclosporin dose. The changes can be reversed by the treatment, except for chronic toxicity.

Imaging findings

For the evaluation of renal complications, Doppler US and/or radionuclide imaging are most commonly used. Imaging

findings, however, are often nonspecific. US findings of acute tubular necrosis, rejection, and cyclosporin toxicity often overlap. Diagnosis should be correlated with clinical and laboratory findings, and renal biopsy is usually needed for confirmation.

In acute rejection, gray-scale US may demonstrate swelling of the transplanted kidney, decreased echogenicity of the renal cortex and medullary pyramids, diminished echogenicity of the renal sinus, and thickening of the wall of the renal pelvis and ureter. Although these morphologic changes are characteristic of allograft rejection, they can also be seen in other causes of allograft dysfunction, including acute tubular necrosis and cyclosporin toxicity.

On color Doppler US, renal blood flow is often diminished and the resistive index (RI) is elevated in patients with acute tubular necrosis, cyclosporin toxicity, and rejection. When vascular resistance within the allograft is markedly increased, it may cause reversal of diastolic flow. It is often seen in patients with acute rejection or renal vein thrombosis but can be seen in any disease with increased vascular resistance of the allograft. Although the elevated RI can also be seen in patients with renal vein thrombosis, urinary tract obstruction, and perirenal fluid collection, an RI value greater than 0.90 is relatively specific for acute rejection. However, using higher RI value as a threshold may result in low sensitivity in diagnosing acute rejection. Because the RI values are nonspecific, serial changes of the RI values are more helpful. The baseline and serial follow-up Doppler studies may improve accuracy in assessing allograft dysfunction.

VASCULAR COMPLICATIONS
Renal artery stenosis

Renal artery stenosis is reported to occur in approximately 10% of renal transplant recipients. It usually occurs in the first year after transplantation. The affected patients may present with allograft dysfunction and hypertension. The most common sites for arterial stenosis are at or just distal to the arterial anastomosis.

Renal vein thrombosis

Renal vein thrombosis is a rare complication of transplantation, occurring in less than 5%. It usually occurs within the first few postoperative days and often presents with swelling and tenderness of the graft. The diagnosis should be suspected when a patient develops nephritic syndrome after transplantation. Once diagnosed, the allograft should be removed immediately.

Arteriovenous fistulas

Intrarenal arteriovenous fistula and pseudoaneurysm most commonly occur following renal biopsy. Although most of these lesions are small and resolve eventually, they may communicate with the collecting system or rupture into the perirenal space. Small and asymptomatic lesions can be carefully followed up, whereas larger lesions usually need to be treated by embolization.

Imaging findings

For the evaluation of vascular complication of the renal allograft, various modalities including color Doppler US, CT angiography, MR angiography, and conventional angiography can be used. Of these, color Doppler US is most commonly used as the first-line imaging modality. Although angiography is the gold standard for detecting vascular abnormalities, it is not commonly used because of its invasiveness.

For the diagnosis of renal artery stenosis of the transplanted kidney, color Doppler US is performed either at the main renal artery or at the intrarenal arteries, as in the native kidneys. At the stenotic segment, focal color aliasing and poststenotic turbulent flow can be seen on color Doppler US. Doppler criteria for significant stenosis at the main artery include a high-frequency shift of more than 7.5 kHz or more than 2 m/sec with distal turbulence. Doppler US of intrarenal arteries may demonstrate a pulsus tardus-parvus waveform (prolonged acceleration time and diminished peak systolic velocity), which is characteristic of significant stenosis of the renal artery. An acceleration time of intrarenal arteries greater than 0.07 second and an acceleration index less than 3 m/sec^2 are considered diagnostic criteria for renal artery stenosis. As CT and MR angiography directly visualize renal arteries in three dimensions, stenotic segment can be well demonstrated using these techniques. For patients with positive Doppler US findings, angiography is often required for both diagnosis and treatment. Renal artery stenosis can be successfully treated in most cases by percutaneous transluminal angioplasty.

US findings of renal vein thrombosis are nonspecific. The allograft is often enlarged and hypoechoic. Doppler US may demonstrate intraluminal echogenic thrombi and absence of flow in the renal vein. Doppler US of the renal artery may demonstrate a high RI and sometimes reversed diastolic flow. Absent venous flow and highly resistive arterial waveform in early postoperative days may suggest the diagnosis of renal vein thrombosis.

Arteriovenous fistula and pseudoaneurysm can be easily depicted on color Doppler US. Arteriovenous fistula is seen as a localized area of high-velocity turbulent flow. The feeding artery may demonstrate a high-velocity, low-resistance waveform, whereas the draining vein may show an arterialized pulsatile waveform. Pseudoaneurysm is seen as a cystic area with internal flow. Doppler US may demonstrate bidirectional flow within the cyst.

UROLOGIC COMPLICATIONS
Hydronephrosis

Immediately following renal transplantation, transient obstruction may occur due to edema at the site of ureteral implantation. Later in the postoperative period ureteral obstruction may be caused by stricture, stone, blood clot, or sloughed papilla as in the native kidney.

Urine leak

Urine leak following renal transplantation most commonly occurs at the ureterovesical anastomosis and the renal pelvis. It

occurs weeks to months following transplantation. It may lead to urinoma and/or urine ascites when the leak is large.

Imaging findings

US can easily detect dilation of the collecting system, although the dilation does not always indicate urinary obstruction. Mild dilation of the collecting system may occur due to volume overload or loss of tone in collecting system after transplantation. Although the use of RI has been reported to be helpful in differentiating obstructive and nonobstructive hydronephrosis, subsequent studies revealed that there is little correlation between RI and the degree of obstruction.

FLUID COLLECTIONS

Various perigraft fluid collections may occur, including hematoma, urinoma, abscess, and lymphocele. The onset of fluid collection may be helpful in differentiating among them. Hematoma and urinoma commonly occur in the early postoperative days, whereas a lymphocele usually occurs later than 4 weeks following transplantation.

Hematoma

Following transplantation, a small amount of perirenal fluid is common and usually represents hematoma or seroma. It often surrounds the allograft and contains internal septa. It resolves spontaneously in several weeks. Hematoma associated with a leak from vascular anastomosis is often large and may displace or compress the allograft.

Urinoma

Urinoma is a rare complication that occurs within 2 weeks following transplantation. The fluid collection is usually located between the allograft and bladder but may occur in the scrotum or thigh. Diminished urine output in an initially functioning allograft suggests urinary leak. Urine ascites may occur when the fluid collection communicates with the peritoneal space.

Lymphocele

Lymphocele is the most common post-transplant fluid collection resulting from lymphatic obstruction due to surgically disrupted lymphatics. It occurs 4 to 8 weeks following transplantation. It is often located between the allograft and bladder and commonly is accompanied by hydronephrosis. When large, it may compress the collecting system or ureter and therefore needs to be treated.

Imaging findings

On US hematomas are often seen as regions of decreased echogenicity but may demonstrate high echogenicity due to clots or cellular debris. Septation is common. CT may demonstrate layering in the cystic lesion. Urinoma is often seen as an anechoic lesion around the allograft or ureter. Leak of intravenous contrast material may be demonstrated on IVU or CT.

Lymphocele is seen as an anechoic lesion, often with multiple fine septations. On Doppler US, it may cause an increase in RIs, particularly when the lesion is very large and compresses the ureter. On CT, lymphocele is seen as a low-attenuated lesion with a CT value of 0 to 20 HU. It does not enhance following administration of intravenous contrast material.

References

1. Dunnick NR, Sandler CM, Newhouse JH, Amis ES Jr: Renal transplantation. In Dunnick NR, Sandler CM, Newhouse JH, Amis ES Jr (eds): Textbook of Uroradiology, 3rd ed. Philadelphia, Lippincott Williams & Wilkins, 2001, pp 242–259.
2. Choyke PL, Becker JA, Zeissman HA: Imaging of the transplanted kidney. In Pollack HM, McClennan BL (eds): Clinical Urography, 2nd ed, vol 3. Philadelphia, WB Saunders, 2000, pp 3091–3118.
3. Quarto diPalo F, Rivolta R, Elli A, et al: Relevance of resistive index ultrasonographic measurement in renal transplantation. Nephron 1996; 73:195.
4. Pozniak MA, Dodd GD, Kelcz F: Ultrasonographic evaluation of renal transplantation. Radiol Clin North Am 1992; 30:1053–1066.
5. Pozniak MA, Kelcz MA, D'Alessandro A, et al: Sonography of renal transplants in dogs: The effect of acute tubular necrosis, cyclosporin nephrotoxicity, and acute rejection on resistive index and renal length. AJR Am J Roentgenol 1992; 158:791–797.
6. Stavros AT, Parker SH, Yakes WF, et al: Segmental stenosis of the renal artery: Pattern recognition of tardus and parvus abnormalities with duplex sonography. Radiology 1992; 184:487–492.
7. Patriquin HB, Lafortune M, Jequier JC, et el: Stenosis of the renal artery: Assessment of slowed systole in the downstream circulation with Doppler sonography. Radiology 1992; 184:479–485.
8. Grenier N, Douws C, Morel D, et al: Detection of vascular complications in renal allografts with color Doppler flow imaging. Radiology 1991; 178:217–223.
9. Perchik JE, Baumgartner BR, Bernadino ME: Renal transplant rejection: Limited value of duplex Doppler sonography. Invest Radiol 1991; 26:422–426.
10. Pozniak MA, Kelcz F, Dodd GD III: Renal transplant ultrasound: Imaging and Doppler. Semin Ultrasound CT MR 1991; 12:319–334.
11. Kaveggia LP, Perrella RR, Grant EG, et al: Duplex Doppler sonography in renal allografts: The significance of reversed flow in diastole. AJR Am J Roentgenol 1990; 155:295–298.
12. Hubsch PJS, Mostbeck G, Barton PP, et al: Evaluation of arteriovenous fistulas and pseudoaneurysms in renal allografts following percutaneous needle biopsy: Color-coded Doppler sonography versus duplex Doppler sonography. J Ultrasound Med 1990; 9:95–100.
13. Meyer M, Paushter D, Steinmuller DR: The use of duplex Doppler ultrasonography to evaluate renal allograft dysfunction. Transplantation 1990; 50:974–978.
14. Allen KS, Jorkasky DK, Arger PH, et al: Renal allografts: Prospective analysis of Doppler sonography. Radiology 1989; 169:371–376.
15. Fleischer AC, Hinton AA, Glick AD, et al: Duplex Doppler sonography of renal transplants: Correlation with histopathology. J Ultrasound Med 1989; 8:89–94.
16. Genkins SM, Sanfilippo FP, Carroll BA: Duplex Doppler sonography of renal transplants: Lack of sensitivity and specificity in establishing pathologic diagnosis. AJR Am J Roentgenol 1989; 152:535–539.
17. Gottlieb RH, Luhmann K, Oates RP: Duplex ultrasound evaluation of normal native kidneys and native kidneys with urinary tract obstruction. J Ultrasound Med 1989; 8:609–611.
18. Middleton WD, Kellman GM, Melson GL, et al: Postbiopsy renal transplant arteriovenous fistulas: Color Doppler versus US characteristics. Radiology 1989; 171:253–257.
19. Platt JF, Rubin JM, Ellis JH: Distinction between obstructive and nonobstructive pyelocaliectasis with duplex Doppler sonography. AJR Am J Roentgenol 1989; 153:997–1000.
20. Snider JF, Hunter DW, Moradian GP, et al: Transplant renal artery stenosis: Evaluation with duplex sonography. Radiology 1989; 172:1027–1030.
21. Taylor KJW, Morse SS, Rigsby CH, et al: Vascular complications in renal allograft: Detections with duplex Doppler US. Radiology 1987; 162:31–38.
22. Noel AW, Velchik MG: Urine extravasation into the scrotum. J Nucl Med 1986; 27:807–809.

Illustrations • Transplanted Kidneys

1. Normal Transplanted Kidney

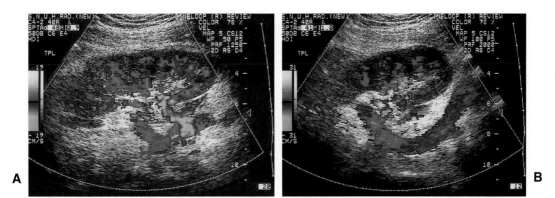

Fig. 1. Normal transplanted kidney in a 47-year-old man. (**A, B,** See also Color Section.)
A, B. Longitudinal (**A**) and transverse (**B**) color Doppler US of the transplant show normal flow in the main renal artery and vein and normal parenchymal vascularity throughout the transplanted kidney.

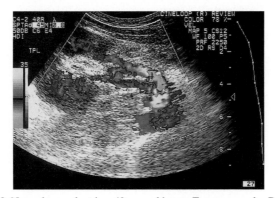

Fig. 2. Normal transplant in a 40-year-old man. Transverse color Doppler US of renal hilum demonstrates normal blood flow in the main renal artery and vein. (See also Color Section.)

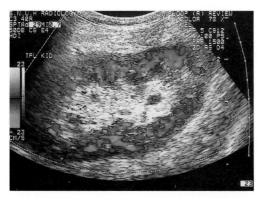

Fig. 3. Normal transplant in a 35-year-old man. Longitudinal color Doppler US demonstrates normal parenchymal vascularity. (See also Color Section.)

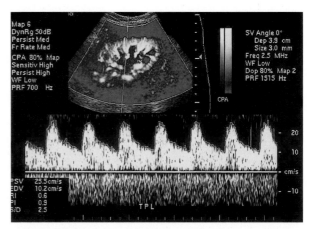

Fig. 4. Power Doppler and spectral Doppler US images of renal allograft in a 34-year-old man. Longitudinal power Doppler US shows normal parenchymal vascularity. Spectral Doppler US of interlobar artery demonstrates normal resistive index of 0.6. (See also Color Section.)

2. Acute Tubular Necrosis

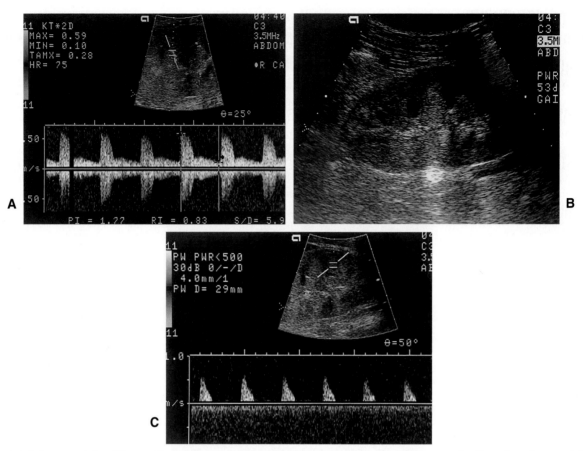

Fig. 1. Acute tubular necrosis in a 29-year-old man with renal allograft. The patient had fever and tenderness on the allograft on the second day after renal transplantation.
A. Spectral Doppler US demonstrates elevated resistive index (0.83). **B.** US performed on the fifth day following transplantation shows mildly swollen allograft with diffusely increased parenchymal echogenicity. **C.** Spectral Doppler US of an interlobar artery performed on the same day demonstrates loss of diastolic flow with resistive index of 1.0.

3. Acute Rejection

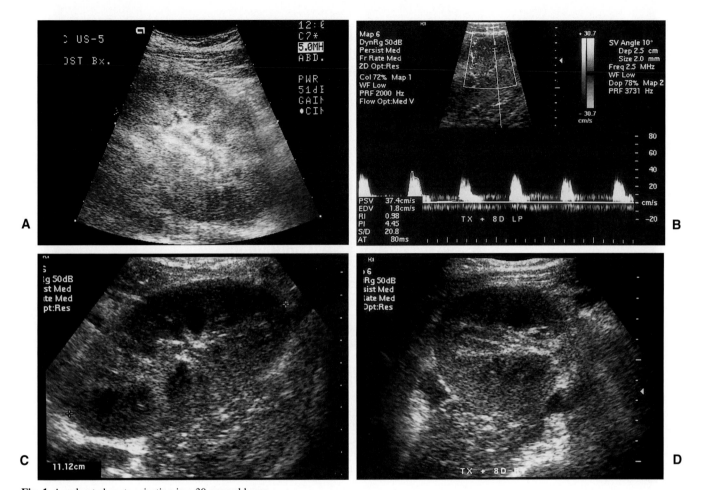

Fig. 1. Accelerated acute rejection in a 30-year-old man.
A. Longitudinal US shows swollen allograft with diffusely increased echogenicity. Biopsy was done on the fourth day after renal transplantation, which confirmed the diagnosis of acute rejection. **B.** Spectral Doppler US of the renal allograft shows sharp peak and weak diastolic flow, suggesting increased tissue resistance, consistent with allograft rejection. **C, D.** Longitudinal (**C**) and transverse (**D**) US images of the renal allograft on the eighth day after renal transplantation. Renal swelling was decreased. Cortical echogenicity also decreased but is still increased compared with that of normal kidney.

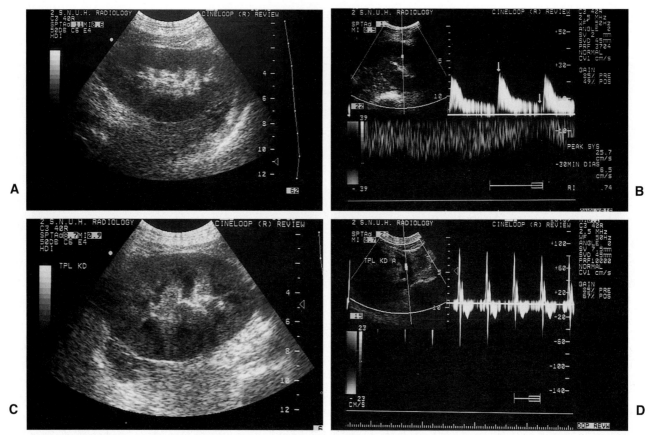

Fig. 2. Acute allograft rejection in a 31-year-old man.
A. Longitudinal US of the renal allograft performed on the seventh day following transplantation shows normal size and parenchymal echogenicity of the allograft. **B.** Spectral Doppler US performed on the same day as **A** shows a slightly elevated resistive index of 0.74. **C.** Longitudinal US performed on the 18th day following transplantation shows swelling of the allograft with decreased echogenicity of the renal sinus and thickening of the urothelium of the renal pelvis, suggesting acute allograft rejection. **D.** Spectral Doppler US shows a markedly increased resistive index.

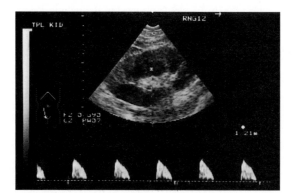

Fig. 3. Acute renal allograft rejection in a 46-year-old man. Spectral Doppler US of interlobar artery shows loss of diastolic flow with a resistive index of 1.0.

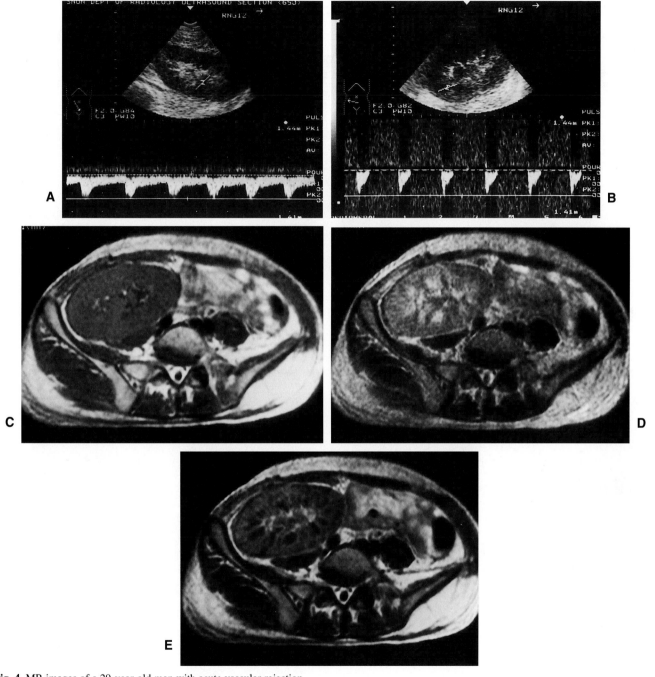

Fig. 4. MR images of a 29-year-old man with acute vascular rejection.
A. Spectral Doppler US performed 2 weeks after transplantation shows normal Doppler spectral pattern and normal resistive index of 0.64. **B.** Spectral Doppler US obtained 3 days after **A** shows a changed Doppler spectral pattern to very high resistance. Diastolic flow is absent, and the resistive index is 1.0. **C.** Transaxial T1-weighted MR image of the renal allograft shows diffuse renal swelling, compressed sinus fat, and loss of normal corticomedullary contrast. **D.** Transaxial T2-weighted MR image of renal allograft shows diffusely increased signal intensity in the renal medulla. Note that the renal sinus fat is compressed and is not well seen. **E.** After administration of intravenous contrast material, the renal cortex shows modest enhancement, whereas the renal medullary pyramids are not well-enhanced, indicating impaired excretory function of the allograft.

4. Chronic Rejection

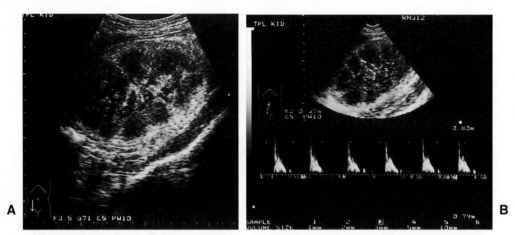

Fig. 1. Chronic renal allograft rejection in a 26-year-old man who had undergone transplantation 3 years earlier.
A. Longitudinal US of the allograft demonstrates increased renal cortical echogenicity and enlarged hypoechoic medullary pyramids. **B.** Spectral Doppler US of an interlobar artery shows an absent diastolic flow with a resistive index of 1.0.

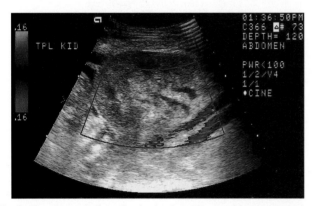

Fig. 2. Chronic renal allograft rejection in a 27-year-old man who had undergone renal transplantation 6 years earlier. Transverse color Doppler US shows diffusely increased parenchymal echogenicity with markedly decreased vascularity, which is suggestive of chronic rejection. (See also Color Section.)

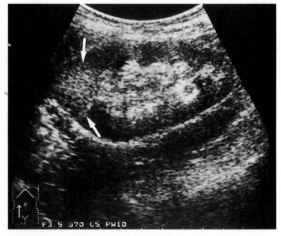

Fig. 3. Chronic rejection in a 43-year-old man who had undergone renal transplantation 3 years earlier. Longitudinal US of the transplanted kidney shows focal echogenic lesion in the upper-polar area *(arrows)*. Biopsy revealed chronic rejection.

5. Vascular Lesions in the Transplanted Kidney

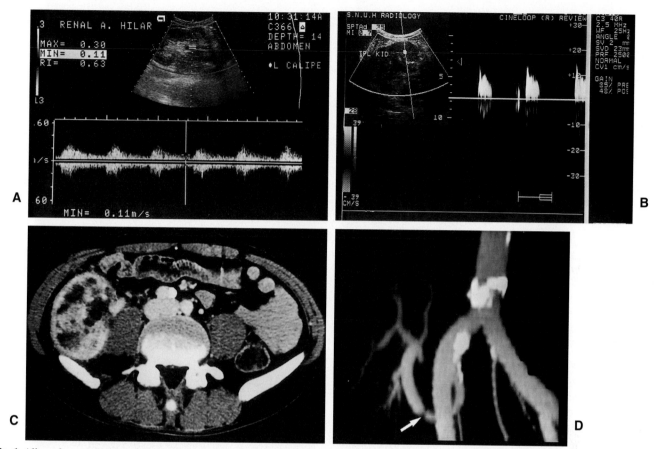

Fig. 1. Allograft renal artery stenosis with chronic rejection in a 33-year-old man who had undergone renal transplantation 5 years earlier.
A. Spectral Doppler US of the transplanted kidney reveals marked spectral broadening and a characteristic pulsus tardus-parvus pattern, which suggests renal artery stenosis. **B.** Spectral Doppler US performed 1 year later shows absent diastolic flows with a resistive index of 1.0. **C.** CT angiography was performed immediately before hemodialysis. Axial CT demonstrates heterogeneous renal parenchymal enhancement, which suggests chronic rejection. **D.** Maximal intensity projection image shows a focal stenosis *(arrow)* of the allograft renal artery at the site of anastomosis with the internal iliac artery.

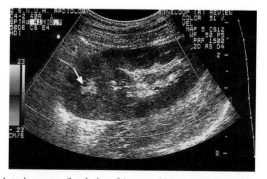

Fig. 2. Arteriovenous fistula in a 31-year-old man with transplant rejection who had undergone renal biopsy 1 month earlier. Color Doppler US of renal allograft demonstrates a hypervascular lesion in the upper portion of the allograft *(arrow)*. Note the turbulence in the lesion, shown as a mosaic pattern of flow signals. (See also Color Section.)

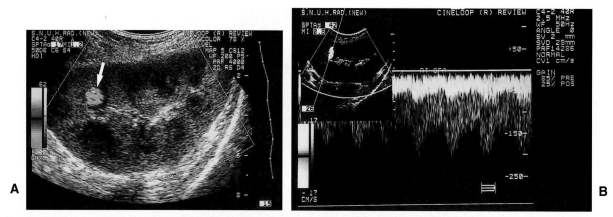

Fig. 3. Pseudoaneurysm in a 29-year-old woman with renal allograft, who had had an allograft biopsy 1 year earlier.
A. Color Doppler US reveals a focal area of high-velocity lesion with aliasing in the upper portion of the transplanted kidney *(arrow)*. (**A,** See also Color Section.) **B.** Spectral Doppler US of the lesion demonstrates a mixed, continuous and pulsatile flow with prominent spectral broadening.

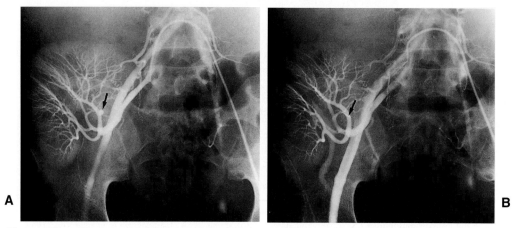

Fig. 4. A 27-year-old man with pseudoaneurysm of the transplant renal artery caused by a previous allograft biopsy.
A. Right iliac arteriography demonstrates a small aneurysm *(arrow)* in the segmental artery of the renal allograft. **B.** Embolization was performed by using a coil *(arrow)*, and postembolization arteriography shows disappeared aneurysm.

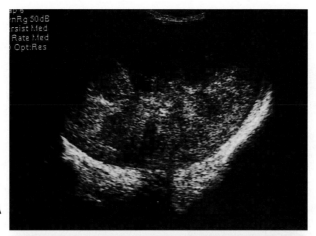

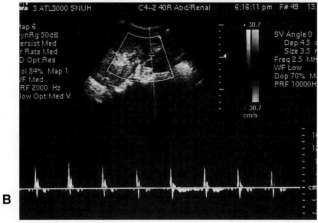

Fig. 5. Thrombosis of the allograft renal vein in a 52-year-old man who had undergone transplantation 4 years earlier.
A. Gray-scale US shows severe swelling of the transplanted kidney with diffusely increased parenchymal echogenicity. Note that the renal sinus is obliterated due to parenchymal swelling. **B.** Spectral Doppler US performed at the main renal artery of the allograft shows a very weak, high-resistance flow pattern. Renal parenchymal blood flow was markedly decreased and therefore Doppler spectrum could not be obtained from the intrarenal arteries. Transplant nephrectomy revealed hemorrhagic infarct of the kidney due to renal vein thrombosis.

6. Periallograft Fluid Collections

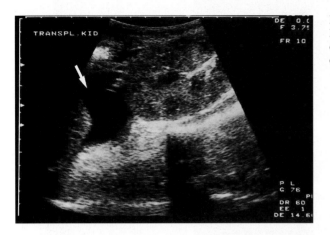

Fig. 1. Perirenal fluid collection in a 30-year-old man with renal transplant. Longitudinal US of the renal allograft shows a small amount of fluid collection *(arrow)* in the superior aspect of the renal allograft. The renal echogenicity is diffusely increased, which is suggestive of allograft rejection.

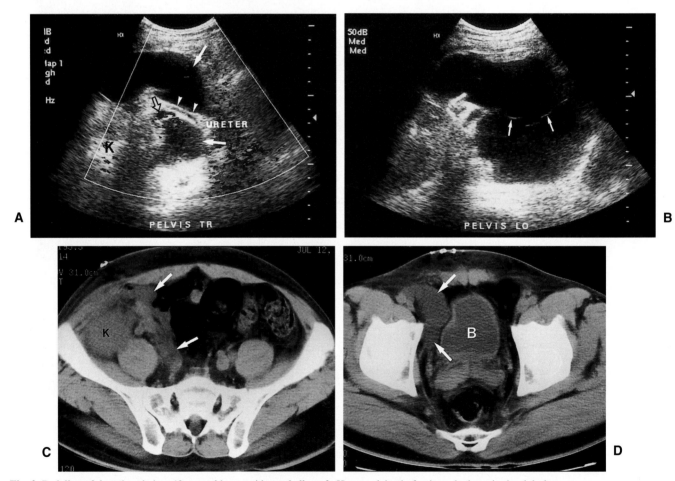

Fig. 2. Periallograft lymphocele in a 43-year-old man with renal allograft. He complained of pain and edema in the right leg.
A. Transverse US at the hilum of renal allograft demonstrates a fluid collection *(arrows)* encircling the ureter *(arrowheads)* and renal vascular pedicle *(open arrow)*. K, transplanted kidney. **B.** A consecutive US image of the fluid collection shows a fine internal septation *(arrows)*. **C.** Nonenhanced CT scan of the upper pelvis shows a small fluid collection *(arrows)* in the anteromedial aspect of the renal allograft (K). **D.** A consecutive nonenhanced CT scan of the lower pelvis shows a fluid collection *(arrows)* in the lateral aspect of the urinary bladder (B), which is a typical location for lymphocele.

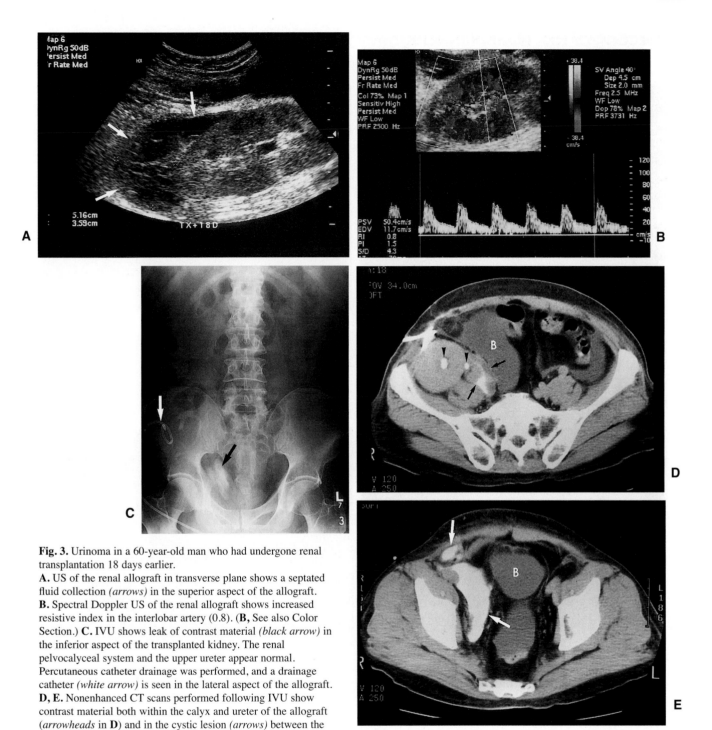

Fig. 3. Urinoma in a 60-year-old man who had undergone renal transplantation 18 days earlier.
A. US of the renal allograft in transverse plane shows a septated fluid collection *(arrows)* in the superior aspect of the allograft.
B. Spectral Doppler US of the renal allograft shows increased resistive index in the interlobar artery (0.8). (**B,** See also Color Section.) **C.** IVU shows leak of contrast material *(black arrow)* in the inferior aspect of the transplanted kidney. The renal pelvocalyceal system and the upper ureter appear normal. Percutaneous catheter drainage was performed, and a drainage catheter *(white arrow)* is seen in the lateral aspect of the allograft.
D, E. Nonenhanced CT scans performed following IVU show contrast material both within the calyx and ureter of the allograft *(arrowheads* in **D)** and in the cystic lesion *(arrows)* between the allograft and bladder (B).

7. Infection of the Transplanted Kidney

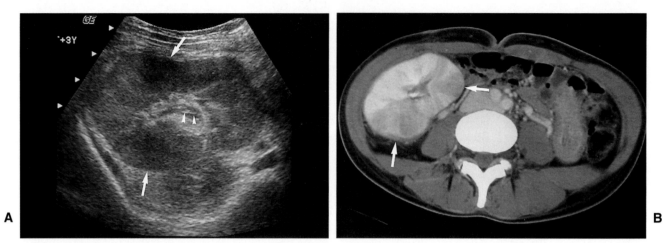

Fig. 1. Acute pyelonephritis in a transplanted kidney in a 30-year-old woman.
A. Transverse US demonstrates hypoechoic areas in both anterior and posterior portions of the kidney *(arrows)*. Near-field parenchymal lesion that is outlined by straight margins may be an artifact, but the lesion in the posterior parenchyma accompanies a bulging contour, which suggests a true lesion. The urothelium is thickened in the renal pelvis *(arrowheads)*. **B.** Contrast-enhanced CT demonstrates multifocal perfusion defects *(arrows)* mostly in the posterior portions of the transplanted kidney.

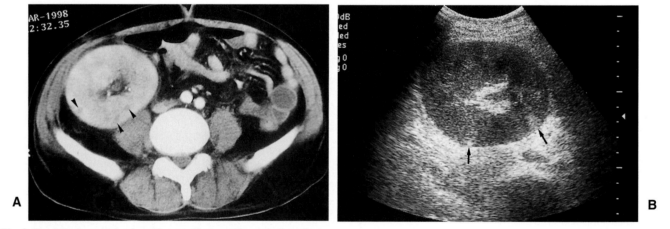

Fig. 2. Candidiasis occurring in a 42-year-old man with renal allograft.
A. Contrast-enhanced CT scan shows diffuse swelling of the renal allograft with heterogeneous enhancement of the renal parenchyma. Note small, low-attenuated lesions in the peripheral renal parenchyma *(arrowheads)*. **B.** Transverse US demonstrates small hyperechoic lesions *(arrows)*. US-guided biopsy revealed *Candida* infection of the transplanted kidney.

8. Miscellaneous Lesions of the Transplanted Kidney

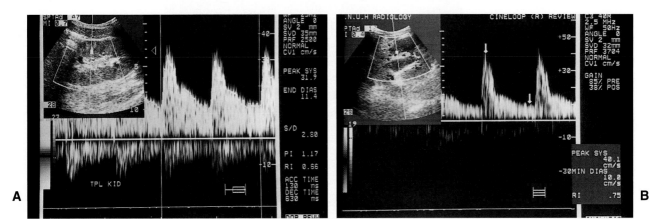

Fig. 1. Ureteral obstruction of the transplanted kidney at anastomosis in a 39-year-old man with renal allograft.
A. Spectral Doppler US of the transplanted kidney shows a normal Doppler spectral pattern and a normal resistive index of 0.66. **B.** Spectral Doppler US performed 1 year later, when the patient complained of decreased amount of urine, shows dilated renal pelvis and an elevated resistive index of 0.77.

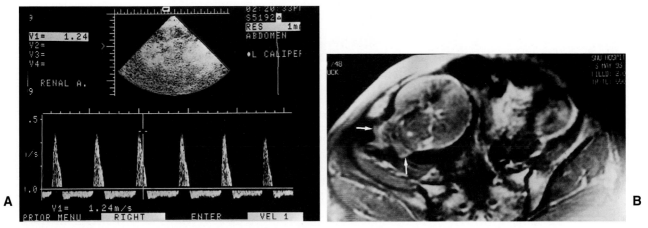

Fig. 2. Postbiopsy rupture of the renal allograft in a 48-year-old woman with allograft rejection.
A. Spectral Doppler US of an interlobar artery shows highly resistive flow and diastolic flow reversal, suggestive of severe vascular compromise.
B. After biopsy of the transplanted kidney, which revealed acute vascular rejection, the patient complained of severe pain at the biopsy site. Contrast-enhanced T1-weighted MR image of the renal allograft reveals rupture of renal allograft with perirenal fluid collection *(arrows)*.

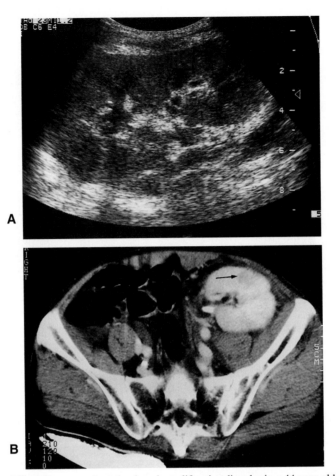

Fig. 3. Post-transplantation lymphoproliferative disorder in a 44-year-old man who had received a renal transplant from a living-unrelated donor 2 months earlier.
A. Longitudinal US of the transplanted kidney shows diffuse enlargement of the kidney with increased renal parenchymal echogenicity. No focal lesions are demonstrated. **B.** Contrast-enhanced CT shows diffuse enlargement of the transplanted kidney with focal low-attenuated lesion *(arrow)*. Renal biopsy revealed post-transplantation lymphoproliferative disorder of polymorphous variant with T-cell lineage, and transplant nephrectomy was performed.

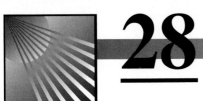

28

Pediatric Urinary Tract Infection and Related Conditions

IN-ONE KIM

Urinary tract infection is defined as a bacterial infection of the renal parenchyma, bladder, or urethra, singly or in combination. The growth of bacterial counts on culture greater than 100,000 colonies per cubic milliliter from the clean, midstream urine establishes the diagnosis. *Acute pyelonephritis* is an acute tubulointerstitial inflammatory disease of the kidney caused by bacterial infection. The underlying conditions of the urinary tract infection are vesicoureteral reflux, structural abnormalities causing obstruction, calculi, and hematogenous spread of the organisms. The most common causative organism is *Escherichia coli*, which comprises more than 80% of the cases. The patients present with nonspecific symptoms such as anorexia, lethargy, vomiting, irritability, fever, diarrhea, or failure to thrive. Acute pyelonephritis is an important cause of morbidity in children, and chronic urinary tract infection can cause hypertension or chronic renal failure.

PATHOPHYSIOLOGY

Urinary tract infection results from the imbalance between the bacterial virulence and host resistance. Presence of fimbria, rapid generation time of the bacteria, and the ability to sequester important nutrients or specific endotoxin enhance the survival or proliferation of the bacteria in the host. Host resistance factors are specific antibodies, unimpeded urinary flow, low density of the bacterial receptors, and anatomic barriers such as ureterovesical junction to prevent reflux or calyceal structures. Unidirectional flow of the urine is one of the most important factors in host resistance to bacterial infection, which is usually compromised by obstruction or reflux resulting from congenital abnormalities.

Obstruction can occur at any site, but the most common site is the ureteropelvic junction. Distal ureteral obstruction can occur functionally at the level of the distal segment of the ureter, often called *primary megaureter*. Ectopic ureterocele associated with the duplicated system and urethral obstruction most commonly due to posterior urethral valve are frequent causes of obstruction causing urinary tract infection.

Vesicoureteral reflux is an important cause of urinary tract infection in children. The reflux provides a pathway for the bacteria to reach the kidney from the bladder. It also causes stagnation of the urine, which enhances proliferation of the bacteria. Primary vesicoureteral reflux is due to maldevelopment or immaturity of the ureterovesical junction, and secondary reflux is frequently due to the presence of bladder

diverticulum at the ureterovesical junction, posterior urethral valve, or voiding disturbance from neurogenic bladder or bladder-sphincter dyssynergia. Parenchymal damage is more closely related to intrarenal reflux.

IMAGING

Imaging evaluation is reasonable for the first occurrence of infection in both sexes. The purposes of imaging are to detect structural or physiologic abnormality, to detect renal scar or reflux nephropathy, for baseline study for the evaluation of the renal growth, and to establish the prognosis. Radiologic techniques for the evaluation of urinary tract infection include voiding cystourethrography (VCU), ultrasonography (US), intravenous urography (IVU), renal cortical scintigraphy, and computed tomography (CT). Usually US is the first modality used to evaluate the structural abnormality of the kidney, and color Doppler study can detect a perfusion abnormality that accompanies acute pyelonephritis. US is useful in complicated renal infections such as abscesses, pyonephrosis, and perirenal fluid collections. IVU can be used to evaluate renal cortical scarring and excretory anatomy, but it is often insensitive in detecting acute renal infection. To detect vesicoureteral reflux, conventional or radionuclide VCU is the first examination. The cystographic study also provides the information regarding the bladder capacity, residual volume, and the presence of bladder-sphincter dyssynergia. Renal cortical scintigraphy is useful in identifying both acute inflammation and scars or reflux nephropathy, and it also provides quantitative information about functional renal tubular mass. CT is a sensitive means of evaluating the renal parenchyma in acute infection or detecting stones or perfusion defects. It is useful in cases in which complications are suspected but the US findings are negative.

ACUTE PYELONEPHRITIS

Acute pyelonephritis is defined as acute bacterial infection of the kidney with acute inflammation usually involving both the renal pelvis and parenchyma. The route of infection is most commonly ascending infection by either reflux or bacterial capability of ascent against the urine flow. The parenchymal component of the infection typically shows wedge-shaped lesions pointing to the papilla. It is tubulointerstitial nephritis accompanying cortical vasoconstriction and edema. Less commonly, hematogenous infection can cause acute pyelonephritis in patients with an

immunocompromised condition, drug abuse, or extrarenal source of infection. *Staphylococcus aureus* is the most common pathogen. The terminology of acute focal nephritis, focal bacterial nephritis, or lobar nephronia is widely used to represent the same condition.

CT is the most sensitive imaging modality in the diagnosis of acute pyelonephritis and suspected complication of renal infection. CT shows renal swelling with streaky, wedge-shaped or round, nonenhancing renal parenchyma. CT also demonstrates the presence of abscess or perirenal extension of the infection or renal scar. US is a good screening tool, but it is less sensitive in demonstrating early changes of inflammation. US shows renal swelling and focal echogenic abnormalities ranging from hypoechoic to hyperechogenic lesions with renal swelling. Color Doppler US also shows abnormally decreased perfusion.

CHRONIC PYELONEPHRITIS

Chronic pyelonephritis is usually caused by focal parenchymal scarring from a previous bacterial infection. It also begins in the medulla as a localized area of fibrosis and scar and results in a retraction of the outer margin and outer pulling of the papilla and calyceal distortion frequently in polar areas. US or IVU demonstrates loss of renal substance as reduced renal thickness at one of the renal poles or retraction of the renal pyramids or distorted calyces. Renal papillary necrosis, which is usually caused by decreased blood flow associated with diabetes, analgesics, or sickle cell disease in an older child or adult, can be confusing due to the loss of medulla, blunting of calyces, and thinning of the parenchyma.

PYONEPHROSIS

Pyonephrosis means infection of the kidney associated with obstruction. The renal parenchyma is the same as in an infected kidney without obstruction, but the content of the pelvocalyceal system shows echogenic materials on US or higher density of urine on CT.

CYSTITIS

Infection of the bladder can be caused by bacteria or virus or drug therapy, particularly with cyclophosphamide. The bladder wall is thickened with an irregular margin in a well-distended state due to edema or spasm that is apparent on US. Masslike lesions mimicking intraluminal tumor and blood clots can be seen in extensive hemorrhagic cystitis. Due to the altered compliance of the bladder wall, vesicoureteral reflux accompanies cystitis.

VESICOURETERAL REFLUX

Vesicoureteral reflux, the most common abnormality underlying urinary tract infection in childhood, is reported to be present in 30% to 40% of children with urinary tract infection. A high incidence of reflux, reportedly about 60%, is found in siblings and descents of the patients. Vesicoureteral reflux is now regarded as a primary phenomenon due to incompetence of the ureteropelvic junction and is not secondary to either obstruction or infection. Rarely reflux can be secondary to a voiding dysfunction.

Normal competence of the ureterovesical junction is due to the valvular mechanism of the submucosal ureteral tunnel and the obliquity and length of the intramural ureter. Reflux is now believed to result from the immaturity of the valvular mechanism, which is one of the rationales of medical suppression therapy, which allows for the maturation of the ureterovesical junction.

Vesicoureteral reflux is considered to be associated with renal scarring, and the correlation is high between the prevalence of scarring and the grade of reflux. The patients with higher grade of reflux are more likely to develop new or progressive scarring after urinary tract infection. Intrarenal reflux has more importance in scar formation, allowing parenchymal access of the microorganism. The two types of renal papillae are well described: simple and compound. Compound papillae are more prone to reflux, which facilitates intrarenal reflux. The compound papillae are mostly present in the polar region, which explains the frequent parenchymal loss of polar region in pyelonephritis. To produce intrarenal reflux, increasingly high pressures are required over the first 12 months of life, which suggests that increasingly effective defenses against intrarenal reflux are developing then. The "big-bang" theory suggests the particular susceptibility to renal scarring in the infancy period. Intrauterine reflux is reported to be a cause of reflux nephropathy even without overt urinary tract infection, and high-grade reflux of sterile urine may interfere with normal renal growth.

In the evaluation of vesicoureteral reflux, IVU and US may be completely normal even with a gross reflux. VCU or radionuclide cystography can be used to diagnose reflux. The grade of reflux is classified according to the extent of reflux and the degree of dilation of the refluxed ureter and pelvocalyceal systems. Radionuclide cystography is usually used for follow-up of known reflux.

VCU is indicated in patients with a urinary tract infection, especially with pyelonephritis, and in those with a sibling or parents with reflux. Prenatally detected hydronephrosis or hydroureter is also an indication for VCU. Changing degree of hydronephrosis during US is highly suggestive of reflux.

During VCU, the presence or absence of reflux, and the degree of reflux should be determined. The site of ureter insertion or coexisting bladder diverticulum, which might be connected with the refluxed ureter, should be carefully scrutinized.

URETEROPELVIC DUPLICATION

Ureteropelvic duplication is thought to be due to premature division of the ureteral bud or the development of two ureteral buds from the same mesonephric (Wolffian) duct. Incomplete duplication is more frequent. The Weigert-Meyer rule applies in complete duplication. Complete duplication has a higher incidence of infection, vesicoureteral reflux, parenchymal scarring, and obstruction. The ureter draining the upper moiety is usually obstructed and upper-pole kidney can be dysplastic. Reflux usually involves the ureter draining the lower moiety.

ECTOPIC URETEROCELE

Ectopic ureterocele is a cystlike protrusion of the dilated submucosal portion of an ectopic ureter into the bladder lumen. It is almost invariably associated with duplication, and the involved ureter is usually from the upper moiety, which is fre-

quently dysplastic. Disproportionately large ureterocele associated with a very tiny upper moiety is described as *ureterocele disproportion*. Ectopic ureterocele is usually unilateral, and in half of the cases, contralateral duplication is present. The ureterocele may fill the base of the bladder and obstruct the entire urinary tract or cause intermittent urethral obstruction. In the lower-pole moiety, vesicoureteral reflux is possible due to interference with the muscular support of the orifice. US demonstrates a dilated upper pole connected with the dilated tortuous ureter terminating in a round, thin-walled, anechoic intravesical ureterocele. Ureterocele might be invisible on VCU due to highly opaque contrast material or ureterocele deformed by bladder filling. Contrast dilution and observation during the early filling phase are important. Ectopic ureterocele frequently causes obstruction and acute infection, and therefore endoscopic incision is usually done to relieve obstruction of the upper moiety. Reflux of the lower moiety might disappear after the ureterocele incision.

ECTOPIC URETER

The primitive ureter arises from the mesonephric duct. The orifice migrates to lie in the bladder concomitant with a caudal migration of the remainder of the duct, which in boys contributes to the formation of the genital tract. Failure of the ureter to separate from the mesonephric duct results in the ureteral orifice being located at some point distal to its normal location, resulting in ureteral ectopia, which is much more frequent in girls.

In girls, ureteral ectopia is usually associated with a duplex kidney, and the upper segment terminates ectopically in the urethra, vestibule, or vagina. The opening is usually distal to the urethral sphincter, causing urinary incontinence. In this situation, upper-pole moiety might be too small to detect radiologically. In case of high suspicion, but where the IVU is not diagnostic, CT is the examination of choice. If the ureter inserts into the urethra at the level of the sphincter, cyclic voiding can demonstrate the reflux. In boys, ectopic ureter opens into the posterior urethra, ejaculatory ducts, seminal vesicles, vas deferens, or rectum, resulting in infection, hydroureteronephrosis, prostatitis, or epididymitis. Incontinence is usually not present in boys.

References

1. Cheon JE, Kim IO, Seok EH, et al: Radiologic findings after endoscopic incision of ureterocele. J Korean Radiol Soc 2001; 44:115–119.
2. Bellah RD, Long FR, Canning DA: Ureterocele eversion with vesicoureteral reflux in duplex kidney: Findings at voiding cystourethrography. AJR Am J Roentgenol 1995; 165:409.
3. Talner LB, Davidson AJ, Lebowitz RL, et al: Acute pyelonephritis: Can we agree on terminology? Radiology 1994; 192:297–305.
4. Ditchfield MR, De Campo JF, Cook DJ, et al: Vesicoureteral reflux: An accurate predictor of acute pyelonephritis in childhood urinary tract infection? Radiology 1994; 190:413–415.
5. Blyth B, Dasserini-Glazel G, Camuffo C, et al: Endoscopic incision of ureteroceles: Intravesical versus ectopic. J Urol 1993; 149:556–560.
6. Rypens F, Avni EF, Bank WO, et al: The ureterovesical junctions in children: Sonographic findings after surgical or endoscopic treatment. AJR Am J Roentgenol 1992; 158:837–842.
7. Zerrin JM, Smith JD, Sanvordenker JK, et al: Sonography of the bladder after ureteral reimplantation. J Ultrasound Med 1992; 11:87–91.
8. Majd M, Rushton HG, Jantausch B, et al: Relationship among vesicoureteral reflux, p-fimbriated *Escherichia coli*, and acute pyelonephritis in children with febrile urinary tract infection. J Pediatr 1991; 119:578–585.
9. Najmaldin A, Burge DM, Atwell JD: Reflux nephropathy secondary to intrauterine vesicoureteral reflux. J Pediatr Surg 1990; 25:387–390.
10. Avni EF, Gansbeke DV, Thoua Y, et al: US demonstration of pyelitis and ureteritis in children. Pediatr Radiol 1988; 18:134–139.
11. Shimada K, Matsui T, Ogino T, et al: Renal growth and progression of reflux nephropathy in children with vesicoureteral reflux. J Urol 1988; 140:1097–1100.
12. Lebowitz RL, Mandell J: Urinary tract infection in children: Putting radiology in its place. Radiology 1987; 165:1–9.
13. Sty JR, Wells RG, Starshak RJ, et al: Imaging in acute renal infection in children. AJR Am J Roentgenol 1987; 148:471–477.
14. Israele V, Darabi A, McCracken GH Jr: The role of bacterial virulence factors and Tamm-Horsfall protein in the pathogenesis of *Escherichia coli* urinary tract infection in children. Am J Dis Child 1987; 141:1230–1234.
15. Lebowitz RL, Olbing H, Parkkulainen KV, et al: International system of radiographic grading of vesicoureteral reflux. Pediatr Radiol 1985; 15:105–109.
16. Glassberg KI, Braren V, Duckett JW, et al: Suggested terminology for duplex systems, ectopic ureters, and ureteroceles. J Urol 1984; 132:1153–1154.

Illustrations • Pediatric Urinary Tract Infection and Related Conditions

1 • Infection of the kidney

2 • Cystitis

3 • Vesicoureteral reflux

4 • Ureterocele

5 • Ureteropelvic duplication

6 • Ectopic ureter

7 • Urethral abnormalities

1. Infection of the Kidney

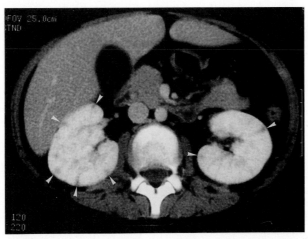

Fig. 1. Renal candidiasis in a 6-year-old boy receiving chemotherapy for acute leukemia. Contrast-enhanced CT shows multifocal, low-attenuated lesions scattered throughout both kidneys *(arrowheads)*. These lesions are seen as wedge-shaped streaks pointing to the hilum.

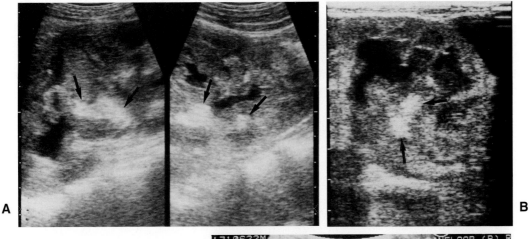

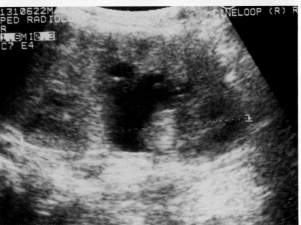

Fig. 2. Renal fungus *(Candida)* ball in an infant after operation for jejunal atresia and strangulation.
A. US of both kidneys shows echogenic materials *(arrows)* occupying the pelvis of both kidneys. **B.** After 3 weeks of antifungal chemotherapy, the fungus ball has resolved partially, but the dilated pelvis and proximal ureter are still impacted with the echogenic materials *(arrows)*. **C.** After 5 weeks of chemotherapy, the fungus ball has nearly completely resolved.

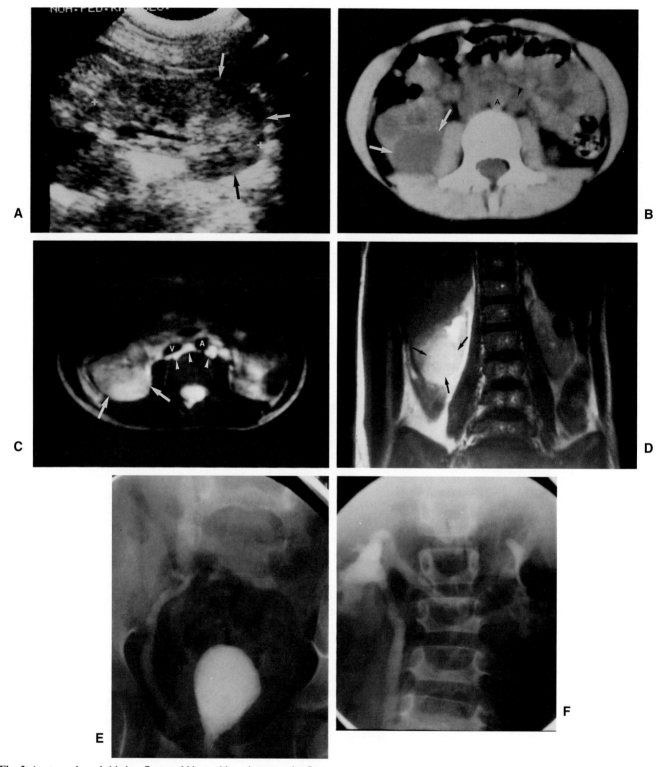

Fig. 3. Acute pyelonephritis in a 7-year-old boy with vesicoureteral reflux.
A. US of the right kidney shows round, echogenic bulging of the lower pole *(arrows)*. **B.** Nonenhanced CT shows round, low-attenuated, masslike lesions in the lower pole of the right kidney *(arrows)*. Multiple, enlarged para-aortic lymph nodes are also seen *(arrowhead)*. A, aorta. **C.** T2-weighted axial MR image shows high-intensity lesion of the right kidney *(arrows)*. Enlarged para-aortic lymph nodes are seen as round, high-intensity lesions *(arrowheads)*. A, aorta; V, inferior vena cava. **D.** Contrast-enhanced coronal MR image shows enhancing, masslike lesion in the lower pole of the right kidney *(arrows)*. A round, low-intensity, masslike lesion is present within the contracted left kidney. **E, F.** VCU shows vesicoureteral reflux in both kidneys. Biopsy of the right lower-polar mass reveals acute pyelonephritis.

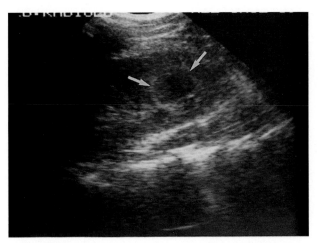

Fig. 4. Renal abscess in a 7-year-old girl. US of the right kidney shows a round, hypoechoic, masslike lesion in the lower pole *(arrows)*. Culture from the aspirate of the lesion revealed *Escherichia coli* infection.

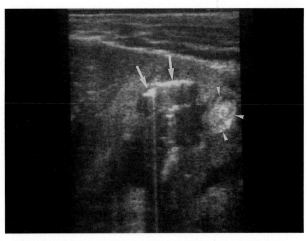

Fig. 5. Emphysematous pyelonephritis in an infant with a cloacal anomaly. US of the kidney shows a linear, hyperechoic lesion *(arrows)* with posterior sonic shadowing and reverberation artifact, suggesting air collection within the dilated calyx. The adjacent calyx is filled with echogenic material *(arrowheads)*.

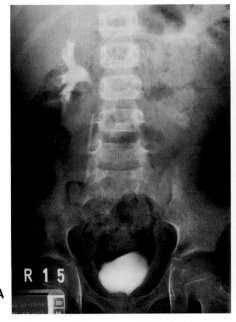

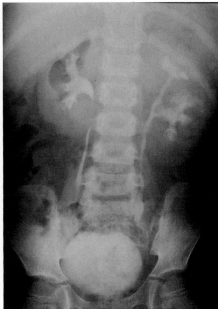

Fig. 6. Renal tuberculosis in a 6-year-old boy.
A. A 15-minute film from IVU shows nonopacification of the left collecting system except localized puddling of contrast material in the lower pole.
B. Delayed radiograph shows irregular, moth-eaten appearance of the calyces and multifocal strictures of the major calyx and the ureter of the left kidney.

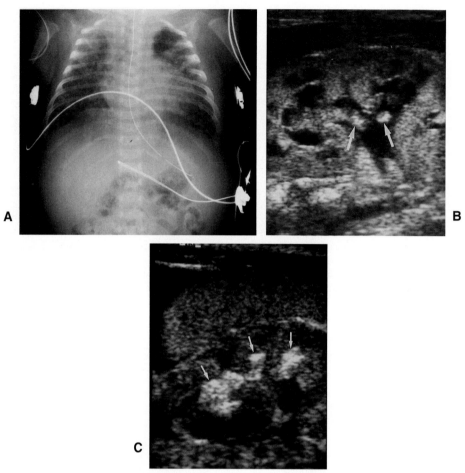

Fig. 7. Renal fungus ball and stone formation complicated by bronchopulmonary dysplasia in a premature infant.
A. Plain radiograph of the chest demonstrates reticulonodular infiltrations in both lungs with uneven hyperaeration suggesting chronic bronchopulmonary dysplasia. Hepatosplenomegaly is also seen. **B.** Echogenic materials within the pelvocalyceal system are probably fungus balls *(arrows)*. Urine culture revealed fungal growth. **C.** Follow-up US shows echogenic materials within the calyces *(arrows)* with posterior shadowing presumed to be stone induced by long-term furosemide (Lasix) therapy.

2. Cystitis

Fig. 1. Hemorrhagic cystitis in a 7-year-old girl with frequency, urgency, hematuria, and dysuria.
A. IVU shows marked irregularity of the bladder wall. The ureterovesical junctions appear as filling defects due to marked thickening of the bladder wall. Anatomy and function of both kidneys are normal. **B.** Delayed radiograph shows decreased bladder capacity with irregular thickening of the wall.

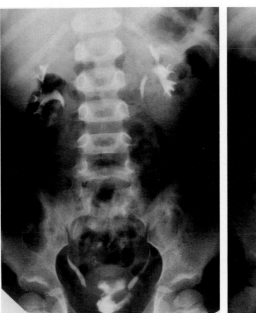

A

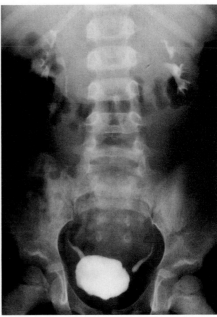

B

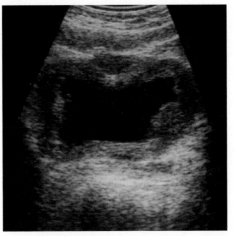

Fig. 2. Acute hemorrhagic cystitis in a 5-year-old boy. US of the bladder shows markedly thickened, lobulated bladder wall.

3. Vesicoureteral Reflux

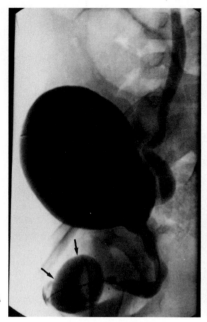

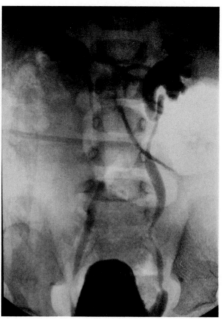

Fig. 1. Grade III–IV vesicoureteral reflux. **A.** VCU shows reflux into the dilated left ureter during voiding. Contrast material distends the glandular prepuce (*arrows*) due to severe phimosis, and the urethra is moderately distended. **B.** Mild clubbing of the calyceal fornices due to reflux is seen in both kidneys.

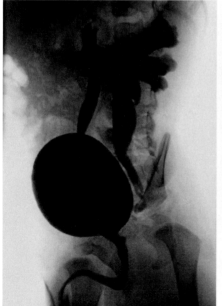

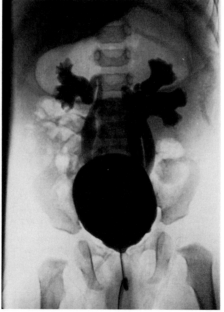

Fig. 2. Grade V vesicoureteral reflux. **A, B.** VCU demonstrates bilateral, high-grade vesicoureteral reflux with dilation of the pelvocalyceal system and ureter. Note incomplete duplication of the left kidney.

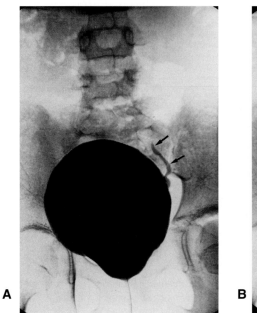

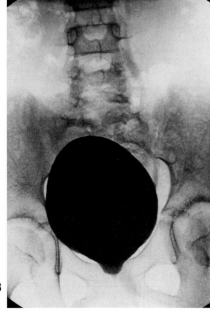

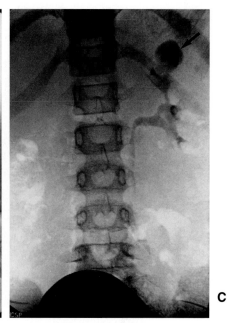

Fig. 3. Vesicoureteral reflux up to the calyceal diverticulum.
A. Filling phase of the VCU demonstrates reflux into the distal portion of the left ureter *(arrows).* **B.** Voiding phase of VCU reveals a reflux into the mildly dilated left ureter. **C.** Refluxed contrast material opacifies the calyces and diverticulum *(arrow)* in the upper pole.

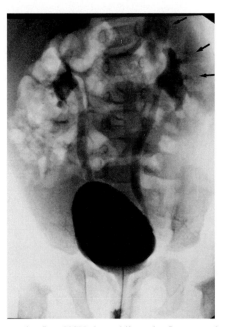

Fig. 4. Intrarenal reflux. VCU shows bilateral reflux up to the calyces, and the opacification of the renal papillae *(arrows)* is demonstrated.

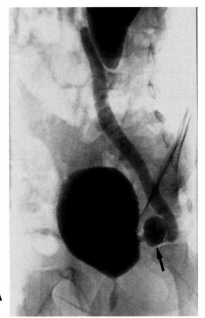

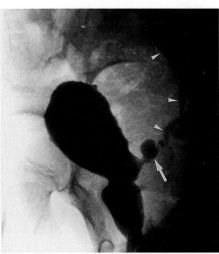

A

B

Fig. 5. Bladder diverticulum with vesicoureteral reflux.
A. Voiding phase of VCU demonstrates bladder diverticulum and severe vesicoureteral reflux. The refluxed ureter inserts into the diverticulum, which is the so-called Hutch diverticulum *(arrow)*.
B. VCU in a 4-year-old girl shows marked distention of the urethra and bladder diverticulum, suggesting urethral obstruction. Ureteral reflux *(arrowheads)* seems to be continuous with the diverticulum *(arrow)*.

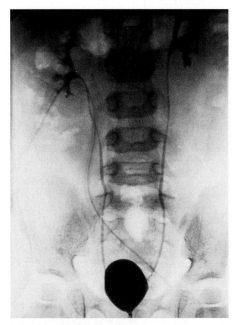

Fig. 6. Vesicoureteral reflux in a patient with chronic renal failure who was undergoing peritoneal dialysis. VCU shows reflux into the nondilated ureter and the pelvocalyces. The reflux is presumed to be caused by decreased compliance of the bladder wall.

4. Ureterocele

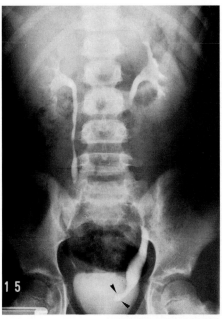

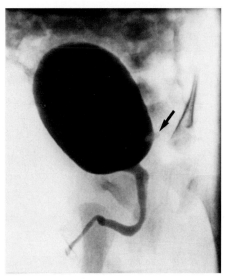

Fig. 2. Ureterocele eversion. On voiding image of the VCU, the partially contrast-filled ureterocele protrudes outward due to the eversion of the ureterocele *(arrow)*.

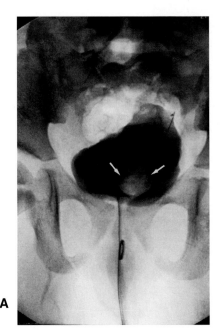

Fig. 1. Simple ureterocele. IVU shows mild dilation of the left distal ureter. The bulbous distal end of the left ureter is outlined by a thin radiolucent wall, which is the so-called cobra-head appearance *(arrowheads)*. Pelvocalyceal systems are normal.

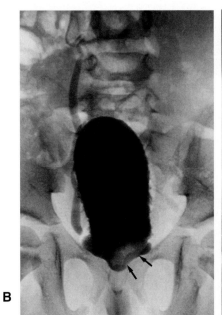

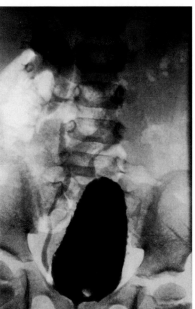

Fig. 3. Ureterocele causing intermittent bladder outlet obstruction.
A. The filling phase of VCU reveals a round filling defect due to ureterocele in the left side *(arrows)*. Slight undulation of the bladder wall suggesting prominent bladder trabeculation. **B.** During voiding, the ureterocele displaced downward *(arrows)* and obstructed the bladder outlet, and the patient suddenly stopped voiding. **C.** The reflux in the right side is most likely due to the bladder outlet obstruction by the ureterocele. Bladder wall trabeculation is evident.

5. Ureteropelvic Duplication

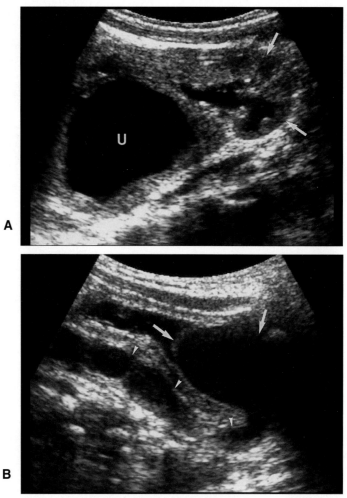

Fig. 1. Renal duplication in a 2-year-old boy with sepsis.
A. Longitudinal US of the kidney reveals duplication of the collecting system and marked hydronephrosis of the upper pole (U) containing echogenic debris, suggesting pyonephrosis. The appearance of the lower pole *(arrows)* is normal. **B.** The longitudinal scan of the bladder demonstrates the ureterocele as a round, cystic mass *(arrows)* that is connected with the dilated ureter *(arrowheads)* draining the upper pole. The wall of the ureter is markedly thickened.

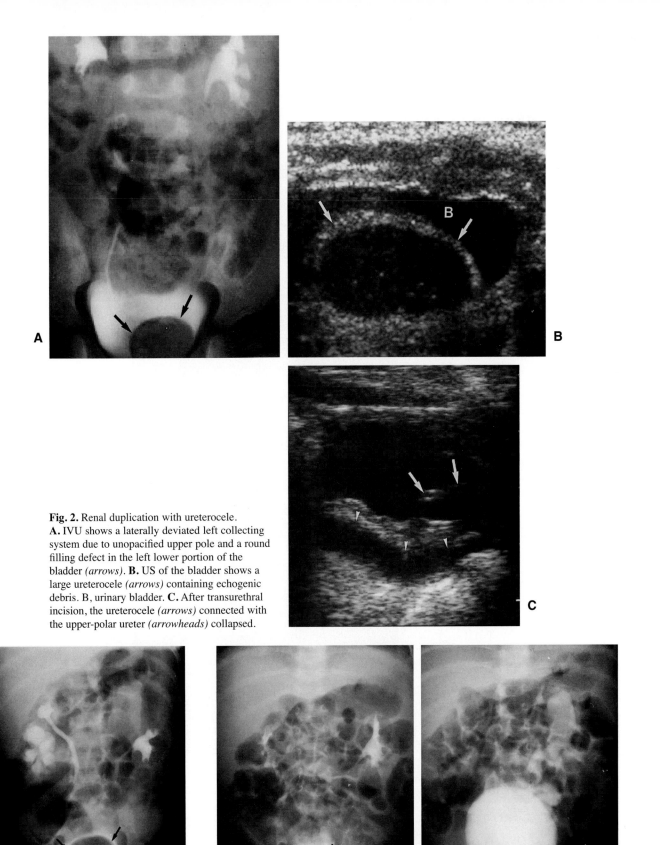

Fig. 2. Renal duplication with ureterocele.
A. IVU shows a laterally deviated left collecting system due to unopacified upper pole and a round filling defect in the left lower portion of the bladder *(arrows)*. **B.** US of the bladder shows a large ureterocele *(arrows)* containing echogenic debris. B, urinary bladder. **C.** After transurethral incision, the ureterocele *(arrows)* connected with the upper-polar ureter *(arrowheads)* collapsed.

Fig. 3. Vesicoureteral reflux into the upper pole after transurethral incision of the ureterocele in an infant with sepsis.
A. IVU shows bilateral duplication and nonfunctioning left upper pole connected with a large ureterocele *(arrows)*. **B.** A 15-minute film of IVU shows collapsed ureterocele after transurethral incision *(arrows)*. **C.** Delayed image of IVU shows reflux into the dilated ureter and pelvocalyces of the upper moiety after transurethral incision.

847

6. Ectopic Ureter

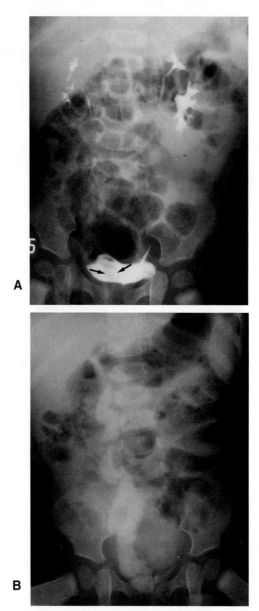

Fig. 1. Dysplastic upper pole with ectopic ureteral insertion in a 15-month-old girl with urinary incontinence.
A. A 15-minute film of IVU shows tubular, radiolucent impression *(arrows)* on the right side of the bladder. **B.** RGU reveals a dilated ureter connected with the collecting system of the dysplastic upper pole. The opening of ectopic ureter was identified at the proximal urethra.

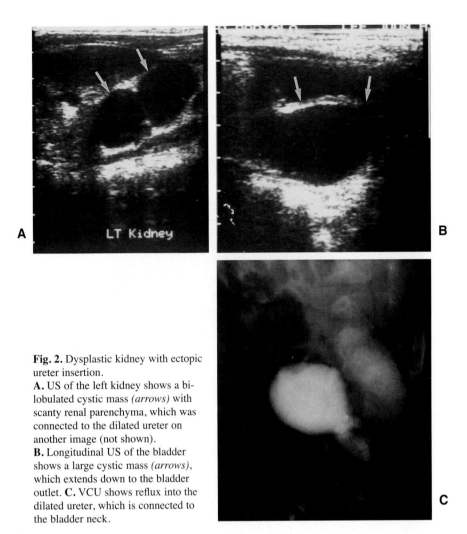

Fig. 2. Dysplastic kidney with ectopic ureter insertion.
A. US of the left kidney shows a bi-lobulated cystic mass *(arrows)* with scanty renal parenchyma, which was connected to the dilated ureter on another image (not shown).
B. Longitudinal US of the bladder shows a large cystic mass *(arrows)*, which extends down to the bladder outlet. **C.** VCU shows reflux into the dilated ureter, which is connected to the bladder neck.

Fig. 3. Dysplastic kidney with ectopic ureteral insertion into the seminal vesicle.
A. VCU shows reflux into the seminal vesicle *(arrows)* and opacification of tortuous linear structure, indicating a rudimentary ureter *(arrowheads)*.
B. Dysplastic right kidney is connected with the refluxed, tortuous, rudimentary ureter *(arrowheads)*. Note prominent bladder trabeculation, left vesicoureteral reflux, and posterior urethral distention, suggesting urethral obstruction.

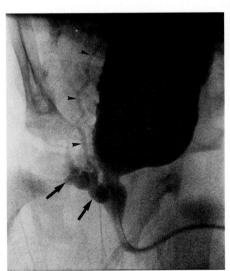

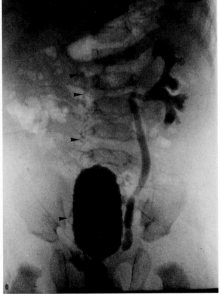

7. Urethral Abnormalities

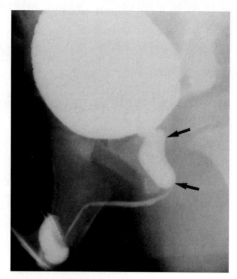

Fig. 1. Posterior urethral valve in a 2-year-old boy with urinary dribbling. VCU shows dilation of the posterior urethra *(arrows)* and accentuation of the bladder trabeculation.

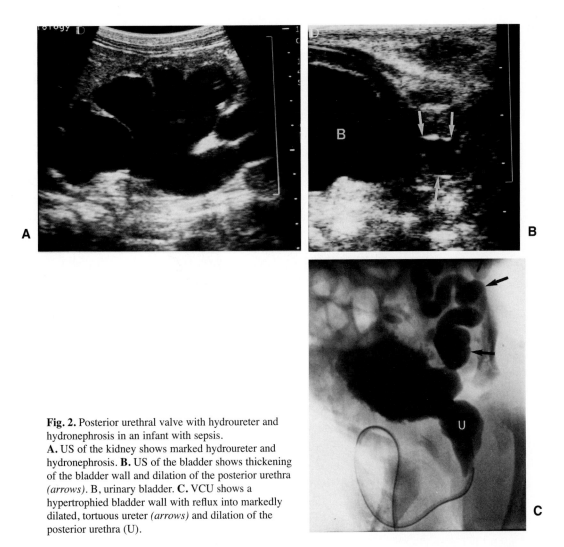

Fig. 2. Posterior urethral valve with hydroureter and hydronephrosis in an infant with sepsis.
A. US of the kidney shows marked hydroureter and hydronephrosis. **B.** US of the bladder shows thickening of the bladder wall and dilation of the posterior urethra *(arrows)*. B, urinary bladder. **C.** VCU shows a hypertrophied bladder wall with reflux into markedly dilated, tortuous ureter *(arrows)* and dilation of the posterior urethra (U).

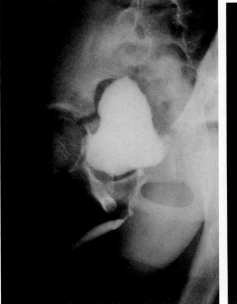

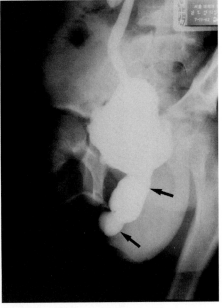

Fig. 3. Posterior urethral valve in 10-year-old boy.
A. Posterior urethral valve is not visualized on RGU. **B.** VCU clearly demonstrates dilation of the posterior urethra *(arrows)*. Note vesicoureteral reflux on the right side.

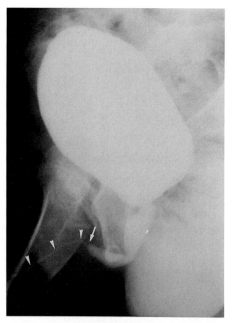

Fig. 4. Anterior urethral valve. VCU shows dilation of the prostatic and bulbous urethra and abrupt decrease of the distal urethral lumen *(arrowheads)* caused by an anterior urethral valve *(arrow)*.

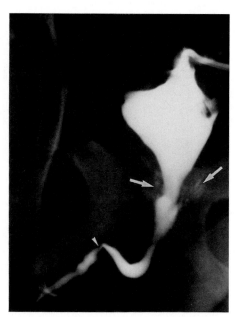

Fig. 5. Reflux into the prostatic ducts in a boy with urethral stricture. Voiding image of cystography shows multiple, fan-shaped, linear filling of contrast material *(arrows)* from the prostatic urethra. A focal stricture *(arrowhead)* is present in the proximal penile urethra.

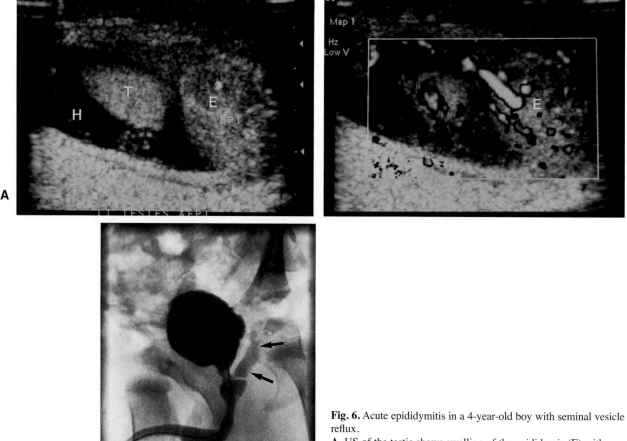

Fig. 6. Acute epididymitis in a 4-year-old boy with seminal vesicle reflux.
A. US of the testis shows swelling of the epididymis (E) with hydrocele (H). T, testis. **B.** Doppler US shows increased blood flow in the enlarged epididymis (E). **C.** VCU demonstrates reflux into the seminal vesicle *(arrows)*.

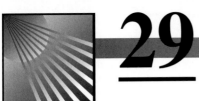

29

Nonvascular Interventions of the Urinary Tract

SEUNG HYUP KIM

PERCUTANEOUS NEPHROSTOMY

Percutaneous nephrostomy (PCN) is a basic uroradiologic interventional technique that provides direct access to the urinary tract to drain an obstructed tract and for further interventional procedures of the tract. It also provides a route for urodynamic study (Whitaker test). It is performed most frequently in the presence of urinary obstruction and has an important role as an emergency procedure in the case of urosepsis secondary to the urinary tract obstruction.

There are no absolute contraindications to PCN, except for a severe bleeding tendency, which requires preprocedural correction. In a patient with urinary infection, care should be taken since excessive manipulation of catheters or overdistention of the renal collecting system may result in septicemia. Antibiotics should be given before and after the procedure in a patient with urinary infection. Sedatives and narcotic analgesics can be used, but with caution, particularly in uremic patients.

The renal anatomy and its relationship to the surrounding organs should be understood to perform PCN successfully and safely. The renal axis parallels the psoas muscle, and the upper poles lie medial and posterior in respect to the lower poles. In a cross section, the kidney is angled about 30 degrees to the coronal plane of the body. Lower-pole posterior calyx is the most appropriate entry site for PCN if it is done for simple external drainage. If further interventional procedures are considered, interpolar or upper-polar calyx can be punctured. PCN can be placed between the 11th and 12th ribs, but puncture above the 11th rib should be avoided since it may injure the lung. The inferior margin of the ribs should be avoided to prevent bleeding from the subcostal vessels as well as pain from nerve and periosteal irritation.

Computed tomography (CT) may be necessary to ensure that the path for PCN will not injure adjacent organs such as liver, spleen, and descending or ascending colon. The risk of significant bleeding decreases when the calyx is entered end-on, thus violating only the small arcuate and interlobular vessels. The risk of damage to the large renal vessels increases when the puncture is done through the infundibulum or the renal pelvis.

The imaging guidance system used to direct the needle for puncture varies depending on equipment availability, patient body habitus, and radiologist's personal preference. After initial puncture, however, fluoroscopy is most widely used to monitor the manipulation of guide wires and catheters. Various types and sizes of PCN catheters can be used based on the viscosity of the urine encountered and underlying abnormality of the urinary tract. Usually 8- to 10-French pigtail-shaped catheters of the self-retaining type are adequate for simple drainage.

The following is the basic technique we are using for PCN:

1. With ultrasonographic (US) observation, the skin entry site is marked and the direction and the depth of needle puncture are decided.
2. Skin is prepared and draped in a sterile fashion.
3. Local anesthesia is applied down to the renal capsule.
4. For localization puncture, a 22-gauge needle is inserted according to the direction and the depth decided at US observation to enter the collecting system. (Continuous US guidance is used with a sterile transducer and guiding system, if necessary.)
5. After aspiration of an adequate amount of urine, the optimal entry site is confirmed by introducing diluted contrast material and air.
6. If the needle is located in the collecting system not appropriate for the tract, the ideal site should be punctured with another needle under fluoroscopic guidance (definitive puncture).
7. A 0.018-inch guide wire is inserted through the puncture needle.
8. Deeper local anesthesia is applied along the guide wire.
9. A coaxial sheath-stiffener system is passed over the guide wire.
10. A 0.038-inch guide wire is introduced through the sheath.
11. The tract is dilated serially using Teflon dilators.
12. A PCN catheter is inserted.
13. The PCN catheter is secured to the skin.

Sometimes a nondilated urinary tract needs to be punctured for PCN for diversion in patients with ureteral injury, most often from gynecologic surgery. In such cases, the collecting system should be opacified by intravenous injection of contrast material, and the puncture is done under fluoroscopic guidance. PCN for transplanted kidney is another special situation. In this situation, the upper-polar or interpolar calyx is usually punctured and a thinner (7- to 8-French) catheter is used. It is important to puncture as far lateral to the kidney as possible to prevent entry into the peritoneal cavity.

Following a PCN, the catheter is changed every 2 or 3 months. Sometimes the catheter locking cannot be released due to encrustation on the locking string. In this situation, a light jerking motion instead of steady pulling may help release the locking. If this maneuver does not work, a sheath is introduced over the catheter; then the catheter can be forcefully pulled into the sheath without injuring the kidney.

Major complications such as septicemia, hemorrhage requiring intervention, pneumothorax/hemothorax, and bowel injury are seen in about 4% of patients undergoing PCN. Gross hematuria is commonly seen after PCN and usually clears within 2 or 3 days. If bleeding does not respond to conservative management, angiography is indicated to identify an arterial trauma such as pseudoaneurysm or arteriovenous fistula, which can then be treated with embolization.

PERCUTANEOUS NEPHROSTOLITHOTOMY

The treatment options for renal calculi include open surgery, percutaneous nephrostolithotomy (PNL), ureteroscopic removal, and extracorporeal shock-wave lithotripsy (ESWL). The development of PNL, ESWL, and ureteroscopy have almost eliminated open stone surgery. The choice of treatment depends on the efficacy, cost, and goals of treatment and the experience and preference of the physician. ESWL is a noninvasive technique and serves as an effective monotherapy for approximately 75% of patients with urinary stones. PNL is ideally suited for complex stones such as staghorn calculi and calculi larger than 2 cm in diameter.

The indications for PNL are the presence of a large stone volume within the kidney; failure of previous ESWL; presence of obstruction distal to a stone; large lower-pole stones in a horseshoe kidney, pelvic kidney, or transplanted kidney; stones in calyceal diverticula or hydrocalycosis; cystine stones; and infected stones.

The puncture technique of PNL is basically the same as that for PCN, but the puncture site should be selected according to the stone shape and location. The localization puncture is done using a 22-gauge needle, and the definitive puncture is usually done with an 18-gauge needle, which permits introduction of a 0.038-inch guide wire. Once the guide wire is positioned, another guide wire is introduced for safety. The tract is dilated and a sheath is introduced to accommodate a nephroscope. The stones are then extracted with fragmentation if necessary. When the stone extraction is completed, the postoperative nephrostomy tube is placed for drainage and tamponade of the tract.

Basically, PNL involves four steps:

1. Creation of a percutaneous access tract, which is the most critical to the success of the whole procedure.
2. Tract dilation up to 30 to 34 French to accommodate a nephroscope.
3. Stone fragmentation and extraction using ultrasonic lithotripsy, forceps, and baskets.
4. Postoperative nephrostomy tube placement.

The entire procedure can be performed in a single session in the operating room using C-arm fluoroscopy, but I prefer a two-session procedure in which access tract creation is done in the radiology department and the remaining procedures in the operating room on the next day. Stones in the proximal ureter can be dislodged into the renal pelvis using a retrograde catheter by catheter-push or flushing and then can be extracted through the nephrostomy tract.

Overall, complications occur in about 20% of patients; they include hemorrhage requiring transfusion, pseudoaneurysm or arteriovenous fistula, urinary tract injury, injury to the adjacent organs, and sepsis.

PERCUTANEOUS DILATION OF THE URINARY TRACT

Although percutaneous dilation is possible in the entire urinary tract from the calyces to the urethra, the ureter is the most common site for percutaneous dilation. The ureteral strictures can be dealt with through either a percutaneous antegrade route or transurethral retrograde route, either under fluoroscopic guidance or using endourologic procedures.

Ureteral strictures are caused by various benign and malignant lesions in and around the ureter. Benign causes include congenital obstruction, which is most common at the ureteropelvic junction, infections such as tuberculosis, postoperative anastomotic strictures following urinary diversion or renal transplantation, iatrogenic causes such as surgical trauma or percutaneous or endourologic procedures, and periureteral causes such as retroperitoneal fibrosis or endometriosis. Malignant lesions causing ureteral obstruction include primary ureteral tumors and secondary lesions, either by direct invasion or metastasis. Ureteral dilation should be considered before surgery for all benign ureteral strictures. However, ureteral dilation is usually not indicated for strictures caused by malignant lesions. Ureteral strictures can be dilated by using various instruments including balloons, catheters, ureteral dilators, electroincision devices, and knives. Knives are used for endourologic procedures. Congenital ureteropelvic junction obstruction is better treated with a combined procedure using a knife and a balloon under endoscopic guidance. Ureteral dilation is usually followed by insertion of a ureteral stent for healing without restenosis.

Results of the percutaneous dilation for benign ureteral strictures are variable. The average success rate is around 50%. Factors affecting the results of balloon dilation are variable and include underlying causes, location, length, duration of strictures, and the presence or absence of associated vascular compromise. Strictures of shorter length and shorter duration have better responses than those of longer length and longer duration. Old, densely fibrotic strictures associated with ischemia appear to be less responsive to dilation; examples are strictures after radical hysterectomy and radiation therapy, strictures at a ureteroenteric anastomosis, and transplantation ureteral strictures. It had been thought that ureteral tuberculosis was likely to cause endarteritis obliterans leading to ischemia, implying that the condition may have a poor response to balloon dilation. However, our experience has shown that the results of ureteral strictures treated with percutaneous dilation and ureteral stenting are promising.

As in all other percutaneous procedures on the urinary tract, percutaneous ureteral dilation should begin with a PCN. Although lower-polar calyx is usually selected in PCN for external drainage, the interpolar calyx is more suitable when ureteral dilation is planned. A catheter with a slightly curved tip

is advanced just above the stenotic lesion, and contrast material is injected for clear documentation of the stenosis. In patients whose ureter has been anastomosed to an ileal or colonic conduit, the ureter can be catheterized in a retrograde fashion through the conduit under fluoroscopic guidance. The stenotic lesion is negotiated with the use of a proper set of a catheter and guide wire, inserted gently and carefully so as not to traumatize the ureter. Then the stenotic lesion is dilated by passing progressively larger-caliber catheters or ureteral dilators or inflating balloons with the appropriate diameter and length. Usually balloon catheters with a diameter of 4 to 10 mm and a length of 3 to 4 cm are used. After dilation, a ureteral stent, either internal or internal-external, is introduced and kept for 3 to 8 weeks to allow the ureter to heal without restenosis.

Sometimes only a guide wire or a thin catheter can be passed but further manipulation is impossible due to very tight stenosis or angulation of the tract. In those cases, one can wait for a few days to let edema, inflammatory changes, or spasm resolve, or one can try to advance the guide wire into the urethra fluoroscopically or try retrograde transurethral retrieval of the guide wire from the bladder either cystoscopically or under fluoroscopy using a guide wire–snare technique. This permits the operator to apply tension on both ends of the guide wire, which keeps the guide wire straight as the dilator or catheter is being advanced through the tight stricture. During this procedure, a catheter should be located in the urethra over the guide wire to protect the urethra from injury. The same technique can be used in patients who have ureteroileostomies.

Causes of failure and common technical problems associated with internal ureteral stent placement include poor angulation of the percutaneous tract, tortuous dilated ureters, tight obstructions, wedging of stent assembly components due to high frictional resistance, and difficulty in positioning of the proximal pigtail. Helpful technical modifications include interpolar rather than lower-polar calyceal access, urinary decompression prior to stenting, and the use of a peel-away sheath.

To evaluate the response of ureteral strictures to percutaneous dilation, follow-up imaging is necessary. Although radionuclide scanning is considered to be the best imaging modality for this purpose, intravenous urography (IVU) and US are also excellent. The interval between follow-up examinations should be individualized.

SCLEROTHERAPY FOR RENAL CYSTS

Benign renal cysts are common in adults and occur in approximately 50% of all patients older than 50 years at autopsy. In the adult, most of the benign renal cysts are simple cortical cysts and, less commonly, parapelvic cysts. Renal cysts vary in size and are frequently multiple. The cause of renal cyst is uncertain, but tubular obstruction with ischemia has been postulated. Rarely renal cysts may shrink and disappear on follow-up examination, but most renal cysts enlarge slowly.

Diagnostic aspiration and cytologic evaluation of renal cysts with radiographic cystogram were once two of the most frequently performed percutaneous interventional procedures, but they have nearly vanished with the advent of US and CT. Today, diagnostic aspiration for renal cyst is performed only rarely, when US or CT cannot definitely establish that a renal cyst is benign. Most of the renal cysts are asymptomatic and

are detected incidentally on US, CT, or IVU performed for unrelated reasons. However, renal cysts may cause symptoms if they become very large or infected or hemorrhagic. They also can cause symptoms due to obstruction of the pelvocalyceal system, pressure atrophy of adjacent parenchyma, and stone formation in obstructed calyces. Rarely, renal cysts may cause renin-dependent hypertension and erythropoietin-related polycythemia vera.

If a renal cyst appears benign and is symptomatic, it can be managed with a combination of percutaneous drainage and sclerotherapy. Simple aspiration of a renal cyst is associated with a high rate of recurrence, that is, between 30% and 80%. This high rate of recurrence is probably due to rapid fluid turnover in the cyst. Various sclerosing agents have been tried to reduce the recurrence following drainage. Those sclerosing agents include hypertonic dextrose solution, hypertonic water-soluble contrast material, iophendylate (Pantopaque), quinacrine, bismuth phosphate, absolute alcohol, tetracycline, minocycline hydrochloride, and morrhuate sodium. They induce sclerosis of the lining of the cyst by chemical irritation. Quinacrine, bismuth phosphate, and iophendylate remain in place after instillation, whereas other agents are removed after therapy. Currently, absolute alcohol is most commonly used due to its rapid and strong sclerosing activity.

The technique and the protocol for sclerotherapy of the renal cyst are variable, and the number of scleroses and intervals between them are also variable. It is usually recommended to insert a small pigtail catheter into the cyst to repeat injection of sclerosing agents until no significant amount of fluid drains from the cyst. Following insertion of a 6- to 8-French catheter, the cyst fluid is aspirated and contrast material is injected to evaluate the appearance of the inner wall of the cyst and to ensure that there is no communication between the cyst cavity and the pelvocalyceal systems. Usually the cyst is replaced with an equal volume of a combination of water-soluble contrast material and air to produce a double-contrast image. Radiographs are taken in multiple projections and various positions of the patient. Then the contrast material is removed as much as possible and 25% to 50% of the cyst volume is replaced with absolute alcohol for 15 to 30 minutes. It is desirable to change the position of the patient every 5 minutes to allow the entire surface of the inner wall of the cyst to make contact with the sclerosing agent. Care must be taken not to overdistend the cyst causing a spill of the sclerosing agent into the surrounding tissue. The procedure should be repeated daily or twice a day according to the amount of the fluid drained. When the amount of drained fluid is less than 5 mL, the catheter is removed. The patient should be followed up with US or other imaging modalities. The procedure can be performed on two or more cysts simultaneously.

If a cystic lesion to be ablated communicates with the renal collecting system (e.g., calyceal diverticulum or hydrocalycosis), a sclerosing agent should not be injected because it may cause fibrotic stricture of the collecting system. Instead, the lesion can be managed by dilation of the narrow neck of the lesion. If a cyst is infected, needle aspiration or percutaneous catheter drainage with antibiotic therapy is usually enough and sclerotherapy is usually not indicated because infection per se has a strong sclerosing effect. If the cyst content is hemorrhagic, it is recommended that sclerotherapy be postponed for several days to wait for the hemorrhagic drainage to

clear and to confirm the absence of malignant cells on cytologic examination.

The results of sclerotherapy for renal cysts are generally excellent. Most of the papers report a 75% to 100% success rate following cyst drainage and sclerotherapy. In the cysts that do not respond well to percutaneous drainage and sclerotherapy, percutaneous marsupialization of the cyst into the renal collecting system can be tried before surgical resection is considered.

Complications associated with the procedure include those related to the cyst puncture and catheter insertion and those caused by the sclerosing agent. The complications that can occur during the cyst puncture and catheter insertion are bleeding (either intracystic or perirenal), arteriovenous fistula, pseudoaneurysm, and infection. The adverse effects of the sclerosing agents include systemic drug reaction and inflammation, fat necrosis, and fibrosis in the retroperitoneum caused by leakage of the sclerosing agents. However, most of these complications can be prevented if the catheter tip is appropriately located and the cyst is not overdistended.

PERCUTANEOUS CATHETER DRAINAGE

Percutaneous catheter drainage (PCD) is a well-accepted technique for draining abdominal and pelvic fluid collections such as abscesses, hematomas, lymphoceles, and peritoneal pseudocysts. Infected tumors also can be drained percutaneously. Some pelvic fluid collections require an approach via transvaginal, transrectal, transperineal, or transgluteal routes. In cases of lymphocele and peritoneal pseudocysts, sclerotherapy is required to prevent recurrence. For sclerotherapy, absolute alcohol is most commonly used, but povidone-iodine solution can be used in lymphocele.

Basic techniques of puncture, guide wire insertion, tract dilation, and catheter placement are identical to those used in PCN. Puncture for transvaginal or transrectal PCD is done under the guidance of endoluminal US. Sometimes it is difficult to dilate the tract transvaginally or transrectally, but it can be performed by using a stiff guide wire or rigid dilators, or by support of an endoluminal US–guiding system. The size and type of the drainage catheter should be selected depending on the nature of the fluid to be drained.

PERCUTANEOUS FOREIGN BODY RETRIEVAL

Various kinds of foreign bodies can be retrieved percutaneously from the urinary tract under fluoroscopic guidance without aid of a nephroscope. The most commonly encountered foreign body in the urinary tract is a malpositioned or fractured ureteral stent. Stones and fungus ball also can be removed percutaneously. Various devices and techniques for retrieval of foreign bodies of the urinary tract have been reported. They include loop snares, baskets, and forceps.

BIOPSIES

Biopsy of masses of the genitourinary tract can be performed by using various types of needles. Various types of biopsy guns have been developed for core biopsy, and they are more commonly used than fine-needle aspiration biopsy in the genitourinary tract. Renal biopsy for confirmation of renal parenchymal disease can be done using a biopsy gun mounted with a 16- to 18-gauge needle. In renal biopsy, care should be taken not to traverse the central renal area since the risk of injury to large vessels is increased when the renal sinus is punctured instead of the peripheral renal cortex. Biopsy of the pelvic lesions, including prostate, seminal tract, and gynecologic, are performed under the guidance of transabdominal or endoluminal US.

Fluoroscopy-guided retrograde brush biopsy has been advocated in patients suspected of having transitional cell carcinoma of the ureter or pelvocalyceal system, but this is not widely used now because of improvement in the ureteroscopic devices.

References

1. Kim HB, Kim SH, Kim YJ, et al: Sclerotherapy of pelvic lymphocele with povidone-iodine and ethanol. J Korean Radiol Soc 1999; 41:147–152.
2. Kim SH: Renal cyst sclerotherapy. In Han MC, Park JH (eds): Interventional Radiology. Seoul, Ilchokak, 1999, pp 620–625.
3. Kim SH: Percutaneous dilatation of the urinary tract. In Han MC, Park JH (eds): Interventional Radiology. Seoul, Ilchokak, 1999, pp 610–619.
4. Lee WJ: Percutaneous nephrolithotripsy. In Han MC, Park JH (eds): Interventional Radiology. Seoul, Ilchokak, 1999, pp 601–609.
5. Lee WJ: Percutaneous nephrostomy. In Han MC, Park JH (eds): Interventional Radiology. Seoul, Ilchokak, 1999, pp 591–600.
6. Fontaine AB, Nijjar A, Rangaraj R: Update on the use of percutaneous nephrostomy/balloon dilation for the treatment of renal transplant leak/obstruction. J Vasc Interv Radiol 1997; 8:649–653.
7. Hanna RM, Dahniya MH: Aspiration and sclerotherapy of symptomatic simple renal cysts: Value of two injections of a sclerosing agent. AJR Am J Roentgenol 1996; 167:781–783.
8. Isaacson S, Pugash RA: Use of a variation of loop snare for manipulation of ureteral stents. AJR Am J Roentgenol 1996; 166:1169–1171.
9. Kwak S, Leef JA, Rosenblum JD: Percutaneous balloon catheter dilatation of benign ureteral strictures: Effect of multiple dilatation procedures on long-term patency. AJR Am J Roentgenol 1995; 165:97–100.
10. Alexander AA, Eschelman DJ, Nazarian LN, et al: Transrectal sonographically guided drainage of deep pelvic abscesses. AJR Am J Roentgenol 1994; 162:1227–1230.
11. Kim SH, Park JH, Han MC: Antegrade balloon dilatation and ureteral stenting for the benign ureteral strictures. J Korean Radiol Soc 1994; 30:57–63.
12. Lu DSK, Papanicolaou N, Girard M, et al: Percutaneous internal ureteral stent placement: Review of technical issues and solutions in 50 consecutive cases. Clin Radiol 1994; 49:256–261.
13. Kim JC, Banner MP, Ramchandani P, et al: Balloon dilation of ureteral strictures after renal transplantation. Radiology 1993; 186:717–722.
14. Kim SH, Yoon HK, Park JH, et al: Tuberculous stricture of the urinary tract: Antegrade balloon dilation and ureteral stenting. Abdom Imaging 1993; 18:186–190.
15. Nosher JL, Siegel R: Percutaneous retrieval of nonvascular foreign bodies. Radiology 1993; 187:649–651.
16. Park JH, Yoon DY, Han JK, et al: Retrieval of intravascular foreign bodies with the snare and catheter capture technique. J Vasc Interv Radiol 1992; 3:581–582.
17. Banner MP, Ramchandani P, Pollack HM: Interventional procedures in the upper urinary tract. Cardiovasc Interv Radiol 1991; 14:267–284.
18. Kim SH, Song IS, Kim JH, et al: Retrieval of a guidewire introducer by catheter capture from the proximal inferior vena cava: Technical note. Cardiovasc Interv Radiol 1991; 14:252–253.
19. Lang EK: Percutaneous infundibuloplasty: Management of calyceal diverticula and infundibular stenosis. Radiology 1991; 181:871–877.
20. van der Kolk HL: Small, deep pelvic abscesses: Definition and drainage guided with an endovaginal probe. Radiology 1991; 181:283–284.
21. van Sonnenberg E, D'Agostino HB, Casola G, et al: Percutaneous abscess drainage: Current concepts. Radiology 1991; 181:617–626.
22. van Sonnenberg E, D'Agostino HB, Casola G, et al: US-guided transvaginal drainage of pelvic abscesses and fluid collections. Radiology 1991; 181:53–56.

23. Banner MP, Amendola MA, Pollack HM: Anastomosed ureters: Fluoroscopically guided transconduit retrograde catheterization. Radiology 1989; 170:45–49.

24. Beckman CF, Roth RA, Bihrle W III: Dilation of benign ureteral strictures. Radiology 1989; 172:437–441.

25. Bush WH, Brannen GE, Lewis GP: Ureteropelvic junction obstruction: Treatment with percutaneous endopyelotomy. Radiology 1989; 171:535–538.

26. Mueller PR, White EM, Glass-Royal M, et al: Infected abdominal tumors: Percutaneous catheter drainage. Radiology 1989; 173:627–629.

27. Sheline M, Amendola MA, Pollack HM, et al: Fluoroscopically guided retrograde brush biopsy in the diagnosis of transitional cell carcinoma of the upper urinary tract: Results in 45 patients. AJR Am J Roentgenol 1989; 153:313–316.

28. Doemeny JM, Banner MP, Shapiro MJ, et al: Percutaneous extraction of renal fungus ball. AJR Am J Roentgenol 1988; 150:1331–1332.

29. Kim SH, Park JH, Han MC, et al: Percutaneous nephrostolithotomy. J Korean Radiol Soc 1988; 24:453–456.

30. Lang EK, Glorioso LW III: Antegrade transluminal dilatation of benign ureteral strictures: Long-term results. AJR Am J Roentgenol 1988; 150:131–134.

31. Shapiro MJ, Banner MP, Amendola MA, et al: Balloon catheter dilation of ureteroenteric strictures: Long-term results. Radiology 1988; 168:385–387.

32. Amis ES Jr, Cronan JJ, Pfister RC: Needle puncture of cystic renal masses: A survey of the Society of Uroradiology. AJR Am J Roentgenol 1987; 148:297–299.

33. Lang EK: Percutaneous nephrostolithotomy and lithotripsy: A multi-institutional survey of complications. Radiology 1987; 162:25–30.

34. Lee WJ, Snyder JA, Smith AD: Staghorn calculi: Endourologic management in 120 patients. Radiology 1987; 165:85–88.

35. Bush WH, Brannen GE, Lewis GP, et al: Upper ureteral calculi: Extraction via percutaneous nephrostomy. AJR Am J Roentgenol 1985; 144:795–799.

36. Banner MP, Pollack HM: Dilatation of ureteral stenoses: Techniques and experience in 44 patients. AJR Am J Roentgenol 1984; 143:789–793.

37. Bush WH, Brannen GE: Parallel-tract push: Adjuvant technique for percutaneous removal of renal calyx calculi. AJR Am J Roentgenol 1984; 143:295–297.

38. Bush WH, Crane RE, Brannen GE: Steerable loop snare for percutaneous retrieval of renal calyx calculi. AJR Am J Roentgenol 1984; 142:367–368.

39. Banner MC, Pollack HM, Ring EJ, et al: Catheter dilatation of benign ureteral strictures. Radiology 1983; 147:427–433.

40. Pollack HM, Banner MP: Replacing blocked or dislodged percutaneous nephrostomy and ureteral stent catheters. Radiology 1982; 145:203–205.

41. Bean WJ: Renal cysts: Treatment with alcohol. Radiology 1981; 138:329–331.

Illustrations • Nonvascular Interventions of the Urinary Tract

1 • Percutaneous nephrostomy

2 • Percutaneous nephrostomy: complications

3 • Ureteral stent placement

4 • Ureteral stent: complications

5 • Percutaneous nephrostolithotomy

6 • Percutaneous nephrostolithotomy in calyceal diverticulum with stones

7 • Percutaneous nephrostolithotomy: complications

8 • Percutaneous ureteroplasty

9 • Sclerotherapy for renal cysts

10 • Percutaneous catheter drainage for pelvic abscess

11 • Ureteral occlusion

12 • Percutaneous stone retrieval under fluoroscopy

13 • Miscellaneous interventions of the urinary tract

1. Percutaneous Nephrostomy

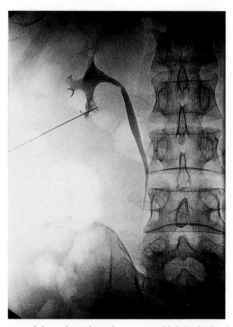

Fig. 1. Puncture of the pelvocalyceal system, which is the basic step in most of the interventional procedures of the urinary tract. A fine needle is inserted into the tip of the lower-polar calyx, and injection of contrast material shows a normal urinary tract. Dilated pelvocalyceal systems are easily punctured with the guidance of US or fluoroscopy, but pelvocalyceal opacification by intravenous injection of contrast material may be helpful in puncturing the nondilated systems.

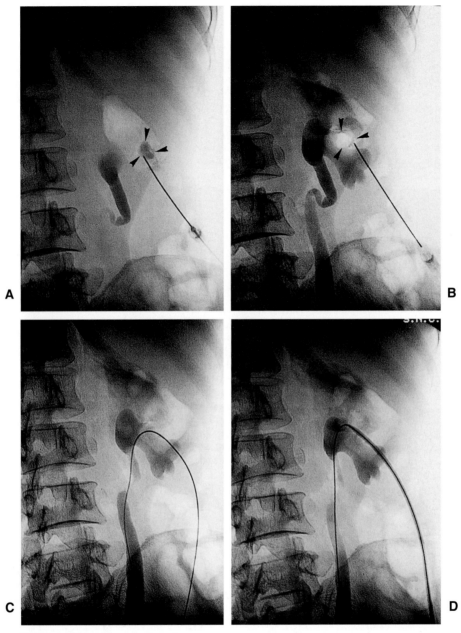

Fig. 2. Techniques of percutaneous nephrostomy.
A. A 22-gauge needle is inserted into the right kidney under the guidance of US and/or fluoroscopy. Contrast material and air are injected to identify the pelvocalyceal systems with the patient in prone position. Note that the needle tip is located in the calyx containing radiopaque contrast material *(arrowheads)*, suggesting anterior location of the calyx. **B.** The needle is inserted again under fluoroscopic guidance into the tip of the posterior calyx containing air *(arrowheads)*. **C.** A guide wire is introduced into the pelvocalyces and ureter. **D.** The tract is dilated over the guide wire up to 10 French.

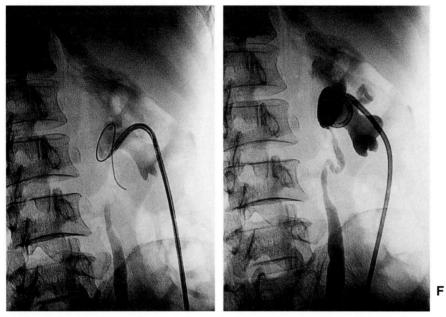

Fig. 2 *Continued.* **E.** A 10-French pigtail catheter is introduced into the renal pelvis. **F.** The guide wire is removed and the nephrostogram is obtained.

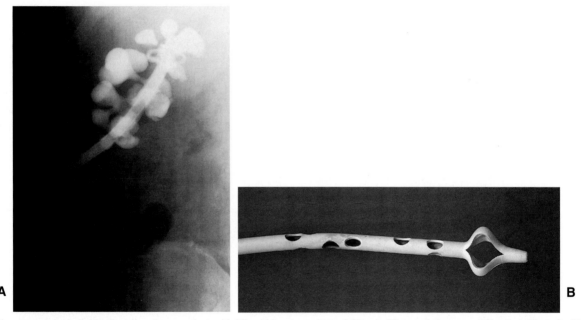

Fig. 3. Nephrostomy tube individually tailored to a patient with idiopathic retroperitoneal fibrosis. The renal sinus was diffusely infiltrated with retroperitoneal fibrosis, and the renal pelvocalyceal systems are so narrowed that the usual pigtail-shaped catheter could not be accommodated in the pelvis. Therefore a Malecot catheter with multiple additional side-holes was used.
A. Nephrostogram shows distorted pelvocalyceal system, which is well opacified and drained by the tube. **B.** Photograph of the Malecot catheter with multiple side-holes. (**B,** See also Color Section.)

2. Percutaneous Nephrostomy: Complications

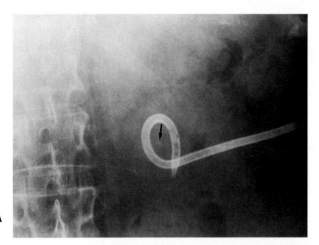

A

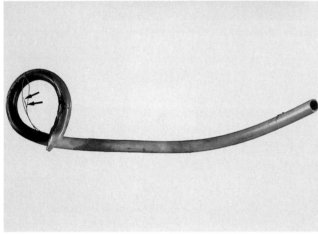

B

Fig. 1. Nephrostomy catheter locked by encrustation on the locking string.
A. The nephrostomy catheter could not be changed because the pigtail of the catheter could not be released. Plain radiograph shows a small calcification *(arrow)* within the loop of the catheter, indicating calcified encrustation on the locking string. **B.** The catheter was removed by introducing a sheath over the catheter. Photograph of the removed catheter shows encrustation on the string of the catheter *(arrows)*. (**B,** See also Color Section.)

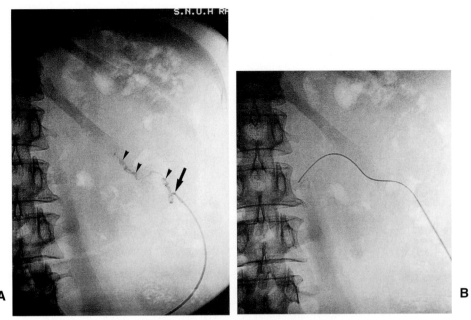

Fig. 2. Reinsertion of nephrostomy catheter after accidental removal of the catheter. Usually the remnant tract is opacified and the tract can be negotiated with a catheter and a floppy guide wire.
A. A small catheter is inserted at the skin opening *(arrow)*, and a tortuous remnant tract *(arrowheads)* is opacified. **B.** A floppy guide wire is inserted into the renal pelvis.

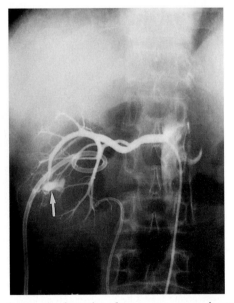

Fig. 3. Pseudoaneurysm formation after percutaneous nephrostomy. There was massive hematuria after nephrostomy, and a selective right renal arteriogram shows a large pseudoaneurysm *(arrow)* near the entry site of the tube into the kidney.

3. Ureteral Stent Placement

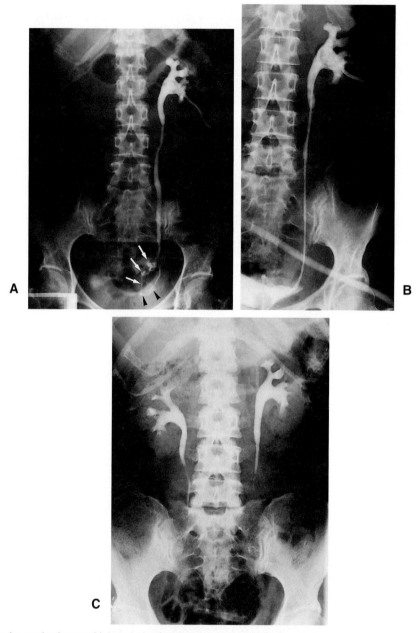

Fig. 1. A 45-year-old woman who received ureteral injury during laparoscopic hysterectomy for uterine myoma.
A. Percutaneous nephrostomy was done, and a nephrostogram shows a fistula *(arrows)* from the left ureter with opacification of the vagina *(arrowheads).* **B.** A ureteral stent was inserted and was kept for 4 weeks. **C.** Follow-up IVU taken 9 months later shows a normal appearance of both urinary tracts.

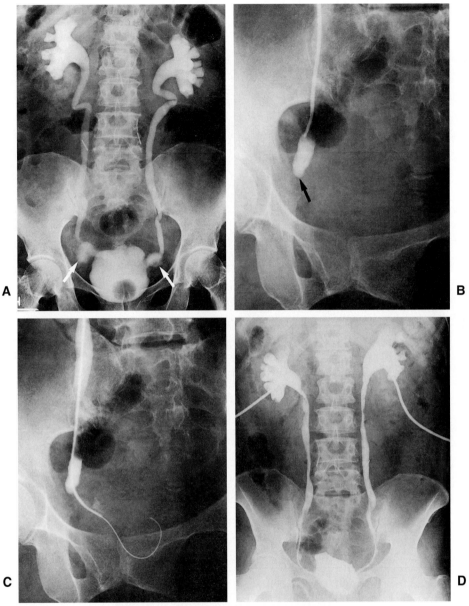

Fig. 2. A 61-year-old woman who underwent radical hysterectomy with pelvic lymph node dissection for uterine cervical carcinoma.
A. IVU taken 7 days after the surgery shows bilateral hydronephrosis and hydroureter and a leak of contrast material from the distal portion of both ureters *(arrows)*. **B.** Percutaneous nephrostomy was done on the left side (patient in prone position), and contrast injection through the catheter shows obstruction of the left ureter *(arrow)*. **C.** The obstructed ureter was negotiated with a curved catheter and a guide wire, and an internal-external ureteral stent was introduced. The same procedure was done on the right urinary tract, and the ureteral stents were kept for 4 weeks. **D.** IVU taken 4 weeks after the procedure shows improved drainage of both urinary tracts, and there is no urine leak in the distal ureters.

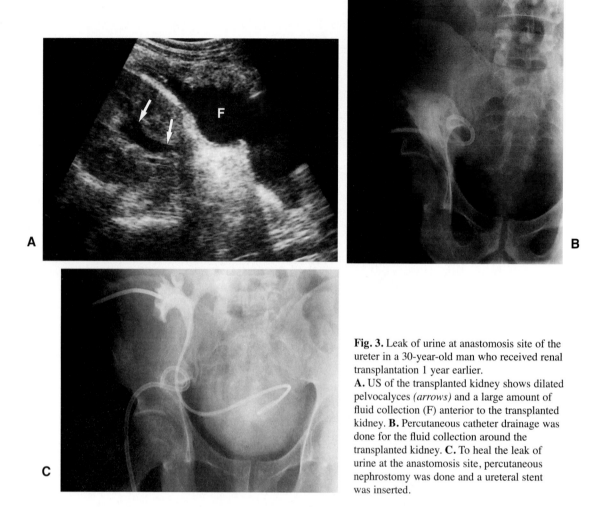

Fig. 3. Leak of urine at anastomosis site of the ureter in a 30-year-old man who received renal transplantation 1 year earlier.
A. US of the transplanted kidney shows dilated pelvocalyces *(arrows)* and a large amount of fluid collection (F) anterior to the transplanted kidney. **B.** Percutaneous catheter drainage was done for the fluid collection around the transplanted kidney. **C.** To heal the leak of urine at the anastomosis site, percutaneous nephrostomy was done and a ureteral stent was inserted.

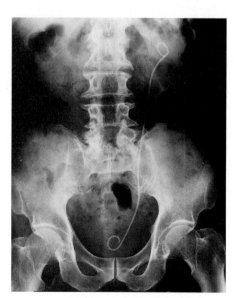

Fig. 4. Double-pigtail ureteral stent in a 68-year-old man who had ureteral obstruction due to prostate cancer with invasion of the urinary bladder. Plain radiograph shows a double-pigtail ureteral stent in the left urinary tract with proximal pigtail in the renal pelvis and distal pigtail in the bladder.

4. Ureteral Stent: Complications

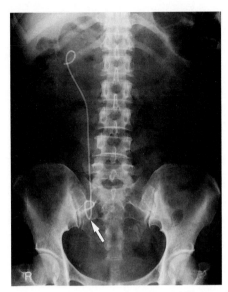

Fig. 1. Malpositioned distal portion of a double-pigtail ureteral stent in a 45-year-old woman. Plain radiograph shows proximally migrated stent with folded distal portion *(arrow)* within the ureter.

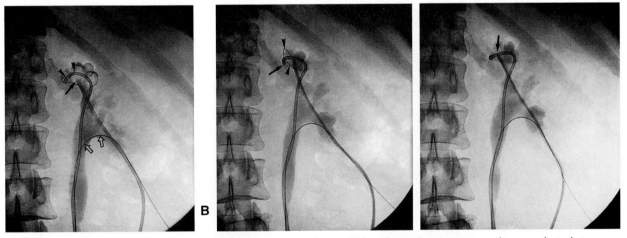

A **B** **C**

Fig. 2. Percutaneous removal of malpositioned ureteral stent in a 36-year-old man. This patient underwent augmentation cystoplasty that was complicated by an anastomotic stricture. Ureteral stenting was performed, but the stent migrated cranially, so percutaneous antegrade removal of the stent was tried by using a loop snare.
A. The lower-pole posterior calyx was punctured and a sheath was introduced with its tip *(arrow)* near the proximal end of the double-pigtail catheter *(arrowheads)*. Note a safety guide wire *(open arrows)*. **B.** A loop snare was opened *(arrowheads)* and the tip of the ureteral stent *(arrow)* was captured. **C.** The tip of the ureteral stent was captured tightly *(arrow)* and was removed. After removal of the stent, a new ureteral stent was introduced over the safety wire.

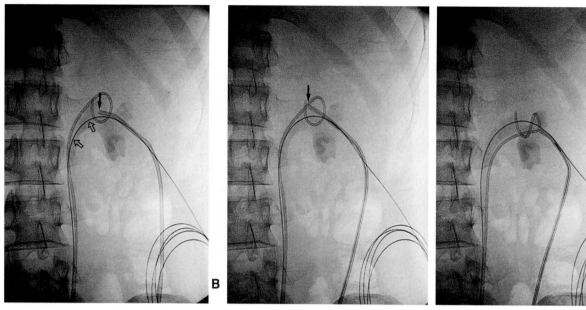

Fig. 3. Percutaneous removal of malpositioned ureteral stent by using a three-pronged retriever.
A. A sheath was introduced through the interpolar calyx with its tip *(arrow)* within the proximal loop of the double-pigtail catheter. Note a safety guide wire *(open arrows)*. **B.** Ureteral stent was captured by the three-pronged retriever *(arrow)*. **C.** Ureteral stent is being removed.

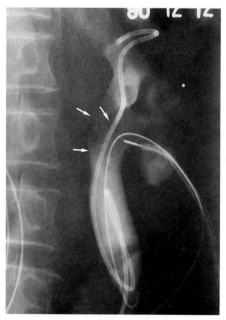

Fig. 4. Another patient with proximally migrated ureteral stent, which was removed by using a three-pronged retriever. The prongs of the retriever are opened *(arrows)* to capture the ureteral stent.

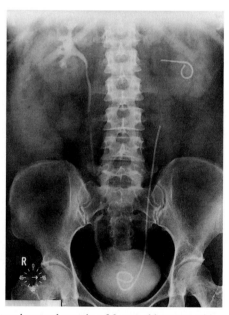

Fig. 5. Fractured ureteral stent in a 36-year-old woman with recurrent uterine cervical carcinoma and ureteral obstruction. IVU taken 3 months after the insertion of the ureteral stent shows a fractured stent and poor opacification of the left urinary tract. The distal portion of the stent was removed cystoscopically, and the proximal segment was removed percutaneously.

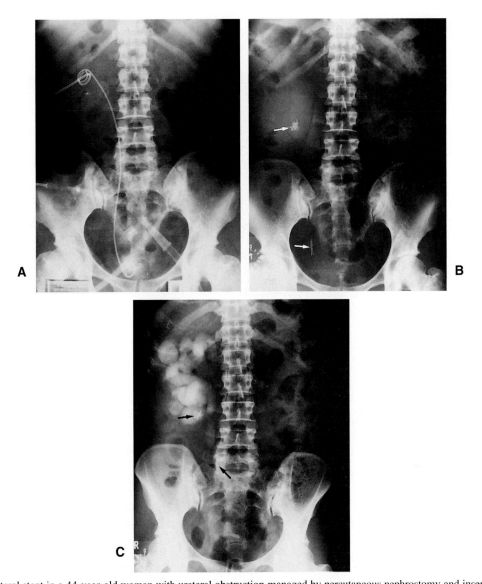

Fig. 6. Fragmented ureteral stent in a 44-year-old woman with ureteral obstruction managed by percutaneous nephrostomy and insertion of the ureteral stent. The patient was then lost to follow-up for 4 years, when she visited the hospital again because of right flank pain.
A. Plain radiograph obtained immediately after insertion of the ureteral stent. A percutaneous nephrostomy catheter was also inserted, but it was kept clamped for 3 days and was removed. **B, C.** IVU taken at the time of revisit after 4 years shows the ureteral stent fragmented into short segments *(arrows)* and distal ureteral obstruction. The stent fragments in the ureter were changing in position during IVU. The patient said that she had urinated the fragments several times. Percutaneous nephrostomy was done. The stent fragments were removed by using a nephroscope and ureteroscope.

5. Percutaneous Nephrostolithotomy

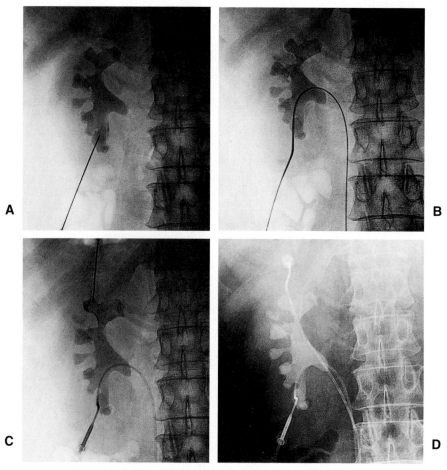

Fig. 1. Tract creation for percutaneous nephrostolithotomy in a 50-year-old man with a staghorn stone.
A. An 18-gauge needle is inserted into the posterior surface of the lower-pole calyx stone. **B.** A floppy guide wire is introduced into the ureter and a sheath is inserted over the guide wire. **C.** Another needle is inserted into the upper-pole calyx stone. **D.** Another sheath is introduced through the upper-pole stone. These procedures were performed in the radiology department. Next day, the tracts were dilated up to 30 French in the operating room, and the stone was removed by using a nephroscope and ultrasonic lithotriptor.

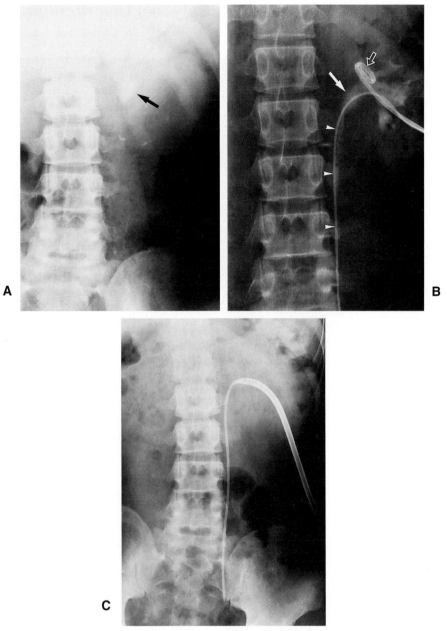

Fig. 2. Percutaneous nephrostolithotomy of the left renal pelvis stone in a 21-year-old man.
A. Plain radiograph shows a radiopaque stone in the left renal pelvis *(arrow)*. **B.** A tract was made through the lower-polar calyx and a sheath was introduced through the stone *(arrow)* into the ureter *(arrowheads)*. A nephrostomy catheter *(open arrow)* was also introduced to the upper-polar calyx for temporary drainage. **C.** The tract was dilated, and the stone was removed by using a nephroscope. After stone removal, a 16-French, tapered nephroureterostomy catheter was introduced for the tamponade of the tract and healing of the ureteropelvic junction where the stone had been located.

6. Percutaneous Nephrostolithotomy in Calyceal Diverticulum with Stones

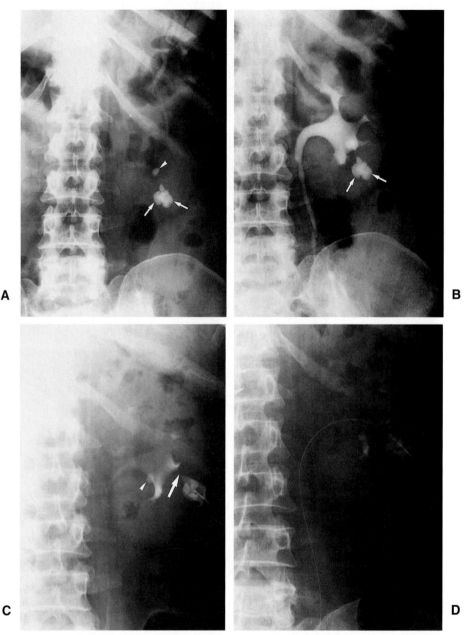

Fig. 1. Percutaneous nephrostolithotomy for stones in a calyceal diverticulum in a 51-year-old woman.
A, B. Plain radiograph **(A)** and IVU **(B)** show multiple, small stones *(arrows)* in the calyceal diverticulum located in the lower-polar region of the left kidney. Contrast material collection in the calyceal diverticulum is not evident. Another small, round calcification *(arrowhead)* is extrarenal calcification, which is evident on **C. C.** A 22-gauge needle was inserted into the calyceal diverticulum, and injection of contrast material shows narrow neck of the diverticulum *(arrow)*. Note that the small, round calcification *(arrowhead)* seen on **A** is extrarenal calcification. **D.** A 0.018-inch floppy guide wire was introduced through the neck of the diverticulum into the renal pelvis and ureter.

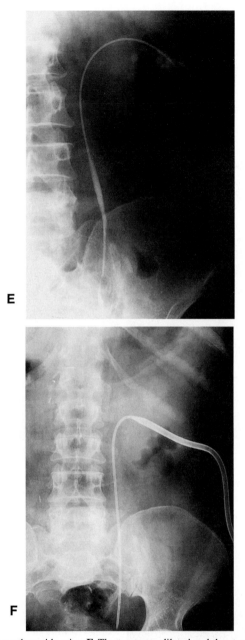

Fig. 1 *Continued.* **E.** A sheath was introduced over the guide wire. **F.** The tract was dilated and the stones were removed by using a nephroscope. The neck of the diverticulum was dilated under nephroscopic control. A 16-French, tapered nephroureterostomy catheter was introduced and then kept for 1 week.

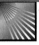

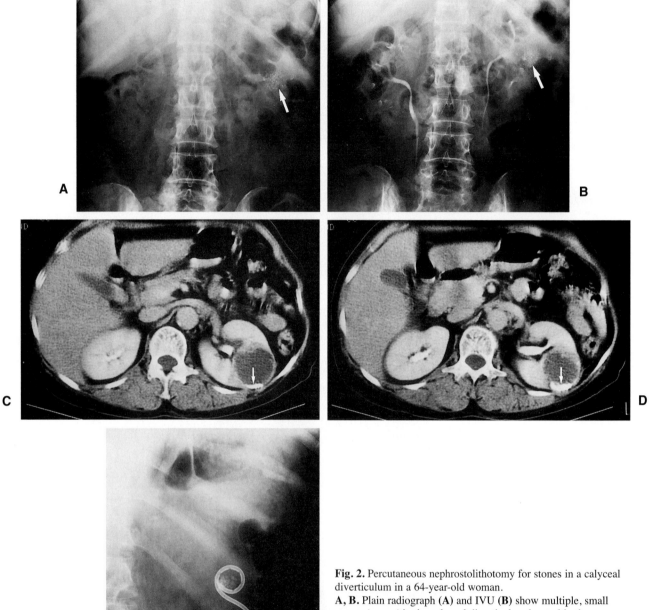

Fig. 2. Percutaneous nephrostolithotomy for stones in a calyceal diverticulum in a 64-year-old woman.
A, B. Plain radiograph **(A)** and IVU **(B)** show multiple, small stones *(arrow)* in the calyceal diverticulum located in the interpolar region of the left kidney. Contrast material collection is not evident in the calyceal diverticulum. **C, D.** Contrast-enhanced CT scans show that the stones *(arrow)* are located in the dependent portion of a large calyceal diverticulum. Collection of contrast material is not seen in the calyceal diverticulum. **E.** The calyceal diverticulum was punctured and a pigtail catheter was left in the diverticulum since the injection of contrast material did not opacify the neck of the diverticulum and the pelvocalyceal systems.

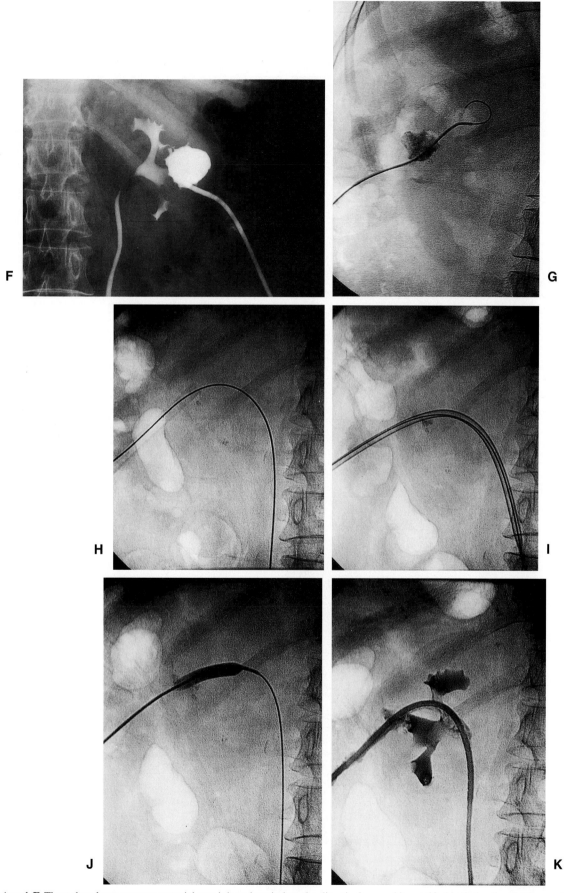

Fig. 2 *Continued*. **F.** Three days later, contrast material was injected again into the diverticulum, and it opacified both the diverticulum and pelvocalyceal systems. **G.** A floppy guide wire was introduced into the pelvocalyceal system through the neck of the diverticulum. **H.** The guide wire and the catheter were introduced into the ureter. **I, J.** The neck of the diverticulum was dilated by using 6- to 10-French long dilators **(I)** and an 8-mm balloon **(J)**. **K.** A 10.2-6.5–French internal-external ureteral stent was introduced into the pelvocalyces and ureter through the calyceal diverticulum and its neck and was kept for 3 weeks.

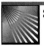
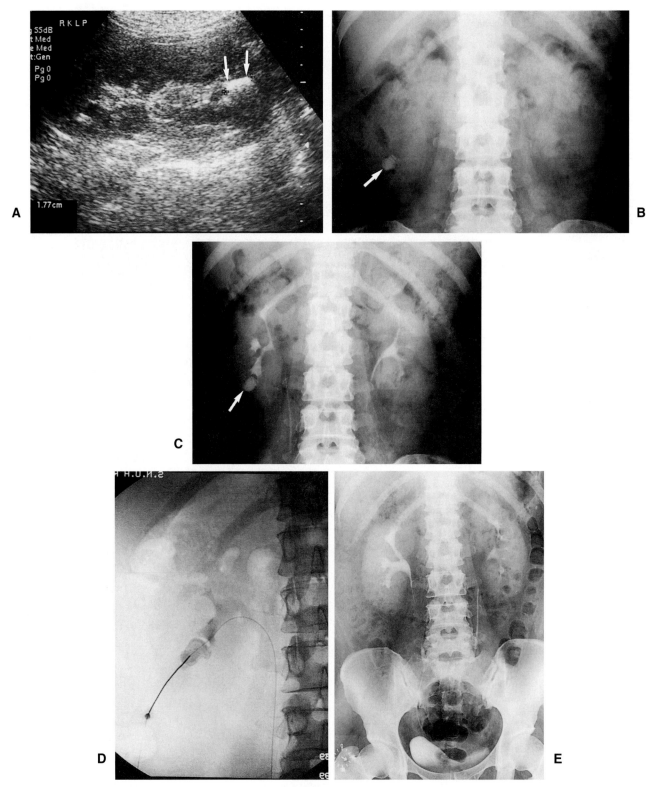

Fig. 3. Percutaneous nephrostolithotomy for stones in a calyceal diverticulum in a 44-year-old woman.
A. US of the right kidney shows an echogenic stone with posterior sonic shadowing in the lower-polar region *(arrows)*. **B, C.** Plain radiograph **(B)** and IVU **(C)** show a calyceal diverticulum containing stones *(arrow)* in the lower pole of the right kidney. **D.** The calyceal diverticulum was punctured and a guide wire was passed through the neck of the diverticulum into the renal pelvis and ureter. The stone was removed and the neck of the diverticulum was dilated. **E.** Follow-up IVU taken 1 year later shows disappeared calyceal diverticulum and normalized right urinary tract.

7. Percutaneous Nephrostolithotomy: Complications

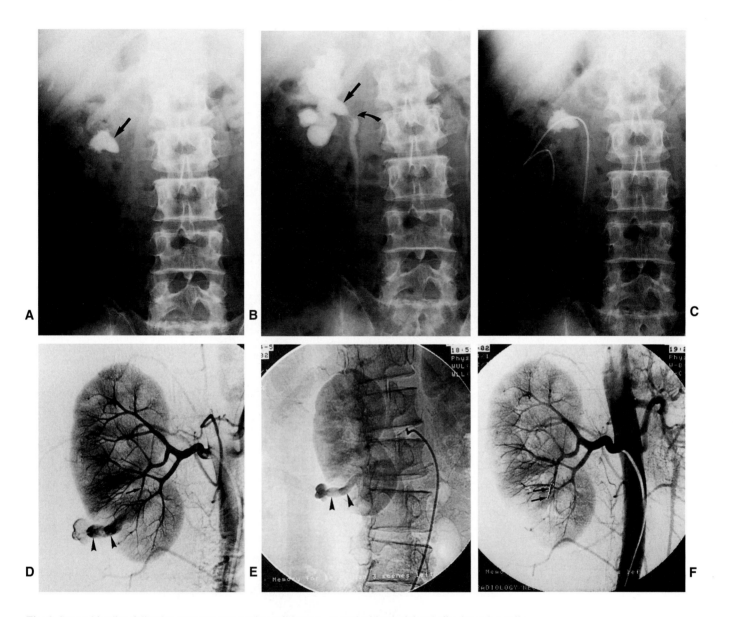

Fig. 1. Severe bleeding following percutaneous nephrostolithotomy treated with arterial embolization using coils.
A. Plain radiograph shows a large stone in the right renal pelvis *(arrow)* as well as small calyceal stones. **B.** IVU shows hydronephrosis due to pelvic stone *(arrow)*. Also note fine nodularities in the proximal ureter *(curved arrow)* adjacent to the stone probably due to mucosal edema. **C.** A percutaneous tract was created and a thin catheter was inserted into the ureter through the stone. Then the tract was dilated and the stones were removed with nephroscopy. After the procedure, severe hematuria and perirenal bleeding occurred and transfusion was required. **D, E.** Right renal arteriograms in oblique projection in arterial **(D)** and nephrographic **(E)** phases show a leak of contrast material from an arterial branch *(arrow in D)* to the lower pole through the tract for percutaneous nephrostolithotomy *(arrowheads)*. **F.** The arterial branch causing bleeding was embolized with coils *(arrows)* and the patient recovered.

8. Percutaneous Ureteroplasty

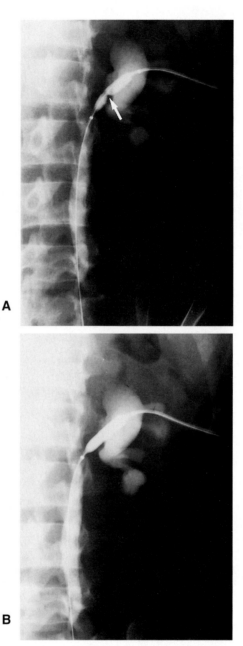

Fig. 1. A 26-year-old man with congenital obstruction of the ureteropelvic junction, which was treated with balloon dilation. **A.** Percutaneous nephrostomy was made and the stenotic ureteropelvic junction was dilated with a 6-mm balloon. Note a waist of the balloon caused by the stenosis *(arrow)*. **B.** The balloon was further inflated and the waist disappeared.

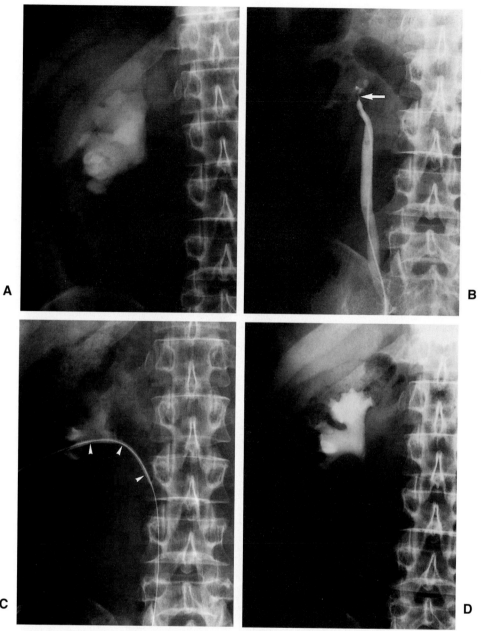

Fig. 2. A 28-year-old man with a stenosis of the right ureteropelvic junction. He had a stone in the right ureteropelvic junction that was treated with extracorporeal shock-wave lithotripsy.
A. IVU before dilation shows marked hydronephrosis of the right kidney. **B.** RGP shows a tight stenosis in the right ureteropelvic junction *(arrow)*.
C. Percutaneous nephrostomy was made and the lesion was dilated serially by using ureteral dilators *(arrowheads)*. **D.** Follow-up IVU taken 10 months after the dilation shows still-remaining but improved hydronephrosis.

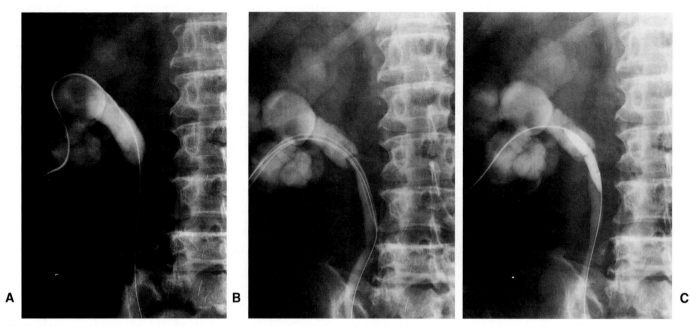

Fig. 3. A 64-year-old man with a proximal ureteral stenosis. He had a history of stone in the right proximal ureter that was treated by surgery 13 years earlier.
A. Percutaneous nephrostomy was created and a guide wire was advanced into the ureter through the stenosis. **B, C.** The stenotic lesion was dilated by using a ureteral dilator (**B**) and an 8-mm balloon (**C**).

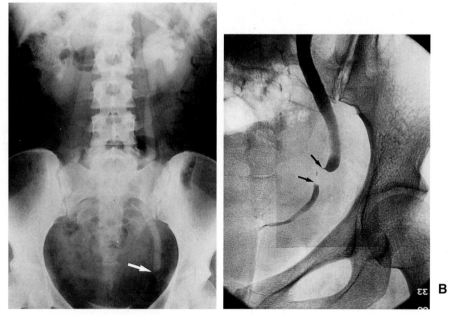

Fig. 4. A 31-year-old woman who received a left ureteral injury during cesarean section. (**A–G,** From Kim SH: Percutaneous dilatation of the urinary tract. In Han MC, Park JH [eds]: Interventional Radiology. Seoul, Ilchokak, 1999, pp 610–619.)
A. Initial IVU shows hydronephrosis and hydroureter with a stricture in the left distal ureter *(arrow)*. **B.** Percutaneous nephrostomy was made and nephrostogram shows a short-segment stricture in the left distal ureter *(arrows)*.

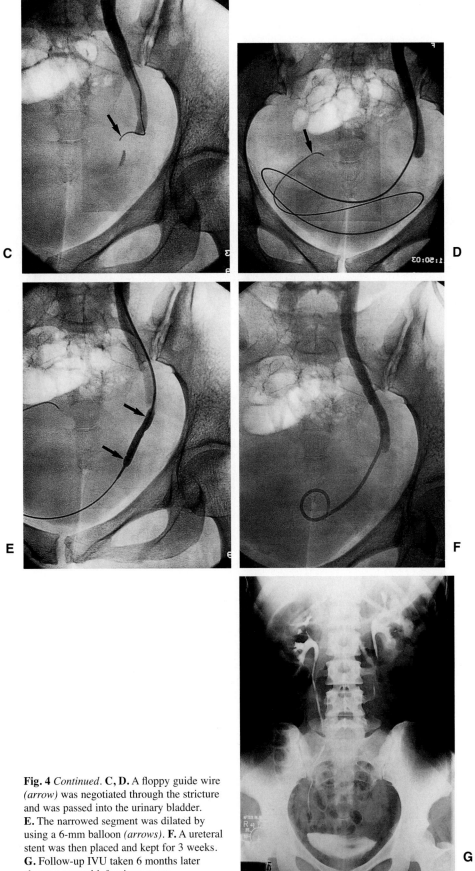

Fig. 4 *Continued.* **C, D.** A floppy guide wire *(arrow)* was negotiated through the stricture and was passed into the urinary bladder. **E.** The narrowed segment was dilated by using a 6-mm balloon *(arrows).* **F.** A ureteral stent was then placed and kept for 3 weeks. **G.** Follow-up IVU taken 6 months later shows a normal left urinary tract.

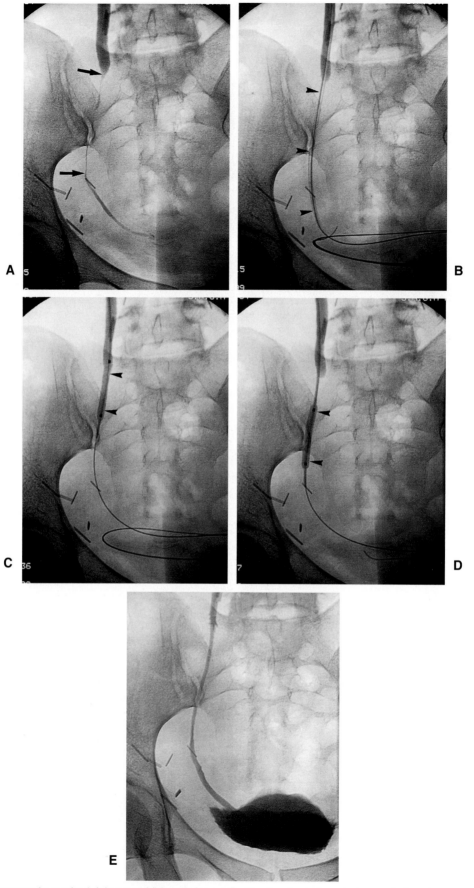

Fig. 5. A 43-year-old woman who received right ureteral injury during a radical hysterectomy for a uterine cervical carcinoma.
A. Percutaneous nephrostomy was performed, and nephrostogram shows a long-segment stricture in the right distal ureter *(arrows)*. **B–D.** The stenosis was dilated by using long ureteral dilators and balloons *(arrowheads)*. **E.** Ureteral stent was placed for 4 weeks, and the follow-up nephrostogram shows a dilated distal ureter without stenosis.

882

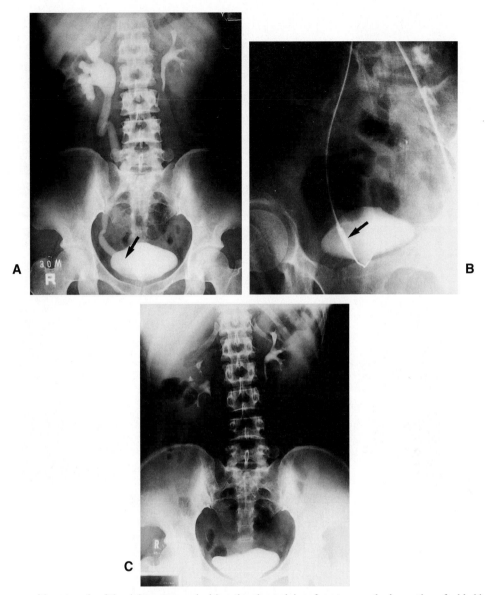

Fig. 6. A 31-year-old woman with a stenosis of the right ureterovesical junction due to injury from transurethral resection of a bladder tumor. The patient did not have a recurrent tumor but had hydronephrosis on the right urinary tract.
A. IVU shows hydronephrosis and hydroureter on the right urinary tract due to a stenosis at the ureterovesical junction *(arrow)*. **B.** Percutaneous nephrostomy was done and the stenotic lesion was dilated by using a 6-mm balloon *(arrow)*. **C.** Follow-up IVU obtained 2 years later shows normalized right urinary tract.

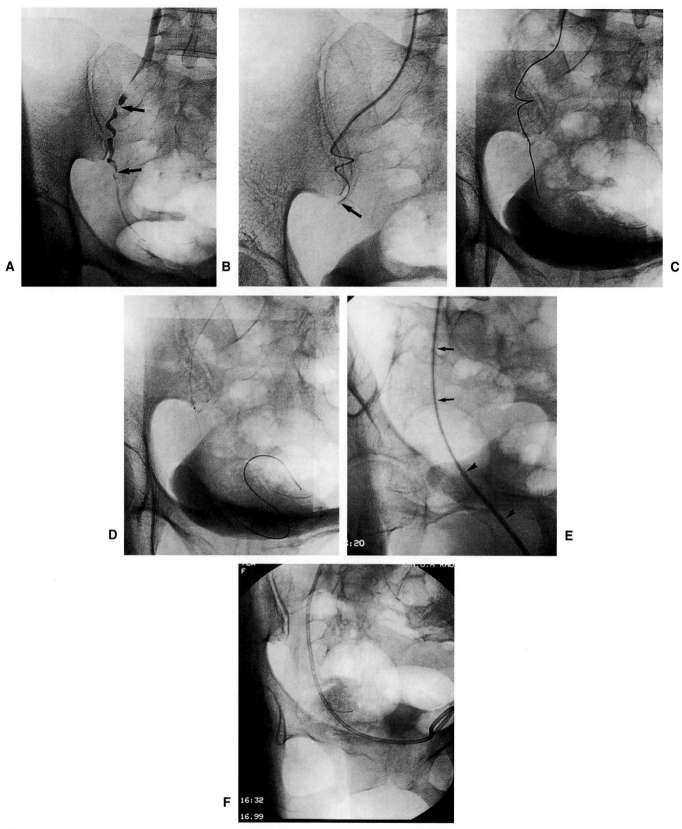

Fig. 7. A 42-year-old woman who had a ureteral stricture that developed after surgery for ovarian cancer.
A. Percutaneous nephrostomy was done, and a nephrostogram shows severe tortuosity of the distal ureter with strictures, probably caused by a severe adhesion *(arrows)*. **B.** The lesion was so tortuous that a guide wire *(arrow)* could not be passed through it. **C, D.** A Microferret infusion catheter system (William Cook Europe) was used, and the lesion could then be negotiated with a 0.016-inch floppy guide wire. **E.** The guide wire was retrieved through the urethra by a guide wire snare, and the lesion was dilated by using ureteral dilators *(arrows)*. Note a catheter introduced over the guide wire to protect the urethra from injury *(arrowheads)*. **F.** A ureteral stent was introduced after dilation.

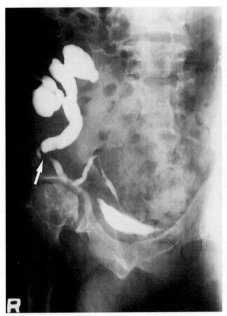
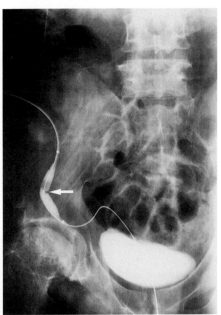

Fig. 8. A 41-year-old man with a stenosis of the ureteral anastomosis site, which developed 1 month after renal transplantation.
A. Percutaneous nephrostomy was done in the transplanted kidney, and a nephrostogram shows a stenosis of the ureter at the ureteroureterostomy site *(arrow)*. **B.** The stenotic lesion was dilated with an 8-mm balloon. Note a small waist in the inflated balloon *(arrow)*.

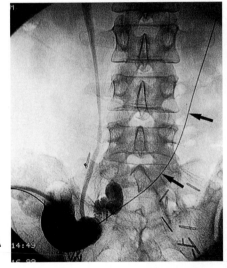
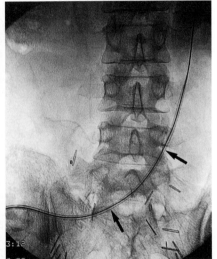
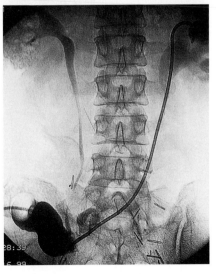

Fig. 9. A 43-year-old man who had an anastomosis stricture that occurred 5 years after radical cystectomy and ileal conduit for bladder cancer. (**A–C,** From Kim SH: Percutaneous dilatation of the urinary tract. In Han MC, Park JH [eds]: Interventional Radiology. Seoul, Ilchokak, 1999, pp 610–619.)
A. Loopogram shows absent reflux of contrast material on the left side due to obstruction at the ureteral anastomosis site. A guide wire *(arrows)* was passed into the left ureter from below with the help of a curved catheter under fluoroscopy. **B.** The narrowed segment was dilated using 8- to 10-French ureteral dilators *(arrows)*. **C.** A ureteral stent was placed in the left ureter.

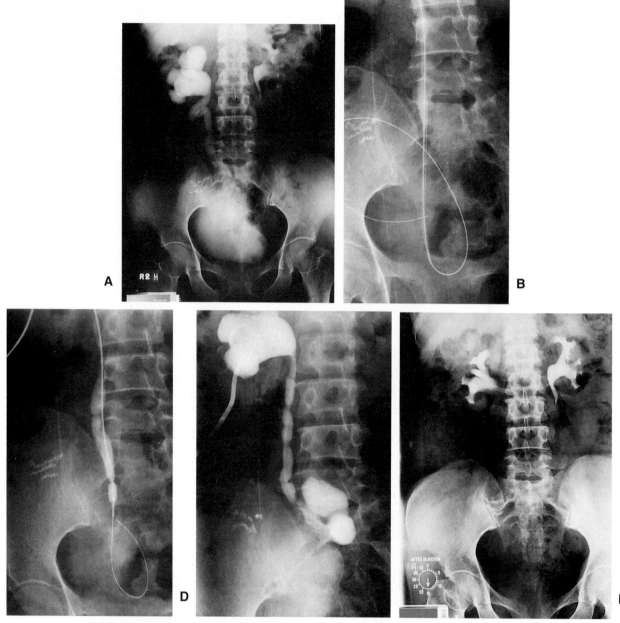

Fig. 10. Improved anastomotic stricture following percutaneous dilation in a 42-year-old man who underwent cystectomy and neobladder formation for congenital incontinence.
A. IVU taken 3 years after surgery shows severe hydronephrosis and hydroureter due to anastomosis stricture. **B, C.** Percutaneous nephrostomy was performed, and the stricture was dilated by using serial dilators up to 10 French (**B**) and an 8-mm balloon (**C**). **D.** After dilation, an internal-external ureteral stent was introduced and kept for 8 weeks. **E.** Follow-up IVU obtained 4 years later shows relieved hydronephrosis and hydroureter of the right urinary tract.

9. Sclerotherapy for Renal Cysts

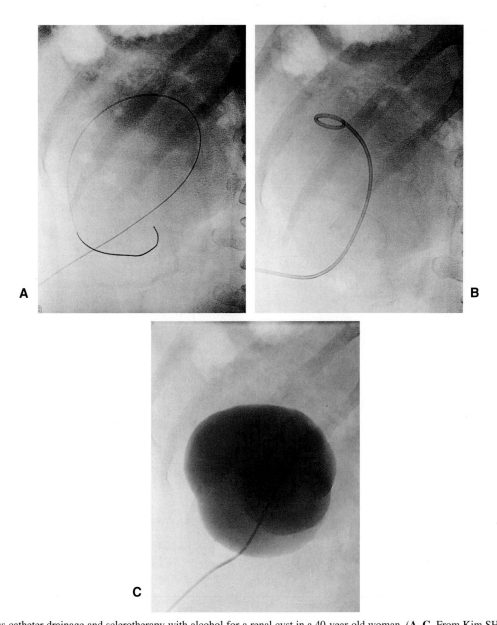

Fig. 1. Percutaneous catheter drainage and sclerotherapy with alcohol for a renal cyst in a 40-year-old woman. (**A–C,** From Kim SH: Renal cyst sclerotherapy. In Han MC, Park JH [eds]: Interventional Radiology. Seoul, Ilchokak, 1999, pp 620–625.)
A. A 22-gauge needle was inserted into the renal cyst and a thin guide wire was introduced. **B.** The tract was dilated and a 7-French pigtail catheter was inserted. **C.** The cyst content was aspirated, and a cystogram was obtained to evaluate the inner wall of the cyst. Then sclerotherapy was done with absolute alcohol, as described in the text.

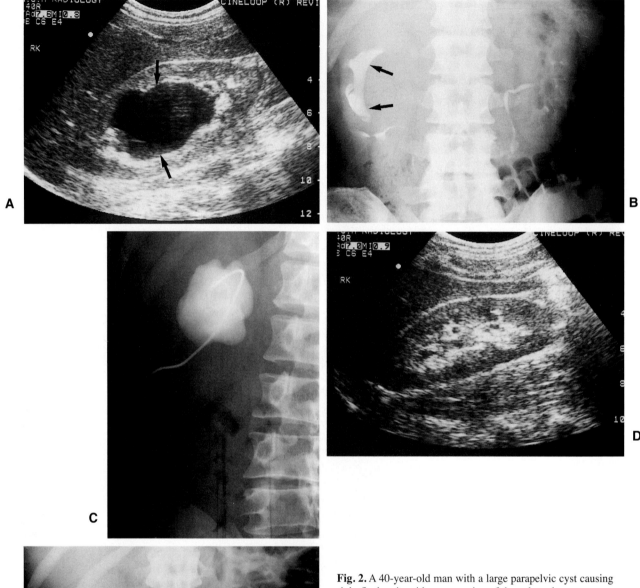

Fig. 2. A 40-year-old man with a large parapelvic cyst causing right flank pain with compression of the pelvocalyces. (**A–E,** From Kim SH: Renal cyst sclerotherapy. In Han MC, Park JH [eds]: Interventional Radiology. Seoul, Ilchokak, 1999, pp 620–625.) **A.** US of the right kidney in longitudinal plane shows a large cyst *(arrows)* in the renal sinus region. **B.** IVU shows compression and deviation of the pelvocalyces due to a parapelvic cyst in the right kidney *(arrows)*. **C.** A 7-French pigtail catheter was inserted into the cyst, and a cystogram shows a lobulated, smooth, inner wall of the cyst. Then sclerotherapy was done with ethanol, as described in the text. **D.** Follow-up US shows that the renal cyst disappeared completely. **E.** Follow-up IVU shows that the pelvocalyceal compression on the right kidney also disappeared. The patient's symptoms also improved.

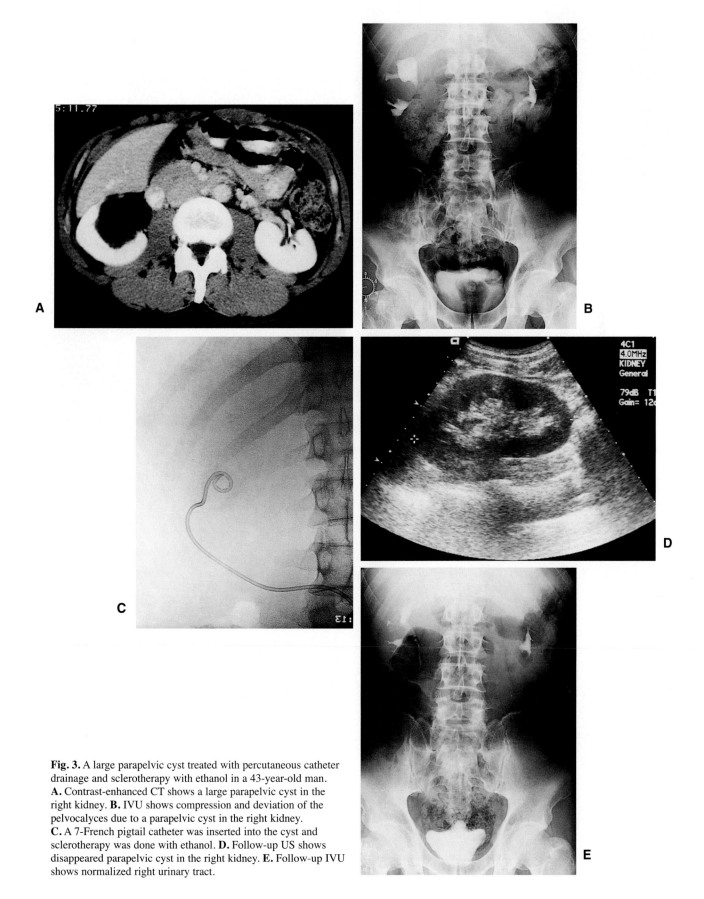

Fig. 3. A large parapelvic cyst treated with percutaneous catheter drainage and sclerotherapy with ethanol in a 43-year-old man.
A. Contrast-enhanced CT shows a large parapelvic cyst in the right kidney. **B.** IVU shows compression and deviation of the pelvocalyces due to a parapelvic cyst in the right kidney.
C. A 7-French pigtail catheter was inserted into the cyst and sclerotherapy was done with ethanol. **D.** Follow-up US shows disappeared parapelvic cyst in the right kidney. **E.** Follow-up IVU shows normalized right urinary tract.

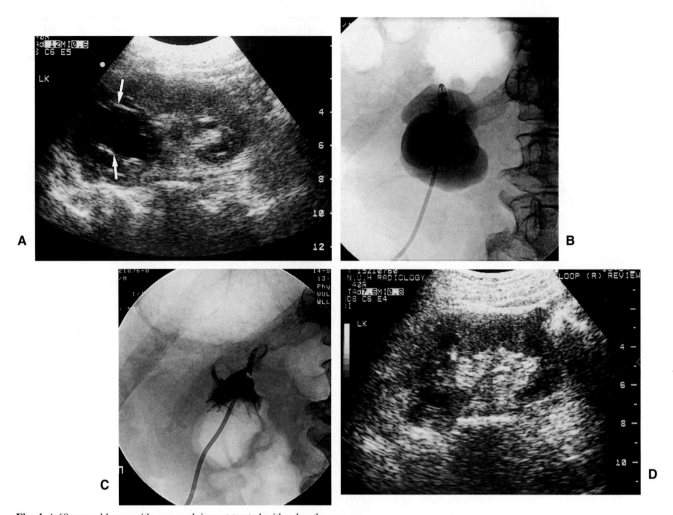

Fig. 4. A 68-year-old man with a parapelvic cyst treated with sclerotherapy.
A. US shows a large parapelvic cyst *(arrows)* in the upper-polar region of the left kidney. **B.** A 7-French catheter was inserted into the cyst and a cystogram shows the lobulated contour of the cyst. Sclerotherapy was done with alcohol, as described in the text. **C.** Cystogram obtained on the second day of sclerotherapy shows collapsed cyst cavity due to adhesion of the inner wall of the cyst. **D.** Follow-up US taken 5 months after sclerotherapy shows completely disappeared cyst.

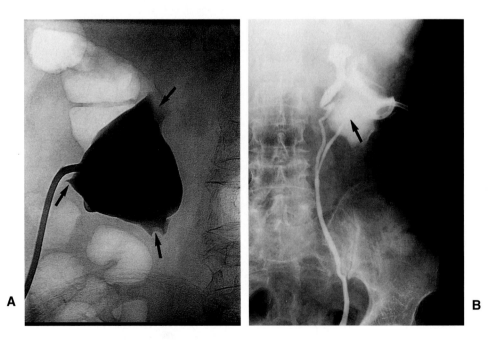

Fig. 5. Erroneous insertion of a catheter into the dilated lower-moiety calyceal system of the partially duplicated left urinary tract in a 55-year-old man. (**A, B,** From Kim SH: Renal cyst sclerotherapy. In Han MC, Park JH [eds]: Interventional Radiology. Seoul, Ilchokak, 1999, pp 620–625.)
A. Cystogram obtained after insertion of a catheter did not reveal communication with the ureter, but the cyst had outer projections with beaks and indentations *(arrows)* that are similar to the calyceal fornices. **B.** RGP was performed, and the cystic lesion was confirmed to be a dilated lower-moiety calyx of the duplicated system associated with obstruction of the ureteropelvic junction *(arrow)*. Cyst sclerotherapy was not performed.

10. Percutaneous Catheter Drainage for Pelvic Abscess

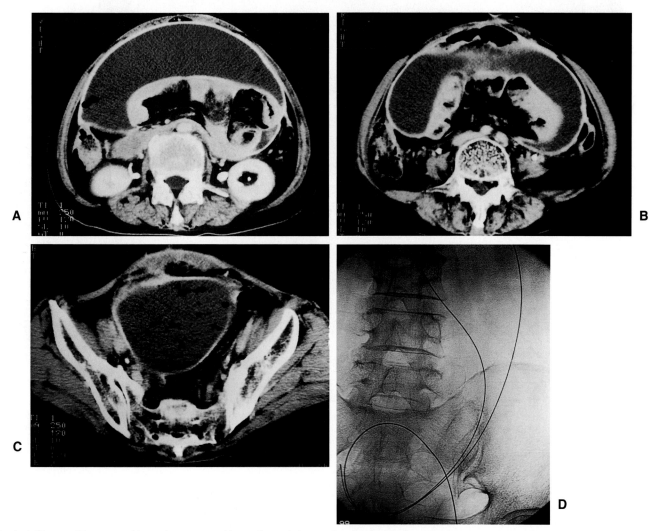

Fig. 1. A 55-year-old woman with ovarian cancer, with a peritoneal abscess that developed after surgery.
A–C. Contrast-enhanced CT scans of the abdomen show fluid collection in the peritoneal cavity. Note thickened, enhancing peritoneum and gas bubbles in the peritoneal fluid. **D.** The abscess was punctured with a needle and a guide wire was passed into the large abscess cavity. A pigtail catheter was introduced into the abscess.

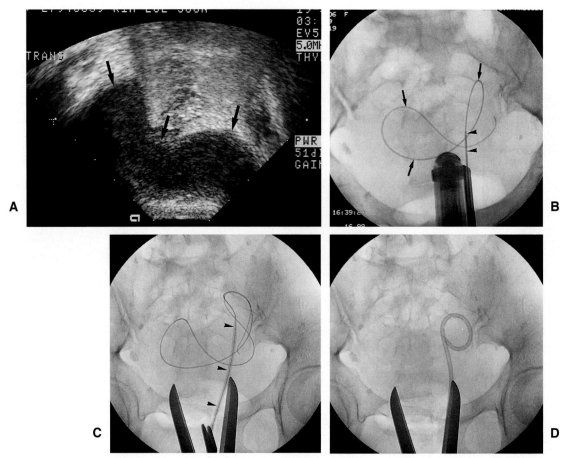

Fig. 2. A 33-year-old woman with a pelvic abscess that occurred following surgery for an ectopic pregnancy. The abscess was drained transvaginally. **A.** Transvaginal US shows a large abscess cavity in the pelvic peritoneal cavity *(arrows)*. **B.** An 18-gauge needle *(arrowheads)* was inserted with the guidance of transvaginal US, and a guide wire *(arrows)* was introduced into the abscess cavity. **C.** The tract was dilated by using 7- to 10-French dilators *(arrowheads)*. **D.** A 10-French pigtail catheter was inserted for drainage.

11. Ureteral Occlusion

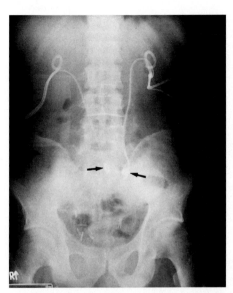

Fig. 1. Bilateral ureteral occlusion for drying up of a urine leak after Miles' surgery for rectal cancer. Bilateral nephrostomy was performed, and occlusion balloons were inflated in the ureters *(arrows)*.

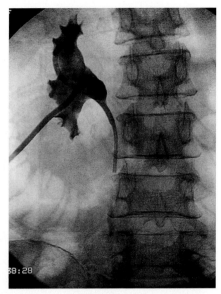

Fig. 2. Use of a cut internal-external ureteral stent for drying up of a urine leak through a vesicovaginal fistula that occurred following hysterectomy in a 50-year-old woman. An internal-external ureteral stent was cut at the proximal ureteral portion and was occluded with a heated needle holder. The cut internal-external stent was positioned in the renal pelvis and proximal ureter. External drainage through this catheter effectively dried up the urine leak.

12. Percutaneous Stone Retrieval under Fluoroscopy

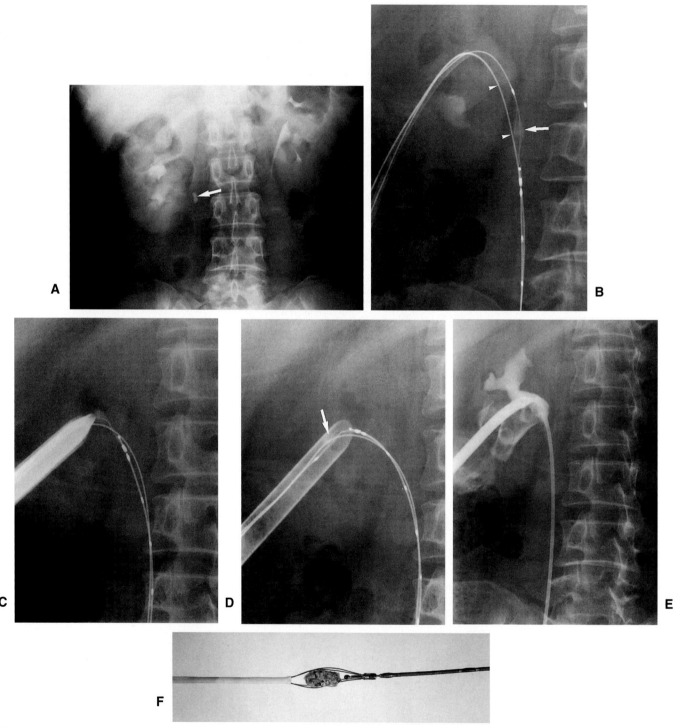

Fig. 1. Percutaneous retrieval of proximal ureteral stone under fluoroscopic guidance in a 47-year-old woman.
A. IVU shows an ovoid stone in the right proximal ureter *(arrow)* with hydronephrosis. **B.** Percutaneous nephrostomy was made, and the stone was captured in the ureteral basket *(arrow)*. Note a safety guide wire *(arrowheads)*. **C.** Then the tract was dilated over the working guide wire and a 26-French sheath was introduced. **D.** The stone *(arrow)* was removed through the sheath. **E.** A ureteral stent was inserted along the safety guide wire and was kept for 2 weeks. **F.** Photograph of the stone in the basket. (**F,** See also Color Section.)

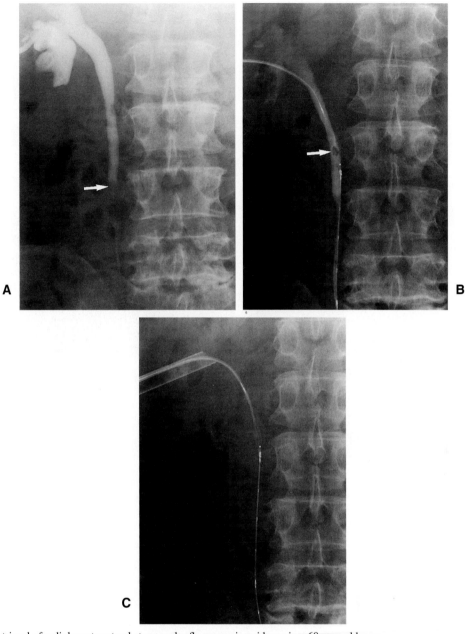

Fig. 2. Percutaneous retrieval of radiolucent ureteral stone under fluoroscopic guidance in a 68-year-old man.
A. Percutaneous nephrostomy was made, and there was an obstructing ureteral stone *(arrow)*. **B.** The stone was captured in the ureteral basket *(arrow)*. **C.** The tract was dilated up to 26 French, and the stone was removed through the sheath.

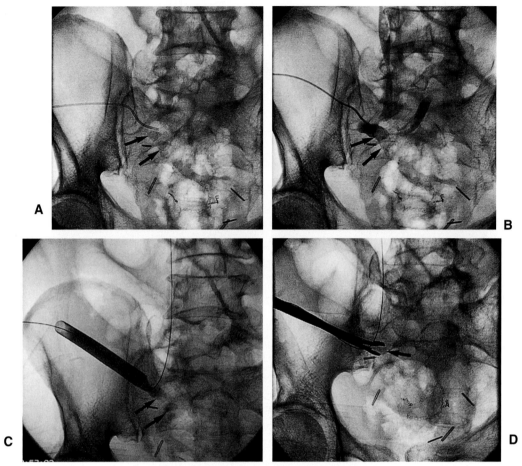

Fig. 3. Retrieval of stones in ileal conduit by using forceps under fluoroscopic guidance.
A. Plain radiograph shows a catheter in the ileal conduit and radiopaque stones *(arrows)* in the conduit. **B.** Loopogram shows reflux of contrast material into both ureters and stones appearing as filling defects *(arrows)* in the conduit. **C.** A guide wire was introduced into the right ureter and a 26-F sheath was introduced into the conduit in front of the stones *(arrows)*. **D.** A stone *(arrow)* was grabbed by a forceps and removed.

13. Miscellaneous Interventions of the Urinary Tract

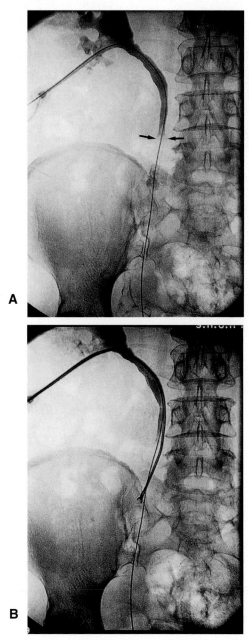

Fig. 1. A 52-year-old woman with diabetes mellitus and candidiasis of the urinary tract. Urinary tract obstruction was managed by percutaneous nephrostomy.
A. Nephrostogram shows obstruction of proximal ureter with widening of the ureteral lumen *(arrows)*. A guide wire was passed through the lesion. **B.** Ureteral tumor was suspected and punch biopsy was done, which did not reveal a tumor.

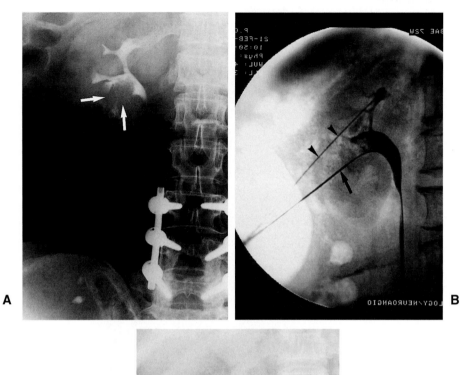

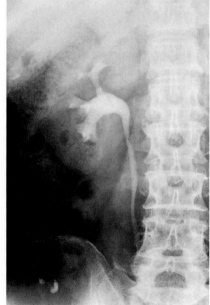

Fig. 2. Management of transitional cell carcinoma involving lower-polar calyx and renal pelvis of the right kidney in a 59-year-old woman. This patient had undergone left nephrectomy 6 years earlier due to a ureteral tumor.
A. IVU shows papillary tumors involving the lower-polar calyx and renal pelvis of the right kidney *(arrows)*. **B.** The upper-polar calyx was punctured with a fine needle *(arrowheads)* and the urinary tract was opacified. Then a second needle *(arrow)* was inserted through the tumor-bearing lower-polar calyx and a guide wire was passed into the renal pelvis and ureter. The tract was dilated and the tumor was resected with nephroscopy. **C.** Follow-up IVU taken 3 months later shows disappeared tumor in the right urinary tract.

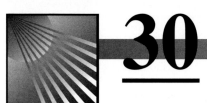

30

Renovascular Interventions

JIN WOOK CHUNG

VASCULAR INTERVENTION FOR RENAL ARTERY STENOSIS

Renovascular hypertension is potentially curable by surgery of nephrectomy, autotransplantation, or bypass graft or, more recently, by radiologic intervention of percutaneous transluminal angioplasty (PTA), intravascular stent placement, and embolization. The purposes of a renal revascularization procedure are to cure or improve renovascular hypertension or renal insufficiency due to renal artery stenosis and to prevent the progression of renal artery stenosis to complete occlusion. Renal PTA or stent should be considered as a treatment option in patients with hemodynamically significant renal artery stenosis and failed medical control of hypertension or loss of renal parenchyma and/or deterioration of renal function during medical treatments.

Although luminal narrowing of 60% to 70% or higher on direct angiography is generally considered as significant stenosis, it is important to determine the physiologic or hemodynamic significance of renal artery stenosis. Captopril renal scan, renal vein renin sampling, Doppler US, and direct measurement of the trans-stenotic pressure gradient are currently used for this purpose. However, none of these are absolutely sensitive or specific in predicting the outcome of PTA or stent placement. They have their own advantages and limitations.

Blood flow through a stenotic renal artery is primarily determined by the length and degree of stenosis. Modification of Poiseuille's law indicates resistance to flow is inversely proportional to the fourth power of the radius:

$$R = \frac{8NL}{\pi r^4}$$

where R = resistance to flow, L = length of stenosis, N = viscosity, π = 3.1416, and r = radius of stenosis.

According to the equation, blood flow through a 70% stenosis may be 5 times greater than the flow through an 80% stenosis and 80 times greater than the flow through a 90% stenosis. Because of this phenomenon, inadequate angioplasties with significant residual stenosis frequently result in remarkable improvement in the renal perfusion and blood pressure control.

In the technique of renal PTA, hydration of the patient before, during, and after the procedure is essential because renal insufficiency due to contrast material is the most common complication. In the patients with compromised renal function, carbon dioxide or gadolinium can be used for angiographic

evaluation. Prior to PTA, blood pressure should be controlled by angiotensin-converting enzyme inhibitors. Aspirin and an antiplatelet agent are started 1 day before the procedure and continued for 3 to 4 months after the procedure. After insertion of an arterial sheath, 3000 to 5000 IU of heparin is administered intravenously. To reduce or prevent arterial spasm during the procedure, 20 mg of nifedipine can be administered sublingually just prior to the procedure. A guiding catheter can facilitate guide wire passage, balloon catheter positioning, and post-PTA angiographic evaluation with the guide wire crossing the lesion in place. Selecting the proper-sized balloon is critical in the safety and effectiveness of PTA. Usually, about a 10% oversized balloon catheter is used for effective dilation.

The Society of Cardiovascular and Interventional Radiology has defined the criteria for technical and clinical success. Technical success is usually defined as the substantial relief of stenosis with residual stenosis less than 20%. Clinical results can be assessed by the effect on blood pressure and improvement of renal function. The patient should be assessed 6 months after PTA. Patients are considered cured of hypertension if the diastolic blood pressure is less than 90 mm Hg without antihypertensive medication. Improvement is defined as diastolic blood pressure (1) less than 90 mm Hg with administration of equal or reduced doses or (2) greater than 90 but less than 110 mm Hg, with at least a 15-mm Hg decrease from measurements obtained before PTA while the patient was receiving a similar or decreased medication regimen. Improvement in renal function is defined as a decrease in serum creatinine to normal levels or 20% below levels obtained before PTA.

Causes of renal artery stenosis and characteristics of lesions affect the results of renal PTA. Atherosclerotic lesions are usually found at the ostium or proximal third of the renal artery as a part of diffuse major arterial disease. They may be complicated by medial dissection and subintimal hemorrhage, calcification, or atheromatous emboli. They tend to be eccentric. Fibromuscular disease tends to occur in young women and involves the more distal main renal artery and branch vessels. According to subtypes of fibromuscular dysplasia, angiographic findings can be different. Medial fibroplasia is the most common subtype, and the pattern of alternating stenosis and aneurysm formation produces the characteristic "beaded" appearance. The other subtypes may appear as nonspecific arterial stenosis. Takayasu's arteritis is a chronic, idiopathic, inflammatory disease that affects the aorta and pulmonary arteries and major aortic branches. It primarily involves the

aorta; therefore, its renal artery involvement usually manifests as smooth narrowing of the proximal third of the renal artery. There is also a strong female preponderance.

Fibromuscular dysplasia shows the best results for PTA. About 40% of patients with fibromuscular dysplasia are cured after PTA and an additional 40% are improved in blood pressure control. In atherosclerotic renal artery stenosis, a short, nonostial, and concentric lesion without calcification is best suited for PTA. Reportedly, 10% to 20% of patients with atherosclerosis are cured after PTA and an additional 40% to 70% are improved in blood pressure control. In Takayasu's arteritis, although small series are reported, the results of PTA seem to be promising. Reported complications of renal PTA are deterioration of renal function, puncture site hematoma or pseudoaneurysm, renal artery spasm, dissection, thrombosis, and perforation.

Renal artery stent placement is indicated when PTA results in elastic recoil with residual stenosis greater than 30% to 50% and a trans-stenotic gradient greater than 20 mm Hg or dissection with flow-compromising intimal flap. In an atherosclerotic renal ostial lesion, renal artery stenosis is frequently caused by an atherosclerotic plaque of the aorta encroaching its origin and, in such circumstance, ballooning alone is inefficient and primary stenting can be indicated. The stent must be as short as possible; therefore, accurate placement of the stent is important. A balloon-expandable stent is usually recommended for precise deployment.

The primary advantages of stent placement over PTA are higher initial technical success rate and larger initial luminal diameter. In a randomized comparative study, the primary 6-month patency rate in primary renal artery stenting (80%) was significantly higher than that in PTA (34%). The primary concern for stent placement is restenosis due to intimal hyperplasia. Restenosis was found in 11% to 33% of patients with a mean follow-up of 6 months to 2 years. Various strategies to prevent or reduce poststent or post-PTA restenosis, including intravascular brachytherapy and drug-releasing stents, are under investigation.

RENAL ARTERY EMBOLIZATION

The most frequent indication for renal embolization is renal injuries, either traumatic or iatrogenic in origin. Iatrogenic conditions that are complications of surgical or interventional procedures include renal biopsy, percutaneous nephrostomy, nephrostolithotomy, partial nephrectomy, and angiographic procedures. Arteriography may show extravasation, arteriovenous fistula with early-draining vein, and pseudoaneurysms with delayed washout as evidence of vascular injury. Those findings indicate a need for embolization.

Renal aneurysm and arteriovenous fistula can be managed with transcatheter embolization. Percutaneous renal ablation can be an alternative to surgical nephrectomy in patients with end-stage renal disease who present with hypertension, pain, or nephrotic syndrome or bleeding and in those who are poor operative candidates.

The indications for transcatheter embolization of renal neoplasms are to relieve symptoms such as hemorrhage, polycythemia, hypercalcemia, and congestive heart failure, to facilitate surgical resection preoperatively, to inhibit tumor growth and to reduce tumor mass, to relieve pain, to stimulate an immune response, and to control metastasis to the residual kidney or a second primary carcinoma in the solitary kidney. In the patients with angiomyolipomas, prophylactic embolotherapy may be considered when the tumor is 4 cm or larger.

Therapeutic embolization of renal cell carcinoma is still a matter of controversy. Most reported survival times of patients after palliative embolization range between 4 and 11 months, depending on tumor stages. Recently, retrospective analysis of 474 patients with renal cell carcinoma who had radical nephrectomy revealed that preoperative embolization significantly prolonged the survival of the patients. In our experience of transcatheter arterial embolization of unresectable renal cell carcinoma with a mixture of ethanol and iodized oil, the median survival period was 23 months in 10 patients with stage III tumor and 7 months in 15 patients with stage IV tumor.

Embolic materials for renal embolization include gelatin sponge particles, stainless-steel coils, microcoils, polyvinyl alcohol particles, and absolute ethanol. In iatrogenic renal injuries, the method of choice is microcatheters with microcoils that enable superselective embolization of small renal arteries without damaging the surrounding renal parenchyma. Absolute ethanol is used in embolotherapy for renal tumors and renal parenchymal ablation in chronic renal failure and/or renovascular hypertension. When absolute ethanol is selected as an embolic material, every effort should be made to prevent reflux and unintentional nontarget embolization. Balloon occlusion technique and adequate opacification of absolute ethanol with contrast material are usually recommended. In renal angiomyolipoma, absolute ethanol opacified with iodized oil can be superselectively delivered to the tumor-feeding arteries under fluoroscopic control to preserve normal renal parenchyma.

References

1. Baumgartner I, von Aesch K, Do DD, et al: Stent placement in ostial and nonostial atherosclerotic renal arterial stenoses: A prospective follow-up study. Radiology 2000; 216:498–505.
2. Soulez G, Oliva VL, Turpin S, et al: Imaging of renovascular hypertension: Respective values of renal scintigraphy, renal Doppler US, and MR angiography. Radiographics 2000; 20:1355–1368.
3. Zielinski H, Szmigielski S, Petrovich Z: Comparison of preoperative embolization followed by radical nephrectomy with radical nephrectomy alone for renal cell carcinoma. Am J Clin Oncol 2000; 23:6–12.
4. Hom D, Eiley D, Lumerman JH, et al: Complete renal embolization as an alternative to nephrectomy. J Urol 1999; 161:24–27.
5. Ree CR: Stents for atherosclerotic renovascular disease. J Vasc Interv Radiol 1999; 10:689–705.
6. Lee W, Kim TS, Chung JW, et al: Renal angiomyolipoma: Embolotherapy with a mixture of alcohol and iodized oil. J Vasc Interv Radiol 1998; 9:255–261.
7. Blum U, Krumme B, Flügel P, et al: Treatment of ostial renal artery stenoses with vascular endoprostheses after unsuccessful balloon angioplasty. N Engl J Med 1997; 336:459–465.
8. Hanks SE, Katz MD: Arteriography and transcatheter embolization in the management of renal trauma. In Baum S, Pentecost MJ (eds): Abram's Angiography. Boston, Little, Brown, 1997, pp 892–899.
9. Matchett WJ, McFarland DR, Russell DK, et al: Azotemia: Gadopentetate dimeglumine as a contrast agent at digital subtraction angiography. Radiology 1996; 201:569–571.
10. Hélénon O, Rody FE, Correas JM, et al: Color Doppler US of renovascular disease in native kidney. Radiographics 1995; 15:833–854.
11. Rene PC, Oliva VL, Bui BT, et al: Renal artery stenosis: Evaluation of Doppler US after inhibition of angiotensin-converting enzyme with captopril. Radiology 1995; 196:675–679.
12. Hawkins IF Jr, Wilcox CS, Kerns SR, et al: CO_2 digital angiography: A safer contrast agent for renal vascular imaging? Am J Kidney Dis 1994; 24:685–694.

13. Park JH, Kim SH, Han JK, et al: Transcatheter arterial embolization of unresectable renal cell carcinoma with a mixture of ethanol and iodized oil. Cardiovasc Intervent Radiol 1994; 17:323–327.

14. Soulen MC, Faykus MH, Shlansky-Goldberg RD, et al: Elective embolization for prevention of hemorrhage from renal angiomyolipomas. J Vasc Interv Radiol 1994; 5:587–591.

15. Zierler RE: Normal arterial physiology. In Strandness DE Jr, van Breda A (eds): Vascular Diseases: Surgical and Interventional Therapy. New York, Churchill Livingstone, 1994, pp 57–64.

16. Itoh K, Tsukamoto E, Nagao K, et al: Captopril renoscintigraphy with Tc-^{99}m DTPA in patients with suspected renovascular hypertension: Prospective and retrospective evaluation. Clin Nucl Med 1993; 18:463–471.

17. Dondi M, Fanti S, De Fabritiis A, et al: Prognostic value of captopril renal scintigraphy in renovascular hypertension. J Nucl Med 1992; 33:2040–2044.

18. Middleton WD: Doppler US evaluation of renal artery stenosis: Past, present, and future. Radiology 1992; 184:307–308.

19. Sharma S, Saxena A, Talwar KK, et al: Renal artery stenosis caused by nonspecific arteritis (Takayasu disease): Results of treatment with percutaneous transluminal angioplasty. AJR Am J Roentgenol 1992; 158:417–422.

20. Roubidoux MA, Dunnick NR, Klotman PE, et al: Renal vein renins: Inability to predict response to revascularization in patients with hypertension. Radiology 1991; 178:819–822.

21. Standards of Practice Committee of the Society of Cardiovascular and Interventional Radiology: Guidelines for percutaneous transluminal angioplasty. Radiology 1990; 177:619–626.

22. Wallace S, Charnsangavej C, Carrasco CH, et al: Renal tumors: Clinical results. In Dondelinger RF, Rossi P, Kurdziel JC, Wallace S (eds): Interventional Radiology. New York, Thieme, 1990, pp 468–477.

23. Park JH, Han MC, Kim SH, et al: Takayasu arteritis: Angiographic findings and results of angioplasty. AJR Am J Roentgenol 1989; 153:1069–1074.

24. Keller FS, Coyle M, Rosch J, et al: Percutaneous renal ablation in patients with end-stage renal disease: Alternative to surgical nephrectomy. Radiology 1986; 159:447–451.

25. Lüscher TF, Greminger P, Kuhlmann U, et al: Renal venous renin determinations in renovascular hypertension: Diagnostic and prognostic value in unilateral renal artery stenosis treated by surgery or percutaneous transluminal angioplasty. Nephron 1986; 44(Suppl 1):17–24.

26. Martin LG, Casarella WJ, Alspaugh JP, et al: Renal artery angioplasty: Increased technical success and decreased complications in the second 100 patients. Radiology 1986; 159:631–634.

27. Tegtmeyer CJ, Sos TA: Techniques of renal angioplasty. Radiology 1986; 161:577–586.

28. Nannie GS, Hawkins IF Jr, Orak JK: Control of hypertension by ethanol renal ablation. Radiology 1983; 148:51–54.

29. Sos TA, Pickering TG, Phil D, et al: Percutaneous transluminal renal angioplasty in renovascular hypertension due to atheroma or fibromuscular dysplasia. N Engl J Med 1983; 309:274–279.

Illustrations • Renovascular Interventions

1 • Renal percutaneous angioplasty in fibromuscular dysplasia

2 • Renal percutaneous angioplasty in atherosclerosis: remodeling

3 • Renal percutaneous angioplasty in atherosclerosis and renal insufficiency: axillary approach

4 • Renal percutaneous angioplasty in Takayasu's arteritis: repeated dilation

5 • Renal percutaneous angioplasty in Takayasu's arteritis: kissing balloon technique

6 • Renal percutaneous angioplasty in solitary kidney

7 • Renal stent placement in atherosclerosis and renal insufficiency: bilateral stenting

8 • Renal stent placement: restenosis and balloon rupture during revision

9 • Renal embolotherapy: postbiopsy bleeding

10 • Renal embolotherapy: guide wire–induced renal perforation

11 • Renal embolotherapy: hemorrhage after percutaneous nephrostolithotomy

12 • Renal embolotherapy: traumatic renal artery aneurysm

13 • Renal embolotherapy: arteriovenous malformation

14 • Renal embolotherapy: uncontrollable hypertension in chronic renal failure

15 • Renal embolotherapy: renal cell carcinoma

16 • Renal embolotherapy: angiomyolipoma

1. Renal Percutaneous Angioplasty in Fibromuscular Dysplasia

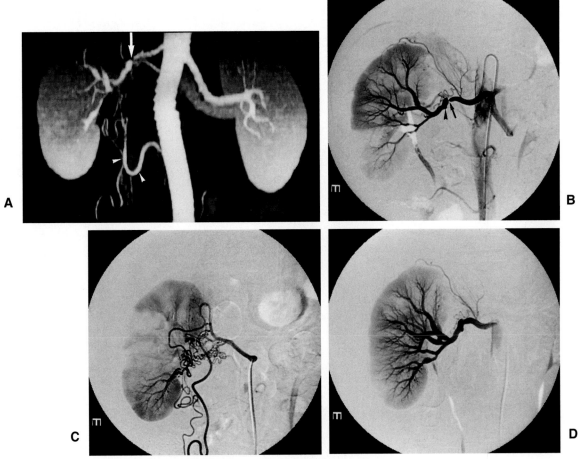

Fig. 1. Successful balloon angioplasty for fibromuscular dysplasia in a 19-year-old man.
A. Spiral CT angiogram shows severe focal stenosis *(arrow)* of the right renal artery and dilated ureteric artery *(arrowheads)*. **B.** Right renal arteriogram shows severe focal stenosis *(arrow)* of the right renal artery at its mid portion with uneven nephrogram due to collateral circulation. Note focal dilation of the renal artery just distal to the stenotic portion *(arrowhead)*. **C.** Selective ureteric arteriogram demonstrates multiple collateral vessels connecting to the intrarenal branches. **D.** After balloon angioplasty, right renal arteriogram shows filling of the entire renal arteries and homogenous nephrogram.

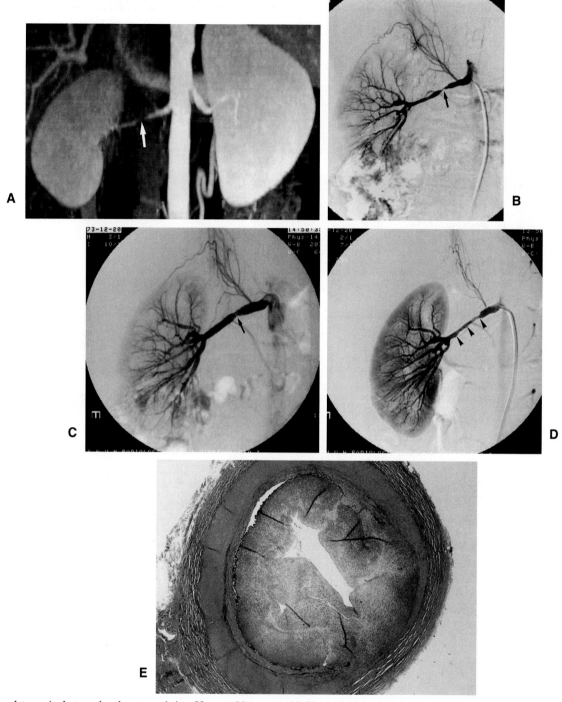

Fig. 2. Incomplete angioplasty and early restenosis in a 22-year-old woman with fibromuscular dysplasia of intimal hyperplasia type.
A. Spiral CT angiogram shows severe focal stenosis *(arrow)* at the mid portion of the right renal artery. Also note the decreased size and delayed arterial perfusion of the right kidney. **B.** Right renal arteriogram shows diffusely narrowed right renal artery at its mid and distal segment with severe focal stenosis at its mid portion *(arrow)*. **C.** Completion arteriogram after balloon dilation reveals residual stenosis of 50% *(arrow)*. **D.** Follow-up arteriogram obtained 10 weeks later shows restenosis of the right renal artery, which extends more distally *(arrowheads)*. The patient twice underwent revision with balloon angioplasty. However, she came back with early recurrence. Finally, aortorenal bypass surgery was performed. **E.** Photomicrograph of the resected renal artery shows prominent circumferential intimal hyperplasia. (**E,** See also Color Section.)

2. Renal Percutaneous Angioplasty in Atherosclerosis: Remodeling

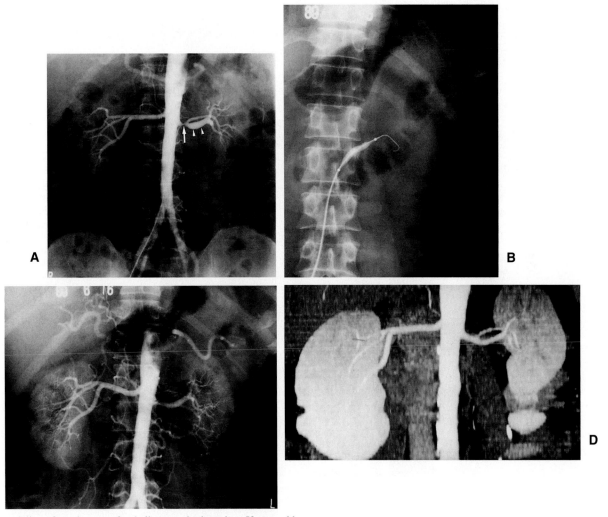

Fig. 1. Remodeling of renal artery after balloon angioplasty in a 52-year-old man.
A. Abdominal aortography shows severe focal stenosis *(arrow)* of the left renal artery just before its branching point, which accompanies poststenotic dilation *(arrowheads)*. **B, C.** After balloon angioplasty, there seems to be considerable residual stenosis of 30% to 40%. **D.** Follow-up CT angiogram taken 5 years later demonstrates a completely normal left renal artery.

3. Renal Percutaneous Angioplasty in Atherosclerosis and Renal Insufficiency: Axillary Approach

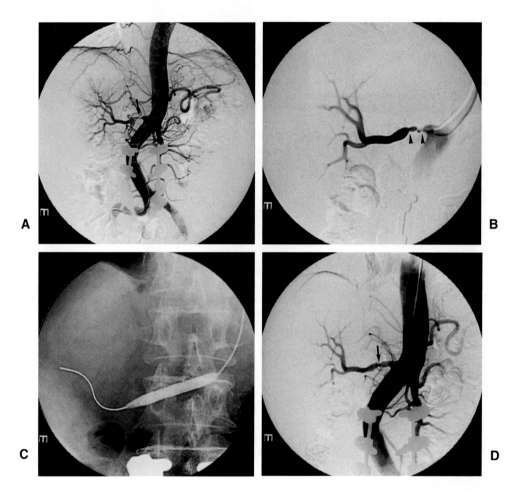

Fig. 1. Renal angioplasty through axillary approach in a 70-year-old man with azotemia.

A. Abdominal aortogram through femoral approach shows right renal artery stenosis *(arrow)*. At that time, the serum creatinine level was 3.3 mg/dL. Because of the tortuosity of the iliac arteries and the aorta, it seems to be difficult to perform renal angioplasty through the femoral approach. **B.** Selective right renal arteriogram via the left axillary artery clearly shows severe focal stenosis *(arrowheads)* of the proximal segment of the right renal artery. **C.** Renal angioplasty was performed using a 6-mm balloon catheter. **D.** Completion aortogram after balloon angioplasty shows relieved renal artery stenosis with residual stenosis of about 30% *(arrow)*. Five years later, the serum creatinine level was 1.2 mg/dL.

2. Renal Percutaneous Angioplasty in Atherosclerosis: Remodeling

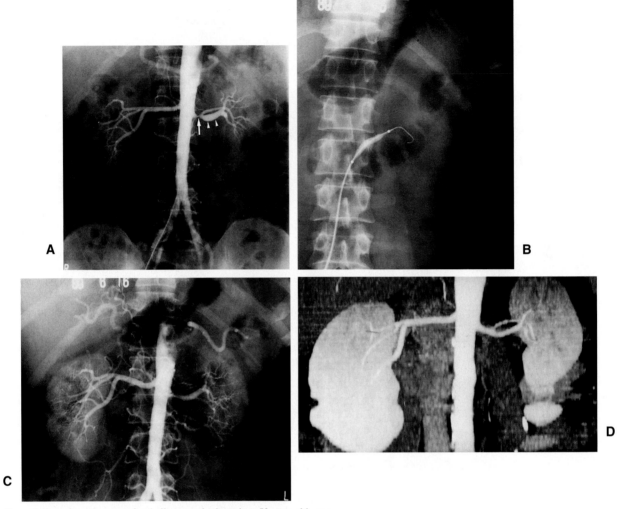

Fig. 1. Remodeling of renal artery after balloon angioplasty in a 52-year-old man.
A. Abdominal aortography shows severe focal stenosis *(arrow)* of the left renal artery just before its branching point, which accompanies poststenotic dilation *(arrowheads)*. **B, C.** After balloon angioplasty, there seems to be considerable residual stenosis of 30% to 40%. **D.** Follow-up CT angiogram taken 5 years later demonstrates a completely normal left renal artery.

3. Renal Percutaneous Angioplasty in Atherosclerosis and Renal Insufficiency: Axillary Approach

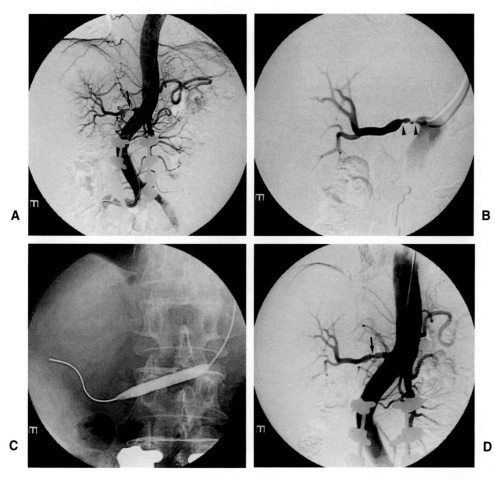

Fig. 1. Renal angioplasty through axillary approach in a 70-year-old man with azotemia.
A. Abdominal aortogram through femoral approach shows right renal artery stenosis *(arrow)*. At that time, the serum creatinine level was 3.3 mg/dL. Because of the tortuosity of the iliac arteries and the aorta, it seems to be difficult to perform renal angioplasty through the femoral approach. **B.** Selective right renal arteriogram via the left axillary artery clearly shows severe focal stenosis *(arrowheads)* of the proximal segment of the right renal artery. **C.** Renal angioplasty was performed using a 6-mm balloon catheter. **D.** Completion aortogram after balloon angioplasty shows relieved renal artery stenosis with residual stenosis of about 30% *(arrow)*. Five years later, the serum creatinine level was 1.2 mg/dL.

4. Renal Percutaneous Angioplasty in Takayasu's Arteritis: Repeated Dilation

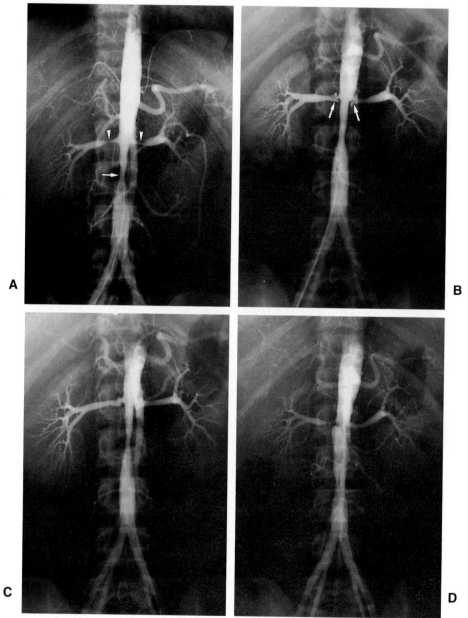

Fig. 1. Repeated PTA of both renal arteries and the aorta and successful long-term result in a 24-year-old woman with Takayasu's arteritis. (**A–H,** From Park JH, Han MC, Kim SH, et al: Takayasu arteritis: Angiographic findings and results of angioplasty. AJR Am J Roentgenol 1989; 153:1069–1074.) **A.** Abdominal aortogram shows smooth segmental narrowing of the infrarenal abdominal aorta *(arrow)*. Proximal portions of both renal arteries show marked stenosis *(arrowheads)*. **B.** Aortogram taken immediately after PTA of bilateral renal arteries with 6-mm balloon catheter shows intimal flaps due to localized dissection at origin of both renal arteries *(arrows)*. **C.** Two months later, follow-up aortogram reveals healing of the dissection of both renal arteries. PTA of the infrarenal abdominal aorta was done with a 12-mm balloon catheter to relieve the weakness of both lower extremities. **D.** Two months later, aortogram shows mild to moderate residual stenosis of the infrarenal abdominal aorta and restenosis of the right renal artery, which was redilated.

Illustration continued on following page

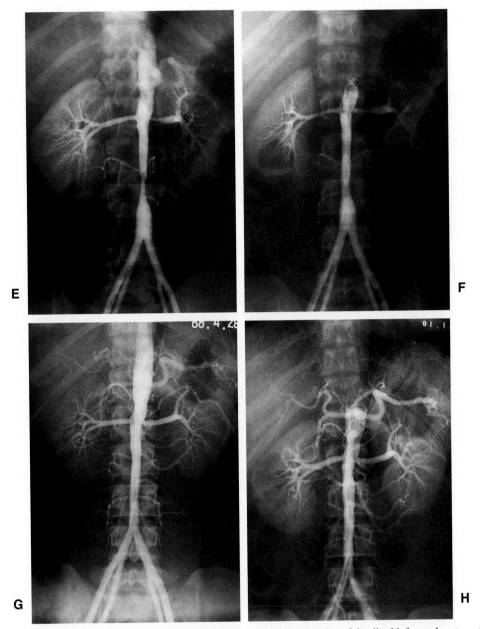

Fig. 1 *Continued*. **E.** Seven months after the initial PTA, follow-up aortogram reveals narrowing of the distal infrarenal aorta and proximal left renal artery. **F.** After PTA of the distal infrarenal aorta and left renal artery, aortogram shows restoration of the lumen of the aorta and renal artery. **G, H.** Follow-up aortograms taken 28 months (**G**) and 6 years (**H**) after initial PTA reveal no evidence of restenosis.

5. Renal Percutaneous Angioplasty in Takayasu's Arteritis: Kissing Balloon Technique

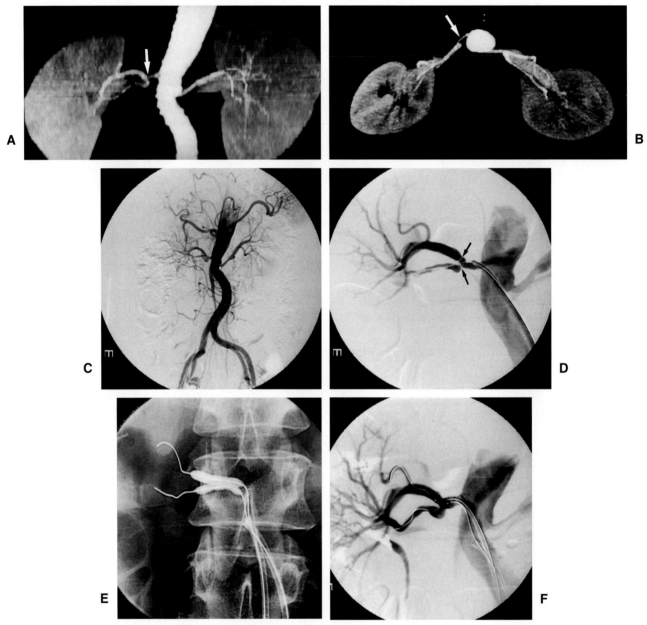

Fig. 1. Renal PTA using a kissing balloon technique in a 49-year-old woman with Takayasu's arteritis.
A, B. Spiral CT angiograms in anteroposterior (**A**) and axial (**B**) projections show bilateral renal artery stenosis, especially severe on the right side *(arrow)*. **C.** Abdominal aortogram shows similar findings. Selective renal vein renin sampling demonstrated the lateralization to the right kidney. **D.** Right renal arteriogram shows not only the stenosis of the short main renal artery but also the membranous or focal stenosis of the proximal portion of its dorsal and ventral divisions *(arrows)*. **E.** Kissing balloon technique was employed, and two coronary balloon catheters (3.5 mm and 3 mm in diameter) were placed in the dorsal and ventral divisions. **F.** Completion arteriogram shows the successful result.

6. Renal Percutaneous Angioplasty in Solitary Kidney

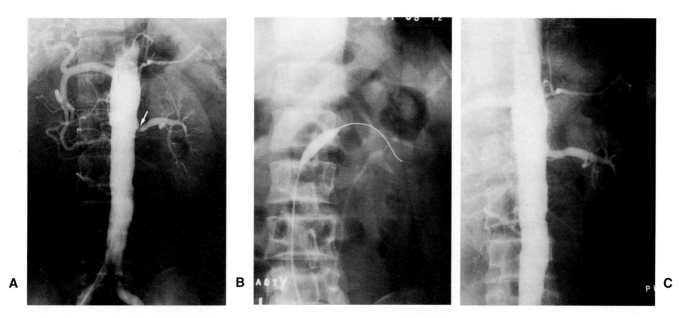

Fig. 1. Renal PTA in a 36-year-old man with solitary kidney.
A. Abdominal aortogram shows severe focal stenosis *(arrow)* at the proximal left renal artery. **B.** Renal angioplasty was performed using a 6-mm balloon catheter. **C.** Completion arteriogram shows the widely patent left renal artery with mild residual stenosis.

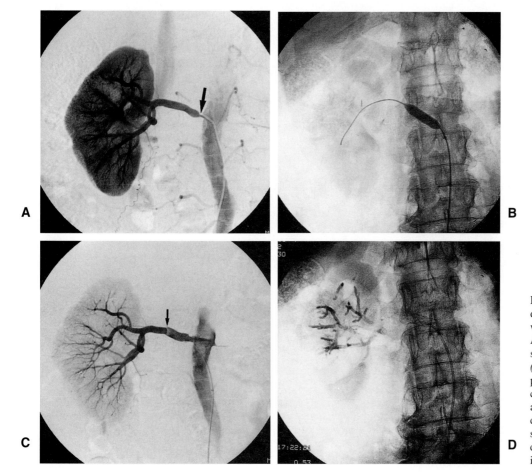

Fig. 2. Renal PTA and severe dissection in a 58-year-old man with solitary kidney.
A. Right renal arteriogram shows severe focal stenosis at its orifice *(arrow)*. **B.** Angioplasty was performed with a 7-mm balloon catheter. **C.** Immediately after angioplasty, severe renal artery dissection occurred *(arrow)*. **D.** In spite of stent placement, the dissection propagated distally and involved intrarenal branches.

7. Renal Stent Placement in Atherosclerosis and Renal Insufficiency: Bilateral Stenting

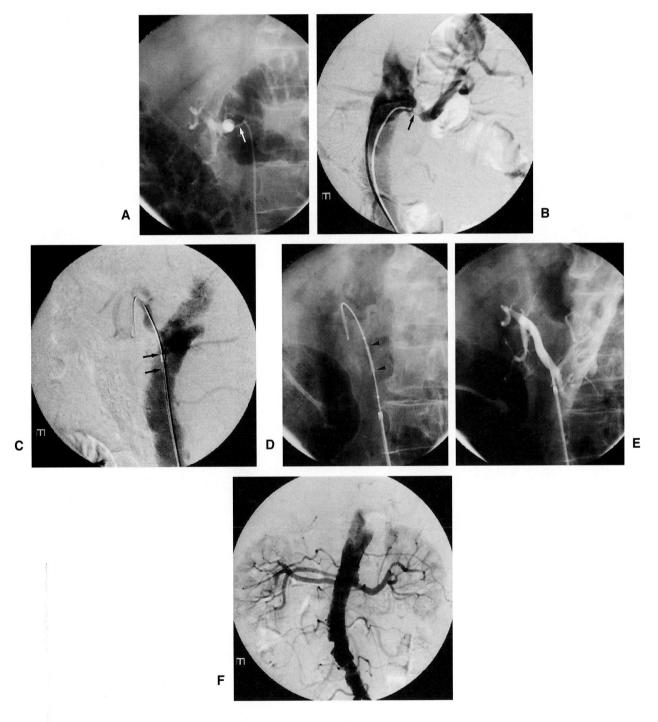

Fig. 1. Stent placement for bilateral renal artery stenosis in a 73-year-old man with azotemia.
A, B. Selective right **(A)** and left **(B)** renal arteriograms show severe focal stenosis at both proximal renal arteries *(arrow)* and poststenotic dilation.
C. After passage of a guide wire through the stenotic segment, a renal guiding catheter was positioned just below the renal orifice *(arrows)*. Because the stiff guide wire straightens the renal artery, it is necessary to perform a renal arteriogram using the guiding catheter. **D.** A balloon-expandable stent *(arrowheads)* mounted on a balloon catheter was placed at the stenotic segment. **E.** Renal arteriogram after stent placement shows successful result.
F. Completion aortogram after bilateral renal stent placement demonstrates widely patent renal arteries. Note the double right renal arteries.

8. Renal Stent Placement: Restenosis and Balloon Rupture during Revision

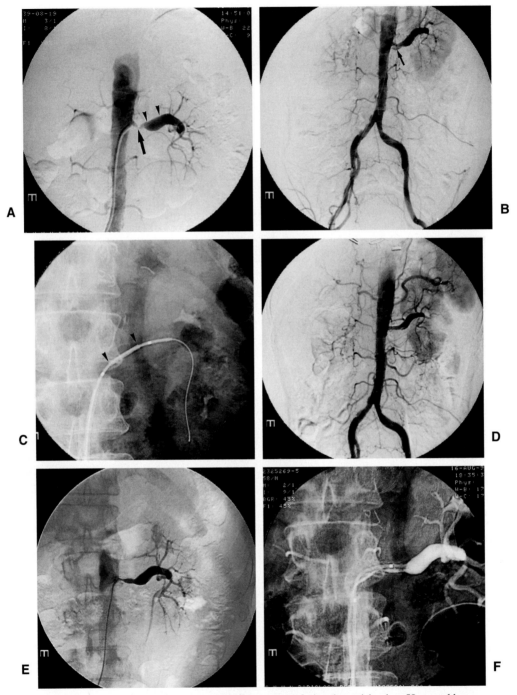

Fig. 1. Restenosis after renal angioplasty and stent placement, and balloon rupture during the revision in a 58-year-old man.
A. Left renal arteriogram shows severe narrowing of the proximal left renal artery *(arrow)* with poststenotic dilation *(arrowheads)*. **B.** After balloon angioplasty, localized subintimal dissection occurred *(arrow)*. **C.** A Palmaz stent *(arrowheads)* was placed in the left renal artery. **D.** Completion aortogram shows the widely patent left renal artery. **E.** Four months later, follow-up angiogram shows restenosis of the left renal artery due to prominent intrastent intimal hyperplasia. The patient underwent revision for the restenosis with balloon angioplasty three times. **F.** At the final attempt, the angioplasty balloon ruptured and was entrapped inside the stent. The ruptured balloon was surgically removed, and aortorenal bypass surgery was performed.

9. Renal Embolotherapy: Postbiopsy Bleeding

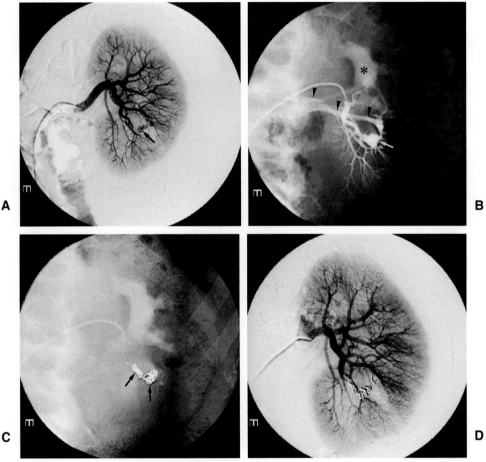

A

B

C

D

Fig. 1. Embolotherapy for hemorrhage after renal biopsy in a 46-year-old man.
A. Left renal arteriogram shows an ill-defined collection of contrast material *(arrow)*. **B.** Selective angiogram using a microcatheter clearly demonstrates a pseudoaneurysm *(arrow)* and arteriovenous shunt. Note early opacification of the renal vein *(arrowheads)* through the shunt. Also note the collection of contrast material in the upper-pole calyx *(asterisk)*. **C.** Feeding arteries supplying the pseudoaneurysm and arteriovenous shunt were embolized with microcoils *(arrows)*. **D.** Postembolization arteriogram shows the disappearance of the pseudoaneurysm and arteriovenous shunt with preservation of normal renal parenchyma.

10. Renal Embolotherapy: Guide Wire–Induced Renal Perforation

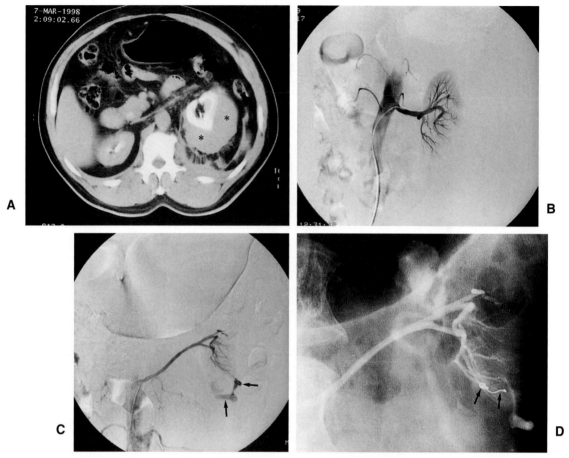

Fig. 1. Guide wire–induced renal perforation during coronary angiography and microcoil embolization in a 62-year-old man.
A. CT scan shows subcapsular hematoma formation *(asterisks)* and delayed accumulation of contrast material in the left renal parenchyma due to parenchymal compression. **B.** Left main renal arteriogram appears normal. **C.** There is an accessory, lower-polar, renal artery with upward direction to explain the renal perforation during blind introduction of a guide wire. Note extravasation of the contrast material *(arrows)*. **D.** Microcoil embolization *(arrows)* was performed with successful cessation of bleeding.

11. Renal Embolotherapy: Hemorrhage after Percutaneous Nephrostolithotripsy

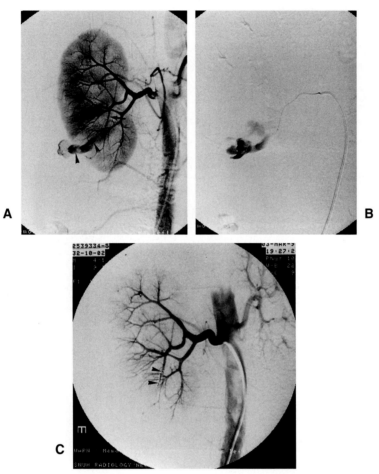

Fig. 1. Embolotherapy for hemorrhage after percutaneous nephrolithotripsy in a 62-year-old man.
A. Right renal arteriogram shows extravasation of contrast material into the perirenal space *(arrowheads)*. **B.** Superselective arteriogram of the feeding artery *(arrow* in **A)** demonstrates brisk hemorrhage. **C.** Completion arteriogram after embolotherapy using microcoils *(arrowheads)* shows cessation of bleeding.

12. Renal Embolotherapy: Traumatic Renal Artery Aneurysm

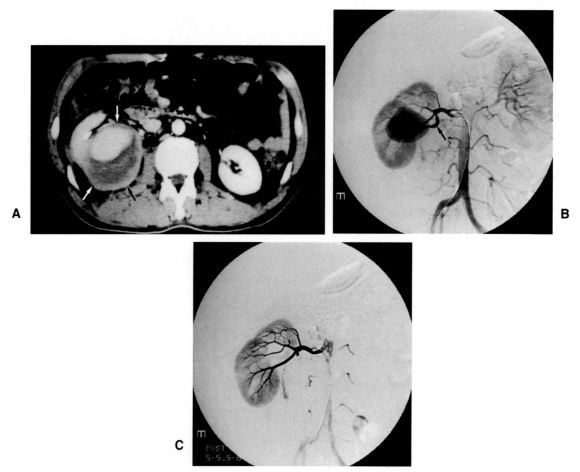

Fig. 1. Traumatic renal artery aneurysm treated by coil embolization in a 47-year-old man.
A. CT scan at the time of admission shows a large intrarenal pseudoaneurysm *(arrows)* with partial thrombosis in the right kidney. **B.** Selective right renal arteriogram reveals a pseudoaneurysm supplied by a single segmental renal artery *(arrow)*. The segmental renal artery was occluded by a stainless-steel coil. **C.** Completion arteriogram shows nonvisualization of the pseudoaneurysm and maintained perfusion of the renal parenchyma.

13. Renal Embolotherapy: Arteriovenous Malformation

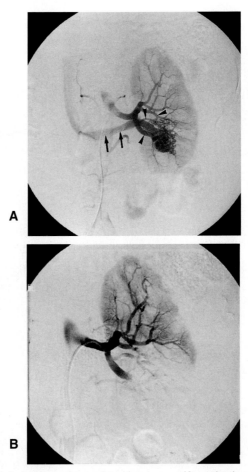

Fig. 1. Embolotherapy for renal arteriovenous malformation in a 43-year-old woman.
A. Left renal arteriogram shows an entangled vascular mass supplied by multiple feeding arteries and early draining renal vein *(arrows)*. Polyvinyl alcohol particles were injected into the feeding arteries *(arrowheads)*. **B.** On postembolization arteriogram, the nidus of the vascular malformation and draining renal vein do not fill.

14. Renal Embolotherapy: Uncontrollable Hypertension in Chronic Renal Failure

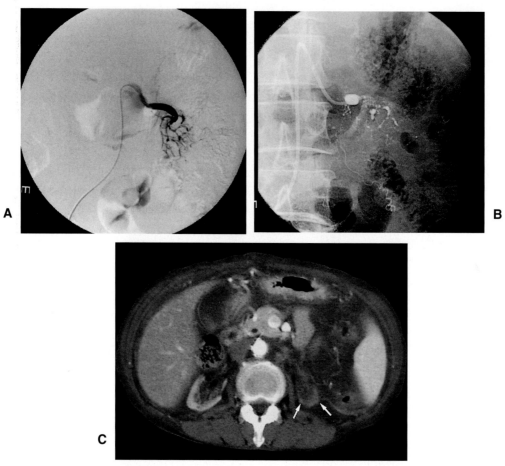

Fig. 1. Renal embolotherapy for uncontrollable hypertension in a 50-year-old woman with chronic renal failure.
A. The patient's initial blood pressure was 160/100 mm Hg in spite of a triple-antihypertensive regimen. Left renal arteriography shows a shrunken left kidney and multifocal stenosis in the intrarenal arteries. **B.** A 3-mL mixture of absolute ethanol–Lipiodol was infused after balloon occlusion of the left renal artery. **C.** Follow-up CT scan shows almost nonopacification of the left renal parenchyma *(arrows)*. After embolotherapy, the patient's blood pressure became controllable with antihypertensive agents.

15. Renal Embolotherapy: Renal Cell Carcinoma

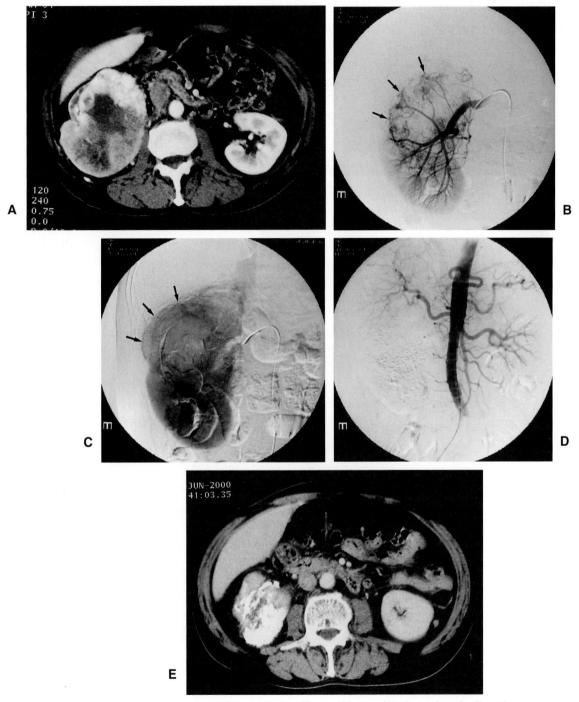

Fig. 1. Renal embolotherapy using an absolute ethanol-Lipiodol mixture in a 65-year-old man with advanced renal cell carcinoma.
A. CT scan shows a large mass replacing the upper half of the right kidney. **B, C.** Selective right renal arteriograms in arterial **(B)** and nephrographic **(C)** phases reveal a hypervascular mass *(arrows)* at the upper pole of the right kidney. A 14-mL mixture of absolute ethanol–Lipiodol was infused after balloon occlusion of the right renal artery. **D.** Completion aortogram shows no antegrade flow in the right renal artery. **E.** As compared with the initial CT, follow-up CT obtained 3 months later demonstrates markedly decreased size of the tumor with persistent retention of high-attenuated Lipiodol.

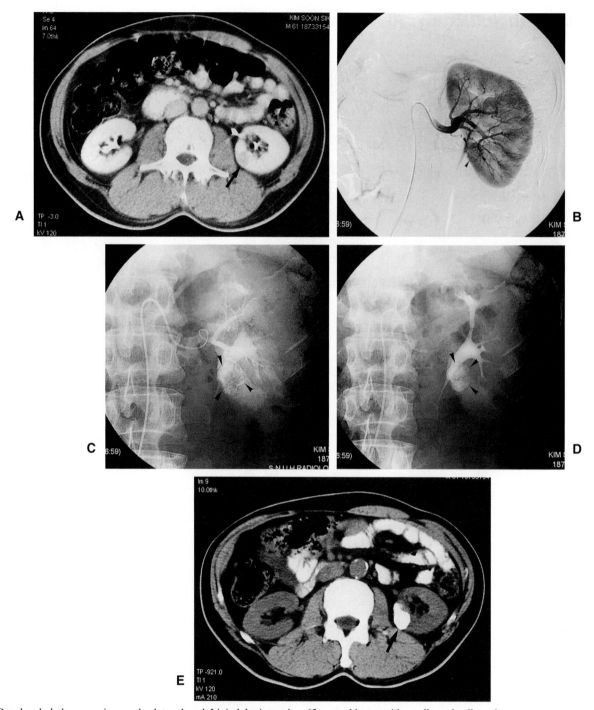

Fig. 2. Renal embolotherapy using an absolute ethanol–Lipiodol mixture in a 62-year-old man with small renal cell carcinoma.
A. CT scan shows a small low-attenuated mass *(arrow)* at the inferomedial aspect of the left kidney. **B, C.** Left renal arteriogram **(B)** and superselective arteriogram using a microcatheter **(C)** reveal tumor hypervascularity *(arrowheads)*. A 2-mL mixture of absolute ethanol–Lipiodol was infused into the tumor-feeding artery using a microcatheter. **D.** Completion simple radiograph shows even accumulation of Lipiodol in the tumor neovasculature with a low-attenuated rim *(arrowheads)* suggesting the presence of a tumor capsule. **E.** Nonenhanced CT scan obtained 4 days later demonstrates homogenous, dense retention of Lipiodol in the tumor *(arrow)*.

16. Renal Embolotherapy: Angiomyolipoma

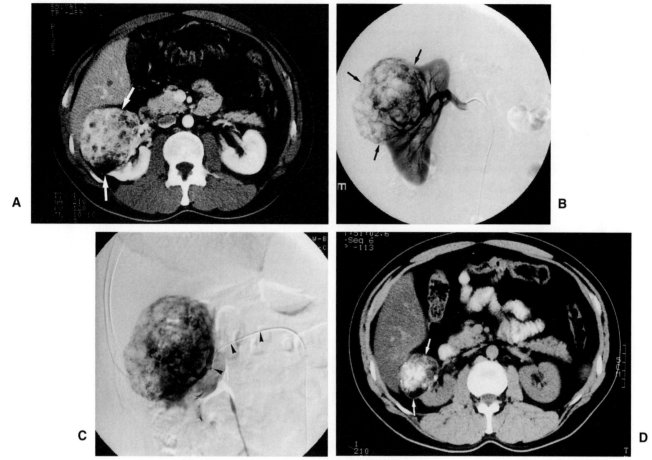

Fig. 1. Embolotherapy for solitary renal angiomyolipoma in a 38-year-old man.
A. CT scan shows a large right renal mass *(arrows)* containing fatty components. **B.** Right renal arteriogram reveals a hypervascular mass *(arrows)*.
C. The tumor-feeding, segmental branch was selectively catheterized with an angled catheter *(arrowheads)* and an 8-mL mixture of absolute ethanol–Lipiodol was infused into it. **D.** Follow-up CT scan obtained 5 months later shows markedly shrunken tumor with Lipiodol uptake *(arrows)* and preserved right renal parenchyma.

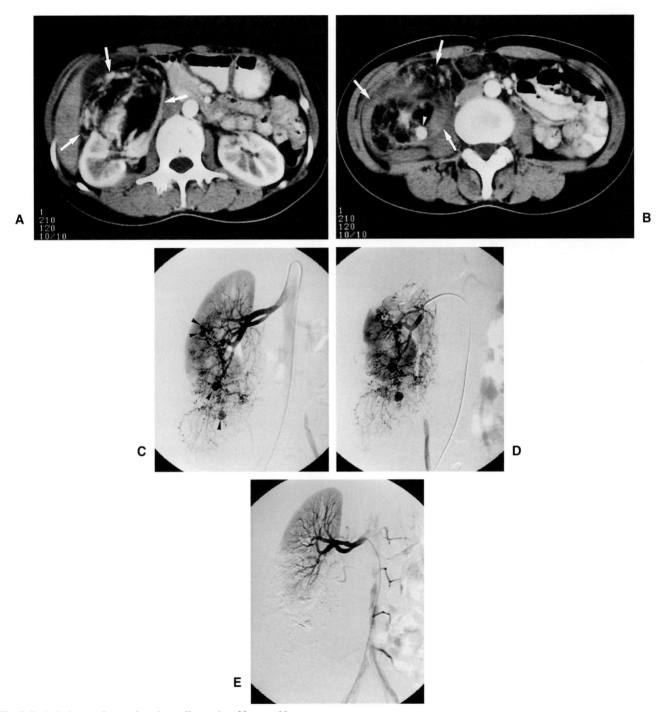

Fig. 2. Embolotherapy for renal angiomyolipoma in a 33-year-old woman.
A, B. Spiral CT scan shows a large mass *(arrows)* containing well-enhancing soft tissue and fatty components. There is a small intratumoral aneurysm *(arrowhead* in **B**). **C.** Right renal arteriogram shows a hypervascular mass in the lower part of right kidney with multiple aneurysms *(arrowheads)* in the tumor vessels. **D.** On selective angiogram of the segmental renal arteries with conventional catheters, the main tumor feeder was identified and embolotherapy was performed by infusing a 14-mL mixture of absolute ethanol–Lipiodol. **E.** Completion renal arteriogram shows disappeared tumor vessels and preserved normal renal parenchyma.

Index

Note: Page numbers followed by f indicate figures;
those followed by t indicate tables.

3

Imaging of Pulmonary Infections

EDITORS

▬ **NESTOR L. MÜLLER, MD, PhD, FRCPC**

Professor and Chairman
Department of Radiology
University of British Columbia
Vancouver, British Columbia, Canada

▬ **TOMÁS FRANQUET, MD, PhD**

Chief, Thoracic Imaging
Associate Professor of Radiology
Department of Radiology
Hospital de Sant Pau
Universitat Autónoma de Barcelona
Barcelona, Spain

▬ **KYUNG SOO LEE, MD**

Professor of Radiology
Department of Radiology
Samsung Medical Center
Sungkyunkwan University School of Medicine
Seoul, Korea

ASSOCIATE EDITOR

▬ **C. ISABELA S. SILVA, MD, PhD**

Thoracic Imaging Research Fellow
Department of Radiology
University of British Columbia
Vancouver General Hospital
Vancouver, British Columbia, Canada

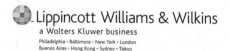
. Lippincott Williams & Wilkins
a Wolters Kluwer business
Philadelphia • Baltimore • New York • London
Buenos Aires • Hong Kong • Sydney • Tokyo

Acquisitions Editor: Lisa McAllister
Developmental Editor: Rebeca Barroso
Managing Editor: Kerry Barrett
Project Manager: Nicole Walz
Manufacturing Manager: Kathleen Brown
Marketing Manager: Angela Panetta
Creative Director: Doug Smock
Cover Designer: Mary Belibasakis
Production Services: Laserwords Private Limited
Printer: Gopsons Papers Limited

Library of Congress Cataloging-in-Publication Data

Müller, Nestor Luiz, 1948-
    Imaging of pulmonary infections / Nestor L. Müller, Tomás Franquet,
Kyung Soo Lee ; associate editor, C. Isabela S. Silva.
        p. ; cm.
    Includes bibliographical references and index.
    ISBN 0-7817-7232-X
    1. Lungs—Diseases—Diagnosis. 2. Lungs—Radiography.
I. Franquet, Tomás. II. Lee, Kyung Soo, MD. III. Silva, C. Isabela S.
IV. Title.
    [DNLM: 1. Lung Diseases—radiography. 2. Diagnosis, Differential.
3. Respiratory Tract Infections—radiography. 4. Tomography, X-Ray
Computed.   WF 600 M9585i 2007]
RC756.M85 2007
616.2′4075—dc22
                                    2006010340

To Alison and Phillip Müller
Salomé, Tomás, Pablo, and Elisa Franquet
Kyung Sook, Joo Hwang, and Joo Young Lee

Contents

Preface

Pulmonary infection is a major cause of morbidity and mortality. Over the last 2 decades, there has been not only an increase in the prevalence of various infections but also the recognition of several important new pathogens. Chest radiograph plays an essential role in the detection of parenchymal abnormalities consistent with pneumonia and in monitoring the response to treatment. Other roles for chest radiography include assessment of disease extent and detection of complications such as cavitation, abscess formation, and pleural effusion. Computed tomography (CT) is a valuable adjunct to chest radiography, particularly in the evaluation of pneumonia in the immunocompromised host, detection of complications such as empyema, and additional or alternative diagnoses, and as a guide to invasive diagnostic or therapeutic procedures.

Imaging of Pulmonary Infections presents a brief, practical approach to the differential diagnosis of pulmonary infections based on their characteristic radiographic and CT manifestations. It discusses the value and limitations of chest radiography, indications for CT, optimal CT technique, and the role of intravenous contrast. The book describes and illustrates the characteristic imaging manifestations of the most common community-acquired pneumonias, nosocomial pneumonias, and the various infections seen in immunocompromised patients. It contains a large number of simple, practical tables that summarize the characteristic manifestations of bacterial, mycobacterial, fungal, and viral infections.

The book is aimed at radiologists, pulmonary medicine physicians, and residents in radiology and pulmonary medicine, as well as internists and family practitioners taking care of patients with respiratory infection. It provides a simple, practical approach to the differential diagnosis of pulmonary infection and summarizes the value and limitations of imaging in the assessment of these patients.

Acknowledgments

We would like to express our gratitude to Ms. Wendy Westman for her superb secretarial assistance and to our colleagues who provided some of the illustrations. In particular, we would like to thank Dr. Joungho Han from the Department of Pathology, Samsung Medical Center, Sungkyunkwan University School of Medicine, Seoul, Korea, for providing several excellent pathology images.

NLM
TF
KSL
CISS

Acknowledgments

We would like to express our gratitude to Mrs. Wendy Worman for her superb secretarial assistance and to our colleagues who provided some of the illustrations. In particular we thank Melanie Cann, Jonathan Pine from the Department of Publishing, Samantha Walker Group, Jonathan Alter in Dermatitis School of Medicine, Mout Belfast, for providing several excellent publishing images.

Pulmonary Infection: Basic Concepts

1

Despite advances in diagnosis and treatment, respiratory tract infection continues to be a major cause of morbidity and mortality. Pneumonia is the leading cause of death due to infectious disease (1). More than 6 million cases of bacterial pneumonia occur each year in the United States and the incidence of pneumonia is increasing. The spectrum of organisms known to cause respiratory infections is broad and constantly increasing as new pathogens are identified, and an increasing number of patients have impaired immunity due to disease or medications. In the United States, it has been estimated that there are 1.1 million cases of community-acquired pneumonia requiring hospitalization each year (1). Nosocomial pneumonia is the most important hospital-acquired infection, being associated with the highest mortality rate of nosocomial infections (2). In addition to direct patient care costs, pneumonia is responsible for >50 million days of restricted activity from work and is the sixth leading cause of death in the United States with a mortality rate of 13.4 per 100,000 (3).

In the last two decades there has been an increase in not only the prevalence of various infections but also the recognition of several important new viral pathogens. These include hantaviruses, human metapneumovirus, avian influenza A viruses, and coronavirus associated with severe acute respiratory syndrome (SARS) (4–11).

PULMONARY HOST DEFENSES

Microorganisms may reach the lower respiratory tract through diverse routes. Although breathed in air contains a myriad of particulate contaminants, some of which are infectious, by far the most common route for bacterial pneumonia is microaspiration from infected oropharyngeal secretions. Aerosolization is an important route of infection for those pathogens believed to be directly inhaled rather than aspirated into the lower respiratory tract, such as *Mycobacterium tuberculosis*, endemic fungi, *Mycoplasma*, *Legionella*, and many respiratory viruses. Gross aspiration occurs in patients with central nervous system disorders affecting swallowing (e.g., seizures, strokes). Hematogenous spread commonly takes place in the setting of endocarditis and intravascular catheter-related infections.

Pulmonary host defense mechanisms include innate or nonspecific (e.g., mechanical barriers and phagocytic defenses) and acquired or specific (e.g., cell-mediated defenses and humoral immunity) mechanisms. Impairment in any of these mechanisms results in reduced ability to clear an infectious inoculum.

Mechanical barriers include the anatomic features of the airways and the mucociliary transport system. Clearance by

mechanical means is influenced by the physical properties of inhaled infectious organisms and particles. Whereas particles >10 μm in diameter are filtered in the upper airways (nasopharynx), particles 5 to 10 μm in diameter may reach the tracheobronchial tree and are cleared by the mucociliary escalator. Only particles between 1 and 2 μm in diameter typically reach the alveoli.

After reaching the distal portions of the lung the ability of infectious organisms to cause progressive infection depends on the balance between the virulence and load of the organism and phagocytic lung defenses (12). Phagocytic functions in the lung are carried out by mononuclear (monocytes, macrophages) and polymorphonuclear (neutrophils, eosinophils) cells (13).

Alveolar macrophages ("big eaters") represent the first line of defense at the level of the alveoli. Macrophages derive from precursors in the bone marrow, and are mobilized to the active focus during active lung infection (13). At the alveolar level, phagocytes are recruited from the interstitium, airways, and blood. Alveolar macrophages have several functions that are important to the host response to bacteria, including bacterial recognition, bacterial phagocytosis, bacterial killing, and the production of inflammatory mediators that are essential for the pulmonary recruitment of leukocytes (13).

Macrophages and monocytes recognize bacteria with a set of cell surface receptors known as *pattern recognition* receptors. Recognition of bacteria by these receptors results in macrophage/monocyte activation and the development of inflammatory response to bacterial pathogens (14, 15).

Impaired alveolar macrophage function occurs in various conditions such as hypoxia, alcoholism, tobacco smoke, and corticosteroid therapy. It is estimated that 20 million individuals in the United States meet the criteria for alcoholism, and between 20% and 40% of patients admitted to large urban hospitals are there because of disease caused by or made worse by alcohol consumption (16, 17). A Canadian group studying pneumonia in >6,000 alcoholics reported a three- and sevenfold increased risk of death in ethanol-abusing men and women, respectively, compared to controls (18).

Failure of mechanical mechanisms such as the mucociliary escalator and phagocytic defenses favors the generation of a humoral immune response specifically directed toward the elimination of extracellular pathogens. The development of specific immune responses in the lungs requires presentation of antigen to CD4$^+$ T lymphocytes.

Pneumonia is more common when host defense is impaired. Defects in phagocytosis or ciliary function, hypogammaglobulinemia, neutropenia, and reduction in CD4$^+$ T lymphocytes can result in increased frequency and severity of pneumonia. In immunocompromised patients, defects in the different components of the immune system predispose the patient to develop specific types of infections (19). Therefore awareness of the immune status of the patient and any underlying abnormality that may affect the immune response is important in the differential diagnosis. For example, functional or anatomic asplenia is an important risk factor for pneumonia, with 80% of cases being due to *Streptococcus pneumoniae*.

CHANGING TRENDS IN PULMONARY INFECTIONS

Diagnosis of pneumonia requires clinical acumen, appropriate microbiologic tests, and imaging. The chest radiograph represents an important initial examination in all patients suspected of having pulmonary infection. In most cases the radiographic findings are suggestive of or consistent with the diagnosis of pneumonia and are sufficiently specific in the proper clinical context to preclude the need for additional imaging (20–23).

The clinician evaluating the patient with a known or suspected diagnosis of pulmonary infection faces a diagnostic challenge because the infection may be caused by a variety of organisms that may present with similar clinical symptoms and signs and result in similar radiographic manifestations. Furthermore, the radiographic manifestations of a given organism may be variable depending on the immunologic status of the patient and the presence of pre- or coexisting lung disease.

The number of immunocompromised patients has increased considerably in the last three decades because of three main phenomena: The acquired immunodeficiency syndrome (AIDS) epidemic, advances in cancer chemotherapy, and expanding solid organ and hematopoietic stem cell transplantation. At the onset of the AIDS epidemic in the early and mid-1980s, there was 50% to 80% mortality for each episode of *Pneumocystis* pneumonia (PCP). Since routine prophylaxis was instituted in 1989, there has been a declining incidence of PCP in the AIDS population (24–26) and a decrease in mortality in mild to moderate cases (27). However, other infections including bacterial pneumonia, fungal infection, cytomegalovirus (CMV), *Mycobacterium Avium-intracellulare* complex (MAC), and tuberculosis remain a significant cause of morbidity and mortality in these patients (24–27). The role of imaging is to identify the presence, location, and extent of pulmonary abnormalities, the course and evolution of pneumonia, the presence of associated complications, and detection of additional or alternative diagnosis.

INTEGRATING CLINICAL AND IMAGING FINDINGS

The most useful imaging modalities for the evaluation of patients with known or suspected pulmonary infection are chest radiography and computed tomography (CT). Imaging examinations should always be interpreted with awareness of the clinical findings including duration of symptoms, presence of fever, cough, dyspnea,

and the presence or absence of leukocytosis (28). Knowledge of whether the patient has community-acquired or nosocomial pneumonia, as well as knowledge of the immune status of the patient, are most helpful in the differential diagnosis and determination of the most likely causative organisms (28, 29). Clinical information can greatly enhance the accuracy of the radiographic diagnosis. For example, the AIDS patient with an acute airspace process who has chills, fever, and purulent sputum probably has pyogenic rather than a *Pneumocystis* pneumonia. In the absence of clinical information, radiologists cannot reliably distinguish between pneumonia and other pulmonary processes (30). Unfortunately, the clinical data and radiographic findings often fail to lead to a definitive diagnosis of pneumonia because there is an extensive number of noninfectious processes associated with febrile pneumonitis, including drug-induced pulmonary disease, acute eosinophilic pneumonia, organizing pneumonia (bronchiolitis obliterans organizing pneumonia [BOOP]), and pulmonary vasculitis that may mimic pulmonary infection (31).

Distinction of localized pneumonia from other pulmonary processes cannot be made with certainty on radiologic grounds (31, 32). Localized pulmonary disease of a lobar or segmental distribution can be produced not only by pneumonia but also by obstructive pneumonitis, hemorrhage, or aspiration of sterile gastric contents. Diagnosis is equally difficult when pneumonia appears as a diffuse pulmonary abnormality. Extensive bilateral abnormalities may be due to bronchopneumonia or due to hydrostatic pulmonary edema, acute respiratory distress syndrome (ARDS), or diffuse pulmonary hemorrhage (33–35).

CHEST RADIOGRAPHY

The American Thoracic Society guidelines recommend that posteroanterior (PA) (and lateral when possible) chest radiographs be obtained whenever pneumonia is suspected in adults (36). The role of chest radiography is as a screening tool for the detection of abnormalities consistent with pneumonia and for monitoring response to therapy. Other roles for chest radiography include assessment of disease extent, detection of complications (i.e., cavitation, abscess formation, pneumothorax, and pleural effusion), detection of additional or alternative diagnoses and, in some cases, guiding invasive diagnostic procedures (see Fig. 1.1).

The most common radiographic manifestations of respiratory infection are foci of consolidation, ground-glass opacities, or reticulonodular opacities (see Fig. 1.2). Other less common radiographic findings include hilar and mediastinal lymphadenopathy, pleural effusion, cavitation, and chest wall invasion. These findings are not specific and may be seen in other conditions. Furthermore any given organism may result in a variety of different patterns of presentation. For example, *Pneumocystis* may result in bilateral ground-glass opacities or consolidation, or, less commonly, focal consolidation, nodules, miliary pattern, or reticulation (36). In up to 10% of patients with proved PCP the chest radiograph is normal (37).

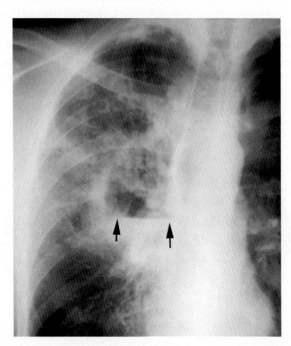

Figure 1.1 Lung abscess. Magnified view of a posteroanterior chest radiograph shows right upper lobe consolidation and a cavity. The cavity has irregular walls and contains an air-fluid level (*arrows*), findings characteristic of lung abscess. The patient was a 43-year-old alcoholic man with staphylococcal pneumonia and lung abscess.

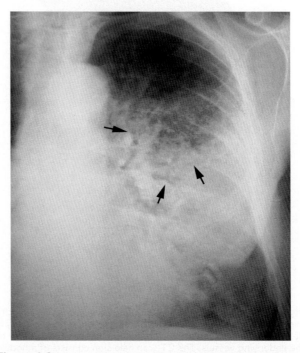

Figure 1.2 Lobar pneumonia. Magnified view of the left lung from a posteroanterior chest radiograph shows extensive left upper lobe consolidation. Air bronchograms (*arrows*) are seen within the consolidation.

COMPUTED TOMOGRAPHY

Computed tomography (CT) is a useful adjunct to conventional radiography in selected cases (30, 32, 38, 39). There is a large literature indicating that CT scan is a sensitive method capable of imaging the lung with excellent spatial resolution and providing anatomic detail similar to that seen by gross pathologic examination. Differences in tissue attenuation and parenchymal changes caused by an acute inflammatory process can be seen readily on CT scan (38, 39). CT scan can also be helpful in the detection, differential diagnosis, and management of patients with pulmonary complications.

Optimal assessment of the parenchyma is obtained with the use of high-resolution CT scan, which allows assessment of the pattern and distribution of abnormalities down to the level of the secondary pulmonary lobule (38). The findings of airspace disease, including airspace nodules, ground-glass opacities, consolidation, air bronchograms, and centrilobular or perilobular distribution, are seen better in CT scan than in conventional radiography (37, 38). Airspace nodules measure 6 to 10 mm in diameter and usually reflect the presence of peribronchiolar consolidation, and therefore are centrilobular in distribution. They are best appreciated in early disease and best seen at the edge of the pathologic process in which consolidation

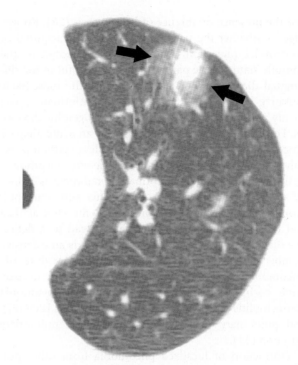

Figure 1.4 Computed tomography (CT) halo sign in angioinvasive aspergillosis. View of the left upper lobe from a high-resolution CT scan (1-mm collimation) shows a nodule surrounded by a halo of ground-glass attenuation ("halo sign") (*arrows*). The patient was a 33-year-old man with acute leukemia and severe neutropenia.

is incomplete. In some circumstances, nodules may be associated with a "halo" of ground-glass attenuation (see Fig. 1.3). In severely neutropenic patients this "halo" sign is highly suggestive of angioinvasive aspergillosis (40) (see Fig. 1.4). However, a similar appearance has been described in other conditions including infection by nontuberculous mycobacteria, *Mucorales*, *Candida*, herpes simplex virus, CMV, Wegener granulomatosis, Kaposi sarcoma, and hemorrhagic metastases (41).

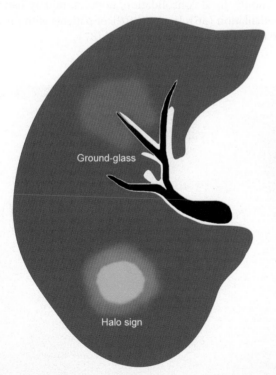

Ground-glass

Halo sign

Figure 1.3 Schematic representation of ground-glass opacity and computed tomography (CT) halo sign. Ground-glass opacity is defined as a hazy increase in attenuation without obscuration of the underlying vessels. The CT scan halo sign consists of a nodule or focal area of consolidation surrounded by a halo of ground-glass attenuation. This sign is seen in a variety of hemorrhagic, inflammatory, and neoplastic nodules (Courtesy of C. Isabela S. Silva, MD, PhD.)

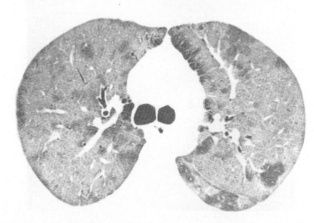

Figure 1.5 Pneumocystis pneumonia. High-resolution computed tomography (CT) image (1-mm collimation) shows extensive bilateral ground-glass opacities. Sparing of some of the secondary lobules results in a geographic appearance. The patient was a 36-year-old man with AIDS.

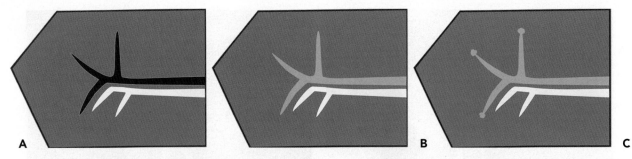

Figure 1.6 Schematic drawing of bronchiolitis and tree-in-bud pattern. The bronchioles and adjacent pulmonary artery are located near the center of the secondary lobule **(A)**. Inflammation of the bronchiolar wall and intraluminal exudate results in linear opacities when the bronchioles are imaged along their long axis or nodular opacities when imaged in cross section. The combination of centrilobular branching linear and nodular opacities is known as the *tree-in-bud* pattern **(B)**. Extension of the inflammatory process into the peribronchiolar parenchyma results in small peribronchiolar nodular opacities and a more prominent "tree-in-bud" pattern **(C)**. (Courtesy of Isabela S. Silva, MD, PhD.)

Ground-glass opacity is defined as hazy increased lung opacity that does not obscure the underlying vascular structures (Fig. 1.3). Ground-glass opacities are a common but nonspecific high-resolution CT scan finding that may result from a variety of interstitial and airspace diseases. Infections that typically present with bilateral ground-glass opacities are *Pneumocystis* and CMV pneumonia (see Fig. 1.5). In AIDS patients the presence of extensive bilateral ground-glass opacities is highly suggestive of PCP. In immunocompromised non-AIDS patients the differential diagnosis includes CMV pneumonia, drug-induced lung disease, pulmonary hemorrhage and organizing pneumonia (42).

A "tree-in-bud" pattern is a characteristic high-resolution CT scan manifestation of infectious bronchiolitis (see Fig. 1.6). It consists of centrilobular branching tubular and nodular structures and reflects the presence of bronchiolar inflammation and filling of the lumen by inflammatory material or mucus (43). This pattern may be seen in a variety of bacterial, mycobacterial, fungal, and viral infections (see Fig. 1.7) (43, 44).

Airspace consolidation, defined as a localized increase in lung attenuation that obscures the underlying vascular structures, may be seen in association with bacterial, fungal, and viral infections (see Fig. 1.8). Focal areas of consolidation secondary to infection in immunocompromised AIDS and non-AIDS patients are most commonly due to bacterial pneumonia (31). Fungal infection needs to be considered particularly in neutropenic patients with hematologic malignancies (42). Parenchymal disease in mycobacterial infection may also appear as patchy nodular areas of consolidation, with or without cavitation (45).

Although CT scan is not recommended for the initial evaluation of patients with pneumonia, it is a valuable adjunct to conventional radiography, being helpful in better characterizing complex pneumonias and in detecting complications (36) (see Fig. 1.9). CT scan is also indicated to rule out underlying lung disease such as lung cancer

Figure 1.7 "Tree-in-bud" pattern in infectious bronchiolitis. Cross-sectional high-resolution computed tomography (CT) (1-mm collimation) image obtained at the level of the lung bases shows centrilobular branching nodular and linear opacities resulting in a "tree-in-bud" appearance (*arrows*). The patient was a 20-year-old woman with recurrent respiratory infections.

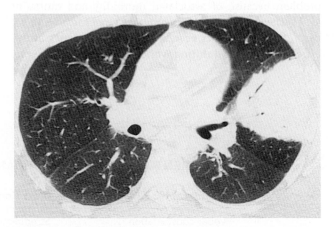

Figure 1.8 Focal consolidation in pneumococcal pneumonia. Computed tomography (CT) image (5-mm collimation) shows a focal area of homogeneous consolidation in the left upper lobe. Note the presence of air bronchograms within the consolidation. The patient was a 53-year-old man. Sputum culture produced a heavy growth of *Streptococcus pneumoniae*. (From Franquet T. Imaging of pneumonia: Trends and algorithms. *Eur Respir J.* 2001;18:196–208, with permission.)

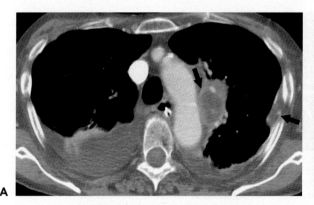
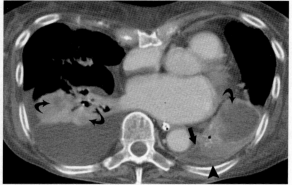

Figure 1.9 Pneumonia with abscess formation and empyema. **A:** Contrast-enhanced computed tomography (CT) image (5-mm collimation) at the level of the aortic arch shows bilateral pleural effusions. Note focal loculations of the left pleural effusion along the lateral chest wall and mediastinum (*straight arrows*) and thickening and enhancement of the visceral and mediastinal pleura suggestive of empyema. **B:** CT image at the level of the left atrium shows bilateral areas of consolidation and pleural effusions. Note focal areas of decreased attenuation (*curved arrows*) in the lower lobes, consistent with lung abscess. Also note thickening and enhancement of the left pleura (*straight arrow*) and increased density of the left extrapleural fat (*arrowhead*), consistent with empyema. The patient was a 88-year-old woman with *Enterococcus* pneumonia, bilateral lower lobe abscesses, and left empyema.

or bronchiectasis in patients with recurrent or nonresolving pneumonia. Several studies have shown that high-resolution CT scan is particularly helpful in the detection, differential diagnosis, and management of immunocompromised patients with pulmonary complications (36–39). These studies have also shown that CT scan may confirm the presence of pneumonia in patients with clinical symptoms and normal or questionable radiographic findings.

COMMUNITY-ACQUIRED PNEUMONIA

Community-acquired pneumonia is a major health care problem because of associated morbidity and mortality (1, 3). The overall rate of pneumonia ranges from 8 to 15 per 1,000 persons per year, with the highest rates at the extremes of age and during winter months (46). Between

485,000 and 1 million patients each year are hospitalized in the United States for treatment of community-acquired pneumonia. The costs of inpatient care exceed outpatient care by a factor of 15 to 20, and comprise most of the estimated $8.4 billion spent annually for care of patients with pneumonia (1, 3, 47, 48).

Hospital admission rates of pneumonia episodes vary from 22% to 51% of patients with community-acquired pneumonia (1). The mortality is higher in less-developed countries, as well as in young and elderly patients. Pulmonary opacities are usually evident on the radiograph within 12 hours of the onset of symptoms. Although radiographic findings do not allow a specific etiologic diagnosis, the radiograph may be helpful in narrowing down the differential diagnosis. In community-acquired pneumonia, diagnosis and disease management most frequently involve chest radiography and generally do not require the use of other imaging modalities (49).

TABLE 1.1
DIFFERENTIAL DIAGNOSIS OF COMMUNITY-ACQUIRED PNEUMONIA

Radiographic Findings	Most Common Organisms
Lobar consolidation	*Streptococcus pneumoniae, Klebsiella pneumoniae*
Round pneumonia	*S. pneumoniae*
Bronchopneumonia	*Staphylococcus aureus*, gram-negative bacilli, anaerobes, *S. pneumoniae*
Interstitial pneumonia	Virus, *Mycoplasma pneumoniae*
Cavity formation	*Mycobacterium tuberculosis, S. aureus*, gram-negative bacilli

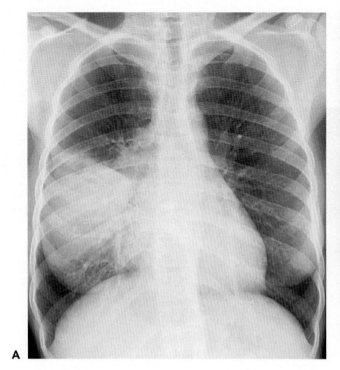
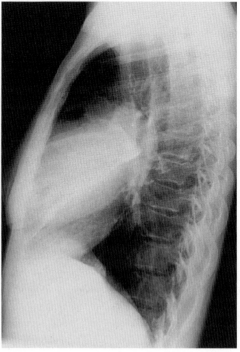

A   B

Figure 1.10 Lobar pneumonia due to *Streptococcus pneumoniae*. Posteroanterior **(A)** and lateral **(B)** chest radiographs show extensive right middle lobe consolidation. The patient was a 29-year-old woman with pneumococcal pneumonia.

The spectrum of causative organisms of community-acquired pneumonia includes gram-positive bacteria such as *S. pneumoniae* (*Pneumococcus*), *Haemophilus influenzae*, and *Staphylococcus aureus*, as well as atypical organisms such as *Mycoplasma pneumoniae*, *Chlamydia pneumoniae*, or *Legionella pneumophila* and viral agents such as influenza A virus and respiratory syncytial viruses (see Table 1.1). *S. pneumoniae* is by far the most common cause of complete lobar consolidation (50–52) (see Fig. 1.10). Other causative agents that produce complete lobar consolidation include *Klebsiella pneumoniae* and other gram-negative bacilli, *L. pneumophila*, *H. influenzae*, and occasionally *M. pneumoniae* (50–53).

A clinical diagnosis of pneumonia can usually be readily established on the basis of clinical signs and symptoms and the radiographic findings. In some cases, community-acquired pneumonia may be difficult to distinguish clinically and radiologically from other entities such as heart failure, pulmonary embolism, and aspiration pneumonia (20, 54).

Radiographically, lobar pneumonia typically appears initially in the lung periphery abutting against the pleura and spreads toward the core portions of the lung. Round pneumonia occurs more frequently in children than in adults and is most commonly caused by *S. pneumoniae* (55) (see Fig. 1.11). In children, active tuberculous and fungal infection also may present with nodular or mass-like opacities (55). Bacterial infections may produce multiple rounded pulmonary nodules or masses, with or without cavitation. This may occur from *Nocardia*, *Aspergillus*, *Legionella*, Q fever, or *M. tuberculosis* infection (55–57).

Bronchopneumonia, which is most commonly caused by *S. aureus* and *H. influenzae*, occurs when infectious organisms, deposited on the epithelium of the bronchi, produce acute bronchial inflammation with epithelial ulcerations and fibrinopurulent exudate formation. As a consequence, the inflammatory reaction rapidly spreads through the airway walls and into the contiguous pulmonary lobules. Radiographically, these inflammatory aggregates cause a typical pattern of multifocal unilateral or bilateral areas of consolidation (see Fig. 1.12). Abscess formation may occur particularly in bronchopneumonia due to *S. aureus* or anaerobes.

Interstitial and/or mixed interstitial and airspace opacities in community-acquired pneumonia are typically due to viruses or *M. pneumoniae* (see Fig. 1.13) (58–60). Up to 30% of all pneumonias in the general population are caused by *M. pneumoniae* (30). During infection, the initial damage is directed toward the mucosa of the bronchioles and later, the peribronchial tissue and interlobular septa become edematous and infiltrated with inflammatory cells.

HOSPITAL-ACQUIRED (NOSOCOMIAL) PNEUMONIA

Nosocomial pneumonia may be defined as one occurring after admission to the hospital, which was neither present

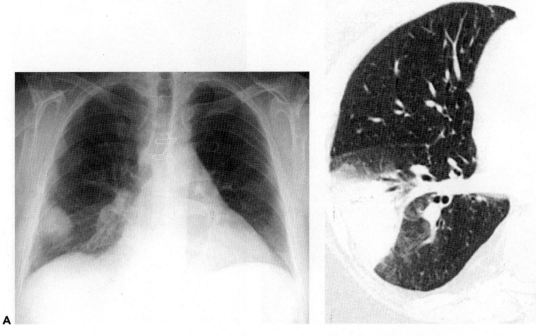

Figure 1.11 Round pneumonia. **A:** Anteroposterior chest radiograph shows a sharply defined rounded opacity in the right lower lung zone. **B:** Computed tomography (CT) image (5-mm collimation) demonstrates mass-like right lower lobe consolidation. The patient was a 58-year-old man with pneumonia due to *Streptococcus pneumoniae*.

nor in a period of incubation at the time of admission (47). Nosocomial pneumonia is the leading cause of death from hospital-acquired infections and an important public health problem. It occurs most commonly among intensive care unit (ICU) patients, predominately in individuals

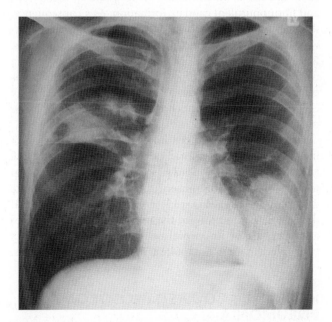

Figure 1.12 Bronchopneumonia. Chest radiograph shows areas of consolidation in the right upper and left lower lobes. The patient was a 23-year-old man with bronchopneumonia due to *Pseudomonas*.

requiring mechanical ventilation (61). The estimated prevalence of nosocomial pneumonia within the ICU setting ranges from 10% to 65%, with case fatality rates of 20% to 55% in most reported series (53,61,62). In patients with ARDS, as many as 55% have secondary pneumonia, and this complication may adversely affect survival (53).

The diagnosis of nosocomial pneumonia is difficult, and the criteria used for surveillance have been based on clinical findings of fever, cough, and the development of purulent sputum in combination with new or progressive opacities on chest radiography. When pneumonia arises in the hospitalized patient, aerobic gram-negative bacilli, particularly *P. aeruginosa* and *Enterobacter* sp., and *S. aureus*, are the major causative organisms (see Fig. 1.14) (63). Other common causes of nosocomial pneumonia are *H. Influenza, S. pneumoniae*, aspiration with anaerobes, *Legionella* sp., and viruses. Respiratory syncytial virus, influenza A and B, and parainfluenza are responsible for >70% of nosocomial viral diseases (63).

ASPIRATION PNEUMONIA

Aspiration pneumonia is particularly common in patients with decreased consciousness, chronic debilitating disease, and with oropharyngeal or airway instrumentation (e.g., patients on tube feeding or on mechanical ventilation). The aspirated material may include sterile gastric secretions, gastric content, or bacteria-laden oropharyngeal secretions

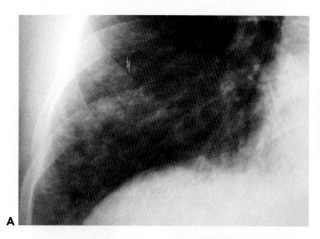
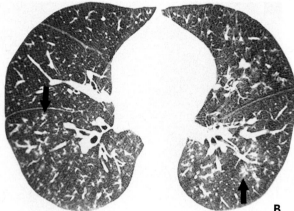

Figure 1.13 Acute bronchiolitis caused by *Mycoplasma pneumoniae*. **A:** Magnified view of the right lower lung zone from a posteroanterior chest radiograph shows a reticulonodular pattern. **B:** High-resolution computed tomography (CT) scan (1-mm collimation) at the level of the inferior pulmonary veins shows multiple bilateral centrilobular nodular and branching linear opacities ("tree-in-bud" pattern) (*arrows*) in both lower lobes. The patient was a previously healthy 24-year-old man. Immunofluorescent microscopy of sputum revealed *M. pneumoniae* organisms.

(see Fig. 1.15). Aspiration of infected oropharyngeal secretions is more common than generally appreciated. Most bacterial pneumonias result from aspiration of infected material from the oropharynx into the lower respiratory tract (54, 64, 65). Alcoholic patients and those with poor oral hygiene are prone to develop pulmonary infections after aspiration. Approximately 90% of infected aspiration pneumonias are caused by anaerobic organisms (66). In hospitalized patients who are colonized with highly virulent organisms, aspirations may overwhelm lung defenses, resulting in the development of pneumonia (1, 67). In the hospitalized patient, the stomach may become colonized

with gram-negative bacteria (67). In these patients, intubation and mechanical ventilation may increase the incidence and size of aspirations, with resultant increase in the development of pneumonia (64, 67). The location of pneumonia depends on the position of the patient when aspiration occurs.

The radiographic manifestations usually consist of bilateral patchy areas of consolidation involving mainly the dependent regions. Because aspiration typically occurs with the patient supine, the areas of consolidation tend to involve mainly the posterior and lateral basal segments of the lower lobes, superior segments of the lower lobes, and posterior segments of the upper lobes. The radiographic manifestations vary somewhat among the various species of gram-negative bacilli. *P. aeruginosa* infection typically results in patchy unilateral or bilateral areas of consolidation (bronchopneumonia); lobar consolidation is uncommon (67). Prolonged clinical course or large aspirations may result in severe necrotizing bronchopneumonia (see Fig. 1.16).

Patients with advanced periodontal disease are at particular risk for development of aspiration pneumonia (66). Radiographic findings include focal or patchy ill-defined areas of consolidation and progressive abscess formation. The opacities are usually unilateral but may involve both lungs.

A distinct form of infection is caused by *Actinomyces israelii*, a low-virulence anaerobic bacteria, that is normally found in the mouth of patients with poor oral hygiene (1). Aspiration of infected material results in a localized or segmental pneumonia, usually in the dependent portions of the lung. If untreated, actinomycosis may invade the chest wall, the mediastinum, or the diaphragm. Radiographically, the disease starts as a localized subsegmental or segmental consolidation. Over a period of weeks to months after the aspiration event, cavitation and pleural effusion (empyema) may occur.

Figure 1.14 Nosocomial pneumonia. Chest radiograph shows extensive asymmetric bilateral airspace consolidation and right pleural effusion. The patient was a 70-year-old man with chronic renal failure with methicillin-resistant *Staphylococcus aureus* (MRSA) nosocomial pneumonia.

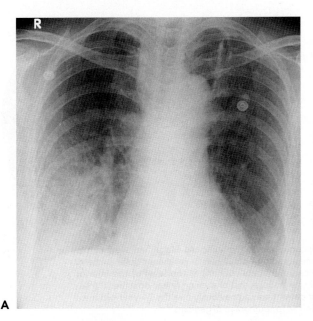

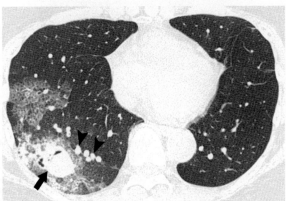

A

B

Figure 1.15 Aspiration pneumonia. **A:** Anteroposterior chest radiograph shows right lower lobe consolidation. Also noted is scarring and volume loss of the left upper lobe due to previous tuberculosis. **B:** High-resolution computed tomography (CT) image (1-mm collimation) demonstrates ground-glass opacities, small foci of consolidation, and abscess (*straight arrow*) in the right lower lobe. The apparent small nodular opacities (*arrowheads*) were shown on sequential images to represent bronchi filled with soft tissue. Bronchoscopy demonstrated filling of the right lower bronchi with aspirated vegetable material. The patient was a 69-year-old woman.

SEPTIC PULMONARY EMBOLISM

Septic pulmonary embolism generally presents with insidious onset of fever, cough, and pulmonary opacities (68). It is seen most commonly in patients with indwelling catheters and in IV drug users; less common causes include pelvic thrombophlebitis and suppurative processes in the head and neck (68). The radiographic manifestations usually consist of bilateral nodular opacities, which are frequently cavitated (see Fig. 1.17). The nodules may be circumscribed or poorly defined and may be associated with patchy areas of consolidation. CT scan demonstrates bilateral nodules most numerous in the peripheral lung regions and lower zones (see Fig. 1.18). The nodules are usually bilateral and may be well circumscribed or poorly defined; they frequently cavitate (68,69). Another common finding on CT scan is the presence of wedge-shaped pleural-based areas of consolidation that may be homogenous or heterogenous and that may cavitate.

PNEUMONIA IN THE IMMUNOCOMPROMISED HOST

Patients with impaired immune function are susceptible to a wide range of infections (see Table 1.2) (25–27). In the last three decades, the AIDS epidemic, advances in the treatment of cancer, organ transplantation, and immunosuppressive therapy have resulted in large numbers of patients with impaired immune system (70–73). Pneumonia is a major clinical problem in these patients. Mildly impaired host immunity, as it occurs in chronic debilitating illness, diabetes mellitus, malnutrition, alcoholism, advanced age, prolonged corticosteroid administration and chronic obstructive lung disease, also may predispose to pulmonary infection (74).

In AIDS patients, infectious causative agents include *Pneumocystis jiroveci* (formerly known as *P. carinii*), *M. tuberculosis*, and MAC, and many of the more common gram-positive and negative bacteria (24, 36, 37). The type and pattern of infection are influenced by the patient's immune status (75). Patients who have >200 CD4 cells per mm^3 are predisposed mainly to bronchial infections and bacterial pneumonia, whereas patients with fewer than 200 CD4 cells per mm^3 are predisposed to opportunistic infections such as *Pneumocystis* (28, 75). The classic radiologic manifestations of PCP consist of bilateral symmetric hazy ground-glass opacities (see Fig. 1.19). These may be diffuse or may involve mainly the perihilar regions, lower lung zones, or upper lung zones. Sparing of portions of lung may result in a characteristic geographic distribution. Advances in the prevention and treatment of PCP have been associated with an increased frequency of different radiographic presentations. A cystic form of PCP, associated with increased risk of spontaneous pneumothorax, has become more prevalent in AIDS patients receiving prophylaxis with aerosolized pentamidine and trimethoprim–sulfamethoxazole (76). Less common radiographic patterns of PCP include parenchymal consolidation, mass

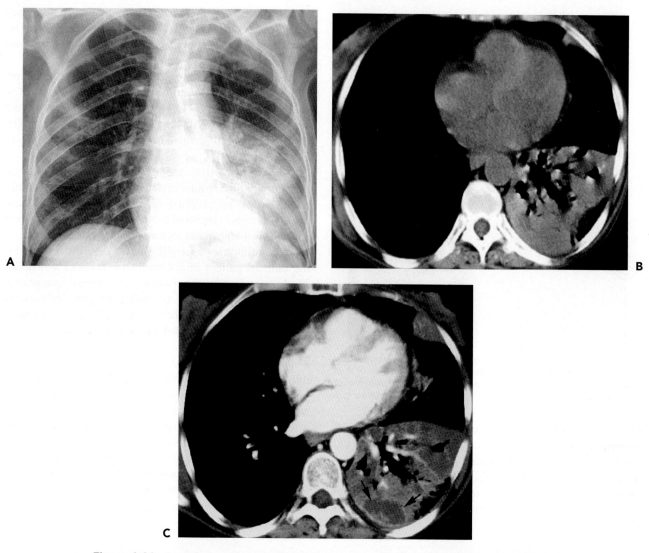

Figure 1.16 Aspiration pneumonia. **A:** Anteroposterior radiograph shows asymmetric bilateral consolidation in the right upper and left lower lung zones. Noncontrast **(B)** and contrast-enhanced **(C)** CT (5-mm collimation) images at the level of lung bases show focal consolidation in lingula and left lower lobe. Hypodense areas (arrows) within the left lower lobe consolidation due to abscess formation are better demonstrated after contrast administration. Also note opacified vessels within the consolidated lung parenchyma and the presence of gas due to necrosis. The patient was a 35-year-old woman. *Staphylococcus aureus* was cultured from a bronchoscopic specimen.

lesions, multiple pulmonary nodules, pleural effusion, and lymph node enlargement (31).

In recent years recurrent episodes of pyogenic airway disease and pneumonia, usually caused by *S. pneumoniae, H. influenzae, P. aeruginosa, Streptococcus viridans, and S. aureus,* have been increasingly recognized (31, 77, 78). The incidence of pyogenic bacterial pneumonia in AIDS patients is five times greater than in the HIV-negative population (31, 79). Recurrent bacterial infections have been included as an AIDS-defining illness in the revised Centers for Disease Control and Prevention (CDC) criteria (80).

After decades of decreasing incidence, tuberculosis has reemerged as an important infection, its increased incidence since the mid-1980s being related to the AIDS epidemic (81, 82). The incidence or tuberculosis in patients with AIDS is 200 to 500 times greater than that in the general population (82, 83). Also increased in these patients is the frequency of nontuberculous mycobacterial infections, most commonly MAC (84). Infection with *M. tuberculosis* or MAC can be acquired through primary infection or secondary to reactivation. The immunosuppressed state associated with AIDS predisposes patients with latent tuberculosis to reactivate their disease. Infection with MAC tends to occur in the late stage of AIDS, when immune deficiency is severe and the CD4 count is <50 cells per mm^3 (84, 85).

Airway involvement has been reported in 10% to 20% of all patients with pulmonary tuberculosis (43, 44, 77, 86). Endobronchial spread results in characteristic centrilobular

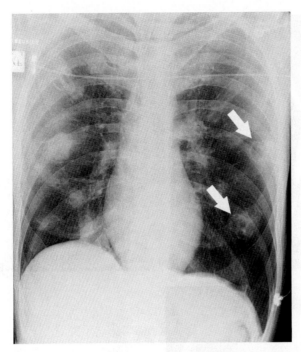

Figure 1.17 Septic pulmonary embolism. Anteroposterior chest radiograph shows bilateral nodules of various sizes, several of which are cavitated (*arrows*). The patient was a 41-year-old male intravenous drug user. Blood cultures grew *Staphylococcus aureus*.

branching linear and nodular opacities ("tree-in-bud" pattern) (44). The combination of patchy areas of consolidation in an upper lobe and a "tree-in-bud" pattern in other lobes is highly suggestive of tuberculosis with endobronchial spread of disease (43, 44). These findings are typically seen in AIDS patients with nearly normal

immune function. In patients with markedly depressed immunity the abnormalities typically resemble primary tuberculosis and consist of patchy areas of consolidation and mediastinal lymphadenopathy.

Approximately 20% of chest radiographs in patients with MAC-related pulmonary disease are normal (87). Radiologic appearances of MAC-related pulmonary disease are similar to tuberculosis, including multifocal patchy consolidation or ill-defined nodules that may cavitate (see Fig. 1.20) (88, 89).

Patients with AIDS are at risk of developing fungal infections, which require intact T-cell function for containment. Fungal pneumonias other than *Pneumocystis* have been increasingly reported in AIDS patients (90–92), most commonly *Cryptococcus* and *Aspergillus* (93). Obstructive bronchopulmonary aspergillosis is a descriptive term for the unusual pattern of a noninvasive form of aspergillosis characterized by the massive intraluminal overgrowth of *Aspergillus* sp., usually *Aspergillus fumigatus*, in patients with AIDS (94, 95). Other fungal infections including *Histoplasma capsulatum* and *Coccidioides immitis* are seen in endemic areas (96, 97).

Patients who have undergone solid organ transplantation have increased susceptibility to infection, the organism being influenced by the degree of immune compromise and time interval since transplantation (71–73). In the immediate postoperative period opportunistic infections are usually not encountered because there is a delay between the onset of the immunosuppressive therapy and the development of immune system dysfunction. Beyond 6 months after transplantation, infections characteristic of patients with defects in cell-mediated immunity (e.g.,

---

TABLE 1.2

DIFFERENTIAL DIAGNOSIS OF INFECTION IN THE IMMUNOCOMPROMISED HOST

Radiologic Findings	Cause of Immunocompromise	Most Common Organisms
Lobar consolidation	AIDS	*Streptoccocus pneumoniae*
	Mild immunosuppression (diabetes, alcoholism, COPD)	*S. pneumoniae*
		Semi-invasive aspergillosis
	Solid organ transplantation	Gram-negative bacilli
		Staphylococcus aureus
Ground-glass opacity	AIDS	*Pneumocystis*
	Hematopoietic stem cell transplantation	Cytomegalovirus
Bronchopneumonia	Neutropenia	*Aspergillus*, bacteria
Interstitial pneumonia	Hematopoietic stem cell transplantation	Cytomegalovirus
	AIDS	*Pneumocystis*
Multiple small nodules	Hematopoietic stem cell transplantation	Cytomegalovirus
	AIDS	Cryptococcosis
Multiple cavitary nodules	Drug addict	*S. aureus*
CT "halo sign"	Neutropenia	Angioinvasive aspergillosis
"Tree-in-bud"	AIDS (CD4 >200 cells/mm^3) Transplantation	Infectious bronchiolitis
		Endobronchial spread of tuberculosis
Lymphadenopathy	AIDS (CD4 <50 cells/mm^3)	*Mycobacterium tuberculosis*

COPD, chronic obstructive pulmonary disease; CT, computed tomography; AIDS, acquired immunodeficiency syndrome.

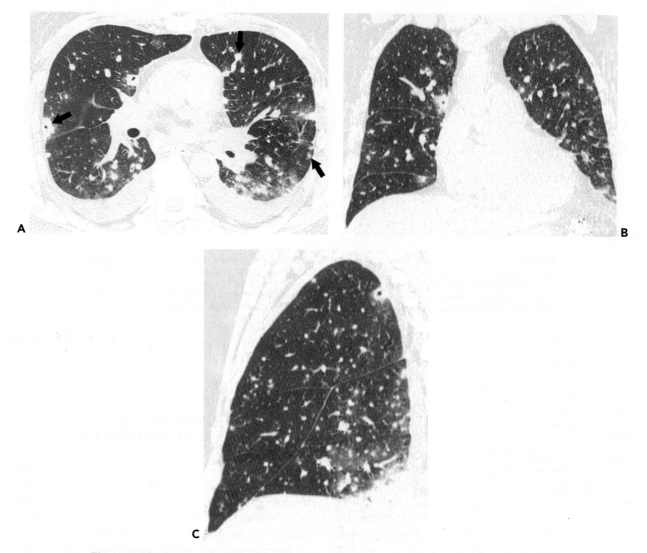

Figure 1.18 Septic pulmonary embolism. **A:** High-resolution computed tomography (CT) image (1-mm collimation) obtained on a multidetector scanner shows bilateral nodules with and without cavitation (*arrows*). The nodules involve mainly the subpleural lung regions. Also noted are small bilateral pleural effusions. Coronal **(B)** and sagittal **(C)** images confirm the predominant subpleural distribution of the nodules. The patient was a 43-year-old man.

Listeria, Nocardia, and fungi) may be a problem (see Fig. 1.21). The organisms that cause infections in recipients of solid organ transplants are different than those seen in hematopoietic stem cell (bone marrow) transplant recipients (98). Compared with hematopoietic stem cell transplant recipients, solid organ transplant patients are immunosuppressed for longer periods (often permanently). In addition, the spectrum of infection is largely determined by the type of transplantation.

Infection rates among lung transplant recipients, occurring in up to 50% of cases, are several fold higher than among recipients of other solid organs (71). During the first month after heart transplantation, gram-negative bacterial pneumonia is particularly common because of prolonged intubation, pulmonary edema, and effects of surgery on lung mechanics (58–60).

Gram-negative bacteria (*Enterobacter* and *Pseudomonas*) and *Staphylococcus* are also a common cause of infection in kidney and liver transplant recipients (71, 99). Bacterial pneumonias are less commonly lethal than viral and fungal infections (99, 100).

CMV is the most common viral pathogen encountered in solid organ and hematopoietic stem cell recipients (71, 98, 101, 102). Primary infection, the most serious, occurs in 50% to 100% of seronegative recipients who receive a graft from a seropositive donor (98). The high-resolution CT scan manifestations of CMV pneumonia usually consist of a variable combination of bilateral ground-glass opacities, areas of consolidation and small centrilobular nodular opacities (see Fig. 1.22).

As many as 40% of patients undergoing hematopoietic stem cell transplantation develop invasive fungal

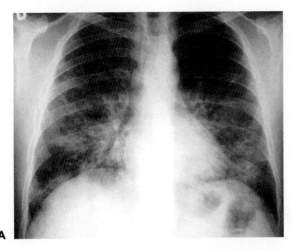

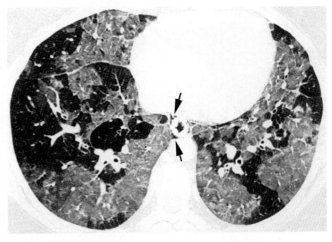

A

B

Figure 1.19 *Pneumocystis* pneumonia in AIDS. **A:** Posteroanterior chest radiograph shows bilateral hazy ground-glass opacities mainly in the middle and lower lung zones. **B:** High-resolution computed tomography (CT) (1-mm collimation) image at the level of lung bases shows bilateral ground-glass opacities interspersed by normal lung parenchyma. Also noted is pneumomediastinum (*arrows*). The patient was a 34-year-old man with acquired immunodeficiency syndrome (AIDS).

disease (103–105). The most common fungi responsible for acute lung disease are *A. fumigatus*, *Candida albicans*, and *Mucorales* (100, 106, 107). Angioinvasive aspergillosis occurs almost exclusively in immunocompromised patients with severe neutropenia (70, 104, 108, 109).

Mildly immunocompromised patients with chronic debilitating illness, diabetes mellitus, malnutrition, alcoholism, advanced age, prolonged corticosteroid administration, and chronic obstructive lung disease are prone to develop a distinct form of aspergillus infection called *semi-invasive* (chronic necrotizing) aspergillosis, characterized histologically by the presence of tissue necrosis and granulomatous inflammation similar to that seen in reactivation of tuberculosis (74). This form of *Aspergillus* infection may be associated with a variety of nonspecific

clinical symptoms such as cough, sputum production, and fever for >6 months (74).

INTERVENTIONAL PROCEDURES IN PATIENTS WITH PNEUMONIA

The only definitive way to reach a specific diagnosis is through demonstration of the organism, that is, by examination of stained smears of sputum, pleural fluid or other biologic material, by culture of respiratory secretions and blood, or by other interventional procedures such as transthoracic fine needle aspiration or biopsy under fluoroscopy or CT scan guidance.

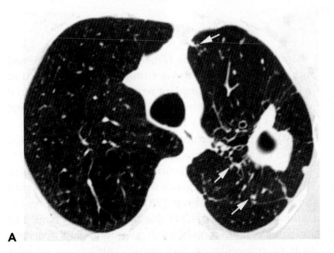

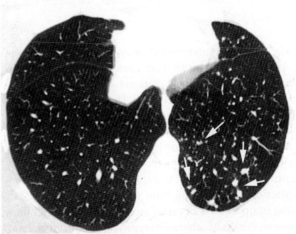

A

B

Figure 1.20 *Mycobacterium avium-intracellulare* complex infection in acquired immunodeficiency syndrome (AIDS). **A, B:** High-resolution computed tomography (CT) (1-mm collimation) images at the level of the upper lobes **(A)** and lung bases **(B)** show a cavitary mass at the left upper lobe and multiple small nodules (*arrows*) in the left upper and lower lobes. Also noted is evidence of emphysema. The patient was a 54-year-old man with AIDS.

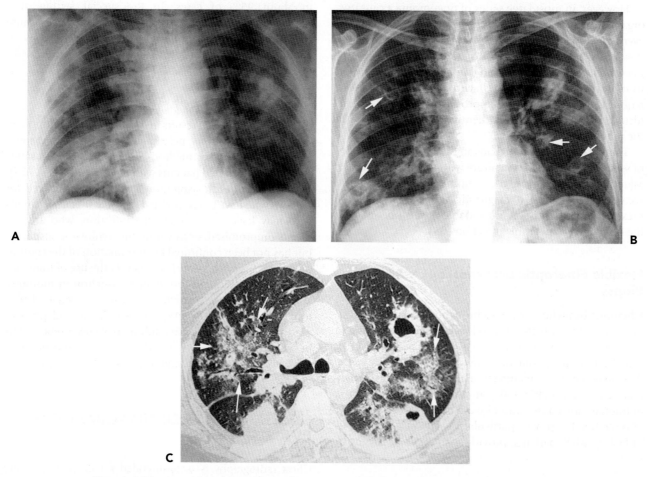

Figure 1.21 Nocardiosis in renal transplant recipient. **A:** Posteroanterior chest radiograph shows bilateral areas of consolidation. **B:** Radiograph 6 days later shows multifocal abscess formation and cavitation (*arrows*). **C:** High-resolution computed tomography (CT) (1-mm collimation) image at the level of the main bronchi shows multiple foci of consolidation, some of which are cavitated. Also noted are patchy bilateral ground-glass opacities with superimposed linear opacities ("crazy-paving" pattern) (*arrows*) and small right pleural effusion. The patient was a 45-year-old man.

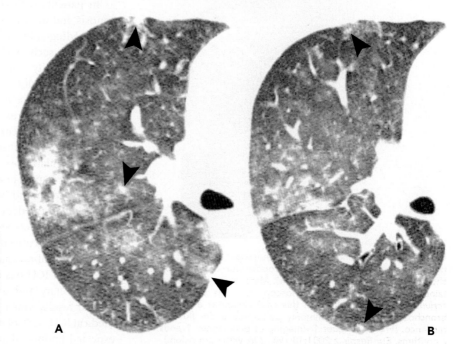

Figure 1.22 Cytomegalovirus pneumonia following hematopoietic stem cell transplant. Views of the right lung from high-resolution computed tomography (CT) (1-mm collimation) image at the level of the bronchus intermedius **(A)** and slightly more caudally **(B)**, show ground-glass opacities, small foci of consolidation, and a few small nodules (*arrowheads*). The patient was a 23-year-old man.

However, in most large series of pneumonia a causative organism cannot be identified in 33% to 45% of patients, even when extensive diagnostic tests are undertaken. Previously healthy patients who are mildly ill because of pneumonia are managed in an empiric fashion. However, in certain circumstances, the lack of a specific organism requires a more aggressive approach in order to obtain histopathologic and cultural identification of the cause of the pulmonary infection.

There has been much debate on the diagnostic accuracy of specimens obtained for culture with various techniques. Material obtained from the sputum or nasopharyngeal secretions have limited diagnostic value because of the presence of normal flora and variable results obtained for the detection of anaerobic infection (95).

Flexible Fiberoptic Bronchoscopy with Lung Biopsy

Fiberoptic bronchoscopy with bronchoalveolar lavage utilizing a protected brush is a well-established technique in the diagnosis of pulmonary infection (see Fig. 1.23) (110). Although this technique may play an important role in the diagnosis of pulmonary infection, the yield of bronchoalveolar lavage is variable and sometimes the diagnosis of a pulmonary infection cannot be established (95, 110, 111). This method has proved particularly useful in the diagnosis of PCP in AIDS patients, providing an etiologic diagnosis

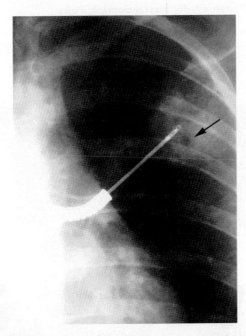

Figure 1.23 Imaging-guided bronchoscopy. Magnified view of the left upper lobe from an anteroposterior chest radiograph shows cavitary consolidation (*arrow*). Material for culture was obtained through fiberoptic bronchoscopy. Cultures grew *Mycobacterium tuberculosis*. Although this case illustrates a radiograph, bronchoscopy is most commonly performed under fluoroscopic guidance. (From Franquet T. Imaging of pneumonia: Trends and algorithms. *Eur Respir J*. 2001;18:196–208, with permission.)

in about 95% of cases. In the special setting of a serious pulmonary process and lack of definable cause with noninvasive methods, fiberoptic bronchoscopy in conjunction with transbronchial lung biopsy is indicated.

Transthoracic Needle Aspiration

Although the reported results in the diagnosis of pulmonary infection are variable, percutaneous fine needle aspiration is an alternative method used to identify causative pathogens in selected patients with pneumonia (112–115). Transthoracic needle aspiration should be considered for patients who have not responded to initial therapy, patients who may have nosocomial superinfection, who are immunocompromised, or in whom tuberculosis is suspected but has not been confirmed by examination of the sputum or gastric lavage. It is not clear whether the use of transthoracic needle aspiration results in a reduction in mortality and morbidity in a cost-effective fashion, compared to a less invasive approach (95). The specificity and positive predictive value of a positive culture have been reported to be as high as 100%, whereas the sensitivity and negative predictive value are 61% and 34% respectively (116).

STRATEGIES FOR OPTIMAL IMAGING EVALUATION

Chest radiography is recommended for all patients with suspected pulmonary infection in order to confirm or exclude the presence of pulmonary abnormalities. Although the chest radiograph does not allow a specific diagnosis it is helpful in narrowing the differential diagnosis and providing guidance for subsequent diagnostic studies.

In patients with community-acquired pneumonia, diagnosis and disease management most frequently rely on chest radiographs and seldom require further diagnostic procedures such as CT scan, bronchoscopy, or biopsy. In the community setting, >90% of patients who develop a segmental or lobar consolidation have either pneumococcal pneumonia or an atypical pneumonia caused by *Mycoplasma* or a virus. In nosocomial pulmonary infection, patchy bronchopneumonia is the most common finding and most likely is caused by one of the gram-negative organisms, particularly *Pseudomonas* or *Klebsiella*. In this particular setting, aspiration pneumonia is always an alternative diagnosis and should be suspected if pneumonia is present bilaterally in the dependent portions of the lungs (20). In ICU patients, there are few studies regarding the accuracy and efficacy of conventional chest radiography. The overall incidence of abnormalities found on chest radiographs in the medical ICU has been reported to be as high as 57% in pulmonary and unstable cardiac patients (117, 118). Similar results were obtained in a study of patients in the medical ICU; 43% of routine chest radiographs showed unexpected findings that influenced therapy (118). CT scan

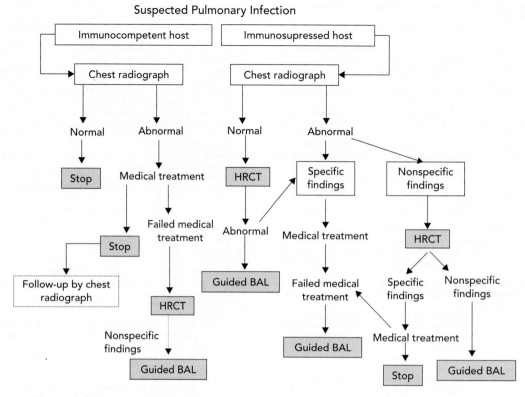

Figure 1.24 Algorithm for evaluation of patients suspected of having pulmonary infection. HRCT, high-resolution computed tomography; BAL, bronchoalveolar lavage.

and invasive diagnostic procedures should be reserved only for complicated cases.

Conversely, management of immunocompromised patients is challenging and difficult because of the diversity of causative organisms. In this group of patients, high-resolution CT scan and invasive procedures are commonly required. High-resolution CT scan can be useful in patients who have respiratory symptoms but normal or questionable radiographic findings, depicting abnormalities not evident on the radiograph and complications and concurrent parenchymal, mediastinal or pleural disease. In addition, high-resolution CT scan is helpful in differentiating infectious from noninfectious acute parenchymal lung disease (39). Specific diagnosis may be made by specimens obtained from bronchoalveolar lavage, bronchial and transbronchial biopsy, or needle aspiration. Under these circumstances, CT scan is useful as a road map toward the region most likely to yield the diagnosis. The algorithm for evaluation of patients suspected of having pulmonary infection is shown in Figure 1.24.

REFERENCES

1. Niederman MS, McCombs JS, Unger AN, et al. The cost of treating community-acquired pneumonia. *Clin Ther*. 1998;20:820–837.
2. Vincent JL, Bihari DJ, Suter PM, et al. The prevalence of nosocomial infection in intensive care units in Europe. Results of the European Prevalence of Infection in Intensive Care (EPIC) Study. EPIC International Advisory Committee. *JAMA*. 1995;274:639–644.
3. Garibaldi RA. Epidemiology of community-acquired respiratory tract infections in adults. Incidence, etiology, and impact. *Am J Med*. 1985; 78:32–37.
4. Bouza E, Munoz P. Introduction: Infections caused by emerging resistant pathogens. *Clin Microbiol Infec*. 2005;11:4.
5. Schwartz DA, Bryan RT, Hughes JM. Pathology and emerging infections–quo vadimus? *Am J Pathol*. 1995;147:1525–1533.
6. Cheney PR. Update on emerging infections from the Centers for Disease Control and Prevention. Hantavirus pulmonary syndrome–Colorado and New Mexico, 1998. *Ann Emerg Med*. 1999;33:121–123.
7. Hammel JM, Chiang WK. Update on emerging infections: News from the Centers for Disease Control and Prevention. Outbreaks of avian influenza A (H5N1) in Asia and interim recommendations for evaluation and reporting of suspected cases–United States, 2004. *Ann Emerg Med*. 2005;45:88–92.
8. Cameron PA, Rainer TH. Update on emerging infections: News from the Centers for Disease Control and Prevention. Update: Outbreak of severe acute respiratory syndrome–worldwide, 2003. *Ann Emerg Med*. 2003;42:110–112.
9. Franquet T, Rodriguez S, Martino R, et al. Human metapneumovirus infection in hematopoietic stem cell transplant recipients: High-resolution computed tomography findings. *J Comput Assist Tomo*. 2005;29:223–227.
10. Hamelin ME, Abed Y, Boivin G. Human metapneumovirus: A new player among respiratory viruses. *Clin Infect Dis*. 2004;38:983–990.
11. Madhi SA, Ludewick H, Abed Y, et al. Human metapneumovirus-associated lower respiratory tract infections among hospitalized human immunodeficiency virus type 1 (HIV-1)-infected and HIV-1-uninfected African infants. *Clin Infect Dis*. 2003;37:1705–1710.
12. Gordon SB, Read RC. Macrophage defences against respiratory tract infections. *Br Med Bull*. 2002;61:45–61.
13. Sibille Y, Reynolds HY. Macrophages and polymorphonuclear neutrophils in lung defense and injury. *Am Rev Respir Dis*. 1990;141:471–501.
14. Aderem A, Ulevitch RJ. Toll-like receptors in the induction of the innate immune response. *Nature*. 2000;406:782–787.
15. Janeway CA Jr, Medzhitov R. Innate immune recognition. *Annu Rev Immunol*. 2002;20:197–216.
16. Happel KI, Bagby GJ, Nelson S. Host defense and bacterial pneumonia. *Semin Respir Crit Care Med*. 2004;25:43–52.
17. Saitz R, Ghali WA, Moskowitz MA. The impact of alcohol-related diagnoses on pneumonia outcomes. *Arch Intern Med*. 1997;157:1446–1452.
18. Schmidt W, De Lint J. Causes of death of alcoholics. *Q J Stud Alcohol*. 1972;33:171–185.
19. Conces DJ Jr. Pulmonary infections in immunocompromised patients who do not have acquired immunodeficiency syndrome: A systematic approach. *J Thorac Imaging*. 1998;13:234–246.

20. Franquet T. Imaging of pneumonia: Trends and algorithms. *Eur Respir J.* 2001;18:196–208.

21. Gharib AM, Stern EJ. Radiology of pneumonia. *Med Clin N Am.* 2001; 85:1461–1491.

22. Tarver RD, Teague SD, Heitkamp DE, et al. Radiology of community-acquired pneumonia. *Radiol Clin N Am.* 2005;43:497–512,viii.

23. Vilar J, Domingo ML, Soto C, et al. Radiology of bacterial pneumonia. *Eur J Radiol.* 2004;51:102–113.

24. Moe AA, Hardy WD. Pneumocystis carinii infection in the HIV-seropositive patient. *Infect Dis Clin N Am.* 1994;8:331–364.

25. Murray JF, Mills J. Pulmonary infectious complications of human immunodeficiency virus infection. Part II. *Am Rev Respir Dis.* 1990;141:1582–1598.

26. Murray JF, Mills J. Pulmonary infectious complications of human immunodeficiency virus infection. Part I. *Am Rev Respir Dis.* 1990;141:1356–1372.

27. Lyon R, Haque AK, Asmuth DM, et al. Changing patterns of infections in patients with AIDS: A study of 279 autopsies of prison inmates and nonincarcerated patients at a university hospital in eastern Texas, 1984–1993. *Clin Infect Dis.* 1996;23:241–247.

28. Shah RM, Kaji AV, Ostrum BJ, et al. Interpretation of chest radiographs in AIDS patients: Usefulness of CD4 lymphocyte counts. *Radiographics.* 1997;17:47–58, discussion 59–61.

29. Hanson DL, Chu SY, Farizo KM, et al. Distribution of CD4+ T lymphocytes at diagnosis of acquired immunodeficiency syndrome-defining and other human immunodeficiency virus-related illnesses. The Adult and Adolescent Spectrum of HIV Disease Project Group. *Arch Intern Med.* 1995;155:1537–1542.

30. Primack SL, Müller NL. High-resolution computed tomography in acute diffuse lung disease in the immunocompromised patient. *Radiol Clin N Am.* 1994;32:731–744.

31. Boiselle PM, Tocino I, Hooley RJ, et al. Chest radiograph interpretation of Pneumocystis carinii pneumonia, bacterial pneumonia, and pulmonary tuberculosis in HIV-positive patients: Accuracy, distinguishing features, and mimics. *J Thorac Imag.* 1997;12:47–53.

32. Janzen DL, Padley SP, Adler BD, et al. Acute pulmonary complications in immunocompromised non-AIDS patients: Comparison of diagnostic accuracy of CT and chest radiography. *Clin Radiol.* 1993;47:159–165.

33. Chastre J, Trouillet JL, Vuagnat A, et al. Nosocomial pneumonia in patients with acute respiratory distress syndrome. *Am J Resp Crit Care Med.* 1998;157:1165–1172.

34. Niederman MS, Fein AM. Sepsis syndrome, the adult respiratory distress syndrome, and nosocomial pneumonia. A common clinical sequence. *Clin Chest Med.* 1990;11:633–656.

35. Seidenfeld JJ, Pohl DF, Bell RC, et al. Incidence, site, and outcome of infections in patients with the adult respiratory distress syndrome. *Am Rev Respir Dis.* 1986;134:12–16.

36. Boiselle PM, Crans CA Jr, Kaplan MA. The changing face of Pneumocystis carinii pneumonia in AIDS patients. *Am J Roentgenol.* 1999;172:1301–1309.

37. Gruden JF, Huang L, Turner J, et al. High-resolution CT in the evaluation of clinically suspected Pneumocystis carinii pneumonia in AIDS patients with normal, equivocal, or nonspecific radiographic findings. *Am J Roentgenol.* 1997;169:967–975.

38. Brown MJ, Miller RR, Müller NL. Acute lung disease in the immunocompromised host: CT and pathologic examination findings. *Radiology.* 1994;190:247–254.

39. Tomiyama N, Müller NL, Johkoh T, et al. Acute parenchymal lung disease in immunocompetent patients: Diagnostic accuracy of high-resolution CT. *Am J Roentgenol.* 2000;174:1745–1750.

40. Kuhlman JE, Fishman EK, Siegelman SS. Invasive pulmonary aspergillosis in acute leukemia: Characteristic findings on CT, the CT halo sign, and the role of CT in early diagnosis. *Radiology.* 1985;157:611–614.

41. Primack SL, Hartman TE, Lee KS, et al. Pulmonary nodules and the CT halo sign. *Radiology.* 1994;190:513–515.

42. Worthy SA, Flint JD, Müller NL. Pulmonary complications after bone marrow transplantation: High-resolution CT and pathologic findings. *Radiographics.* 1997;17:1359–1371.

43. Im JG, Itoh H, Lee KS, et al. CT-pathology correlation of pulmonary tuberculosis. *Crit Rev Diagn Imag.* 1995;36:227–285.

44. Aquino SL, Gamsu G, Webb WR, et al. Tree-in-bud pattern: Frequency and significance on thin section CT. *J Comput Assist Tomo.* 1996;20:594–599.

45. Primack SL, Logan PM, Hartman TE, et al. Pulmonary tuberculosis and Mycobacterium avium-intracellulare: A comparison of CT findings. *Radiology.* 1995;194:413–417.

46. Niederman MS, Bass JB Jr., Campbell GD, et al. Guidelines for the initial management of adults with community-acquired pneumonia: Diagnosis, assessment of severity, and initial antimicrobial therapy. American Thoracic Society. Medical Section of the American Lung Association. *Am Rev Respir Dis.* 1993;148:1418–1426.

47. Finch RG, Woodhead MA. Practical considerations and guidelines for the management of community-acquired pneumonia. *Drugs.* 1998;55:31–45.

48. Jokinen C, Heiskanen L, Juvonen H, et al. Incidence of community-acquired pneumonia in the population of four municipalities in eastern Finland. *Am J Epidemiol.* 1993;137:977–988.

49. Tanaka N, Matsumoto T, Kuramitsu T, et al. High resolution CT findings in community-acquired pneumonia. *J Comput Assist Tomo.* 1996;20:600–608.

50. Cameron DC, Borthwick RN, Philp T. The radiographic patterns of acute mycoplasma pneumonitis. *Clin Radiol.* 1977;28:173–180.

51. Dietrich PA, Johnson RD, Fairbank JT, et al. The chest radiograph in legionnaires' disease. *Radiology.* 1978;127:577–582.

52. Kantor HG. The many radiologic facies of pneumococcal pneumonia. *Am J Roentgenol.* 1981;137:1213–1220.

53. American Thoracic Society. Hospital-acquired pneumonia in adults: Diagnosis, assessment of severity, initial antimicrobial therapy, and preventive strategies. A consensus statement, American Thoracic Society, November 1995. *Am J Resp Crit Care Med.* 1996;153:1711–1725.

54. Franquet T, Gimenez A, Roson N, et al. Aspiration diseases: Findings, pitfalls, and differential diagnosis. *Radiographics.* 2000;20:673–685.

55. Eggli KD, Newman B. Nodules, masses, and pseudomasses in the pediatric lung. *Radiol Clin N Am.* 1993;31:651–666.

56. Kwong JS, Müller NL, Godwin JD, et al. Thoracic actinomycosis: CT findings in eight patients. *Radiology.* 1992;183:189–192.

57. Quagliano PV, Das Narla L. Legionella pneumonia causing multiple cavitating pulmonary nodules in a 7-month-old infant. *Am J Roentgenol.* 1993;161:367–368.

58. Ettinger NA, Trulock EP. Pulmonary considerations of organ transplantation. Part I. *Am Rev Respir Dis.* 1991;143:1386–1405.

59. Ettinger NA, Trulock EP. Pulmonary considerations of organ transplantation. Part 3. *Am Rev Respir Dis.* 1991;144:433–451.

60. Ettinger NA, Trulock EP. Pulmonary considerations of organ transplantation. Part 2. *Am Rev Respir Dis.* 1991;144:213–223.

61. Ibrahim EH, Ward S, Sherman G, et al. A comparative analysis of patients with early-onset vs late-onset nosocomial pneumonia in the ICU setting. *Chest.* 2000;117:1434–1442.

62. Kollef MH. The prevention of ventilator-associated pneumonia. *N Engl J Med.* 1999;340:627–634.

63. Taylor GD, Buchanan-Chell M, Kirkland T, et al. Bacteremic nosocomial pneumonia. A 7-year experience in one institution. *Chest.* 1995;108:786–788.

64. DePaso WJ. Aspiration pneumonia. *Clin Chest Med.* 1991;12:269–284.

65. Marom EM, McAdams HP, Erasmus JJ, et al. The many faces of pulmonary aspiration. *Am J Roentgenol.* 1999;172:121–128.

66. Bartlett JG, Finegold SM. Anaerobic infections of the lung and pleural space. *Am Rev Respir Dis.* 1974;110:56–77.

67. Unger JD, Rose HD, Unger GF. Gram-negative pneumonia. *Radiology.* 1973;107:283–291.

68. Cook RJ, Ashton RW, Aughenbaugh GL, et al. Septic pulmonary embolism: Presenting features and clinical course of 14 patients. *Chest.* 2005;128:162–166.

69. Iwasaki Y, Nagata K, Nakanishi M, et al. Spiral CT findings in septic pulmonary emboli. *Eur J Radiol.* 2001;37:190–194.

70. Cunningham I. Pulmonary infections after bone marrow transplant. *Semin Respir Infect.* 1992;7:132–138.

71. Fishman JA, Rubin RH. Infection in organ-transplant recipients. *N Engl J Med.* 1998;338:1741–1751.

72. Herman SJ. Radiologic assessment after lung transplantation. *Radiol Clin N Am.* 1994;32:663–678.

73. Maurer JR, Tullis DE, Grossman RF, et al. Infectious complications following isolated lung transplantation. *Chest.* 1992;101:1056–1059.

74. Franquet T, Müller NL, Gimenez A, et al. Semiinvasive pulmonary aspergillosis in chronic obstructive pulmonary disease: Radiologic and pathologic findings in nine patients. *Am J Roentgenol.* 2000;174:51–56.

75. Haramati LB, Jenny-Avital ER, Alterman DD. Effect of HIV status on chest radiographic and CT findings in patients with tuberculosis. *Clin Radiol.* 1997;52:31–35.

76. Chow C, Templeton PA, White CS. Lung cysts associated with Pneumocystis carinii pneumonia: Radiographic characteristics, natural history, and complications. *Am J Roentgenol.* 1993;161:527–531.

77. McGuinness G. Changing trends in the pulmonary manifestations of AIDS. *Radiol Clin N Am.* 1997;35:1029–1082.

78. Tamm M, Traenkle P, Grilli B, et al. Pulmonary cytomegalovirus infection in immunocompromised patients. *Chest.* 2001;119:838–843.

79. Padley SP, King LJ. Computed tomography of the thorax in HIV disease. *Eur Radiol.* 1999;9:1556–1569.

80. Centers for Disease Control (CDC). Proceedings of the 1992 international symposium on public health surveillance. Atlanta, Georgia, April 22–24, 1992. *MMWR Morb Mortal Wkly Rep.* 1992;41(Suppl):1–218.

81. Aronchick JM. Pulmonary infections in cancer and bone marrow transplant patients. *Semin Roentgenol.* 2000;35:140–151.

82. Leung AN. Pulmonary tuberculosis: The essentials. *Radiology.* 1999;210: 307–322.

83. Logan PM, Finnegan MM. Pulmonary complications in AIDS: CT appearances. *Clin Radiol.* 1998;53:567–573.

84. Fishman JE, Schwartz DS, Sais GJ. Mycobacterium kansasii pulmonary infection in patients with AIDS: Spectrum of chest radiographic findings. *Radiology.* 1997;204:171–175.

85. MacGregor RR. Tuberculosis: From history to current management. *Semin Roentgenol.* 1993;28:101–108.

86. Im JG, Itoh H, Shim YS, et al. Pulmonary tuberculosis: CT findings–early active disease and sequential change with antituberculous therapy. *Radiology.* 1993;186:653–660.

87. Marinelli DL, Albelda SM, Williams TM, et al. Nontuberculous mycobacterial infection in AIDS: Clinical, pathologic, and radiographic features. *Radiology.* 1986;160:77–82.
88. Erasmus JJ, McAdams HP, Farrell MA, et al. Pulmonary nontuberculous mycobacterial infection: Radiologic manifestations. *Radiographics.* 1999;19:1487–1505.
89. Miller WT Jr. Spectrum of pulmonary nontuberculous mycobacterial infection. *Radiology.* 1994;191:343–350.
90. Stansell JD. Pulmonary fungal infections in HIV-infected persons. *Semin Respir Infect.* 1993;8:116–123.
91. Stansell JD. Fungal disease in HIV-infected persons: Cryptococcosis, histoplasmosis, and coccidioidomycosis. *J Thorac Imag.* 1991;6:28–35.
92. Stansell JD, Osmond DH, Charlebois E, et al. Predictors of Pneumocystis carinii pneumonia in HIV-infected persons. Pulmonary Complications of HIV Infection Study Group. *Am J Resp Crit Care Med.* 1997;155:60–66.
93. Sider L, Westcott MA. Pulmonary manifestations of cryptococcosis in patients with AIDS: CT features. *J Thorac Imag.* 1994;9:78–84.
94. Miller WT Jr, Sais GJ, Frank I, et al. Pulmonary aspergillosis in patients with AIDS. Clinical and radiographic correlations. *Chest.* 1994;105:37–44.
95. Sanchez-Nieto JM, Torres A, Garcia-Cordoba F, et al. Impact of invasive and noninvasive quantitative culture sampling on outcome of ventilator-associated pneumonia: A pilot study. *Am J Resp Crit Care Med.* 1998;157:371–376.
96. Sarosi GA, Johnson PC. Progressive disseminated histoplasmosis in the acquired immunodeficiency syndrome: A model for disseminated disease. *Semin Respir Infect.* 1990;5:146–150.
97. Sarosi GA, Johnson PC. Disseminated histoplasmosis in patients infected with human immunodeficiency virus. *Clin Infect Dis.* 1992;14(Suppl 1):S60–S67.
98. Kotloff RM, Ahya VN, Crawford SW. Pulmonary complications of solid organ and hematopoietic stem cell transplantation. *Am J Resp Crit Care Med.* 2004;170:22–48.
99. Fishman JE, Rabkin JM. Thoracic radiology in kidney and liver transplantation. *J Thorac Imag.* 2002;17:122–131.
100. Bag R. Fungal pneumonias in transplant recipients. *Curr Opin Pulm Med.* 2003;9:193–198.
101. Kang EY Jr, Patz EF, Müller NL. Cytomegalovirus pneumonia in transplant patients: CT findings. *J Comput Assist Tomo.* 1996;20:295–299.
102. Nakhleh RE, Bolman RM 3rd, Henke CA, et al. Lung transplant pathology. A comparative study of pulmonary acute rejection and cytomegaloviral infection. *Am J Surg Pathol.* 1991;15:1197–1201.
103. Paterson DL, Singh N. Invasive aspergillosis in transplant recipients. *Medicine.* 1999;78:123–138.
104. Denning DW. Invasive aspergillosis. *Clin Infect Dis.* 1998;26:781–803, quiz 804–785.
105. Sable CA, Donowitz GR. Infections in bone marrow transplant recipients. *Clin Infect Dis.* 1994;18:273–281, quiz 282–274.
106. Heussel CP, Kauczor HU, Ullmann AJ. Pneumonia in neutropenic patients. *Eur Radiol.* 2004;14:256–271.
107. Franquet T, Müller NL, Lee KS, et al. Pulmonary candidiasis after hematopoietic stem cell transplantation: Thin-section CT findings. *Radiology.* 2005;236:332–337.
108. Kuhlman JE, Fishman EK, Burch PA, et al. CT of invasive pulmonary aspergillosis. *Am J Roentgenol.* 1988;150:1015–1020.
109. Leung AN, Gosselin MV, Napper CH, et al. Pulmonary infections after bone marrow transplantation: Clinical and radiographic findings. *Radiology.* 1999;210:699–710.
110. Jolis R, Castella J, Puzo C, et al. Diagnostic value of protected BAL in diagnosing pulmonary infections in immunocompromised patients. *Chest.* 1996;109:601–607.
111. Castellino RA, Blank N. Etiologic diagnosis of focal pulmonary infection in immunocompromised patients by fluoroscopically guided percutaneous needle aspiration. *Radiology.* 1979;132:563–567.
112. Haverkos HW, Dowling JN, Pasculle AW, et al. Diagnosis of pneumonitis in immunocompromised patients by open lung biopsy. *Cancer.* 1983;52:1093–1097.
113. Hwang SS, Kim HH, Park SH, et al. The value of CT-guided percutaneous needle aspiration in immunocompromised patients with suspected pulmonary infection. *Am J Roentgenol.* 2000;175:235–238.
114. Johnston WW. Percutaneous fine needle aspiration biopsy of the lung. A study of 1,015 patients. *Acta Cytol.* 1984;28:218–224.
115. Perlmutt LM, Johnston WW, Dunnick NR. Percutaneous transthoracic needle aspiration: A review. *Am J Roentgenol.* 1989;152:451–455.
116. Dorca J, Manresa F, Esteban L, et al. Efficacy, safety, and therapeutic relevance of transthoracic aspiration with ultrathin needle in nonventilated nosocomial pneumonia. *Am J Resp Crit Care Med.* 1995;151:1491–1496.
117. Strain DS, Kinasewitz GT, Vereen LE, et al. Value of routine daily chest x-rays in the medical intensive care unit. *Crit Care Med.* 1985;13:534–536.
118. Greenbaum DM, Marschall KE. The value of routine daily chest x-rays in intubated patients in the medical intensive care unit. *Crit Care Med.* 1982;10:29–30.

Bacterial Pneumonia

Pneumonia is a common cause of morbidity and mortality. In the United States there are an estimated 4 million cases of community-acquired pneumonia annually, resulting in approximately 600,000 hospitalizations (1, 2). A meta-analysis of the prognosis and outcome of 33,148 patients who had community-acquired pneumonia showed an overall mortality rate of approximately 14% (3). The mortality varies considerably in specific groups of patients. The mortality rate in patients not requiring hospitalization is approximately 0.1% (1). However, reported mortality rates in patients who have pneumonia of sufficient severity to require hospitalization range from 4% to almost 40% (3–5). Pneumonia develops in approximately 0.5% to 1.0% of hospitalized patients (nosocomial pneumonia) (6). Mortality in such patients is higher, being estimated at approximately 30% (7, 8). In one prospective multicenter study of 2,402 patients in intensive care units (ICUs), 163 (6.8%) of the patients developed nosocomial pneumonia; 75.5% ($n = 123$) of all patients with nosocomial pneumonia were on assisted ventilation (9). One hundred sixty three patients, who were admitted to the ICU during the same period but had no evidence of pneumonia, were used as a control group. For the patients with pneumonia the mean length of stay in the ICU and hospital was significantly longer than in controls, and their mortality five times greater (9).

A diagnosis of pneumonia is usually made on the basis of the clinical history and radiographic findings. Clinical symptoms include fever, cough, and purulent sputum (10). It is important to note, however, that the signs and symptoms of pneumonia may be milder or even absent in the elderly (11). The etiology of pneumonia can be established from sputum, bronchoscopy specimens, blood culture, or fine-needle aspiration. Identification of the bacterial etiology from sputum specimens requires appropriate measures to ensure collection of good quality sputum specimen by avoiding contamination by upper airway flora (11). Unless these measures are taken, sputum Gram stain and culture have low sensitivity and specificity in the diagnosis (12). When purulent sputum uncontaminated by upper airway secretions can be obtained prior to the institution of antibiotics, sputum examination can have a sensitivity of up to 85% in the diagnosis of bacteremic pneumococcal pneumonia (13). Protected brush specimens obtained at bronchoscopy have a sensitivity of 50% to 80% (14, 15) and a specificity >80% (14, 16). Bronchoalveolar lavage (BAL), including protected lavage with quantitative culture of distal lung secretions, has a sensitivity and specificity similar to that of protected brush specimens (17, 18). Blood cultures have poor sensitivity but a high specificity and are of prognostic importance in patients with pneumonia (11). Percutaneous fine-needle aspiration of the lung has only occasionally been used for the identification of pathogens in patients with pneumonia (19–21). In most cases when noninvasive techniques, such as sputum examination and cultures, are nondiagnostic, the patients are treated empirically. However, fine-needle biopsy may be useful in selected patients with aggressive nosocomial infections and in immunosuppressed patients (22, 23). Positive cultures from needle aspiration have specificity and positive predictive value of 100%, but a relatively low sensitivity

and negative predictive values (approximately 60% to 70% and 30% to 40%, respectively) (23, 24).

COMMUNITY-ACQUIRED PNEUMONIA

The most commonly identified pathogen in community-acquired pneumonia is *Streptococcus pneumoniae*, which accounts for approximately 35% of identified organisms (25, 26). Between 2% and 8% of patients have *Haemophilus influenzae* infection (27). Most of the remaining cases seen in the outpatient setting are caused by *Mycoplasma pneumoniae*, *Chlamydia pneumoniae*, and viruses (2, 28, 29). Anaerobic bacteria are an uncommon cause of community-acquired pneumonia. However, anaerobic bacteria have been isolated in approximately 20% to 35% of patients requiring hospitalization for pneumonia (30). Similarly, community-acquired *Staphylococcus aureus* pneumonia is uncommon and usually follows the influenza virus infection. However, *S. aureus* pneumonia is often associated with bacteremia and high mortality and should be considered in all severely ill patients admitted to the ICU for the management of pneumonia (31). *Legionella* species account for <2% of cases of pneumonia but its prevalence is higher in patients sick enough to require hospitalization and admission to the ICU (32). Gram-negative enteric organisms are an uncommon cause of community-acquired pneumonia, but should be considered in severely ill patients, especially those who are older, who have aspirated or who have significant underlying disease (33, 34).

NOSOCOMIAL PNEUMONIA

Hospital-acquired (nosocomial) pneumonia is defined as pneumonia occurring 48 hours or more after admission (35). Bacteria are the most frequently identified cause. The most common organisms early in the hospital course (within the first 4 days) are *S. pneumoniae*, *Moraxella catarrhalis*, *S. aureus*, and *H. influenzae* (36). Most pneumonias that develop 5 or more days after hospitalization are caused by enteric gram-negative organisms, most commonly *Enterobacter* species, *Escherichia coli*, *Klebsiella* species, and *Proteus* species, or by *S. aureus* (35). Pneumonia is particularly common after surgery and in patients undergoing mechanical ventilation. Pneumonia may occur in up to 18% of patients who have undergone surgery (37) and up to 25% to 50% of patients undergoing mechanical ventilation (38–40). Nosocomial bacterial pneumonia is often difficult to recognize because the clinical criteria are nonspecific and bilateral areas of consolidation are often present secondary to acute respiratory distress syndrome (ARDS). In one investigation, nosocomial bacterial pneumonia was found histologically at autopsy in 58% of patients with ARDS, in 36% of whom it was unsuspected (41).

The etiology of nosocomial pneumonia is influenced by the presence of specific risk factors. For example, anaerobic bacteria are more likely to be found in patients who develop pneumonia after aspiration or who have poor dentition or altered consciousness (42). *Pseudomonas aeruginosa* infection should be considered in patients who have received corticosteroids or broad-spectrum antibiotics, who have had a prolonged stay in the ICU, or who have underlying bronchiectasis (43). Prolonged hospitalization or prior use of antibiotics also favors the development of nosocomial pneumonia caused by antibiotic-resistant organisms, such as methicillin-resistant *S. aureus*, *Acinetobacter* species, *Serratia marcescens*, and *P. aeruginosa* (44).

Radiologic Manifestations of Bacterial Pulmonary Infection

Bacterial pulmonary infection is usually acquired through the tracheobronchial tree, most commonly by aspiration

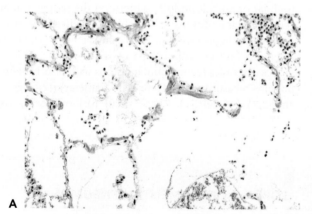
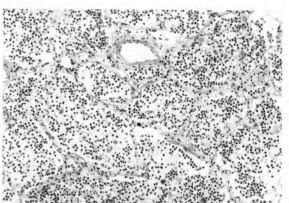

A

B

Figure 2.1 Lobar pneumonia. Photomicrographs show early **(A)** and advanced **(B)** stages of lobar pneumonia caused by *Streptococcus pneumoniae*. In **(A)**, the airspaces are filled with edema fluid; only occasional neutrophils are evident. In **(B)**, neutrophils predominate. The abundant fluid produced in the early stage of the disease flows relatively easily from airspace to airspace, resulting in the homogeneous consolidation seen grossly. Note that alveolar septa are intact in both stages of the disease, that is, there is no evidence of irreversible tissue damage. (From Müller NL, Fraser RS, Lee KS, et al. *Diseases of the lung. Radiologic and pathologic correlations.* Philadelphia, PA: Lippincott Williams & Wilkins; 2003.)

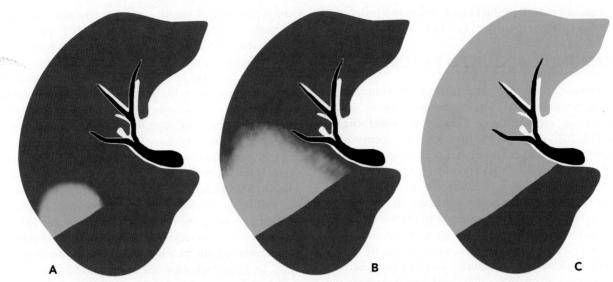

A   B   C

Figure 2.2 Progression of consolidation in lobar pneumonia. The consolidation usually occurs initially in the periphery of the lung adjacent to the visceral pleura or interlobar fissure **(A)**. The infection spreads across segmental boundaries to occupy a confluent portion of the parenchyma **(B)**. The area of consolidation abutting an interlobar fissure is sharply defined. The margins of the consolidation spreading to the remaining parenchyma tend to have ill-defined margins (ground-glass opacities on computed tomography scan) because the pneumonia initially results in only partial filling of the airspaces. The bronchi usually remain patent, resulting in an air bronchogram **(C)**. (Courtesy of C. Isabela S. Silva, MD, PhD.)

or inhalation of microorganisms, or, occasionally, by direct physical implantation from an infected source, such as a bronchoscope (45). Pulmonary infection may also occur through the pulmonary vasculature, typically in association with an extrapulmonary focus of infection such as endocarditis. The organisms responsible for the infection may be found free in the blood (sepsis) or may be associated with thrombus (septic emboli).

Bacteria result in two main types of pneumonia: Lobar (nonsegmental) pneumonia and bronchopneumonia (lobular pneumonia). Other manifestations include abscess formation, pneumatocele, septic embolism, pleural effusion, and empyema.

Lobar (nonsegmental) pneumonia is characterized histologically by the filling of alveolar airspaces by an exudate of edema fluid and neutrophils (see Fig. 2.1) (46). The consolidation usually begins in the periphery of the lung adjacent to the visceral pleura and spreads centripetally through interalveolar pores (pores of Kohn) and small airways (46). The airspace filling typically extends across pulmonary segments (nonsegmental consolidation), sometimes to involve the entire lobe (see Fig. 2.2). Lobar pneumonia is characterized on the radiograph and on computed tomography (CT) scan by the presence of homogeneous airspace consolidation involving adjacent segments of a lobe (see Fig. 2.3 and Table 2.1). The consolidation tends to occur initially in the periphery of the lung beneath the visceral pleura and usually abuts an interlobar fissure. The consolidation spreads centrally across segmental boundaries and may eventually involve the entire lobe. The bronchi usually remain patent, resulting in air bronchograms within the

areas of consolidation. On high-resolution CT scan, areas of ground-glass opacities denoting incomplete filling of alveoli can often be seen adjacent to the airspace consolidation (see Fig. 2.4) (47, 48). Most cases of lobar pneumonia are caused by bacteria, most commonly by *S. pneumoniae* and less commonly by *Klebsiella pneumoniae*, *Legionella pneumophila*, *H. influenzae*, and *M. Tuberculosis* (11, 49).

Bronchopneumonia (lobular pneumonia) is characterized histologically by predominantly peribronchiolar inflammation (see Fig. 2.5) (46). This peribronchiolar inflammation is initially reflected by the presence of a small nodular or reticulonodular pattern on the radiograph and centrilobular nodules and branching opacities (tree-in-bud pattern) on high-resolution CT scan (see Fig. 2.6). Further extension into the adjacent parenchyma results in patchy airspace nodules (centrilobular lesions with poorly defined margins measuring 4 to 10 mm in diameter) (see Figs. 2.6 and 2.7) (46, 50, 51). These small foci of disease may

TABLE 2.1
LOBAR (NONSEGMENTAL) PNEUMONIA

Consolidation crosses segmental boundaries
Affects predominantly one lobe
Most common organisms
   Streptococcus pneumoniae
   Klebsiella pneumoniae
   Legionella pneumophila

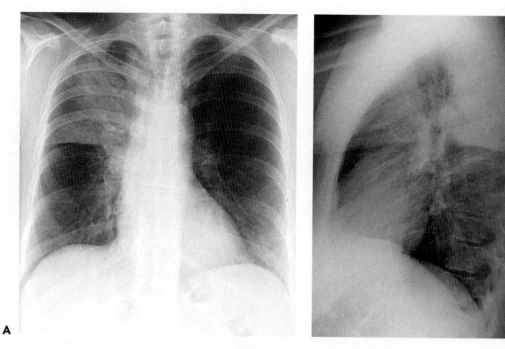

Figure 2.3 Lobar pneumonia. Posteroanterior **(A)** and lateral **(B)** chest radiographs show extensive consolidation in the right upper lobe. The consolidation crosses segmental boundaries, has well-defined margins where it abuts the interlobar fissures and poorly defined margins elsewhere. The patient was a 50-year-old woman with pneumococcal pneumonia.

progress to lobular, subsegmental, or segmental areas of consolidation (see Figs. 2.6 and 2.8 and Table 2.2). The areas of consolidation may be patchy or confluent, involve one or more segments of a single lobe, and may be multilobar, unilateral, or bilateral (51). Confluence of pneumonia in adjacent lobules and segments may result in a pattern simulating lobar pneumonia; distinction from the latter can be made in most cases by the presence of segmental or lobular distribution of the abnormalities in other areas. Cavitation is common particularly in patients with extensive consolidation (22). Because it involves the airways, bronchopneumonia frequently results in loss of volume of the affected segments or lobes. Air bronchograms are seldom evident on the radiograph but can frequently be seen on high-resolution CT scan.

Characteristic manifestations of bronchopneumonia on high-resolution CT scan include centrilobular nodules and branching linear opacities, airspace nodules, and multifocal lobular areas of consolidation (see Fig. 2.9) (46–48). The nodular and branching linear opacities result in an appearance resembling a tree-in-bud and reflect the presence of inflammatory exudate in the lumen and walls of membranous and respiratory bronchioles and the lung parenchyma immediately adjacent to them (46). The nodules seen in bronchopneumonia usually measure 4 to 10 mm in diameter and have poorly defined margins. Although these nodular opacities are often referred to as "acinar shadows," they reflect the presence of peribronchiolar areas of consolidation and not acinar consolidation (46, 50). Therefore the term *airspace nodules* is preferable. The most

common causative organisms of bronchopneumonia are *S. aureus, H. influenzae, P. aeruginosa,* and anaerobic bacteria (11, 22, 47).

It should be noted that the radiologic pattern is influenced by the presence of underlying disease such as emphysema and age, and immunologic status of the patient (52). It is also important to keep in mind that the radiographic manifestations are often delayed. This is particularly important in nosocomial infections in patients whose chest radiographs are often performed within hours of the onset of symptoms, a time when the pneumonia may not yet be apparent on the radiograph (22). Radiographic abnormalities may be particularly delayed in patients with neutropenia (53). In one study of 175 consecutive patients with gram-negative pneumonia who were neutropenic following antineoplastic chemotherapy, 70 episodes of pneumonia were initially diagnosed clinically, in the absence of radiographically detectable disease (53). In 27 of these 70 episodes, pneumonia was evident on a follow-up radiograph. In 25 of 57 patients with no radiographically detectable infiltrates, the diagnosis of pneumonia was established at autopsy (53). The radiographic appearance of a visible pneumonic infiltrate may be delayed not only in patients with neutropenia but also in those with functional defects of granulocytes due to diabetes, alcoholism, and uremia (22). CT scan, particularly high-resolution CT scan, has been shown to be more sensitive than the radiograph in the detection of subtle abnormalities and may show findings suggestive of pneumonia up to 5 days earlier than chest radiographs (54).

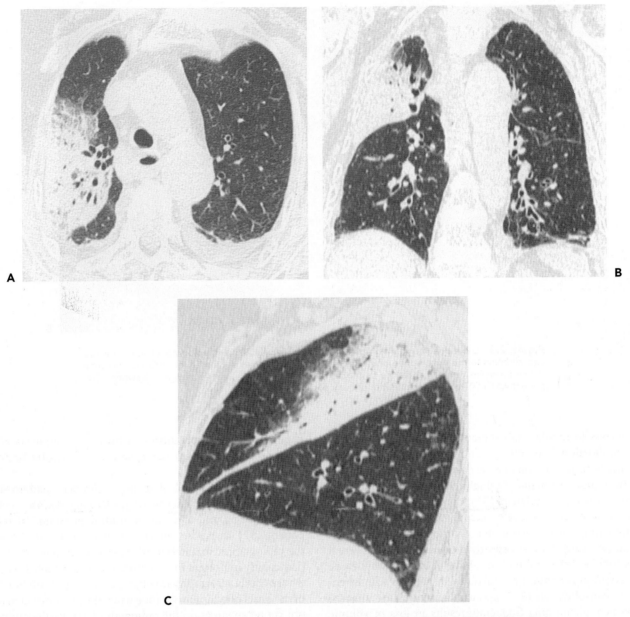

A

B

C

Figure 2.4   Lobar pneumonia. High-resolution computed tomography (CT) scan (1-mm collimation) **(A)** obtained in a multidetector CT scanner shows airspace consolidation in the right upper lobe. Note the presence of patent bronchi within the consolidation (air bronchogram) and the presence of ground-glass opacities at the boundary of the consolidation and normal lung. Coronal **(B)** and sagittal **(C)** reformations show that the consolidation crosses segmental boundaries and involves the apical, posterior and, to a lesser extent, anterior segments of the right upper lobe.

High-resolution CT scan allows a better depiction of the pattern and distribution of pneumonia than the radiograph (48, 55) but is seldom required in the evaluation of patients with suspected or proved bacterial pneumonia. CT scan is recommended, however, in patients with clinical suspicion of infection and normal or nonspecific radiographic findings, in the assessment of suspected complications of pneumonia or suspicion of an underlying lesion such as pulmonary carcinoma (22, 56). CT scan is also indicated in patients with pneumonia and persistent or recurrent pulmonary opacities (22).

Lung abscess is defined as a localized necrotic cavity containing pus (57). It usually represents an inflammatory mass, the central part of which has undergone purulent liquefactive necrosis (11). The most common cause of lung abscess is aspiration (57). Abscesses occur most commonly in the posterior segment of an upper lobe or the superior segment of a lower lobe (57). However, they may also be present predominantly or exclusively in the anterior lung regions (see Fig. 2.10). Lung abscesses usually measure 2 to 6 cm in diameter, although they may become larger measuring up to 12 cm in diameter (57). Abscesses often

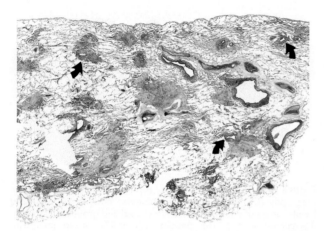

Figure 2.5 Acute bronchopneumonia. Low magnification photomicrograph shows several small foci of consolidation located around the lumens of small bronchioles (*arrows*). (From Müller NL, Fraser RS, Lee KS, et al. *Diseases of the lung. Radiologic and pathologic correlations*. Philadelphia, PA: Lippincott Williams & Wilkins; 2003.)

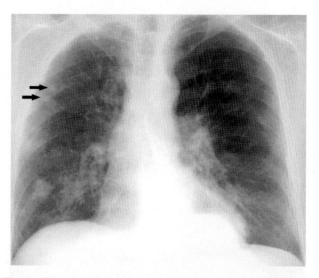

Figure 2.7 Bronchopneumonia. Chest radiograph shows poorly defined nodular opacities (*arrows*) in the right upper lobe and small bilateral foci of consolidation. Also noted is a large hiatus hernia with an air–fluid level. The patient was a 37-year-old man with *Escherichia coli* pneumonia.

erode into an airway, resulting in drainage of necrotic material and the formation of a cavity (see Fig. 2.10). Pulmonary abscesses may develop in the course of known pneumonia or may be the initial manifestation of the disease. The radiologic manifestations consist of single or multiple masses that are often cavitated (see Table 2.3). In one review of the radiographic findings in 50 patients, the internal margins of the abscesses were smooth in 88% and shaggy in 12% (58). Air–fluid levels were present in 72% and adjacent parenchymal consolidation in 48%. Maximal wall thickness was equal to or <4 mm in 4%

of cases, between 5 and 15 mm in 82%, and >15 mm in 14%. CT scan typically demonstrates low-attenuation central region or cavitation and rim enhancement following intravenous administration of contrast (Fig. 2.10) (59, 60). Common causes of lung abscess include anaerobic bacteria (most commonly *Fusobacterium nucleatum* and Bacteroides species), *S. aureus, P. aeruginosa,* and *K. pneumoniae* (57, 61).

Occasionally pneumonia may result in extensive necrosis (necrotizing pneumonia). Radiologic manifestations

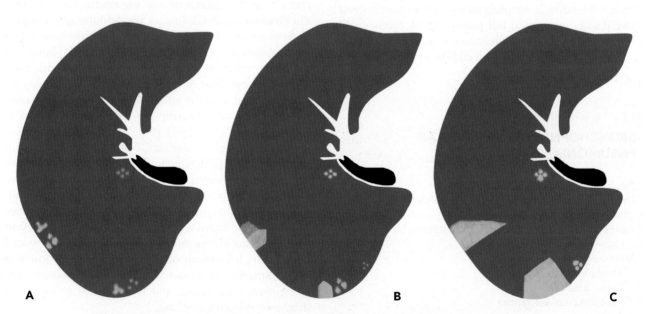

Figure 2.6 Progression of bronchopneumonia. The organisms may initially involve mainly the bronchioles resulting in centrilobular nodules and branching opacities (tree-in-bud pattern) **(A)**. The consolidation initially involves the peribronchiolar regions. It progresses to become lobular, subsegmental or segmental **(B and C)**. It is usually multifocal and patchy but the consolidation typically does not cross segmental boundaries. (Courtesy of C. Isabela S. Silva, MD, PhD.)

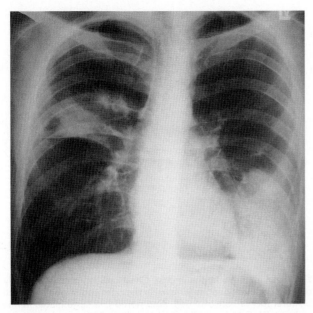

Figure 2.8 Bronchopneumonia. Chest radiograph shows areas of consolidation in the right upper and left lower lobes. The patient was a 23-year-old man with bronchopneumonia.

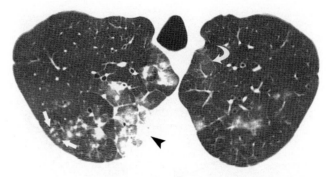

Figure 2.9 Bronchopneumonia. High-resolution computed tomography (CT) scan shows centrilobular nodules (*arrows*) and lobular areas of consolidation (*arrowhead*) and ground-glass opacity (*curved arrow*). The patient was a 53-year-old man with bronchopneumonia.

consist initially of small lucencies within an area of consolidated lung, usually developing within lobar consolidation associated with enlargement of the lobe and outward bulging of the fissure (bulging fissure sign) (62) (see Fig. 2.11). The lucencies rapidly coalesce into a large cavity containing fluid and sloughed lung (see Fig. 2.12).

Pneumatocele is a thin-walled, gas-filled space that usually develops in association with infection (11). It presumably results from drainage of a focus of necrotic lung parenchyma followed by check-valve obstruction of the airway subtending it, enabling air to enter the parenchymal space during inspiration but preventing its egress during expiration (63). The complication is caused most often by *S. aureus* in infants and children and *Pneumocystis jiroveci* in

TABLE 2.2

BRONCHOPNEUMONIA (LOBULAR PNEUMONIA)

Patchy, inhomogeneous consolidation
Lobular, subsegmental, segmental consolidation
Usually involves several lobes
Centrilobular nodules and tree-in-bud pattern on
   high-resolution CT scan
Most common organisms
   Staphylococcus aureus
   Escherichia coli
   Pseudomonas aeruginosa
   Anaerobes
   Haemophilus influenzae

CT, computed tomography.

patients who have acquired immunodeficiency syndrome (AIDS) (52, 64). Pneumatoceles typically increase in size over days or weeks, may result in pneumothorax, and usually resolve over weeks or months (see Fig. 2.13).

Septic emboli to the lungs originate in a variety of sites, including cardiac valves (endocarditis), peripheral veins (thrombophlebitis), and venous catheters or pacemaker wires. The common feature in all these sites is endothelial damage associated with the formation of friable thrombus-containing organisms (usually bacteria) (52). Turbulence of flowing blood results in the detachment of small fragments of thrombus that are carried to the pulmonary arteries. Septic embolism is characterized radiologically by the presence of nodules that usually measure 1 to 3 cm in diameter and that are frequently cavitated (see Fig. 2.14). The cavitation reflects the necrosis associated with the organisms and the neutrophilic exudate. On cross-sectional CT images the nodules often appear to have a vessel leading into them. This has been called the *feeding vessel* (see Fig. 2.15) (65, 66). Multiplanar and maximum intensity projection (MIP) reformations have shown however that in most patients the pulmonary arteries course around the nodule and that vessels appearing to enter the nodule usually are pulmonary veins draining the nodule (Fig. 2.15) (67). Dodd et al. performed multidetector high-resolution CT scan in 14 patients with septic embolism (67). Ninety-three nodules (40%) showed a vessel that appeared to enter the nodule on transverse images, but the vessel was shown to pass around the nodule on multiplanar reconstructions and/or MIPs. Forty-four nodules (19%) showed a central vessel entering the lesion on all imaging planes. All of these vessels could be traced back to the left atrium on transverse images, consistent with pulmonary vein branches. The "feeding vessel" sign is therefore a misnomer and is of limited value in the diagnosis of septic embolism.

Occlusion of pulmonary arteries by septic emboli or thrombus may result in hemorrhage and/or infarction and less well-defined or wedge-shaped foci of disease. These subpleural wedge-shaped areas of consolidation,

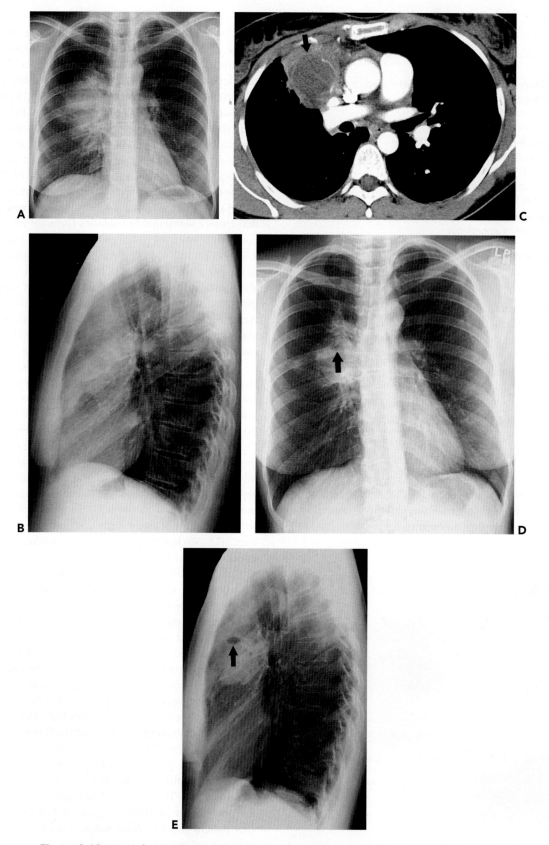

Figure 2.10   Lung abscess. Posteroanterior **(A)** and lateral **(B)** chest radiographs show dense right upper airspace consolidation. Contrast-enhanced computed tomography (CT) scan **(C)** demonstrates large focal area of decreased attenuation with rim enhancement (*arrow*) characteristic of lung abscess. Posteroanterior **(D)** and lateral **(E)** chest radiographs 3 weeks later show decreased size of lung abscess and development of cavitation with fluid level (*arrows*). The patient was a 43-year-old woman with lung abscess secondary to *Haemophilus aphrophilus*.

TABLE 2.3
LUNG ABSCESS

Inflammatory mass with central purulent necrosis
Frequently cavitate
Smooth or shaggy inner margins
Air–fluid levels common
Maximal wall thickness usually <15 mm
Low-attenuation central region and rim enhancement on CT
    scan
Most common organisms
    Anaerobic bacteria
    Staphylococcus aureus
    Pseudomonas aeruginosa

CT, computed tomography.

often with central areas of necrosis or frank cavitation, are often difficult to identify on the radiograph but are commonly seen on CT scan (66). Septic emboli are seen most commonly in intravenous drug users and in patients with central venous lines.

AEROBIC BACTERIA

Gram-positive Cocci

Streptococcus Pneumoniae

S. pneumoniae (pneumococcus) is the most commonly identified pathogenic organism in patients admitted to the hospital for pneumonia, accounting for approximately 40%

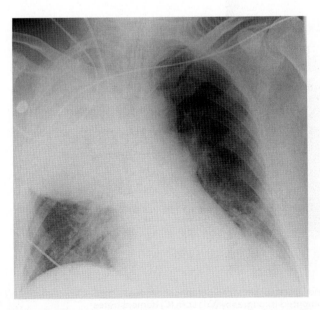

Figure 2.11 Bulging fissure sign. Posteroanterior chest radiograph shows dense right upper lobe airspace consolidation with downward bulging of the minor fissure. The patient was a 66-year-old man with pneumococcal pneumonia.

of all isolated species (27, 68). Risk factors for the development of pneumococcal pneumonia include the extremes of age (69–71), chronic heart or lung disease (70, 71), immunosuppression (70, 71), alcoholism (72), institutionalization (73, 74), and prior splenectomy (75). The characteristic clinical presentation is abrupt in onset, with fever, chills, cough, and pleuritic chest pain. In the elderly, these classic features of disease may be absent, and pneumonia may be confused with or confounded by other common medical problems, such as congestive heart failure, pulmonary thromboembolism, or malignancy (74, 76).

The characteristic radiographic pattern of acute pneumococcal pneumonia consists of homogeneous consolidation that crosses segmental boundaries (nonsegmental) but involves only one lobe (lobar pneumonia) (see Figs. 2.16 and 2.17 and Table 2.4) (11). Because the consolidation begins in the peripheral airspaces of the lung, it almost invariably abuts against a visceral pleural surface, either interlobar or over the convexity of the lung (11). Occasionally, infection is manifested as a spherical focus of consolidation that simulates a mass (round pneumonia); this pattern is seen more commonly in children than in adults (see Fig. 2.18) (77).

Although homogeneous lobar consolidation is the most characteristic radiographic manifestation of acute pneumococcal pneumonia, other patterns are not uncommon. In one prospective study of 30 patients with *S. pneumoniae*, 20 (67%) had lobar consolidation (lobar pneumonia), 6 (20%) had patchy areas of consolidation (bronchopneumonia), and 4 (13%) had mixed airspace and reticulonodular opacities (see Figs. 2.19 and 2.20) (78). In another review of 132 patients who had severe community-acquired pneumonia treated in the ICU, 28 (65%) of 43 patients with *S. pneumoniae* pneumonia had typical lobar consolidation, and 35% had bronchopneumonia; none had reticular or reticulonodular opacities (79).

Complications, such as cavitation and pneumatocele formation, are rare. It is probable that many of these are related to mixed infections; associated anaerobic microorganisms in particular are likely to be undetected because of lack of appropriate culture methods (80). Pleural effusion is evident on posteroanterior and lateral radiographs in approximately 10% of patients overall (81); effusion is present in approximately 30% of patients who have severe pneumonia requiring treatment in the ICU (79), and in 50% of patients with bacteremia (82). Lymphadenopathy is seldom evident on the radiograph but is commonly seen on CT scan (83). In one study of 35 adults hospitalized with pneumococcal pneumonia, intrathoracic lymphadenopathy was present on CT scan in 19 (54%) patients (83). The lymphadenopathy was ipsilateral to the pneumonia in 100% of patients (19 of 19 patients). One patient also had contralateral lymphadenopathy. Comorbidities included HIV infection ($n = 15$); smoking ($n = 21$); emphysema ($n = 5$); hepatitis C ($n = 5$); and diabetes ($n = 3$). None of the differences in the prevalence of lymphadenopathy among the subgroups was statistically significant.

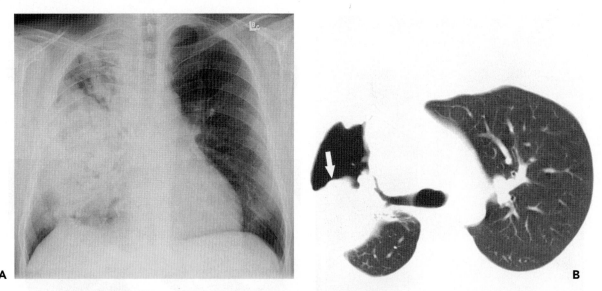

Figure 2.12 Necrotizing pneumonia. Chest radiograph **(A)** shows inhomogeneous and dense consolidation in the right lung. Computed tomography (CT) **(B)** image shows a large cavity and sloughed lung within the cavity (*arrow*). The patient was a 42-year-old alcoholic man with necrotizing pneumonia secondary to *Klebsiella pneumoniae* and anaerobic organisms.

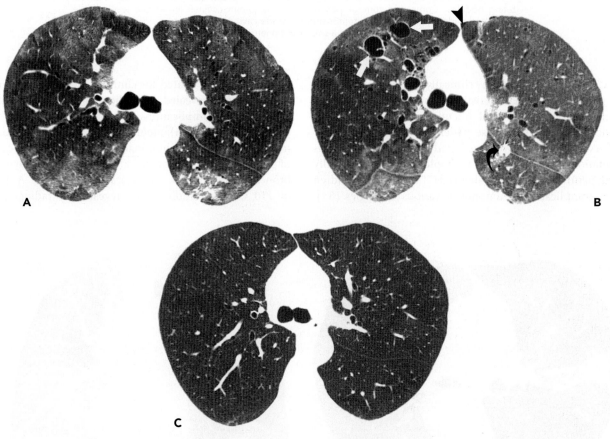

Figure 2.13 Pneumatoceles. High-resolution computed tomography (CT) image at the level of the main bronchi **(A)** shows extensive bilateral ground-glass opacities. High-resolution CT scan image at the same level 1 month later **(B)** shows several pneumatoceles (*straight arrows*) in the right upper lobe. Also noted is a small left pneumothorax (*arrowhead*) and a left chest tube in the major fissure (*curved arrow*). The patient was a 55-year-old woman who developed *Pneumocystis* pneumonia while undergoing treatment for nonHodgkin lymphoma. The pneumonia resolved but no follow-up images immediately following resolution of the pneumonia were available. High-resolution CT scan image 3 years later **(C)** demonstrates resolution of the pneumatoceles.

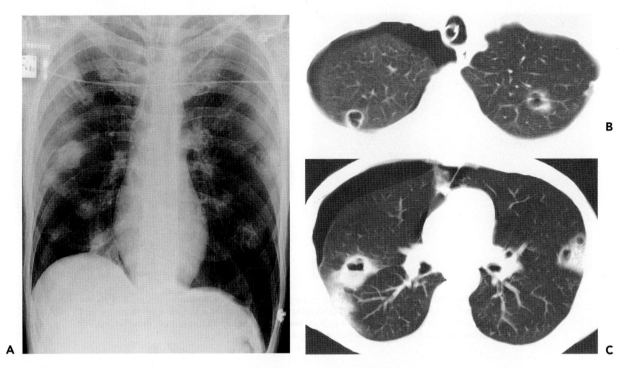

Figure 2.14 Septic embolism. Posteroanterior chest radiograph **(A)** shows several bilateral cavitating nodules. Computed tomography (CT) images (5-mm collimation) at the level of the upper **(B)** and middle **(C)** lung zones demonstrate that the cavitating nodules are located mainly in the subpleural lung regions. Also noted is a small right pneumothorax.

CT scan seldom adds any clinically relevant information in patients with characteristic radiographic and clinical findings of pneumococcal pneumonia and therefore is seldom warranted in these patients. CT scan is helpful, however, in patients with suspected complications such as cavitation, empyema, and bronchopleural fistula. Donnelly et al. performed contrast-enhanced CT scans in 56 children with complicated pneumonia of various etiologies (84).

CT scans were evaluated for clinically significant findings that were not revealed by radiography including lung parenchymal complications (cavitary necrosis, abscess, bronchopleural fistula), pleural complications (loculation, malpositioned chest tube), inaccurate estimation of cause of chest opacity on radiography (pleural vs. parenchymal), bronchial obstruction, or pericardial effusion. A total of 110 CT scan findings, not revealed by radiography,

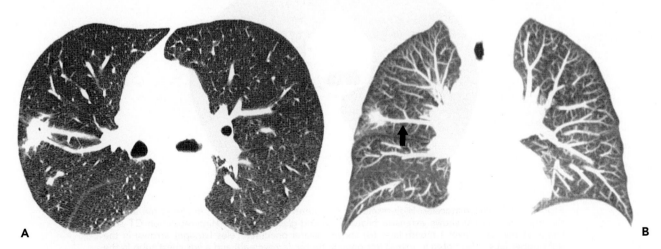

Figure 2.15 Feeding vessel sign. Cross-sectional high-resolution computed tomography (CT) image **(A)** shows two vessels apparently coursing into a nodule ("feeding vessel sign"). Coronal maximum intensity projection image **(B)** demonstrates that the only vessel in close contact with the nodule is a draining vein (*arrow*).

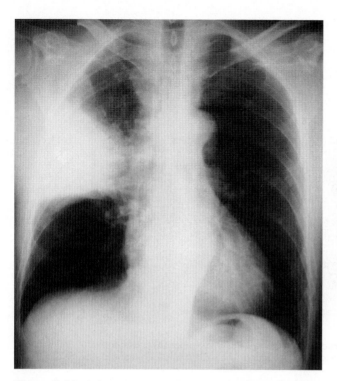

Figure 2.16 Lobar pneumonia due to *Streptococcus pneumoniae*. Chest radiograph shows nonsegmental right upper lobe consolidation. The patient was a 71-year-old man with pneumococcal pneumonia.

were seen including 40 parenchymal complications, 37 pleural complications, 20 inaccurate estimations of cause of chest opacity on radiography, and 13 pericardial effusions. All CT scans showed at least one significant finding not seen on radiography (84). Hodina et al. reviewed the radiographs and CT scan images of nine children admitted in the pediatric ICU for persistent or progressive pneumonia, respiratory distress, or sepsis despite adequate antibiotic therapy, including four patients with *S. pneumoniae* pneumonia (85). Chest radiographs showed consolidations in eight of the nine patients. On CT scan examination, cavitary necrosis was localized to one lobe in two patients, and seven patients showed multilobar or bilateral areas of cavitary necrosis. In three of the nine patients the cavitary necrosis was initially shown on CT scan and visualization by chest radiography was delayed by a time span varying from 5 to 9 days. Parapneumonic effusions were shown by chest radiography in three patients and by CT scan in five patients. Bronchopleural fistulae, present in three patients, were only seen on CT scan. The authors concluded that CT scan allows a better assessment of the presence of pulmonary and pleural complications in children with necrotizing pneumonia and allows an earlier diagnosis of this rapidly progressing condition (85).

Staphylococcus Aureus

S. aureus is an uncommon cause of community-acquired pneumonia, accounting for only approximately 3% of all

cases (25–27). It is, however, an important cause of nosocomial pneumonia, especially in the ICU. In this setting, *S. aureus* is one of the more common pathogenic organisms, being found in 15% or more of all cases (86–89). Of particular importance is the dramatic increase of the incidence of methicillin-resistant *Staphylococcus aureus* (MRSA) infections in recent years in patients admitted to the ICU and the associated increase in morbidity and mortality (90).

Bacteremic *S. aureus* pneumonia is found most commonly in ICU patients and in intravenous drug users (91). In one prospective study of 134 cases, 80% of primary staphylococcal pneumonias were nosocomial and 68% of the overall cases were in patients in the ICU; 72% of the patients with community-acquired *S. aureus* pneumonia were intravenous drug users (91).

The clinical presentation of *S. aureus* pneumonia usually is abrupt, with fever, pleuritic chest pain, cough, and expectoration of purulent yellow or brown sputum, sometimes streaked with blood (11). The characteristic pattern of presentation pathologically and radiologically is as a bronchopneumonia (lobular pneumonia) (see Table 2.5) (46). *S. aureus* bronchopneumonia, like other bronchopneumonias, is characterized histologically by predominantly peribronchiolar inflammation (46). This results in poorly defined 4 to 10 mm-diameter nodules (airspace nodules) (see Fig. 2.21). The airway involvement in *S. aureus* bronchopneumonia is easier to see on high-resolution CT scan than on the radiograph (92). It is manifested on high-resolution CT scan by centrilobular nodular and branching

---

TABLE 2.4
STREPTOCOCCUS PNEUMONIAE (PNEUMOCOCCAL) PNEUMONIA

Most common cause of community-acquired pneumonia
  (40% of cases)
Risk factors: Old age, chronic heart or lung disease
Most common radiologic presentation
  Homogeneous lobar (nonsegmental) consolidation
  Consolidation abuts visceral pleural surface
Less common presentation
  Patchy unilateral or bilateral consolidation
    (bronchopneumonia)
  Spherical focus of consolidation (round pneumonia)
  Dense consolidation with bulging of interlobar fissure
Other findings
  Pleural effusion: Approximately 10% of cases
  Lymphadenopathy: Approximately 50% of cases on CT
    scan
Main value of CT scan: Evaluation of patients with
  suspected cavitation or empyema

CT, computed tomography.

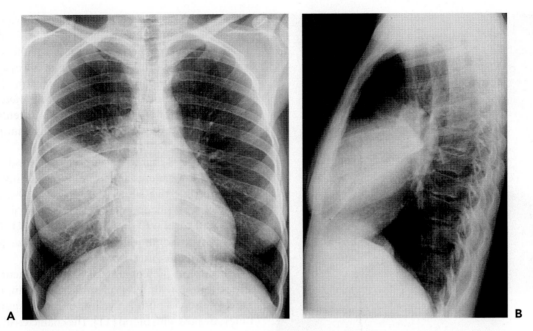

Figure 2.17   Lobar pneumonia due to *Streptococcus pneumoniae*. Posteroanterior **(A)** and lateral **(B)** chest radiographs show extensive right middle lobe consolidation. The patient was a 29-year-old woman with pneumococcal pneumonia.

linear opacities (tree-in-bud pattern) seen in approximately 40% of patients with staphylococcal pneumonia (see Fig. 2.22) (47, 92). The peribronchiolar inflammation usually progresses rapidly to lobular, subsegmental, or segmental areas of consolidation, which may be patchy or confluent. The pneumonia is bilateral in approximately 40% of patients. Depending on the severity of involvement, the process may be patchy or homogeneous; the latter represents confluent bronchopneumonia

(see Fig. 2.23). Because an inflammatory exudate fills the airways, segmental atelectasis may accompany the consolidation, and air bronchograms are seldom evident on the radiograph (46).

In a review of the radiographic abnormalities of 26 adults with community-acquired staphylococcal pneumonia, 14 (54%) had homogeneous consolidation, 12 (46%) had patchy consolidation, and 2 (8%) had a mixed picture (51). The consolidation involved a single lobe

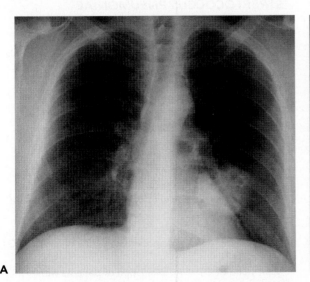
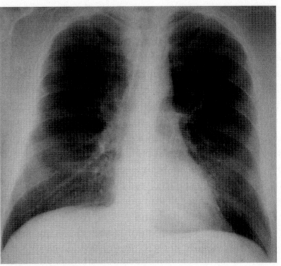

Figure 2.18   Round pneumonia due to *Streptococcus pneumoniae*. Chest radiograph **(A)** shows a round area of consolidation mimicking a mass in the left lower lobe. Chest radiograph 1 week later **(B)** shows almost complete resolution of the airspace consolidation. The patient was a 50-year-old man with pneumococcal pneumonia.

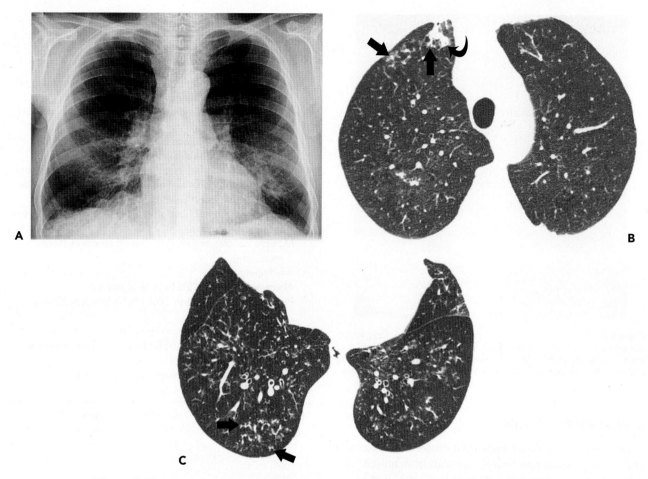

Figure 2.19 Bronchiolitis and bronchopneumonia due to *Streptococcus pneumoniae*. Chest radiograph **(A)** shows bilateral reticulonodular pattern involving mainly the lower lung zones. High-resolution computed tomography (CT) scan image at the level of the aortic arch **(B)** demonstrates centrilobular nodules (*straight arrows*) and small foci of consolidation (*curved arrow*) in the right upper lobe. High-resolution CT image at the level of the lung bases **(C)** shows bilateral centrilobular nodules and branching opacities (tree-in-bud pattern) (*arrows*). The findings are consistent with bronchiolitis and early bronchopneumonia. The patient was a 70-year-old man with pneumococcal pneumonia.

in 36% of cases, more than one lobe in 54%, and was bilateral in 35%. In a second series of 31 adults, 15 (60%) had multilobar consolidation and 12 (39%) had bilateral pneumonia (93); the consolidation involved predominantly or exclusively the lower lobes in 16 patients (64%). Abscesses develop in 15% to 30% of patients (51, 93). The abscesses are usually solitary and typically have an irregular shaggy inner wall. Pneumatocele formation also is common, occurring in approximately 50% of children (94) and 15% of adults (51). Pneumatoceles usually appear during the first week of the pneumonia and disappear spontaneously within weeks (95) or months (96). Spontaneous pneumothorax, which is presumably secondary to ruptured pneumatoceles, occurs in approximately 10% of adults and 30% of children (51). Pleural effusions occur in 30% to 50% of patients; of these, approximately half represent empyemas (see Fig. 2.24) (51, 93).

In pneumonia related to hematogenous spread of organisms (septic embolism), the radiologic appearance is one of multiple nodules or masses throughout the lungs (see Fig. 2.25). Sometimes the nodules have poorly defined borders or are confluent. Abscesses may erode into bronchi and produce air-containing cavities, frequently with fluid levels (97) (Fig. 2.14). On CT scan, most abnormalities are in a subpleural location. In 40% to 70% of patients cross-sectional CT scan images appear to show a vessel coursing into the nodule ("feeding vessel" sign) (65–67). MIP reformations have shown, however, that in most patients the pulmonary arteries course around the nodule and that vessels appearing to enter the nodule usually are draining pulmonary veins (Fig. 2.15) (67). Most nodules eventually cavitate. Septic infarcts also frequently result in subpleural wedge-shaped areas of consolidation; these were reported in 11 (73%) of 15 patients in one series (65). The wedge-shaped areas of consolidation are usually multiple and are seen together with nodules. In one series of 14 patients with septic emboli, the patients had a total of 233 nodules and 91 wedge-shaped opacities (67).

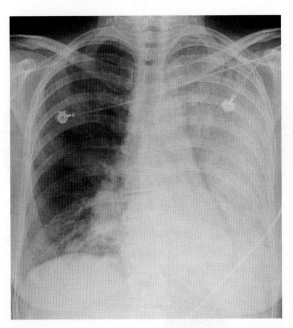

Figure 2.20 Extensive bilateral pneumonia due to *Streptococcus pneumoniae.* Chest radiograph shows diffuse consolidation of the left lung and patchy foci of consolidation in the right lung. The patient was a 49-year-old woman with pneumococcal pneumonia.

TABLE 2.5
***STAPHYLOCOCCUS AUREUS* PNEUMONIA**

Approximately 3% of community-acquired pneumonias and 15% of nosocomial pneumonias
Risk factors: Intravenous drug users and patients in the ICU
Most common radiologic presentation
    Patchy unilateral (60%) or bilateral (40%) consolidation (bronchopneumonia)
    Airspace nodules (4–10 mm diameter) commonly present
    Centrilobular nodules and tree-in-bud pattern on CT scan
Less common presentation
    Homogeneous consolidation (usually represents confluent bronchopneumonia)
    Multiple nodules and wedge-shaped opacities (septic embolism)
Other findings
    Abscess formation: 15% to 30% of patients
    Pneumatocele formation: 50% of children and 15% of adults
    Pneumothorax: 30% of children and 15% of adults
    Pleural effusion: 30% to 50% of cases (half of these are empyemas)
Main value of CT scan: Evaluation of patients with suspected cavitation or empyema

ICU, intensive care unit; CT, computed tomography.

Gram-negative Bacilli

Gram-negative bacilli are important causes of nosocomial and, under certain conditions, community-acquired lung infection. More than 50% of ventilator-associated pneumonias are caused by these organisms; when only lung superinfection is considered, they are responsible for about two thirds of cases (88, 89).

Klebsiella Pneumoniae

K. pneumoniae accounts for 1% to 5% of all cases of community-acquired pneumonia and approximately 15% of cases of nosocomial pneumonia (9, 98). Acute pneumonia caused by *K. pneumoniae* occurs predominantly in men, many of whom are chronic alcoholics (99) or have underlying chronic bronchopulmonary disease (5). The onset of acute pneumonia usually is abrupt, with prostration, fever, productive cough, dyspnea, and pleuritic chest pain (5).

Community-acquired *Klebsiella* pneumonia, similar to pneumococcal pneumonia, typically presents as a lobar pneumonia (see Fig. 2.26 and Table 2.6). The consolidation usually begins in the periphery of the lung adjacent to the visceral pleura and spreads centripetally through interalveolar pores (pores of Kohn) and small airways (46). The airspace filling typically extends across pulmonary segments (nonsegmental consolidation), resulting in homogeneous lobar consolidation with air bronchograms (92). Compared with pneumococcal pneumonia, acute *Klebsiella* pneumonia has a greater tendency to result in a voluminous inflammatory exudate leading to lobar expansion with resultant bulging of interlobar fissures and

a greater tendency for abscess and cavity formation (see Fig. 2.27) (92, 100, 101). Bulging of interlobar fissures has been reported in approximately 30% of patients who have *Klebsiella* pneumonia, compared with 10% or less of patients with pneumococcal pneumonia (100, 101). Because of the greater prevalence of pneumococcal pneumonia, lobar expansion in any patient is more likely to be due to *S. pneumoniae* than to *Klebsiella.* Pleural effusion is seen in 60% to 70% of cases (100, 102). Occasionally, acute *Klebsiella* pneumonia undergoes only partial resolution and progresses to a chronic phase with cavitation and persistent positive cultures; in this circumstance, the radiographic picture simulates that seen in tuberculosis.

The pattern of lobar (nonsegmental) airspace consolidation is seen more commonly in patients who have community-acquired rather than nosocomial *Klebsiella* pneumonia (92). Approximately 75% of patients with community-acquired infection have lobar pneumonia, most commonly involving the right upper lobe (103). By contrast, in one study of 15 patients who had *Klebsiella* infection, 13 of whom were considered to have hospital-acquired pneumonia, consolidation confined to one lobe occurred in 7 of 15 patients, patchy bilateral consolidation consistent with bronchopneumonia occurred in 7, and patchy unilateral consolidation occurred in 1 (102); none of the 15 patients developed lobar expansion or cavitation.

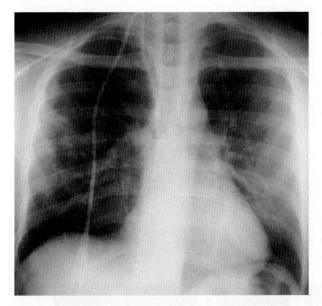

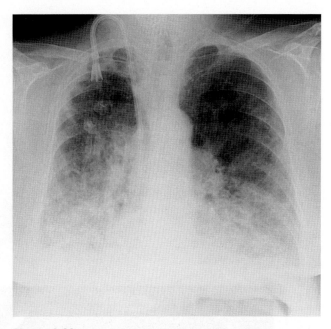

Figure 2.21 Bronchopneumonia due to *Staphylococcus aureus*. Chest radiograph shows poorly defined small nodular opacities and small foci of consolidation in the right mid lung zone. Also note the presence of central venous line. The patient was a 33-year-old immunocompromised man with *Staphylococcus aureus* bronchopneumonia.

Figure 2.23 Bronchopneumonia due to *Staphylococcus aureus*. Chest radiograph shows bilateral poorly defined nodular opacities and patchy areas of consolidation. Also noted is a central venous line. The patient was a 70-year-old man with methicillin-resistant *Staphylococcus aureus* pneumonia.

Complications of *Klebsiella* pneumonia include abscess formation, parapneumonic effusion, and empyema. Moon et al. reviewed the CT scan findings in 11 patients with complicated *Klebsiella* pneumonia (100). In all patients the parenchymal consolidation included enhancing homogeneous areas and poorly marginated low-density areas with multiple small cavities, suggesting necrotizing pneumonia. In nine patients scattered enhancing structures presumably representing atelectatic lung and pulmonary vessels were

noted within necrotic areas of consolidated lung. Eight patients had pleural effusion and five demonstrated diffuse pleural enhancement suggestive of empyema. Follow-up CT scan in three patients with necrotizing pneumonia showed slow resolution from the periphery to the center and residual scarring on follow-up CT scan at 2 to 3 months (100). Rarely, *Klebsiella* pneumonia may result in bronchopleural fistula. A single case of bronchobiliary

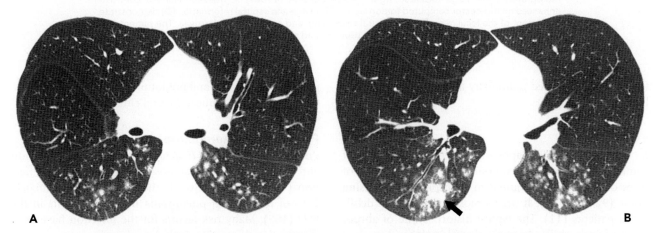

Figure 2.22 Bronchiolitis and bronchopneumonia due to *Staphylococcus aureus*. High-resolution computed tomography (CT) scan image at the level of the bronchus intermedius **(A)** shows centrilobular nodular opacities in the superior segment of the lower lobes. High-resolution CT scan image at a slightly more caudal level **(B)** shows bilateral centrilobular nodular opacities and a small focus of consolidation (*arrow*) in right lower lobe. The findings are consistent with bronchiolitis and early bronchopneumonia. The patient was a 38-year-old woman with *Staphylococcus aureus* pneumonia.

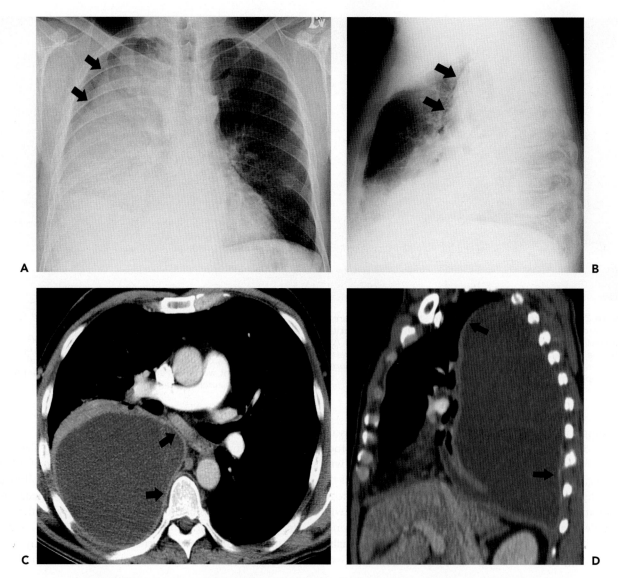

Figure 2.24 Empyema due to *Staphylococcus aureus*. Posteroanterior **(A)** and lateral **(B)** chest radiographs show large loculated right pleural effusion (*arrows*). Cross-sectional **(C)** contrast-enhanced multidetector computed tomography (CT) image and sagittal reformation **(D)** demonstrate the extent of the loculated effusion, pleural thickening, and enhancement (*arrows*). The patient was a 44-year-old man and an intravenous drug user. He had no radiologic evidence of septic embolism.

fistula with combined pulmonary and liver abscesses has been described (104).

Escherichia Coli

E. coli accounts for approximately 4% of cases of community-acquired pneumonia and 5% to 20% of cases of pneumonia acquired in a hospital or a nursing home (92, 105, 106). It occurs most commonly in debilitated patients (11). The typical history is one of abrupt onset of fever, chills, dyspnea, pleuritic pain, and productive cough in a patient with preexisting chronic disease (92).

The radiographic manifestations usually are those of bronchopneumonia (see Fig. 2.28); rarely a pattern of lobar pneumonia may be seen (see Table 2.7) (107). The pneumonia tends to be severe (106). Involvement usually is multilobar and predominately in the lower lobes. Cavitation is uncommon. Pleural effusion is common.

Pseudomonas Aeruginosa

Pneumonia caused by *P. aeruginosa* is the most common and most lethal form of nosocomial pulmonary infection (108). The organism is the cause of approximately 20% of nosocomial pneumonia in adult patients in the ICU (109). Many risk factors for the infection have been identified in this setting, including chronic obstructive pulmonary disease (COPD) (relative risk, 29.9), mechanical ventilation longer than 8 days (relative risk, 8.1), and prior use of antibiotics (relative risk, 5.5) (110). Risk factors noted in other studies include the use of corticosteroids, malnutrition, and prolonged hospitalization (35).

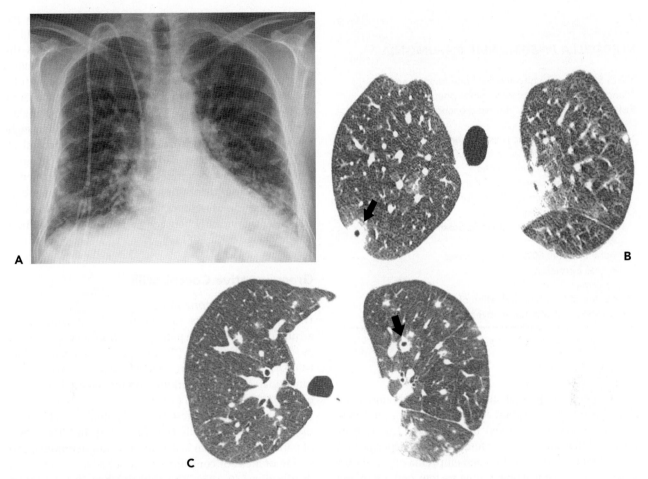

Figure 2.25 Septic embolism due to *Staphylococcus aureus*. Chest radiograph **(A)** shows numerous bilateral nodules of various sizes. Also noted is a central venous line. High-resolution computed tomography (CT) images at the level of the lung apices **(B)** and aortic arch **(C)** demonstrate bilateral cavitating (*arrows*) and noncavitating nodules. The patient was a 43-year-old man with positive blood cultures for *Staphylococcus aureus*.

Although *P. aeruginosa* pneumonia is generally a nosocomial infection, it is sometimes community acquired (111). The clinical presentation is typically abrupt, with chills, fever, severe dyspnea, and productive cough. Pleural pain is uncommon. The organism is an important cause of chronic airway colonization and pneumonia in patients who have cystic fibrosis.

The radiologic manifestations of *P. aeruginosa* pneumonia are usually those of bronchopneumonia, consisting of multifocal bilateral areas of consolidation (see Fig. 2.29 and Table 2.8) (112). These areas may be lobular, subsegmental, or segmental in distribution and patchy or confluent (112). The consolidation frequently involves all lobes (112), although it tends to involve predominantly the lower lobes. Less common radiographic manifestations include lobar consolidation with or without bulging fissure (see Fig. 2.30), multiple nodular opacities (see Fig. 2.31) (113), and (occasionally) a reticular pattern (112).

The reported incidence of abscess formation in acute *P. aeruginosa* pneumonia is variable (112, 114). In one review of 56 patients who had ventilator-associated

P. aeruginosa documented at bronchoscopy (112), 12 patients (23%) developed cavitation (in two, evident on CT scan but not on chest radiograph). The cavities may be small or large (112), may be single or multiple, and may have thin or thick walls (112). Pneumatocele formation was reported in 4 of 56 patients in one series (112).

Unilateral or bilateral pleural effusions, usually small, were identified on chest radiography in 16 (84%) of 19 patients in one early study (115) but in only 13 (23%) of 56 patients in a more recent series (112). Empyema is seen in a small percentage of cases (112); rarely, enlargement of the cardiopericardial silhouette occurs secondary to purulent pericarditis (116).

Winer-Muram et al. reviewed the radiographic manifestations of ventilator-associated *P. aeruginosa* pneumonia in 56 patients (112). In eight patients in whom CT scan was performed, CT scan results were compared with radiographic findings. Twenty-six patients with ARDS had diffuse bilateral confluent opacities; 30 patients without ARDS had multifocal opacities. In 13 patients, cavities were detected at chest radiography, CT scan, or both. Seven of

TABLE 2.6
KLEBSIELLA PNEUMONIAE PNEUMONIA

1% to 5% of community-acquired pneumonias and approximately 15% of nosocomial pneumonias

Risk factors: Alcoholism, chronic bronchopulmonary disease, ICU patients

Most common radiologic presentation
  Community-acquired pneumonia: Homogeneous lobar (nonsegmental) consolidation
  Nosocomial pneumonia: Multifocal unilateral (60%) or bilateral (40%) consolidation (bronchopneumonia)

Other common findings
  Bulging of interlobar fissures: Approximately 30% of patients
  Pleural effusion: 60% to 70% of cases
  Abscess formation
  Empyema

Main value of CT scan: Evaluation of patients with suspected cavitation or empyema

ICU, intensive care unit; CT, computed tomography.

29 patients with pleural abnormalities had empyema. CT scan provided important additional information (presence of cavities or effusions) in four cases. The authors concluded that the radiologic findings are nonspecific and that the frequencies of cavities and empyema of ventilator-associated *P. aeruginosa* pneumonia are low, perhaps owing to prompt diagnosis and therapy (112).

Shah et al. reviewed the CT scan findings in 28 patients with nosocomial *P. aeruginosa* pneumonia (117). All patients had consolidation; in 82% of patients the consolidation involved multiple lobes. Nodular opacities were present in 14 (50%), including centrilobular nodules and tree-in-bud pattern in 9 (64%) and larger, randomly distributed nodules in 5 (36%) patients. Ground-glass opacities were seen in nine (31%) and necrosis in eight (29%). Thirteen (46%) patients had bilateral pleural effusions and five (18%) had unilateral pleural effusions. Coexistent positive respiratory cultures were identified in 13 patients. The distribution of consolidation, frequency and distribution of nodules, and frequency of necrosis did not differ significantly between patients with and without other positive cultures (117).

Gram-negative Coccobacilli

Haemophilus Influenzae

H. influenzae accounts for 5% to 20% of community-acquired pneumonias in patients in whom an organism can be identified successfully (79,118,119). Risk factors include COPD (120), alcoholism, diabetes mellitus, anatomic or functional asplenia, immunoglobulin defect (121, 122), old age (123), and AIDS (124).

The radiologic manifestations of pulmonary *H. influenzae* infection are variable (see Table 2.9). In 50% to 60% of patients, the pattern is that of bronchopneumonia, consisting of areas of consolidation in a patchy or segmental distribution (79, 125). The consolidation may be unilateral or bilateral and tends to involve mainly the lower

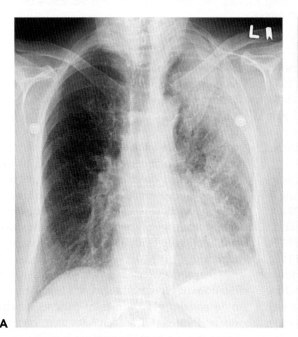
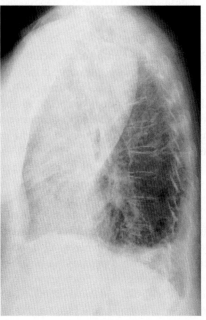

A   B

Figure 2.26 Lobar pneumonia due to *Klebsiella pneumoniae*. Posteroanterior **(A)** and lateral **(B)** chest radiographs show extensive left upper lobe consolidation and small left pleural effusion. The patient was a 73-year-old woman with *K. pneumoniae* pneumonia.

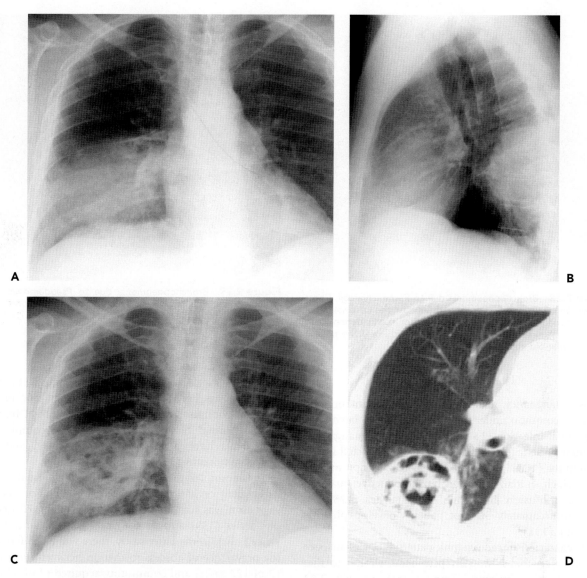

Figure 2.27 *Klebsiella pneumoniae* pneumonia and abscess formation. Posteroanterior **(A)** and lateral **(B)** chest radiographs show dense area of consolidation in right lower lobe. Chest radiograph **(C)** and 5-mm collimation computed tomography (CT) scan of the right lung **(D)** 3 days later demonstrate abscess formation and multiple cavities. The patient was a 53-year-old man with *K. pneumoniae* pneumonia.

lobes (79, 125). In 30% to 50% of patients, the pattern is that of lobar consolidation similar to that of *S. pneumoniae*; this pattern may be seen alone or in combination with a pattern of bronchopneumonia (79, 125). A small nodular or reticulonodular pattern, by itself or in combination with airspace consolidation, occurs in 15% to 30% of cases (see Fig. 2.32) (79, 125). High-resolution CT scan in these patients shows a diffuse micronodular pattern with numerous bilateral centrilobular nodules measuring <5 mm in diameter (Fig. 2.32) (126). This pattern reflects the presence of cellular bronchiolitis (126). Cavitation has been reported in 15% or less of cases (79, 125) and pleural effusion in approximately 50% (125, 127); empyema is uncommon.

Legionella Species

The precise incidence of *L. pneumophila* pneumonia (Legionnaires disease) is unknown. Prospective studies on consecutive patients hospitalized with pneumonia show an incidence of 2% to 25% (128, 129). Among patients who have nosocomial pneumonia, the reported incidence of *Legionella* species has varied from 1% to 40% (129). In our experience *Legionella* pneumonia is relatively uncommon, accounting for <5% of patients hospitalized with community-acquired pneumonia and <5% of cases of nosocomial pneumonia.

Legionnaires disease shows a propensity for older men, the male-to-female ratio being of the order of 2 or 3:1 (130). Most cases occur in patients with preexisting

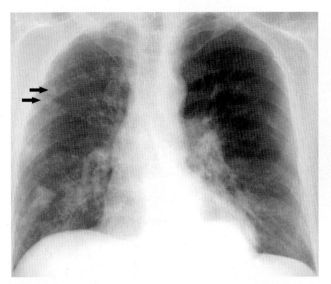

Figure 2.28 Bronchopneumonia due to *Escherichia coli*. Chest radiograph shows poorly defined nodular opacities (*arrows*) in the right upper lobe and small bilateral foci of consolidation. Also noted is a large hiatus hernia with an air–fluid level. The patient was a 37-year-old man with *E. coli* pneumonia.

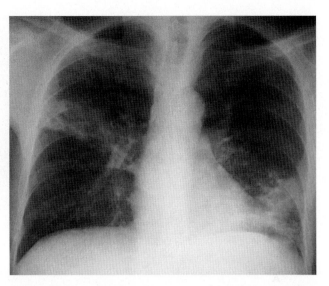

Figure 2.29 Bronchopneumonia due to *Pseudomonas*. Chest radiograph shows patchy areas of consolidation and poorly defined nodular opacities in the right upper and left lower lobes. The patient was a 40-year-old man with *Pseudomonas* pneumonia.

disease. Malignancy, renal failure, and transplantation are the most common underlying conditions associated with nosocomial infection (131, 132); COPD and malignancy are often present in patients who become infected in the community (133). The usual presenting symptoms are fever; cough, initially dry and later productive; malaise; myalgia; confusion; headaches; and diarrhea (128, 129, 131). Approximately 30% of patients develop pleuritic chest pain (131).

The characteristic radiographic pattern is one of airspace consolidation that is initially peripheral, similar to that seen in acute *S. pneumoniae* pneumonia (see Fig. 2.33 and Table 2.10). In many cases, the area of consolidation subsequently enlarges to occupy all or a large portion of a lobe (lobar pneumonia) or to involve contiguous lobes or to become bilateral (134–136). Progression of the pneumonia usually is rapid (134), most of a lobe becoming involved within 3 or 4 days, often despite the institution of appropriate antibiotic therapy (137). No difference has been found in the radiographic findings between community-acquired and nosocomial infection in the normal host (128, 136); immunocompromised individuals have a high rate of cavitation and hilar lymphadenopathy (138).

In immunocompetent patients, abscess formation with subsequent cavitation is infrequent (139). For example, cavitation was identified in only 3 (4%) of 70 cases in one series (139) and 9 (6%) of 154 cases in a second series (136). In the latter study, there was no difference in the prevalence of abscess formation between nosocomial (7 of 122 cases) and community-acquired (2 of 32 cases) pneumonia (136). By contrast, cavitation is seen commonly

---

TABLE 2.7

ESCHERICHIA COLI PNEUMONIA

4% of community-acquired pneumonias and 5% to 20% of nosocomial pneumonias
Risk factors: Debilitated patients
Most common radiologic presentation
    Multifocal unilateral or bilateral consolidation
    (bronchopneumonia)
Other common finding
    Pleural effusion

TABLE 2.8

PSEUDOMONAS AERUGINOSA PNEUMONIA

20% of nosocomial pneumonias
Risk factors: COPD, mechanical ventilation, prior use of
    antibiotics
Most common radiologic presentation
    Multifocal bilateral consolidation (bronchopneumonia)
    Commonly involves all lobes
    CT scan commonly shows centrilobular nodules and
    tree-in-bud pattern
Other common findings
    Abscess formation: Approximately 20% of cases
    Pleural effusion: Approximately 60% of cases

COPD, chronic obstructive pulmonary disease; CT, computed tomography.

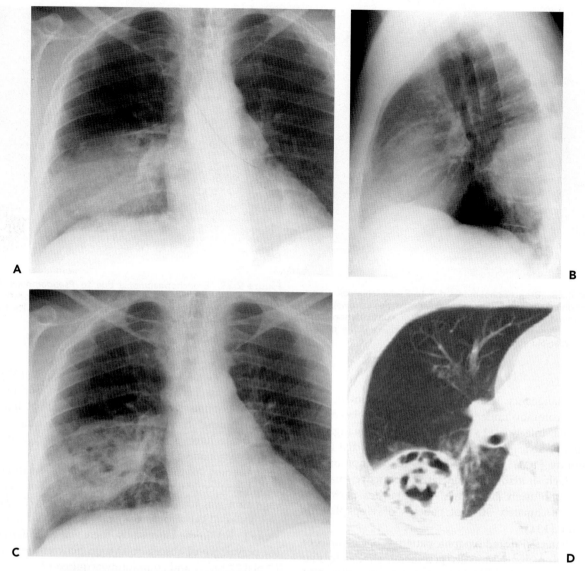

Figure 2.27 *Klebsiella pneumoniae* pneumonia and abscess formation. Posteroanterior **(A)** and lateral **(B)** chest radiographs show dense area of consolidation in right lower lobe. Chest radiograph **(C)** and 5-mm collimation computed tomography (CT) scan of the right lung **(D)** 3 days later demonstrate abscess formation and multiple cavities. The patient was a 53-year-old man with *K. pneumoniae* pneumonia.

lobes (79, 125). In 30% to 50% of patients, the pattern is that of lobar consolidation similar to that of *S. pneumoniae*; this pattern may be seen alone or in combination with a pattern of bronchopneumonia (79, 125). A small nodular or reticulonodular pattern, by itself or in combination with airspace consolidation, occurs in 15% to 30% of cases (see Fig. 2.32) (79, 125). High-resolution CT scan in these patients shows a diffuse micronodular pattern with numerous bilateral centrilobular nodules measuring <5 mm in diameter (Fig. 2.32) (126). This pattern reflects the presence of cellular bronchiolitis (126). Cavitation has been reported in 15% or less of cases (79, 125) and pleural effusion in approximately 50% (125, 127); empyema is uncommon.

Legionella Species

The precise incidence of *L. pneumophila* pneumonia (Legionnaires disease) is unknown. Prospective studies on consecutive patients hospitalized with pneumonia show an incidence of 2% to 25% (128, 129). Among patients who have nosocomial pneumonia, the reported incidence of *Legionella* species has varied from 1% to 40% (129). In our experience *Legionella* pneumonia is relatively uncommon, accounting for <5% of patients hospitalized with community-acquired pneumonia and <5% of cases of nosocomial pneumonia.

Legionnaires disease shows a propensity for older men, the male-to-female ratio being of the order of 2 or 3:1 (130). Most cases occur in patients with preexisting

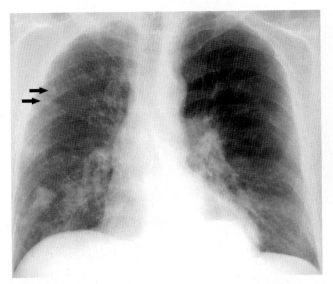

Figure 2.28   Bronchopneumonia due to *Escherichia coli*. Chest radiograph shows poorly defined nodular opacities (*arrows*) in the right upper lobe and small bilateral foci of consolidation. Also noted is a large hiatus hernia with an air–fluid level. The patient was a 37-year-old man with *E. coli* pneumonia.

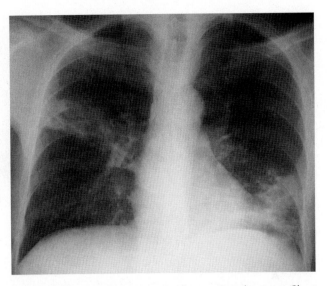

Figure 2.29   Bronchopneumonia due to *Pseudomonas*. Chest radiograph shows patchy areas of consolidation and poorly defined nodular opacities in the right upper and left lower lobes. The patient was a 40-year-old man with *Pseudomonas* pneumonia.

disease. Malignancy, renal failure, and transplantation are the most common underlying conditions associated with nosocomial infection (131, 132); COPD and malignancy are often present in patients who become infected in the community (133). The usual presenting symptoms are fever; cough, initially dry and later productive; malaise; myalgia; confusion; headaches; and diarrhea (128, 129, 131). Approximately 30% of patients develop pleuritic chest pain (131).

The characteristic radiographic pattern is one of airspace consolidation that is initially peripheral, similar to that seen in acute *S. pneumoniae* pneumonia (see Fig. 2.33 and Table 2.10). In many cases, the area of consolidation subsequently enlarges to occupy all or a large portion of a lobe (lobar pneumonia) or to involve contiguous lobes or to become bilateral (134–136). Progression of the pneumonia usually is rapid (134), most of a lobe becoming involved within 3 or 4 days, often despite the

institution of appropriate antibiotic therapy (137). No difference has been found in the radiographic findings between community-acquired and nosocomial infection in the normal host (128, 136); immunocompromised individuals have a high rate of cavitation and hilar lymphadenopathy (138).

In immunocompetent patients, abscess formation with subsequent cavitation is infrequent (139). For example, cavitation was identified in only 3 (4%) of 70 cases in one series (139) and 9 (6%) of 154 cases in a second series (136). In the latter study, there was no difference in the prevalence of abscess formation between nosocomial (7 of 122 cases) and community-acquired (2 of 32 cases) pneumonia (136). By contrast, cavitation is seen commonly

TABLE 2.7
ESCHERICHIA COLI PNEUMONIA

4% of community-acquired pneumonias and 5% to 20% of nosocomial pneumonias
Risk factors: Debilitated patients
Most common radiologic presentation
  Multifocal unilateral or bilateral consolidation (bronchopneumonia)
Other common finding
  Pleural effusion

TABLE 2.8
PSEUDOMONAS AERUGINOSA PNEUMONIA

20% of nosocomial pneumonias
Risk factors: COPD, mechanical ventilation, prior use of antibiotics
Most common radiologic presentation
  Multifocal bilateral consolidation (bronchopneumonia)
  Commonly involves all lobes
  CT scan commonly shows centrilobular nodules and tree-in-bud pattern
Other common findings
  Abscess formation: Approximately 20% of cases
  Pleural effusion: Approximately 60% of cases

COPD, chronic obstructive pulmonary disease; CT, computed tomography.

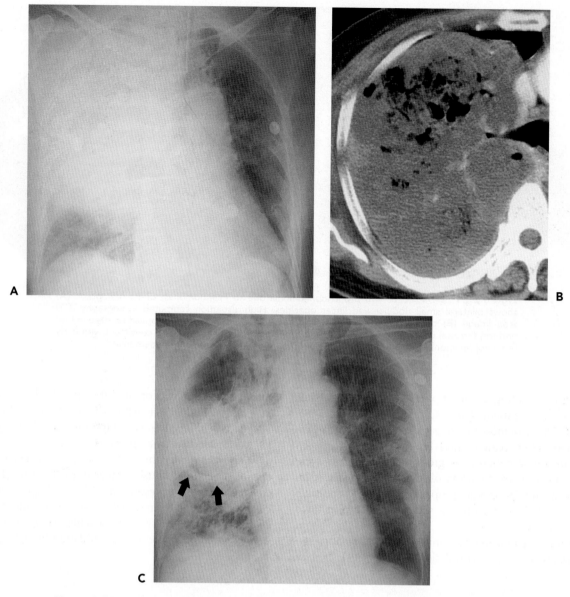

Figure 2.30 Severe pneumonia due to *Pseudomonas*. Chest radiograph **(A)** shows dense right upper lobe consolidation with bulging of the right minor fissure. View of the right lung from a contrast-enhanced computed tomography (CT) scan **(B)** shows low attenuation and decreased vascularity of the right lung consistent with necrotizing pneumonia and contralateral shift of the mediastinum. Chest radiograph 1 week later **(C)** demonstrates large right upper lobe cavity immediately above the level of the bulging minor fissure (*arrows*). The patient was a 49-year-old man with *Pseudomonas* pneumonia.

in immunocompromised patients (140, 141). In one series of 10 patients who had received renal transplants, cavitation was identified in 7, the interval between the first evidence of infection and cavitation ranging from 4 to 14 days (142). Pleural effusion may occur at the peak of the illness; it was described in 35% to 63% of cases in two series (131, 135).

Occasionally, the focus of *Legionella* pneumonia is round or oval, simulating a mass (round pneumonia) (see Fig. 2.34) (143). Single or multiple nodules, which sometimes undergo rapid growth, may be seen in addition

to consolidation involving part or all of one or more lobes (144). Most investigators have found the radiographic pattern associated with infection by various *Legionella* species to be similar to that of *L. pneumophila* (145–147).

In most patients with *Legionella* pneumonia, the diagnosis of pneumonia can be made on the basis of the clinical and radiographic findings, and CT scan adds little additional information. CT scan may be helpful, however, in patients with complicated pneumonia and in patients with normal or nonspecific radiographic findings. In one study of eight patients with mild *Legionella* pneumonia, the

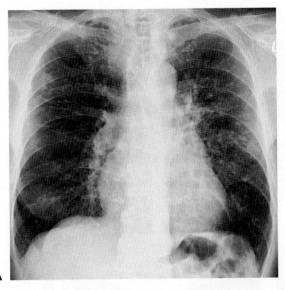
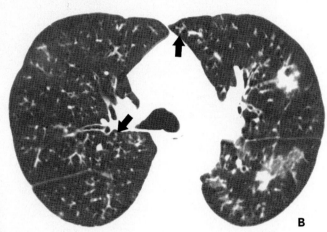

Figure 2.31 Bronchiolitis and bronchopneumonia due to *Pseudomonas*. Chest radiograph **(A)** shows bilateral small nodular and linear opacities. High-resolution computed tomography (CT) scan image **(B)** demonstrates centrilobular small nodular and branching opacities (tree-in-bud pattern) (*arrows*) consistent with bronchiolitis and small foci of consolidation consistent with early bronchopneumonia. The patient was a 68-year-old man with *Pseudomonas* pneumonia.

main clinical finding was fever of no >38 degrees Celsius; only 4 of the 8 patients had respiratory symptoms (148). Chest CT scan demonstrated peripheral airspace consolidation in seven patients and ground-glass opacities in seven; in 6 of 7 patients the ground-glass opacities were located adjacent to the areas of consolidation. The consolidation and ground-glass opacities involved multiple segments. Pleural effusion was seen on CT scan in three patients (148).

Pulmonary abnormalities may persist long after the acute phase of Legionnaires disease (138, 149). In one study of 122 survivors of an outbreak of Legionnaires disease among individuals who visited a flower exhibition, 57% still had respiratory symptoms including dyspnea 13 to 19 months after recovery from *Legionella* pneumonia (149). Thirty-three of these patients had reduced carbon monoxide diffusing capacity of the lung (DLCO) and underwent high-resolution CT scan. High-resolution CT scan demonstrated residual parenchymal abnormalities in 21 patients including linear opacities in all 21 patients, subsegmental or segmental consolidation in eight (38%),

---

TABLE 2.9
***HAEMOPHILUS INFLUENZAE* PNEUMONIA**

5% to 20% of community-acquired pneumonias
Risk factors: COPD, alcoholism, old age
Most common radiologic presentation
    50% to 60%: Patchy unilateral or bilateral consolidation (bronchopneumonia)
    30% to 40%: Homogeneous lobar (nonsegmental) consolidation
Less common findings:
    Small nodular pattern with tree-in-bud pattern on CT scan
    Spherical consolidation (round pneumonia)
    Cavitation: Up to 15% of cases
    Pleural effusion: 50% of cases

COPD, chronic obstructive pulmonary disease; CT, computed tomography.

TABLE 2.10
***LEGIONELLA PNEUMOPHILA* PNEUMONIA (LEGIONNAIRES DISEASE)**

2% to 25% of community-acquired pneumonias requiring hospitalization
Risk factors: Elderly, man, malignancy, organ transplantation
Most common radiologic presentation
    Homogeneous lobar (nonsegmental) consolidation
    Progresses to involve multiple lobes
Less common findings:
    Spherical consolidation (round pneumonia)
    Single or multiple nodular or mass-like areas of consolidation
Complications:
    Cavitation: particularly in immunocompromised patients
    Hilar lymphadenopathy: In immunocompromised patients
    Pleural effusion: 35% to 60% of cases

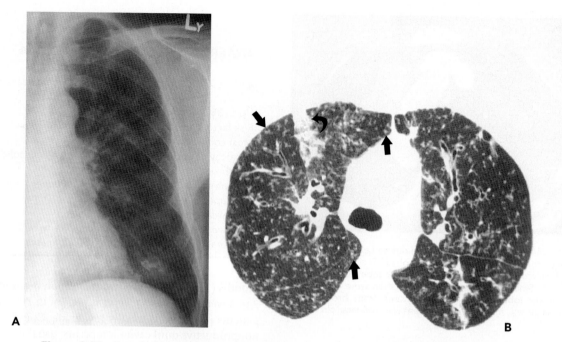

Figure 2.32 Bronchiolitis and bronchopneumonia due to *Haemophilus influenza*. View of the left lung from chest radiograph **(A)** shows poorly defined small nodular opacities. High-resolution computed tomography (CT) image at the level of the tracheal carina **(B)** demonstrates centrilobular nodules (*straight arrows*) consistent with bronchiolitis and lobular areas of consolidation (*curved arrow*) reflecting the presence of bronchopneumonia. The patient was a 50-year-old man with *H. influenza* pneumonia.

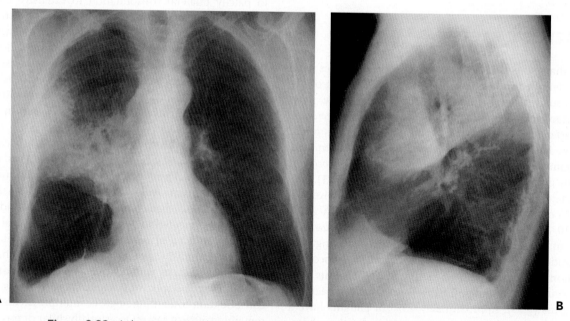

Figure 2.33 Lobar pneumonia due to *Legionella pneumophila*. Posteroanterior **(A)** and lateral **(B)** chest radiographs show right upper lobe consolidation and small right pleural effusion. The patient was a 77-year-old man with *legionella* pneumonia.

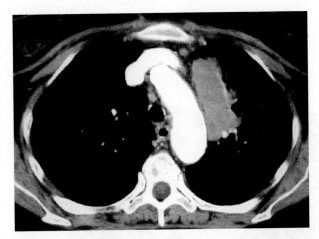

Figure 2.34 Mass-like consolidation due to *Legionella micdadei* Contrast-enhanced computed tomography (CT) scan image shows dense focal consolidation in the left upper lobe adjacent to the aortic arch. Small focal areas of consolidation were also present in the lower lobes (not shown). Cultures from bronchoscopy specimens grew *L. micdadei*. The patient was a 66-year-old woman.

bronchiectasis or bronchiolectasis in seven (33%), and cysts in four (19%). The need for mechanical ventilation during the acute phase of Legionnaires disease, delayed initiation of adequate antibiotic therapy, and COPD were identified as risk factors for the persistence of lung abnormalities (149).

ANAEROBIC BACTERIA

More than 30 genera and 200 species of anaerobes have been identified in human infection; such infection of the lung usually is polymicrobial (150). Among the most important agents are the gram-negative bacilli *Bacteroides*, *Fusobacterium*, *Porphyromonas*, and *Prevotella*; the gram-positive bacilli *Actinomyces*, *Eubacterium*, and *Clostridium*; the gram-positive cocci *Peptostreptococcus* and *Peptococcus*; and the gram-negative cocci *Veillonella* (42, 151–153).

Anaerobic bacteria are isolated in approximately 20% to 35% of all patients admitted to hospital with pneumonia (30, 154) and are second only to *S. pneumoniae* as a cause of community-acquired pneumonia requiring hospitalization (11). They also are important in nosocomial infection; for example, in one study of 159 patients with nosocomial pneumonia 59 (35%) were due to anaerobic organisms (155). Approximately 25% of patients have a history of impaired consciousness associated with such factors as general anesthesia, acute cerebrovascular accident, epileptic seizure, drug ingestion, or alcoholism (156, 157). The clinical features of anaerobic pulmonary infection are variable, ranging from simple aspiration to acute, severe, necrotizing pneumonias to chronic infections presenting as lung abscess or empyema (158). The clinical symptoms may be acute with fever, cough, and pleuritic chest pain resembling *S. pneumoniae* pneumonia (159) or may have an insidious protracted course over several weeks or even

TABLE 2.11

ANAEROBIC BACTERIAL PNEUMONIA

20% to 35% of community-acquired pneumonias requiring hospitalization
Up to 35% of nosocomial pneumonias
Risk factors: Impaired consciousness of any cause
Most common radiologic presentation
  Patchy or confluent unilateral or bilateral consolidation (bronchopneumonia)
  Involves mainly posterior segment of upper lobe and superior segment of lower lobe
Complications:
  Abscess formation and cavitation: 20% to 60% of cases
  Pleural effusion and empyema: 50% of cases

months (11). Overall, the mean duration is approximately 2 to 3 weeks (160, 161). Fever is present in 70% to 80% of patients (157) but is usually low grade. Cough is initially nonproductive until cavitation occurs, usually 7 to 10 days or more after the onset of pneumonia (11, 156); in 40% to 75% of cases the expectoration is putrid (157, 160). Foul-smelling sputum always indicates the presence of anaerobic organisms (11).

The radiographic pattern is that of bronchopneumonia ranging from localized segmental areas of consolidation to patchy bilateral consolidation to extensive confluent multilobar consolidation (see Table 2.11). The distribution of pneumonia from aspiration of material contaminated by anaerobic organisms reflects gravitational flow. The posterior segments of the upper lobes or superior segments of the lower lobes tend to be involved with aspiration in the recumbent position and the basal segments of the lower lobes are involved when aspiration occurs in an erect patient (see Figs. 2.35 and 2.36) (61, 160).

Cavitation has been reported in 20% to 60% of cases (see Fig. 2.37) (159, 162). In one study of 69 patients, approximately 50% had pulmonary parenchymal abnormalities, 30% had empyema without apparent parenchymal abnormalities, and 20% had combined parenchymal and pleural disease at presentation (162). The parenchymal abnormalities consisted of consolidation without cavitation in approximately 50% of cases and lung abscess (defined as a circumscribed cavity with relatively little surrounding consolidation) or necrotizing pneumonia (defined as areas of consolidation containing single or multiple cavities) in the remaining 50% of cases. Occasionally, hilar or mediastinal lymph node enlargement is associated with an abscess, a combination of findings that may resemble that seen in patients who have pulmonary carcinoma (163).

NOCARDIA SP

Nocardia are aerobic gram-positive bacilli found in the soil and distributed throughout the world (57). The most

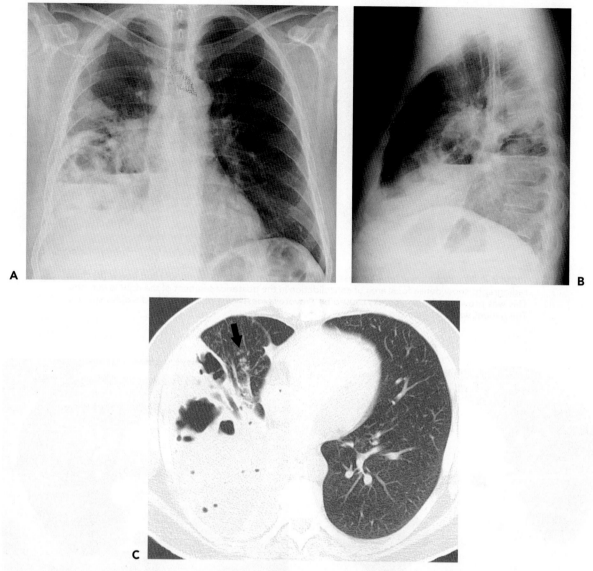

Figure 2.35 Necrotizing right lower lobe pneumonia due to anaerobes. Posteroanterior **(A)** and lateral **(B)** chest radiographs show areas of consolidation and several air–fluid levels within the right lower lobe. Less extensive consolidation is evident in the right middle lobe. Computed tomography (CT) image **(C)** confirms the radiographic findings and also demonstrates a few centrilobular nodules in the right middle lobe (*arrow*). The patient was a 50-year-old man with pneumonia due to anaerobic organisms.

common pathogen is *N. asteroides*, which accounts for approximately 80% of pulmonary infections; less common pathogens are *N. brasiliensis* and *N. otitidiscaviarum* (57) Nocardiosis is more common in men than in women (male-to-female ratio 2:1 to 3:1) and in immunocompromised patients, particularly those with lymphoma (164, 165), those who have undergone organ transplant (166, 167), those on corticosteroid therapy (168) and those with AIDS (169) but can also produce infection in patients with no concurrent abnormality (168).

The most common clinical symptoms are low-grade fever, productive cough, and weight loss often with exacerbations and remissions over periods of days to weeks (57). In most cases the clinical course is chronic,

with a duration of symptoms before diagnosis of 3 weeks or more (168).

The most frequent radiographic manifestation of pulmonary nocardiosis consists of homogeneous nonsegmental airspace consolidation that is usually peripheral, abuts the adjacent pleura, and is often extensive (see Table 2.12) (57,92,170). Less commonly the consolidation may be patchy and inhomogeneous (see Fig. 2.38) (92). The consolidation tends to involve multiple lobes and shows no predilection for the lower lobes (170). Multifocal peripheral nodules or masses with irregular margins may also be seen (171, 172). Cavitation is common, seen in one third or more of patients, and may occur within areas of consolidation, nodular opacities, or masses (see

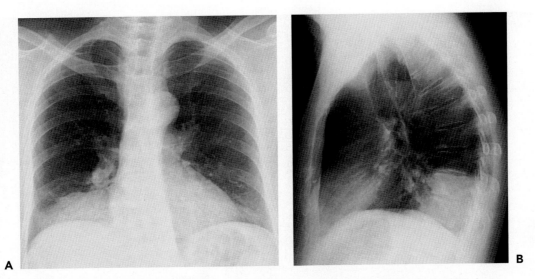

Figure 2.36 Right lower lobe abscess due to anaerobes. Posteroanterior **(A)** and lateral **(B)** chest radiographs show dense focal area of consolidation in the posterior segment of the right lower lobe. This was proved to be an abscess caused by *Prevotella loescheii* a pigmented bacteroides species. The patient was a 61-year-old man.

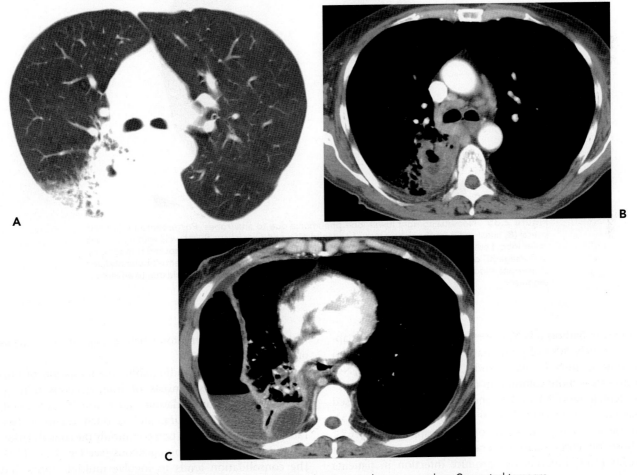

Figure 2.37 Right lower lobe pneumonia and empyema due to anaerobes. Computed tomography (CT) image (5-mm collimation) at the level of the main bronchi photographed at lung windows **(A)** shows right lower lobe consolidation and cavitation consistent with abscess formation. CT scan image photographed at mediastinal windows **(B)** better demonstrates the right lower lobe abscess. Also noted are several normal-sized paratracheal lymph nodes. CT image at a more caudal level **(C)** shows right empyema. The air–fluid level was related to the presence of a chest tube (not shown). Cultures grew various species of anaerobes. The patient was a 57-year-old woman.

TABLE 2.12
NOCARDIA ASTEROIDES PNEUMONIA

Uncommon
Risk factors: Male, immunocompromised patients
Most common radiologic presentation
  Homogeneous peripheral multilobar (nonsegmental)
    consolidation
  CT scan frequently demonstrates localized areas of low
    attenuation within the consolidation due to abscess
    formation
Less common presentation
  Patchy unilateral or bilateral consolidation
    (bronchopneumonia)
  Multifocal irregular peripheral nodules or masses
Complications:
  Cavitation: 35% of cases
  Pleural effusion: Common

CT, computed tomography.

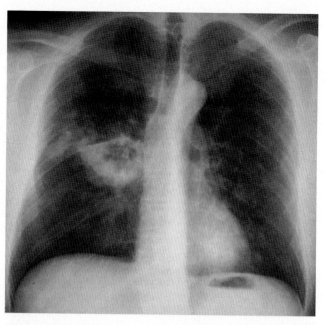

Figure 2.39 Bronchopneumonia and abscess formation due to *Nocardia*. Chest radiograph shows cavitating mass in the right hilar region and nodular opacities and foci of consolidation in the right upper lobe. The patient was a 52-year-old woman with proved pulmonary nocardiosis.

Figs. 2.38 and 2.39). In one series of 12 cases, cavitation was the most common radiographic manifestation, occurring within a consolidated lobe in three patients and within a solitary mass in four (173). Pleural effusion is common and empyema may occur (170). Evidence of chest wall involvement is seldom seen on the radiograph (92). Extension to the pericardium or mediastinum occurs occasionally (170, 174).

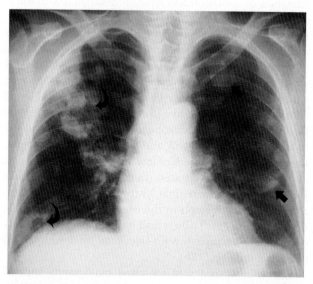

Figure 2.38 Bronchopneumonia and abscess formation due to *Nocardia*. Chest radiograph shows patchy areas of consolidation, focal nodular and mass-like opacities (*straight arrows*) and evidence of cavitation (*curved arrows*). The patient was a 58-year-old man with proved pulmonary nocardiosis. (Case courtesy of Dr. Jim Barrie, University of Alberta Medical Centre.)

CT scan may be helpful in assessing the extent of the disease and as a guide to obtain material for a definitive diagnosis (171, 172). In one review of the CT scan findings in five patients, the predominant abnormality consisted of multifocal areas of consolidation (172). Localized areas of low attenuation with rim enhancement suggestive of abscess formation were present within the areas of consolidation in three patients and cavitation in one patient. Variable sized pulmonary nodules were identified in three patients (see Fig. 2.40). Pleural involvement was present in all cases, including pleural effusion in four, empyema in one, and pleural thickening in four. Chest wall extension was identified in three patients.

ACTINOMYCES SP

Actinomyces sp. are anaerobic filamentous bacteria (57). The most common pathogen is *A. israelii*. The organism is a normal inhabitant of the human oropharynx and is frequently found in dental caries and at gingival margins of individuals who have poor oral hygiene (175). In most cases, the disease is believed to be acquired by the spread of organisms from these sites (11). Most patients are alcoholics (176).

Actinomycosis is a chronic granulomatous infection characterized by suppuration, sulfur granules, abscess formation, and sinus tracts (57). The initial clinical manifestations of pulmonary involvement are nonproductive cough and low-grade fever (11). With progression of the disease the cough becomes productive of purulent and, in

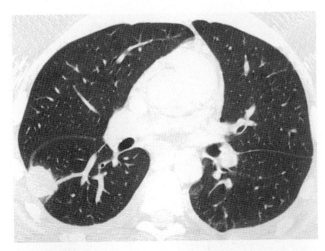

Figure 2.40 Right lower lobe nodule due to *Nocardia*. Computed tomography (CT) image shows right lower lobe nodule. Needle biopsy demonstrated *Nocardia*. The patient was a 42-year-old man.

TABLE 2.13

***ACTINOMYCES ISRAELII* PNEUMONIA**

Uncommon
Risk factors: Poor oral hygiene, alcoholism
Most common radiologic presentation
  Unilateral, peripheral, and patchy consolidation
  Mainly lower lobe
  CT scan frequently demonstrates areas of low
    attenuation within the consolidation due to abscess
    formation
  CT scan frequently demonstrates thickening of the
    pleura adjacent to the consolidation
Less common presentation
  Mass-like consolidation
Complications:
  Extension to the pleura with thickening, effusion, and
    empyema
  Extension to the mediastinum, pericardium and chest
    wall (uncommon)

CT, computed tomography.

---

many cases, blood-streaked sputum. Pleuritic chest pain commonly develops as the infection spreads to the pleura and chest wall (11).

The most characteristic radiographic manifestation of pulmonary actinomycosis consists of unilateral, peripheral, and patchy consolidation (see Fig. 2.41 and Table 2.13) (59, 176). The consolidation tends to involve mainly the lower lobes (176). Another common manifestation of pulmonary actinomycosis is as a mass, sometimes cavitated, that simulates pulmonary carcinoma (see Fig. 2.42) (92, 177). Patients with chronic pleuropulmonary actinomycosis may develop extensive fibrosis (92). Pleural effusion occasionally is the only radiographic manifestation (178). In patients with pulmonary actinomycosis pleural effusion usually represents empyema (see Fig. 2.43).

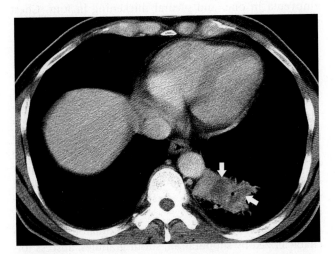

Figure 2.41 Left lower lobe consolidation and abscess due to actinomycosis. Image from contrast-enhanced computed tomography (CT) scan shows focal left lower lobe consolidation with foci of low attenuation (*arrows*) consistent with abscess formation. The patient was a 49-year-old man with pulmonary actinomycosis.

Mediastinal and pericardial involvement may occur but is uncommon (179). Chest wall involvement, frequently seen in the past, is now uncommon (59, 176). The manifestations of chest wall involvement include a soft tissue mass and rib abnormalities and are better seen on CT scan than on the radiograph (176, 180).

The characteristic manifestations of pulmonary actinomycosis on CT scan consist of focal or patchy areas of consolidation frequently containing central areas of low attenuation or cavitation and typically associated with thickening of the adjacent pleura (Figs. 2.41 and 2.42) (59, 176). Kwong et al. reviewed the chest radiographs and CT scans in eight patients with pulmonary actinomycosis (176). Airspace consolidation, seen on the radiograph and CT scan in all patients, was present in the lower lobes in seven patients (88%) and upper lobes in three (38%). Pleural effusion was present in five (62%). Pleural thickening adjacent to the airspace consolidation was identified on the radiograph in four (50%) and on CT scan in all eight. Cavitation or central areas of low attenuation not apparent on the radiograph were seen on the CT scan in five cases (62%). Hilar or mediastinal lymphadenopathy was identified on the radiograph in three cases (38%) and on the CT scan in six (75%). Chest wall invasion occurred in only one case (12%); there was no associated rib destruction or periosteal reaction (176).

Cheon et al. reviewed the chest radiographs and CT scans in 22 patients with pulmonary actinomycosis (59). In all patients the abnormalities were unilateral and had an average diameter of 6.5 cm (range, 2 to 12 cm). CT scan demonstrated patchy airspace consolidation ($n = 20$) or a mass ($n = 2$). Fifteen (75%) of the 20 patients with airspace

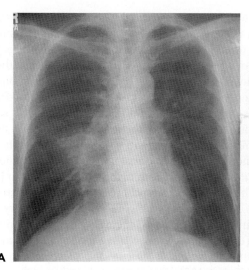
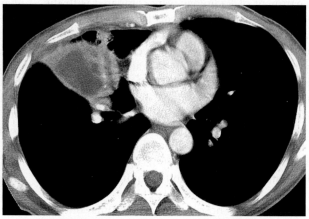

Figure 2.42   Right middle lobe abscess due to actinomycosis. Chest radiograph **(A)** shows a dense area of consolidation in the right middle lobe. Image from contrast-enhanced computed tomography (CT) scan **(B)** demonstrates large focal area of decreased attenuation within the right middle lobe consistent with abscess formation. The patient was a 40-year-old man with pulmonary actinomycosis.

consolidation had central areas of low attenuation within the consolidation. Thirteen of the 15 patients underwent contrast medium–enhanced CT scan. Ten (77%) of the 13 patients showed ring-like rim enhancement around the central areas of low attenuation. Focal pleural thickening adjacent to the areas of consolidation was seen in 16 patients (73%). Correlation of CT scan with histologic findings in patients who underwent lobectomy showed that the central low-attenuation areas in the CT scan represented abscesses with sulfur granules or a dilated bronchus that contained inflammatory cells and *Actinomyces* colonies.

Figure 2.43   Pneumonia and right empyema due to actinomycosis. Contrast-enhanced computed tomography (CT) scan image demonstrates focal areas of consolidation in the right middle lobe and lingula. Also noted are a loculated right pleural effusion, right pleural thickening, and enhancement (*arrows*), proved to be a right empyema due to actinomycosis. The left pleural effusion was shown to be a transudate. The patient was a 34-year-old man.

Peripheral enhancement of the low-attenuation areas represented the wall of the microabscess or increased vascularity within granulation tissue in the surrounding parenchyma (59).

CLINICAL UTILITY AND LIMITATIONS OF CHEST RADIOGRAPHY AND COMPUTED TOMOGRAPHY SCAN

A. Sensitivity and Specificity of Chest Radiography in the Detection of Pneumonia

In most patients with bacterial pulmonary infection, a confident diagnosis of pneumonia can be made on the basis of clinical, radiographic, and laboratory findings. The chest radiograph has a high sensitivity and specificity in the detection and exclusion of community-acquired pneumonia (78). It is currently believed that pulmonary opacities usually become visible radiographically within 12 hours after the onset of the symptoms of pneumonia (22). This time frame should allow detection of pulmonary abnormalities radiographically in most cases of community-acquired pneumonia (22). However, the interobserver agreement in the diagnosis of community-acquired pneumonia is only fair to good for experienced radiologists, and poor to fair for inexperienced radiologists and residents, respectively (181, 182). In one prospective multicenter study of 272 patients with suspected community-acquired pneumonia, two staff radiologists agreed on the presence of pulmonary abnormalities in 79% of patients and its absence in 6% (181). In a second study, a radiologic panel diagnosed pneumonia in 21 of 319 adult patients with acute respiratory infections (182). The agreements between the panel and three independent interpreters, two residents

in radiology, and one senior chest physician, were assessed. Also the reports given by the specialist in radiology at the Department of Radiology were compared with the panel's evaluation. The κ-agreements between the panel's interpretations and those by the Department of Radiology and the consultant in chest medicine were 0.71 and 0.72, respectively, and the corresponding κ-values between the residents and the panel was only 0.50. The proportion of agreement when pneumonia was diagnosed was 0.56 between the panel and the Department of Radiology, and 0.59 between the panel and the chest consultant, compared to 0.36 between the panel and the residents. These studies demonstrate the difficulty in recognizing the radiologic manifestations of community-acquired pneumonia and the importance of experience (182).

The recognition of nosocomial pneumonia on the chest radiograph is even more difficult than that of community-acquired pneumonia. These patients are often referred for chest radiography within hours of the onset of symptoms, a time in which they may not have any visible radiographic abnormality (22). Hospitalized patients are also likely to have decreased immune response that may further delay the development of radiographically visible opacities. These include particularly patients with severe neutropenia (53, 183). One group of investigators assessed 195 episodes of pneumonia in 175 consecutive patients who were neutropenic following antineoplastic chemotherapy (53). In these patients, 70 episodes of pneumonia were initially diagnosed clinically, in the absence of radiographically detectable disease. In 27 of the 70 episodes, parenchymal opacities were subsequently seen on follow-up chest radiography. In 25 of 57 patients with no radiographically detectable infiltrates, the diagnosis of pneumonia was established at autopsy (53). The authors found a positive correlation between the neutrophil count and the presence of radiographic abnormalities (53).

CT scan, particularly high-resolution CT scan, has a greater sensitivity than radiography in demonstrating the presence of pulmonary abnormalities. It can therefore be helpful in patients with suspected pneumonia and normal or questionable radiographic abnormalities (22, 54). High-resolution CT scan is particularly helpful in patients with neutropenia. Heussel et al. prospectively evaluated 87 patients with febrile neutropenia that persisted for >2 days despite empiric antibiotic treatment (54). The patients had a total of 146 prospective examinations. If findings on chest radiographs were normal ($n = 126$) or nonspecific ($n = 20$), high-resolution CT scan was performed. Findings on chest radiographs were nonspecific for pneumonia in 20 (14%) of 146 cases; high-resolution CT scan in all these 20 cases were suggestive of pneumonia. Microorganisms were detected in 11 of these 20 cases. In 70 (48%) of 146 cases the chest radiographs were normal but high-resolution CT scan showed findings suggestive of pneumonia. Microorganisms were detected in 30 of these 70 cases. In 22 (31%) of these 70 cases, an opacity was observed on the chest radiograph approximately 5 days after the CT scan study. Only 3 (5%)

of 56 pneumonias occurred within 7 days after a normal high-resolution CT scan ($p < 0.005$). The authors concluded that when high-resolution CT scan shows findings suggestive of pneumonia in patients with neutropenia, the probability of pneumonia being detected on chest radiographs during the 7-day follow-up is 31%, whereas the probability is only 5% if the findings on the prior CT scan are normal. On the basis of the results of their study, they recommended that all patients with neutropenia with fever of unknown origin and normal findings on chest radiographs should be examined with high-resolution CT scan (54).

The detection of nosocomial pneumonia is particularly difficult in patients with concomitant pulmonary abnormalities such as ARDS, edema, hemorrhage, interstitial lung disease, or atelectasis. These abnormalities may mimic pneumonia and also obscure the presence of pneumonia (22, 184, 185). Wunderink et al. evaluated the last chest radiograph prior to autopsy in 69 ventilated patients (185). Pneumonia was present in 24 (35%) of the 69 autopsies. Stepwise logistic regression analysis showed that the presence of air bronchograms was the only radiographic finding that correlated with pneumonia in the total group, correctly predicting 64% of pneumonias. In patients without ARDS, the presence of air bronchograms or areas of consolidation correlated with pneumonia, whereas in patients with ARDS, no radiographic finding correlated with the presence of pneumonia. In only 30% of cases was there an increase in the areas of consolidation as compared to prior radiographs due to pneumonia (185). Winer-Muram et al. assessed the diagnostic accuracy of bedside chest radiography for ARDS, pneumonia, or both in 40 patients receiving mechanical ventilation (184). Diagnosis of pneumonia was based on culture of specimens obtained by fiber-optic bronchoscopy with protected specimen brushing and BAL. The overall diagnostic accuracy was 0.84 for ARDS and 0.52 for pneumonia. Review of previous radiographs and knowledge of clinical data did not enhance diagnostic accuracy for ARDS or pneumonia. Presence of ARDS resulted in an increase in false-negative results because the diffuse areas of increased consolidation in ARDS obscured the radiographic features of pneumonia. The authors concluded that chest radiography is of limited value for the diagnosis of pneumonia in patients receiving mechanical ventilation.

CT scan is only slightly superior to radiography in the diagnosis of pneumonia in patients with ARDS (186). In one study CT scans were obtained within 1 week of bronchoscopic sampling in 31 patients receiving mechanical ventilation for ARDS (186). CT scans were rated for pneumonia independently by four radiologists who were unaware of the clinical diagnosis. The diagnostic accuracy was only fair, with only 70% true-negative ratings and 59% true-positive ratings. No single CT scan finding reliably identified the presence of pneumonia (186).

As noted in the preceding text, both radiography and CT scan have limitations in the diagnosis of pneumonia. The main value of and indications for CT scan are in the evaluation of patients with clinical suspicion of pneumonia

and normal or nonspecific radiographic findings, in the assessment of suspected complications of pneumonia or suspicion of an underlying lesion such as pulmonary carcinoma (22, 56). CT scan is also indicated in patients with persistent or recurrent pulmonary opacities (22). Several groups of investigators have shown that CT scan may demonstrate the presence of pneumonia in patients with normal radiographs and complications such as cavitation and empyema that may not be evident on the radiograph (48, 56).

B. Accuracy of Chest Radiography and CT Scan in Determining the Specific Etiology of Pneumonia

The distinction of bacterial from viral community-acquired pneumonias is important because it has therapeutic management implication. However, identification of a specific bacterial organism is less important because most recent therapeutic guidelines recommend combining antibiotic regimens covering both typical and atypical bacteria (22).

Chest radiography is of limited value in determining the specific etiology of pneumonia (47, 56, 187). Levy et al. assessed the value of initial noninvasive bacteriologic and radiologic investigations in 420 patients with community-acquired pneumonia (78). They demonstrated that segmental and lobar areas of consolidation were caused by bacteria in over 90% of cases, whereas most of the diffuse interstitial or mixed abnormalities were due to viral, atypical bacterial, or tuberculous infections. No finding allowed a specific diagnosis of any given organism. Fang et al. compared the radiographic, clinical, and laboratory features of typical bacterial pneumonia with the findings of patients with atypical bacterial pneumonia in a prospective study of 359 adults with community-acquired pneumonia, and found no parameters that could reliably differentiate these groups (188).

Tanaka et al. (48) assessed the value of high-resolution CT scan in the distinction of bacterial and atypical community-acquired pneumonia. The study included 32 patients, 18 with bacterial pneumonia and 14 with atypical pneumonia (mycoplasma pneumonia [$n = 12$], chlamydia pneumonia [$n = 1$], and influenza viral pneumonia [$n = 1$]). Bacterial pneumonia frequently presented with airspace consolidation and segmental distribution (72%) that tended to locate at the middle and outer zones of the lung. Atypical pneumonia frequently presented with centrilobular opacities (64%), airspace nodules (71%), airspace consolidation and ground-glass opacities in a lobular distribution (57% and 86%, respectively), and a tendency of the lesions to involve the inner third of the lung in addition to the middle and outer thirds (86%). There was, however, considerable overlap of the findings; no CT scan pattern allowed reliable distinction of bacterial from atypical pneumonia.

Tomiyama et al. (189) assessed the high-resolution CT scans of 90 immunocompetent patients with acute parenchymal lung diseases including 19 with bacterial pneumonia, 13 with mycoplasmal pneumonia, 21 with acute interstitial pneumonia, 18 with hypersensitivity pneumonitis, 10 with acute eosinophilic pneumonia, and 9 with pulmonary hemorrhage. Two independent observers made a correct first-choice diagnosis in an average of 55 (61%) of 90 cases. Correct first-choice diagnosis was made in 50% of cases of bacterial pneumonia and 62% of mycoplasmal pneumonia compared to 90% cases of acute interstitial pneumonia, 72% of hypersensitivity pneumonitis, 30% of acute eosinophilic pneumonia, and 28% of pulmonary hemorrhage. Overall, CT scan findings allowed distinction between infectious and noninfectious causes in 81 (90%) of 90 cases. Centrilobular branching structures were identified in 69% of patients with mycoplasmal pneumonia and 34% of patients with bacterial pneumonia, and were less commonly seen in the other diseases. Centrilobular nodules were found in most patients with mycoplasmal pneumonia (96% of interpretations), hypersensitivity pneumonitis (81% of interpretations), and bacterial pneumonia (61% of interpretations), and were found less commonly in the other entities. In patients with mycoplasmal pneumonia and bacterial pneumonia, the centrilobular nodules were patchy in distribution, whereas in patients with hypersensitivity pneumonitis they were diffuse. Segmental distribution was found in all patients with mycoplasmal pneumonia and in 76% of patients with bacterial pneumonia. A combination of airspace consolidation, centrilobular nodules, and segmental distribution was found in 85% of patients with mycoplasmal pneumonia, 45% of those with bacterial pneumonia, and in only a small percentage of cases with noninfectious acute pulmonary disease (189). These results suggest that in patients with acute lung disease the presence of centrilobular branching opacities (tree-in-bud pattern), patchy distribution of centrilobular nodules, segmental consolidation, or ground-glass opacities are highly suggestive of pneumonia but that there is considerable overlap between the CT scan findings of bacterial and mycoplasma pneumonia.

Reittner et al. (47) assessed the high-resolution CT scan findings in 114 patients with pneumonia, including 58 immunocompetent and 56 immunocompromised patients. The pneumonias were due to bacterial infection ($n = 35$), M. pneumoniae ($n = 28$), Pneumocystis ($n = 22$), fungi ($n = 20$), and viruses ($n = 9$). The bacterial pneumonias, only assessed in immunocompetent patients, were due to S. pneumoniae ($n = 14$), S. aureus ($n = 16$), P. aeruginosa ($n = 3$), or K. pneumoniae ($n = 2$). All Pneumocystis, fungal, and viral pneumonias in the study were in immunocompromised patients. The most common high-resolution CT scan manifestations of bacterial pneumonia were consolidation seen in 30 (85%) patients and ground-glass opacities seen in 11 (35%) patients. The consolidation had a segmental distribution in 24 (80%) and a nonsegmental distribution in 6 (20%). Lobular areas of consolidation were seen associated with segmental consolidation in 11 patients and centrilobular nodules in 6 patients. The ground-glass opacities had a nonsegmental distribution

and were usually seen adjacent to areas of consolidation. By comparison, airspace consolidation was seen in 22 of 28 (79%) patients and ground-glass opacities in 24 (86%) patients with *Mycoplasma* pneumonia. The consolidation in *Mycoplasma* pneumonia was nonsegmental in 15 (68%) and lobular or segmental in the remaining cases. The ground-glass opacities were nonsegmental in 13 (54%) patients and lobular in 11 (45%). Centrilobular nodules were present in 24 (96%) patients. Patients with *Pneumocystis* pneumonia were most likely to have ground-glass opacities (95% of cases) and least likely to have consolidation (9%) and centrilobular nodules (none in 22 patients). The ground-glass opacities in patients with *Pneumocystis* pneumonia were bilateral, symmetric, and extensive. The other types of pneumonia were associated with more focal areas of ground-glass opacities, usually adjacent to areas of airspace consolidation (47).

In the study by Reittner et al. (47) there was no significant difference in the prevalence of ground-glass opacities between bacterial, mycoplasmal, viral, and fungal pneumonias. In 11 of 24 (45%) patients with *M. pneumoniae* pneumonia the ground-glass opacities showed a lobular distribution. This distribution of ground-glass opacities was not seen in other forms of pneumonia. Small nodules were seen more commonly in patients with *M. pneumoniae* pneumonia (24 of 28 patients, 86%) than in bacterial pneumonias (6 of 35 patients, 17%; $p <0.01$, chi-square test), and were not seen in patients with *Pneumocystis* pneumonia. However, there was no significant difference in the prevalence of nodules between *M. pneumoniae* (25 of 28 patients, 89%), viral (7 of 9 patients, 78%), and fungal pneumonias (13 of 20 patients, 65%). The authors concluded that there is considerable overlap between the high-resolution CT scan features of the various types of pneumonia. The presence of extensive areas of ground-glass opacities with absence of airspace consolidation is highly suggestive of *Pneumocystis* pneumonia and the combination of centrilobular nodules and lobular areas of ground-glass opacities is most suggestive of *M. pneumoniae* pneumonia. Other causes of pneumonia could not be distinguished on the basis of pattern or distribution of abnormalities on high-resolution CT scan (47).

REFERENCES

1. Fine MJ, Auble TE, Yealy DM, et al. A prediction rule to identify low-risk patients with community-acquired pneumonia. *N Engl J Med.* 1997;336:243–250.
2. Marrie TJ, Peeling RW, Fine MJ, et al. Ambulatory patients with community-acquired pneumonia: The frequency of atypical agents and clinical course. *Am J Med.* 1996;101:508–515.
3. Fine MJ, Smith MA, Carson CA, et al. Prognosis and outcomes of patients with community-acquired pneumonia. A meta-analysis. *JAMA.* 1996;275:134–141.
4. Kaplan V, Angus DC, Griffin MF, et al. Hospitalized community-acquired pneumonia in the elderly: Age- and sex-related patterns of care and outcome in the United States. *Am J Respir Crit Care Med.* 2002;165:766–772.
5. Leeper KV Jr. Severe community-acquired pneumonia. *Semin Respir Infect.* 1996;11:96–108.
6. Craven DE, Steger KA. Nosocomial pneumonia in mechanically ventilated adult patients: Epidemiology and prevention in 1996. *Semin Respir Infect.* 1996;11:32–53.
7. Bassin AS, Niederman MS. New approaches to prevention and treatment of nosocomial pneumonia. *Semin Thorac Cardiovasc Surg.* 1995;7:70–77.
8. Hubmayr RD, Burchardi H, Elliot M, et al. Statement of the 4th International Consensus Conference in Critical Care on ICU-Acquired Pneumonia—Chicago, Illinois, May 2002. *Intensive Care Med.* 2002;28:1521–1536.
9. Alp E, Guven M, Yildiz O, et al. Incidence, risk factors and mortality of nosocomial pneumonia in intensive care units: A prospective study. *Ann Clin Microbiol Antimicrob.* 2004;3:17.
10. Heckerling PS, Tape TG, Wigton RS, et al. Clinical prediction rule for pulmonary infiltrates. *Ann Intern Med.* 1990;113:664–670.
11. Fraser RS, Colman N, Müller NL, et al. *Synopsis of diseases of the chest.* Philadelphia, PA: Elsevier Saunders; 2005.
12. Ewig S, Schlochtermeier M, Goke N, et al. Applying sputum as a diagnostic tool in pneumonia: Limited yield, minimal impact on treatment decisions. *Chest.* 2002;121:1486–1492.
13. Gleckman R, DeVita J, Hibert D, et al. Sputum gram stain assessment in community-acquired bacteremic pneumonia. *J Clin Microbiol.* 1988;26:846–849.
14. Chastre J, Fagon JY, Bornet-Lecso M, et al. Evaluation of bronchoscopic techniques for the diagnosis of nosocomial pneumonia. *Am J Respir Crit Care Med.* 1995;152:231–240.
15. Torres A, el-Ebiary M, Padro L, et al. Validation of different techniques for the diagnosis of ventilator-associated pneumonia. Comparison with immediate postmortem pulmonary biopsy. *Am J Respir Crit Care Med.* 1994;149:324–331.
16. Marquette CH, Copin MC, Wallet F, et al. Diagnostic tests for pneumonia in ventilated patients: Prospective evaluation of diagnostic accuracy using histology as a diagnostic gold standard. *Am J Respir Crit Care Med.* 1995;151:1878–1888.
17. Jourdain B, Joly-Guillou ML, Dombret MC, et al. Usefulness of quantitative cultures of BAL fluid for diagnosing nosocomial pneumonia in ventilated patients. *Chest.* 1997;111:411–418.
18. Meduri GU, Wunderink RG, Leeper KV, et al. Management of bacterial pneumonia in ventilated patients. Protected bronchoalveolar lavage as a diagnostic tool. *Chest.* 1992;101:500–508.
19. Scott JA, Hall AJ. The value and complications of percutaneous transthoracic lung aspiration for the etiologic diagnosis of community-acquired pneumonia. *Chest.* 1999;116:1716–1732.
20. Torres A, Jimenez P, Puig de la Bellacasa J, et al. Diagnostic value of nonfluoroscopic percutaneous lung needle aspiration in patients with pneumonia. *Chest.* 1990;98:840–844.
21. Ishida T, Hashimoto T, Arita M, et al. Efficacy of transthoracic needle aspiration in community-acquired pneumonia. *Intern Med.* 2001;40:873–877.
22. Herold CJ, Sailer JG. Community-acquired and nosocomial pneumonia. *Eur Radiol.* 2004;14(suppl 3):E2–20.
23. Sanchez-Nieto JM, Torres A, Garcia-Cordoba F, et al. Impact of invasive and noninvasive quantitative culture sampling on outcome of ventilator-associated pneumonia: A pilot study. *Am J Respir Crit Care Med.* 1998;157:371–376.
24. Dorca J, Manresa F, Esteban L, et al. Efficacy, safety, and therapeutic relevance of transthoracic aspiration with ultrathin needle in nonventilated nosocomial pneumonia. *Am J Respir Crit Care Med.* 1995;151:1491–1496.
25. Ruiz M, Ewig S, Marcos MA, et al. Etiology of community-acquired pneumonia: Impact of age, comorbidity, and severity. *Am J Respir Crit Care Med.* 1999;160:397–405.
26. Woodhead M. Community-acquired pneumonia in Europe: Causative pathogens and resistance patterns. *Eur Respir J Suppl.* 2002;36:20s–27s.
27. Macfarlane J. An overview of community acquired pneumonia with lessons learned from the British Thoracic Society Study. *Semin Respir Infect.* 1994;9:153–165.
28. Maartens G, Lewis SJ, de Goveia C, et al. 'Atypical' bacteria are a common cause of community-acquired pneumonia in hospitalised adults. *S Afr Med J.* 1994;84:678–682.
29. Porath A, Schlaeffer F, Lieberman D. The epidemiology of community-acquired pneumonia among hospitalized adults. *J Infect.* 1997;34:41–48.
30. Kato T, Uemura H, Murakami N, et al. Incidence of anaerobic infections among patients with pulmonary diseases: Japanese experience with transtracheal aspiration and immediate bedside anaerobic inoculation. *Clin Infect Dis.* 1996;23(suppl 1):S87–S96.
31. Soler N, Torres A, Ewig S, et al. Bronchial microbial patterns in severe exacerbations of Chronic Obstructive Pulmonary Disease (COPD) requiring mechanical ventilation. *Am J Respir Crit Care Med.* 1998;157:1498–1505.
32. El-Solh AA, Sikka P, Ramadan F, et al. Etiology of severe pneumonia in the very elderly. *Am J Respir Crit Care Med.* 2001;163:645–651.
33. Leroy O, Santre C, Beuscart C, et al. A five-year study of severe community-acquired pneumonia with emphasis on prognosis in patients admitted to an intensive care unit. *Intensive Care Med.* 1995;21:24–31.
34. Leroy O, Vandenbussche C, Coffinier C, et al. Community-acquired aspiration pneumonia in intensive care units. Epidemiological and prognosis data. *Am J Respir Crit Care Med.* 1997;156:1922–1929.
35. Hospital-acquired pneumonia in adults: Diagnosis, assessment of severity, initial antimicrobial therapy, and preventive strategies. A consensus statement, American Thoracic Society, November 1995. *Am J Respir Crit Care Med.* 1996;153:1711–1725.
36. Craven DE, Steger KA. Epidemiology of nosocomial pneumonia. New perspectives on an old disease. *Chest.* 1995;108:1S–16S.

37. Baker AM, Meredith JW, Haponik EF. Pneumonia in intubated trauma patients. Microbiology and outcomes. *Am J Respir Crit Care Med.* 1996;153:343–349.

38. Chastre J, Trouillet JL, Vuagnat A, et al. Nosocomial pneumonia in patients with acute respiratory distress syndrome. *Am J Respir Crit Care Med.* 1998;157:1165–1172.

39. Craven DE. Epidemiology of ventilator-associated pneumonia. *Chest.* 2000;117:186S–187S.

40. Markowicz P, Wolff M, Djedaini K, et al. ARDS Study Group. Multicenter prospective study of ventilator-associated pneumonia during acute respiratory distress syndrome. Incidence, prognosis, and risk factors. *Am J Respir Crit Care Med.* 2000;161:1942–1948.

41. Andrews CP, Coalson JJ, Smith JD, et al. Diagnosis of nosocomial bacterial pneumonia in acute, diffuse lung injury. *Chest.* 1981;80:254–258.

42. Dore P, Robert R, Grollier G, et al. Incidence of anaerobes in ventilator-associated pneumonia with use of a protected specimen brush. *Am J Respir Crit Care Med.* 1996;153:1292–1298.

43. Talon D, Mulin B, Rouget C, et al. Risks and routes for ventilator-associated pneumonia with Pseudomonas aeruginosa. *Am J Respir Crit Care Med.* 1998;157:978–984.

44. Trouillet JL, Chastre J, Vuagnat A, et al. Ventilator-associated pneumonia caused by potentially drug-resistant bacteria. *Am J Respir Crit Care Med.* 1998;157:531–539.

45. Nelson KE, Larson PA, Schraufnagel DE, et al. Transmission of tuberculosis by flexible fiberbronchoscopes. *Am Rev Respir Dis.* 1983;127:97–100.

46. Müller NL, Fraser RS, Lee KS, et al. *Diseases of the lung: Radiologic and pathologic correlations.* Philadelphia, PA: Lippincott Williams & Wilkins; 2003.

47. Reittner P, Ward S, Heyneman L, et al. Pneumonia: High-resolution CT findings in 114 patients. *Eur Radiol.* 2003;13:515–521.

48. Tanaka N, Matsumoto T, Kuramitsu T, et al. High resolution CT findings in community-acquired pneumonia. *J Comput Assist Tomogr.* 1996;20:600–608.

49. Franquet T. Imaging of pneumonia: Trends and algorithms. *Eur Respir J.* 2001;18:196–208.

50. Itoh H, Tokunaga S, Asamoto H, et al. Radiologic-pathologic correlations of small lung nodules with special reference to peribronchiolar nodules. *Am J Roentgenol.* 1978;130:223–231.

51. Macfarlane J, Rose D. Radiographic features of staphylococcal pneumonia in adults and children. *Thorax.* 1996;51:539–540.

52. Fraser RS, Müller NL, Colman N, et al. *Diagnosis of diseases of the chest.* Philadelphia, PA: WB Saunders; 1999.

53. Zornoza J, Goldman AM, Wallace S, et al. Radiologic features of gram-negative pneumonias in the neutropenic patient. *Am J Roentgenol.* 1976;127:989–996.

54. Heussel CP, Kauczor HU, Heussel G, et al. Early detection of pneumonia in febrile neutropenic patients: Use of thin-section CT. *Am J Roentgenol.* 1997;169:1347–1353.

55. Janzen DL, Padley SP, Adler BD, et al. Acute pulmonary complications in immunocompromised non-AIDS patients: Comparison of diagnostic accuracy of CT and chest radiography. *Clin Radiol.* 1993;47:159–165.

56. Vilar J, Domingo ML, Soto C, et al. Radiology of bacterial pneumonia. *Eur J Radiol.* 2004;51:102–113.

57. Travis WD, Colby TV, Koss MN, et al. *Non-neoplastic disorders of the lower respiratory tract.* Washington, DC: Armed Forces Institute of Pathology; 2002.

58. Groskin SA, Panicek DM, Ewing DK, et al. Bacterial lung abscess: A review of the radiographic and clinical features of 50 cases. *J Thorac Imaging.* 1991;6:62–67.

59. Cheon JE, Im JG, Kim MY, et al. Thoracic actinomycosis: CT findings. *Radiology.* 1998;209:229–233.

60. Stark DD, Federle MP, Goodman PC, et al. Differentiating lung abscess and empyema: Radiography and computed tomography. *Am J Roentgenol.* 1983;141:163–167.

61. Mori T, Ebe T, Takahashi M, et al. Lung abscess: Analysis of 66 cases from 1979 to 1991. *Intern Med.* 1993;32:278–284.

62. Penner C, Maycher B, Long R. Pulmonary gangrene. A complication of bacterial pneumonia. *Chest.* 1994;105:567–573.

63. Quigley MJ, Fraser RS. Pulmonary pneumatocele: Pathology and pathogenesis. *Am J Roentgenol.* 1988;150:1275–1277.

64. Feuerstein I, Archer A, Pluda JM, et al. Thin-walled cavities, cysts, and pneumothorax in Pneumocystis carinii pneumonia: Further observations with histopathologic correlation. *Radiology.* 1990;174:697–702.

65. Huang RM, Naidich DP, Lubat E, et al. Septic pulmonary emboli: CT-radiographic correlation. *Am J Roentgenol.* 1989;153:41–45.

66. Kuhlman JE, Fishman EK, Teigen C. Pulmonary septic emboli: Diagnosis with CT. *Radiology.* 1990;174:211–213.

67. Dodd J, Souza CA, Müller NL. *High-resolution helical multidetector CT in pulmonary septic embolism: Evaluation of the feeding vessel sign.* In press.

68. Porath A, Schlaeffer F, Pick K, et al. Pneumococcal community-acquired pneumonia in 148 hospitalized adult patients. *Eur J Clin Microbiol Infect Dis.* 1997;16:863–870.

69. Sankilampi U, Herva E, Haikala R, et al. Epidemiology of invasive Streptococcus pneumoniae infections in adults in Finland. *Epidemiol Infect.* 1997;118:7–15.

70. Klugman KP, Feldman C. Streptococcus pneumoniae respiratory tract infections. *Curr Opin Infect Dis.* 2001;14:173–179.

71. Marrie TJ. Pneumococcal pneumonia: Epidemiology and clinical features. *Semin Respir Infect.* 1999;14:227–236.

72. Koivula I, Sten M, Makela PH. Risk factors for pneumonia in the elderly. *Am J Med.* 1994;96:313–320.

73. Haglund LA, Istre GR, Pickett DA, et al. Pneumococcus Study Group. Invasive pneumococcal disease in central Oklahoma: Emergence of high-level penicillin resistance and multiple antibiotic resistance. *J Infect Dis.* 1993;168:1532–1536.

74. Loeb M. Pneumonia in the elderly. *Curr Opin Infect Dis.* 2004;17:127–130.

75. Bisno AL, Freeman JC. The syndrome of asplenia, pneumococcal sepsis, and disseminated intravascular coagulation. *Ann Intern Med.* 1970;72:389–393.

76. Musgrave T, Verghese A. Clinical features of pneumonia in the elderly. *Semin Respir Infect.* 1990;5:269–275.

77. Hershey CO, Panaro V. Round pneumonia in adults. *Arch Intern Med.* 1988;148:1155–1157.

78. Levy M, Dromer F, Brion N, et al. Community-acquired pneumonia. Importance of initial noninvasive bacteriologic and radiographic investigations. *Chest.* 1988;93:43–48.

79. Moine P, Vercken JB, Chevret S, et al. French Study Group for Community-Acquired Pneumonia in the Intensive Care Unit. Severe community-acquired pneumonia. Etiology, epidemiology, and prognosis factors. *Chest.* 1994;105:1487–1495.

80. Leatherman JW, Iber C, Davies SF. Cavitation in bacteremic pneumococcal pneumonia. Causal role of mixed infection with anaerobic bacteria. *Am Rev Respir Dis.* 1984;129:317–321.

81. Brewin A, Arango L, Hadley WK, et al. High-dose penicillin therapy and pneumococcal pneumonia. *JAMA.* 1974;230:409–413.

82. Lippmann ML, Goldberg SK, Walkenstein MD, et al. Bacteremic pneumococcal pneumonia. A community hospital experience. *Chest.* 1995;108:1608–1613.

83. Stein DL, Haramati LB, Spindola-Franco H, et al. Intrathoracic lymphadenopathy in hospitalized patients with pneumococcal pneumonia. *Chest.* 2005;127:1271–1275.

84. Donnelly LF, Klosterman LA. The yield of CT of children who have complicated pneumonia and noncontributory chest radiography. *Am J Roentgenol.* 1998;170:1627–1631.

85. Hodina M, Hanquinet S, Cotting J, et al. Imaging of cavitary necrosis in complicated childhood pneumonia. *Eur Radiol.* 2002;12:391–396.

86. al-Ujayli B, Nafziger DA, Saravolatz L. Pneumonia due to Staphylococcus aureus infection. *Clin Chest Med.* 1995;16:111–120.

87. Spencer RC. Predominant pathogens found in the European Prevalence of Infection in Intensive Care Study. *Eur J Clin Microbiol Infect Dis.* 1996;15:281–285.

88. George DL. Epidemiology of nosocomial pneumonia in intensive care unit patients. *Clin Chest Med.* 1995;16:29–44.

89. Rello J, Quintana E, Ausina V, et al. Incidence, etiology, and outcome of nosocomial pneumonia in mechanically ventilated patients. *Chest.* 1991;100:439–444.

90. Sista RR, Oda G, Barr J. Methicillin-resistant Staphylococcus aureus infections in ICU patients. *Anesthesiol Clin North America.* 2004;22:405–435.

91. Gonzalez C, Rubio M, Romero-Vivas J, et al. Staphylococcus aureus bacteremic pneumonia: Differences between community and nosocomial acquisition. *Int J Infect Dis.* 2003;7:102–108.

92. Müller NL, Fraser RS, Colman N, et al. *Radiologic diagnosis of diseases of the chest.* Philadelphia, PA: WB Saunders; 2001.

93. Kaye MG, Fox MJ, Bartlett JG, et al. The clinical spectrum of Staphylococcus aureus pulmonary infection. *Chest.* 1990;97:788–792.

94. Chartrand SA, McCracken GH Jr. Staphylococcal pneumonia in infants and children. *Pediatr Infect Dis.* 1982;1:19–23.

95. Dines DE. Diagnostic significance of pneumatocele of the lung. *JAMA.* 1968;204:1169–1172.

96. Flaherty RA, Keegan JM, Sturtevant HN. Post-pneumonic pulmonary pneumatoceles. *Radiology.* 1960;74:50–53.

97. Naraqi S, McDonnell G. Hematogenous staphylococcal pneumonia secondary to soft tissue infection. *Chest.* 1981;79:173–175.

98. Bouza E, Cercenado E. Klebsiella and enterobacter: Antibiotic resistance and treatment implications. *Semin Respir Infect.* 2002;17:215–230.

99. Jong GM, Hsiue TR, Chen CR, et al. Rapidly fatal outcome of bacteremic Klebsiella pneumoniae pneumonia in alcoholics. *Chest.* 1995;107:214–217.

100. Moon WK, Im JG, Yeon KM, et al. Complications of Klebsiella pneumonia: CT evaluation. *J Comput Assist Tomogr.* 1995;19:176–181.

101. Barnes DJ, Naraqi S, Igo JD. The diagnostic and prognostic significance of bulging fissures in acute lobar pneumonia. *Aust NZJ Med.* 1988;18:130–133.

102. Korvick JA, Hackett AK, Yu VL, et al. Klebsiella pneumonia in the modern era: Clinicoradiographic correlations. *South Med J.* 1991;84:200–204.

103. Schmidt AJ, Stark P. Radiographic findings in Klebsiella (Friedlander's) pneumonia: The bulging fissure sign. *Semin Respir Infect.* 1998;13:80–82.

104. Frobe M, Kullmann F, Scholmerich J, et al. Bronchobiliary fistula associated with combined abscess of lung and liver. *Med Klin (Munich).* 2004;99:391–395.

105. Crossley KB, Thurn JR. Nursing home-acquired pneumonia. *Semin Respir Infect.* 1989;4:64–72.

106. Marrie TJ, Fine MJ, Obrosky DS, et al. Community-acquired pneumonia due to Escherichia coli. *Clin Microbiol Infect.* 1998;4:717–723.

107. Jaffey PB, English PW II, Campbell GA, et al. Escherichia coli lobar pneumonia: Fatal infection in a patient with mental retardation. *South Med J.* 1996;89:628–630.

108. Dunn M, Wunderink RG. Ventilator-associated pneumonia caused by Pseudomonas infection. *Clin Chest Med.* 1995;16:95–109.

109. Maloney SA, Jarvis WR. Epidemic nosocomial pneumonia in the intensive care unit. *Clin Chest Med.* 1995;16:209–223.

110. Rello J, Ausina V, Ricart M, et al. Risk factors for infection by Pseudomonas aeruginosa in patients with ventilator-associated pneumonia. *Intensive Care Med.* 1994;20:193–198.

111. Pennington JE, Reynolds HY, Carbone PP. Pseudomonas pneumonia. A retrospective study of 36 cases. *Am J Med.* 1973;55:155–160.

112. Winer-Muram HT, Jennings SG, Wunderink RG, et al. Ventilator-associated Pseudomonas aeruginosa pneumonia: Radiographic findings. *Radiology.* 1995;195:247–252.

113. Iannini PB, Claffey T, Quintiliani R. Bacteremic Pseudomonas pneumonia. *JAMA.* 1974;230:558–561.

114. McHenry MC, Hawk WA. Bacteremia caused by gram-negative bacilli. *Med Clin North Am.* 1974;58:623–638.

115. Unger JD, Rose HD, Unger GF. Gram-negative pneumonia. *Radiology.* 1973;107:283–291.

116. Tirdel GB, Gibbons GH, Fishman RS. Pneumonia with an enlarged cardiac silhouette. *Chest.* 1996;109:1380–1382.

117. Shah RM, Wechsler R, Salazar AM, et al. Spectrum of CT findings in nosocomial Pseudomonas aeruginosa pneumonia. *J Thorac Imaging.* 2002;17:53–57.

118. Gomez J, Banos V, Ruiz Gomez J, et al. Prospective study of epidemiology and prognostic factors in community-acquired pneumonia. *Eur J Clin Microbiol Infect Dis.* 1996;15:556–560.

119. Mundy LM, Auwaerter PG, Oldach D, et al. Community-acquired pneumonia: Impact of immune status. *Am J Respir Crit Care Med.* 1995;152: 1309–1315.

120. Johnson SR, Thompson RC, Humphreys H, et al. Clinical features of patients with beta-lactamase producing Haemophilus influenzae isolated from sputum. *J Antimicrob Chemother.* 1996;38:881–884.

121. Gillis S, Dann EJ, Berkman N, et al. Fatal Haemophilus influenzae septicemia following bronchoscopy in a splenectomized patient. *Chest.* 1993;104:1607–1609.

122. Trollfors B, Claesson B, Lagergard T, et al. Incidence, predisposing factors and manifestations of invasive Haemophilus influenzae infections in adults. *Eur J Clin Microbiol.* 1984;3:180–184.

123. Rello J, Rodriguez R, Jubert P, et al. Study Group for Severe Community-Acquired Pneumonia. Severe community-acquired pneumonia in the elderly: Epidemiology and prognosis. *Clin Infect Dis.* 1996;23:723–728.

124. Falco V, Fernandez de Sevilla T, Alegre J, et al. Bacterial pneumonia in HIV-infected patients: A prospective study of 68 episodes. *Eur Respir J.* 1994;7:235–239.

125. Pearlberg J, Haggar AM, Saravolatz L, et al. Hemophilus influenzae pneumonia in the adult. Radiographic appearance with clinical correlation. *Radiology.* 1984;151:23–26.

126. Lee KS, Kim TS, Han J, et al. Diffuse micronodular lung disease: HRCT and pathologic findings. *J Comput Assist Tomogr.* 1999;23:99–106.

127. Wallace RJ Jr, Musher DM, Martin RR. Hemophilus influenzae pneumonia in adults. *Am J Med.* 1978;64:87–93.

128. Porath A, Schlaeffer F, Lieberman D, et al. Legionella species community-acquired pneumonia. A review of 56 hospitalized adult patients. *Chest.* 1996;109:1243–1249.

129. Roig J, Domingo C, Morera J. Legionnaires' disease. *Chest.* 1994;105:1817–1825.

130. Davis GS, Winn WC Jr, Beaty HN. Legionnaires disease. Infections caused by Legionella pneumophilia and Legionella-like organisms. *Clin Chest Med.* 1981;2:145–166.

131. Kirby BD, Snyder KM, Meyer RD, et al. Legionnaires' disease: Report of sixty-five nosocomially acquired cases of review of the literature. *Medicine (Baltimore).* 1980;59:188–205.

132. Prodinger WM, Bonatti H, Allerberger F, et al. Legionella pneumonia in transplant recipients: A cluster of cases of eight years' duration. *J Hosp Infect.* 1994;26:191–202.

133. Helms CM, Viner JP, Weisenburger DD, et al. Sporadic Legionnaires' disease: Clinical observations on 87 nosocomial and community-acquired cases. *Am J Med Sci.* 1984;288:2–12.

134. Dietrich PA, Johnson RD, Fairbank JT, et al. The chest radiograph in legionnaires' disease. *Radiology.* 1978;127:577–582.

135. Kroboth FJ, Yu VL, Reddy SC, et al. Clinicoradiographic correlation with the extent of Legionnaire disease. *Am J Roentgenol.* 1983;141:263–268.

136. Pedro-Botet ML, Sabria-Leal M, Haro M, et al. Nosocomial and community-acquired Legionella pneumonia: Clinical comparative analysis. *Eur Respir J.* 1995;8:1929–1933.

137. Storch GA, Sagel SS, Baine WB. The chest roentgenogram in sporadic cases of Legionnaires' disease. *JAMA.* 1981;245:587–590.

138. Coletta FS, Fein AM. Radiological manifestations of Legionella/Legionella-like organisms. *Semin Respir Infect.* 1998;13:109–115.

139. Fairbank JT, Mamourian AC, Dietrich PA, et al. The chest radiograph in Legionnaires' disease. Further observations. *Radiology.* 1983;147:33–34.

140. Meenhorst PL, Mulder JD. The chest X-ray in Legionella pneumonia (Legionnaires' disease). *Eur J Radiol.* 1983;3:180–186.

141. Mirich D, Gray R, Hyland R. Legionella lung cavitation. *Can Assoc Radiol J.* 1990;41:100–102.

142. Moore EH, Webb WR, Gamsu G, et al. Legionnaires' disease in the renal transplant patient: Clinical presentation and radiographic progression. *Radiology.* 1984;153:589–593.

143. Carter JB, Wolter RK, Angres G, et al. Nodular Legionnaire disease. *Am J Roentgenol.* 1981;137:612–613.

144. Pope TL Jr, Armstrong P, Thompson R, et al. Pittsburgh pneumonia agent: Chest film manifestations. *Am J Roentgenol.* 1982;138:237–241.

145. Mehta P, Patel JD, Milder JE. Legionella micdadei (Pittsburgh pneumonia agent). Two infections with unusual clinical features. *JAMA.* 1983; 249:1620–1623.

146. Muder RR, Reddy SC, Yu VL, et al. Pneumonia caused by Pittsburgh pneumonia agent: Radiologic manifestations. *Radiology.* 1984;150:633–637.

147. Rudin JE, Wing EJ. A comparative study of Legionella micdadei and other nosocomial acquired pneumonia. *Chest.* 1984;86:675–680.

148. Yagyu H, Nakamura H, Tsuchida F, et al. Chest CT findings and clinical features in mild Legionella pneumonia. *Intern Med.* 2003;42:477–482.

149. Jonkers RE, Lettinga KD, Pels Rijcken TH, et al. Abnormal radiological findings and a decreased carbon monoxide transfer factor can persist long after the acute phase of Legionella pneumophila pneumonia. *Clin Infect Dis.* 2004;38:605–611.

150. Brooks GF, Butel JS, Ornston LN. *Jawetz, Melnick & Adelberg's medical microbiology.* Norwalk, CT: Appleton & Lange; 1995.

151. Bartlett JG. Anaerobic bacterial infections of the lung and pleural space. *Clin Infect Dis.* 1993;16(suppl 4):S248–S255.

152. Brook I, Frazier EH. Aerobic and anaerobic microbiology of empyema. A retrospective review in two military hospitals. *Chest.* 1993;103:1502–1507.

153. Marina M, Strong CA, Civen R, et al. Bacteriology of anaerobic pleuropulmonary infections: Preliminary report. *Clin Infect Dis.* 1993;16(suppl 4):S256–S262.

154. Pollock HM, Hawkins EL, Bonner JR, et al. Diagnosis of bacterial pulmonary infections with quantitative protected catheter cultures obtained during bronchoscopy. *J Clin Microbiol.* 1983;17:255–259.

155. Bartlett JG, O'Keefe P, Tally FP, et al. Bacteriology of hospital-acquired pneumonia. *Arch Intern Med.* 1986;146:868–871.

156. Bartlett JG, Gorbach SL, Finegold SM. The bacteriology of aspiration pneumonia. *Am J Med.* 1974;56:202–207.

157. Gopalakrishna KV, Lerner PI. Primary lung abscess; analysis of 66 cases. *Cleve Clin Q.* 1975;42:3–13.

158. Verma P. Laboratory diagnosis of anaerobic pleuropulmonary infections. *Semin Respir Infect.* 2000;15:114–118.

159. Bartlett JG. Anaerobic bacterial pneumonitis. *Am Rev Respir Dis.* 1979; 119:19–23.

160. Bartlett JG, Finegold SM. Anaerobic infections of the lung and pleural space. *Am Rev Respir Dis.* 1974;110:56–77.

161. Gorbach SL, Bartlett JG. Anaerobic infections. *N Engl J Med.* 1974;290: 1177–1184.

162. Landay MJ, Christensen EE, Bynum LJ, et al. Anaerobic pleural and pulmonary infections. *Am J Roentgenol.* 1980;134:233–240.

163. Rohlfing BM, White EA, Webb WR, et al. Hilar and mediastinal adenopathy caused by bacterial abscess of the lung. *Radiology.* 1978;128:289–293.

164. Pinkhas J, Oliver I, De Vries A, et al. Pulmonary nocardiosis complicating malignant lymphoma successfully treated with chemotherapy. *Chest.* 1973;63:367–370.

165. Young LS, Armstrong D, Blevins A, et al. Nocardia asteroides infection complicating neoplastic disease. *Am J Med.* 1971;50:356–367.

166. Bach MC, Adler JL, Breman J, et al. Influence of rejection therapy on fungal and Nocardial infections in renal-transplant recipients. *Lancet.* 1973; 1:180–184.

167. Krick JA, Stinson EB, Remington JS. Nocardia infection in heart transplant patients. *Ann Intern Med.* 1975;82:18–26.

168. Menendez R, Cordero PJ, Santos M, et al. Pulmonary infection with Nocardia species: A report of 10 cases and review. *Eur Respir J.* 1997; 10:1542–1546.

169. Coker RJ, Bignardi G, Horner P, et al. Nocardia infection in AIDS: A clinical and microbiological challenge. *J Clin Pathol.* 1992;45:821–822.

170. Feigin DS. Nocardiosis of the lung: Chest radiographic findings in 21 cases. *Radiology.* 1986;159:9–14.

171. Raby N, Forbes G, Williams R. Nocardia infection in patients with liver transplants or chronic liver disease: Radiologic findings. *Radiology.* 1990;174:713–716.

172. Yoon HK, Im JG, Ahn JM, et al. Pulmonary nocardiosis: CT findings. *J Comput Assist Tomogr.* 1995;19:52–55.

173. Grossman CB, Bragg DG, Armstrong D. Roentgen manifestations of pulmonary nocardiosis. *Radiology.* 1970;96:325–330.

174. Balikian JP, Herman PG, Kopit S. Pulmonary nocardiosis. *Radiology.* 1978;126:569–573.

175. Suzuki JB, Delisle AL. Pulmonary actinomycosis of periodontal origin. *J Periodontol.* 1984;55:581–584.

176. Kwong JS, Müller NL, Godwin JD, et al. Thoracic actinomycosis: CT findings in eight patients. *Radiology.* 1992;183:189–192.

177. Hsieh MJ, Liu HP, Chang JP, et al. Thoracic actinomycosis. *Chest.* 1993; 104:366–370.

178. Coodley EL, Yoshinaka R. Pleural effusion as the major manifestation of actinomycosis. *Chest*. 1994;106:1615–1617.
179. Morgan DE, Nath H, Sanders C, et al. Mediastinal actinomycosis. *Am J Roentgenol*. 1990;155:735–737.
180. Webb WR, Sagel SS. Actinomycosis involving the chest wall: CT findings. *Am J Roentgenol*. 1982;139:1007–1009.
181. Albaum MN, Hill LC, Murphy M, et al. Interobserver reliability of the chest radiograph in community-acquired pneumonia. PORT Investigators. *Chest*. 1996;110:343–350.
182. Melbye H, Dale K. Interobserver variability in the radiographic diagnosis of adult outpatient pneumonia. *Acta Radiol*. 1992;33:79–81.
183. Donowitz GR, Harman C, Pope T, et al. The role of the chest roentgenogram in febrile neutropenic patients. *Arch Intern Med*. 1991;151:701–704.
184. Winer-Muram HT, Rubin SA, Ellis JV, et al. Pneumonia and ARDS in patients receiving mechanical ventilation: Diagnostic accuracy of chest radiography. *Radiology*. 1993;188:479–485.
185. Wunderink RG, Woldenberg LS, Zeiss J, et al. The radiologic diagnosis of autopsy-proven ventilator-associated pneumonia. *Chest*. 1992;101:458–463.
186. Winer-Muram HT, Steiner RM, Gurney JW, et al. Ventilator-associated pneumonia in patients with adult respiratory distress syndrome: CT evaluation. *Radiology*. 1998;208:193–199.
187. Tew J, Calenoff L, Berlin BS. Bacterial or nonbacterial pneumonia: Accuracy of radiographic diagnosis. *Radiology*. 1977;124:607–612.
188. Fang GD, Fine M, Orloff J, et al. New and emerging etiologies for community-acquired pneumonia with implications for therapy. A prospective multicenter study of 359 cases. *Medicine (Baltimore)*. 1990;69:307–316.
189. Tomiyama N, Müller NL, Johkoh T, et al. Acute parenchymal lung disease in immunocompetent patients: Diagnostic accuracy of high-resolution CT. *Am J Roentgenol*. 2000;174:1745–1750.

Pulmonary Tuberculosis

3

Tuberculosis (TB) is a chronic, recurrent, contagious infection caused by *Mycobacterium tuberculosis*. It is a major cause of morbidity and mortality worldwide. It is estimated that in 2006 active pulmonary TB will develop in >10 million individuals and will lead to >2 million deaths (1–3). Most cases occur in southeast Asia and Africa. Of the estimated 8.8 million new cases in 2003, 3 million occurred in southeast Asia, 2.4 million in Africa, 439,000 in Europe and 370,000 in the Americas (4). The incidence in the Americas is lowest in Canada and in the United States. During 2004, a total of 14,511 confirmed TB cases (4.9 cases per 100,000 population) were reported in the United States (5). Slightly >half (54%) of the US cases were foreign-born persons (5).

Patients with active pulmonary TB may be asymptomatic, have mild or progressive dry cough, or present with multiple symptoms including fever, fatigue, weight loss, night sweats, and cough producing bloody sputum. It is estimated that each patient with active disease will infect on average between 10 and 15 people every year (4). Many of the cases of active TB are not recognized. It is likely that the World Health Organization 2005 target to detect at least 70% of all estimated sputum smear-positive cases worldwide and to treat at least 85% of them successfully was not met (6).

DEVELOPMENT OF INFECTION

M. tuberculosis is an aerobic, nonmotile, non–spore-forming rod that is highly resistant to drying, acid, and alcohol. It is transmitted from person to person through droplet nuclei containing the organism and is spread mainly by coughing. The contagiousness of a patient with TB increases with the greater extent of the disease, the presence of cavitation, the frequency of coughing, and the virulence of the organism (7). The risk of developing active TB is greatest in patients with altered host cellular immunity. These include extremes of age, malnutrition, cancer, immunosuppressive therapy, human immunodeficiency virus (HIV) infection, end stage renal disease, and diabetes.

PATHOGENESIS

Inhaled mycobacteria are phagocytized by alveolar macrophages, where the organisms multiply and eventually kill the cells. Interaction of macrophages with T lymphocytes results in differentiation of macrophages into epithelioid histiocytes (7). The epithelioid histiocytes aggregate into small clusters resulting in granulomas. After several weeks, granulomas are well formed, and their central portions undergo necrosis (7). As the disease progresses, individual necrotic foci tend to enlarge and coalesce. The rapid

178. Coodley EL, Yoshinaka R. Pleural effusion as the major manifestation of actinomycosis. *Chest.* 1994;106:1615–1617.
179. Morgan DE, Nath H, Sanders C, et al. Mediastinal actinomycosis. *Am J Roentgenol.* 1990;155:735–737.
180. Webb WR, Sagel SS. Actinomycosis involving the chest wall: CT findings. *Am J Roentgenol.* 1982;139:1007–1009.
181. Albaum MN, Hill LC, Murphy M, et al. Interobserver reliability of the chest radiograph in community-acquired pneumonia. PORT Investigators. *Chest.* 1996;110:343–350.
182. Melbye H, Dale K. Interobserver variability in the radiographic diagnosis of adult outpatient pneumonia. *Acta Radiol.* 1992;33:79–81.
183. Donowitz GR, Harman C, Pope T, et al. The role of the chest roentgenogram in febrile neutropenic patients. *Arch Intern Med.* 1991;151:701–704.
184. Winer-Muram HT, Rubin SA, Ellis JV, et al. Pneumonia and ARDS in patients receiving mechanical ventilation: Diagnostic accuracy of chest radiography. *Radiology.* 1993;188:479–485.
185. Wunderink RG, Woldenberg LS, Zeiss J, et al. The radiologic diagnosis of autopsy-proven ventilator-associated pneumonia. *Chest.* 1992;101:458–463.
186. Winer-Muram HT, Steiner RM, Gurney JW, et al. Ventilator-associated pneumonia in patients with adult respiratory distress syndrome: CT evaluation. *Radiology.* 1998;208:193–199.
187. Tew J, Calenoff L, Berlin BS. Bacterial or nonbacterial pneumonia: Accuracy of radiographic diagnosis. *Radiology.* 1977;124:607–612.
188. Fang GD, Fine M, Orloff J, et al. New and emerging etiologies for community-acquired pneumonia with implications for therapy. A prospective multicenter study of 359 cases. *Medicine (Baltimore).* 1990;69:307–316.
189. Tomiyama N, Müller NL, Johkoh T, et al. Acute parenchymal lung disease in immunocompetent patients: Diagnostic accuracy of high-resolution CT. *Am J Roentgenol.* 2000;174:1745–1750.

Pulmonary Tuberculosis

3

Tuberculosis (TB) is a chronic, recurrent, contagious infection caused by *Mycobacterium tuberculosis*. It is a major cause of morbidity and mortality worldwide. It is estimated that in 2006 active pulmonary TB will develop in >10 million individuals and will lead to >2 million deaths (1–3). Most cases occur in southeast Asia and Africa. Of the estimated 8.8 million new cases in 2003, 3 million occurred in southeast Asia, 2.4 million in Africa, 439,000 in Europe and 370,000 in the Americas (4). The incidence in the Americas is lowest in Canada and in the United States. During 2004, a total of 14,511 confirmed TB cases (4.9 cases per 100,000 population) were reported in the United States (5). Slightly >half (54%) of the US cases were foreign-born persons (5).

Patients with active pulmonary TB may be asymptomatic, have mild or progressive dry cough, or present with multiple symptoms including fever, fatigue, weight loss, night sweats, and cough producing bloody sputum. It is estimated that each patient with active disease will infect on average between 10 and 15 people every year (4). Many of the cases of active TB are not recognized. It is likely that the World Health Organization 2005 target to detect at least 70% of all estimated sputum smear-positive cases worldwide and to treat at least 85% of them successfully was not met (6).

DEVELOPMENT OF INFECTION

M. tuberculosis is an aerobic, nonmotile, non–spore-forming rod that is highly resistant to drying, acid, and alcohol. It is transmitted from person to person through droplet nuclei containing the organism and is spread mainly by coughing. The contagiousness of a patient with TB increases with the greater extent of the disease, the presence of cavitation, the frequency of coughing, and the virulence of the organism (7). The risk of developing active TB is greatest in patients with altered host cellular immunity. These include extremes of age, malnutrition, cancer, immunosuppressive therapy, human immunodeficiency virus (HIV) infection, end stage renal disease, and diabetes.

PATHOGENESIS

Inhaled mycobacteria are phagocytized by alveolar macrophages, where the organisms multiply and eventually kill the cells. Interaction of macrophages with T lymphocytes results in differentiation of macrophages into epithelioid histiocytes (7). The epithelioid histiocytes aggregate into small clusters resulting in granulomas. After several weeks, granulomas are well formed, and their central portions undergo necrosis (7). As the disease progresses, individual necrotic foci tend to enlarge and coalesce. The rapid

bacillary growth phase is arrested with the development of cell-mediated immunity and delayed-type hypersensitivity at 2 to 10 weeks after the initial infection (8, 9). The initial focus of parenchymal disease is termed the *Ghon focus*. The Ghon focus may be microscopic or large enough to be visible radiologically. It either enlarges as the disease progresses or, much more commonly, undergoes healing. Healing may result in a visible scar that may be dense and contain foci of calcification. However, usually there is residual central necrotic material. Although the disease at this stage is inactive, the encapsulated necrotic areas contain viable organisms and are a potential focus for reactivation in later life (7).

During the early stage of infection, organisms commonly spread through lymphatic channels to regional hilar and mediastinal lymph nodes and through the bloodstream to more distant sites in the body. The combination of the Ghon focus and affected lymph nodes is known as the *Ranke complex* (7). The course of the disease in lymph nodes is similar to that in the parenchyma, consisting initially of granulomatous inflammation and necrosis followed by fibrosis and calcification. However, the inflammatory reaction is usually much greater in lymph nodes resulting in radiologically visible lymphadenopathy. Hematogenous dissemination in primary TB is probably common but seldom results in miliary disease (7).

The initial infection is usually clinically silent. Development of specific immunity is usually adequate to limit further multiplication of the bacilli (10). Some of the bacilli remain dormant and viable for many years. This condition, known as *latent TB infection*, may be detectable only by means of a positive purified protein derivative tuberculin skin test or by the presence of radiologically identifiable calcification at the site of the primary lung infection or in regional lymph nodes (11). In approximately 5% of infected individuals immunity is inadequate and clinically active disease develops within 1 year of infection, a condition known as *progressive primary TB* (8). Risk factors for progressive primary disease include immunosuppression (especially HIV infection), extremes of age, or a large inoculation of mycobacteria. For most infected individuals, however, TB remains clinically and microbiologically latent for many years.

In approximately 5% of the infected population, endogenous reactivation of latent infection develops many years after the initial infection (8). Such reactivation is frequently associated with malnutrition, debilitation, or immunosuppression (12). Postprimary TB tends to involve predominantly the apical and posterior segments of the upper lobes and the superior segments of the lower lobes. This localization is likely due to a combination of relatively higher oxygen tension and impaired lymphatic drainage in these regions (7, 11). As distinct from primary TB, in which healing is the rule, postprimary TB tends to progress. The main abnormalities are progressive extension of inflammation and necrosis, frequently with the development of communication with the airways and

cavity formation (7). Endobronchial spread of necrotic material from a cavity may result in tuberculous infection in the same lobe or in other lobes. Hematogenous dissemination may result in miliary TB. Although most cases of postprimary TB probably result from reactivation of organisms in a focus acquired during the primary infection in some cases, postprimary TB may result from reinfection by new organisms.

RADIOLOGIC MANIFESTATIONS

Patients who develop the disease after initial exposure are considered to have primary TB. Patients who develop the disease as a result of reactivation of a previous focus of TB or because of reinfection are considered to have postprimary (reactivation) TB. Traditionally, it was believed that the clinical, pathologic, and radiologic manifestations of postprimary TB were quite distinct from those of primary TB. However, more recent studies based on DNA fingerprinting suggest that the radiographic features are often similar in patients who apparently have primary disease and those who have postprimary TB (13). Time from acquisition of infection to development of clinical disease does not reliably predict the radiographic appearance of TB. The only independent predictor of radiographic appearance is the integrity of the host immune response (13). Patients with normal response tend to show parenchymal granulomatous inflammation with slowly progressive nodularity and cavitation whereas patients with immunodeficiency have a tendency to develop lymphadenopathy. Because these results are preliminary and because the vast majority of published data are based on the traditional concept of primary and postprimary disease, we follow the traditional outline in this book.

PRIMARY TUBERCULOSIS

The initial parenchymal focus of TB (Ghon focus) may enlarge and result in an area of airspace consolidation (see Fig. 3.1) or, more commonly, undergo healing by transformation of the granulomatous tissue into mature fibrous tissue. Such healing is often accompanied by dystrophic calcification of the necrotic tissue. Spread of organisms to the regional lymph nodes results in granulomatous inflammatory reaction and lymph node enlargement (see Figs. 3.1 and 3.2). The combination of the Ghon focus and affected nodes is known as the *Ranke complex*.

Primary TB occurs most commonly in children, but is being seen with increasing frequency in adults (see Figs. 3.1–3.3) (12, 14). There is considerable difference in the prevalence of radiologic findings in children compared to that in adults (see Table 3.1). The most common abnormality in children consists of lymph node enlargement, which is seen in 90% to 95% of cases (15, 16). The lymphadenopathy is usually unilateral and located in the hilum or paratracheal region. On CT scan, the enlarged

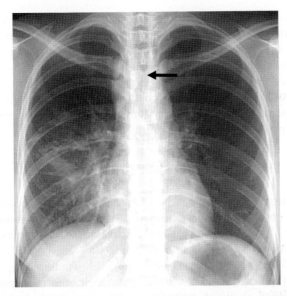

Figure 3.1 Primary tuberculosis with consolidation and lymphadenopathy in a 26-year-old woman. Posteroanterior chest radiograph shows airspace consolidation in the right middle and lower lung zones. Also note right paratracheal lymphadenopathy with associated focal tracheal narrowing (*arrow*).

nodes frequently have focal areas of low attenuation and show peripheral (rim) enhancement (Fig. 3.2) (17, 18). The former corresponds to the central necrotic portion of the node and the latter to the surrounding vascular rim of granulomatous inflammatory tissue. The enlarged nodes can compress the adjacent bronchi and result in atelectasis, which is usually lobar and right-sided.

Airspace consolidation, related to parenchymal granulomatous inflammation and usually unilateral, is evident radiographically in approximately 70% of children with primary TB (15). It shows no predilection for any particular lung zone (15). As compared to children, adults who have primary TB are less likely to have lymph node enlargement (10% to 30% of patients) and more likely to have parenchymal consolidation (approximately 90% of patients) (Fig. 3.3) (19, 20). The parenchymal consolidation in primary TB is most commonly homogeneous but may also be patchy, linear, nodular, or mass-like (21). Parenchymal consolidation in adults may involve predominantly or exclusively the upper or lower lung zones (21). Pleural effusion is seen in 5% to 10% of children and 30% to 40% of adults with primary TB (15, 17, 20). The pleural

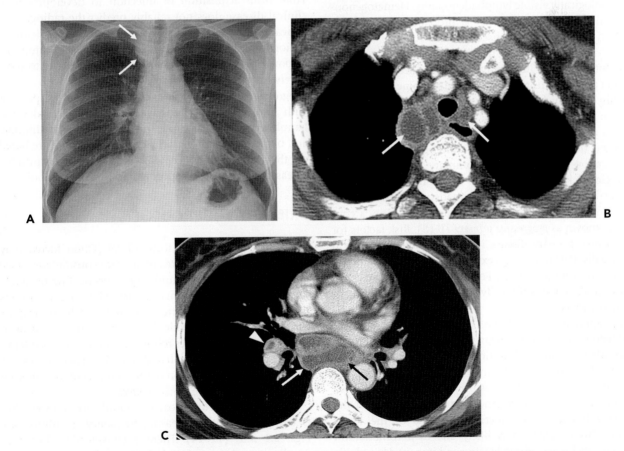

Figure 3.2 Primary tuberculosis with lymphadenopathy in a 38-year-old woman. **A:** Chest radiograph shows mediastinal widening in the right paratracheal region (*arrows*). **B:** Computed tomography (CT) image (5-mm collimation) scan obtained at the level of the great vessels shows enlarged bilateral paratracheal lymph nodes (*arrows*) with central necrotic low attenuation and peripheral rim enhancement. **C:** CT image at the level of the right hilum demonstrates enlarged lymph nodes in the subcarinal region (*arrows*) and right hilum (*arrowhead*) with the same characteristics as those described in (**B**).

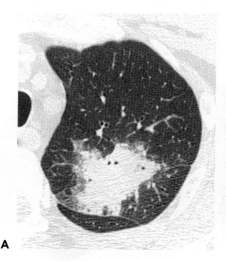
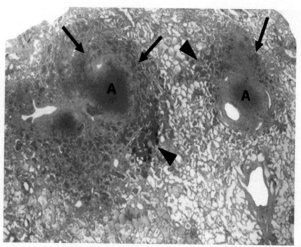

Figure 3.3 Primary tuberculosis in a 45-year-old woman with neutropenia following bone marrow transplantation. **A:** High-resolution computed tomography (CT) image (1-mm collimation) at the level of the thoracic inlet shows consolidation and adjacent ground-glass opacity in the left upper lobe. **B:** Photomicrograph of wedge biopsy specimen from the left upper lobe demonstrates lung microabscesses **(A)** surrounded by a layer (*arrows*) of epithelioid histiocytes, the two components of the granulomatous inflammatory reaction of tuberculosis. Also note fibrinous exudates (*arrowheads*) in alveolar spaces surrounding necrotic granulomas.

effusion is usually unilateral and on the same side as the primary focus of TB. The effusion may be large and present in patients without evidence of parenchymal disease on chest radiographs (20).

POSTPRIMARY TUBERCULOSIS

Postprimary TB typically involves mainly the apical and posterior segments of the upper lobes and/or the superior segments of the lower lobes (see Figs. 3.4 and 3.5) (7, 21, 22). As with primary disease, the postprimary form is characterized histologically by necrotizing granulomatous inflammation. Coalescence and enlargement of multiple foci of inflammation result in progressive consolidation. Destruction of lung parenchyma and scarring result in a nodular appearance (Fig. 3.4). Extension into an airway is followed by the drainage of necrotic material and the formation of one or more cavities (Fig. 3.5). Endobronchial spread results in the formation of additional foci of tuberculous disease in other regions of the lungs (see Figs. 3.4–3.6).

The most common radiographic manifestation of postprimary TB consists of focal or patchy heterogenous consolidation involving the apical and posterior segments of the upper lobes and the superior segments of the lower lobes (see Table 3.2) (Figs. 3.4–3.6) (21, 22). Another common finding is the presence of poorly defined nodules and linear opacities (fibronodular pattern of TB).

TABLE 3.1
PRIMARY TUBERCULOSIS

Most common in children; increasing incidence in adults

Main Radiologic Manifestations

a. Children
   Hilar and/or mediastinal lymphadenopathy: 90%–95% of cases
   Airspace consolidation: 70%
   Consolidation may involve upper or lower lung zones
   Pleural effusion: 5%–10%
   Miliary disease: 3%
b. Adults
   Hilar and/or mediastinal lymphadenopathy: 10%–30% of cases
   Airspace consolidation: 90%
   Consolidation may involve upper or lower lung zones
   Pleural effusion: 30%–40%
   Miliary disease: 5%

TABLE 3.2
POSTPRIMARY TUBERCULOSIS

Characteristic Manifestations on Chest Radiography

Apical and posterior segment of upper lobe predominance
Poorly defined focal or patchy consolidation
Nodular pattern with scarring (fibronodular pattern)

Common Associated Findings

Cavitation: 20%–45%
Nodules 4–10 mm in diameter, away from primary focus: 20%–25%
Hilar and/or mediastinal lymphadenopathy: 5%–10%
Pleural effusion: 15%–25%

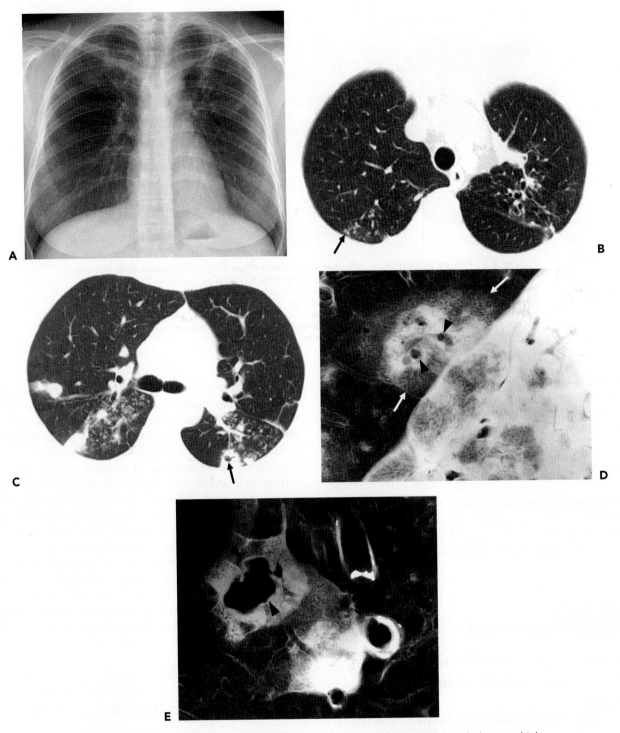

Figure 3.4 Postprimary tuberculosis in a 33-year-old woman. **A:** Chest radiograph shows multiple variable-sized nodules with poorly defined margins in both upper lung zones. **B:** Computed tomography (CT) image (2.5-mm collimation) obtained at the level of the great vessels shows tree-in-bud opacities (*arrow*) in the right upper lobe. Also note bronchiectasis and reticulation in the left upper lobe due to previous tuberculous infection. **C:** CT image obtained at the level of the main bronchi shows cavitating nodule (*arrow*) in the left lower lobe, bilateral noncavitating nodules and tree-in-bud opacities. **D:** Contact radiograph and surface photograph of sliced lung specimen obtained from a different patient who died of endobronchial spread of tuberculosis show lobular consolidation (*arrows*) and 2- to 3-mm diameter centrilobular cavities (*arrowheads*). Lobular consolidation consists of loose periphery and compact center. Microscopic examination (not shown) revealed caseation necrosis at the dense center and nonspecific inflammation at loose periphery. **E:** Contact radiograph of lung specimen obtained from an area adjacent to that in **(D)** demonstrates consolidation in a secondary pulmonary lobule containing larger necrotic cavity (*arrowheads*). Cavitation may begin at the lobular center, followed by coalescence of small cavities, resulting in a larger cavity. (Courtesy of Dr. Im J.-G. Seoul, Korea: Department of Radiology, Seoul National University Hospital.)

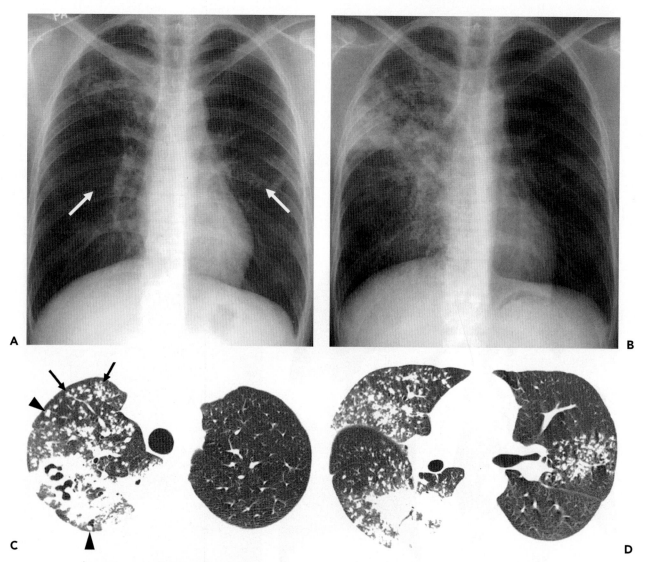

Figure 3.5 Postprimary tuberculosis with progression of disease in a 30-year-old man with multidrug resistant tuberculosis. **A:** Initial chest radiograph obtained shows consolidation containing cavity in right upper lobe and several nodules (*arrows*) in both lungs. **B:** Follow-up radiograph obtained 2 months after, **(A)** demonstrates markedly increased extent of disease in both lungs with consolidation and nodules. **C:** High-resolution computed tomography (CT) image (1-mm collimation) obtained at the level of the thoracic inlet and at a similar time as **(B)** shows consolidation containing several cavities in the posterior segment of the right upper lobe. Also noted are branching nodular and linear opacities (tree-in-bud pattern) (*arrows*) and centrilobular small nodules (*arrowheads*). **D:** CT scan obtained at the level of bronchus intermedius demonstrates nodules in the right lower lobe and small centrilobular nodules and tree-in-bud opacities in both lungs. **E:** CT scan obtained at a level similar to that in, and 1 month after, **(C)** shows progression of disease with diffuse right upper lobe cavitary consolidation and nodules. **F:** CT scan obtained at a level similar to that in, and 1 month after, **(D)** demonstrates multifocal bilateral consolidation containing cavities. Also note several bilateral small centrilobular nodules (*arrowheads*). **G:** Coronal reformation (2-mm collimation) image shows extent of tuberculous lesions consisting of multifocal cavitary consolidation, nodules, small centrilobular nodules, and tree-in-bud opacities. **H:** Photomicrograph of right pneumonectomy pathologic specimen demonstrates abscesses (A) containing yellow creamy necrotic materials, consolidation, nodules, small nodules of centrilobular location, and nodular branching lesions (*arrows*). Branching suggests that lesions are centered on airways. **I:** Sagittal section of contact radiograph of autopsy specimen in a different patient, who died of endobronchial spread of tuberculosis, shows parenchymal consolidation of several contiguous secondary pulmonary lobules, branching small centrilobular nodules (*arrows*), and nonbranching centrilobular nodules (*arrowheads*). These branching centrilobular nodules manifest as tree-in-bud opacities on high-resolution CT scans. (Courtesy of Dr. Im J.-G. Seoul, Korea: Department of Radiology, Seoul National University Hospital.)

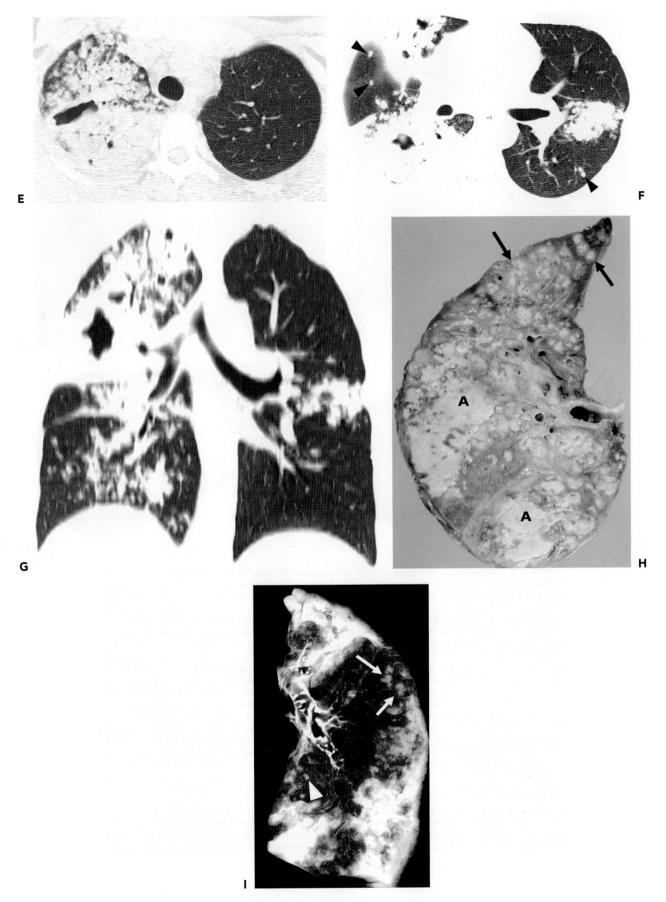

Figure 3.5 *(continued).*

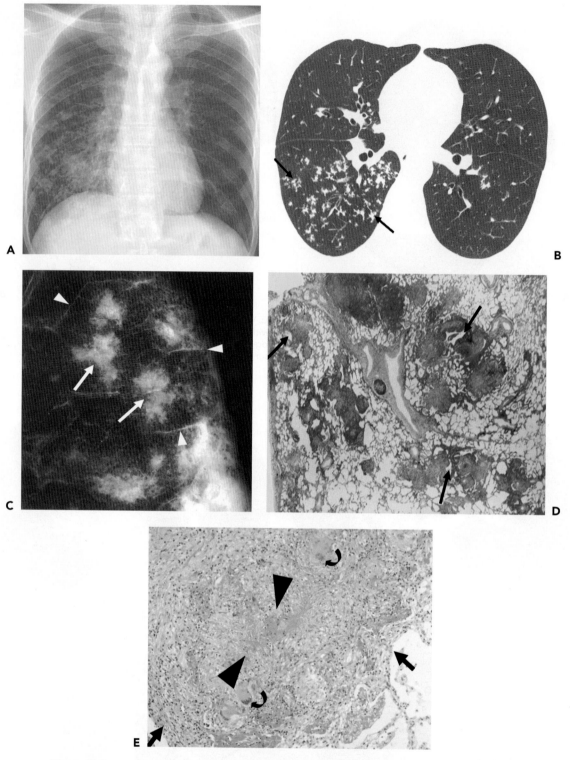

Figure 3.6 Endobronchial spread of tuberculosis in a 49-year-old man. **A:** Chest radiograph shows small nodules in the right middle and lower lung zones and to a lesser extent in the left mid–lung zone. **B:** High-resolution computed tomography (CT) image (1-mm collimation) at the level of basal trunks shows tree-in-bud opacities (*arrows*) mainly in the superior segment of the right lower lobe. **C:** Magnified view of the contact radiograph of pneumonectomy specimen obtained from the site of endobronchial spread of tuberculosis in another patient shows poorly defined branching centrilobular nodules (*arrows*). Also note interlobular septa (*arrowheads*) demarcating secondary pulmonary lobules. (Courtesy of Dr. Im J.-G., Seoul, Korea: Department of Radiology, Seoul National University Hospital.) **D:** Photomicrograph obtained from branching centrilobular nodules demonstrates relatively well-circumscribed lesions, adjacent to small membranous bronchioles (*arrows*). **E:** Magnified view of one of the lesions shows granuloma (*arrows*) with central necrosis (*arrowheads*). Also note multinucleated giant cells (*curved arrows*).

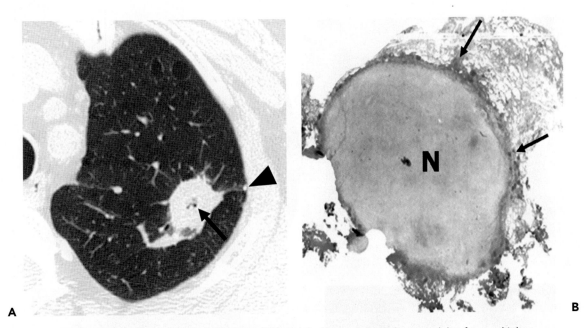

Figure 3.7 Tuberculoma in a 67-year-old man. **A:** View of the left upper lobe from a high-resolution CT scan (1-mm collimation) shows nodule with central cavitation (*arrow*) and surrounding smaller satellite nodules (*arrowhead*). **B:** Photomicrograph of surgical specimen demonstrates a well-defined granuloma with central necrosis (N) and surrounding thin layer of epithelioid histiocytes and lymphocytes (*arrows*).

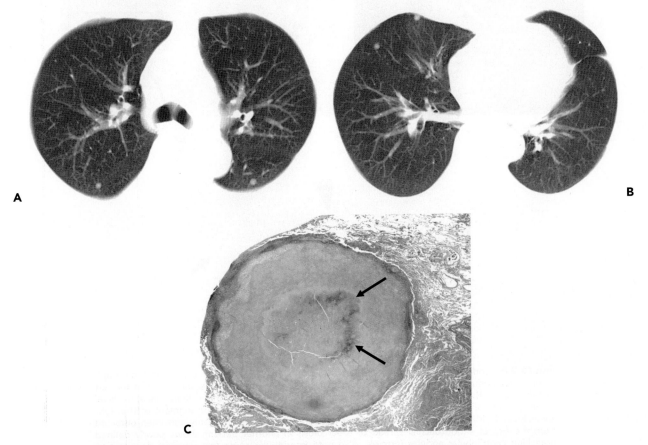

Figure 3.8 Multiple small tuberculomas in a 66-year-old man. **A** and **B:** Computed tomography (CT) images (7-mm collimation) at the level of the tracheal carina **(A)** and right inferior pulmonary vein **(B)** show several small nodules in both lungs. **C:** Photomicrograph of biopsy specimen of one of the nodules shows a well-demarcated granuloma with central necrosis and calcification (*arrows*).

In one review of the radiographic features of 158 patients with postprimary TB, approximately 55% presented with consolidation, 25% with a fibronodular pattern, and 5% with a mixed pattern (22). Single or multiple cavities are evident radiographically in 20% to 45% of patients (20–22). Air–fluid levels are seen in 10% to 20% of tuberculous cavities (20, 22). In approximately 85% of patients the cavities involve the apical and/or posterior segment of the upper lobes and in approximately 10% the superior segments of the lower lobes (21). Endobronchial spread, manifested as 4 to 10 mm diameter nodules distant from the site of the cavity, is evident radiographically in 10% to 20% of cases (22, 23).

In approximately 5% of patients with postprimary TB the main manifestation is a tuberculoma, defined as a sharply marginated round or oval lesion measuring 0.5 to 4.0 cm in diameter (21, 22). Histologically, the central part of the tuberculoma consists of caseous material and the periphery of epithelioid histiocytes and multinucleated giant cells and a variable amount of collagen (see Figs. 3.7 and 3.8). Tuberculomas usually occur in the upper lobes; approximately 80% are single and 20% are multiple. Satellite nodules histologically identical to the larger focus of disease and measuring 1 to 5 mm in diameter are present in most cases. Tuberculomas are most commonly smoothly marginated; however, fibrosis related to vessels, interlobular septa or lung parenchyma adjacent to the nodule may result in spiculated margins (13, 14, 24). Calcification within the nodule or satellite nodule around the periphery of the dominant nodule is present in 20% to 30% of cases (Fig. 3.8). Cavitation within the dominant nodule or the surrounding satellite nodules may also be seen. Following intravenous administration of contrast, tuberculomas often show ring-like or curvilinear enhancement on CT scan. The latter corresponds histologically to the fibrous tissue/granulomatous inflammatory tissue capsule, whereas the nonenhancing area corresponds to the central necrotic material (24).

Hilar or mediastinal lymphadenopathy is uncommon in postprimary TB, being seen in approximately 5% to 10% of patients (20, 22). Pleural effusion, typically unilateral, occurs in 15% to 20% of patients (25). Although pleural effusion is usually associated with parenchymal abnormalities, it may be the only radiologic manifestation of TB. Pleural effusion can be caused by rupture of a tuberculous cavity into the pleural space. This may result in the formation of tuberculous empyema and, occasionally, a bronchopleural fistula with pleural air–fluid level (26).

COMPUTED TOMOGRAPHY FINDINGS OF PULMONARY TUBERCULOSIS

The most common CT scan findings of postprimary pulmonary TB are centrilobular nodules and branching linear and nodular opacities (tree-in-bud pattern), patchy or lobular areas of consolidation, and cavitation (see Table 3.3) (Figs. 3.4–3.6) (14, 27, 28). The centrilobular nodules and tree-in-bud pattern reflect the presence of endobronchial spread and are due to the presence of caseation necrosis and granulomatous inflammation filling and surrounding terminal and respiratory bronchioles and alveolar ducts (Figs. 3.4–3.6) (27, 29). Coalescence of small nodules or clustering of small nodules leads to the formation of a large nodule (see Fig. 3.9). Most tuberculous cavities are thick-walled, but thin-walled cavities are also common, particularly in patients undergoing treatment.

TABLE 3.3

POSTPRIMARY PULMONARY TUBERCULOSIS

Characteristic Manifestations on CT Scan

Apical and posterior segment of upper lobe predominance
2–4 mm diameter centrilobular nodules: 90%–95% of patients
Tree-in-bud pattern: 70%–80%
Patchy or lobular consolidation: 50%–60%
5–10 mm diameter nodules: 60%–70%
Cavitation: 60%–70%

Common Associated Findings

Bronchovascular distortion: 20%
Hilar and/or mediastinal lymphadenopathy: 30%
Nodes typically have low attenuation center and rim enhancement
Pleural effusion: 20%–30%

CT, computed tomography.

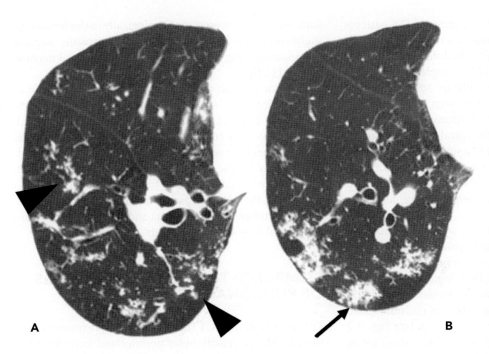

A

B

Figure 3.9 Confluence of small nodules in endobronchial spread of pulmonary TB in a 75-year-old woman. **A** and **B:** Views of the right lung from high-resolution computed tomography (CT) scans (1-mm collimation) obtained at the levels of basal trunks **(A)** and segmental bronchi **(B)**, respectively, show tree-in-bud opacities (*arrowheads*) and confluence of small nodules (*arrow*).

Im et al. (28) assessed the CT scan findings in 29 patients with newly diagnosed pulmonary TB and 12 patients with recent reactivation. The most common abnormality on CT scan was the presence of 2 to 4 mm diameter centrilobular nodules and/or branching linear structures (tree-in-bud pattern) seen in 95% of patients. Other common findings included cavitary nodules (69% of patients), lobular consolidation (52% of patients), interlobular septal thickening (34% of patients), and bronchovascular distortion (17% of patients). Findings of endobronchial spread of TB were often present in the absence of cavitation. Mediastinal lymph node enlargement was seen in 9 of 29 (31%) patients who had newly diagnosed disease. In 11 of 12 patients with recent reactivation TB, CT scan clearly differentiated old fibrotic lesions from new active lesions by demonstrating centrilobular nodules or a tree-in-bud pattern. Patients having follow-up high-resolution CT scan during treatment showed a gradual decrease in lobular consolidation. Most of the centrilobular nodular and branching opacities disappeared within 5 months after the start of treatment. On the other hand, bronchovascular distortion, fibrosis, emphysema, and bronchiectasis increased on follow-up scans (28).

Hatipoglu et al. (30) compared high-resolution CT scan findings in 32 patients who had newly diagnosed active pulmonary TB and 34 patients who had inactive disease. Findings seen only in patients who had active TB included centrilobular nodules (91% of patients), tree-in-bud pattern (71% of patients), nodules 5 to 8 mm in diameter (69% of patients), and consolidation (44% of patients). Cavitation was present in 50% of patients who had active TB and 12% of patients who had inactive disease (30). Poey et al. (31) performed high-resolution

CT scan before and after 6 months of antituberculosis treatment in 27 patients with postprimary pulmonary TB. Centrilobular nodules and poorly marginated nodules were present only before treatment. Reticular pattern (intralobular and septal thickening) and fibrosis were seen both before and after treatment (31).

Hilar and mediastinal lymph node enlargement is commonly seen on CT scan in patients who have active TB (32, 33). In the study by Im et al. (28) mediastinal lymph node enlargement was seen on high-resolution CT scan in 9 of 29 (31%) patients who had newly diagnosed disease, and in 2 of 12 (17%) patients who had reactivation. Enlarged lymph nodes in patients with active TB typically show central areas of low attenuation on contrast-enhanced CT scan, with peripheral rim enhancement (17). Moon et al. (34) assessed the role of CT scan in the diagnosis of tuberculous mediastinal lymphadenitis in 37 patients who had active disease and 12 patients who had inactive disease. In the 37 patients who had active disease, mediastinal lymph nodes ranged in size from 1.5 to 6.7 cm (mean, 2.8 ± 1.0 cm), and all had central low attenuation and peripheral rim enhancement. Foci of calcification were seen within the lymph nodes in seven patients (19%). In the 12 patients who had inactive disease, the nodes were usually smaller than nodes in patients who had active disease, and they appeared homogeneous without low-attenuation areas. Calcifications within the nodes were seen in 10 of the 12 (83%) patients who had inactive disease. Low-attenuation areas within the lymph nodes in patients who had active TB corresponded pathologically to areas of caseous necrosis. In all the 25 patients followed up after treatment, enlarged mediastinal nodes decreased in size and low-attenuation areas within the nodes disappeared (34).

MILIARY TUBERCULOSIS

Miliary spread of TB can occur in both primary and postprimary disease (35). In the latter situation, it may be seen in association with typical parenchymal changes as described in the preceding text or may be the only pulmonary abnormality. Each focus of miliary infection results in local granulomas, which, when well developed, consist of a region of central necrosis surrounded by a relatively well-delimited rim of epithelioid histiocytes and fibrous tissue (see Fig. 3.10). The characteristic radiographic and high-resolution CT scan findings consist of 1 to 3 mm diameter nodules randomly distributed throughout both lungs (Figs. 3.10 and 3.11) (35, 36). Thickening of interlobular septa and fine intralobular networks are frequently evident (Fig. 3.11) (28).

COMPLICATIONS AND SEQUELAE OF TUBERCULOSIS

Pulmonary TB may result in a number of complications and sequelae (see Table 3.4) (26, 37, 38). Parenchymal and

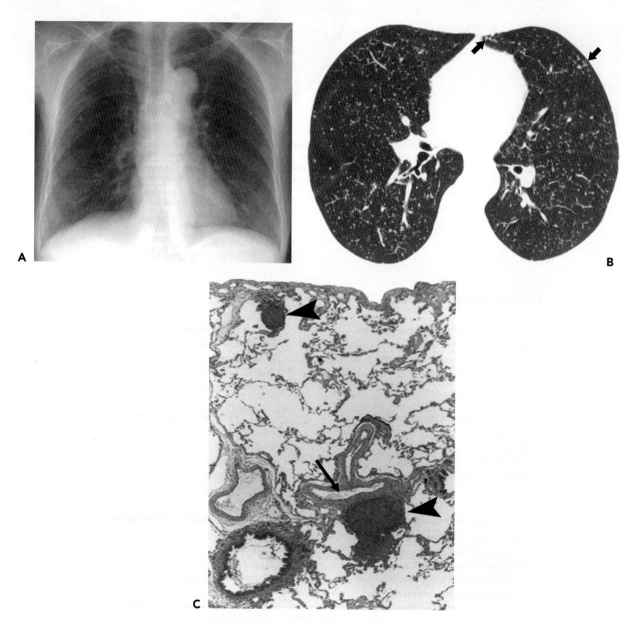

Figure 3.10 Miliary tuberculosis in a 65-year-old woman. **A:** Chest radiograph shows miliary nodular opacities. **B:** High-resolution computed tomography (CT) image (1-mm collimation) shows randomly distributed bilateral small nodules. Also note tree-in-bud opacities (*arrows*). **C:** Photomicrograph of surgical biopsy specimen shows granulomas (*arrowheads*) along the arteriole (*arrow*) and in the alveolar wall.

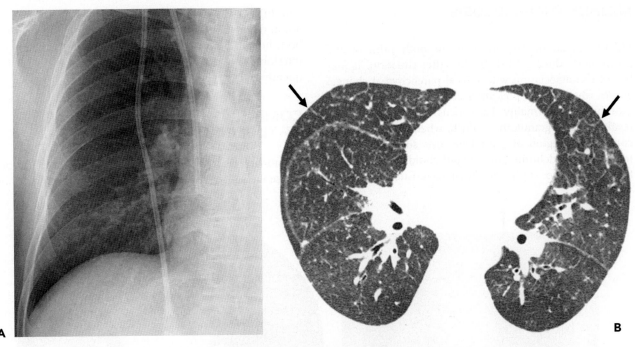

Figure 3.11 Miliary tuberculosis in a 40-year-old man with chronic myeloid leukemia. **A:** Targeted view of the right lung from a chest radiograph shows millet-sized nodules. A central venous line is in place for chemotherapy. **B:** High-resolution computed tomography (CT) image (1-mm collimation) at the level of the right middle lobar bronchus shows bilateral small nodules in random distribution. Also note interlobular septal thickening (*arrows*).

TABLE 3.4
COMPLICATIONS AND SEQUELAE OF TUBERCULOSIS

Parenchymal Complications
Acute respiratory distress syndrome
Extensive lung destruction and cicatrization
Multiple cystic lung lesions
Aspergilloma

Airway Complications
Bronchiectasis
Bronchiolitis obliterans
Tracheobronchial stenosis
Broncholithiasis

Vascular Complications
Pulmonary and bronchial arteritis and
   thrombosis
Bronchial artery pseudoaneurysm
Pulmonary artery pseudoaneurysm
   (Rasmussen aneurysm)

Mediastinal Complications
Esophagomediastinal fistula
Esophagobronchial fistula
Fibrosing mediastinitis
Constrictive pericarditis

Pleural Complications
Pleurisy
Empyema
Fibrothorax
Pneumothorax
Bronchopleural fistula

Chest Wall Complications
Osteomyelitis
Chondritis
Spondylitis
Empyema necessitatis

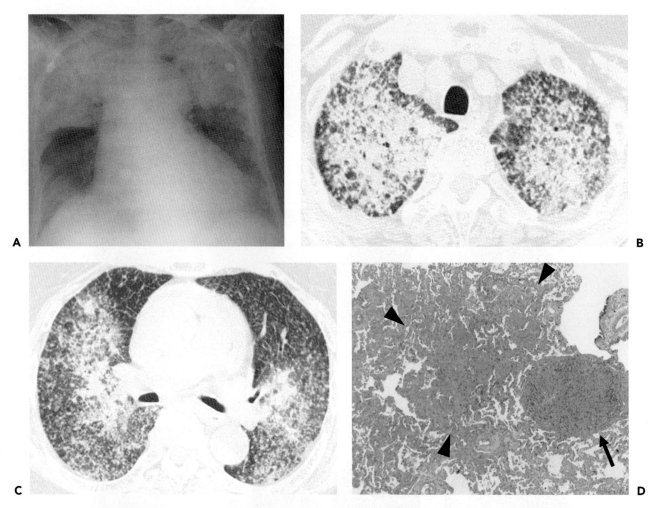

Figure 3.12 Pulmonary tuberculosis presenting as acute respiratory distress syndrome (ARDS) in a 69-year-old woman. **A:** Chest radiograph shows extensive bilateral upper lobe consolidation and diffuse miliary nodules. Also note the ground-glass opacity in lower lung zones and cardiomegaly. **B:** High-resolution computed tomography (CT) image (1-mm collimation) at the level of the great vessels shows airspace consolidation, ground-glass opacities, and numerous bilateral randomly distributed small nodules. **C:** CT image at the level of the distal left main bronchus demonstrates small nodules of random distribution, interlobular septal thickening, and patchy parenchymal opacities. **D:** Photomicrograph of surgical biopsy specimen demonstrates multiple discrete granulomas (*arrow*). Also noted is the diffuse alveolar wall thickening due to fibroblastic proliferation and lymphocytic infiltration (*arrowheads*) consistent with the organizing stage of diffuse alveolar damage.

airway complications include acute respiratory distress syndrome (ARDS) (see Fig. 3.12) (39–41), extensive lung destruction and cicatrization, multiple cystic lung lesions (see Fig. 3.13), aspergilloma (see Fig. 3.14), bronchiectasis, tracheobronchial stenosis (see Figs. 3.15 and 3.16), and broncholithiasis (see Fig. 3.17) (26, 38). The radiologic manifestations of ARDS secondary to TB include extensive bilateral ground-glass opacities or consolidation superimposed on findings of miliary or endobronchial spread of TB (Fig. 3.12). Multiple cystic lesions may develop in patients recovering from ARDS or in patients with extensive consolidation due to TB (42). The cystic lesions may resemble pneumatoceles or bullae (Fig. 3.13). They may resolve over several months or persist (42).

Vascular complications of postprimary tuberculosis include pulmonary and bronchial arteritis and thrombosis, bronchial artery pseudoaneurysm (see Fig. 3.18), and Rasmussen aneurysm (see Fig. 3.19) (26). Rasmussen aneurysm is a pseudoaneurysm that results from weakening of the pulmonary artery wall by adjacent cavitary TB. Mediastinal complications include esophagomediastinal or esophagobronchial fistula (see Fig. 3.20), constrictive pericarditis, and fibrosing mediastinitis (see Fig. 3.21) (26). Pleural complications include tuberculous pleurisy and empyema, empyema necessitatis, fibrothorax, pneumothorax, and bronchopleural fistula (26, 37). Empyema necessitatis results from leakage of tuberculous empyema through the parietal pleura with discharge of its contents into the subcutaneous tissues of the chest wall or, less commonly,

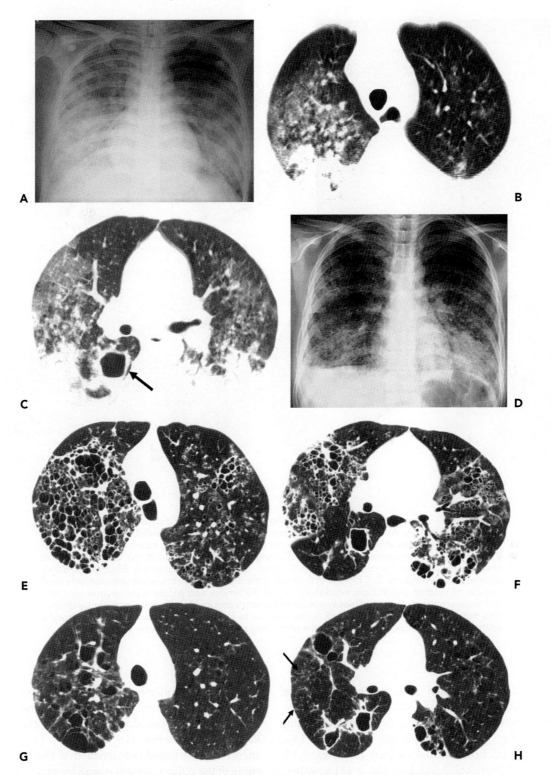

Figure 3.13 Tuberculosis resulting in reversible cystic lung lesions in a 26-year-old woman. **A:** Chest radiograph shows extensive bilateral airspace consolidation. Endotracheal and nasogastric tubes are in place. **B** and **C:** Computed tomography (CT) images (7-mm collimation) at the level of the distal trachea **(A)** and distal main bronchi **(B)**, respectively, show bilateral ground-glass opacities and patchy consolidation. Also note small nodules in both lungs and a thin-walled cavity (*arrow* in **C**) in the superior segment of the right lower lobe. **D:** Chest radiograph obtained 1 month after **(A)** shows multiple small cystic lesions in both lungs along with patchy ground-glass opacities, areas of consolidation, and right pleural effusion. **E** and **F:** CT scans obtained at levels similar to those in, and 1 month after, **(B)** and **(C)**, respectively, with the patient on treatment for tuberculosis, show extensive bilateral cystic changes. Parenchymal opacities and the small nodules have improved in the interval. **G** and **H:** CT scans obtained at levels similar to those in, and 4 months after, **(E)** and **(F)**, respectively, show decreased extent of cystic lesions and parenchymal opacities. A few small nodules and tree-in-bud opacities are still present (*arrows* in **H**).

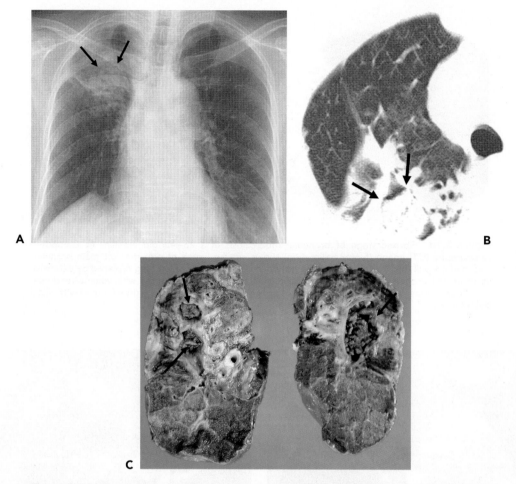

Figure 3.14 Aspergilloma in a 61-year-old woman. **A:** Chest radiograph shows right upper lobe volume loss and cavity with air-crescent sign (*arrows*) surrounding a soft tissue opacity. **B:** Computed tomography (CT) image (5-mm collimation) at the level of the aortic arch shows dense right upper lobe consolidation and scarring. A cavity containing a mass with adjacent crescent of air (air–crescent sign) (*arrows*) is present within the consolidation. **C:** Photomicrograph of gross pathologic specimen demonstrates well-circumscribed cavities filled with tan-colored material (*arrows*) consistent with aspergillomas.

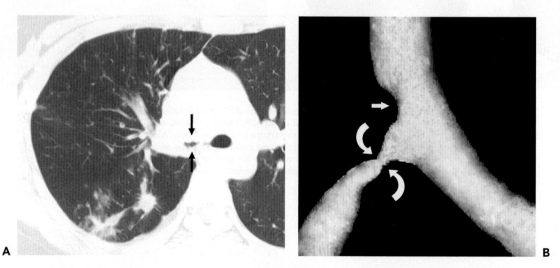

Figure 3.15 Active bronchial tuberculosis in a 34-year-old woman. **A:** View of the right lung from a computed tomography (CT) scan (5-mm collimation) shows marked luminal narrowing of right main bronchus (*arrows*) and wall thickening. Also note variable-sized nodules and parenchymal opacity representing parenchymal tuberculosis. **B:** Three-dimensional airway image obtained with shaded-surface display technique demonstrates irregular narrowing of distal trachea (*straight arrow*) and right main bronchus (*curved arrows*) along with obliterated right upper lobar bronchus.

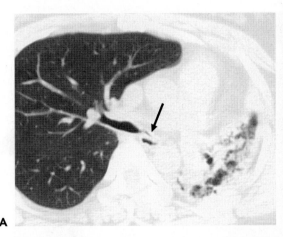
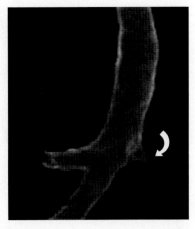

Figure 3.16 Fibrotic stage of bronchial tuberculosis in a 28-year-old woman. **A:** Computed tomography (CT) image (5-mm collimation) shows slit-like lumen of proximal left main bronchus and marked wall thickening (*arrow*). Also note decreased volume of left lung replaced by extensive scarring and bronchiectasis. **B:** Three-dimensional airway image obtained with volume-rendering technique demonstrates rat-tail narrowing of proximal left main bronchus (*curved arrow*) with distal obliteration.

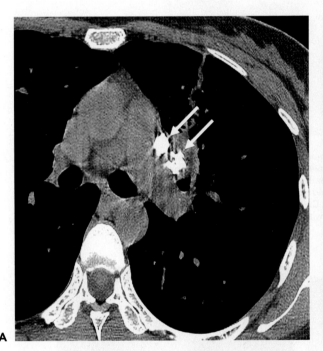
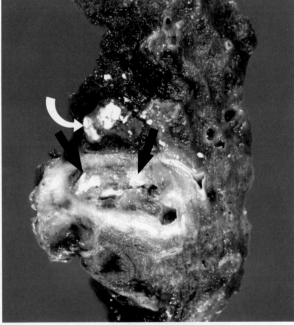

Figure 3.17 Broncholithiasis in a 44-year-old woman. **A:** High-resolution computed tomography (CT) image (1-mm collimation) photographed using soft tissue windows at the level of distal main bronchi shows calcified lymph nodes (*arrows*) in aortopulmonary window. Also noted are obstruction of anterior segmental bronchus of left upper lobe and partial atelectasis of corresponding segment. **B:** Resected left upper lobe shows bronchial wall fibrosis and luminal obstruction by inflammatory exudates and granulation tissue. Calcified debris is evident in airway lumen (*straight arrows*) and peribronchial lymph nodes (*curved arrow*).

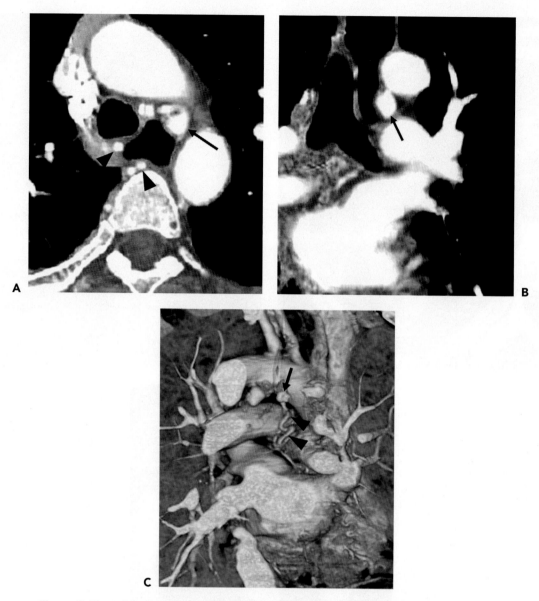

Figure 3.18 Left bronchial artery pseudoaneurysm in a 31-year-old man with chronic tuberculosis in both upper lobes. Patient had undergone right bronchial artery embolization previously. **A:** Computed tomography (CT) image (1.25-mm collimation) at the level of azygos arch shows aneurysmal dilatation (*arrow*) of left bronchial artery. Also note enlarged branches of right bronchial artery (*arrowheads*) and calcified lymph nodes in right lower paratracheal area. **B:** Coronal reconstruction CT image (2-mm collimation) shows aneurysmal dilatation (*arrow*) of left bronchial artery, which arises from the aortic arch. **C:** Volume-rendering image shows pseudoaneurysm (*arrow*) and hypertrophied left bronchial artery (*arrowheads*) distal to it.

pericardium, vertebral column, or esophagus (37). The main chest wall complications are tuberculous osteomyelitis and chondritis, tuberculous spondylitis, and empyema necessitatis (see Fig. 3.22) (26, 37).

TUBERCULOSIS IN ACQUIRED IMMUNODEFICIENCY SYNDROME

HIV infection is the strongest known risk factor for progression from latent to active TB (43). Of the estimated 42 million people infected with HIV worldwide, >25%

have active TB (43). Most patients live in countries with limited health care resources in Africa and Asia. The incidence of TB in these countries is increasing (44). Immune restoration induced by Highly Active Anti-Retroviral Therapy (HAART) in developed countries has considerably improved the prognosis of HIV-positive patients and reduced the prevalence of opportunistic infection and TB in these patients. However, HIV-associated TB continues to occur in countries where HAART is widely used and is seen in patients on antiretroviral treatment (45). Furthermore, HAART may result in the paradoxical worsening of TB manifestations in patients

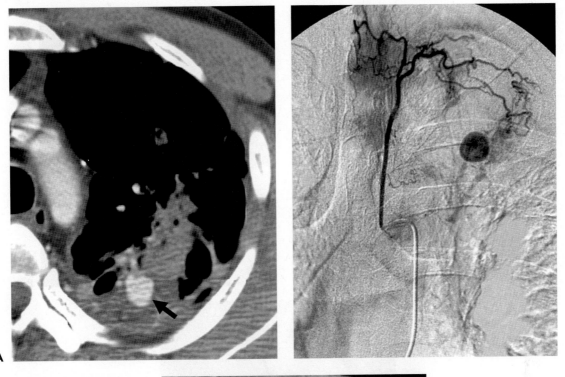

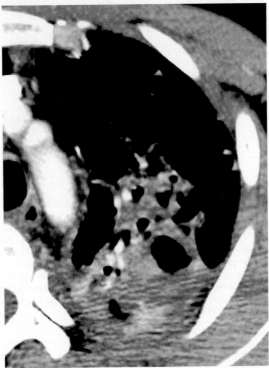

Figure 3.19   Pulmonary artery pseudoaneurysm (Rasmussen aneurysm) in a 33-year-old man. **A:** Computed tomography (CT) image (5-mm collimation) at the level of aortic arch shows cavitary left upper lobe consolidation containing contrast-enhancing round vascular structure (*arrow*). **B:** Left intercostal arteriogram shows retrograde filling of round vascular structure observed on CT scan, through intercostal artery–pulmonary artery shunting. **C:** Follow-up CT scan obtained at a level similar to that in **(A)** after treatment shows disappearance of enhancing vascular structure in left upper lobe.

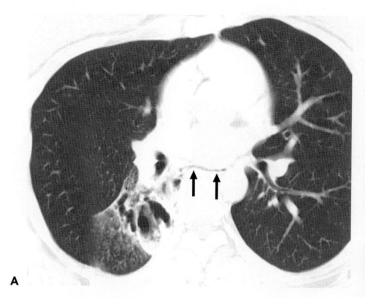
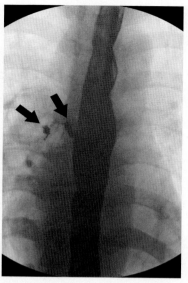

Figure 3.20 Esophagobronchial fistula complicating tuberculous lymphadenitis in a 26-year-old woman with history of cough associated with food intake. **A:** Computed tomography (CT) image (5-mm collimation) at the level of the left basal trunk shows cavitary consolidation and small nodules in the superior segment of the right lower lobe. Also note the tubular air-filled structure (*arrows*) between esophagus and right lung parenchyma, indicating the presence of a fistulous tract between esophagus and right lower lobe airways. **B:** Esophagogram demonstrates a fistulous connection between esophagus and the airway in right lung (*arrows*).

with Immune Reconstitution Inflammatory Syndrome (IRIS) (44, 46).

The manifestations of TB in AIDS patients are influenced by the degree of immunosuppression and by whether the patient is receiving HAART. The radiologic manifestations are reviewed in Chapter 7.

UTILITY OF CT IN TUBERCULOSIS

Chest radiographs play a major role in the diagnosis and management of patients with TB. However, the radiographs may be normal or show only mild or nonspecific findings in patients with active disease (20, 47). Common causes of a missed diagnosis of TB are failure to recognize hilar and mediastinal lymphadenopathy as a manifestation of primary disease in adults, overlooking of mild parenchymal abnormalities in patients with postprimary disease, and failure to recognize that an upper lobe nodule or mass surrounded by small nodular opacities or scarring may represent TB (20). The sensitivity of radiography is particularly low in patients with disseminated disease. For instance, in one study that included the chest radiographs of 71 patients with miliary TB, three independent observers recognized the presence of miliary disease in only 42 to 49 of the 71 patients (sensitivity, 59% to 69%) (35).

CT scan is more sensitive than chest radiography in the detection and characterization of both subtle parenchymal disease and mediastinal lymphadenopathy (28, 36, 47, 48). In patients clinically suspected of having TB with normal

or equivocal radiographic abnormalities, the increased sensitivity of CT scan may allow prompt diagnosis before results of culture are obtained. In one study of 41 consecutive children with confirmed TB, eight (20%) had the diagnosis suggested only on CT scan. The findings on CT scan in these eight patients with no apparent abnormalities on chest radiographs included low-attenuation lymph nodes with rim enhancement, calcifications, and nodules of bronchogenic spread or miliary disease in patients with no abnormalities evident on the radiograph (47). In 15 patients (37%), CT scans provided information that altered clinical management.

CT scan, especially high-resolution CT scan is particularly helpful in the detection of small foci of cavitation in areas of confluent pneumonia and in areas of dense nodularity and scarring (28, 49). For example, in one study of 41 patients who had active TB, high-resolution CT scan showed cavities in 58%, whereas chest radiographs showed cavities in only 22% (28).

High-resolution CT scan is also helpful in detecting the presence of diffuse lung involvement when the chest radiographs are normal or show only questionable or minimal abnormalities (14, 28, 50).

High-resolution CT scan is more sensitive than radiography in demonstrating the presence of miliary disease and endobronchial spread of TB, a finding that is highly suggestive of active disease (36, 49). Endobronchial spread of TB is characterized by the presence of centrilobular nodules and tree-in-bud pattern distant from the primary site of infection. Lee et al. (51) assessed the utility of CT scan in the evaluation of pulmonary TB in 188 patients. A tentative

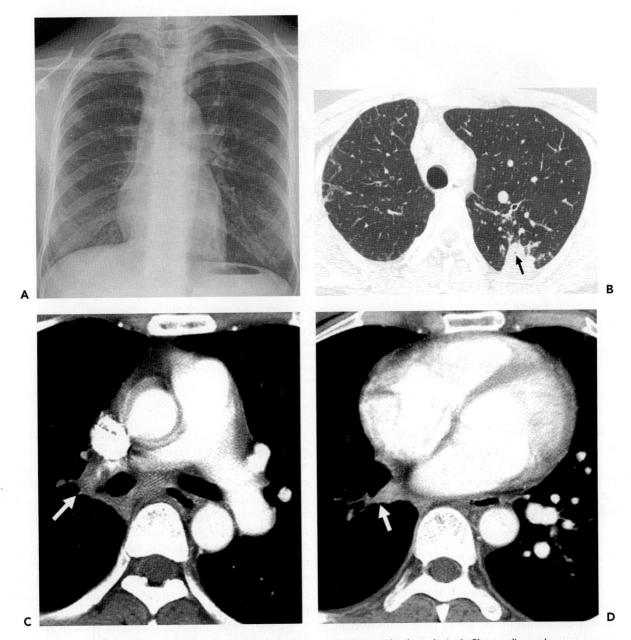

Figure 3.21   Fibrosing mediastinitis in a 34-year-old woman with tuberculosis. **A:** Chest radiograph shows nodular opacities in left upper lobe. Also note decreased right lung volume. **B:** High-resolution computed tomography (CT) image (1-mm collimation) at the level of the distal trachea shows a subpleural nodule containing a small cavity (*arrow*) in the left upper lobe and surrounding small nodules and branching nodular lesions. Also note decreased volume of the right lung and interlobular septal thickening. The septal thickening was due to venous congestion secondary to severe stenosis of the right pulmonary veins by fibrosing mediastinitis. **C:** CT image (5-mm collimation) at the level of the distal left main bronchus shows narrowing of right interlobar pulmonary artery due to mediastinal fibrosis (*arrow*). **D:** CT image at the ventricular level shows marked narrowing of the right inferior pulmonary vein without contrast filling (*arrow*).

diagnosis of active TB on CT scan was based on the pattern of parenchymal abnormalities and the presence of cavitation or evidence of endobronchial spread. A total of 133 of 146 patients (91%) with TB were correctly identified on CT scan as having pulmonary TB, whereas 32 of 42 patients (76%) without TB were correctly excluded. The main causes of misdiagnosis of TB were lung cancer and bacterial pneumonia. Active TB was correctly identified on CT scan in 71 of 89 (80%) patients and inactive disease in 51 of 57 (89%) patients (51).

CT scan is also helpful in the evaluation of pleural complications, including tuberculous effusion, empyema, and bronchopleural fistula, and may demonstrate pleural disease not evident on chest radiography (49, 52).

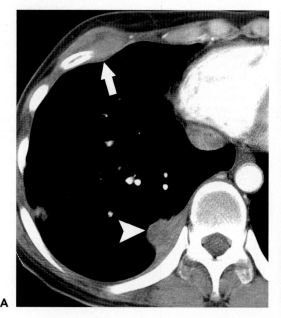
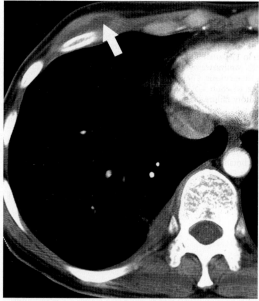

Figure 3.22   Pleural and chest wall tuberculosis in a 35-year-old woman. **A:** View of the right chest from a contrast enhanced computed tomography (CT) (5-mm collimation) at the level of the suprahepatic inferior vena cava shows a subpleural nodule (*arrowhead*) in the right lower lobe, small right pleural effusion and focal soft tissue thickening (*arrow*) of the right anterior chest wall. **B:** CT scan obtained 10 mm below that in **(A)** demonstrates right pleural effusion, and lentiform right chest wall lesion showing central low attenuation (*arrow*) consistent with focal tuberculous chest wall abscess.

REFERENCES

1. Cegielski JP, Chin DP, Espinal MA, et al. The global tuberculosis situation. Progress and problems in the 20th century, prospects for the 21st century. *Infect Dis Clin N Am.* 2002;16:1–58.
2. Corbett EL, Watt CJ, Walker N, et al. The growing burden of tuberculosis: Global trends and interactions with the HIV epidemic. *Arch Intern Med.* 2003; 163:1009–1021.
3. Tufariello JM, Chan J, Flynn JL. Latent tuberculosis: Mechanisms of host and bacillus that contribute to persistent infection. *Lancet Infect Dis.* 2003; 3:578–590.
4. World Health Organization. *Fact sheet No 104. Tuberculosis.* http://www.who.int/mediacentre/factsheets/fs104, Revised April 2005 Accessed September 7, 2005.
5. Centers for Disease Control and Prevention (CDC). Trends in tuberculosis–United States, 2004. *MMWR Morb Mortal Wkly Rep.* 2005;54:245–249.
6. Gupta R, Espinal MA, Raviglione MC. Tuberculosis as a major global health problem in the 21st century: A WHO perspective. *Semin Respir Crit Care Med.* 2004;25:245–253.
7. Fraser RS, Colman N, Müller NL, et al. *Synopsis of diseases of the chest.* Philadelphia, PA: Elsevier, WB Saunders; 2005.
8. American Thoracic Society. Diagnostic standards and classification of tuberculosis. *Am Rev Respir Dis.* 1990;142:725–735.
9. Medlar EM. The behavior of pulmonary tuberculous lesions; a pathological study. *Am Rev Tuberc.* 1955;71:1–244.
10. Ellner JJ. Review: The immune response in human tuberculosis–implications for tuberculosis control. *J Infect Dis.* 1997;176:1351–1359.
11. MacGregor RR. Tuberculosis: From history to current management. *Semin Roentgenol.* 1993;28:101–108.
12. Geng E, Kreiswirth B, Burzynski J, et al. Clinical and radiographic correlates of primary and reactivation tuberculosis: A molecular epidemiology study. *JAMA.* 2005;293:2740–2745.
13. Jones BE, Ryu R, Yang Z, et al. Chest radiographic findings in patients with tuberculosis with recent or remote infection. *Am J Respir Crit Care Med.* 1997; 156:1270–1273.
14. Lee KS, Song KS, Lim TH, et al. Adult-onset pulmonary tuberculosis: Findings on chest radiographs and CT scans. *Am J Roentgenol.* 1993;160:753–758.
15. Leung AN, Müller NL, Pineda PR, et al. Primary tuberculosis in childhood: Radiographic manifestations. *Radiology.* 1992;182:87–91.
16. Weber AL, Bird KT, Janower ML. Primary tuberculosis in childhood with particular emphasis on changes affecting the tracheobronchial tree. *Am J Roentgenol.* 1968;103:123–132.
17. Im JG, Song KS, Kang HS, et al. Mediastinal tuberculous lymphadenitis: CT manifestations. *Radiology.* 1987;164:115–119.
18. Pombo F, Rodriguez E, Mato J, et al. Patterns of contrast enhancement of tuberculous lymph nodes demonstrated by computed tomography. *Clin Radiol.* 1992;46:13–17.
19. Choyke PL, Sostman HD, Curtis AM, et al. Adult-onset pulmonary tuberculosis. *Radiology.* 1983;148:357–362.
20. Woodring JH, Vandiviere HM, Fried AM, et al. Update: The radiographic features of pulmonary tuberculosis. *Am J Roentgenol.* 1986;146:497–506.
21. Leung AN. Pulmonary tuberculosis: The essentials. *Radiology.* 1999;210: 307–322.
22. Krysl J, Korzeniewska-Koesela M, Müller NL, et al. Radiologic features of pulmonary tuberculosis: An assessment of 188 cases. *Can Assoc Radiol J.* 1994; 45:101–107.
23. Hadlock FP, Park SK, Awe RJ, et al. Unusual radiographic findings in adult pulmonary tuberculosis. *Am J Roentgenol.* 1980;134:1015–1018.
24. Murayama S, Murakami J, Hashimoto S, et al. Noncalcified pulmonary tuberculomas: CT enhancement patterns with histologic correlation. *J Thorac Imag.* 1995;10:91–95.
25. Epstein DM, Kline LR, Albelda SM, et al. Tuberculous pleural effusions. *Chest.* 1987;91:106–109.
26. Kim HY, Song KS, Goo JM, et al. Thoracic sequelae and complications of tuberculosis. *Radiographics.* 2001;21:839–858, discussion 859–860.
27. Im JG, Itoh H, Lee KS, et al. CT-pathology correlation of pulmonary tuberculosis. *Crit Rev Diagn Imag.* 1995;36:227–285.
28. Im JG, Itoh H, Shim YS, et al. Pulmonary tuberculosis: CT findings—early active disease and sequential change with antituberculous therapy. *Radiology.* 1993;186:653–660.
29. Lee JY, Lee KS, Jung KJ, et al. Pulmonary tuberculosis: CT and pathologic correlation. *J Comput Assist Tomo.* 2000;24:691–698.
30. Hatipoglu ON, Osma E, Manisali M, et al. High resolution computed tomographic findings in pulmonary tuberculosis. *Thorax.* 1996;51:397–402.
31. Poey C, Verhaegen F, Giron J, et al. High resolution chest CT in tuberculosis: Evolutive patterns and signs of activity. *J Comput Assist Tomor.* 1997;21:601–607.
32. Codecasa LR, Besozzi G, De Cristofaro L, et al. Epidemiological and clinical patterns of intrathoracic lymph node tuberculosis in 60 human immunodeficiency virus-negative adult patients. *Monaldi Arch Chest Dis.* 1998; 53:277–280.
33. Lee KS, Im JG. CT in adults with tuberculosis of the chest: Characteristic findings and role in management. *Am J Roentgenol.* 1995;164:1361–1367.
34. Moon WK, Im JG, Yeon KM, et al. Mediastinal tuberculous lymphadenitis: CT findings of active and inactive disease. *Am J Roentgenol.* 1998; 170:715–718.
35. Kwong JS, Carignan S, Kang EY, et al. Miliary tuberculosis. Diagnostic accuracy of chest radiography. *Chest.* 1996;110:339–342.

36. McGuinness G, Naidich DP, Jagirdar J, et al. High resolution CT findings in miliary lung disease. *J Comput Assist Tomo.* 1992;16:384–390.

37. Choi JA, Hong KT, Oh YW, et al. CT manifestations of late sequelae in patients with tuberculous pleuritis. *Am J Roentgenol.* 2001;176:441–445.

38. Kim Y, Lee KS, Yoon JH, et al. Tuberculosis of the trachea and main bronchi: CT findings in 17 patients. *Am J Roentgenol.* 1997;168:1051–1056.

39. Agarwal MK, Muthuswamy PP, Banner AS, et al. Respiratory failure in pulmonary tuberculosis. *Chest.* 1977;72:605–609.

40. Choi D, Lee KS, Suh GY, et al. Pulmonary tuberculosis presenting as acute respiratory failure: Radiologic findings. *J Comput Assist Tomo.* 1999; 23:107–113.

41. Levy H, Kallenbach JM, Feldman C, et al. Acute respiratory failure in active tuberculosis. *Crit Care Med.* 1987;15:221–225.

42. Ko KS, Lee KS, Kim Y, et al. Reversible cystic disease associated with pulmonary tuberculosis: Radiologic findings. *Radiology.* 1997;204:165–169.

43. Bock N, Reichman LB. Tuberculosis and HIV/AIDS: Epidemiological and clinical aspects (World Perspective). *Semin Respir Crit Care Med.* 2004;25: 337–344.

44. Aaron L, Saadoun D, Calatroni I, et al. Tuberculosis in HIV-infected patients: A comprehensive review. *Clin Microbiol Infec.* 2004;10:388–398.

45. Girardi E, Antonucci G, Vanacore P, et al. Tuberculosis in HIV-infected persons in the context of wide availability of highly active antiretroviral therapy. *Eur Respir J.* 2004;24:11–17.

46. Shelburne SA 3rd, Hamill RJ. The immune reconstitution inflammatory syndrome. *AIDS Rev.* 2003;5:67–79.

47. Kim WS, Moon WK, Kim IO, et al. Pulmonary tuberculosis in children: Evaluation with CT. *Am J Roentgenol.* 1997;168:1005–1009.

48. Pastores SM, Naidich DP, Aranda CP, et al. Intrathoracic adenopathy associated with pulmonary tuberculosis in patients with human immunodeficiency virus infection. *Chest.* 1993;103:1433–1437.

49. Sharma SK, Mukhopadhyay S, Arora R, et al. Computed tomography in miliary tuberculosis: Comparison with plain films, bronchoalveolar lavage, pulmonary functions and gas exchange. *Australas Radiol.* 1996;40: 113–118.

50. Kuhlman JE, Deutsch JH, Fishman EK, et al. CT features of thoracic mycobacterial disease. *Radiographics.* 1990;10:413–431.

51. Lee KS, Hwang JW, Chung MP, et al. Utility of CT in the evaluation of pulmonary tuberculosis in patients without AIDS. *Chest.* 1996;110:977–984.

52. Hulnick DH, Naidich DP, McCauley DI. Pleural tuberculosis evaluated by computed tomography. *Radiology.* 1983;149:759–765.

Nontuberculous Mycobacterial Pulmonary Disease

4

Nontuberculous mycobacteria (NTM) are mycobacteria other than *Mycobacterium tuberculosis* and *Mycobacterium leprae*. Previous names for this group of organisms included "environmental mycobacteria," "atypical mycobacteria," or "mycobacteria other than tuberculosis" (1, 2). Unlike *M. tuberculosis*, which is an obligate human pathogen with no environmental reservoir, NTM are commonly isolated from environmental sources such as water and soil (3, 4). An increasing number of NTM have been recognized to be affecting the lung. Although the incidence of disseminated *Mycobacterium avium* complex (MAC) infections in patients with human immunodeficiency virus (HIV) has decreased in recent years with the use of highly active antiretroviral treatments (HAART), the rate of pulmonary NTM infection in other immunocompromised and nonimmunocompromised patients is increasing (5).

NTM have been traditionally classified into four groups on the basis of growth rates, colony morphology, and pigmentation (Runyon Classification System) (6). Groups I, II, and III are slow growers, requiring a time similar to that required by *M. tuberculosis* to grow in culture, whereas Group IV organisms are rapid growers that grow well in routine bacteriologic media in <7 days. The slow growers are further differentiated according to their ability to produce yellow pigment (3) (see Table 4.1).

The Runyon classification system has been primarily a tool for microbiologists, and has allowed easier identification of individual NTM species by mycobacterial laboratories. However, it has become less relevant in recent years because of advances in mycobacteriology, including more rapid culture techniques, DNA probes, and high-pressure liquid chromatography. In addition, this system is of little value to clinicians because the organisms in a particular Runyon class may cause different patterns of disease. A more appropriate grouping for these organisms is currently based on the type of clinical disease they produce: Pulmonary disease, lymphadenopathy, cutaneous disease, and disseminated disease (2, 3).

EPIDEMIOLOGY

Most NTM are environmentally ubiquitous and have been recovered from water and soil. It is generally accepted that most human infection is due to environmental NTM (2, 3). Person-to-person transmission of infection is rare and isolation of infected individuals is therefore not required. Although contact with environmental mycobacteria is

TABLE 4.1

CLASSIFICATION OF MYCOBACTERIAL SPECIES COMMONLY CAUSING HUMAN DISEASE

Mycobacterium tuberculosis complex
   Mycobacterium tuberculosis
   Mycobacterium bovis
   Mycobacterium africanum
Mycobacterium leprae
Nontuberculous mycobacteria
   Slowly growing mycobacteria
      Mycobacterium kansasii (Photochromogens, Runyon group I)
      Mycobacterium marinum
      Mycobacterium gordonae (Scotochromogens, Runyon group II)
      Mycobacterium scrofulaceum
      Mycobacterium avium complex (Nonchromogens, Runyon group III)
         Mycobacterium avium
         Mycobacterium intracellulare
      Mycobacterium terrae complex
      Mycobacterium ulcerans
      Mycobacterium xenopi
   Rapidly growing mycobacteria (Runyon group IV)
      Mycobacterium fortuitum
      Mycobacterium chelonae
      Mycobacterium abscessus

common, overt disease is uncommon because of the low virulence of these organisms. Disease usually develops in immunocompromised patients, in patients with preexisting lung disease, and only occasionally in otherwise apparently healthy persons (5).

There is considerable geographic variability in the prevalence of NTM disease and in the mycobacterial species responsible for it. Overall, the most common NTM resulting in pulmonary disease is the MAC (5). The second most common NTM pathogen is *Mycobacterium kansasii* in the United States and Japan and *Mycobacterium xenopi* in Canada and Europe, except for Scandinavia and areas of northern Europe, where *Mycobacterium malmoense* is second to MAC (7, 8).

DIAGNOSTIC CRITERIA

Unlike *M. tuberculosis*, NTM are not obligate pathogens. Accordingly, the isolation of an NTM species from a respiratory sample is not sufficient evidence for the presence of NTM lung disease. The diagnosis of pulmonary NTM disease is based on clinical, radiographic, and bacteriologic criteria (1–3). The necessary clinical criterion is the presence of compatible symptoms and signs, with the

reasonable exclusion of other etiologies of pulmonary disease. However, the signs and symptoms of NTM lung disease are variable and nonspecific. Clinical manifestations include chronic cough, fever, chills, night sweats, dyspnea on exertion, hemoptysis, and weight loss (5). NTM infection of the lungs often occurs in the context of preexisting lung disease, especially chronic obstructive pulmonary disease, bronchiectasis, pneumoconiosis, and previous tuberculosis. As a result, the clinical manifestations of NTM lung disease are often similar to those of the underlying disease (3).

The radiographic criteria required for diagnosis are the presence of consolidation, cavitation, or multiple nodules at plain chest radiography or high-resolution computed tomography (CT). The radiographic manifestations are variable, depending on the presence or absence of underlying disease, and on the NTM species (see Table 4.2).

In 1997, the American Thoracic Society issued a revised statement of diagnostic criteria for NTM lung disease (1, 2) (see Table 4.3), and in 2000, the British Thoracic Society

TABLE 4.2

RADIOLOGIC FINDINGS OF NONTUBERCULOUS MYCOBACTERIAL PULMONARY DISEASE

Species	Radiographic Findings

Mycobacterium avium complex	Upper lobe cavitary form
	  Thin-walled upper lobe cavities
	  Apical pleural thickening
	Nodular bronchiectatic form
	  Bilateral nodular or reticulonodular opacities
	  Centrilobular nodules and tree-in-bud pattern on CT scan
	  Bronchiectasis mainly in right middle lobe and lingula

Mycobacterium kansasii	Thin-walled upper lobe cavities
Mycobacterium abscessus *Mycobacterium fortuitum* *Mycobacterium chelonae*	Reticulonodular pattern Cavitation in approximately 15% Multiple small nodules Multi-focal bronchiectasis, Focal areas of consolidation on CT scan

CT, computed tomography.

TABLE 4.3

AMERICAN THORACIC SOCIETY CRITERIA FOR THE DIAGNOSIS OF NONTUBERCULOUS MYCOBACTERIAL PULMONARY DISEASE

Clinical criteria
1. Compatible symptoms and signs
2. Reasonable exclusion of other disease

Radiologic criteria
1. Plain chest radiography
   Infiltrates with or without nodules (persistent for ≥2 mo or progression)
   Cavitation
   Nodules alone (multiple)
2. High-resolution CT scan
   Multiple small nodules
   Multifocal bronchiectasis with or without small lung nodules

Bacteriologic criteria
If three sputum/bronchial wash results are available from the previous 12 mo:
1. Three positive cultures with negative acid-fast bacilli smear results, or
2. Two positive cultures and one positive acid-fast bacilli smear

If only one bronchial wash is available:
1. Positive culture with a 2+, 3+, or 4+ acid-fast bacilli smear, or 2+, 3+, or 4+ growth on solid media

If sputum/bronchial wash evaluations are nondiagnostic or another disease cannot be excluded:
1. Transbronchial or lung biopsy yielding nontuberculous mycobacteria, or
2. Biopsy showing mycobacterial histopathologic features (granulomatous inflammation or acid-fast bacilli smear) and one or more sputa or bronchial washing procedures positive for nontuberculous mycobacterium, even in low numbers

CT, computed tomography.

published guidelines for the management of NTM disease (2). According to the British guidelines, which has less strict diagnostic criteria than those of the American Thoracic Society statement, NTM pulmonary disease is diagnosed when positive cultures develop from specimens of sputum obtained at least 7 days apart (two separate positive cultures) from a patient whose chest radiograph suggests mycobacterial infection and who may or may not have clinical symptoms or signs.

The American Thoracic Society diagnostic criteria put greater emphasis on multiple cultures using at least three sputum samples, the use of bronchoscopy with bronchial washing, transbronchial lung biopsy, and high-resolution CT scan, especially in patients without cavitation. These criteria were considered by some investigators as being primarily designed for use in the United States, where the incidence of tuberculosis is low and the relative

incidence of NTM pulmonary disease is high (9). In developing countries, where the incidence of pulmonary tuberculosis is much higher than that of NTM pulmonary disease, the initiation of presumptive antituberculous treatment, especially in smear-positive patients prior to identification of isolates, is common practice (9). With empirical first-line antituberculous treatment, early sputum conversion to culture negativity would be expected in some cases of NTM pulmonary disease, reducing the likelihood of further positive culture of isolates. In general, evidence of disease, such as consistent pulmonary opacities on chest radiographs and the repeated isolation of multiple colonies of the same strain of NTM in the absence of other pathogens, is sufficient for the diagnosis of NTM pulmonary disease.

Because NTM pulmonary disease can be indolent, appropriate follow-up is essential to determine the significance of potentially pathogenic NTM isolated from sputum. Delays in diagnosis are frequent, and radiographs may remain unchanged for years. In one study, there was an average interval of 6.4 years before radiographic change was apparent (10). When NTM cultures are positive, stable findings at chest radiographs, especially at relatively short intervals, are not sufficient grounds to exclude infection. In the absence of lung biopsy, months to years of clinical, radiographic, and microbiologic follow-up of certain patients may be required to reliably determine the significance of NTM respiratory isolates (3).

LABORATORY METHODS

The methods of acid-fast staining and culture currently used for *M. tuberculosis* are acceptable for most NTM species. The appearance of NTM at microscopy is generally indistinguishable from that of *M. tuberculosis*, and the American Thoracic Society has recommended that samples should be inoculated onto at least one solid medium (Lowenstein–Jensen or Middlebrook 7H10 and 7H11) and into a liquid culture system (BACTEC, MGIT, ESP); the latter allows more rapid culture and isolation of a greater range of species than does the use of solid media alone (3).

NTM are identified by their pattern of pigmentation, growth characteristics, microscopic appearance, and biochemical reactions. More rapid discriminating systems are being developed, and include DNA probes, high-performance liquid chromatography, polymerase chain reaction restriction enzyme analysis, and 16S ribosomal ribonucleic acid (rRNA) gene sequence analysis (2,3).

Susceptibility testing of NTM is more difficult and more controversial than that of *M. tuberculosis*. In general, the results of standard susceptibility tests are of little or no value in predicting clinical efficacy in NTM infections, and the provision of *in vitro* susceptibility results to clinicians is likely to be more confusing than helpful (2,3). Both the American Thoracic Society and the British Thoracic Society

have recommended that routine testing of the susceptibility of NTM to antituberculous drugs be discouraged (2, 3).

MYCOBACTERIUM AVIUM COMPLEX

MAC is the most commonly isolated and most clinically important pulmonary NTM pathogen, and includes the two species *Mycobacterium avium* and *Mycobacterium intra-cellulare*. The fact that they are distinct, however, has no clinical or prognostic value for individual patients. They are therefore considered together as MAC.

MAC pulmonary disease occurs in patients with chronic lung disease, with deficient cellular immunity, with AIDS, and also with increasing frequency in persons without apparent underlying disease. Early studies showed that patients with chronic lung disease or deficient cellular immunity accounted for >50% of cases of MAC pulmonary disease, whereas patients without predisposing factors accounted for approximately 25% of the total number of

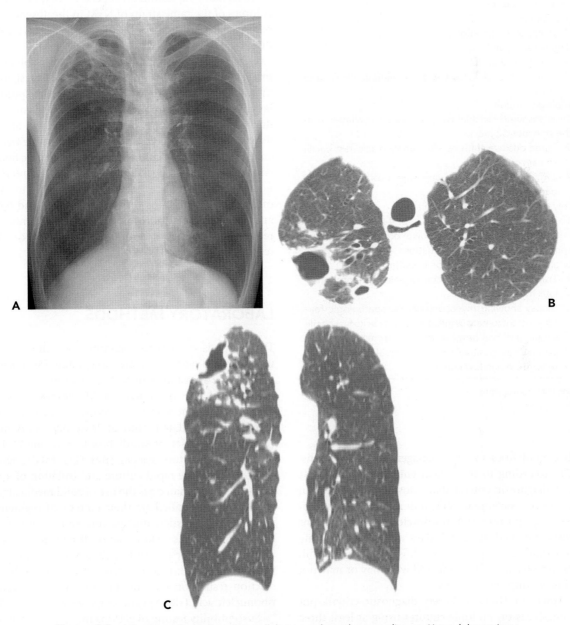

Figure 4.1 *Mycobacterium avium–intracellulare* complex pulmonary disease. Upper lobe cavitary form. **A:** Chest radiograph shows thin-walled cavities in the right upper lung zone and reticulonodular opacities in both upper zones. Also note the poorly defined parenchymal opacity in the right middle lung zone. **B:** Computed tomography (CT) image (2.5-mm collimation) at the level of great vessels shows bronchiectasis, two cavitary lesions, and several small nodules in the right upper lobe. **C:** Coronal reformation (2-mm collimation) shows a large thin-walled cavity, small nodules, and bronchiectasis in right upper lobe. Also note the nodular ground-glass opacity in the left upper lobe and nodule and bronchiectasis in the left lung base. The patient was a 48-year-old man.

HIV-negative cases (11). More recent studies have shown a steady increase in the incidence of MAC pulmonary disease in persons without underlying predisposing condition that currently accounts for >50% of cases of MAC pulmonary infection in HIV-negative cases (12).

The symptoms and signs of MAC lung disease are variable and nonspecific. Moreover, the natural history of MAC pulmonary disease in patients who are HIV-negative is unpredictable. Some patients show a stable clinical and radiographic picture for years, while others demonstrate a relatively rapid progression of the disease. This feature

appears to relate in part to the existence of two main types of clinical disease and presentation.

The two main patterns of MAC pulmonary disease are the upper lobe cavitary form (see Figs. 4.1 and 4.2) and the nodular bronchiectatic form (3) (see Fig. 4.3). The former is usually seen in white, middle-aged or elderly men who smoke or abuse alcohol. Common underlying pulmonary disorders include chronic obstructive pulmonary disease, previous tuberculosis, and silicosis. Chest radiography frequently demonstrates apical cavitary changes similar to those seen in postprimary

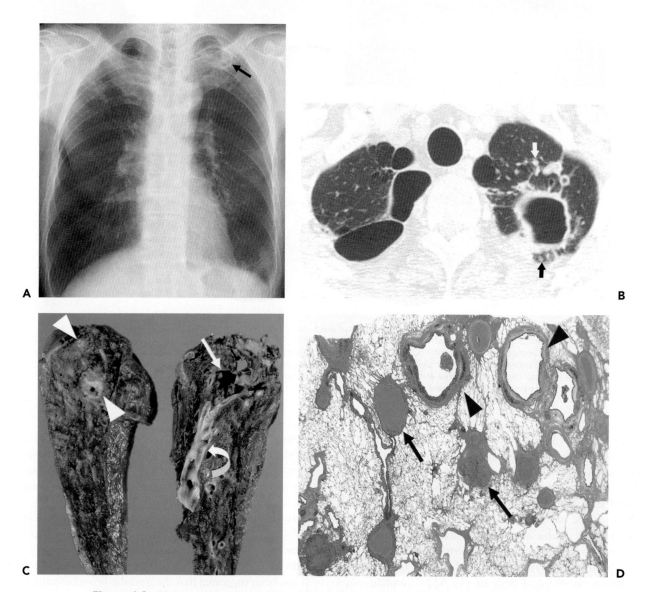

Figure 4.2 *Mycobacterium avium–intracellulare* complex pulmonary disease. Upper lobe cavitary form. **A:** Chest radiograph shows a thin-walled cavity (*arrow*) in the left upper lobe and reticulonodular opacities in the right upper lobe. Also note the bullae in the right apex. **B:** Computed tomography (CT) image (2.5-mm collimation) at the level of great vessels shows thin-walled cavity and nodules (*arrows*) in the left upper lobe. Also note the bullae in both apices. **C:** Photomicrograph of the left upper lobectomy specimen demonstrates several thin-walled cavities (*straight arrow*), variable-sized granulomas (*arrowheads*), and bronchiectasis (*curved arrow*). **D:** Histologic section shows granulomas with central caseation necrosis (*arrows*) along bronchioles. Also note the ectatic bronchi with thick walls (*arrowheads*). The patient was a 54-year-old man.

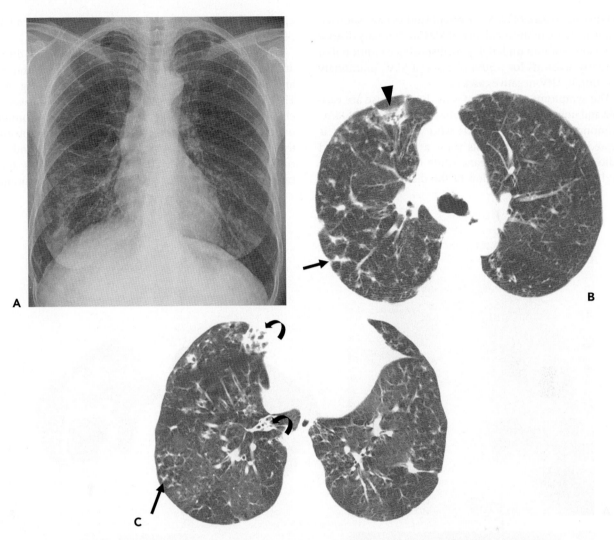

Figure 4.3 *Mycobacterium avium–intracellulare* complex pulmonary disease. Nodular bronchiectatic form. **A:** Chest radiograph shows asymmetric bilateral reticulonodular opacities. **B** and **C:** Computed tomography (CT) images (2.5-mm collimation) at the level of the main bronchi **(B)** and suprahepatic inferior vena cava **(C)**, respectively, demonstrate centrilobular small nodules and branching opacities (tree-in-bud pattern) (*straight arrows*), parenchymal opacities (*arrowhead* in **B**), and bronchiectasis (*curved arrows* in **C**).

tuberculosis (13–15). Cavitation is common and frequently associated with apical pleural thickening. The cavities are usually thin-walled (16, 17) (Figs. 4.1 and 4.2). Endobronchial spread of disease is common and manifests as unilateral or bilateral small ill-defined nodules on chest radiograph. High-resolution CT scan shows the nodules to be centrilobular and frequently associated with branching opacities (tree-in-bud pattern). Upper lobe fibrosis with volume loss and traction bronchiectasis occurs in one-third of patients (13–15). Lymphadenopathy and pleural effusion are uncommon. This form of disease is generally progressive, and if left untreated, can lead to extensive lung destruction and eventually, death (3).

The second pattern of presentation, known as the *nodular bronchiectatic form* (1), is typically indolent and occurs predominantly in nonsmoking middle-aged or elderly women who present with chronic cough and sputum production. Most of these patients have no history of previous or underlying lung disease (11, 18). In addition, the radiographic findings are quite distinct from those of the classic upper lobe cavitary form of the disease. The characteristic radiographic findings are bilateral nodular or reticulonodular opacities particularly in the right middle lobe, and lingula (11, 18) (see Fig. 4.3). The apical pattern resembling reactivated tuberculosis is not present. It has been suggested that the nodular bronchiectatic form may result from habitual voluntary suppression of cough leading to the development of nonspecific inflammatory processes in these poorly draining lung regions and subsequent growth of MAC (18). Because this form is seen particularly in elderly women and may be related to their fastidiousness, this pattern of presentation is commonly referred to as Lady Windermere syndrome (18).

Most patients with the nodular bronchiectatic form of MAC infection have underlying bronchiectasis, which becomes colonized by the organism (19). The characteristic high-resolution CT scan findings consist of multifocal small (<5 mm) centrilobular nodules and branching opacities (tree-in-bud pattern) and bronchiectasis that may be diffuse or involve predominantly or exclusively the right middle lobe and lingula (17, 20–22). Transbronchial

or surgical lung biopsy specimens show granulomatous inflammation, suggesting lung tissue invasion by the organisms (23) (see Fig. 4.4). Histopathologically the CT findings have been shown to reflect the presence of bronchiolectasis and bronchiolar and peribronchiolar inflammation with or without granuloma formation (24, 25) (see Fig. 4.5). Both the high-resolution CT scan and the pathologic findings are considered to be due to the

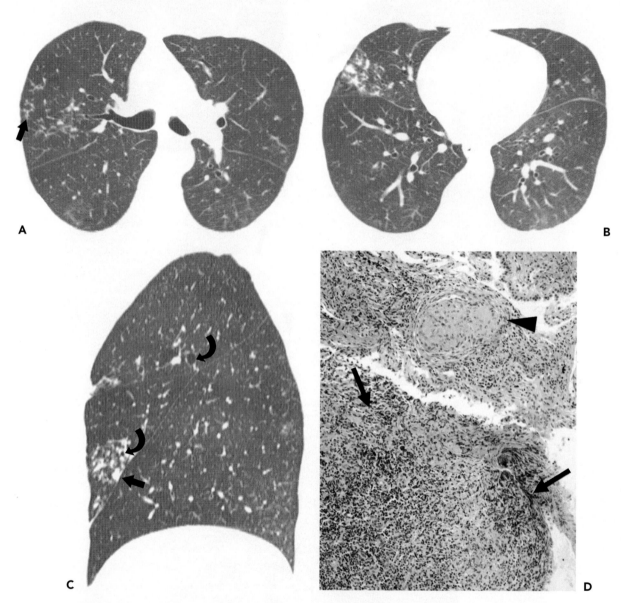

Figure 4.4 *Mycobacterium avium–intracellulare* complex pulmonary disease. Nodular bronchiectatic form. **A:** High-resolution computed tomography (CT) (1-mm collimation) image obtained on a multidetector CT scanner at the level of the anterior and posterior segmental bronchi of the right upper lobe shows multiple small nodules and branching centrilobular opacities (tree-in-bud pattern) (*straight arrow*) in the right upper lobe. **B:** High-resolution CT image at a more caudal level shows multiple small nodules and branching centrilobular opacities (tree-in-bud pattern) in the right middle lobe and nodular ground-glass opacity in lingula. **C:** Sagittal reformation shows multiple small nodules (*straight arrow*) and branching centrilobular opacities in the right middle lobe and small opacities in the right upper lobe. Also noted is bronchiectasis (*curved arrows*) in the right upper and middle lobes. **D:** Photomicrograph of lung specimen obtained by transbronchial lung biopsy in a different patient with similar CT scan findings shows infiltration with lymphocytes and bronchiolar mural granulomas (*arrows*). Also note a small granuloma (*arrowhead*) in the peribronchiolar interstitium.

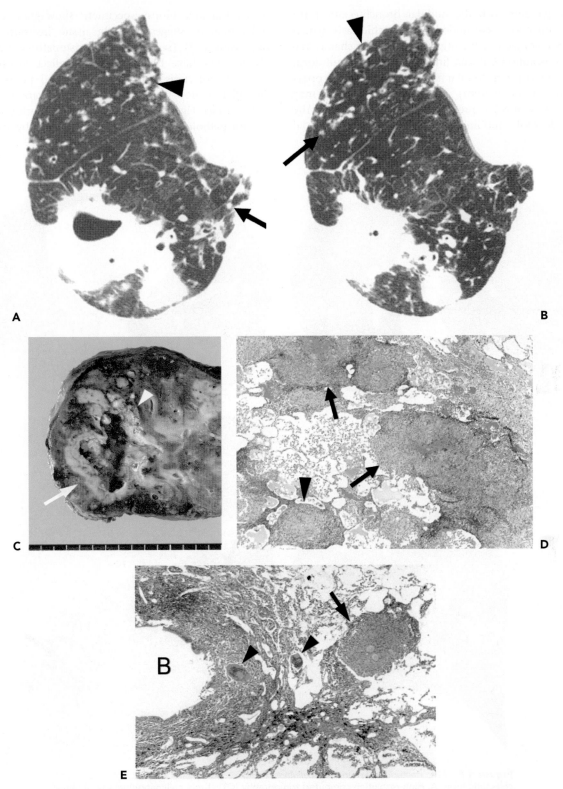

Figure 4.5 *Mycobacterium avium–intracellulare* complex infection. **A** and **B:** Images of the right lung 10 mm apart from a Computed tomography (CT) scan (2.5-mm collimation) at the level of the suprahepatic inferior vena cava show cavitary consolidation, large nodule, small nodules (*arrows*), and branching centrilobular opacities (tree-in-bud pattern) (*arrowheads*). **C:** Right lower lobectomy specimen shows several granulomas with caseating material, one of which contains central necrotic cavity (*arrow*). Bronchial wall destruction (*arrowhead*) due to inflammation and granulomatous reaction is also apparent. **D:** Photomicrograph of histopathologic specimen shows granulomas (*arrows*) in bronchiolar wall and small granuloma (*arrowhead*) in alveolar wall. **E:** Magnified view demonstrates well-defined granuloma (*arrow*) adjacent to inflamed bronchiole **(B)**. Also note Langerhans type giant cells (*arrowheads*). The patient was a 52-year-old woman.

presence of mycobacterial disease, rather than colonization (3).

In the nodular bronchiectatic pattern of presentation, isolation of MAC from sputum specimens is less consistent than in the upper lobe cavitary form of the disease. Sputum may be intermittently positive or show only low numbers of organisms. Because of high false-negative rates of sputum cultures in such a population, up to 45% of patients may require bronchoscopic lavage fluid for culture or lung biopsy for diagnosis of active MAC infection (26). This low sensitivity of sputum cultures may result from the noncavitary nature of the disease.

In some patients, the condition initially involves the presence of small peripheral nodules with the subsequent development of more small nodules and bronchiectasis in the adjacent parenchyma (23, 27) (see Fig. 4.6). Moore demonstrated the progression of existing bronchiectasis as well as the formation of new areas of bronchiectasis on serial CT scan examinations (28). Such results strongly suggest that in some patients at least, bronchiectasis may not only be a predisposing condition for MAC infection but may also be caused by the disease.

The nodular bronchiectatic form of MAC disease tends to progress much more slowly than the cavitary form.

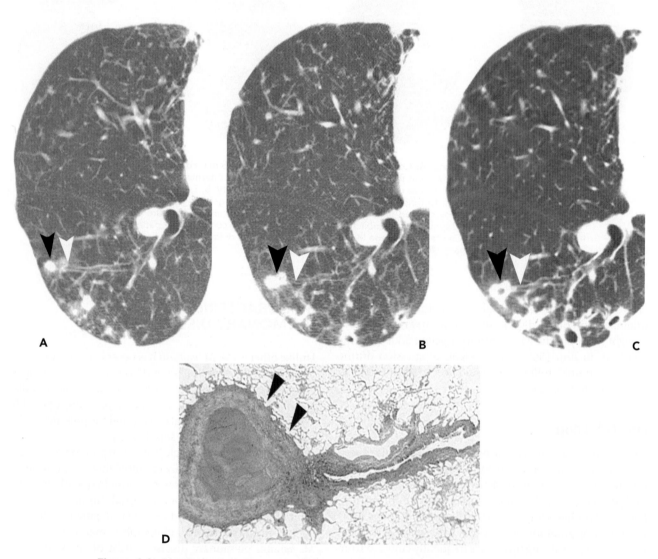

Figure 4.6 *Mycobacterium avium–intracellulare* complex disease. **A:** Computed tomography (CT) image (2.5-mm collimation) at the level of the right basal trunk shows multiple small centrilobular nodules in the right lung. Also note the dilated bronchus (*white arrowhead*) coursing toward a nodule (*black arrowhead*) in right lower lobe. **B:** CT scan obtained at a level similar to and 6 months after that of (**A**) demonstrates increased size and early cavitation of the small nodule (*black arrowhead*) in contact with a dilated bronchus (*white arrowhead*). Cavitating nodules are also seen posteriorly. **C:** CT scan obtained 17 months after (**A**) demonstrates increased size of the cavitating nodule (*black arrowhead*) in contact with a dilated bronchus (*white arrowhead*). Also note other enlarged cavitating nodules posteriorly. **D:** Photomicrograph shows a granuloma (*arrowheads*) containing central caseation necrosis, connected to inflamed peripheral bronchus. The patient was a 57-year-old man.

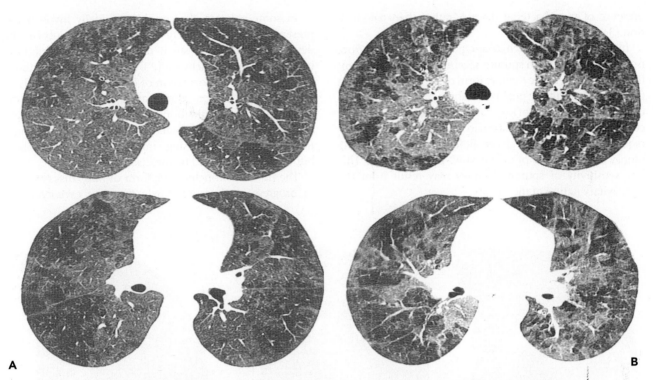

A

B

Figure 4.7 Hot tub lung. **A:** Computed tomography (CT) images (1.5-mm collimation) obtained at end of maximal inspiration at levels of the aortic arch and bronchus intermedius show bilateral ground-glass opacities and areas of decreased attenuation and vascularity. **B:** Expiratory CT images obtained at levels similar to those of **(A)** demonstrate patchy bilateral ground-glass opacities and air-trapping. Lung biopsy showed findings of hypersensitivity pneumonitis, but culture of biopsy material demonstrated growth of *Mycobacterium avium–intracellulare* complex. The patient was a 49-year-old woman. (Courtesy of H. Page McAdams, MD, Department of Radiology, Duke University Medical Center, Durham, NC, USA.)

However, eventually it may lead to respiratory failure. In the original report of this disease, the condition was progressive in eight (38%) of the 21 immunocompetent adult patients involved. In four (50%) of the eight, progression during the longitudinal follow-up period led to death due to respiratory failure (11).

Hot Tub Lung

Hot tub lung refers to hypersensitivity pneumonitis caused by aerosolized and inhaled MAC organisms from a hot tub, which provides an ideal environment for the growth of bacteria (29, 30). Patients present with bronchitis, fever, and flu-like symptoms. Lung biopsy specimens show noncaseating granulomas typical of hypersensitivity pneumonitis (31). MAC organisms are frequently cultured from biopsy specimens or from bronchoalveolar lavage fluid. Chest radiograph shows diffuse reticular or fine nodular opacities (29, 30). High-resolution CT scan shows findings of subacute hypersensitivity pneumonitis with extensive bilateral ground-glass opacities and poorly defined centrilobular nodules (29, 30, 32) (see Fig. 4.7). Patients usually recover uneventfully when they are removed from exposure (32–34).

MYCOBACTERIUM KANSASII PULMONARY DISEASE

Unlike other NTM, *M. kansasii* has never been found in soil or natural water supplies, but has been discovered in piped water systems in cities where it is endemic. *M. kansasii* disease is concentrated in urban areas, supporting a possible association between clinical disease and the presence of the organism in potable water supplies (3).

The clinical and radiologic features of pulmonary disease caused by *M. kansasii* usually resemble those of pulmonary tuberculosis. *M. kansasii* presents more frequently in older men; a history of cigarette smoking and chronic obstructive pulmonary disease is found in >50% of patients (35).

The most common radiographic manifestations of *M. kansasii* pulmonary disease consist of single or multiple upper lobe cavities and endobronchial spread to other lobes. The cavities tend to have thinner walls and less surrounding parenchymal infiltration than in tuberculosis (9, 36) (see Fig. 4.8). The differences are not sufficient to permit differential diagnosis on the basis of the radiographic findings alone, even though the presence of pleural effusion or lower lobe involvement makes *M. kansasii* infection very unlikely (37). Most patients have

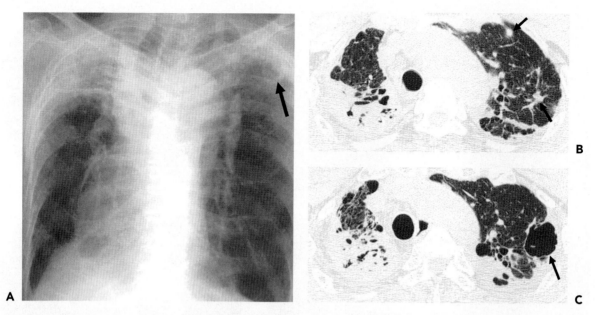

Figure 4.8 *Mycobacterium kansasii* pulmonary disease. **A:** Chest radiograph shows bilateral upper lobe reticulonodular opacities and upper lobe volume loss with marked cephalad retraction of the hila. A thin-walled cavity (*arrow*) is present in the left upper lobe. Also note the right apical pleural thickening and emphysematous overinflation in the remaining lungs. **B:** Computed tomography (CT) image (2.5-mm collimation) at the level of the aortic arch shows dense right upper lobe consolidation containing air bronchograms. Also note nodules (*arrows*), reticulation, and pleural and fissural thickening in both hemithoraces. **C:** CT scan obtained 15 mm caudal to **(B)** demonstrates additional finding of thin-walled cavity (arrow) in the left upper lobe. The patient was a 78-year-old man.

evidence of emphysema on high-resolution CT scan (38). A less common form of presentation consists of bilateral nodules, usually well circumscribed and measuring <1 cm in diameter (14). Most patients with this form of presentation have bronchiectasis, which may be diffuse or involve predominantly or exclusively the right middle lobe and lingula. The findings in this group of patients therefore resemble those of MAC.

RAPIDLY GROWING MYCOBACTERIAL PULMONARY DISEASE

Most clinical pulmonary disease is due to three clinically relevant species of rapidly growing mycobacteria: *Mycobacterium abscessus*, *Mycobacterium fortuitum*, and *Mycobacterium chelonae*. Among the pulmonary diseases these cause, *M. abscessus* (formerly *Mycobacterium chelonae*, subspecies *abscessus*) is responsible for approximately 80% of isolates and *M. fortuitum* for 15% (39, 40).

Most patients with rapidly growing mycobacterial pulmonary disease are middle-aged or older, female, and nonsmokers (39). Only approximately 20% of patients have underlying disorders, including prior mycobacterial infection, gastroesophageal disorders with chronic vomiting, and bronchiectasis (39, 40). As in other forms of NTM lung disease, symptoms are indolent and diagnosis is usually not established until >2 years after the onset of symptoms (39).

The most frequent patterns seen at chest radiography are reticulonodular opacities (see Fig. 4.9). Cavitation occurs in only 15% of patients (41) (see Fig. 4.10). The disease is typically multilobar and bilateral, with slight upper lobe predominance (39, 42, 43). The most common high-resolution CT scan findings are multifocal bronchiectasis, small nodules (<5 mm) and branching centrilobular lesions (tree-in-bud pattern), focal areas of consolidation, and bronchial wall thickening, and are similar to those reported for MAC pulmonary disease (26, 43).

In most patients with *M. abscessus*, the disease progresses very slowly, and some patients show little radiographic change over a period of years. Although the disease is slowly progressive it may eventually result in respiratory failure and death (14%) (40).

There is considerable overlap in common CT scan findings of MAC and *M. abscessus* pulmonary diseases (44). No significant difference is found in the presence of small nodules, tree-in-bud pattern, and bronchiectasis. However, lobar volume loss, large nodules, airspace consolidation, and thin-walled cavity are more frequently seen in MAC than in *M. abscessus* infection (see Figs. 4.11 and 4.12). The upper lobe cavitary form (Fig. 4.10) is more frequent in the MAC (37%) group than in *M. abscessus* (14%) ($p = 0.029$), whereas the nodular bronchiectatic form (see Fig. 4.13) is more frequent in the *M. abscessus* group (81% vs. 53% in MAC) ($p = 0.012$). Although there is no sex difference in MAC infection, women are more frequently affected than men in *M. abscessus* infection (44).

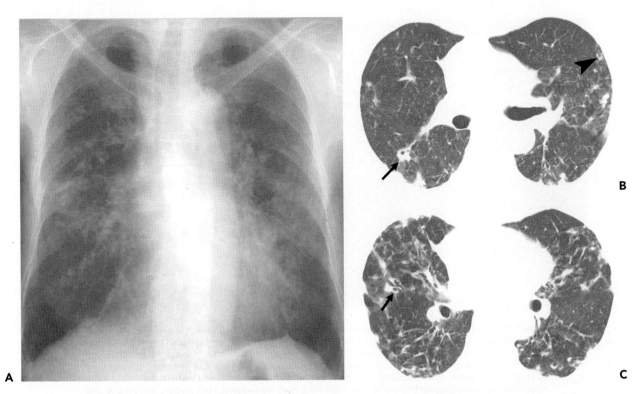

Figure 4.9 *Mycobacterium abscessus* pulmonary disease. Nodular bronchiectatic form. **A:** Chest radiograph shows bilateral nodular and mild reticular opacities in middle lung zones. **B:** Computed tomography (CT) image (2.5-mm collimation) at the level of the bronchus intermedius shows bilateral small nodules, a cavitating nodule (*arrow*), tree-in-bud opacities (*black arrowhead*), and small nodules. **C:** CT image at the level of the basal trunks demonstrates bilateral variable-sized small nodules and bronchiectasis (*arrow*). The patient was a 64-year-old woman.

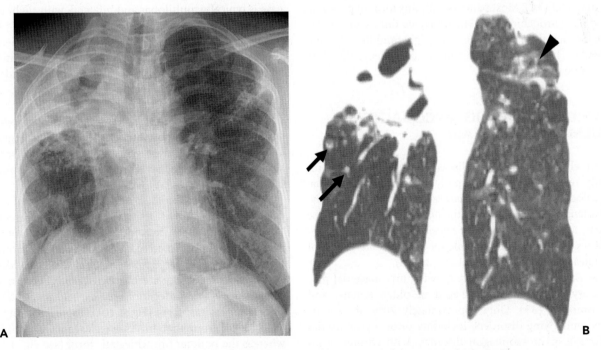

Figure 4.10 *Mycobacterium abscessus* pulmonary disease. Upper lobe cavitary form. **A:** Chest radiograph shows a large cavitary lesion in the right upper lobe and marked right upper lobe volume loss. Also note the nodular and reticular opacities in the right middle and lower zones and left upper lung zone. **B:** Coronal reformation (2-mm collimation) image shows large cavitary consolidation and decreased volume of right upper lobe. Also note small nodular opacities (*arrows*) and patchy ground-glass opacities (*arrowhead*). The patient was a 38-year-old woman.

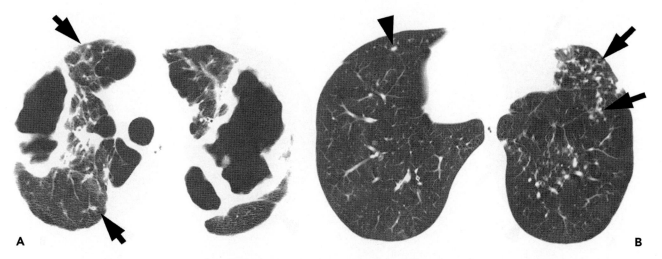

Figure 4.11 *Mycobacterium avium–intracellulare* complex pulmonary disease. **A:** Computed tomography (CT) image (2.5-mm collimation) at the level of the great vessels shows multiple large cavities in both lung apices. Also note several bilateral small nodules (*arrows*). **B:** CT image at the level of the suprahepatic inferior vena cava shows multiple small nodules and branching centrilobular opacities (tree-in-bud pattern) (*arrows*) in the lingula and left lower lobe. A small nodule is also seen in the right middle lobe (*arrowhead*). The patient was a 66-year-old man.

COMPLICATIONS

Patients with bronchiectasis, either prior to or secondary to NTM, are at increased risk of developing bacterial superinfection and growth of Aspergillus, which may result in aspergilloma formation or in semi-invasive aspergillosis. Extensive bronchiectasis with associated bronchial artery hypertrophy may result in severe hemoptysis.

Disseminated NTM infection with positive blood cultures, usually MAC, is seen most commonly in patients with AIDS (45). NTM disease in AIDS is identified mainly in markedly immunosuppressed patients (CD4 count <50 per mm^3). Diagnosis is made even with negative radiographic findings, if sputum, bronchoalveolar lavage fluid, or blood cultures are positive for NTM. The most common radiologic manifestation of intrathoracic disease in these patients is mediastinal or hilar lymphadenopathy. Small scattered nodules, miliary nodules, or mass-like lesions are uncommon (13, 14) (see Chapter 7).

Disseminated NTM disease may also occur in immunosuppressed non-AIDS patients. Risk factors include transplantation, lymphoproliferative disorders, and corticosteroid or other immunosuppressive drug therapy. Radiologic manifestations are varied and include extensive mediastinal or hilar lymphadenopathy, scattered heterogeneous pulmonary opacities, cavitation, and miliary nodules (13, 14) (see Fig. 4.14).

DIFFERENTIAL DIAGNOSIS

Upper lobe cavitary form of MAC pulmonary disease shows similar radiologic features of postprimary pulmonary tuberculosis with cavitary lesions. However, when multiple cavities are present on imaging studies, pulmonary tuberculosis, particularly multidrug-resistant tuberculosis, is the primary diagnostic choice rather than nontuberculous mycobacterial disease. The nodular bronchiectatic form of NTM pulmonary disease should be differentiated from other causes of extensive bronchiectasis including ciliary dyskinesia, cystic fibrosis, allergic bronchopulmonary aspergillosis, and diffuse panbronchiolitis. In NTM pulmonary disease, bronchiectasis is almost always associated with tree-in-bud opacities and asymmetric distribution, and is often accompanied by volume loss, most commonly in the right middle lobe and lingula (21, 25).

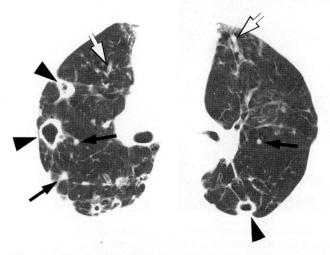

Figure 4.12 *Mycobacterium avium–intracellulare* complex pulmonary disease. Computed tomography (CT) image (2.5-mm collimation) at the level of the bronchus intermedius shows multiple bilateral cavitary nodules (*arrowheads*). Also note small nodules (*arrows*) and bronchiectasis (*open arrows*). The patient was a 69-year-old woman.

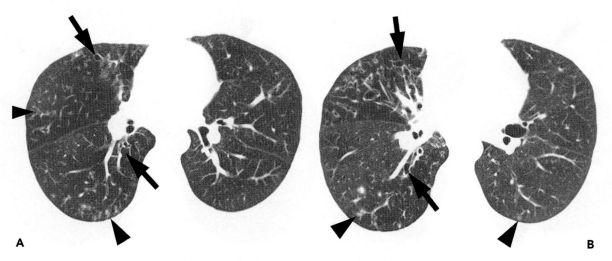

Figure 4.13 *Mycobacterium abscessus* pulmonary disease. **A:** Computed tomography (CT) image (2.5-mm collimation) at the level of the proximal lower lobe bronchus shows bronchiectasis (*arrows*) and tree-in-bud opacities (*arrowheads*) in the right lung. **B:** CT scan obtained at the level of the basal trunks shows bronchiectasis (*arrows*) and tree-in-bud opacities (*arrowheads*) in both lungs. The patient was a 45-year-old woman.

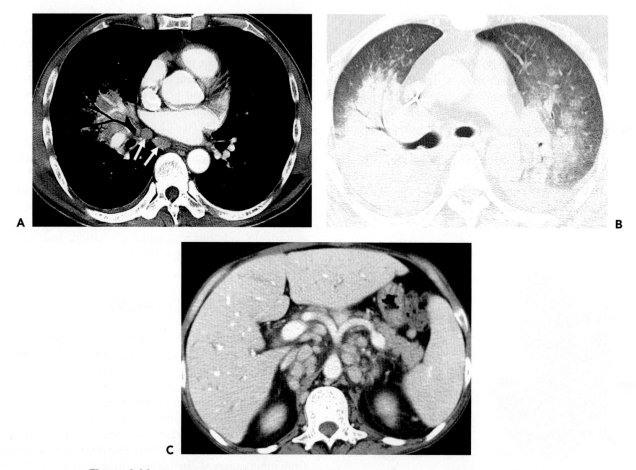

Figure 4.14 Disseminated *Mycobacterium avium–intracellulare* complex infection. **A:** Mediastinal window image with contrast enhanced computed tomography (CT) scan (5-mm collimation) obtained at the level of the left atrium shows parenchymal consolidation with air bronchograms in the right middle lobe. Also note enlarged right hilar and subcarinal lymph nodes (*arrows*) and small right pleural effusion. **B:** Follow-up CT scan obtained at the level of the right upper lobar bronchus 6 months after **(A)** shows extensive bilateral consolidation and new left pleural effusion. **C:** CT scan obtained at the level of the celiac axis and 8 months after **(A)** demonstrates enlarged abdominal lymph nodes. The patient was a 49-year-old man receiving corticosteroid treatment for primary adrenal insufficiency.

UTILITY OF COMPUTED TOMOGRAPHY SCAN

Several studies have demonstrated that the presence of bilateral well-defined small nodules and tree-in-bud pattern associated with bronchiectasis involving mainly the right middle lobe and lingula on high-resolution CT scan is suggestive of MAC pulmonary infection (16, 21, 22). However, these CT scan findings are not 100% specific for MAC pulmonary infection. Similar findings have been reported in patients with tuberculosis and pulmonary infections caused by various NTM organisms including *M. kansasii*, and *M. xenopi*, and rapidly growing mycobacteria such as *M. abscessus*, *M. fortuitum*, and *M. chelonae* (42, 43). Two studies showed that only approximately 50% of patients with such CT scan features have MAC pulmonary infection (22, 24). In a recent study by Koh et al. (21), approximately one-third of patients with bilateral well-defined small nodules and tree-in-bud pattern associated with bronchiectasis on high-resolution CT scan had NTM pulmonary infection; the most common organisms being MAC and *M. abscessus*.

REFERENCES

1. Medical Section of the American Lung Association. Diagnosis and treatment of disease caused by nontuberculous mycobacteria. This official statement of the American Thoracic Society was approved by the board of directors, March 1997. *Am J Respir Crit Care Med.* 1997;156:S1–25.
2. British Thoracic Society. Management of opportunistic mycobacterial infections: Joint tuberculosis committee guidelines. *Thorax.* 1999;55:210–218.
3. American Thoracic Society. Diagnosis and treatment of disease caused by nontuberculous mycobacteria. *Am Rev Respir Dis.* 1990;142:940–953.
4. Wolinsky E. Nontuberculous mycobacteria and associated diseases. *Am Rev Respir Dis.* 1979;119:107–159.
5. Wagner D, Young LS. Nontuberculous mycobacterial infections: A clinical review. *Infection.* 2004;32:257–270.
6. Runyon EH. Anonymous mycobacteria in pulmonary disease. *Med Clin North Am.* 1959;43:273–290.
7. O'Brien RJ, Geiter LJ, Snider DE Jr. The epidemiology of nontuberculous mycobacterial diseases in the United States. Results from a national survey. *Am Rev Respir Dis.* 1987;135:1007–1014.
8. Tsukamura M, Kita N, Shimoide H, et al. Studies on the epidemiology of nontuberculous mycobacteriosis in Japan. *Am Rev Respir Dis.* 1988;137:1280–1284.
9. Corbett EL, Blumberg L, Churchyard GJ, et al. Nontuberculous mycobacteria: Defining disease in a prospective cohort of South African miners. *Am J Respir Crit Care Med.* 1999;160:15–21.
10. Woodring JH, Vandiviere HM, Melvin IG, et al. Roentgenographic features of pulmonary disease caused by atypical mycobacteria. *South Med J.* 1987;80:1488–1497.
11. Prince DS, Peterson DD, Steiner RM, et al. Infection with Mycobacterium avium complex in patients without predisposing conditions. *N Engl J Med.* 1989;321:863–868.
12. Wallace RJ Jr, Zhang Y, Brown BA, et al. Polyclonal Mycobacterium avium complex infections in patients with nodular bronchiectasis. *Am J Respir Crit Care Med.* 1998;158:1235–1244.
13. Erasmus JJ, McAdams HP, Farrell MA, et al. Pulmonary nontuberculous mycobacterial infection: Radiologic manifestations. *Radiographics.* 1999;19:1487–1505.
14. Miller WT Jr. Spectrum of pulmonary nontuberculous mycobacterial infection. *Radiology.* 1994;191:343–350.
15. Christensen EE, Dietz GW, Ahn CH, et al. Pulmonary manifestations of Mycobacterium intracellularis. *Am J Roentgenol.* 1979;133:59–66.
16. Lynch DA, Simone PM, Fox MA, et al. CT features of pulmonary Mycobacterium avium complex infection. *J Comput Assist Tomogr.* 1995;19:353–360.
17. Primack SL, Logan PM, Hartman TE, et al. Pulmonary tuberculosis and Mycobacterium avium-intracellulare: A comparison of CT findings. *Radiology.* 1995;194:413–417.
18. Reich JM, Johnson RE. Mycobacterium avium complex pulmonary disease presenting as an isolated lingular or middle lobe pattern. The Lady Windermere syndrome. *Chest.* 1992;101:1605–1609.
19. Ahn CH, McLarty JW, Ahn SS, et al. Diagnostic criteria for pulmonary disease caused by Mycobacterium kansasii and Mycobacterium intracellulare. *Am Rev Respir Dis.* 1982;125:388–391.
20. Hartman TE, Swensen SJ, Williams DE. Mycobacterium avium-intracellulare complex: Evaluation with CT. *Radiology.* 1993;187:23–26.
21. Koh WJ, Lee KS, Kwon OJ, et al. Bilateral bronchiectasis and bronchiolitis at thin-section CT: Diagnostic implications in nontuberculous mycobacterial pulmonary infection. *Radiology.* 2005;235:282–288.
22. Swensen SJ, Hartman TE, Williams DE. Computed tomographic diagnosis of Mycobacterium avium-intracellulare complex in patients with bronchiectasis. *Chest.* 1994;105:49–52.
23. Tanaka E, Amitani R, Niimi A, et al. Yield of computed tomography and bronchoscopy for the diagnosis of Mycobacterium avium complex pulmonary disease. *Am J Respir Crit Care Med.* 1997;155:2041–2046.
24. Fujita J, Ohtsuki Y, Suemitsu I, et al. Pathological and radiological changes in resected lung specimens in Mycobacterium avium intracellulare complex disease. *Eur Respir J.* 1999;13:535–540.
25. Jeong YJ, Lee KS, Koh WJ, et al. Nontuberculous mycobacterial pulmonary infection in immunocompetent patients: Comparison of thin-section CT and histopathologic findings. *Radiology.* 2004;231:880–886.
26. Huang JH, Kao PN, Adi V, et al. Mycobacterium avium-intracellulare pulmonary infection in HIV-negative patients without preexisting lung disease: Diagnostic and management limitations. *Chest.* 1999;115:1033–1040.
27. Kim TS, Koh WJ, Han J, et al. Hypothesis on the evolution of cavitary lesions in nontuberculous mycobacterial pulmonary infection: Thin-section CT and histopathologic correlation. *Am J Roentgenol.* 2005;184:1247–1252.
28. Moore EH. Atypical mycobacterial infection in the lung: CT appearance. *Radiology.* 1993;187:777–782.
29. Marchetti N, Criner K, Criner GJ. Characterization of functional, radiologic and lung function recovery post-treatment of hot tub lung. A case report and review of the literature. *Lung.* 2004;182:271–277.
30. Rickman OB, Ryu JH, Fidler ME, et al. Hypersensitivity pneumonitis associated with Mycobacterium avium complex and hot tub use. *Mayo Clin Proc.* 2002;77:1233–1237.
31. Marras TK, Wallace RJ Jr, Koth LL, et al. Hypersensitivity pneumonitis reaction to Mycobacterium avium in household water. *Chest.* 2005;127:664–671.
32. Pham RV, Vydareny KH, Gal AA. High-resolution computed tomography appearance of pulmonary Mycobacterium avium complex infection after exposure to hot tub: Case of hot-tub lung. *J Thorac Imaging.* 2003;18:48–52.
33. Embil J, Warren P, Yakrus M, et al. Pulmonary illness associated with exposure to Mycobacterium-avium complex in hot tub water. Hypersensitivity pneumonitis or infection? *Chest.* 1997;111:813–816.
34. Kahana LM, Kay JM, Yakrus MA, et al. Mycobacterium avium complex infection in an immunocompetent young adult related to hot tub exposure. *Chest.* 1997;111:242–245.
35. Johanson WG Jr, Nicholson DP. Pulmonary disease due to Mycobacterium kansasii. An analysis of some factors affecting prognosis. *Am Rev Respir Dis.* 1969;99:73–85.
36. Christensen EE, Dietz GW, Ahn CH, et al. Radiographic manifestations of pulmonary Mycobacterium kansasii infections. *Am J Roentgenol.* 1978;131:985–993.
37. Evans AJ, Crisp AJ, Hubbard RB, et al. Pulmonary Mycobacterium kansasii infection: Comparison of radiological appearances with pulmonary tuberculosis. *Thorax.* 1996;51:1243–1247.
38. Hollings NP, Wells AU, Wilson R, et al. Comparative appearances of non-tuberculous mycobacteria species: A CT study. *Eur Radiol.* 2002;12:2211–2217.
39. Griffith DE, Girard WM, Wallace RJ Jr. Clinical features of pulmonary disease caused by rapidly growing mycobacteria. An analysis of 154 patients. *Am Rev Respir Dis.* 1993;147:1271–1278.
40. Wallace RJ Jr, Swenson JM, Silcox VA, et al. Spectrum of disease due to rapidly growing mycobacteria. *Rev Infect Dis.* 1983;5:657–679.
41. Wallace RJ Jr. Diagnostic and therapeutic consideration in patients with pulmonary disease due to the rapidly growing mycobacteria. *Semin Respir Infect.* 1986;1:230–233.
42. Han D, Lee KS, Koh WJ, et al. Radiographic and CT findings of nontuberculous mycobacterial pulmonary infection caused by Mycobacterium abscessus. *Am J Roentgenol.* 2003;181:513–517.
43. Hazelton TR, Newell JD Jr, Cook JL, et al. CT findings in 14 patients with Mycobacterium chelonae pulmonary infection. *Am J Roentgenol.* 2000;175:413–416.
44. Chung MJ, Lee KS, Koh WJ, et al. Thin-section CT findings of nontuberculous mycobacterial pulmonary diseases: Comparison between Mycobacterium avium-intracellulare complex and mycobacterium abscessus infection. *J Korean Med Sci.* 2005;20:777–783.
45. Topics in pulmonary medicine symposium: Mycobacterial disease in AIDS. In highlights: ATS symposia summaries and topics. *Am Rev Respir Dis.* 1987;136:1027–1030.

Viruses, Mycoplasma, and Chlamydia

5

Viruses, mycoplasma, and chlamydia are common and important causes of lower respiratory tract infection and may result in tracheobronchitis, bronchiolitis, and pneumonia. Viral pneumonia in adults can be divided into two broad categories: So-called atypical pneumonia in otherwise normal hosts and viral pneumonia in immunocompromised patients (1). Atypical pneumonia can be due to viruses, mycoplasma, and chlamydia. Viruses account for approximately 10% to 20% of community-acquired pneumonias (2–4). Most viral pneumonias in immunocompetent adults are due to influenza virus; other common viral etiologies include respiratory syncytial virus (RSV) and adenovirus. Immunocompromised hosts are particularly susceptible to pneumonias caused by cytomegalovirus (CMV) and herpes viruses.

Infection by viruses, mycoplasma, and chlamydia is usually acquired through the airways. Because the organisms replicate within tissue cells, the most prominent histologic changes are seen in the epithelium and adjacent interstitial tissue (5). Bronchiolitis is manifested histologically by a neutrophilic exudate in the airway lumen and a predominantly mononuclear infiltrate in its wall (see Fig. 5.1) (5). Parenchymal involvement is typically that of bronchopneumonia. It initially involves the lung adjacent to the terminal and respiratory bronchioles resulting in poorly defined peribronchiolar airspace nodules of 4 to

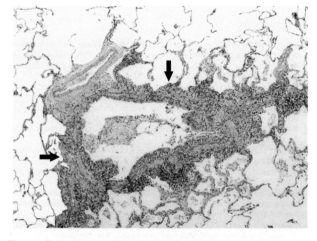

Figure 5.1 Bronchiolitis due to *Mycoplasma pneumoniae*. Histologic section demonstrates inflammation of the bronchiolar wall (*arrows*) and presence of intraluminal exudate. The adjacent parenchyma is normal (Hematoxylin and Eosin stain original magnification × 25). Serologic tests were positive for *Mycoplasma pneumoniae*. (From Müller NL and Miller RR. Diseases of the bronchioles. *Radiology*. 1995;196:3–12, with permission.)

10 mm diameter (see Fig. 5.2). The pneumonia typically extends from a peribronchiolar distribution to involve the entire secondary lobule resulting in lobular consolidation, a characteristic histologic feature of bronchopneumonia (see Fig. 5.3) (5).

The bronchiolar and peribronchiolar inflammation is initially reflected by the presence of a small nodular or reticulonodular pattern on the radiograph and centrilobular nodules and branching opacities (tree-in-bud pattern) on high-resolution computed tomography (CT) scan (see Fig. 5.4) (1, 5–7). Bronchiolitis may be associated with partial airway obstruction resulting in areas of air

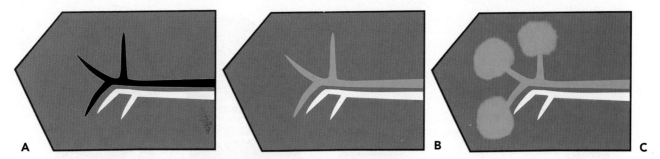

Figure 5.2   Bronchiolitis: Distribution in relation to the secondary pulmonary lobule. The bronchioles and adjacent pulmonary artery are located near the center of the secondary pulmonary lobule **(A)**. Inflammation of the bronchiolar wall and intraluminal exudate results in linear opacities when the bronchioles are imaged along their long axis or nodular opacities when imaged in cross-section **(B)**. Extension of the inflammatory process into the parenchyma results in 4 to 10 mm diameter centrilobular nodular opacities **(C)**. (Courtesy of C. Isabela S. Silva, MD, PhD.)

trapping and hyperinflation. Airway obstruction may be the predominant or the only clinical and radiologic finding of bronchiolitis in infants and young children but is relatively uncommon in adults (1, 5–7). Extension of the inflammatory process into the adjacent parenchyma results in 4 to 10 mm diameter centrilobular airspace nodules. These small foci of disease may progress to lobular, subsegmental, or segmental areas of consolidation characteristic of bronchopneumonia (see Fig. 5.5) (1, 5–7). Partial filling of the airspaces results in ground-glass opacities (Fig. 5.5).

While some organisms, such as RSV and *Mycoplasma pneumoniae*, typically cause bronchiolitis, others, such as influenza virus may result in rapidly progressive pneumonia, particularly in the elderly and in immunocompromised patients (5). Histologically, the lungs in these patients show

diffuse alveolar damage (DAD), characterized by interstitial lymphocyte infiltration, airspace hemorrhage and edema, type II cell hyperplasia, and hyaline membrane formation (5, 8). The radiologic findings include homogeneous or patchy unilateral or bilateral airspace consolidation and ground-glass opacities (1, 9, 10).

VIRUSES

RNA Viruses

Influenza Virus

Influenza can occur as pandemics or epidemics, or sporadically in individuals or small clusters of patients. It has been estimated that influenza results in symptomatic

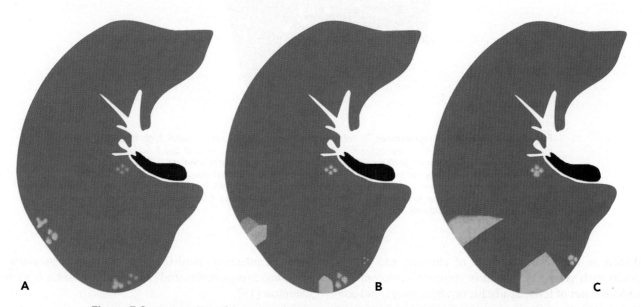

Figure 5.3   Progression of bronchopneumonia. The organisms may initially involve mainly the bronchioles, resulting in centrilobular nodules and branching opacities (tree-in-bud pattern) **(A)**. Progression to bronchopneumonia results in lobular, subsegmental, and segmental areas of consolidation **(B** and **C)**. The consolidation is usually multifocal and patchy but the consolidation typically does not cross the segmental boundaries. (Courtesy of C. Isabela S. Silva, MD, PhD.)

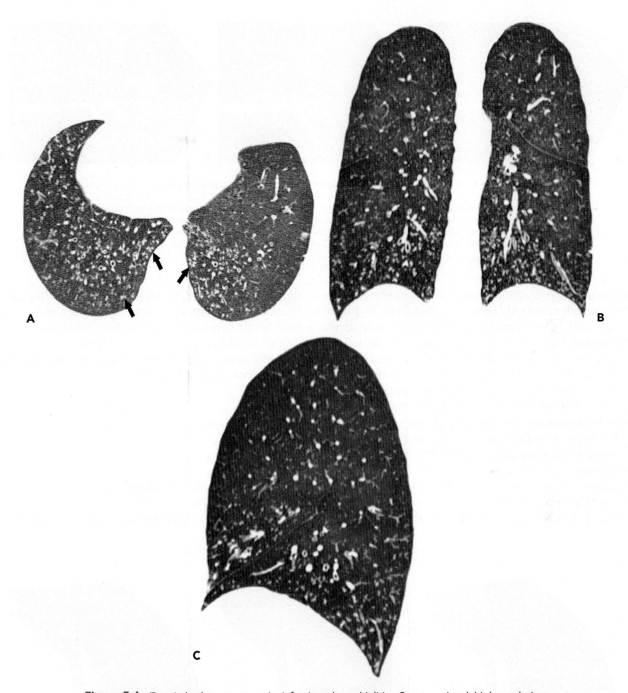

Figure 5.4 Tree-in-bud appearance in infectious bronchiolitis. Cross-sectional high-resolution computed tomography (CT) (1-mm collimation) image obtained at the level of the lung bases **(A)** on a multidetector CT scanner shows centrilobular branching nodular and linear opacities resulting in a tree-in-bud appearance (*arrows*). Coronal reformation **(B)** shows that the abnormalities involve almost exclusively the lower lung zones. Sagittal reformation **(C)** shows involvement of the right lower lobe and, to a lesser extent, right middle lobe. The patient was a 20-year-old woman with recurrent respiratory infections.

disease in approximately 20% of children and 5% of adults each year (11). The most common symptoms are sudden onset of fever, headache, myalgia, cough, and sore throat (12). Pneumonia is an uncommon but potentially severe complication of influenza infection. Although it may be caused by the virus itself (usually type A and occasionally type B organisms) (13, 14) superimposed

bacterial infection, particularly by *Staphylococcus aureus*, *Streptococcus pneumoniae*, and *Haemophilus influenza*, is more common (15).

Primary influenza viral pneumonia occurs most commonly in the elderly and in patients with cardiopulmonary disease (15). The clinical manifestations in these patients typically include high fever, tachypnea, and

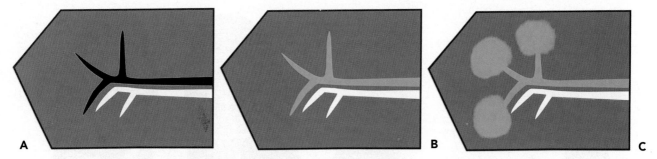

Figure 5.2 Bronchiolitis: Distribution in relation to the secondary pulmonary lobule. The bronchioles and adjacent pulmonary artery are located near the center of the secondary pulmonary lobule **(A)**. Inflammation of the bronchiolar wall and intraluminal exudate results in linear opacities when the bronchioles are imaged along their long axis or nodular opacities when imaged in cross-section **(B)**. Extension of the inflammatory process into the parenchyma results in 4 to 10 mm diameter centrilobular nodular opacities **(C)**. (Courtesy of C. Isabela S. Silva, MD, PhD.)

trapping and hyperinflation. Airway obstruction may be the predominant or the only clinical and radiologic finding of bronchiolitis in infants and young children but is relatively uncommon in adults (1, 5–7). Extension of the inflammatory process into the adjacent parenchyma results in 4 to 10 mm diameter centrilobular airspace nodules. These small foci of disease may progress to lobular, subsegmental, or segmental areas of consolidation characteristic of bronchopneumonia (see Fig. 5.5) (1, 5–7). Partial filling of the airspaces results in ground-glass opacities (Fig. 5.5).

While some organisms, such as RSV and *Mycoplasma pneumoniae*, typically cause bronchiolitis, others, such as influenza virus may result in rapidly progressive pneumonia, particularly in the elderly and in immunocompromised patients (5). Histologically, the lungs in these patients show

diffuse alveolar damage (DAD), characterized by interstitial lymphocyte infiltration, airspace hemorrhage and edema, type II cell hyperplasia, and hyaline membrane formation (5, 8). The radiologic findings include homogeneous or patchy unilateral or bilateral airspace consolidation and ground-glass opacities (1, 9, 10).

VIRUSES

RNA Viruses

Influenza Virus

Influenza can occur as pandemics or epidemics, or sporadically in individuals or small clusters of patients. It has been estimated that influenza results in symptomatic

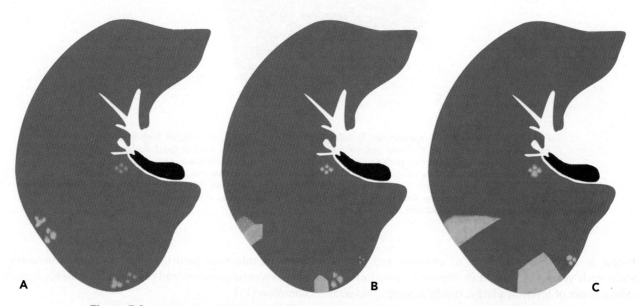

Figure 5.3 Progression of bronchopneumonia. The organisms may initially involve mainly the bronchioles, resulting in centrilobular nodules and branching opacities (tree-in-bud pattern) **(A)**. Progression to bronchopneumonia results in lobular, subsegmental, and segmental areas of consolidation **(B and C)**. The consolidation is usually multifocal and patchy but the consolidation typically does not cross the segmental boundaries. (Courtesy of C. Isabela S. Silva, MD, PhD.)

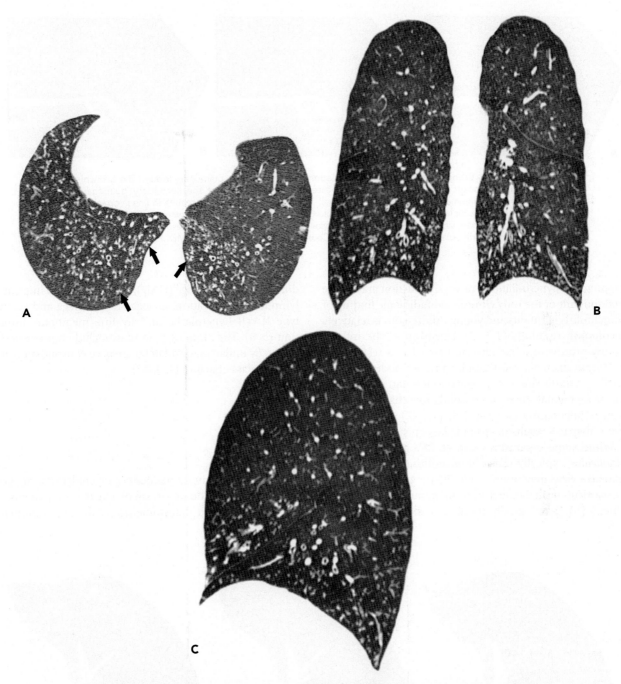

Figure 5.4 Tree-in-bud appearance in infectious bronchiolitis. Cross-sectional high-resolution computed tomography (CT) (1-mm collimation) image obtained at the level of the lung bases **(A)** on a multidetector CT scanner shows centrilobular branching nodular and linear opacities resulting in a tree-in-bud appearance (*arrows*). Coronal reformation **(B)** shows that the abnormalities involve almost exclusively the lower lung zones. Sagittal reformation **(C)** shows involvement of the right lower lobe and, to a lesser extent, right middle lobe. The patient was a 20-year-old woman with recurrent respiratory infections.

disease in approximately 20% of children and 5% of adults each year (11). The most common symptoms are sudden onset of fever, headache, myalgia, cough, and sore throat (12). Pneumonia is an uncommon but potentially severe complication of influenza infection. Although it may be caused by the virus itself (usually type A and occasionally type B organisms) (13, 14) superimposed

bacterial infection, particularly by *Staphylococcus aureus*, *Streptococcus pneumoniae*, and *Haemophilus influenza*, is more common (15).

Primary influenza viral pneumonia occurs most commonly in the elderly and in patients with cardiopulmonary disease (15). The clinical manifestations in these patients typically include high fever, tachypnea, and

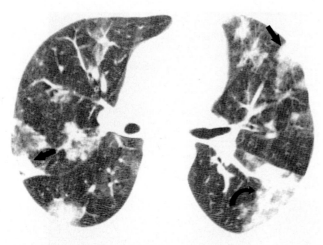

Figure 5.5 Lobular and subsegmental consolidation in viral pneumonia. High-resolution computed tomography (CT) (1-mm collimation) image obtained at the level of the bronchus intermedius shows lobular (*straight arrows*) and subsegmental (*curved arrow*) areas of consolidation. The patient was a 52-year-old man who developed cytomegalovirus pneumonia following liver transplantation. (From Franquet et al. *Am J Roentgenol.* 2003;181:1059–1063, with permission.)

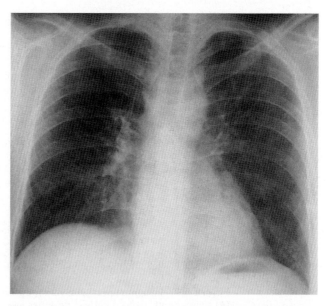

Figure 5.6 Influenza pneumonia with reticulonodular pattern. Posteroanterior chest radiograph shows mild reticulonodular pattern in the middle and upper lung zones. The patient was a 30-year-old man with recurrent respiratory infections.

cyanosis developing within 1 day of the onset of influenza illness (15). Mortality in patients with primary influenza pneumonia is high (15). Pneumonia due to superimposed bacterial infection also occurs most commonly in the elderly and in patients with underlying pulmonary disease (15). Clinically, these patients initially present with typical influenza symptoms. The symptoms appear to be improving when the clinical course is complicated by recrudescence of fever and development of chills, pleuritic chest pain, and productive cough (15). The clinical symptoms in these patients tend to be milder than symptoms in those with primary influenza pneumonia and the mortality is lower (15). In one review of the clinical findings and complications in 35 patients hospitalized with influenza (10), approximately 90% of patients had serious comorbid illnesses, most commonly chronic respiratory or heart disease or diabetes. Seventeen patients developed pneumonia; these patients tended to be older (mean age 63 years) and had a higher incidence of chronic lung disease than those without pneumonia. Shortness of breath was the only symptom that distinguished patients with pneumonia from those with an upper respiratory tract illness alone. Respiratory test results and/or blood culture results were positive in five patients (29%); *S. aureus* was isolated in all five patients and *S. pneumoniae* in one patient. Ten of the patients with pneumonia (59%) were admitted to the intensive care unit (ICU) and five patients (29%) died (10).

The most common radiographic manifestations of influenza pneumonia include extensive bilateral reticular or reticulonodular opacities with or without superimposed areas of consolidation (see Fig. 5.6 and Table 5.1) (1, 10, 15). Less commonly, patients with primary influenza pneumonia may present with focal areas of consolidation,

usually in the lower lobes, without apparent reticular or reticulonodular opacities (see Fig. 5.7) (10, 15, 16). Serial radiographs may show poorly defined, patchy or nodular areas of consolidation, 1 to 2 cm in diameter, which become rapidly confluent (1, 16). Pleural effusion is uncommon. The radiologic abnormalities usually resolve in approximately 3 weeks (16).

Kim et al. evaluated the high-resolution CT scan findings of influenza virus pneumonia in two immunocompetent patients and reported that both lungs had areas of multifocal peribronchovascular or subpleural consolidation (1). In one patient, some of the areas of consolidation had

---

TABLE 5.1
INFLUENZA VIRUS

Symptomatic disease (influenza): 20% of children and 5% of adults each year

Primary influenza virus pneumonia is uncommon

    Risk factors: Old age, cardiopulmonary disease

    Most common radiologic manifestations:

        Bilateral reticular or reticulonodular opacities

        Focal areas of consolidation that may become confluent

Secondary bacterial pneumonia is relatively common

    Risk factors: Old age, cardiopulmonary disease

    Most common radiologic manifestations:

        Patchy unilateral or bilateral consolidation (bronchopneumonia)

        Lobular, subsegmental or segmental distribution

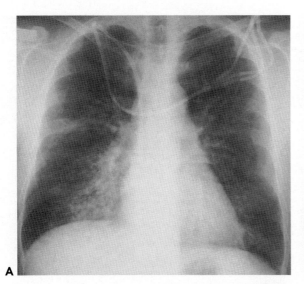
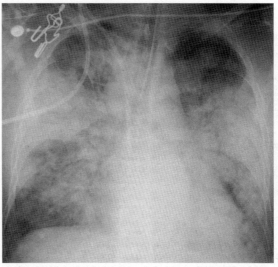

A   B

Figure 5.7   Influenza pneumonia with progression over 1 week. Posteroanterior chest radiograph
(A) shows poorly defined nodular opacities and small areas of consolidation in the right middle and
lower lung zones. Chest radiograph 1 week later **(B)** demonstrates extensive bilateral consolidation
and poorly defined nodular opacities. Also noted are endotracheal tube and central venous line. The
patient was a 44-year-old man with influenza pneumonia.

a lobular distribution and were associated with airspace
nodules. The other patient showed diffuse ground-glass
opacities with irregular linear areas of increased attenuation. Tanaka et al. reported the high-resolution CT scan
findings of influenza virus pneumonia in one immunocompetent patient as consisting of bilateral ground-glass
opacities in a lobular distribution (17).

The manifestations of secondary bacterial pneumonia
are those of bronchopneumonia and include lobular,
subsegmental, or segmental unilateral or bilateral areas
of consolidation (10, 15, 16).

Influenza infection in the immunocompromised host
usually presents with similar clinical findings as in the normal host. However, there is a greater prevalence of severe
disease particularly in patients with acquired immunodeficiency syndrome (AIDS) (15, 18). Oikonomou et al.
described the radiographic and high-resolution CT scan
findings of influenza pneumonia in four immunocompromised patients with hematologic malignancies (9). The
most common finding on the chest radiographs was the
presence of patchy, poorly defined areas of consolidation.
The consolidation was bilateral in three patients and unilateral in one. Two patients had ill-defined small nodules
and patchy ground-glass opacities evident on the radiograph. The findings on high-resolution CT scan included
patchy ground-glass opacities, focal areas of consolidation, centrilobular nodules, and a tree-in-bud pattern (see
Fig. 5.8). The centrilobular nodules measured 2 to 9 mm
in diameter and were bilateral and asymmetric in distribution. The tree-in-bud pattern was limited to small areas
of the parenchyma and was asymmetric and bilateral in
distribution. The extent of abnormalities seen on high-
resolution CT scan was greater than that apparent on the
radiograph (9).

Respiratory Syncytial Virus

RSV is a common cause of upper and lower respiratory
tract infection in infants and small children (16). Infection in adults is usually mild and limited to the upper
respiratory tract; however, pneumonia can occur, particularly, in the elderly or chronically ill patients in nursing
homes or hospital (19–21) and in immunocompromised
individuals (22, 23).

The radiographic findings in infants and children include bronchial wall thickening, peribronchial opacities,

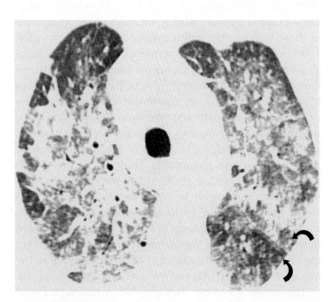

Figure 5.8   Influenza pneumonia. High-resolution computed
tomography (CT) (1-mm collimation) scan at the level of the aortic arch demonstrates extensive bilateral ground-glass opacities,
patchy areas of consolidation, and several centrilobular nodules
(*arrows*). The patient was a 61-year-old woman with influenza
pneumonia.

TABLE 5.2
RESPIRATORY SYNCYTIAL VIRUS

Infection common in infants and children; uncommon in
adults
RSV bronchiolitis
    Risk factors: Infants and young children
    Most common radiologic manifestations:
        Hyperinflation
        Bronchial wall thickening, peribronchial opacities
RSV pneumonia
    Risk factors: Infants, young children, elderly, chroni-
    cally ill patients
    Most common radiologic manifestations:
        Patchy bilateral consolidation (bronchopneumonia)
        Lobular, subsegmental or segmental distribution
        Centrilobular nodules and tree-in-bud pattern on
           high-resolution CT scan

RSV, respiratory syncytial virus; CT, computed tomography.

and perihilar linearity (see Table 5.2) (16, 24). Other common findings include hyperinflation (reflecting the presence of acute bronchiolitis) and patchy bilateral consolidation (reflecting the presence of bronchopneumonia) (see Fig. 5.9) (16, 24). In one review of the radiographic manifestations of RSV lower respiratory tract infection in 108 children in the 1 day to 10 years age-group, the main findings included normal chest radiograph (30%), central consolidation (32%), or peribronchial thickening (26%) (25). Other findings included hyperinflation (11%), lobar consolidation (6%), patchy segmental consolidation (6%), and pleural effusion (6%).

The radiographic findings of RSV pneumonia in adults usually consist of patchy bilateral areas of consolidation (26). Less commonly, the patients may present with a bilateral reticulonodular pattern (26). The main high-resolution CT scan findings are centrilobular nodules and branching nodular opacities (tree-in-bud pattern), reflecting the presence of bronchiolitis, and multifocal ground-glass opacities or areas of consolidation, due to bronchopneumonia. Expiratory CT scan may show air trapping (see Fig. 5.10). In one review of 20 patients who had RSV pneumonia after allogeneic bone marrow transplantation, the predominant high-resolution CT scan findings included small centrilobular nodules (10 of 20, 50%), multifocal areas of airspace consolidation and multifocal ground-glass opacities (6 of 20, 30%), and bronchial wall thickening (6 of 20, 30%) (see Fig. 5.11) (27). The centrilobular nodules were 1 to 5 mm in diameter and in half the cases were associated with branching nodular and linear opacities resulting in a tree-in-bud pattern. The abnormalities were bilateral and asymmetric in distribution in 13 patients, bilateral and symmetric in 2 patients, and unilateral in 1 patient (27). In a review of the high-resolution CT scan findings in ten patients with RSV infection after lung transplantation (28), the main abnormalities included ground-glass opacities seen in seven of ten patients, airspace consolidation in five, and centrilobular nodular and branching linear opacities (tree-in-bud pattern) in four patients (28).

Hantaviruses

Hantaviruses are a group of viruses that cause two characteristic symptom complexes: Hemorrhagic fever with

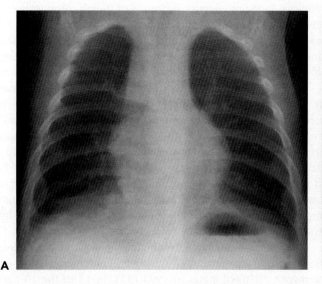
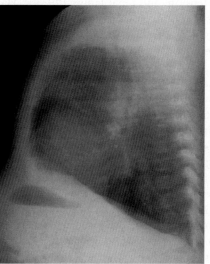

A   **B**

Figure 5.9 Respiratory syncytial virus (RSV) bronchiolitis. Posteroanterior **(A)** and lateral **(B)** chest radiographs show hyperinflation with decreased vascularity at the lung bases and flattening of the diaphragm. The patient was a 3-month-old girl with RSV bronchiolitis. (Case courtesy of Dr. Eric Effman, Children's Hospital and Medical Center, Seattle, Washington.)

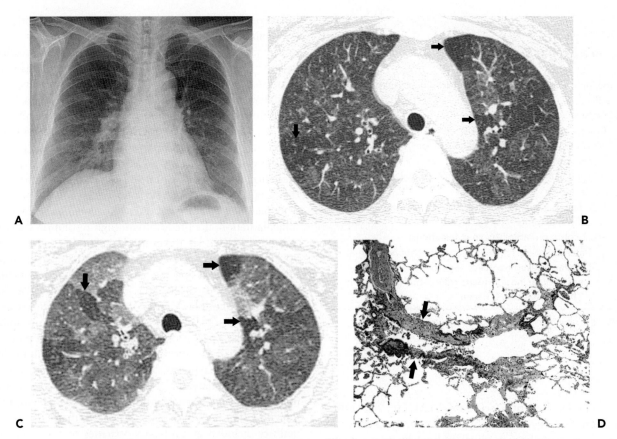

Figure 5.10   Respiratory syncytial virus (RSV) bronchiolitis. Posteroanterior chest radiograph **(A)** shows no obvious abnormality. Inspiratory high-resolution computed tomography (CT) (1-mm collimation) image **(B)** demonstrates localized areas of decreased attenuation and vascularity (*arrows*). Expiratory high-resolution CT image **(C)** at the same level as (B) demonstrates areas of air trapping (*arrows*). Biopsy specimen **(D)** demonstrates bronchiolitis obliterans (*arrows*). The patient was a 53-year-old woman with RSV bronchiolitis.

renal syndrome and hantavirus pulmonary syndrome. Hemorrhagic fever with renal syndrome is characterized by fever, hypotension, and renal failure (29, 30). Hantavirus pulmonary syndrome is characterized by the presence of respiratory distress from noncardiogenic edema (1). The most common organism responsible for the hantavirus pulmonary syndrome in North America is the Sin Nombre virus (31).

The natural reservoirs of the Hantaviruses are wild rodents and deer mice (29, 32). The organism is believed to be transmitted to humans by inhalation of dried rodent excreta associated with outdoor activities in rural areas, such as cleaning barns and harvesting rice. Increased contact between humans and rodent reservoirs has resulted in an increase prevalence of Hantavirus infections in the last two decades (32). A number of cases of hantavirus pulmonary syndrome have been described in North and South America and in Asia (31, 32).

Hantavirus pulmonary syndrome develops 9 to 35 days after exposure to the virus. It is characterized by three stages. The initial stage is the prodromal phase, which is followed by the cardiopulmonary and convalescent phases. The prodromal phase is manifested by a flu-like

illness with myalgia, fever, headache, cough, vomiting, and diarrhea (30). This is followed within 3 to 6 days by progressive shortness of breath, progressive respiratory insufficiency, respiratory failure, and shock (30). Histologically, the cardiopulmonary phase is characterized by interstitial and airspace edema, mild to moderate interstitial infiltrates of lymphocytes, and epithelial necrosis with destruction of type I cells and hyaline membranes (1, 33).

The radiographic manifestations include interstitial edema with or without rapid progression to airspace disease (see Table 5.3) (1, 30, 34). The airspace disease shows a central or bibasilar distribution (see Fig. 5.12). In most patients the radiologic manifestations of hantavirus pulmonary syndrome are consistent with those of noncardiogenic pulmonary edema. However, renal failure may result in findings of interstitial and airspace hydrostatic pulmonary edema and cardiomegaly (see Fig. 5.13) (1).

Ketai et al. described the radiographic manifestations in 16 patients seen during an epidemic in the southwestern United States in 1993 (33). In 13 of the 16 patients, the initial chest radiographs showed findings consistent with those of interstitial pulmonary edema, including septal (Kerley B) lines, hilar indistinctness, and peribronchial

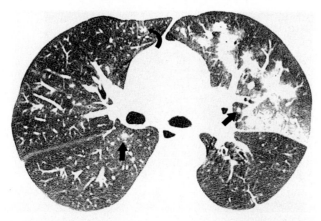

Figure 5.11 Respiratory syncytial virus (RSV) pneumonia. High-resolution computed tomography (CT) scan at the level of bronchus intermedius shows ground-glass opacities and dense focal areas of consolidation in left upper lobe. Note centrilobular nodular opacities (*straight arrows*) in left upper and right lower lobes. Centrilobular branching nodular opacities (tree-in-bud pattern, curved arrow) are present in the right upper lobe. The patient was a 40-year-old man with chronic myelogenous leukemia and respiratory syncytial virus pneumonia. (From Gasparetto EL, Escuissato DL, Marchiori E, et al. High-resolution CT findings of respiratory syncytial virus pneumonia after bone marrow transplantation. *Am J Roentgenol.* 2004;182:1133–1137, with permission.)

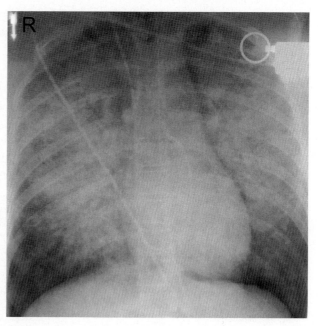

Figure 5.12 Hantavirus pulmonary syndrome. Chest radiograph shows extensive bilateral consolidation with relative sparing of the peripheral regions and lung bases. The patient presented with respiratory failure and developed acute respiratory distress syndrome. The infection was presumably related to contact with deer mice. The patient was a 31-year-old woman.

cuffing. In the three patients who had normal radiographs at presentation, findings consistent with interstitial pulmonary edema developed within 48 hours. Within 48 hours of admission, 11 patients developed extensive airspace consolidation. The distribution was bibasilar or perihilar in ten patients and predominantly peripheral in one patient. The time to resolution of the radiographic findings in the nine patients who survived ranged from 5 days to >3 weeks. Pleural effusions were present on the initial chest radiographs in two patients and developed within 48 hours in nine other patients. The effusions were small in five patients and large in six patients (33).

Boroja et al. (34) described the radiographic findings in 20 patients and identified two different patterns of presentation. Thirteen (65%) patients presented with fulminant clinical and radiographic findings and required intensive care support. The radiographic findings in these patients included interstitial edema with rapid progression to bilateral airspace consolidation. Six (46%) of these 13 patients died within a few days of presentation. The second group (7 of 20, 35%) presented with mild clinical symptoms. The radiographic findings included mild interstitial edema and minimal airspace consolidation that resolved in a mean time of 8 days. None of the patients in the second group died. Seventy-five percent (15 of 20) of the patients had small bilateral pleural effusions. One patient had a small right-sided pleural effusion, and three patients had no pleural effusion. Nineteen of the 20 patients (95%) lived or worked in rural communities or had contact with deer mice or deer mice droppings (34).

Severe Acute Respiratory Syndrome Coronavirus

The severe acute respiratory syndrome (SARS) coronavirus is the cause of SARS, which is a new infectious disease that first emerged in the Guangdong province in southern China, in November 2002 (35, 36). SARS rapidly spread from China to affect patients in a number of countries around the world. Within approximately 8 months, the global cumulative total of the cases was 8,422 with 916 deaths (case fatality rate of 11%) (35).

The natural reservoir of the organism is believed to be wild animals such as raccoon-dogs, ferrets, and civets (36). The disease is transmitted by droplets or direct inoculation

---

TABLE 5.3

HANTAVIRUS

Infection results from exposure to wild rodents and deer mice

Risk factors: Outdoor activities in rural areas

Most common radiologic manifestations:

    Septal (Kerley B) lines

    Hilar indistinctness

    Peribronchial cuffing

    Rapid progression to airspace consolidation

    Consolidation predominantly perihilar or in lower lobes

    Pleural effusion

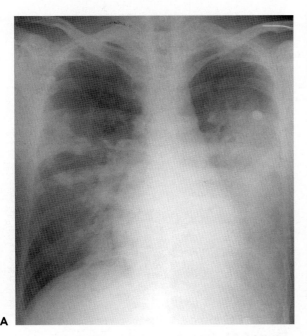
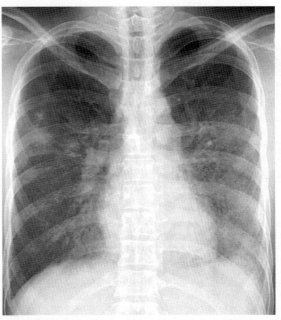

Figure 5.13 Hantavirus hemorrhagic fever with renal syndrome. Chest radiograph **(A)** shows extensive asymmetric bilateral consolidation. The patient presented with fever, oliguria, and shortness of breath. Chest radiograph 1 week later **(B)** when the patient was on hemodialysis for renal failure demonstrates considerable improvement but residual interstitial pulmonary edema. The patient was a 21-year-old man.

from contact with infected surfaces (35). The mean incubation period was 6.4 days (range 2 to 10). The duration between onset of symptoms and hospitalization was 3 to 5 days (35). Presenting symptoms include fever, chills, dry cough, myalgia, and headache (37). These can progress to clinical, radiologic, and pathologic features of ARDS. Laboratory findings include lymphopenia, evidence of disseminated intravascular coagulation, and elevated blood levels of lactate dehydrogenase (LDH) and creatine kinase (37).

Histologic assessment of autopsy specimens showed that the predominant pattern of lung injury was DAD. The histology varied according to the duration of illness. Cases of 10 or fewer days' duration demonstrated acute-phase DAD. Cases of >10 days' duration exhibited organizing-phase DAD, type II pneumocyte hyperplasia, and, frequently, superimposed bacterial bronchopneumonia (38).

The most common radiologic manifestations include focal unilateral or multifocal unilateral or bilateral areas of consolidation (see Figs. 5.14 and 5.15 and Table 5.4) (39–41). The consolidation tends to involve predominantly the peripheral lung regions and the middle and lower lung zones (39–41). Less common radiographic findings include focal or diffuse ground-glass opacities and, rarely, lobar consolidation (see Fig. 5.16) (39–41). The extent of parenchymal abnormalities on chest radiography correlates inversely with the oxygen saturation ($r = -0.67, p <0.001$) (42).

Approximately 20% to 40% of patients with SARS have normal radiographs at presentation (39, 41). High-resolution CT scan demonstrates parenchymal abnormalities in virtually all these patients (see Fig. 5.17) (39, 40, 43). The most common high-resolution CT scan findings

include focal, multifocal or diffuse ground-glass opacities or areas of consolidation (see Figs. 5.17–5.19) (40, 43, 44). Interlobular septal and intralobular interstitial thickening is often seen superimposed on the ground-glass opacities ("crazy-paving" pattern) (43, 44). High-resolution

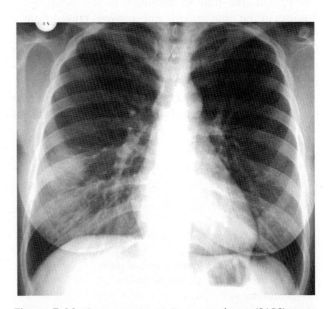

Figure 5.14 Severe acute respiratory syndrome (SARS) coronavirus pneumonia. Chest radiograph obtained at hospital admission shows ill-defined hazy increased density (ground-glass opacity) in right middle lung zone. The patient was a 29-year-old woman with SARS coronavirus pneumonia. (From Müller NL, Ooi GC, Khong PL, et al. Severe acute respiratory syndrome: Radiographic and CT findings. *Am J Roentgenol.* 2003;181:3–8, with permission.)

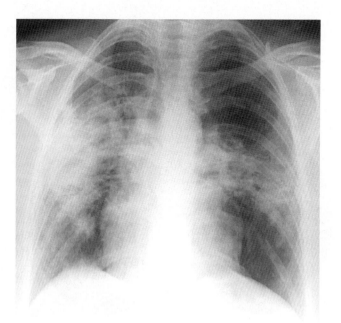

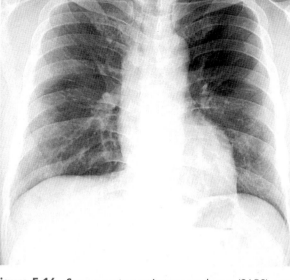

Figure 5.15 Severe acute respiratory syndrome (SARS) coronavirus pneumonia. Chest radiograph shows asymmetric bilateral consolidation involving mainly the middle lung zones. The patient was a 44-year-old woman with SARS coronavirus pneumonia.

Figure 5.16 Severe acute respiratory syndrome (SARS) coronavirus pneumonia. Chest radiograph shows subtle bilateral ground-glass opacities, with relative sparing of left upper lobe. The patient was a 48-year-old man with SARS coronavirus pneumonia. (From Müller NL, Ooi GC, Khong PL, et al. Severe acute respiratory syndrome: Radiographic and CT findings. *Am J Roentgenol.* 2003;181:3–8, with permission.)

CT scan findings such as branching nodular and linear opacities (tree-in-bud pattern) (44), hilar and mediastinal lymphadenopathy (44), and pleural effusion commonly seen in other pneumonias are uncommon in patients with SARS (43, 44).

DNA Viruses

Adenovirus

Adenovirus infection accounts for 5% to 10% of all respiratory illnesses in children (45, 46). It may result in pharyngitis, laryngotracheobronchitis, bronchiolitis, and

pneumonia. In most children the adenovirus infection is mild. In a small percentage of patients it may result in severe bronchopneumonia, respiratory failure, and death (47). Follow-up of children with severe adenovirus pneumonia may show residual sequelae, most commonly bronchiolitis obliterans, bronchiectasis, and unilateral hyperlucent lung (Swyer-James-MacLeod syndrome) (40, 47–49, 51). Sequelae are more common following adenovirus pneumonia than after other childhood pneumonias (52). Although less common than during childhood, adenovirus may result in lower respiratory tract infection and pneumonia in non-immunocompromised (2, 53) and immunocompromised adults (54, 55). Adenovirus infection in immunocompromised patients is often severe and can be fatal (54).

The histologic findings of mild adenovirus pneumonia consist of interstitial inflammatory cell infiltration (56). Severe pneumonia is characterized by the presence of patchy areas of hemorrhagic consolidation, necrotic changes with DAD, and areas of overinflation or atelectasis (57). The main symptoms of adenovirus bronchiolitis and pneumonia are fever, cough, and shortness of breath; approximately 25% of patients present with wheezing (45).

The radiographic manifestations of adenovirus bronchiolitis in infants and children are similar to those of RSV bronchiolitis and include bronchial wall thickening, peribronchial infiltrates, and perihilar linearity (see Table 5.5). The radiographic and CT manifestations of adenovirus bronchopneumonia in children and adults include patchy bilateral areas of consolidation in a lobular or segmental distribution (see Fig. 5.20) (1, 7). Other common findings

---

TABLE 5.4

SEVERE ACUTE RESPIRATORY SYNDROME CORONAVIRUS

Infection transmitted by droplets or direct inoculation
Pandemic in 2003; sporadic cases since
Most common radiologic manifestations:
    Focal or multifocal unilateral or bilateral consolidation
    Mainly peripheral lung regions
    Middle and lower lung zones
    Chest radiograph initially normal in 20% to 40% of cases
    High-resolution CT scan usually abnormal when radiograph normal
        graph normal
    Tree-in-bud pattern and pleural effusion typically absent

CT, computed tomography.

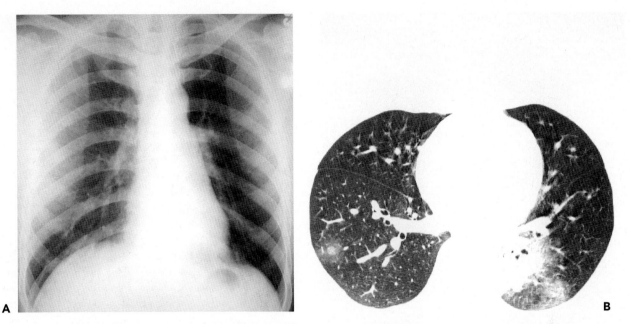

Figure 5.17 Severe acute respiratory syndrome (SARS) coronavirus pneumonia. Chest radiograph **(A)** acquired at hospital admission shows no obvious abnormality. High-resolution computed tomography (CT) scan **(B)** obtained on the same day as **(A)** shows focal area of consolidation in superior segment of left lower lobe with adjacent ground-glass opacification. Subpleural ground-glass opacification is also present in the contralateral lung. The patient was a 27-year-old man with SARS coronavirus pneumonia. (From Müller NL, Ooi GC, Khong PL, et al. Severe acute respiratory syndrome: Radiographic and CT findings. *Am J Roentgenol.* 2003;181:3–8, with permission.)

in children include hyperinflation and lobar atelectasis (1). Sequelae of adenovirus bronchopneumonia in children include bronchiectasis, bronchiolitis obliterans, and unilateral hyperlucent lung (Swyer-James-MacLeod syndrome).

The findings of adenovirus pneumonia in adults have been described mainly in immunocompromised patients. In one review of the radiographic findings in five adults who developed adenovirus pneumonia following lung transplantation, the abnormalities included heterogeneous opacities, focal mass-like consolidation, homogeneous opacity, and pleural effusion (58). In three of the five patients, subsequent radiographs showed progression to diffuse homogeneous parenchymal consolidation; in the remaining two patients the findings were milder and rapidly improved (58). High-resolution CT scan in one immunocompetent adult with adenoviral bronchopneumonia showed patchy bilateral ground-glass opacities in a lobular and segmental distribution (53).

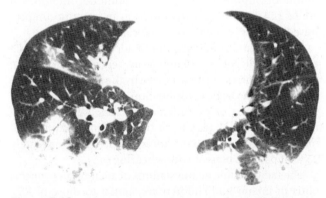

Figure 5.18 Severe acute respiratory syndrome (SARS) coronavirus pneumonia. High-resolution computed tomography (CT) image at the level of the lower lung zones shows bilateral airspace consolidation involving mainly the subpleural lung regions. The patient was a 48-year-old woman with SARS coronavirus pneumonia. (From Müller NL, Ooi GC, Khong PL, et al. High-resolution CT findings of severe acute respiratory syndrome at presentation and after admission. *Am J Roentgenol.* 2004;182:39–44, with permission.)

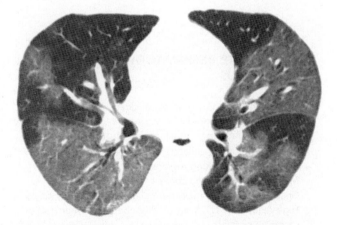

Figure 5.19 Severe acute respiratory syndrome (SARS) coronavirus pneumonia. High-resolution computed tomography (CT) scan shows extensive bilateral ground-glass opacities. The patient was a 48-year-old man with SARS coronavirus pneumonia (same patient in Figure 5.16).

TABLE 5.5
ADENOVIRUS

Infection common in children; relatively uncommon in
adults
Adenovirus bronchiolitis
   Risk factors: Infants and young children
   Most common radiologic manifestations:
      Hyperinflation
      Bronchial wall thickening
      Peribronchial infiltrates
Adenovirus pneumonia
   Risk factors: Infants and young children; immunocom-
   promised adults
   Most common radiologic manifestations:
      Patchy bilateral consolidation
      Lobular, subsegmental, segmental distribution
      Hyperinflation common in infants and young
         children
Sequelae of adenovirus bronchopneumonia in childhood
   Bronchiectasis
   Bronchiolitis obliterans

Herpes Simplex Virus

Herpes simplex virus pneumonia is an uncommon infection seen almost exclusively in patients who are immunocompromised or in whom airways have been traumatized
from intubation, burns, or smoke inhalation (1, 59–61).
The virus may spread to the lung by aspiration or extension
of oropharyngeal infection into the lower respiratory system or by hematogenous spread in patients with sepsis (62).

   The histologic features of herpes simplex lower respiratory tract infection include focal or diffuse ulcers in the
tracheobronchial epithelium with or without associated

necrotizing bronchopneumonia (1, 63). The airway lesion
is characterized histologically by epithelial necrosis and
ulceration. Pneumonia is characterized by alveolar necrosis
and a proteinaceous exudate with a variable polymorphonuclear inflammatory response (1, 64).

   The radiographic manifestations usually include patchy
bilateral subsegmental or segmental ground-glass opacities
or consolidation (see Table 5.6) (1, 60). Other common
findings include reticular opacities, poorly defined nodular
opacities (airspace nodules), and pleural effusions (see
Fig. 5.21) (65–67). Aquino et al. reviewed the radiographic
findings in 23 patients (1, 60). The abnormalities included
patchy subsegmental and segmental areas of ground-glass
opacity and consolidation seen in all patients and pleural
effusions seen in 12 patients (1, 60). Umans et al. reviewed
the radiographic findings in 14 patients with herpes
simplex virus pneumonia (67). The chest radiographs
in 12 patients showed lung opacification, predominantly
lobar or more extensive and always bilateral. Most patients
presented with a mixed airspace and interstitial pattern
of opacities, but 11 of 14 showed at least one focus of
airspace consolidation. Lobar, segmental, or subsegmental
atelectasis was present in seven patients, and unilateral or
bilateral pleural effusion in eight patients. Two patients
had normal radiographs.

   Common findings on CT scan include multifocal
subsegmental and segmental ground-glass opacities, focal
areas of consolidation, and pleural effusion (Fig. 5.21) (60).
High-resolution CT scan commonly demonstrates small
centrilobular nodules in addition to ground-glass opacities
and foci of consolidation (68, 69).

Varicella-zoster Virus

Varicella-zoster virus causes two distinct clinical manifestations: (i) Chickenpox (varicella), representing primary
and usually disseminated disease in previously uninfected

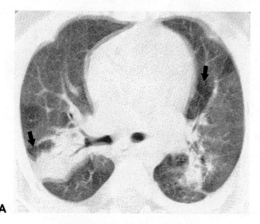
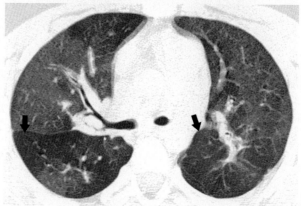

A   B

Figure 5.20 Adenovirus bronchopneumonia. Computed tomography (CT) image at the level of
the right upper lobe bronchus in a male infant **(A)** shows patchy bilateral consolidation and small
foci of decreased attenuation and vascularity. High-resolution CT image obtained at the same
level as **(A)** 4 years later demonstrates extensive bilateral areas of decreased attenuation and
vascularity consistent with bronchiolitis obliterans **(B)**. The patient was a young child with adenovirus
bronchopneumonia.

TABLE 5.6

HERPES SIMPLEX VIRUS PNEUMONIA

Seen almost exclusively in immunocompromised patients
  Most common radiologic manifestations:
    Patchy bilateral consolidation
    Lobular, subsegmental, or segmental distribution
    Reticular opacities
    Pleural effusion
  High-resolution CT scan findings:
    Lobular, subsegmental, or segmental consolidation or
      ground-glass opacities
    Centrilobular nodules and tree-in-bud pattern

CT, computed tomography.

Varicella (chickenpox) is a common infection of childhood typically affecting children aged 2 to 8 years (71). Data from Europe and North America have shown that the incidence of chickenpox in adults has doubled in the last two decades and that approximately 7% of adults are susceptible to the disease (71). Most cases of varicella pneumonia occur in very young children or adults (72,73). Predisposing conditions include underlying malignancy, particularly leukemia and lymphoma, and other causes of immunodeficiency (74). Overall, approximately 1 in 400 children with varicella develop pneumonia (71). Adults who develop chickenpox are at much greater risk of developing pneumonia, the reported incidence ranging from 5% to 50% (71,75,76). A report of 110 chest radiographs from 114 US army recruits who developed varicella during basic training showed that 18 (16%) had radiographic evidence of pneumonia (77).

Varicella pneumonia usually presents 1 to 6 days after the onset of the rash and is associated with fever, cough, dyspnea, and occasionally with pleuritic chest pain (71). Histologic features of varicella-zoster virus pneumonia include endothelial damage in small blood vessels, with focal hemorrhagic necrosis, mononuclear infiltration of alveolar walls, and fibrinous exudates in the alveoli (71). These can progress to DAD (1,70). With recovery from the

individuals, and (ii) zoster (shingles), representing reactivation of a latent virus, typically as unilateral skin eruptions along a nerve path often accompanied by severe neuralgia (70). Although either form may be associated with pneumonia, most cases of pneumonia occur in relation to chickenpox (70).

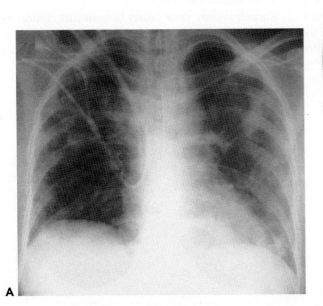
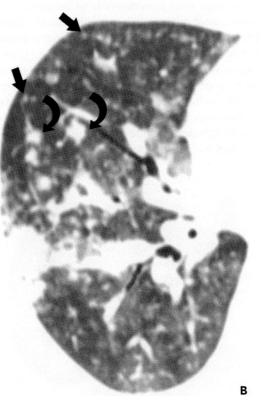

Figure 5.21 Herpes simplex virus pneumonia. Chest radiograph **(A)** shows patchy bilateral consolidation and poorly defined nodular opacities. Central venous line and nasogastric tube are in place. View of the right lung on a computed tomography (CT) scan **(B)** demonstrates foci of consolidation, small centrilobular nodules (*straight arrows*), and 5 to 10 mm diameter nodules (*curved arrows*). The patient was a 42-year-old woman with herpes simplex virus pneumonia following hematopoietic stem cell transplantation.

TABLE 5.7
VARICELLA PNEUMONIA

Occurs in small percentage of young children and adults
with varicella
  Risk factors: Leukemia, lymphoma, immunodeficiency
  Most common radiologic manifestations:
    Reticular opacities
    Multiple ill-defined 5 to 10 mm diameter nodules
    Multifocal areas of consolidation
  High-resolution CT scan findings:
    Numerous small nodular opacities
    Some with halo of ground-glass attenuation
    Patchy ground-glass opacities

CT, computed tomography.

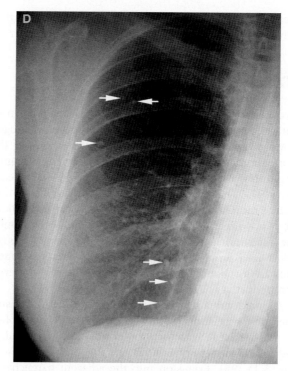

Figure 5.22 Calcified nodules due to previous varicella pneumonia. View of the right lung from a chest radiograph shows multiple, small, calcified nodules (*arrows*). The patient was a 33-year-old woman with previous varicella virus pneumonia.

initial disease, spherical nodules are often seen, scattered randomly throughout the lungs (1). Histologically, the nodules are composed of an outer fibrous capsule enclosing areas of hyalinized collagen or necrotic tissue (1, 70).

Chest radiographic findings of varicella-zoster virus pneumonia typically include reticular opacities or multiple ill-defined nodules measuring 5 to 10 mm in diameter (see Table 5.7) (1, 71, 78). The nodules may be confluent and progress to extensive airspace consolidation. The nodules usually resolve within a week of the disappearance of the skin lesions. Occasionally, the lesions may calcify and persist as numerous, well-defined, randomly scattered, 2- to 3-mm densely calcified nodules (see Fig. 5.22) (70). In one survey of 463 individuals who had a history of chickenpox as adults, only 8 (1.7%) had residual calcified nodules (79). Hilar lymphadenopathy and pleural effusion may be seen but are uncommon (70). The hilar lymph nodes do not calcify (70).

High-resolution CT scan usually shows 1- to 10-mm well-defined or ill-defined nodules diffusely present throughout both lungs (78, 80) or, less commonly, in a patchy asymmetric distribution (see Fig. 5.23). Other findings include nodules with a surrounding halo of ground-glass opacity, patchy ground-glass opacities, and coalescence of nodules. These findings disappear concurrently with healing of skin lesions after antiviral chemotherapy (80).

Cytomegalovirus

CMV infection is common, with 40% to 100% of adults being seropositive for the virus (81). Most patients with CMV infection are asymptomatic, the only sequela being the presence of latent virus as a potential source of reinfection. CMV is an uncommon cause of community-acquired pneumonia (82). In one study of 443 patients with community-acquired pneumonia, only 4 (0.9%) were caused by CMV (83, 84). Pneumonia is much more frequent

in immunocompromised patients, particularly in those with organ transplantation (82, 85, 86) for example, CMV pneumonia occurs in 2% of patients with autologous stem cell transplantation and in 10% to 40% of patients with allogeneic transplantation (87, 88) (see Chapter 8). The incidence of CMV pneumonia in patients with AIDS has

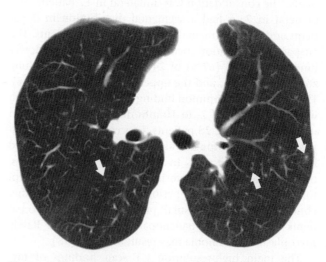

Figure 5.23 Varicella pneumonia. Computed tomography (CT) image (5-mm collimation) shows small nodules (*arrows*) involving mainly the left lung. The patient was a 30-year-old man who developed varicella pneumonia following double lung transplantation.

decreased dramatically since the introduction of highly active antiretroviral therapy (HAART) (89) (see Chapter 7).

MYCOPLASMA PNEUMONIAE

Mycoplasma are bacteria that lack a cell wall and grow in an extracellular location (90). The most important pathogen is *Mycoplasma pneumoniae. M. pneumoniae* is one of the more common causes of community-acquired pneumonia, accounting for approximately 10% to 15% of overall cases (91, 92) and up to 50% of cases in specific groups, such as military recruits (93). Infections occur throughout the year, with a peak during the autumn and early winter. The infection is transmitted person to person through aerosolized droplets. The typical case begins insidiously after an incubation period of 9 to 21 days with fever, nonproductive cough, headache, and malaise (94).

The predominant histologic abnormality in mycoplasma pneumonia is bronchiolitis (5, 95). The bronchiolitis is characterized by a neutrophil-rich luminal exudate and an inflammatory infiltrate in the bronchiolar wall (Fig. 5.1) (95). Extension into the adjacent parenchyma results in peribronchiolar inflammation, and lobular and segmental areas of consolidation. Less common histologic manifestations include DAD, organizing pneumonia, bronchiolitis obliterans, and bronchiectasis (49, 90, 95).

The most common radiographic manifestations are a reticulonodular pattern and/or patchy areas of consolidation (see Table 5.8) (6, 96, 97). The reticulonodular pattern may be unilateral or bilateral (see Figs. 5.24 and 5.25). The consolidation tends to involve mainly the lower lobes (see Fig. 5.26). Reittner et al. reviewed the radiographic and high-resolution CT scan findings in 28 patients with *M. pneumoniae* pneumonia (6). The most common radiographic abnormality was the presence of focal areas of airspace consolidation seen in 24 of the 28 (85%) patients. The consolidation was unilateral in 17 patients and bilateral in 7; it had a segmental distribution in 9 patients and a nonsegmental distribution in 15 patients. The airspace consolidation involved predominantly the lower lung zones in 16 (67%) of 24 patients, the middle lung zones in 5 (21%), and the upper lung zones in 3 (13%). The second most common finding on the chest radiograph was the presence of 2- to 10-mm diameter nodules, seen in 14 (50%) of the 28 patients. Less common abnormalities included peribronchovascular thickening ($n = 5$), and linear opacities ($n = 3$). In 3 (11%) of the 28 patients, the chest radiographs were interpreted as normal except for the presence of mild peribronchial thickening. Other abnormalities included small pleural effusions in two patients and hilar lymphadenopathy in three (6). Rarely mycoplasma pneumonia may result in ARDS (98).

The main high-resolution CT scan findings of mycoplasma pneumonia include centrilobular nodular and branching opacities (tree-in-bud pattern) in a patchy distribution (see Fig. 5.27), areas of lobular or segmental

TABLE 5.8
***MYCOPLASMA PNEUMONIAE* PNEUMONIA**

Accounts for 10% to 15% of cases of community-acquired pneumonia
Most common in children and young adults
Most common radiologic manifestations:
    Patchy bilateral ground-glass opacities
    Patchy bilateral areas of consolidation
    Most commonly lower lobes

High-resolution CT scan findings:
    Bilateral lobular ground-glass opacities
    Bilateral lobular or segmental consolidation
    Centrilobular nodules and branching opacities
    (tree-in-bud pattern)

CT, computed tomography.

ground-glass opacity or consolidation (Fig. 5.26), and thickening of the bronchovascular bundles (6, 99). In the study by Reittner et al. (6) the most common abnormalities on high-resolution CT scan included nodules seen in 25 (89%) patients, ground-glass opacities in 24 (85%), areas of airspace consolidation in 22 (75%), and interlobular septal thickening seen in six (21%). The nodules measured between 2 and 10 mm in diameter and had a predominantly centrilobular and/or peribronchovascular distribution and involved mainly the lower lung zones. The areas of consolidation involved the lower lobes in 14

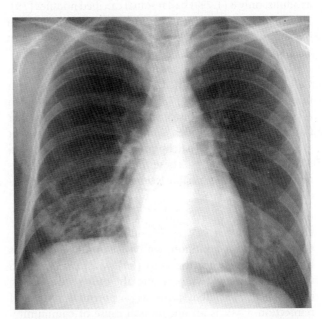

Figure 5.24 Mycoplasma pneumonia. Chest radiograph shows poorly defined nodular opacities in the right lower lung zone. The patient was a 30-year-old woman with *Mycoplasma pneumoniae* pneumonia.

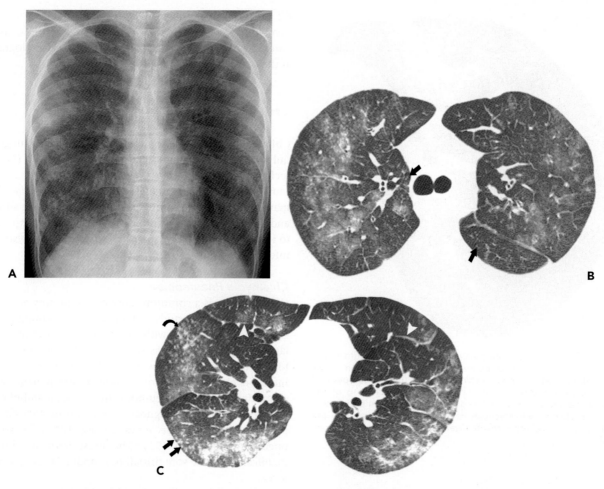

Figure 5.25 Mycoplasma pneumonia. Chest radiograph **(A)** shows bilateral reticulonodular pattern. High-resolution computed tomography (CT) image at the level of the main bronchi **(B)** demonstrates bilateral ground-glass opacities and centrilobular nodules (*arrows*). High-resolution CT scan at the level of the basal segmental bronchi **(C)** shows centrilobular nodules (*straight arrows*), branching opacities (tree-in-bud pattern) (*curved arrow*), ground-glass opacities, small foci of consolidation, and mild thickening of the interlobular septa (*arrowheads*). The patient was a 20-year-old man with *Mycoplasma pneumoniae* pneumonia.

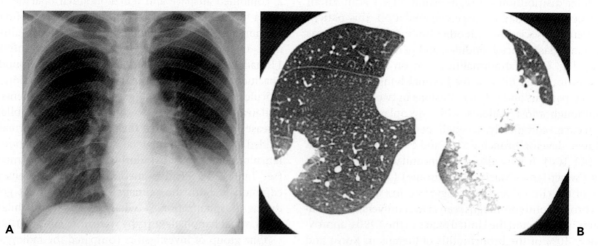

Figure 5.26 Mycoplasma pneumonia. Chest radiograph **(A)** shows extensive consolidation in the left lower lung zone, mild consolidation in the right lower lung zone, and small left pleural effusion. High-resolution computed tomography (CT) scan **(B)** demonstrates extensive consolidation and several small nodules in the left lower lobe, lobular consolidation in the right lower lobe, and small left pleural effusion. The patient was a 27-year-old woman with *Mycoplasma pneumoniae* pneumonia.

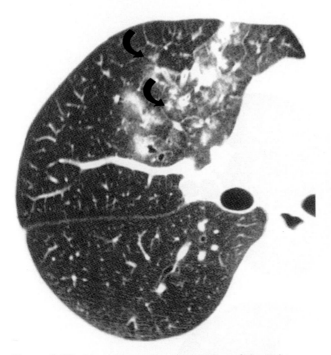

Figure 5.27 Mycoplasma pneumonia. View of the right upper lobe on high-resolution computed tomography (CT) scan shows centrilobular nodules and branching opacities (tree-in-bud pattern) (*arrows*), lobular ground-glass opacities, mild thickening of the interlobular septa, and small foci of consolidation. The patient was a 36-year-old man with *Mycoplasma pneumoniae* pneumonia. (Case courtesy of Dr. Takeshi Johkoh, Osaka University Medical School, Osaka, Japan.)

patients, the middle lobe or lingula in 3, and the upper lobes in 2; in the remaining 3 patients, more than one lobe was involved. The consolidation was predominantly subpleural in five patients, predominantly peribronchovascular in four, and random in five; eight patients had both subpleural and peribronchovascular areas of consolidation. In 13 (59%) patients, the areas of consolidation had a lobular distribution on high-resolution CT scan. In all 22 patients who had airspace consolidation, this pattern was seen in association with other findings including areas of ground-glass opacity, nodules, and peribronchovascular thickening. Other abnormalities seen on high-resolution CT scan included hilar or mediastinal lymphadenopathy in seven patients and pleural effusions in two patients (6).

Although most patients with mycoplasma pneumonia recover completely, a small percentage, particularly children, develop bronchiectasis and bronchiolitis obliterans (49, 100). It may also result in unilateral hyperlucent lung (Swyer-James-MacLeod syndrome) (101). In one review of the clinical and radiologic findings of 31 children with bronchiolitis obliterans seen at four university medical centers in Korea and the United States in the 1990s, approximately 30% of the bronchiolitis obliterans in Korea and 20% in the United States were secondary to mycoplasma pneumonia (49). The high-resolution CT scan findings in these patients included areas of decreased attenuation and vascularity, bronchiectasis, and air trapping on expiratory

CT scan. The areas affected by these abnormalities, usually involving two or more lobes, corresponded to the areas of parenchymal abnormalities seen on the chest radiograph at the time of pneumonia (100).

CHLAMYDIA

Chlamydia are obligate intracellular bacteria that can grow only in host cells and not in artificial culture media (90). It includes three organisms, *Chlamydia trachomatis* that may cause pneumonia in infants, *Chlamydia pneumoniae* that may cause mild pneumonia in children and young adults, and *Chlamydia psittaci*, a zoonosis associated with exposure to infected birds (mainly parrots), that can cause systemic infection and pneumonia (psittacosis) (90).

Chlamydia Pneumoniae
C. pneumoniae is a common cause of community-acquired pneumonia. In one study of 65 patients presenting to the emergency department with a principal symptom of cough lasting longer than 2 weeks and <3 months, 13 (20%) were found to have serologic evidence of recent *C. pneumoniae* infection (102). In a second study of 507 patients with community-acquired pneumonia treated in an ambulatory setting, an etiologic diagnosis was made in 48% of the patients; *C. pneumoniae* accounted for 12% of cases of pneumonia in them (92). The most frequent clinical manifestations are sore throat, nonproductive cough, and fever.

Radiographic manifestations have been described in one series of 55 adults hospitalized for community-acquired pneumonia (102). On the basis of serologic criteria, the patients were categorized as having acute primary (17 patients [31%]) or recurrent (38 patients [69%]) infection. Findings in the first group included airspace consolidation in 11 patients, reticulonodular opacities in 2, combined airspace and reticulonodular opacities in 3, and a normal radiograph in 1 patient. The consolidation was unilateral in 12 patients, lobar in 9, and multifocal in 3. Of the 38 patients who had recurrent infection, 11 had airspace consolidation; 14 had reticulonodular opacities; 6 had a combination of consolidation and reticulonodular opacities. Fourteen of the 38 patients had unilateral abnormalities, and 24 patients had bilateral disease. In both the groups, the radiographic abnormalities tended to progress to bilateral areas of consolidation and reticulonodular opacities during the course of infection (see Table 5.9). Small to medium pleural effusions were common in both the primary and the recurrent groups during hospitalization. Cavitary disease and hilar or mediastinal lymphadenopathy were uncommon (102).

One group of investigators compared the radiographic manifestations of *C. pneumoniae* with those of *S. pneumoniae* (103). The patients were divided into three groups: 24 patients with serologic evidence of *C. pneumoniae* only; 8 patients with combined *C. pneumoniae* and *S. pneumoniae*

TABLE 5.9
***CHLAMYDIA PNEUMONIAE* PNEUMONIA**

Accounts for 10% to 20% of cases of community-acquired pneumonia
Most common radiologic manifestations:
  Patchy unilateral or bilateral areas of consolidation (bronchopneumonia)
  Reticular opacities
  Combination of consolidation and reticular opacities
  Small pleural effusion

TABLE 5.10
***CHLAMYDIA PSITTACI* PNEUMONIA (PSITTACOSIS, ORNITHOSIS)**

Risk factors: Contact with infected parrots, parakeets, or poultry
Most common radiologic manifestations:
  Unilateral segmental or lobar areas of consolidation
  Ground-glass opacities
  Reticular pattern radiating from the hila

infection; and 13 patients with infection caused by *S. pneumoniae* only. Bronchopneumonia was observed in 21 (88%) of the group with *C. pneumoniae* and 10 (77%) of the group with *S. pneumoniae* ($p = 0.67$). Lobar or sublobar (airspace) pneumonia was seen in seven (29%) of the patients with *C. pneumoniae* compared to seven (54%) with pneumonia caused by *S. pneumoniae*. In the combined group, bronchopneumonia was seen as frequently as in the group with *C. pneumoniae*, and airspace involvement was seen as frequently as in the group with *S. pneumoniae*. The authors concluded that radiographic findings cannot be used to differentiate pneumonia caused by *C. pneumoniae* from that caused by *S. pneumoniae* (103).

Okada et al. compared the clinical and CT scan findings of 40 patients with *C. pneumoniae* pneumonia and 42 patients with mycoplasma pneumonia (104). The clinical findings of these two etiologic agents were similar. Chest CT scan findings in patients with *C. pneumoniae* pneumonia consisted mainly of ground-glass opacities ($n = 38$) and airspace consolidation ($n = 28$); 12 had pleural effusion.

Airspace consolidation and pleural effusions were significantly more frequent than in patients with *M. pneumoniae* pneumonia. Centrilobular nodules and bronchial wall thickening on the other hand were significantly less common than in patients with *M. pneumoniae* pneumonia.

Chlamydia Psittaci (Psittacosis, Ornithosis)

Psittacosis is usually acquired by exposure to infected birds, most commonly parrots, parakeets, and poultry (70). Infection usually occurs when an person inhales the bacteria, usually from dried bird droppings from infected birds. Patients with *C. psittaci* pneumonia present after an incubation period of 1 to 2 weeks with fever, malaise, myalgia, headache, dry cough, dyspnea, and pleuritic chest pain (90).

The radiographic manifestations include homogeneous ground-glass opacities, a patchy reticular pattern radiating from the hila or involving the lung bases, and segmental or lobar areas of consolidation (see Fig. 5.28 and Table 5.10) (105–107). In patients with severe pneumonia, the clinical and radiologic findings may resemble those of pneumococcal pneumonia (108). Hilar lymphadenopathy may occur (107).

CLINICAL UTILITY AND LIMITATIONS OF CHEST RADIOGRAPHY AND COMPUTED TOMOGRAPHY SCAN

A. Sensitivity and specificity of chest radiography in the detection of viral pneumonia

The chest radiograph has high sensitivity and specificity in the detection and exclusion of community-acquired pneumonia (109). However, the interobserver agreement in the diagnosis of community-acquired pneumonia is only fair to good for experienced radiologists, and poor to fair for inexperienced radiologists and residents (110, 111). Furthermore, there is poor agreement between radiologists in the assessment of the predominant pattern of pneumonia, whether consistent with lobar pneumonia, bronchopneumonia, or atypical/viral pneumonia. In one prospective multicenter study of 272 patients with suspected community-acquired pneumonia, two staff radiologists

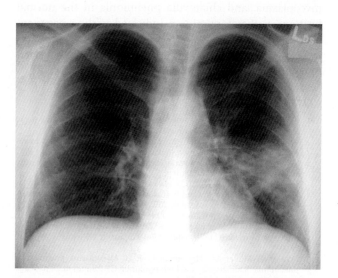

Figure 5.28 Psittacosis. Posteroanterior chest radiograph shows focal consolidation in the lingula. The patient was a 37-year-old man with *Chlamydia psittaci* pneumonia.

agreed on the presence or absence of pulmonary abnormalities in 85% of cases (kappa 0.37) (110). For the 224 patients with abnormalities identified by both radiologists, there was further agreement that the abnormalities consistent of consolidation in 96% of patients and reticulonodular (interstitial) in no patients. Among the 210 patients with consolidation, both radiologists classified the consolidation as lobar in 75% and as bronchopneumonia in 2.4%. The authors concluded that experienced radiologists show fair to good interobserver agreement in identifying the presence of parenchymal abnormalities in patients with community-acquired pneumonia but show poor agreement in determining the pattern of abnormality (110).

CT scan, particularly high-resolution CT scan, has a greater sensitivity than radiography in demonstrating the presence of pulmonary abnormalities. It can therefore be helpful in patients with suspected pneumonia and with normal or questionable radiographic abnormalities (112). It is seldom warranted, however, in patients with suspected viral pneumonia except in immunocompromised hosts.

B. Accuracy of chest radiography and CT scan in determining the specific etiology of pneumonia

Chest radiography is of limited value in determining the specific etiology of pneumonia (99, 109, 113). Levy et al. assessed the value of initial noninvasive bacteriologic and radiologic investigations in 420 patients with community-acquired pneumonia (109). They demonstrated that segmental and lobar areas of consolidation were caused by bacteria in over 90% of cases, whereas the majority of diffuse interstitial or mixed abnormalities were due to viral, atypical bacterial, or tuberculous infections. No finding allowed a specific diagnosis of any given organism.

Tanaka et al. (17) assessed the value of high-resolution CT scan in distinguishing bacterial pneumonia from atypical community-acquired pneumonia. The study included 32 patients, 18 with bacterial pneumonia and 14 with atypical pneumonia (mycoplasma pneumonia [$n = 12$], chlamydia pneumonia [$n = 1$], and influenza viral pneumonia [$n = 1$]). Bacterial pneumonia frequently showed airspace consolidation with segmental distribution (72%) that tended to locate at the middle and outer zones of the lung. Atypical pneumonia frequently showed centrilobular opacities (64%), airspace nodules (71%), airspace consolidation and ground-glass opacity in a lobular distribution (57% and 86%, respectively), and tendency of the lesions to involve the inner third of the lung in addition to the middle and outer thirds (86%). There was however considerable overlap of the findings and no CT scan pattern allowed reliable distinction of bacterial from atypical pneumonia.

Tomiyama et al. (114) assessed the high-resolution CT scans of 90 immunocompetent patients with acute parenchymal lung diseases including 19 with bacterial pneumonia, 13 with mycoplasmal pneumonia, 21 with acute interstitial pneumonia, 18 with hypersensitivity pneumonitis, 10 with acute eosinophilic pneumonia, and 9 with pulmonary hemorrhage. Two independent observers made a correct first-choice diagnosis in an average of 55 (61%) of 90 cases. Correct first-choice diagnosis was made in 50% of cases of bacterial pneumonia and 62% of mycoplasmal pneumonia compared to 90% cases of acute interstitial pneumonia, 72% of hypersensitivity pneumonitis, 30% of acute eosinophilic pneumonia, and 28% of pulmonary hemorrhage. Overall, CT scan findings allowed distinction between infectious and noninfectious causes in 81 (90%) of 90 cases. Centrilobular branching structures were identified in 69% of patients with mycoplasmal pneumonia and in 34% of patients with bacterial pneumonia, and were less commonly seen in the other diseases. Centrilobular nodules were found in most patients with mycoplasmal pneumonia (96% of interpretations), hypersensitivity pneumonitis (81% of interpretations), and bacterial pneumonia (61% of interpretations), and were found less commonly in patients with other entities. In patients with mycoplasmal pneumonia and bacterial pneumonia, the centrilobular nodules were patchy in distribution, whereas in those with hypersensitivity pneumonitis they were diffuse. Segmental distribution was found in all patients with mycoplasmal pneumonia and in 76% of patients with bacterial pneumonia. A combination of airspace consolidation, centrilobular nodules, and segmental distribution was found in 85% of patients with mycoplasmal pneumonia, 45% of those with bacterial pneumonia, and in only a small percentage of cases with noninfectious acute pulmonary disease (114). These results suggest that in patients with acute lung disease the presence of centrilobular branching opacities (tree-in-bud pattern), patchy unilateral or asymmetric bilateral distribution of centrilobular nodules, and segmental consolidation or ground-glass opacities is highly suggestive of pneumonia but that there is considerable overlap between the CT scan findings of bacterial and mycoplasma pneumonia.

The various studies show that CT scan adds limited additional diagnostic information in the diagnosis of viral, mycoplasma, and chlamydia pneumonia in the normal host and is therefore seldom indicated in the assessment of these patients. CT scan, however, is often helpful and indicated in immunocompromised patients with suspected or complicated viral pneumonia (see Chapters 7 and 8).

REFERENCES

1. Kim EA, Lee KS, Primack SL, et al. Viral pneumonias in adults: Radiologic and pathologic findings. *Radiographics*. 2002;22 Spec No:S137–149.
2. de Roux A, Marcos MA, Garcia E, et al. Viral community-acquired pneumonia in nonimmunocompromised adults. *Chest*. 2004;125:1343–1351.
3. Jokinen C, Heiskanen L, Juvonen H, et al. Microbial etiology of community-acquired pneumonia in the adult population of 4 municipalities in eastern Finland. *Clin Infect Dis*. 2001;32:1141–1154.
4. Macfarlane J, Holmes W, Gard P, et al. Prospective study of the incidence, etiology and outcome of adult lower respiratory tract illness in the community. *Thorax*. 2001;56:109–114.
5. Müller NL, Fraser RS, Lee KS, et al. *Diseases of the lung: Radiologic and pathologic correlations*. Philadelphia, PA: Lippincott Williams & Wilkins; 2003.
6. Reittner P, Müller NL, Heyneman L, et al. Mycoplasma pneumoniae pneumonia: Radiographic and high-resolution CT features in 28 patients. *Am J Roentgenol*. 1999;174:37–41.
7. Han BK, Son JA, Yoon HK, et al. Epidemic adenoviral lower respiratory tract infection in pediatric patients: Radiographic and clinical characteristics. *Am J Roentgenol*. 1998;170:1077–1080.

8. Yeldandi AV, Colby TV. Pathologic features of lung biopsy specimens from influenza pneumonia cases. *Hum Pathol.* 1994;25:47–53.
9. Oikonomou A, Müller NL, Nantel S. Radiographic and high-resolution CT findings of influenza virus pneumonia in patients with hematologic malignancies. *Am J Roentgenol.* 2003;181:507–511.
10. Oliveira EC, Marik PE, Colice G. Influenza pneumonia: A descriptive study. *Chest.* 2001;119:1717–1723.
11. Nicholson KG, Wood JM, Zambon M. Influenza. *Lancet.* 2003;362:1733–1745.
12. Shorman M, Moorman JP. Clinical manifestations and diagnosis of influenza. *South Med J.* 2003;96:737–739.
13. Glezen WP. Viral pneumonia as a cause and result of hospitalization. *J Infect Dis.* 1983;147:765–770.
14. Nolan TF Jr, Goodman RA, Hinman AR, et al. Morbidity and mortality associated with influenza B in the United States, 1979–1980. A report from the center for disease control. *J Infect Dis.* 1980;142:360–362.
15. Khater F, Moorman JP. Complications of influenza. *South Med J.* 2003;96:740–743.
16. Fraser RS, Müller NL, Colman N, et al. *Diagnosis of diseases of the chest.* Philadelphia, PA: WB Saunders; 1999.
17. Tanaka N, Matsumoto T, Kuramitsu T, et al. High resolution CT findings in community-acquired pneumonia. *J Comput Assist Tomogr.* 1996;20:600–608.
18. Safrin S, Rush JD, Mills J. Influenza in patients with human immunodeficiency virus infection. *Chest.* 1990;98:33–37.
19. Morales F, Calder MA, Inglis JM, et al. A study of respiratory infections in the elderly to assess the role of respiratory syncytial virus. *J Infect.* 1983;7:236–247.
20. Sorvillo FJ, Huie SF, Strassburg MA, et al. An outbreak of respiratory syncytial virus pneumonia in a nursing home for the elderly. *J Infect.* 1984;9:252–256.
21. Falsey AR, Hennessey PA, Formica MA, et al. Respiratory syncytial virus infection in elderly and high-risk adults. *N Engl J Med.* 2005;352:1749–1759.
22. Parham DM, Bozeman P, Killian C, et al. Cytologic diagnosis of respiratory syncytial virus infection in a bronchoalveolar lavage specimen from a bone marrow transplant recipient. *Am J Clin Pathol.* 1993;99:588–592.
23. van Dissel JT, Zijlmans JM, Kroes AC, et al. Respiratory syncytial virus, a rare cause of severe pneumonia following bone marrow transplantation. *Ann Hematol.* 1995;71:253–255.
24. Osborne D. Radiologic appearance of viral disease of the lower respiratory tract in infants and children. *Am J Roentgenol.* 1978;130:29–33.
25. Kern S, Uhl M, Berner R, et al. Respiratory syncytial virus infection of the lower respiratory tract: Radiological findings in 108 children. *Eur Radiol.* 2001;11:2581–2584.
26. Lerida A, Marron A, Casanova A, et al. Respiratory syncytial virus infection in adult patients hospitalized with community-acquired pneumonia. *Enferm Infecc Microbiol Clin.* 2000;18:177–181.
27. Gasparetto EL, Escuissato DL, Marchiori E, et al. High-resolution CT findings of respiratory syncytial virus pneumonia after bone marrow transplantation. *Am J Roentgenol.* 2004;182:1133–1137.
28. Ko JP, Shepard JA, Sproule MW, et al. CT manifestations of respiratory syncytial virus infection in lung transplant recipients. *J Comput Assist Tomogr.* 2000;24:235–241.
29. Butler JC, Peters CJ. Hantaviruses and Hantavirus pulmonary syndrome. *Clin Infect Dis.* 1994;19:387–394; quiz 395.
30. Khan AS, Khabbaz RF, Armstrong LR, et al. Hantavirus pulmonary syndrome: The first 100 US cases. *J Infect Dis.* 1996;173:1297–1303.
31. Moolenaar RL, Breiman RF, Peters CJ. Hantavirus pulmonary syndrome. *Semin Respir Infect.* 1997;12:31–39.
32. Miedzinski L. Community-acquired pneumonia: New facets of an old disease–Hantavirus pulmonary syndrome. *Respir Care Clin N Am.* 2005;11:45–58.
33. Ketai LH, Williamson MR, Telepak RJ, et al. Hantavirus pulmonary syndrome: Radiographic findings in 16 patients. *Radiology.* 1994;191:665–668.
34. Boroja M, Barrie JR, Raymond GS. Radiographic findings in 20 patients with Hantavirus pulmonary syndrome correlated with clinical outcome. *Am J Roentgenol.* 2002;178:159–163.
35. Chan-Yeung M, Xu RH. SARS: Epidemiology. *Respirology.* 2003;8(suppl):S9–14.
36. Poon LL, Guan Y, Nicholls JM, et al. The aetiology, origins, and diagnosis of severe acute respiratory syndrome. *Lancet Infect Dis.* 2004;4:663–671.
37. Hui DS, Sung JJ. Severe acute respiratory syndrome. *Chest.* 2003;124:12–15.
38. Franks TJ, Chong PY, Chui P, et al. Lung pathology of severe acute respiratory syndrome (SARS): A study of 8 autopsy cases from Singapore. *Hum Pathol.* 2003;34:743–748.
39. Grinblat L, Shulman H, Glickman A, et al. Severe acute respiratory syndrome: Radiographic review of 40 probable cases in Toronto, Canada. *Radiology.* 2003;228:802–809.
40. Müller NL, Ooi GC, Khong PL, et al. Severe acute respiratory syndrome: Radiographic and CT findings. *Am J Roentgenol.* 2003;181:3–8.
41. Wong KT, Antonio GE, Hui DS, et al. Severe acute respiratory syndrome: Radiographic appearances and pattern of progression in 138 patients. *Radiology.* 2003;228:401–406.
42. Ooi CG, Khong PL, Lam B, et al. Severe acute respiratory syndrome: Relationship between radiologic and clinical parameters. *Radiology.* 2003;229:492–499.
43. Wong KT, Antonio GE, Hui DS, et al. Thin-section CT of severe acute respiratory syndrome: Evaluation of 73 patients exposed to or with the disease. *Radiology.* 2003;228:395–400.
44. Müller NL, Ooi GC, Khong PL, et al. High-resolution CT findings of severe acute respiratory syndrome at presentation and after admission. *Am J Roentgenol.* 2004;182:39–44.
45. Chen HL, Chiou SS, Hsiao HP, et al. Respiratory adenoviral infections in children: A study of hospitalized cases in southern Taiwan in 2001–2002. *J Trop Pediatr.* 2004;50:279–284.
46. Rocholl C, Gerber K, Daly J, et al. Adenoviral infections in children: The impact of rapid diagnosis. *Pediatrics.* 2004;113:e51–e56.
47. Chuang YY, Chiu CH, Wong KS, et al. Severe adenovirus infection in children. *J Microbiol Immunol Infect.* 2003;36:37–40.
48. Bateman ED, Hayashi S, Kuwano K, et al. Latent adenoviral infection in follicular bronchiectasis. *Am J Respir Crit Care Med.* 1995;151:170–176.
49. Kim CK, Kim SW, Kim JS, et al. Bronchiolitis obliterans in the 1990s in Korea and the United States. *Chest.* 2001;120:1101–1106.
50. Simila S, Linna O, Lanning P, et al. Chronic lung damage caused by adenovirus type 7: A ten-year follow-up study. *Chest.* 1981;80:127–131.
51. Spigelblatt L, Rosenfeld R. Hyperlucent lung: Long-term complication of adenovirus type 7 pneumonia. *Can Med Assoc J.* 1983;128:47–49.
52. Farng KT, Wu KG, Lee YS, et al. Comparison of clinical characteristics of adenovirus and non-adenovirus pneumonia in children. *J Microbiol Immunol Infect.* 2002;35:37–41.
53. Motallebi M, Mukunda BN, Ravakhah K. Adenoviral bronchopneumonia in an immunocompetent adult: Computed tomography and pathologic correlations. *Am J Med Sci.* 2003;325:285–287.
54. Pham TT, Burchette JL Jr, Hale LP. Fatal disseminated adenovirus infections in immunocompromised patients. *Am J Clin Pathol.* 2003;120:575–583.
55. Raboni SM, Nogueira MB, Tsuchiya LR, et al. Respiratory tract viral infections in bone marrow transplant patients. *Transplantation.* 2003;76:142–146.
56. Kawai T, Fujiwara T, Aoyama Y, et al. Diffuse interstitial fibrosing pneumonitis and adenovirus infection. *Chest.* 1976;69:692–694.
57. Becroft DM. Histopathology of fatal adenovirus infection of the respiratory tract in young children. *J Clin Pathol.* 1967;20:561–569.
58. Matar LD, McAdams HP, Palmer SM, et al. Respiratory viral infections in lung transplant recipients: Radiologic findings with clinical correlation. *Radiology.* 1999;213:735–742.
59. Schuller D, Spessert C, Fraser VJ, et al. Herpes simplex virus from respiratory tract secretions: Epidemiology, clinical characteristics, and outcome in immunocompromised and nonimmunocompromised hosts. *Am J Med.* 1993;94:29–33.
60. Aquino SL, Dunagan DP, Chiles C, et al. Herpes simplex virus 1 pneumonia: Patterns on CT scans and conventional chest radiographs. *J Comput Assist Tomogr.* 1998;22:795–800.
61. Graham BS, Snell JD Jr. Herpes simplex virus infection of the adult lower respiratory tract. *Medicine (Baltimore).* 1983;62:384–393.
62. Ramsey PG, Fife KH, Hackman RC, et al. Herpes simplex virus pneumonia: Clinical, virologic, and pathologic features in 20 patients. *Ann Intern Med.* 1982;97:813–820.
63. Byers RJ, Hasleton PS, Quigley A, et al. Pulmonary herpes simplex in burns patients. *Eur Respir J.* 1996;9:2313–2317.
64. Nash G, Foley FD. Herpetic infection of the middle and lower respiratory tract. *Am J Clin Pathol.* 1970;54:857–863.
65. Brown MJ, Miller RR, Müller NL. Acute lung disease in the immunocompromised host: CT and pathologic examination findings. *Radiology.* 1994;190:247–254.
66. Janzen DL, Padley SP, Adler BD, et al. Acute pulmonary complications in immunocompromised non-AIDS patients: Comparison of diagnostic accuracy of CT and chest radiography. *Clinical Radiology.* 1993;47:159–165.
67. Umans U, Golding RP, Duraku S, et al. Herpes simplex virus 1 pneumonia: Conventional chest radiograph pattern. *Eur Radiol.* 2001;11:990–994.
68. Weller TH. Varicella and herpes zoster. Changing concepts of the natural history, control, and importance of a not-so-benign virus. *N Engl J Med.* 1983;309:1434–1440.
69. Gasparetto EL, Escuissato DL, Inoue C, et al. Herpes simplex virus type 2 pneumonia after bone marrow transplantation: High-resolution CT findings in 3 patients. *J Thorac Imaging.* 2005;20:71–73.
70. Fraser RS, Colman N, Müller NL, et al. *Synopsis of diseases of the chest.* Philadelphia, PA: Elsevier Saunders; 2005.
71. Mohsen AH, McKendrick M. Varicella pneumonia in adults. *Eur Respir J.* 2003;21:886–891.
72. Jura E, Chadwick EG, Josephs SH, et al. Varicella-zoster virus infections in children infected with human immunodeficiency virus. *Pediatr Infect Dis J.* 1989;8:586–590.
73. Locksley RM, Flournoy N, Sullivan KM, et al. Infection with varicella-zoster virus after marrow transplantation. *J Infect Dis.* 1985;152:1172–1181.
74. Charles RE, Katz RL, Ordonez NG, et al. Varicella-zoster virus infection with pleural involvement. A cytologic and ultrastructural study of a case. *Am J Clin Pathol.* 1986;85:522–526.
75. Mohsen AH, Peck RJ, Mason Z, et al. Lung function tests and risk factors for pneumonia in adults with chickenpox. *Thorax.* 2001;56:796–799.
76. Wilkins EG, Leen CL, McKendrick MW, et al. Management of chickenpox in the adult. A review prepared for the UK Advisory Group on chickenpox

on behalf of the British Society for the Study of Infection. *J Infect.* 1998;36(suppl 1):49–58.

77. Weber DM, Pellecchia JA. Varicella pneumonia: Study of prevalence in adult men. *JAMA.* 1965;192:572–573.

78. Frangides CY, Pneumatikos I. Varicella-zoster virus pneumonia in adults: Report of 14 cases and review of the literature. *Eur J Intern Med.* 2004; 15:364–370.

79. Brunton FJ, Moore ME. A survey of pulmonary calcification following adult chicken-pox. *Br J Radiol.* 1969;42:256–259.

80. Kim JS, Ryu CW, Lee SI, et al. High-resolution CT findings of varicella-zoster pneumonia. *Am J Roentgenol.* 1999;172:113–116.

81. Marrie TJ, Janigan DT, Haldane EV, et al. Does cytomegalovirus play a role in community-acquired pneumonia? *Clin Invest Med.* 1985;8:286–295.

82. Ho M. Epidemiology of cytomegalovirus infections. *Rev Infect Dis.* 1990; 12(suppl 7):S701–S710.

83. Ettinger NA, Bailey TC, Trulock EP, et al. Washington University Lung Transplant Group. Cytomegalovirus infection and pneumonitis. Impact after isolated lung transplantation. *Am Rev Respir Dis.* 1993;147:1017–1023.

84. Meyers JD, Flournoy N, Thomas ED. Nonbacterial pneumonia after allogeneic marrow transplantation: A review of ten years' experience. *Rev Infect Dis.* 1982;4:1119–1132.

85. Austin JHM, Schulman LL, Mastrobattista JD. Pulmonary infection after cardiac transplantation: Clinical and radiologic considerations. *Radiology.* 1989;172:259–265.

86. Olliff JF, Williams MP. Radiological appearances of cytomegalovirus infections. *Clin Radiol.* 1989;40:463–467.

87. Coy DL, Ormazabal A, Godwin JD, et al. Imaging evaluation of pulmonary and abdominal complications following hematopoietic stem cell transplantation. *Radiographics.* 2005;25:305–317; discussion 318.

88. Konoplev S, Champlin RE, Giralt S, et al. Cytomegalovirus pneumonia in adult autologous blood and marrow transplant recipients. *Bone Marrow Transplant.* 2001;27:877–881.

89. Drew WL. Cytomegalovirus disease in the highly active antiretroviral therapy era. *Curr Infect Dis Rep.* 2003;5:257–265.

90. Travis WD, Colby TV, Koss MN, et al. *Non-neoplastic disorders of the lower respiratory tract.* Washington, DC: Armed Forces Institute of Pathology; 2002.

91. Amundson DE, Weiss PJ. Pneumonia in military recruits. *Mil Med.* 1994; 159:629–631.

92. Marrie TJ, Poulin-Costello M, Beecroft MD, et al. Etiology of community-acquired pneumonia treated in an ambulatory setting. *Respir Med.* 2005; 99:60–65.

93. Ali NJ, Sillis M, Andrews BE, et al. The clinical spectrum and diagnosis of Mycoplasma pneumoniae infection. *Q J Med.* 1986;58:241–251.

94. Marrie TJ, Beecroft M, Herman-Gnjidic Z, et al. Symptom resolution in patients with Mycoplasma pneumoniae pneumonia. *Can Respir J.* 2004; 11:573–577.

95. Rollins S, Colby T, Clayton F. Open lung biopsy in Mycoplasma pneumoniae pneumonia. *Arch Pathol Lab Med.* 1986;110:34–41.

96. Cameron DC, Borthwick RN, Philp T. The radiographic patterns of acute mycoplasma pneumonitis. *Clin Radiol.* 1977;28:173–180.

97. Putman CE, Curtis AM, Simeone JF, et al. Mycoplasma pneumonia. Clinical and roentgenographic patterns. *Am J Roentgenol Radium Ther Nucl Med.* 1975;124:417–422.

98. Van Bever HP, Van Doorn JW, Demey HE. Adult respiratory distress syndrome associated with Mycoplasma pneumoniae infection. *Eur J Pediatr.* 1992;151:227–228.

99. Reittner P, Ward S, Heyneman L, et al. Pneumonia: High-resolution CT findings in 114 patients. *Eur Radiol.* 2003;13:515–521.

100. Kim CK, Chung CY, Kim JS, et al. Late abnormal findings on high-resolution computed tomography after Mycoplasma pneumonia. *Pediatrics.* 2000;105:372–378.

101. Stokes D, Sigler A, Khouri NF, et al. Unilateral hyperlucent lung (Swyer-James syndrome) after severe Mycoplasma pneumoniae infection. *Am Rev Respir Dis.* 1978;117:145–152.

102. McConnell CT Jr, Plouffe JF, File TM, et al. Radiographic appearance of Chlamydia pneumoniae (TWAR strain) respiratory infections. CBPIS Study Group. Community-based Pneumonia Incidence Study. *Radiology.* 1994;192:819–824.

103. Kauppinen MT, Lahde S, Syrjala H. Roentgenographic findings of pneumonia caused by Chlamydia pneumoniae. A comparison with streptococcus pneumonia. *Arch Intern Med.* 1996;156:1851–1856.

104. Okada F, Ando Y, Wakisaka M, et al. Chlamydia pneumoniae pneumonia and Mycoplasma pneumoniae pneumonia: Comparison of clinical findings and CT findings. *J Comput Assist Tomogr.* 2005;29:626–632.

105. Barrett PK, Greenberg MJ. Outbreak of ornithosis. *Br Med J.* 1966;5507: 206–207.

106. Heddema ER, Kraan MC, Buys-Bergen HE, et al. A woman with a lobar infiltrate due to psittacosis detected by polymerase chain reaction. *Scand J Infect Dis.* 2003;35:422–424.

107. Stenstrom R, Jansson E, Wager O. Ornithosis pneumonia with special reference to roentgenological lung findings. *Acta Med Scand.* 1962;171: 349–356.

108. Goupil F, Pelle-Duporte D, Kouyoumdjian S, et al. Severe pneumonia with a pneumococcal aspect during an ornithosis outbreak. *Presse Med.* 1998;27:1084–1088.

109. Levy M, Dromer F, Brion N, et al. Community-acquired pneumonia. Importance of initial noninvasive bacteriologic and radiographic investigations. *Chest.* 1988;93:43–48.

110. Albaum MN, Hill LC, Murphy M, et al. Interobserver reliability of the chest radiograph in community-acquired pneumonia. PORT Investigators. *Chest.* 1996;110:343–350.

111. Melbye H, Dale K. Interobserver variability in the radiographic diagnosis of adult outpatient pneumonia. *Acta Radiol.* 1992;33:79–81.

112. Herold CJ, Sailer JG. Community-acquired and nosocomial pneumonia. *Eur Radiol.* 2004;14(suppl 3):E2–20.

113. Tew J, Calenoff L, Berlin BS. Bacterial or nonbacterial pneumonia: Accuracy of radiographic diagnosis. *Radiology.* 1977;124:607–612.

114. Tomiyama N, Müller NL, Johkoh T, et al. Acute parenchymal lung disease in immunocompetent patients: Diagnostic accuracy of high-resolution CT. *Am J Roentgenol.* 2000;174:1745–1750.

Fungal and Parasitic Infection

6

Fungal and parasitic infections are an increasingly frequent cause of pulmonary disease worldwide. Increased risk for the development of infection has resulted because of expanding population in endemic areas; increased travel to endemic areas; and increased numbers of immunocompromised patients (1). A high index of suspicion is required to diagnose fungal and parasitic infection, particularly in patients who do not reside in endemic areas.

The most common endemic mycosis in North America is histoplasmosis; other relatively common endemic mycoses are coccidioidomycosis and blastomycosis (1, 2). Although most of these infections in nonimmunocompromised persons are self-limited, some patients can develop severe pneumonitis, as well as various forms of chronic pulmonary infection. Paracoccidioidomycosis (South American blastomycosis) is endemic in South America, and it carries a high mortality rate in countries such as Brazil (3).

Several mycoses are ubiquitous but almost exclusively affect predisposed persons, particularly immunocompromised patients. These mycoses include cryptococcosis, aspergillosis, candidiasis, and mucormycosis, and those caused by *Pneumocystis jiroveci*. The number of persons at risk for developing pulmonary infection from these organisms continues to grow (4, 5). In this chapter we focus on the radiologic manifestations of pulmonary mycoses and parasitic infestations seen in nonimmunocompromised persons. Infections in immunocompromised patients are discussed in Chapters 7 and 8.

FUNGI

Histoplasmosis

Histoplasmosis is caused by the dimorphic fungus *Histoplasma capsulatum*. It is endemic in the Mississippi and Ohio river valleys in the United States, the St. Lawrence river valley in Canada, and South America (1). The manifestations of pulmonary disease are quite varied. The most common pathologic abnormality is focal granulomatous inflammation, necrosis, and fibrosis, identical to that of tuberculosis. This disease is usually too limited in extent to be visible on chest radiography and is not recognized clinically. Occasionally, enlargement or coalescence of several inflammatory foci results in single or multiple poorly defined areas of airspace consolidation (6). In most patients, ipsilateral hilar lymph node enlargement is evident on the radiograph.

A much more common clinical presentation is that of a solitary nodule seen on chest radiography or computed tomography (CT) scan in an asymptomatic patient (see Table 6.1). The nodule corresponds histologically to an

TABLE 6.1
HISTOPLASMOSIS

Histoplasma capsulatum

Endemic areas: Central and eastern United States and Canada

Most common radiologic findings

    Solitary lung nodule (histoplasmoma)

        1–3 cm diameter

        Soft-tissue density or calcified

    Hilar and mediastinal lymph node calcification

Other manifestations

    Heavy exposure: Multiple nodules 1–4 cm in diameter

    Chronic histoplasmosis: Upper lobe consolidation and cavitation

    Fibrosing mediastinitis

    Broncholithiasis

    Miliary disease: In immunocompromised patient

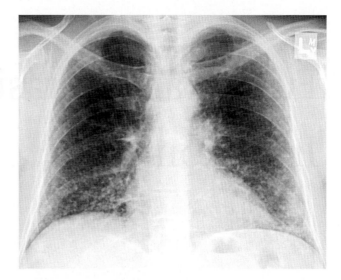

Figure 6.2 Multiple bilateral nodules due to acute histoplasmosis. Chest radiograph shows numerous well-defined bilateral nodules. The patient was a 56-year-old man who developed cough and shortness of breath following heavy exposure to histoplasmosis while exploring a contaminated cave.

encapsulated focus of necrotizing granulomatous inflammation that develops in the same manner as the Ghon focus of tuberculosis. Nodules that have been present for more than a few months frequently show central (target) or diffuse calcification as a result of dystrophic calcification of the necrotic material (see Fig. 6.1). Calcified nodules are frequently associated with calcified hilar and mediastinal lymph nodes (6). The scenarios described in the preceding text are often unassociated with a clear history of exposure to a source of infection. Exposure to a relatively large number of organisms, such as during excavation of a contaminated work site or while exploring contaminated caves, may result in symptoms and multiple areas of

consolidation or diffuse nodular opacities on chest radiograph and CT scan (see Figs. 6.2 and 6.3). Disseminated disease with a miliary or diffuse reticulonodular pattern occurs mainly in immunocompromised patients (6, 7).

Chronic histoplasmosis is an uncommon manifestation of this disease, being seen in approximately 1 of 2,000 exposed individuals (1). It occurs almost exclusively in patients with chronic obstructive lung disease and results in chronic upper lobe consolidation, often with cavitation, resembling tuberculosis (see Fig. 6.4). Like the latter condition, healing frequently results in upper lobe scarring,

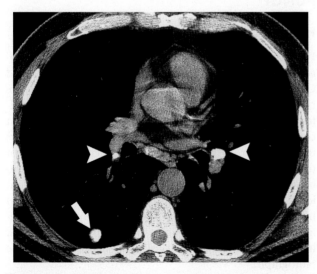

Figure 6.1 Calcified nodule and lymph nodes due to previous histoplasmosis. High-resolution computed tomography (CT) image shows calcified nodule (*arrow*) in right lower lobe and calcified right and left hilar (*arrowheads*) and subcarinal lymph nodes. The patient was a 54-year-old asymptomatic man.

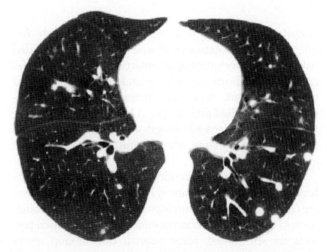

Figure 6.3 Multiple bilateral nodules due to acute histoplasmosis. High-resolution (1.3-mm collimation) computed tomography (CT) image shows multiple well-defined bilateral nodules. The patient was a 37-year-old man who developed cough and shortness of breath 1 week after heavy exposure to histoplasmosis while exploring a contaminated cave.

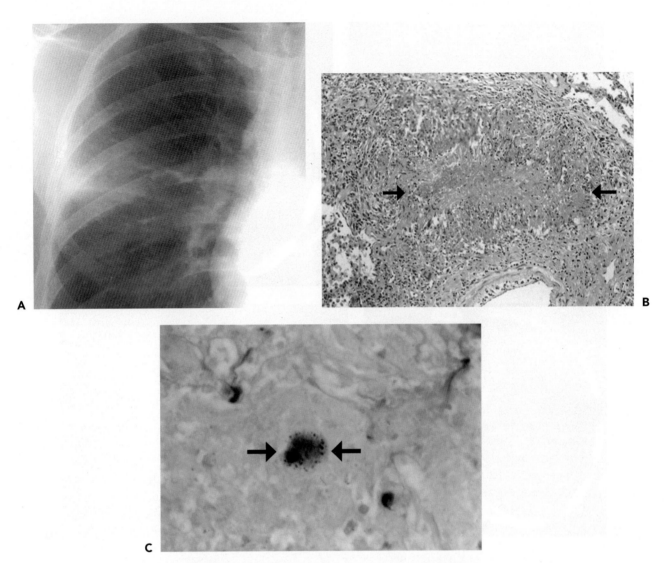

Figure 6.4 Histoplasmosis. **A:** View of right upper lung zone from a chest radiograph shows mild airspace consolidation. **B:** Photomicrograph of pathologic specimen shows necrotizing granulomatous inflammation (*arrows*), with surrounding chronic inflammatory cell infiltration and fibrosis. **C:** Photomicrograph with Gomori methenamine silver staining shows fungal organism (*arrows*) consistent with *Histoplasma capsulatum*. The patient was a 28-year-old man who presented with right chest pain. (Courtesy of Dr. Sang Jin Kim, Department of Radiology, Yonsei University Yongdong Severance Hospital, Seoul, Korea.)

volume loss, and pleural thickening. Calcification of hilar and mediastinal nodes is commonly seen. The nodes may erode into the lumen of adjacent bronchi and result in broncholithiasis (6, 7).

Mediastinal lymph node involvement may occur in any form of histoplasmosis. Such nodes may be enlarged or normal in size and are usually well circumscribed. In some patients, however, the inflammatory process extends into the adjacent mediastinum, resulting in fibrosing mediastinitis. Histologic examination in such cases shows dense fibrous tissue containing variable numbers of mononuclear inflammatory cells and granulomas. Organisms may be difficult to identify. The typical radiologic manifestation consists of a focal paratracheal mass of calcified lymph nodes frequently associated with partial or complete obstruction of the superior vena cava (6, 7).

Coccidioidomycosis

Coccidioidomycosis is caused by inhalation of spores of the dimorphic fungus *Coccidioides immitis*. It is endemic in southwestern United States and northern Mexico. Several patterns of this disease can be seen (see Table 6.2). Acute (primary) infection results in bronchopneumonia, initially associated with a predominantly neutrophilic exudate and subsequently with granulomatous inflammation. In most patients, the reaction is mild and the radiograph is normal. Approximately 40% of patients are symptomatic and have

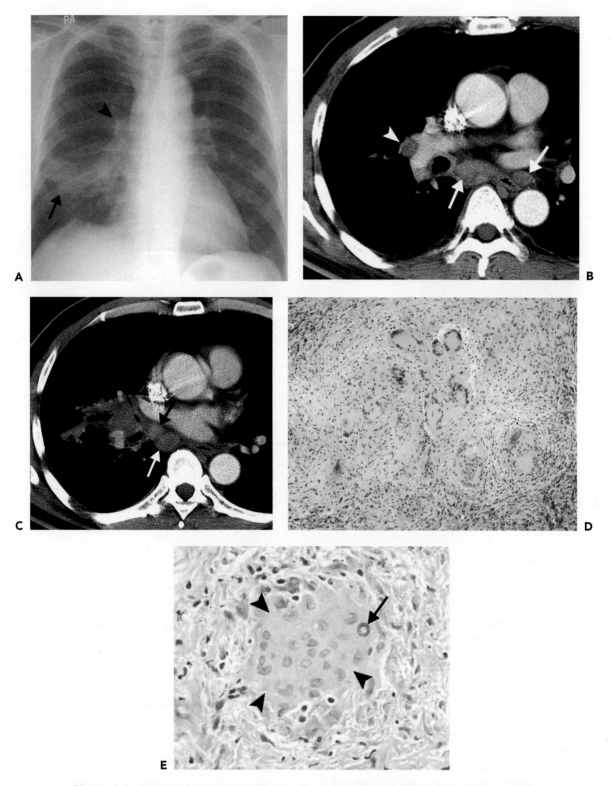

Figure 6.5 Coccidioidomycosis. **A:** Chest radiograph shows consolidation in right lower lung zone (*arrow*) and right hilar enlargement (*arrowhead*). **B:** Mediastinal window of contrast-enhanced computed tomography (CT) (5-mm collimation) scan obtained at the level of bronchus intermedius shows enlarged right hilar (*arrowhead*), subcarinal, and paraesophageal lymph nodes (*arrows*). **C:** CT scan obtained at the level of the right middle lobe bronchus shows parenchymal consolidation in the right middle lobe and enlarged subcarinal lymph nodes (*arrows*). **D:** Photomicrograph of the surgical biopsy specimen shows granulomatous inflammation and fibrosis with infiltration of multinucleated giant cells, eosinophils, and lymphocytes (Hematoxylin and Eosin stain, ×100). **E:** Photomicrograph shows a yeast form developing a spherule of *Coccidioides immitis* (*arrow*), which is engulfed by a multinucleated giant cell (*arrowheads*). The periodic acid-Schiff stain highlights its thick yeast wall (Periodic acid-Schiff stain, ×400). The patient was a 58-year-old man with a 1 month history of dyspnea and fever.

TABLE 6.2
COCCIDIOIDOMYCOSIS

Coccidioides immitis
Endemic areas: Southwestern United States and northern
   Mexico
Most common radiologic findings
   Primary coccidioidomycosis
      1. Single or multiple foci of airspace consolidation
   Chronic pulmonary coccidioidomycosis
      1. Solitary lung nodule 1–3 cm in diameter
      2. 10%–15% cavitate, thick-walled or thin-walled
        (grape skin)
Other manifestations
   Lymphadenopathy in 20% of cases
   Miliary disease: In immunocompromised patient

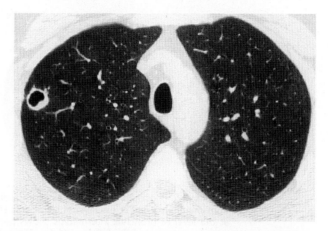

Figure 6.7 Coccidioidomycosis. High-resolution computed to-mography (CT) image (1.5-mm collimation) shows thin-walled cav-ity in right upper lobe. The diagnosis of coccidioidomycosis was made at surgical resection. The patient was a 44-year-old man who developed coccidioidomycosis following travel to an endemic area.

patchy areas of consolidation evident on the radiograph (see Fig. 6.5). Associated hilar lymph node enlargement is seen in 20% of cases. The consolidation usually resolves over several weeks (8).

Chronic pulmonary coccidioidomycosis is radiologically characterized by nodules or cavities (see Figs. 6.6 and 6.7). Most are discovered incidentally in asymptomatic patients; approximately 25% can be seen to result from incomplete resolution of acute bronchopneumonia (see Fig. 6.8). In most patients the nodules or cavities are solitary and measure 2 to 4 cm in diameter. They may be thin walled ("grape skin") or thick walled (8) and

usually have homogeneous attenuation on CT scan (9). Histologically, the lesions correspond to foci of necrotizing granulomatous inflammation. Although sharply delimited by a well-developed fibrous capsule most often, inflammation surrounding the necrotic tissue can result in adjacent ill-defined areas of consolidation (9).

This disease is rarely progressive but occasionally may result in unilateral or bilateral upper lobe consolidation, sometimes associated with single or multiple cavities, resembling reactivation tuberculosis. Disseminated disease

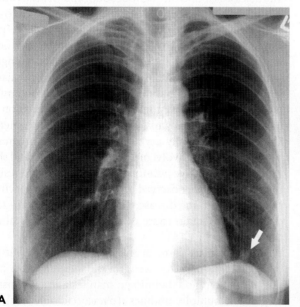

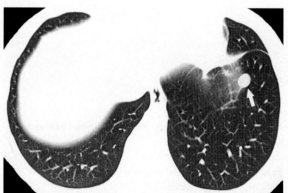

Figure 6.6 Coccidioidomycosis. **A:** Chest radiograph shows smoothly marginated left lower lobe nodule (*arrow*). **B:** Computed tomography (CT) image confirms the presence of left lower lobe nodule (*arrow*). The diagnosis of coccidioidomycosis was made at surgical resection. The patient was a 48-year-old woman with no symptoms related to the nodule.

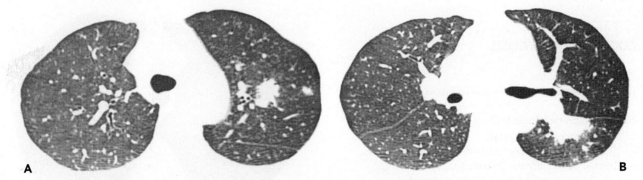

Figure 6.8 Coccidioidomycosis. **A:** High-resolution computed tomography (CT) (1-mm collimation) image obtained at the level of aortic arch shows nodules in left upper lobe. **B:** CT scan image at the level of bronchus intermedius shows peribronchial consolidation and small nodules in the superior segment of the left lower lobe. The patient was a 30-year-old doctor who worked in her clinical laboratory on fungus cultures. (Courtesy of Dr. Jin Sung Lee, Department of Radiology, Asan Medical Center, University of Ulsan, Seoul, Korea.)

is most commonly seen in immunocompromised patients and is usually manifested radiologically as a diffuse reticulonodular pattern or miliary nodules.

Blastomycosis

Blastomycosis is caused by the dimorphic fungus *Blastomyces dermatitidis*. The disease occurs most commonly in the central and southeastern United States (endemic areas include the Ohio, Mississippi, and Missouri river valleys, particularly in Wisconsin) and southern Canada (mainly Quebec, Ontario, and Manitoba) (1). Patients with the disease usually present with symptoms of acute pneumonia, including abrupt onset of fever, chills, productive cough, and pleuritic chest pain. Arthralgias and myalgias are common and erythema nodosum develops occasionally.

The most common radiographic findings consist of acute airspace consolidation, observed in 25% to 75% of patients (see Table 6.3 and Fig. 6.9). The consolidation is patchy or confluent and may be subsegmental, segmental, or nonsegmental (10–12). Cavitation may be seen in up to 50% of patients with airspace consolidation (11).

TABLE 6.3
BLASTOMYCOSIS

Blastomyces dermatitidis
Endemic areas: Central and southeastern United States and
   southern Canada
Most common radiologic findings
   Patchy or confluent acute airspace consolidation
   Single or multiple masses
   Cavitation in up to 50% of patients
Other manifestations
   Pleural effusion in 10%–15% of patients
   Miliary disease: In immunocompromised patient

The second most common presentation, observed in approximately 30% of patients, is solitary or multiple masses (see Fig. 6.10). Clinically overwhelming infection may result in miliary dissemination. Pleural effusion is present in 10% to 15% of patients. Hilar or mediastinal lymph node enlargement is relatively uncommon. There is poor correlation between the radiologic abnormalities and the clinical presentation (10, 12).

Paracoccidioidomycosis (South American Blastomycosis)

Paracoccidioidomycosis (South American blastomycosis) is caused by the dimorphic fungus *Paracoccidioides brasiliensis*. The disease is found throughout South and Central America including Mexico (3). South American blastomycosis is seen more frequently in men, and most patients range from 25 to 45 years in age. The infection usually occurs in farmers, manual laborers, and other workers engaged in rural occupations and is probably caused by inhalation, which results in primary pneumonia and secondary systemic dissemination. Animal-to-human transmission and person-to-person transmission have not been documented. The disease is usually asymptomatic but can progress to severe pulmonary involvement, leading to cough and shortness of breath. Active pulmonary involvement and residual fibrotic lesions are observed in 80% and 60%, respectively, of patients with the disease. The lungs are the main target organ and the main cause of morbidity and mortality in these patients (13, 14).

In the primary form of the disease, transient airspace consolidation may be seen in the middle lung zone. The most common radiologic manifestation consists of single or multiple nodules (paracoccidioidomas) that may be single or multiple (see Table 6.4). Progressive pulmonary disease may resemble tuberculosis; however, the lower lobes are more frequently involved than the upper lobes, and cavitations are less common. Hilar

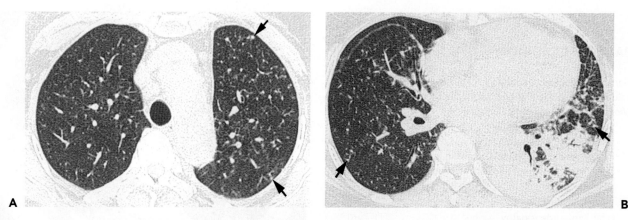

Figure 6.9 Blastomycosis in a 69-year-old woman. **A:** High-resolution (1-mm collimation) computed tomography (CT) image at the level of the aortic arch shows small centrilobular nodules (*arrows*) in the left upper lobe. **B:** CT scan obtained at the level of the basal trunk demonstrates areas of consolidation in the left lower lobe. Also note tree-in-bud opacities (*arrows*) in both lower lobes.

lymph node enlargement can occur by itself or in association with parenchymal involvement. High-resolution CT scan findings consist of multiple variable-sized nodules, cavitation, centrilobular opacities, peribronchovascular interstitial thickening, intralobular lines, and traction bronchiectasis (see Fig. 6.11). These abnormalities are usually bilateral and symmetric (15). A reversed CT halo sign (central ground-glass opacity surrounded by a crescent or ring of consolidation) is seen in 10% of patients with active *P. brasiliensis* infection (see Fig. 6.12) (16). The areas of ground-glass opacity in these patients correspond to the presence of inflammatory infiltrates in the alveolar

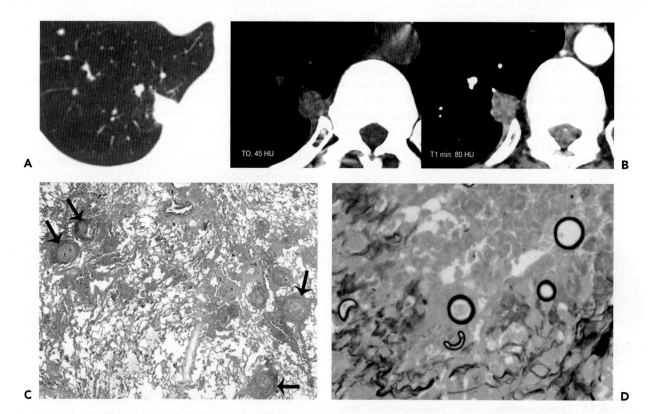

Figure 6.10 Blastomycosis. **A:** View of the right lower lobe from a computed tomography (CT) image (2.5-mm collimation) shows triangular nodule in right lower lobe. **B:** Dynamic CT scans obtained at similar level to **(A)** demonstrate marked and persistent enhancement suggesting active inflammatory nodule. **C:** Photomicrograph of wedge resection specimen demonstrates foci of granulomatous inflammation (*arrows*). **D:** Photomicrograph with Gomori methenamine silver staining reveals yeast forms of *Blastomyces dermatitidis*. The patient was a 69-year-old woman.

TABLE 6.4
PARACOCCIDIOIDOMYCOSIS

Paracoccidioides brasiliensis
Endemic areas: Central and South America
Most common radiologic findings
    Single or multiple nodules
    Commonly cavitated
    Progressive consolidation, scarring, and cavitation
    May resemble tuberculosis but tends to involve mainly lower lobes
Other manifestations
    Hilar lymphadenopathy
    Disseminated disease: In immunocompromised patient

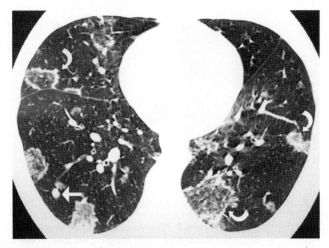

Figure 6.12 Paracoccidioidomycosis with reverse halo sign. High-resolution computed tomography (CT) image shows bilateral focal ground-glass opacities surrounded by a crescent or ring of consolidation (reversed halo sign) (*curved arrows*). Also note the patchy ground-glass opacities without surrounding consolidation and right lower lobe nodule (*straight arrow*). The patient was a 45-year-old man. (From Gasparetto EL, Escuissato DL, Davaus T, et al. Reversed halo sign in pulmonary paracoccidioidomycosis. *Am J Roentgenol.* 2005;184:1932–1934, with permission.)

septa, and the peripheral consolidation reflects the presence of areas of intra-alveolar inflammatory infiltrates without organizing pneumonia (16).

Cryptococcosis

Cryptococcosis is caused by *Cryptococcus neoformans,* which is commonly distributed in soil, especially that containing pigeon and avian droppings. Infection is acquired by inhaling spores of fungus. The lungs, central nervous system, blood, skin, bone, joints, and prostate are the most commonly involved sites.

Cryptococcosis occurs predominantly in immunocompromised patients (17) but can also be seen in the normal host. The incidence in the United States increased considerably in the 1980s in relation to the AIDS epidemic but decreased after 1990, before highly active antiretroviral therapy (HAART) became available, and further thereafter (17). Although cryptococcosis and other opportunistic

fungal infections in persons with AIDS are no longer a major problem in developed countries, they are a major cause of morbidity and mortality in developing countries (4).

The spectrum of pulmonary cryptococcosis depends on the host's defenses. In the immunocompetent host, cryptococcal infections are commonly localized to the lung and the patients are asymptomatic. In the immunocompromised patient, cryptococcal infections often cause symptomatic pulmonary infections and often disseminate to the central nervous system, skin, and bones.

Approximately one third of patients are asymptomatic. Symptoms range from mild cough and low-grade fever to acute presentation with high fever and severe shortness of breath. The disease can spread rapidly throughout the lungs and disseminate to extrapulmonary sites, especially the meninges in immunocompromised patients.

Histopathologically, immunocompetent patients show granulomatous response, such as noncaseating granulomas or extensive caseation. In immunocompromised patients, intact alveolar spaces become filled with yeasts. The radiologic findings include solitary or multiple nodular opacities (see Fig. 6.13), segmental or lobar consolidation (see Fig. 6.14), hilar and mediastinal lymphadenopathy, and pleural effusion (see Table 6.5). Cavitation is seen in approximately 10% to 15% of cases (18–20). The radiologic manifestations are influenced by the patient's age and immune status. Immunocompetent patients tend to present with nodules or masses (18, 19, 21), younger patients are more likely to present with cavitation (18), and immunocompromised patients are more likely to have airspace consolidation, lymphadenopathy, pleural effusion, and disseminated disease (22–24).

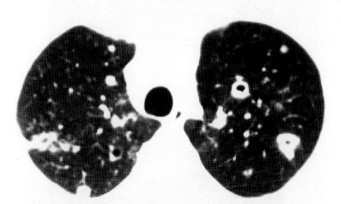

Figure 6.11 Paracoccidioidomycosis. High-resolution computed tomography (CT) image (1.5-mm collimation) shows several cavitated nodules in the upper lobes and focal ground-glass opacities. Fine needle aspiration of one of the nodules demonstrated *Paracoccidioides brasiliensis.* The patient was a 52-year-old man. (Case courtesy of Dr. Arthur Soares Souza Jr., Instituto de Radiodiagnostico Rio Preto, Sao Paulo, Brazil.)

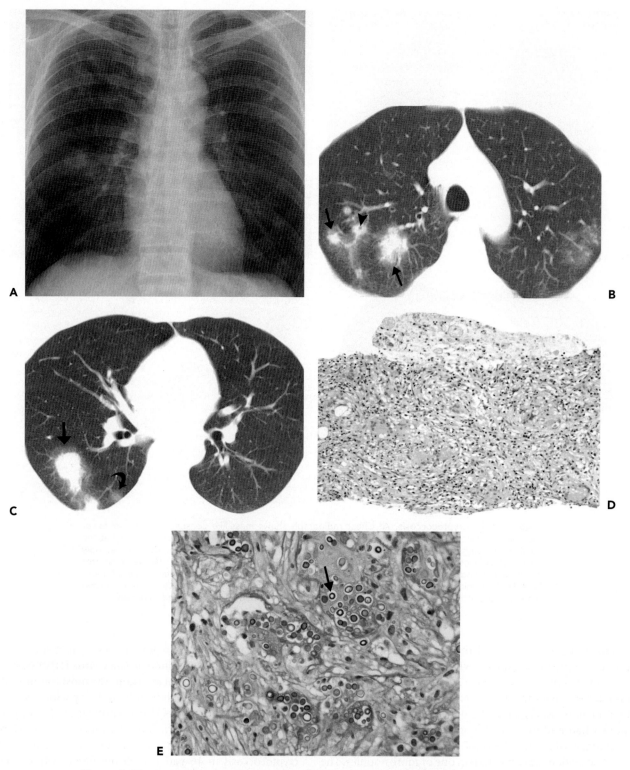

Figure 6.13   Cryptococcosis. **A:** Chest radiograph shows multiple bilateral poorly defined nodular opacities. **B:** Computed tomography (CT) image (5-mm collimation) at the level of the aortic arch shows multiple bilateral variable-sized nodules. Some nodules demonstrate a surrounding halo of ground-glass attenuation (CT halo sign) (*straight arrows*) and one of nodules in the right upper lobe shows cavitation (*arrowhead*). **C:** CT scan obtained at the level of the right inferior pulmonary vein shows nodules with CT halo sign (*straight arrow*) and nodular area of ground-glass opacity (*curved arrow*) in the superior segment of the right lower lobe. **D:** Photomicrograph of core biopsy specimen from one of the nodules in the right lung demonstrates irregular foci of granulomatous inflammation consisting of epithelioid histiocytes and multinucleated giant cells (Hematoxylin and Eosin, ×40). **E:** Magnified view shows many yeast forms of spherical-shaped cryptococci surrounded by wide clear spaces representing unstained capsules (*arrow*) (Periodic acid-Schiff stain, x400). The patient was a 37-year-old immunocompetent man with chronic cough.

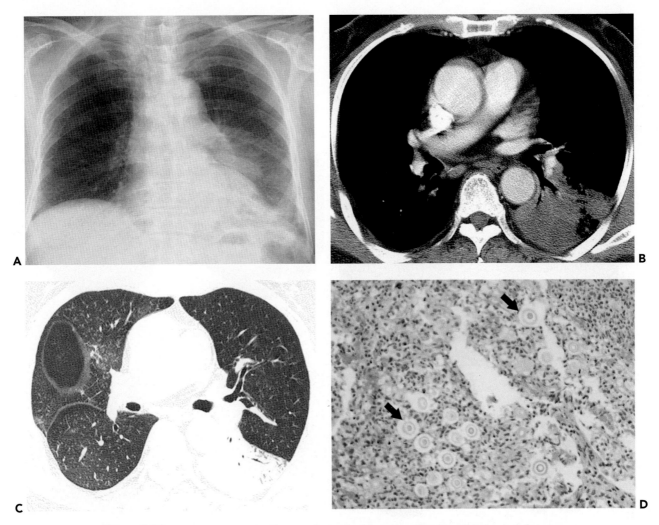

Figure 6.14 Cryptococcosis. **A:** Chest radiograph shows mass-like consolidation in left lower lobe. **B:** Contrast-enhanced computed tomography (CT) image (5-mm collimation) obtained at the level of the right middle lobe bronchus shows left lower lobe consolidation. **C:** Lung window image of high-resolution CT scan (1-mm collimation) obtained at similar level to (**B**) demonstrates consolidation and air bronchograms in left lower lobe. Also note ground-glass opacities in right upper lobe. **D:** Photomicrograph of the transbronchial lung biopsy specimen shows acute inflammation and many cryptococci (*arrows*) with wide unstained capsules. The patient was a 74-year-old man.

Fox and Müller reviewed the CT scan findings in 12 immunocompetent patients with pulmonary cryptococcosis (18). Ten (83%) of the 12 patients had pulmonary nodules or masses and 2 patients had nonsegmental consolidation with associated cavitation. Four patients had single and six had multiple nodules or masses ranging from 5 to >50 mm in diameter. Three of the ten patients with nodules had evidence of cavitation in one or more nodules. The distribution of parenchymal changes was predominately in the lower lobe in approximately 60% of cases, upper lobe in 20%, and middle lobe or lingula in 20%. Two patients had hilar or mediastinal lymphadenopathy; none had any pleural abnormality. All six patients older than the median age of 44 years demonstrated only one or two peripheral nodules. By contrast, all six patients presenting with cavitary disease, consolidation, or greater than two nodules were younger than the median age of 44 (18).

Friedman et al. (25) reported chest radiographic findings of 14 human immunodeficiency virus (HIV)-positive patients with cryptococcal infection. The most common abnormalities consisted of reticulonodular opacities ($n = 9$), focal or widespread airspace consolidation ($n = 7$), or ground-glass opacities ($n = 6$). Lacomis et al. (26) reviewed the radiographic and CT scan manifestations of cryptococcosis in 46 patients, all but one of whom were immunocompromised because of HIV infection, organ transplantation, or other causes. In most patients the abnormalities were bilateral and consisted of patchy irregular or mass-like airspace opacities or lobar or segmental consolidation. Approximately 50% of patients had nodules or masses. Pleural effusions were seen in approximately 30% of patients and lymph node enlargement in 25% of cases. The lymph node enlargement was mild (1 to 1.5 cm) and never occurred as a single abnormality. The

TABLE 6.5
CRYPTOCOCCOSIS

Cryptococcus neoformans
Worldwide distribution
May affect healthy host
Most common radiologic findings
    Single or multiple nodules 1–5 cm in diameter
Other manifestations
    Airspace consolidation: Mainly in immunocompromised patients
    Cavitation, particularly in young adults and immunocompromised patients
    Lymphadenopathy: Mainly in immunocompromised patients
    Disseminated disease: In immunocompromised patients

TABLE 6.6
ASPERGILLOMA

Aspergillus fumigatus
Ubiquitous organisms
Fungus colonizes cavity or ectatic airway
Most commonly in patients with previous tuberculosis or sarcoidosis
Most common radiologic findings
    Round or oval intracavitary mass
    Separated from the wall by an airspace (air-crescent sign)
    Moves when the patient changes position
    Adjacent pleural thickening

combination of findings consisting of consolidation, nodules, and effusions or lymph node enlargement was more frequent than a single abnormality. There was no difference in the radiographic appearances of pulmonary disease between HIV-infected patients and other immunocompromised individuals. In most patients (92%), CT scan provided either additional information on the extent of disease or improved characterization of the disease process. CT scan confirmed a general trend for a peripheral distribution of the disease in all groups that correlates with the pathologically recognized spread of cryptococcus in the subpleural alveoli (26).

Aspergillosis

Several species of *Aspergillus* may result in pulmonary disease. By far the most common human pathogen is *Aspergillus fumigatus*. Infection is usually acquired by inhalation of the organisms that are ubiquitous in the environment. Pulmonary aspergillosis is virtually always seen in individuals who have some underlying abnormality—structural abnormality in the lung (such as a cavity), atopy, or deficiency of the inflammatory or immunologic response. The pathologic and radiologic manifestations of the disease can be divided into three main forms: Aspergilloma, allergic bronchopulmonary aspergillosis (ABPA), and invasive aspergillosis. The last named is in turn subdivided into angioinvasive, bronchopneumonic (airway-invasive), and chronic necrotizing ("semi-invasive") forms (27).

Aspergilloma

Aspergilloma (fungus ball) is a conglomeration of intertwined fungal hyphae admixed with mucus and cellular debris within a pulmonary cavity or ectatic bronchus. The most common underlying cause is tuberculosis, with approximately 25% to 50% of patients having a history of this

disease. Other common predisposing conditions include sarcoidosis, bronchiectasis of any cause, and chronic cavities of any cause.

Radiologically, mycetomas present as a solid, round or oval mass of soft-tissue density within a spherical or ovoid cavity (see Table 6.6 and Fig. 6.15). Typically, the mass is separated from the wall of the cavity by an airspace, resulting in the distinctive air-crescent sign. The fungus ball usually moves when the patient changes position. The most characteristic finding of aspergilloma on CT scan consists of an ovoid or round soft-tissue intracavitary mass (see Figs. 6.15 and 6.16). CT scan may also demonstrate fungal fronds situated on the cavity wall that intersect with each other and form an irregular sponge-like network, before developing into the mature fungus ball. Occasionally, the mycelial mass grows to fill the cavity completely, obliterating the airspace necessary for its radiographic identification. Mycetomas may demonstrate small nodular, peripheral, or extensive areas of calcification. Fungal organisms are almost always identified histologically only in the lumen of the cavity. Focal ulceration of the epithelium lining the wall, possibly as a result of secreted toxins, is common. The ulceration may result in bleeding from the often markedly enlarged bronchial arteries located in the cavity wall (see Fig. 6.17).

Allergic Bronchopulmonary Aspergillosis

ABPA is an uncommon pulmonary disorder seen almost exclusively in asthmatic patients. The pathogenesis is uncertain but is believed to involve both type I and type III allergic reactions (27). It has been postulated that in asthmatic patients, inhaled *Aspergillus* spores have a propensity to germinate and proliferate in the proximal airways, which often show evidence of asthma-associated mucosal injury (28). The resulting fungal hyphae apparently induce increased mucus production and additional mucosal injury, eventually resulting in bronchiectasis (27).

Pathologically, segmental and proximal subsegmental bronchi are dilated and distended with mucus that

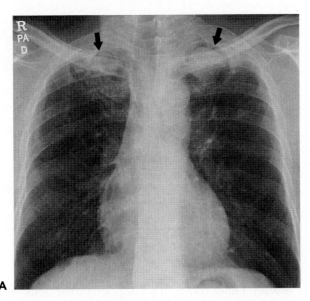

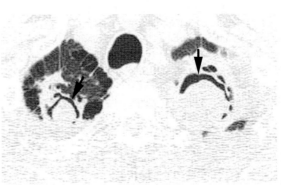

Figure 6.15 Bilateral upper lobe aspergillomas. **A:** Chest radiograph shows focal masses with surrounding air-crescent sign (*arrows*) in both apices and apical pleural thickening. Also note the nodular and reticular opacities in both upper lobes related to previous tuberculosis. **B:** High-resolution computed tomography (CT) image (1-mm collimation) shows aspergillomas with surrounding air crescent (*arrows*). Also noted are dense scarring, bronchiectasis, and emphysema. The patient was a 65-year-old man who had previously had tuberculosis.

contains numerous eosinophils and scattered, typically fragmented fungal hyphae (27). The adjacent bronchial wall shows fibrosis and chronic inflammation with abundant eosinophils (see Fig. 6.18). Although there may be focal ulceration of the airway epithelium, tissue invasion by the fungus is not seen. Bronchioles distal to the ectatic bronchi may also be distended with mucus or their

epithelium may be replaced by a granulomatous inflammatory infiltrate and their lumens filled by necrotic debris (bronchocentric granulomatosis). Patchy filling of alveolar airspaces by eosinophils (eosinophilic pneumonia) may be seen in the adjacent lung parenchyma (29).

The earliest radiographic manifestation consists of a fleeting foci of consolidation that reflect eosinophilic

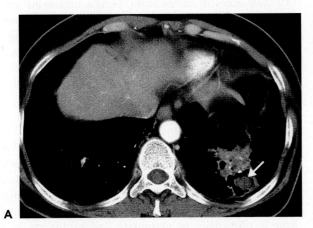

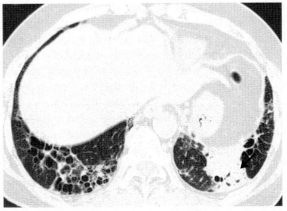

Figure 6.16 Lower lobe aspergilloma. **A:** Computed tomography (CT) image (5-mm collimation) at the level of the diaphragm shows low-attenuation aspergilloma (*arrow*) in a dilated left lower lobe bronchus. Surrounding consolidation was due to hemorrhage. **B:** Lung window image of high-resolution CT scan (1-mm collimation) obtained at a level similar to (**A**) demonstrates a fungus ball with air-crescent sign (*arrow*) and the surrounding parenchymal hemorrhage in the left lower lobe. Also note the underlying pulmonary fibrosis with honeycombing, reticulation, and ground-glass opacities in lung bases. The patient was a 55-year-old man with idiopathic pulmonary fibrosis.

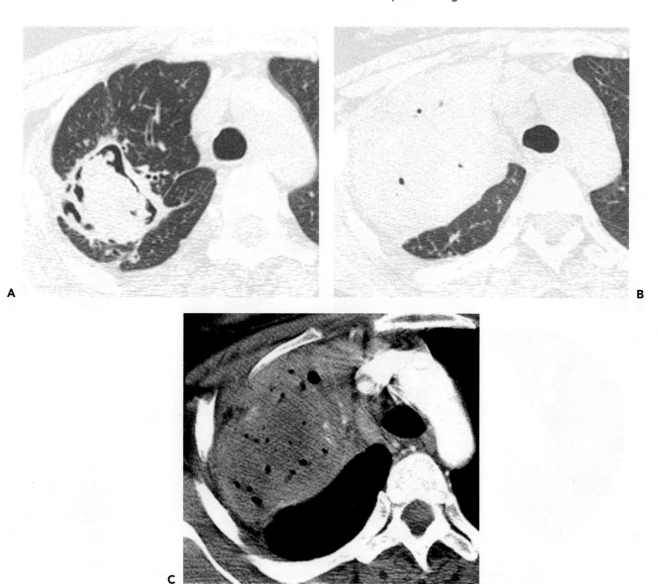

Figure 6.17   Aspergilloma and pulmonary hemorrhage. **A:** Lung window image of high-resolution computed tomography (CT) scan (1-mm collimation) obtained at the level of the aortic arch shows an intracavitary fungus ball with surrounding air-crescent sign in the right upper lobe. Also note small nodules and bronchiectasis around the aspergilloma cavity. **B:** CT scan obtained at a level similar to and 3 months after **(A)** demonstrates extensive right upper lobe consolidation. **C:** Mediastinal window of contrast-enhanced CT image shows intracavitary and surrounding parenchymal hemorrhage, confirmed at surgery. The patient was a 30-year-old woman who had had tuberculosis.

parenchymal infiltration (see Table 6.7 and Fig. 6.18) (27). With progression of the disease and the development of bronchiectasis and mucoid impaction, branching Y- and V-shaped ("gloved-finger") opacities can be seen, mainly involving the central regions of the upper lobes (see Figs. 6.18 and 6.19). High-resolution CT scan shows varicose or cystic bronchiectasis mainly involving segmental and subsegmental upper lobe bronchi (27, 30). Other findings include mucoid impaction and centrilobular nodules, the latter reflecting the presence of dilated bronchioles filled with mucus or necrotic debris. In approximately 30% of

cases, the mucous plugs have high attenuation, presumably because of the presence of calcium salts (31).

Semi-Invasive Pulmonary Aspergillosis

Semi-invasive pulmonary aspergillosis is a locally progressive chronic granulomatous form of aspergillosis that occurs in the setting of mild immunologic suppression. This unusual form of pulmonary aspergillosis clinically resembles a number of other chronic pulmonary diseases including tuberculosis, actinomycosis, and histoplasmosis (32). The patients are usually middle-aged and have

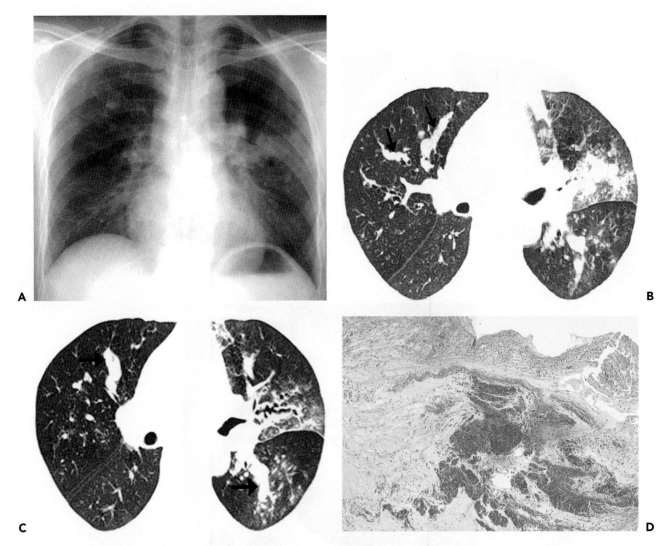

Figure 6.18 Allergic bronchopulmonary aspergillosis. **A:** Chest radiograph shows multifocal bilateral consolidation and poorly defined nodular opacities. **B** and **C:** High-resolution computed tomography (CT) images (1-mm collimation) at the level of the distal left main bronchus **(B)** and lingular bronchus **(C)** show parenchymal consolidation, bronchiectasis, mucus plugging (*arrows*), and bilateral small centrilobular nodules and branching opacities (tree-in-bud pattern). **D:** Photomicrograph of the transbronchial lung biopsy specimen demonstrates mucus plug containing mucin and numerous eosinophils. The patient was a 41-year-old asthmatic man with chronic cough, fever, and dyspnea.

poor nutrition because of alcoholism, diabetes mellitus, chronic granulomatous disease, or connective tissue disorders. Pulmonary abnormalities resulting in lowered defense mechanisms of the lung such as chronic obstructive lung disease, previous surgery, radiation therapy, pulmonary infarction, or pneumoconiosis are often present (32). Clinical symptoms include cough, the presence of sputum, fever, weight loss, and hemoptysis, usually progressing over several months (see chapter 8).

Gross lung specimens show ill-defined consolidation and fibrosis containing single or multiple thick-walled cavities or ectatic bronchi. Histologically, there is often a mixture of fibrosis and acute or organizing pneumonia. Foci of necrotizing granulomatous inflammation containing

fungal hyphae may be seen in the parenchyma or in relation to large or small airways (bronchocentric granulomatosis) (see Fig. 6.20).

Gefter et al. (33) reviewed the radiographic manifestations of semi-invasive pulmonary aspergillosis in five patients. The abnormalities consisted of consolidation or progressive cystic infiltrates subsequently forming a thick-walled cavity and aspergilloma (see Fig. 6.20 and Table 6.8). The findings mainly involved the upper lobes and were frequently associated with adjacent pleural thickening. The CT scan findings are variable, ranging from findings of bronchopneumonia to cavitary consolidation containing an aspergilloma (Fig. 6.20) (32). The main feature distinguishing chronic necrotizing pulmonary aspergillosis

ALLERGIC BRONCHOPULMONARY ASPERGILLOSIS

Aspergillus fumigatus
Ubiquitous organisms
Hypersensitivity reaction in patients with asthma
Most common radiologic findings
    Mucoid impaction: Finger-like, Y- or V-shaped bifurcating
        opacities
    Segmental and subsegmental (central) bronchiectasis
    Predominately upper lobe involvement
Other findings:
    Increased attenuation in 30% of cases of
        mucoid impaction
    Patchy, fleeting areas of airspace consolidation

from aspergilloma is the presence of tissue invasion and destruction.

Invasive Pulmonary Aspergillosis

Invasive aspergillosis is the most common opportunistic pulmonary fungal infection. The major risk factors for invasive aspergillosis include severe or prolonged neutropenia (absolute neutrophil count <500 per μL), prolonged corticosteroid therapy, graft versus host disease after allogenic hematopoietic stem cell transplantation, and late-stage AIDS (see chapters 7 and 8). Infection begins when aerosolized spores are inhaled into the distal airways and airspaces. In the absence of an effective host immune response, the spores mature into hyphae that can invade the pulmonary arteries. This results in pulmonary arterial thrombosis, hemorrhage, lung necrosis, and systemic dissemination (34–36).

Clinical symptoms include fever, cough, and dyspnea. Symptoms suggestive of pulmonary embolism including pleuritic chest pain and hemoptysis may also occur.

The radiologic manifestations include multiple, ill-defined, 1- to 3-cm diameter nodules mainly involving the peripheral lung regions and the lower lobes (see Table 6.9). The nodules gradually coalesce into larger masses or areas of consolidation (see Fig. 6.21). An early CT scan finding (best seen on thin-section images) is a rim of ground-glass opacity surrounding the nodules (CT halo sign) (see Fig. 6.22) (35, 36). This finding is nonspecific and has also been described in patients with tuberculosis, mucormycosis, and Wegener granulomatosis. In the appropriate clinical setting, however, the CT halo sign is highly suggestive of angioinvasive aspergillosis. Cavitation in the nodules or masses occurs in 40% of affected patients and often results in an air-crescent sign (34). The intracavitary content in invasive aspergillosis consists of infarcted lung tissue, which usually occurs after granulocyte recovery and tends to indicate a good prognosis. Segmental, lobar, or diffuse pulmonary consolidation may occur. Pleural effusion is uncommon, and lymphadenopathy is rare. Chest wall or mediastinal invasion may be seen, and systemic dissemination to the central nervous system, kidney, and

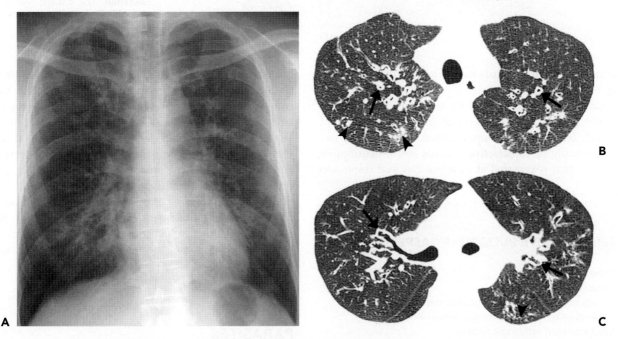

Figure 6.19 Allergic bronchopulmonary aspergillosis. **A:** Chest radiograph shows poorly defined perihilar opacities. **B** and **C:** High-resolution computed tomography (CT) scan (1-mm collimation) images at levels of the aortic arch **(B)** and main bronchi **(C)** demonstrate central bronchiectasis (*arrows*) and small nodules (*arrowheads*). The patient was a 33-year-old asthmatic man with chronic cough.

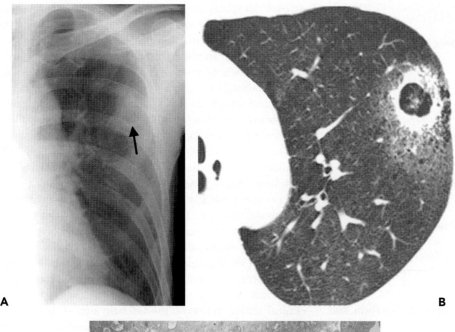

A

B

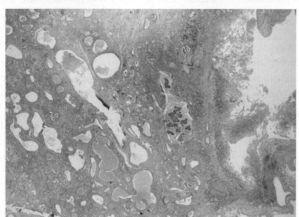

C

Figure 6.20 Chronic necrotizing aspergillosis (semi-invasive aspergillosis). **A:** Chest radiograph shows focal parenchymal opacity containing a central air-filled cystic lesion (*arrow*) in the left upper lung zone. **B:** High-resolution computed tomography (CT) image (1-mm collimation) at the level of the aortic arch demonstrates consolidation and surrounding ground-glass opacity in left upper lobe. Also note presence of emphysema. **C:** Photomicrograph shows a necrotizing granuloma with cavitation. The patient was a 53-year-old man with diabetes and emphysema.

gastrointestinal tract occurs in 25% to 50% of patients (see Fig. 6.23)

Airway-invasive aspergillosis accounts for approximately 15% to 30% of cases of invasive disease (37). As with bacterial bronchopneumonia, it is characterized histologically by liquefactive necrosis and a neutrophilic infiltrate that is centered at membranous and respiratory

bronchioles. Vascular infiltration and coagulative necrosis are usually absent or minimal in extent. The most common radiographic presentation consists of patchy unilateral or bilateral areas of consolidation (see Fig. 6.24). High-resolution CT scan demonstrates centrilobular nodules and branching linear opacities (tree-in-bud pattern), and patchy areas of consolidation, often in a peribronchial distribution (Fig. 6.24). Histologically, these findings correspond to the foci of necrotizing bronchitis and bronchiolitis, typically associated with a neutrophilic inflammatory reaction. *Aspergillus* organisms can be seen to infiltrate the airway walls and adjacent parenchyma (37).

TABLE 6.8

SEMI-INVASIVE PULMONARY ASPERGILLOSIS

Aspergillus fumigatus
Ubiquitous organisms
Locally progressive chronic granulomatous form
Patients with mild immunosuppression
Most common radiologic findings
    Progressive focal or patchy consolidation
    Often with cavity formation, resembling tuberculosis
    May develop intracavitary aspergilloma
    Mainly involves the upper lobes

PARASITES

Parasites are organisms living in or on another living organism, obtaining part or all of their organic nutriment from that organism and causing some degree of

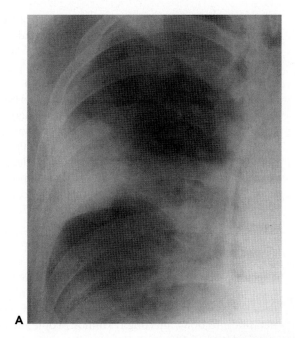

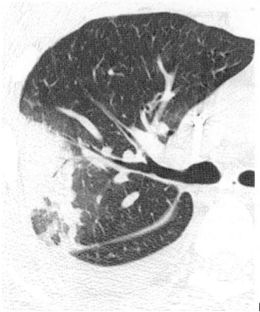

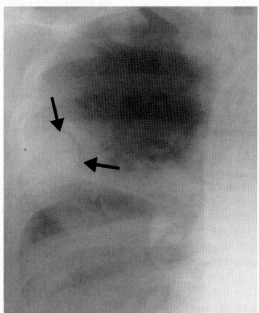

Figure 6.21 Angioinvasive pulmonary aspergillosis. **A:** Chest radiograph shows pleural-based airspace consolidation in right upper lobe. A central venous line is in place. **B:** View of right lung from high-resolution computed tomography (CT) scan (1-mm collimation) at the level of the right upper lobar bronchus demonstrates focal consolidation and surrounding halo of ground-glass attenuation (CT halo sign) in right upper lobe. **C:** Chest radiograph obtained 6 days after **(A)** with recovery from neutropenia demonstrates air crescent (*arrows*) within area of airspace consolidation. The patient was a 30-year-old man with acute myelogenous leukemia.

damage to their host. Parasitic infestations are common in developing countries, particularly in tropical and subtropical regions. In industrialized countries, pulmonary disease due to parasites is seen in individuals who have traveled to endemic areas and in recent immigrants.

Parasites that most commonly result in pulmonary disease include protozoa (e.g., amebiasis), nematodes (e.g.,

ascariasis, strongyloides, and toxocariasis), cestodes (e.g., echinococcosis), and trematodes (e.g., schistosomiasis, paragonimiasis).

Amebiasis

Amebiasis is a protozoan infection caused by *Entamoeba histolytica*. It is estimated to affect approximately 1% of

TABLE 6.9
INVASIVE PULMONARY ASPERGILLOSIS

Aspergillus fumigatus
Ubiquitous organisms
Immunocompromised patients with severe neutropenia
Two main forms: Angioinvasive and airway invasive (bronchopneumonia)
Radiologic manifestations of angioinvasive aspergillosis
    Multiple nodules
    Poorly defined margins on chest radiograph
    Commonly have ground-glass halo on HRCT
    Segmental consolidation
    Cavitation and air-crescent sign usually in recovery phase
Radiologic manifestations of airway-invasive aspergillosis
    Bronchiolitis and bronchopneumonia
    Centrilobular nodules and branching opacities (tree-in-bud pattern)
    Patchy unilateral or asymmetric bilateral consolidation

HRCT, high-resolution computed tomography.

the world's population and to result in 40,000 to 110,000 deaths annually. The infestation is acquired by ingestion of cysts that become trophozoites in the colon (38). The prevalence of infection is highest in highly populated areas, areas with poor sanitation, and the tropics. In the United States, amebiasis is more common in rural areas and in areas of low socioeconomic status.

The most common extraintestinal manifestations of amebiasis are liver abscess and pleuropulmonary involvement (see Table 6.10). Pleuropulmonary infection may result from direct extension from a liver abscess or, less commonly, from aspiration or hematogenous dissemination. Pleuropulmonary extension occurs in 6% to 40% of patients with amebic liver abscess.

Pleural effusion is a common finding in the setting of an amebic liver abscess (see Fig. 6.25). Such effusion can either

be sterile, as in inflammatory pleural reactions, or represent an empyema if the hepatic abscess ruptures and traverses the diaphragm. Classically, the elevation of the right hemidiaphragm precedes the visualization of pleural or pulmonary lesions. Airspace consolidation and cavitation are frequently seen. Drainage of the abscess into a bronchus may result in hepatobronchial or bronchobiliary fistula. Invasion of the inferior vena cava occurs occasionally and may result in pulmonary thromboembolism. Pericarditis and effusion may result from an acute inflammatory reaction or abscess drainage to the pericardium from the liver (38–41). Parenchymal lesions that are discontinuous with the diaphragm have been reported.

Ascariasis

The nematode *Ascaris lumbricoides* is acquired by ingesting food or fluids contaminated with feces. The infection is distributed worldwide and is one of the most common parasitic infections, affecting 1.3 billion people and causing approximately 1,550 deaths per year. Parasites migrate from the small intestine to the pulmonary circulation, where they mature and cause destruction of capillaries and alveolar walls with subsequent edema, hemorrhage, and epithelial cell desquamation, causing chemotaxis of neutrophils and eosinophils (38).

Patients complain of fever, cough, and expectoration and may have peripheral blood eosinophilia. The diagnosis is confirmed by identifying larvae in the sputum or eggs in the stool (42).

Chest radiograph and CT scan demonstrate migratory, patchy airspace opacities that characteristically clear within 10 days (see Table 6.11). Lobar consolidation and alveolar hemorrhage have also been described (42, 43).

Strongyloidiasis

Humans are the primary host of *Strongyloides stercoralis*, a microscopic nematode with infective larvae that invade the lungs and small intestine by migrating from

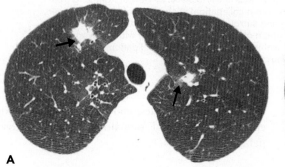
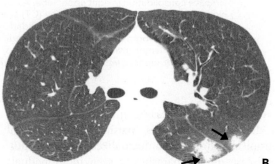

Figure 6.22 Angioinvasive pulmonary aspergillosis. **A** and **B:** High-resolution computed tomography (CT) images (1-mm collimation) at the levels of the great vessels **(A)** and main bronchi **(B)** show bilateral nodules with irregular margins and surrounding ground-glass opacities (CT halo sign) (*arrows*). The patient was a 27-year-old man with acute myelogenous leukemia and neutropenia.

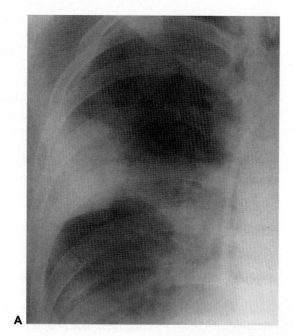

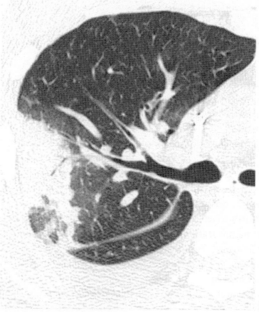

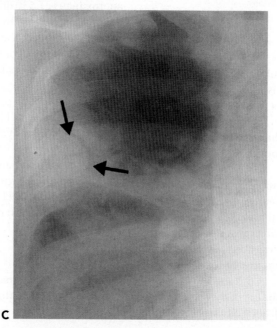

Figure 6.21 Angioinvasive pulmonary aspergillosis. **A:** Chest radiograph shows pleural-based airspace consolidation in right upper lobe. A central venous line is in place. **B:** View of right lung from high-resolution computed tomography (CT) scan (1-mm collimation) at the level of the right upper lobar bronchus demonstrates focal consolidation and surrounding halo of ground-glass attenuation (CT halo sign) in right upper lobe. **C:** Chest radiograph obtained 6 days after **(A)** with recovery from neutropenia demonstrates air crescent (*arrows*) within area of airspace consolidation. The patient was a 30-year-old man with acute myelogenous leukemia.

damage to their host. Parasitic infestations are common in developing countries, particularly in tropical and subtropical regions. In industrialized countries, pulmonary disease due to parasites is seen in individuals who have traveled to endemic areas and in recent immigrants.

Parasites that most commonly result in pulmonary disease include protozoa (e.g., amebiasis), nematodes (e.g.,

ascariasis, strongyloides, and toxocariasis), cestodes (e.g., echinococcosis), and trematodes (e.g., schistosomiasis, paragonimiasis).

Amebiasis

Amebiasis is a protozoan infection caused by *Entamoeba histolytica*. It is estimated to affect approximately 1% of

TABLE 6.9
INVASIVE PULMONARY ASPERGILLOSIS

Aspergillus fumigatus
Ubiquitous organisms
Immunocompromised patients with severe neutropenia
Two main forms: Angioinvasive and airway invasive (bronchopneumonia)
Radiologic manifestations of angioinvasive aspergillosis
    Multiple nodules
    Poorly defined margins on chest radiograph
    Commonly have ground-glass halo on HRCT
    Segmental consolidation
    Cavitation and air-crescent sign usually in recovery phase
Radiologic manifestations of airway-invasive aspergillosis
    Bronchiolitis and bronchopneumonia
    Centrilobular nodules and branching opacities (tree-in-bud pattern)
    Patchy unilateral or asymmetric bilateral consolidation

HRCT, high-resolution computed tomography.

the world's population and to result in 40,000 to 110,000 deaths annually. The infestation is acquired by ingestion of cysts that become trophozoites in the colon (38). The prevalence of infection is highest in highly populated areas, areas with poor sanitation, and the tropics. In the United States, amebiasis is more common in rural areas and in areas of low socioeconomic status.

The most common extraintestinal manifestations of amebiasis are liver abscess and pleuropulmonary involvement (see Table 6.10). Pleuropulmonary infection may result from direct extension from a liver abscess or, less commonly, from aspiration or hematogenous dissemination. Pleuropulmonary extension occurs in 6% to 40% of patients with amebic liver abscess.

Pleural effusion is a common finding in the setting of an amebic liver abscess (see Fig. 6.25). Such effusion can either

be sterile, as in inflammatory pleural reactions, or represent an empyema if the hepatic abscess ruptures and traverses the diaphragm. Classically, the elevation of the right hemidiaphragm precedes the visualization of pleural or pulmonary lesions. Airspace consolidation and cavitation are frequently seen. Drainage of the abscess into a bronchus may result in hepatobronchial or bronchobiliary fistula. Invasion of the inferior vena cava occurs occasionally and may result in pulmonary thromboembolism. Pericarditis and effusion may result from an acute inflammatory reaction or abscess drainage to the pericardium from the liver (38–41). Parenchymal lesions that are discontinuous with the diaphragm have been reported.

Ascariasis

The nematode *Ascaris lumbricoides* is acquired by ingesting food or fluids contaminated with feces. The infection is distributed worldwide and is one of the most common parasitic infections, affecting 1.3 billion people and causing approximately 1,550 deaths per year. Parasites migrate from the small intestine to the pulmonary circulation, where they mature and cause destruction of capillaries and alveolar walls with subsequent edema, hemorrhage, and epithelial cell desquamation, causing chemotaxis of neutrophils and eosinophils (38).

Patients complain of fever, cough, and expectoration and may have peripheral blood eosinophilia. The diagnosis is confirmed by identifying larvae in the sputum or eggs in the stool (42).

Chest radiograph and CT scan demonstrate migratory, patchy airspace opacities that characteristically clear within 10 days (see Table 6.11). Lobar consolidation and alveolar hemorrhage have also been described (42, 43).

Strongyloidiasis

Humans are the primary host of *Strongyloides stercoralis*, a microscopic nematode with infective larvae that invade the lungs and small intestine by migrating from

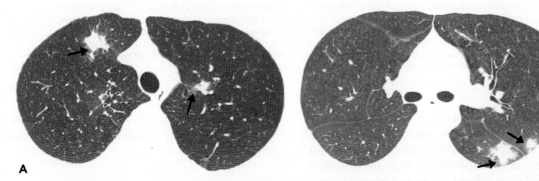

Figure 6.22 Angioinvasive pulmonary aspergillosis. **A** and **B:** High-resolution computed tomography (CT) images (1-mm collimation) at the levels of the great vessels **(A)** and main bronchi **(B)** show bilateral nodules with irregular margins and surrounding ground-glass opacities (CT halo sign) (*arrows*). The patient was a 27-year-old man with acute myelogenous leukemia and neutropenia.

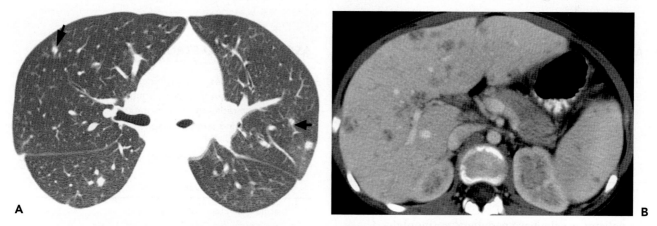

Figure 6.23 Disseminated aspergillosis. **A:** High-resolution computed tomography (CT) image (1-mm collimation) at the level of the right upper lobar bronchus shows bilateral small nodules. Some nodules (*arrows*) demonstrate CT halo sign. **B:** Mediastinal window image of enhanced CT scan (5-mm collimation) obtained at the level of the porta hepatis shows multiple small low-attenuation nodules in the liver and spleen. Liver biopsy reveals fungal organisms compatible with *Aspergillus*. The patient was a 12-year-old girl with acute lymphoblastic leukemia.

the soil through the skin (38). A chronic pathway of continuous autoinfection can lead to a massive and life-threatening parasitic infestation (hyperinfection syndrome), especially in patients with AIDS and in those who are receiving corticosteroid therapy, in whom mortality may exceed 70% (44). This parasite is found in all

tropical and subtropical regions. Approximately 35 million people are infected worldwide (38). The highest infection rates in the United States are in the Southeast and Puerto Rico.

Clinical manifestations include pneumonia, bronchospasm or bronchitis, abdominal pain, and diarrhea.

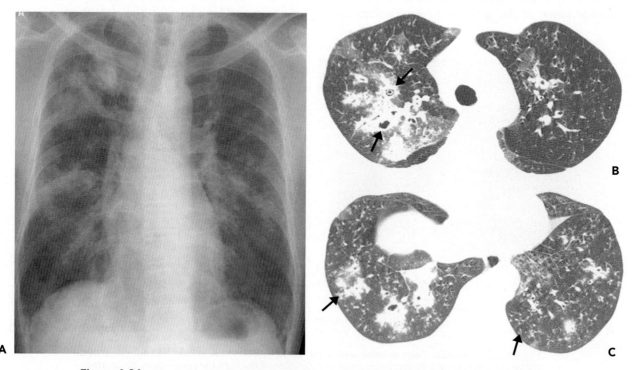

Figure 6.24 Airway-invasive aspergillosis. **A:** Chest radiograph shows multifocal bilateral nodular opacities. **B:** High-resolution computed tomography (CT) image (1-mm collimation) at the level of the aortic arch shows cavitating nodular opacities (*arrows*), focal areas of consolidation, and ground-glass opacities. **C:** CT scan obtained at the level of the liver dome shows parenchymal opacities, small centrilobular nodules, and tree-in-bud opacities (*arrows*). The patient was a 49-year-old man.

TABLE 6.10
AMEBIASIS

Entamoeba histolytica
Endemic areas: Tropical regions, areas of poor sanitation
Most common extraintestinal manifestations
    Liver abscess
    Elevation of the right hemidiaphragm
    Pleural effusion
    Consolidation and atelectasis in the right lower lobe

The patients usually have peripheral eosinophilia. Hyperinfection occurs in severely immunocompromised patients, in whom eosinophilia may be absent. Definitive diagnosis is made by identifying the larvae in the sputum (44–47).

Imaging findings include ill-defined, patchy, migratory airspace consolidation that typically resolves within 1 to 2 weeks (Table 6.11). Hyperinfection syndrome can manifest with extensive pneumonia, alveolar hemorrhage, and acute respiratory distress syndrome (ARDS) (see Fig. 6.26). A miliary pattern has also been described (48). Pleural effusion and secondary superimposed bacterial infection with cavitation and abscess formation may also be seen (44).

Toxocariasis

Human visceral and ocular toxocariasis is caused by nematode larvae of the genus *Toxocara*. *Toxocara canis*,

TABLE 6.11
ASCARIASIS AND STRONGYLOIDIASIS

Ascaris lumbricoides, Strongyloides stercoralis
Endemic areas: Southeast Asia, South America, and Africa
Most common radiologic manifestation
    Patchy, fleeting areas of airspace consolidation
Rarely
    Strongyloides hyperinfection in immunocompromised patient
    Miliary pattern, ARDS

ARDS, acute respiratory distress syndrome.

an intestinal parasite of dogs, foxes, and other canids, has a worldwide distribution and is the main cause of toxocariasis and visceral larva migrans (49, 50).

Visceral larva migrans is acquired by ingesting embryonated *Toxocara* eggs. The larvae, hatched from the eggs in the intestine, invade the intestinal wall and disseminate through the portal blood stream to the liver, and then to various organs, including the brain, heart, and lungs. Lung involvement is common and manifests as patchy migratory pulmonary opacities that represent eosinophilic infiltrates (51).

Because they do not develop or grow in humans (humans being accidental hosts, not definitive hosts), *Toxocara* larvae only migrate through the viscera and give rise to visceral larva migrans. Therefore, the eggs or mature

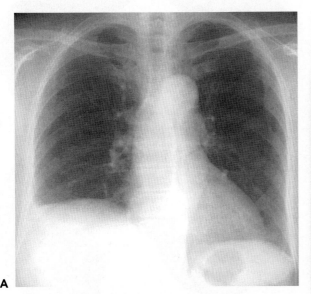

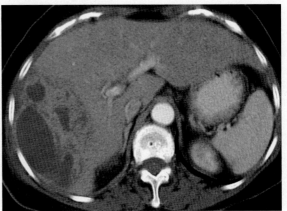

A   **B**

Figure 6.25 Amebic liver abscess and right pleural effusion. **A:** Chest radiograph shows obliteration of the right costophrenic angle and elevation of the right hemidiaphragm. **B:** Contrast-enhanced computed tomography (CT) scan (5-mm collimation) at the level of the porta hepatis demonstrates multiloculated low-attenuation lesion in the right lobe of the liver. Fine needle aspiration demonstrated amebic abscess. The patient was a 61-year-old woman.

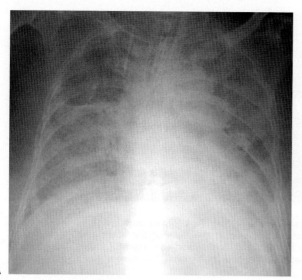
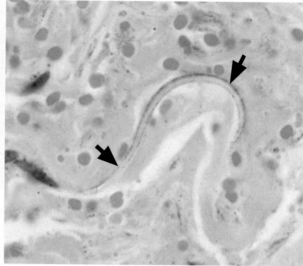

Figure 6.26 *Strongyloides stercoralis* hyperinfection. **A:** Chest radiograph shows diffuse bilateral consolidation. Central venous line and endotracheal tube are in place. The patient was a 70-year-old diabetic woman who presented with diarrhea and vomiting and had multiple hemorrhagic petechiae in abdomen and thorax. **B:** Photomicrograph of the skin lesion biopsy demonstrates larva (*arrows*).

adults are not seen. The definite diagnosis can be made only by demonstrating the larvae. However, the diagnosis is difficult because the larvae are only 0.02 mm in size. In practice, the diagnosis is usually made by enzyme-linked immunosorbent assay (ELISA) using an antigen of *T. canis*.

In patients with positive ELISA test result for *T. canis* and peripheral blood eosinophilia, the chest radiograph is abnormal in about half the cases and chest CT scan is abnormal in approximately three fourths of cases. Pulmonary visceral larva migrans of *T. canis* most commonly presents with poorly defined nodules without zonal predominance on chest radiographs. High-resolution CT scan demonstrates multiple unilateral or bilateral nodules with surrounding halo or nodular areas of ground-glass opacity. The abnormalities show transient and migratory nature on sequential studies. The presence of parenchymal abnormalities on imaging studies appears to be proportional to the peripheral blood eosinophil counts. Hepatic involvement with multiple low-attenuation nodules of eosinophilic abscess is commonly seen in association with the pulmonary findings (see Fig. 6.27) (52–55).

Echinococcosis (Hydatid Disease)

The most common cause of human hydatid disease is *Echinococcus granulosus*. It occurs in two forms, pastoral and sylvatic. The former is the more common form and is seen predominantly in the Middle East, South America, and Russia. The latter is seen in Alaska and northern Canada. The intermediate hosts of the pastoral variety are sheep, cows, horses, and pigs, and the definite hosts are dogs. The intermediate hosts of the sylvatic are moose, deer, elk,

caribou, and bison, and the definite hosts are dogs, wolves, arctic foxes, and coyotes (56).

Humans acquire the disease by direct contact with definite hosts or by ingestion of eggs present in water, food, or soil (56). In the duodenum the eggs hatch into larvae that pass through the portal system to the liver, where most are trapped. Most of those that escape are in turn trapped in the pulmonary alveolar capillaries. In both the liver and the lung, the larvae develop into cysts that are typically spherical or oval in shape. The cysts are surrounded by a pericyst consisting of fibrous tissue containing a nonspecific chronic inflammatory infiltrate. The surrounding lung usually shows compressive atelectasis. The cyst itself consists of a laminated outer membrane (the exocyst) and a thin inner layer of cells (the endocyst) that produce intracystic fluid and larval protoscoleces. Daughter cysts may develop directly from the exocyst or from free protoscoleces. A multicystic structure may result from serial cyst formation over several generations.

The radiologic manifestations consist of sharply marginated, spherical or oval masses 1 to 20 cm in diameter that are surrounded by the normal lung (see Table 6.12) (57, 58). On high-resolution CT scan, the cysts are found to have homogeneous water density (see Fig. 6.28) (38, 59). Multiple cysts are seen in 20% to 30% of patients. When there is communication between the cyst and the airways, air may enter the space between the pericyst and exocyst and produce a thin crescent of air around the periphery of the cyst (air-crescent sign). When there is communication between the airways and the inner portion of the cyst through the endocyst, expulsion of the contents

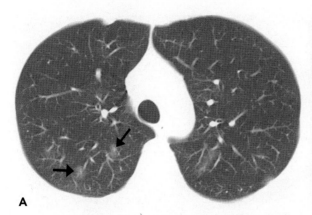

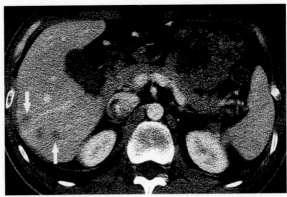

Figure 6.27 Visceral larva migrans with *Toxocara canis* infection. **A:** Lung window image of computed tomography (CT) scan (2.5-mm collimation) obtained at the level of the aortic arch shows multiple bilateral small nodules with a halo sign (*arrows*). **B:** Contrast-enhanced CT image (5-mm collimation) demonstrates intrahepatic low-attenuation nodules (*arrows*). The patient was a 36-year-old man.

of the cyst produces an air-fluid level. The cyst fluid may spill into the surrounding lung, causing an inflammatory reaction that leads to parenchymal consolidation. After the cyst has ruptured into the bronchial tree, the collapsed endocyst/exocyst may be contrasted with surrounding air, resulting in the classic water-lily sign.

Schistosomiasis

Schistosomiasis is caused by flukes of the class Trematoda including *Schistosoma mansoni*, *Schistosoma japonicum*, and *Schistosoma hematobium*. The disease occurs in areas inhabited by the intermediate host, the snail. Infestation by *S. mansoni* and *S. hematobium* is endemic in the Middle East (Egypt and parts of Saudi Arabia) and in large areas

of central and southern Africa. *S. mansoni* is also found in the Caribbean islands and in South America, particularly in Brazil. *S. japonicum* is predominant in China, Japan, and the Philippines. Schistosomiasis affects 150 to 200 million people worldwide and results in 500,000 deaths each year (38).

The larvae, acquired by drinking, swimming, or working in freshwater containing the infective cercariae, travel through the venous circulation to the pulmonary capillaries, by means of which they reach the systemic circulation. They then traverse the mesenteric vessels into the intrahepatic portal vein. After developing into adolescent worms in the portal venous system, they move upstream to the superior mesenteric, inferior mesenteric, or visceral venules. The male and female worms copulate in these vessels, and the females then migrate to smaller venous channels in the submucosa and mucosa of the bowel and bladder and lay their eggs. Many of these eggs are extruded into the bowel and bladder lumens and excreted in feces or urine. These eggs reach freshwater and develop into larvae, which enter the snails (60).

Tissue damage (inflammatory reaction and fibrosis) occurs as a result of a reaction to the antigens derived from the eggs. Such damage may be localized to the gastrointestinal or vesical mucosa. However, some eggs are also released directly into venous blood. In cases of *S. mansoni* and *S. japonicum*, release usually occurs into the portal system with deposition in the liver. With *S. hematobium*, release occurs into the inferior vena cava with direct embolization to the lungs. Eggs of the former two species may also reach the lungs through portal–systemic vein anastomoses once the liver has become cirrhotic as a result of *Schistosoma*-related fibrosis. Once they reach the lungs, most embolized eggs become impacted in small pulmonary arteries and arterioles, after which they are extruded into the surrounding perivascular tissue. The eggs incite an inflammatory reaction and fibrosis, which if widespread results in obliterative arteritis and pulmonary hypertension (60).

TABLE 6.12
ECHINOCOCCOSIS (HYDATID DISEASE)

Echinococcus granulosus
Pastoral variety: Intermediate host is mainly sheep
  Endemic areas: Southeastern Europe, Middle East, South America, Australia
Sylvatic variety: Intermediate host is mainly moose, deer, and elk
  Endemic areas: Northern Canada, Alaska
Most common radiologic findings
  Single or multiple nodules or masses
  Smoothly marginated
  Water density on computed tomography
Other manifestations
  Air-crescent sign (when cyst communicates with bronchus)
  Water-lily sign (when cyst membrane floats in residual fluid)

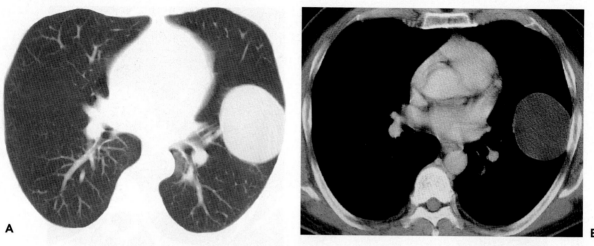

Figure 6.28 Hydatid cyst. **A:** Computed tomography (CT) image (7-mm collimation) shows smoothly marginated mass in the left lung. **B:** Contrast-enhanced CT scan photographed at mediastinal window settings demonstrates that the lesion has water density consistent with the cyst. The patient was a 51-year-old man with surgically proven hydatid cyst.

Pulmonary involvement is divided into early and late forms. In acute schistosomiasis (Katayama fever), which can be seen during the migration of larvae through the lungs, chest radiograph or CT scan shows patchy parenchymal consolidation consistent with eosinophilic pneumonia (60). Small nodular lesions with poorly defined borders or, less commonly, a reticulonodular pattern or bilateral diffuse ground-glass opacities may be seen.

Chronic pulmonary disease results from granulomatous reaction to eggs deposited in the pulmonary vasculature, which leads to intimal fibrosis, pulmonary hypertension,

and cor pulmonale. Radiography and CT scan show cardiomegaly and enlarged central pulmonary arteries (61, 62). Diagnosis is made by identifying eggs in stool or urine samples or at rectal biopsy.

Paragonimiasis

Paragonimiasis is caused by flukes of the genus *Paragonimus*; the most frequent etiologic agent is *Paragonimus westermani*. Humans typically acquire the disease by ingesting raw or undercooked crabs or crayfish infected with the

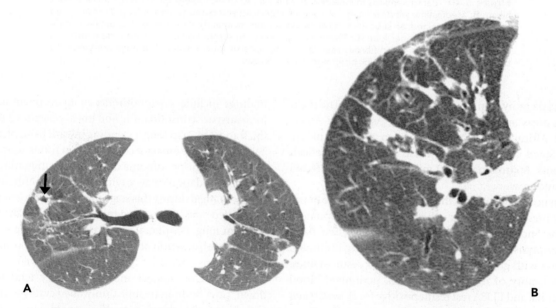

Figure 6.29 Paragonimiasis manifesting as cyst, nodules, and linear opacities. **A:** High-resolution computed tomography (CT) image (1-mm collimation) at the level of the right upper lobar bronchus shows a cystic lesion (*arrow*) and linear opacities in the right upper lobe and a nodule in the left upper lobe. **B:** View of the right lung from CT scan performed at the level of the right inferior pulmonary vein demonstrates a nodule in the right lower lobe and linear opacities in the right middle lobe. The patient was a 41-year-old woman.

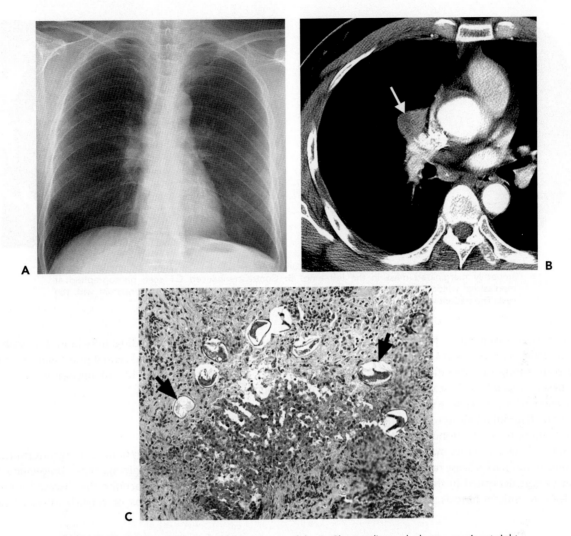

Figure 6.30 Paragonimiasis manifesting as a nodule. **A:** Chest radiograph shows prominent right hilum. **B:** Mediastinal window image of contrast-enhanced computed tomography (CT) scan (5-mm collimation) obtained at subcarinal level shows an approximately 2.6-cm low-attenuation nodule (*arrow*) in the right upper lobe. **C:** Photomicrograph of the surgical biopsy specimen demonstrates a chronic inflammatory and fibrous reaction to the eggs of *Paragonimus*. The eggs are yellow to brown and oval and have a thick birefringent shell (*arrows*).

metacercaria or by drinking contaminated water. The main endemic areas are East Asia, Southeast Asia, Latin America, and Africa. Many cases have been reported in the United States among Indo-Chinese and Latin-American immigrants. Approximately 20 million people are infected in endemic areas.

The major target organ is the lung, followed by the brain. Patients present with fever, chest pain, and respiratory symptoms including chronic cough, pleuritic chest pain, and hemoptysis. Parasites induce inflammatory infiltrates, sometimes with granuloma formation, and cystic cavities. Previous history of ingesting raw crab, peripheral blood eosinophilia, and ELISA test result positive for *P. westermani* enable a diagnosis of the disease (38).

Pleuropulmonary manifestations depend on the stage of the disease. The early stage of infection is characterized by the migration of a juvenile worm and the late stage by the formation of cysts around the worm. Early findings include pneumothorax or hydropneumothorax, focal airspace consolidation, and linear opacities 2 to 4 mm thick and 3 to 7 cm long, extending inward from pleura (see Table 6.13). The airspace consolidation is due to exudative or hemorrhagic pneumonia caused by the migrating worm. The consolidation may cavitate. Contrast-enhanced CT scans obtained during this stage may show hypoattenuating fluid-filled cysts surrounded by dense consolidation in the adjacent lung. Peripheral atelectasis may also be observed, caused by obstruction of small airways by the worm. Linear opacities are caused by the migration of juvenile worms. As these worms mature into adults, they tend to settle down. Later findings include thin-walled cysts (worm cysts) (see Fig. 6.29), dense mass-like consolidation, nodules (Figs. 6.29 and 6.30), or bronchiectasis. On CT scans round low-attenuation cystic lesions (5 to 15 mm in diameter), filled with either fluid or air, are characteristically seen within the consolidation (63, 64).

TABLE 6.13
PARAGONIMIASIS

Paragonimus westermani

Endemic areas: Southeast Asia, South America, Western Africa

Most common radiologic findings

    Focal areas of consolidation

    Single or multiple nodules

    Single or multiple 0.5–5 cm diameter cystic lesions

    Fluid or air-filled cystic lesions on CT scan

CT, computed tomography

REFERENCES

1. Goldman M, Johnson PC, Sarosi GA. Fungal pneumonias. The endemic mycoses. *Clin Chest Med.* 1999;20:507–519.
2. Cano MV, Hajjeh RA. The epidemiology of histoplasmosis: A review. *Semin Respir Infect.* 2001;16:109–118.
3. Simoes LB, Marques SA, Bagagli E. Distribution of paracoccidioidomycosis: Determination of ecologic correlates through spatial analyses. *Med Mycol.* 2004;42:517–523.
4. Richardson MD. Changing patterns and trends in systemic fungal infections. *J Antimicrob Chemother.* 2005;56(suppl 1):i5–i11.
5. Spellberg B, Edwards J Jr, Ibrahim A. Novel perspectives on mucormycosis: Pathophysiology, presentation, and management. *Clin Microbiol Rev.* 2005;18:556–569.
6. Conces DJ Jr. Histoplasmosis. *Semin Roentgenol.* 1996;31:14–27.
7. Gurney JW, Conces DJ. Pulmonary histoplasmosis. *Radiology.* 1996;199:297–306.
8. Batra P, Batra RS. Thoracic coccidioidomycosis. *Semin Roentgenol.* 1996;31:28–44.
9. Kim KI, Leung AN, Flint JD, et al. Chronic pulmonary coccidioidomycosis: Computed tomographic and pathologic findings in 18 patients. *Can Assoc Radiol J.* 1998;49:401–407.
10. Halvorsen RA, Duncan JD, Merten DF, et al. Pulmonary blastomycosis: Radiologic manifestations. *Radiology.* 1984;150:1–5.
11. Sheflin JR, Campbell JA, Thompson GP. Pulmonary blastomycosis: Findings on chest radiographs in 63 patients. *Am J Roentgenol.* 1990;154:1177–1180.
12. Winer-Muram HT, Beals DH, Cole FH Jr. Blastomycosis of the lung: CT features. *Radiology.* 1992;182:829–832.
13. Blotta MH, Mamoni RL, Oliveira SJ, et al. Endemic regions of paracoccidioidomycosis in Brazil: A clinical and epidemiologic study of 584 cases in the southeast region. *Am J Trop Med Hyg.* 1999;61:390–394.
14. Tobon AM, Agudelo CA, Osorio ML, et al. Residual pulmonary abnormalities in adult patients with chronic paracoccidioidomycosis: Prolonged follow-up after itraconazole therapy. *Clin Infect Dis.* 2003;37:898–904.
15. Funari M, Kavakama J, Shikanai-Yasuda MA, et al. Chronic pulmonary paracoccidioidomycosis (South American blastomycosis): High-resolution CT findings in 41 patients. *Am J Roentgenol.* 1999;173:59–64.
16. Gasparetto EL, Escuissato DL, Davaus T, et al. Reversed halo sign in pulmonary paracoccidioidomycosis. *Am J Roentgenol.* 2005;184:1932–1934.
17. Friedman GD, Jeffrey Fessel W, Udaltsova NV, et al. Cryptococcosis: The 1981–2000 epidemic. *Mycoses.* 2005;48:122–125.
18. Fox DL, Müller NL. Pulmonary cryptococcosis in immunocompetent patients: CT findings in 12 patients. *Am J Roentgenol.* 2005;185:622–626.
19. Lindell RM, Hartman TE, Nadrous HF, et al. Pulmonary cryptococcosis: CT findings in immunocompetent patients. *Radiology.* 2005;236:326–331.
20. Murayama S, Sakai S, Soeda H, et al. Pulmonary cryptococcosis in immunocompetent patients: HRCT characteristics. *Clin Imaging.* 2004;28:191–195.
21. Zinck SE, Leung AN, Frost M, et al. Pulmonary cryptococcosis: CT and pathologic findings. *J Comput Assist Tomogr.* 2002;26:330–334.
22. Feigin DS. Pulmonary cryptococcosis: Radiologic-pathologic correlates of its three forms. *Am J Roentgenol.* 1983;141:1262–1272.
23. Khoury MB, Godwin JD, Ravin CE, et al. Thoracic cryptococcosis: Immunologic competence and radiologic appearance. *Am J Roentgenol.* 1984;141:893–896.
24. Miller KD, Mican JA, Davey RT. Asymptomatic solitary pulmonary nodules due to cryptococcus neoformans in patients infected with human immunodeficiency virus. *Clin Infect Dis.* 1996;23:810–812.
25. Friedman EP, Miller RF, Severn A, et al. Cryptococcal pneumonia in patients with the acquired immunodeficiency syndrome. *Clin Radiol.* 1995;50:756–760.
26. Lacomis JM, Costello P, Vilchez R, et al. The radiology of pulmonary cryptococcosis in a tertiary medical center. *J Thorac Imaging.* 2001;16:139–148.
27. Franquet T, Müller NL, Gimenez A, et al. Spectrum of pulmonary aspergillosis: Histologic, clinical, and radiologic findings. *Radiographics.* 2001;21:825–837.
28. Bromley IM, Donaldson K. Binding of Aspergillus fumigatus spores to lung epithelial cells and basement membrane proteins: Relevance to the asthmatic lung. *Thorax.* 1996;51:1203–1209.
29. Thompson BH, Stanford W, Galvin JR, et al. Varied radiologic appearances of pulmonary aspergillosis. *Radiographics.* 1995;15:1273–1284.
30. Ward S, Heyneman L, Lee MJ, et al. Accuracy of CT in the diagnosis of allergic bronchopulmonary aspergillosis in asthmatic patients. *Am J Roentgenol.* 1999;173:937–942.
31. Logan PM, Müller NL. High-attenuation mucous plugging in allergic bronchopulmonary aspergillosis. *Can Assoc Radiol J.* 1996;47:374–377.
32. Kim SY, Lee KS, Han J, et al. Semiinvasive pulmonary aspergillosis: CT and pathologic findings in six patients. *Am J Roentgenol.* 2000;174:795–798.
33. Gefter WB, Weingrad TR, Epstein DM, et al. "Semi-invasive" pulmonary aspergillosis: A new look at the spectrum of Aspergillus infections of the lung. *Radiology.* 1981;140:313–321.
34. Kim MJ, Lee KS, Kim J, et al. Crescent sign in invasive pulmonary aspergillosis: Frequency and related CT and clinical factors. *J Comput Assist Tomogr.* 2001;25:305–310.
35. Kuhlman JE, Fishman EK, Siegelman SS. Invasive pulmonary aspergillosis in acute leukemia: Characteristic findings on CT, the CT halo sign, and the role of CT in early diagnosis. *Radiology.* 1985;157:611–614.
36. Won HJ, Lee KS, Cheon JE, et al. Invasive pulmonary aspergillosis: Prediction at thin-section CT in patients with neutropenia–a prospective study. *Radiology.* 1998;208:777–782.
37. Logan PM, Primack SL, Miller RR, et al. Invasive aspergillosis of the airways: Radiographic, CT, and pathologic findings. *Radiology.* 1994;193:383–388.
38. Martinez S, Restrepo CS, Carrillo JA, et al. Thoracic manifestations of tropical parasitic infections: A pictorial review. *Radiographics.* 2005;25:135–155.
39. Ibarra-Perez C. Thoracic complications of amebic abscess of the liver: Report of 501 cases. *Chest.* 1981;79:672–677.
40. Landay MJ, Setiawan H, Hirsch G, et al. Hepatic and thoracic amoebiasis. *Am J Roentgenol.* 1980;135:449–454.
41. Shamsuzzaman SM, Hashiguchi Y. Thoracic amebiasis. *Clin Chest Med.* 2002;23:479–492.
42. Zumla AI, James DG. Immunologic aspects of tropical lung disease. *Clin Chest Med.* 2002; 23:283–308.
43. Barrett-Connor E. Parasitic pulmonary disease. *Am Rev Respir Dis.* 1982;126:558–563.
44. Chu E, Whitlock WL, Dietrich RA. Pulmonary hyperinfection syndrome with strongyloides stercoralis. *Chest.* 1990;97:1475–1477.
45. Davidson RA. Infection due to strongyloides stercoralis in patients with pulmonary disease. *South Med J.* 1992;85:28–31.
46. Simpson WG, Gerhardstein DC, Thompson JR. Disseminated strongyloides stercoralis infection. *South Med J.* 1993;86:821–825.
47. Woodring JH, Halfhill H II, Reed JC. Pulmonary strongyloidiasis: Clinical and imaging features. *Am J Roentgenol.* 1994;162:537–542.
48. Krysl J, Müller NL, Miller RR, et al. Patient with miliary nodules and diarrhea. *Can Assoc Radiol J.* 1991;42:363–366.
49. Gillespie SH. The epidemiology of Toxocara canis. *Parasitol Today.* 1988;4:180–182.
50. Glickman LT, Schantz PM. Epidemiology and pathogenesis of zoonotic toxocariasis. *Epidemiol Rev.* 1981;3:230–250.
51. Glickman L, Schantz P, Dombroske R, et al. Evaluation of serodiagnostic tests for visceral larva migrans. *Am J Trop Med Hyg.* 1978;27:492–498.
52. Chong S, Lee KS, Lim JH, et al. Pulmonary visceral larva migrans of Toxocara canis in adults: Radiographic and high-resolution CT findings. *Am J Roentgenol.* 2006;submitted.
53. Inoue K, Inoue Y, Arai T, et al. Chronic eosinophilic pneumonia due to visceral larva migrans. *Intern Med.* 2002;41:478–482.
54. Roig J, Romeu J, Riera C, et al. Acute eosinophilic pneumonia due to toxocariasis with bronchoalveolar lavage findings. *Chest.* 1992;102:294–296.
55. Sane AC, Barber BA. Pulmonary nodules due to Toxocara canis infection in an immunocompetent adult. *South Med J.* 1997;90:78–79.
56. Bhatia G. Echinococcus. *Semin Respir Infect.* 1997;12:171–186.
57. Beggs I. The radiology of hydatid disease. *Am J Roentgenol.* 1985;145:639–648.
58. Sadrieh M, Dutz W, Navabpoor MS. Review of 150 cases of hydatid cyst of the lung. *Dis Chest.* 1967;52:662–666.
59. Saksouk FA, Fahl MH, Rizk GK. Computed tomography of pulmonary hydatid disease. *J Comput Assist Tomogr.* 1986;10:226–232.
60. Schwartz E. Pulmonary schistosomiasis. *Clin Chest Med.* 2002;23:433–443.
61. Phillips JF, Cockrill H, Jorge E, et al. Radiographic evaluation of patients with schistosomiasis. *Radiology.* 1975;114:31–37.
62. Schwartz E, Rozenman J, Perelman M. Pulmonary manifestations of early schistosome infection among nonimmune travelers. *Am J Med.* 2000;109:718–722.
63. Im JG, Whang HY, Kim WS, et al. Pleuropulmonary paragonimiasis: Radiologic findings in 71 patients. *Am J Roentgenol.* 1992;159:39–43.
64. Mukae H, Taniguchi H, Matsumoto N, et al. Clinicoradiologic features of pleuropulmonary Paragonimus westermani on Kyusyu Island, Japan. *Chest.* 2001;120:514–520.

Acquired Immunodeficiency Syndrome

Respiratory infections are a major cause of morbidity and mortality in patients with acquired immunodeficiency syndrome (AIDS) (1). It is estimated that >70% of patients with AIDS will suffer at least one pulmonary infection during the course of their illness (2). The type of pulmonary infection occurring in an human immunodeficiency virus (HIV)-infected patient depends on the stage of the HIV infection, history of prior infection, virulence of the infecting organism, and other host-related factors, such as the disease exposure and geographic location (3–5).

Immunosuppression associated with HIV infection increases the susceptibility to a variety of pulmonary infections, which represent at least 65% of all AIDS-defining illnesses (see Table 7.1) (2). The risk of pulmonary infection is influenced by the patient's immune status, being greatest at a CD4 lymphocyte count of <200 cells per mm^3 (2, 6, 7). Opportunistic lung infections seldom occur in patients with >200 CD4 lymphocytes per mm^3. HIV-positive patients with >500 CD4 lymphocytes per mm^3 are only mildly immunocompromised and are at increased risk only for bronchial infections and bacterial pneumonia. However, patients with <200 CD4 lymphocytes per mm^3 are predisposed to pulmonary infections caused by a variety of opportunistic and nonopportunistic pathogens, including *Pneumocystis* pneumonia (PCP), nontuberculous mycobacterial infection, and recurrent bacterial pneumonia. At CD4 lymphocyte counts <100 cell per mm^3, and especially at CD4 lymphocyte counts <50 cell per mm^3, the patients are prone to pulmonary infection by endemic fungi and cytomegalovirus (CMV) (7, 8), and to develop disseminated infection by *Mycobacterium avium-intracellulare* complex (MAC).

The most common organisms causing pulmonary infection in HIV-positive patients are gram-positive and gram-negative bacteria, *Pneumocystis jiroveci* (previously known as *P. carinii*), *Mycobacterium tuberculosis*, and MAC (9–11). A resurgence of tuberculosis has been seen worldwide, largely related to the AIDS epidemic (12).

In recent years, there have been changing patterns in the epidemiology and treatment of HIV infection (9).

TABLE 7.1

INFECTIONS IN PATIENTS WITH ACQUIRED IMMUNODEFICIENCY SYNDROME

Risk and type of infection are influenced by the patient's immune status
CD4 lymphocyte count >500 cells/mm^3:
 Risk low
 Most common infection: Bacterial pneumonia
CD4 lymphocyte count <500 cells/mm^3:
 Increased risk of infection
CD4 lymphocyte count 200–500 cells/mm^3:
 Mainly bacterial infection and tuberculosis
CD4 lymphocyte count <200 cell/mm^3:
 Pneumocystis pneumonia, MAC
CD4 lymphocyte count <100 cell/mm^3:
 Endemic fungi, cytomegalovirus, disseminated MAC

MAC, *Mycobacterium avium-intracellulare* complex.

The introduction of highly active antiretroviral therapy (HAART) and the use of prophylactic antibiotics has been associated with a dramatic reduction in the number of HIV-positive patients presenting with respiratory infections (13). HAART has resulted in a decrease in the viral load, an increase in the mean CD4 lymphocyte count causing reduction of the morbidity and mortality from opportunistic infection, and a considerable increase in survival rates (13). However, pulmonary parenchymal complications remain the main cause of morbidity and mortality in these patients (14). Early diagnosis and treatment of these complications is important to improve survival.

In most patients with AIDS, a confident diagnosis of the pulmonary complications can be made from a combination of clinical, radiographic, and laboratory findings (15). However, 5% to 10% of patients with AIDS and pulmonary disease have normal or questionable radiographic findings (6). High-resolution computed tomography (CT) scan is more sensitive than radiography in demonstrating parenchymal abnormalities in patients with AIDS and is superior to the radiograph in the differential

TABLE 7.2

BACTERIAL INFECTIONS IN ACQUIRED IMMUNODEFICIENCY SYNDROME

Commonest cause of pulmonary infection
Common organisms:
 Streptococcus pneumoniae
 Haemophilus influenzae
 Pseudomonas aeruginosa
 Streptococcus viridans
 Staphylococcus aureus

TABLE 7.3

RADIOGRAPHIC FINDINGS OF BACTERIAL INFECTIONS IN ACQUIRED IMMUNODEFICIENCY SYNDROME

Lobar or "rounded" pneumonia: *Pneumococcus*
Bronchopneumonia (unilateral or bilateral):
 Staphylococcus, Pseudomonas, Klebsiella, Enterobacter, and *Haemophilus*
Pyogenic airways infection: *Pseudomonas*
Cavitation: *Pseudomonas, Staphylococcus*, and septic embolism
Pneumothorax: Septic embolism

diagnosis of the pulmonary complications seen in these patients (9, 14, 16).

BACTERIA

Bacterial pneumonia and pyogenic bronchitis are the commonest causes of pulmonary infection in patients with AIDS, being particularly frequent among intravenous drug users and smokers (17, 18). Bacterial pneumonias are most commonly due to *Streptococcus pneumoniae, Haemophilus influenzae, Pseudomonas aeruginosa, Streptococcus viridans*, and *Staphylococcus aureus* (see Table 7.2) (1, 2, 17, 19). In an autopsy-based study of 233 HIV-positive patients with pulmonary complications, bacterial pneumonia due to *P. aeruginosa* and *S. aureus* was the most frequent pulmonary complication (4, 20). *S. pneumoniae* has been identified as the leading cause of community-acquired bacterial pneumonia in HIV-positive patients seen at all levels of CD4

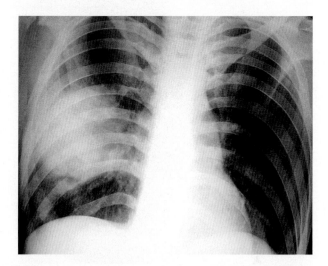

Figure 7.1 Rounded pneumonia due to *Streptococcus pneumoniae*. Anteroposterior chest radiograph shows mass-like consolidation with poorly defined margins in the right upper lobe. The patient was a 34-year-old man with acquired immunodeficiency syndrome. (From Franquet T. Respiratory infection in the AIDS and immunocompromised patient. *Eur Radiol.* 2004;14(suppl 3):E21–E33 with permission.)

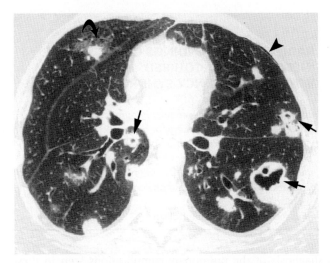

Figure 7.2 Septic embolism. High-resolution computed tomography (CT) image (1-mm collimation) shows multiple bilateral nodules. Some of the nodules are cavitated (*straight arrows*) and one has a surrounding halo of ground-glass attenuation (CT halo sign) (*curved arrow*). Also noted is small left pneumothrox (*arrow head*). The patient, a 36-year-old man, was an intravenous drug user with acquired immunodeficiency syndrome.

lymphocyte count (21, 22). The incidence of *S. pneumoniae* infection in HIV-positive individuals is 5 to 18 times greater than that in the general population, and the development of *S. pneumoniae* septicemia is 100 times greater (23).

Nosocomial pneumonias among HIV-positive patients are indistinguishable from those occurring in other hospitalized patients (24). As reported by Afessa et al. (4),

P. aeruginosa is a common cause of both community-acquired and nosocomial bacterial pneumonia in hospitalized patients with HIV, especially in those with low leukocyte and CD4 lymphocyte counts.

The diagnosis of bacterial infection in patients with AIDS may be established by the combination of clinical, radiographic, and microbiologic findings (see Table 7.3). Respiratory symptoms are common and patients can present with dyspnea, cough, and, less commonly, pleuritic chest pain. A productive cough with purulent sputum suggests a bacterial infection, whereas a nonproductive cough and dyspnea are more characteristic of PCP or other fungal infections. Patients with pneumonia may be febrile, tachycardic, and tachypneic.

The most common chest radiographic features of pneumonia include single or multiple areas of focal consolidation, in either a patchy or lobar distribution (25). Lobar pneumonia is characterized by the spread of bacteria and inflammatory exudates between the alveolar airspaces and crossing segmental boundaries (nonsegmental consolidation), a pattern seen most commonly in *S. pneumoniae* pneumonia. A rounded appearance (rounded pneumonia) may also be seen, particularly in *S. pneumoniae* pneumonia (see Fig. 7.1) (22, 25–27). Bronchopneumonia, characterized by patchy unilateral or bilateral consolidation, can result from a variety of gram-positive and gram-negative bacteria, most commonly *Staphylococcus, Streptococcus, Pseudomonas, Klebsiella, Enterobacter,* and *Haemophilus* species. HIV-positive patients who are intravenous drug users have an increased prevalence of cavitated *P. aeruginosa*

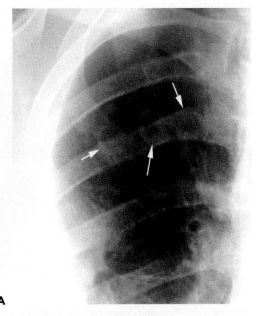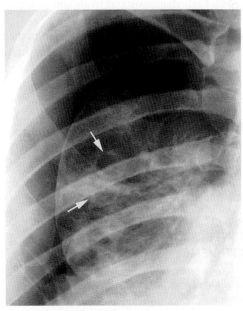

A   **B**

Figure 7.3 Septic embolism and pneumothorax. **A:** Magnified view of the right upper chest on a posteroanterior radiograph shows multiple thin-walled cysts in the right upper lobe (*arrows*). Also noted is a right pleural effusion. **B:** Image obtained 48 hours after **(A)** shows a right-sided pneumothorax. Cystic lesions are still visible in the right upper lobe (*arrows*). The patient, a 29-year-old man, was an intravenous drug abuser with acquired immunodeficiency syndrome, staphylococcal endocarditis, and septic embolism.

pneumonia, recurrent staphylococcal infections, and septic emboli (see Fig. 7.2). These various infections may be associated with complications such as pneumothorax and empyema (see Fig. 7.3) (25, 28).

Although a focal consolidation is highly suggestive of bacterial pneumonia, differentiation from atypical patterns of opportunistic infections is often impossible on the basis of radiographic findings. Conversely, atypical patterns, including bilateral diffuse opacities, are not uncommon manifestations of bacterial pneumonia (14, 27, 29, 30). Uncomplicated bacterial pneumonia may have a clinical and radiographic response to antibiotic therapy, which is similar to immunocompetent individuals undergoing treatment for community-acquired pneumonia (14, 27, 29, 30).

Pyogenic airway diseases, including infectious bronchitis and bronchiolitis, are seen with increasing frequency in HIV-positive patients (31, 32). They are characterized histologically by inflammation of the bronchi and bronchioles and the presence of an inflammatory exudate and mucus in airway lumen (33, 34). Chest radiographs are usually normal or may show subtle bronchial wall thickening, presenting as "tram tracks." CT scan is of limited value in the assessment of bronchitis but is often helpful in the diagnosis of bronchiolitis and early bronchopneumonia. The characteristic high-resolution CT scan findings of infectious bronchiolitis and bronchopneumonia include a "tree-in-bud" pattern characterized by: (a) small centrilobular nodular opacities representing bronchioles

impacted with inflammatory material and peribronchiolar inflammation being seen in cross-section, (b) branching linear opacities corresponding to abnormal bronchioles being seen along their long axis, and (c) focal areas of consolidation due to bronchopneumonia (see Fig. 7.4) (34).

Nosocomial pneumonias in AIDS are indistinguishable from those occurring in other hospitalized patients.

MYCOBACTERIA

Mycobacterium tuberculosis

Mycobacterium tuberculosis remains an important respiratory pathogen in HIV-positive patients. After decades of decreasing incidence, tuberculosis has reemerged as an important infection worldwide (35). The main factor responsible for the significant increase of tuberculosis since the mid-1980s has been the increased prevalence of HIV infection. The incidence of tuberculosis in patients with AIDS is 200 to 500 times greater than that of the general population (36, 37). HIV infection is the strongest known risk factor for progression from latent to active tuberculosis (38). Of the estimated 42 million individuals infected with HIV worldwide, >25% have active tuberculosis (38). Most of these patients live in countries with limited health care resources in Africa and Asia. The incidence of tuberculosis in these countries is increasing (24).

The manifestations of tuberculosis in patients with AIDS are influenced by the degree of immunosuppression (see Table 7.4) (5). The radiologic findings in patients with mild

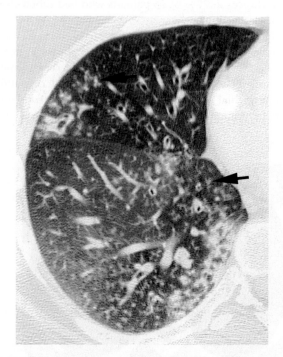

Figure 7.4 Bacterial bronchiolitis. View of the right lower lung zone on a high-resolution computed tomography (CT) scan (1-mm collimation) shows centrilobular branching nodules ("tree-in-bud" pattern) (*arrows*) and small poorly defined areas of consolidation. The patient was a 28-year-old woman with acquired immunodeficiency syndrome who presented with fever and persistent productive cough.

TABLE 7.4
TUBERCULOSIS IN ACQUIRED IMMUNODEFICIENCY SYNDROME

Incidence: 200 to 500 times that of the general population
Influenced by the degree of immunosuppression
Most common radiologic presentation:
>200 CD4 cells/mm^3: Findings similar to postprimary disease in the healthy host
    Focal areas of consolidation
    Nodules
    Mainly in apical and posterior segments of the upper lobes
    Cavitation: 20%–25% of patients
    Lymph node enlargement: 10% of cases
<200 CD4 cells/mm^3: Findings similar to primary tuberculosis
    Hilar and/or mediastinal lymph node enlargement
    Evident on the radiograph in 30% to 60% of patients
    Evident on CT scan in 70% to 90% of patients
    Decreased attenuation and rim enhancement on CT scan
    Focal or patchy areas of consolidation

CT, computed tomography.

immunosuppression (>200 CD4 cells per mm³) are usually similar to those of postprimary disease in the healthy host (39–41). The abnormalities include focal areas of consolidation and nodular opacities involving mainly the apical and posterior segments of the upper lobes. Cavitation occurs in approximately 20% of patients and lymph node enlargement in 10%. In patients with severe immunosuppression (CD4 lymphocyte count <200 per mm³) the findings tend to resemble those of primary tuberculosis (36, 41). The predominant abnormalities include hilar and/or mediastinal lymph node enlargement and airspace consolidation. Enlarged hilar and/or mediastinal nodes are evident on the radiograph in 30% to 60% of patients and on CT scan in 70% to 90% (36, 37, 42). The enlarged nodes usually have decreased attenuation on CT scan and often show rim enhancement following intravenous administration of contrast (see Fig. 7.5) (42, 43). The decreased number of T lymphocytes and deficient delayed-type hypersensitivity reaction in patients with AIDS result in impaired ability to form granulomas, kill the bacilli, and localize the disease. Therefore these patients have increased prevalence of miliary tuberculosis (see Fig. 7.6) (36).

Although the chest radiograph plays an important role in the diagnosis of tuberculosis it may be normal in up to 15% of patients with AIDS and sputum culture-positive disease (44, 45). Furthermore, the radiograph may fail to demonstrate characteristic findings of tuberculosis in patients with active disease. In a retrospective study of 133 patients with AIDS who had culture-positive tuberculosis, chest radiographs failed to suggest the correct diagnosis in 32% of cases (44). Tuberculosis could not be diagnosed when radiographs appeared normal (13% of cases), showed minimal radiographic abnormalities, such as linear opacities or calcified granulomas, or showed atypical patterns of disease, such as diffuse opacities mimicking PCP. High-resolution CT scan may demonstrate parenchymal abnormalities in patients with normal radiographs and

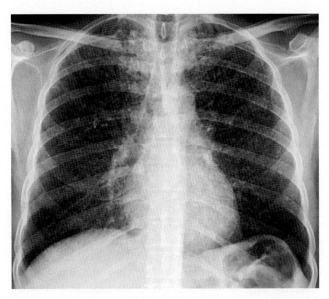

Figure 7.6 Miliary tuberculosis. Posteroanterior chest radiograph shows numerous bilateral 2 to 4 mm diameter nodules. The patient was a 50-year-old man with acquired immunodeficiency syndrome and miliary tuberculosis.

characteristic findings in patients with nonspecific radiographic findings. Hartman et al. (46) assessed the accuracy of CT scan interpretation in 102 patients with AIDS who had proven intrathoracic disease. On CT scan, mycobacterial infection was correctly suggested as the first choice of diagnosis in 44% of patients, and was among the top three choices in 77% of 26 patients who had tuberculosis or MAC infection.

Similar to the radiograph, high-resolution CT scan in patients with AIDS and tuberculosis shows a greater prevalence of mediastinal lymph node enlargement and miliary spread and lower prevalence of cavitation, endobronchial spread of infection and consolidation than in nonimmunocompromised patients (37, 47, 48).

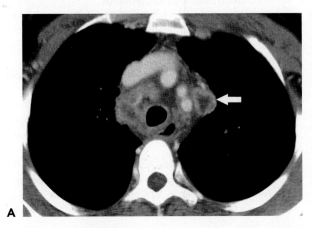
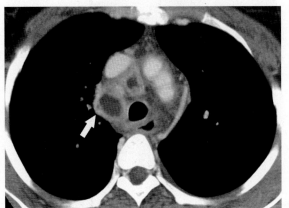

Figure 7.5 Tuberculous lymphadenopathy. Contrast-enhanced computed tomography (CT) images at the level of the great vessels **(A)** and slightly more caudally **(B)** show several enlarged mediastinal lymph nodes. The enlarged nodes have decreased attenuation and show rim enhancement (*arrows*). The patient was a 39-year-old woman with acquired immunodeficiency syndrome.

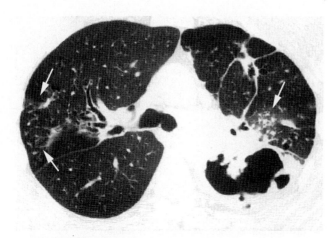

Figure 7.7 Cavitary tuberculosis. High-resolution computed tomography (CT) scan (1-mm collimation) at the level of the carina shows a large cavity in the superior segment of the left lower lobe. Also note bilateral centrilobular nodules and branching linear structures (*arrows*). The findings are characteristic of reactivation tuberculosis with endobronchial spread. The patient was a 39-year-old man with acquired immunodeficiency syndrome.

Leung et al. (47) compared the CT scan findings of 42 HIV-positive and 42 HIV-negative patients who had pulmonary tuberculosis. Findings seen with significantly lower frequency in HIV-positive patients compared to HIV-negative patients were cavitation (19% vs. 55%), consolidation (43% vs. 69%), and endobronchial spread (57% vs. 90%) resulting in centrilobular nodular opacities and "tree-in-bud" pattern (see Figs. 7.7 and 7.8) (49). Conversely, a miliary pattern was seen in 17% of HIV-positive patients and in none of the negative ones (see Fig. 7.9). Laissy et al. (37) compared the conventional and high-resolution CT scan findings in 29 HIV-positive and 47 HIV-negative patients who had newly diagnosed pulmonary tuberculosis. HIV-positive patients demonstrated

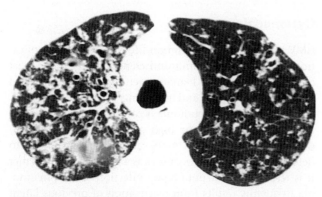

Figure 7.8 Endobronchial spread of tuberculosis. High-resolution computed tomography (CT) image (1-mm collimation) shows numerous bilateral centrilobular nodules and extensive branching linear and nodular opacities ("tree-in-bud" pattern). Also note bilateral bronchiectasis. The patient was a 45-year-old man with acquired immunodeficiency syndrome. (From Franquet T. Respiratory infection in the AIDS and immunocompromised patient. *Eur Radiol.* 2004;14(suppl 3):E21–E33, with permission.)

significantly lower frequency of cavitation (24% vs. 49%). Cavitation was seen in only 13% of HIV-positive patients who had <200 CD4 T cells per mm^3 compared to 50% of HIV-positive patients who had 200 or more CD4 T cells per mm^3. On the other hand, lymphadenopathy was significantly more common in patients who had <200 CD4 T cells per mm^3 (70% vs. 33%).

Mycobacterium avium-intracellulare Complex

MAC accounts for most nontuberculous mycobacterial infections seen in patients with AIDS (50–52). MAC infection usually results from primary exposure rather than reactivation of latent organisms. It tends to occur in the late stage of AIDS, when immune deficiency is severe and the CD4 lymphocyte count drops below 50 cells per mm^3 (53).

Diagnosis of pulmonary nontuberculous mycobacterial infection is often difficult because isolation of the organism from sputum or bronchoalveolar lavage (BAL) fluid may be the result of airway colonization rather than infection (53). The diagnosis may be established from the combination of positive culture of sputum or BAL fluid, appropriate clinical and radiologic findings, and a therapeutic response. Approximately 20% of chest radiographs in patients with MAC-related pulmonary disease are normal (50). The most common findings include mediastinal or hilar lymphadenopathy. The pulmonary manifestations, when present, resemble those of tuberculosis and include multifocal patchy areas of consolidation or ill-defined nodules that may cavitate (see Fig. 7.10) (50, 53, 54). Pleural effusions are more common in MAC than in tuberculosis but miliary disease is rare (53).

Immune Reconstitution Inflammatory Syndrome

The radiographic and CT scan manifestations of tuberculosis in HIV-positive patients have changed considerably since the introduction of HAART (13). Because HAART results in partial restoration of cell-mediated immunity, patients with AIDS receiving HAART are more likely to show a pattern resembling postprimary tuberculosis. Busi Rizzi et al. (13) reviewed the chest radiographs in 209 HIV-infected patients with culture-confirmed pulmonary tuberculosis. CT images were also reviewed in 42 patients whose chest radiographs were normal or showed only questionable abnormalities. Postprimary pattern became more frequent after 1996 when HAART came into clinical use, being seen in 82% (27/33) of patients receiving HAART compared to 44% (77/176) of patients not on HAART (p <0.001). A primary pattern was significantly more frequent (p <0.001) in patients with more severe immunosuppression (CD4 lymphocyte <200 per mm^3) (13).

Although HAART has resulted in a marked decrease in the frequency of opportunistic infections among HIV-infected individuals, some HAART-treated patients exhibit

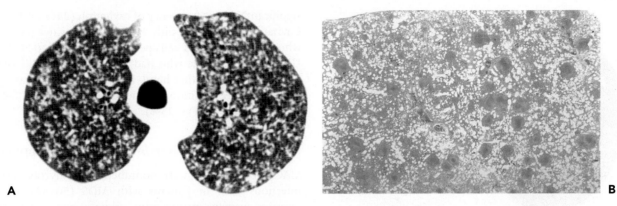

A   B

Figure 7.9 Miliary tuberculosis. **A:** High-resolution computed tomography (CT) scan (1-mm collimation) shows numerous small nodules in random distribution. **B:** Photomicrograph of whole-mount, low-power histologic section demonstrates multiple granulomas with necrotic centers (hematoxylin and eosin ×40). The patient was a 42-year-old woman with acquired immunodeficiency syndrome. (From Marchiori E, Müller NL, Soares Souza A Jr, et al. Pulmonary disease in patients with AIDS: High-resolution CT and pathologic findings. *Am J Roentgenol.* 2005;184:757–764, with permission.)

paradoxical clinical deterioration, despite satisfactory control of viral replication and improvement in CD4 lymphocyte counts (55, 56). This clinical deterioration, known as immune reconstitution inflammatory syndrome (IRIS) or immune restoration syndrome (57), is a result of an exuberant inflammatory response (55, 56). In this condition, previously subclinical infections become clinically manifested or preexisting infections clinically deteriorate. IRIS is most frequently associated with mycobacterial infections and results in clinical deterioration of patients with tuberculosis and MAC infection (55, 56, 58). Treatment includes continuation of therapy for tuberculosis or MAC, continuation of effective HAART, and use of anti-inflammatory agents. Although the clinical

manifestations of IRIS are sometimes dramatic, and result in substantial morbidity, most patients improve with therapy (55, 56, 59).

The radiologic findings of IRIS in patients with mycobacterial infection include development of marked lymphadenopathy and increase in extent of the parenchymal abnormalities (see Fig. 7.11) (55, 56, 59). Buckingham et al. (59) reviewed the radiologic findings in five HIV-infected patients with IRIS due to mycobacterial infection. The clinical and radiologic deterioration occurred between 10 days and 7 months after starting HAART. Chest radiographic abnormalities due to IRIS included marked mediastinal lymphadenopathy in three of the five patients (with associated tracheal narrowing in two patients) and new pulmonary opacities in four patients, one of whom developed pleural effusion (59).

VIRUSES

Cytomegalovirus

CMV pneumonia is a common life-threatening complication seen in immunocompromised patients. It occurs most commonly following hematopoietic stem cell and solid organ transplantation and in patients with AIDS (14, 60).

Although CMV pneumonia is common in patients with advanced AIDS (61), the high prevalence (almost 90%) of CMV in patients with AIDS often makes it difficult to determine whether the organism is a bystander or whether it is responsible for pulmonary infection. CMV pneumonia frequently results from reactivation of previous latent infection and usually occurs in patients with CD4 counts <50 cells per mm^3. The manifestations of CMV pneumonia depend on the severity of the infection that results in varying degrees of inflammation, hemorrhage, diffuse alveolar damage, and fibrosis. The radiographic manifestations include a reticular or reticulonodular pattern, ground-glass

Figure 7.10 *Mycobacterium avium*-intracellulare complex (MAC) infection. High-resolution computed tomography (CT) image (1-mm collimation) at the level of the aortic arch shows 1.5-cm diameter right upper lobe nodule (*straight arrow*) and several small centrilobular nodules (*curved arrows*). Also noted are focal areas of scarring and emphysema. The patient was a 48-year-old man with acquired immunodeficiency syndrome and pulmonary MAC infection.

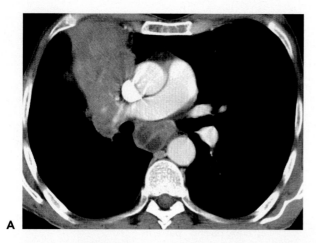
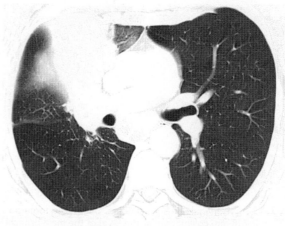

A   B

Figure 7.11   Immune reconstitution inflammatory syndrome **A:** Contrast-enhanced computed tomography (CT) scan (5-mm collimation) shows enlarged low attenuation subcarinal lymph nodes with rim enhancement. Also noted is right hilar lymphadenopathy and obstructive pneumonitis of the anterior segment of the right upper lobe. **B:** Lung window settings better demonstrate the obstructive pneumonitis. Note lack of air bronchogram consistent with complete bronchial obstruction by the enlarged right hilar nodes. (Case courtesy of Dr. Jen Ellis, Department of Radiology, St. Paul's Hospital, Vancouver, Canada.)

opacities, airspace consolidation, or a combination of these patterns (see Table 7.5 and Fig. 7.12) (62). There is no radiographic finding characteristic enough to allow differentiation of CMV pneumonia from other infections (63–65). McGuinness et al. (60) described the high-resolution CT scan findings in 21 patients with AIDS and CMV pneumonia. The most common abnormalities consisted of ground-glass opacities, dense airspace consolidation, and discrete pulmonary nodules or masses (see Figs. 7.13 and 7.14). This pattern differs from that seen in immunocompromised non-AIDS patients who seldom develop dense consolidation or masses (63, 65).

FUNGI

Patients with AIDS are at risk of developing fungal infections, which require intact T cell function for containment.

Fungal pneumonias other than PCP have been increasingly reported in patients with AIDS (66, 67), the most common ones being *Cryptococcus* and *Aspergillus* (68). Other fungal infections including *Histoplasma capsulatum* and *Coccidioides immitis* are seen in endemic areas (69, 70).

Pneumocystis jiroveci (carinii) (Pneumocystis pneumonia)

Pneumocystis organisms are unicellular organisms that encompass multiple species that are host-specific and currently classified as fungi. The *Pneumocystis* that infects humans does not infect animals and was recently renamed

TABLE 7.5

VIRAL INFECTIONS IN ACQUIRED IMMUNODEFICIENCY SYNDROME

Cytomegalovirus pneumonia is common in
    patients with advanced AIDS
CD4 counts below 50 cells/mm^3
Most common radiologic presentations:
    Reticular or reticulonodular pattern
    Ground-glass opacities
    Airspace consolidation
    Combination of these patterns

AIDS, acquired immunodeficiency syndrome.

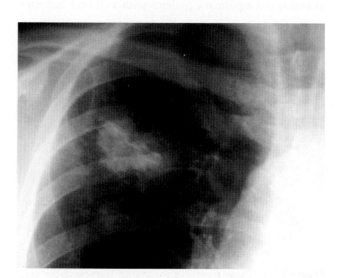

Figure 7.12   Cytomegalovirus pneumonia. View of the right upper lobe on anteroposterior chest radiograph shows focal airspace consolidation. The patient was a 34-year-old man with acquired immunodeficiency syndrome.

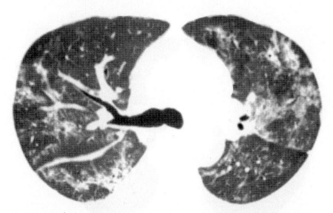

Figure 7.13 Cytomegalovirus pneumonia. Computed tomography (CT) image (8-mm collimation) at the level of the main bronchi shows extensive bilateral ground-glass opacities and several poorly defined focal areas of consolidation. Also noted are several small centrilobular nodules. The patient was a 43-year-old man with acquired immunodeficiency syndrome and cytomegalovirus pneumonia.

P. jiroveci. P. carinii on the other hand infects only rats. *P. jiroveci* is a common cause of life-threatening opportunistic infection in patients with AIDS (67). Most patients have CD4 counts of <100 cells per mm³ at the time of diagnosis of their first episode of PCP (1).

Clinical symptoms include nonproductive cough, shortness of breath, and hypoxia in room air. Abnormal chest radiographs have been reported in up to 90% of patients with suspected PCP. The characteristic radiographic manifestations consist of symmetric bilateral ground-glass opacities (see Table 7.6). These may be diffuse but tend to involve mainly the perihilar regions or middle and lower lung zones (see Figs. 7.15 and 7.16) (11, 12). Disease progression may result in predominantly perihilar or diffuse bilateral airspace consolidation. High-resolution CT scan is the imaging modality of choice to evaluate symptomatic patients with a clinical suspicion

TABLE 7.6
PNEUMOCYSTIS *JIROVECI* PNEUMONIA

Chest radiograph

    Bilateral symmetric ground-glass opacities or fine reticulonodular pattern

    Tends to involve mainly the perihilar regions

    May be diffuse or involve mainly the lower or upper lung zones

High-resolution CT scan:

    Bilateral symmetric ground-glass opacities

    May be patchy or diffuse

    Superimposed fine linear pattern may be present ("crazy paving" pattern)

Other manifestations:

    Cystic lesions (pneumatoceles) in approximately 30% of cases

    Focal or confluent areas of parenchymal consolidation

    Reticular pattern

    Nodules or multiple small nodules

    Pneumothorax

CT, computed tomography.

for PCP, who have normal or equivocal chest radiographs (11, 12, 71). The most common high-resolution CT scan manifestation of PCP consists of patchy or confluent, symmetric, bilateral ground-glass opacities (see Figs. 7.16 to 7.18) (6, 8, 10, 11, 71–73).

The ground-glass opacities and areas of consolidation reflect the presence of alveolar filling by a foamy exudate, constituted mainly of surfactant, fibrin, and cellular debris. The organisms are typically seen as small

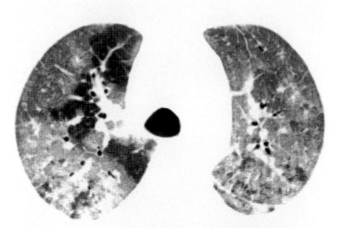

Figure 7.14 Cytomegalovirus pneumonia. High-resolution computed tomography (CT) image (2-mm collimation) at the level of the aortic arch shows extensive bilateral ground-glass opacities and small foci of consolidation. The patient was a 29-year-old man with acquired immunodeficiency syndrome.

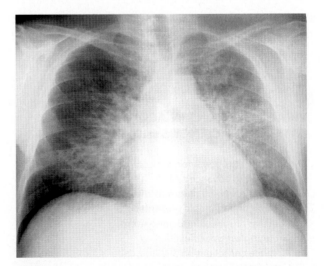

Figure 7.15 *Pneumocystis* pneumonia. Posteroanterior chest radiograph shows bilateral symmetric perihilar ground-glass opacities and reticulonodular pattern. The patient was a 36-year-old man with acquired immunodeficiency syndrome.

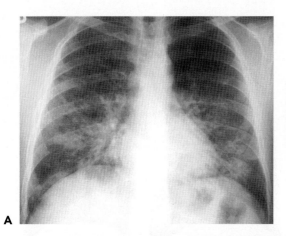
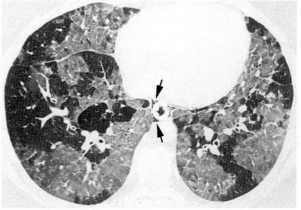

Figure 7.16 *Pneumocystis* pneumonia. **A:** Posteroanterior chest radiograph shows bilateral hazy ground-glass opacities mainly in the middle and lower lung zones. **B:** High-resolution computed tomography (CT) scan (1-mm collimation) at the level of lung bases shows bilateral ground-glass opacities interspersed by normal lung parenchyma. Also noted is pneumomediastinum (*arrows*). The patient was a 34-year-old man with acquired immunodeficiency syndrome.

"bubbles" within this foamy exudate (6, 19, 28, 74). Interstitial edema or cellular infiltration may result in septal and intralobular lines. The combination of ground-glass opacities and superimposed septal and intralobular linear opacities results in a pattern known as "crazy paving" (26, 75).

Advances in the prevention and treatment of *Pneumocystis* infection have resulted in an increased frequency of atypical radiologic manifestations including multiple pulmonary nodules, parenchymal consolidation, interlobular septal thickening, intralobular linear opacities, mass lesions, pleural effusion, and lymph node enlargement (see Figs. 7.19 and 7.20) (9, 29, 30, 46, 76, 77).

Nodules in PCP reflect the presence of granulomatous inflammation consisting of clusters of epithelioid histiocytes

and multinucleated giant cells (6, 19, 28, 74). Rarely, these granulomas may undergo necrosis and cavitate.

A cystic form of PCP has been described in 10% to 30% of patients with AIDS, being particularly common in patients receiving prophylaxis with aerosolized pentamidine and trimethoprim-sulfamethoxazole (9). The cysts usually have thin walls, tend to involve mainly the upper lobes, and may be unilateral or bilateral (see Figs 7.21 and 7.22). Patients with cysts have an increased propensity to develop pneumothorax (see Fig. 7.23) (6, 19, 28). The cysts usually represent pneumatoceles. Less commonly they result from tissue invasion by *Pneumocystis* followed by necrosis (74). Occasionally, PCP may result in interstitial fibrosis. This can be mild or severe and is manifested on CT scan by the presence of irregular linear opacities, traction bronchiectasis, and traction bronchiolectasis (see Fig. 7.24) (19, 29, 30).

Although the high-resolution CT scan findings are not specific for PCP, the presence of bilateral ground-glass opacities in an HIV-positive patient allows a presumptive diagnosis to be made and early treatment to be instituted before microbiologic confirmation becomes available (12).

Aspergillus fumigatus (Aspergillosis)

Several species of fungi may cause airway and pulmonary disease in HIV-positive patients, but most cases are due to *Aspergillus fumigatus*. The histologic, clinical, and radiologic manifestations of pulmonary aspergillosis are determined by the number and virulence of the organisms and the patient's immune response (78–80). Opportunistic *Aspergillus* infections account for 0.1% to 0.5% of pulmonary infections seen in patients with AIDS (81). The incidence has significantly increased in recent years because of the prolonged survival of patients with very

Figure 7.17 *Pneumocystis* pneumonia. High-resolution computed tomography (CT) scan (1-mm collimation) at the level of inferior pulmonary veins shows patchy bilateral ground-glass opacities. The chest radiography was normal. The patient was a 40-year-old man with acquired immunodeficiency syndrome. (From Franquet T. Respiratory infection in the AIDS and immunocompromised patient. *Eur Radiol.* 2004;14(suppl 3):E21–E33, with permission.)

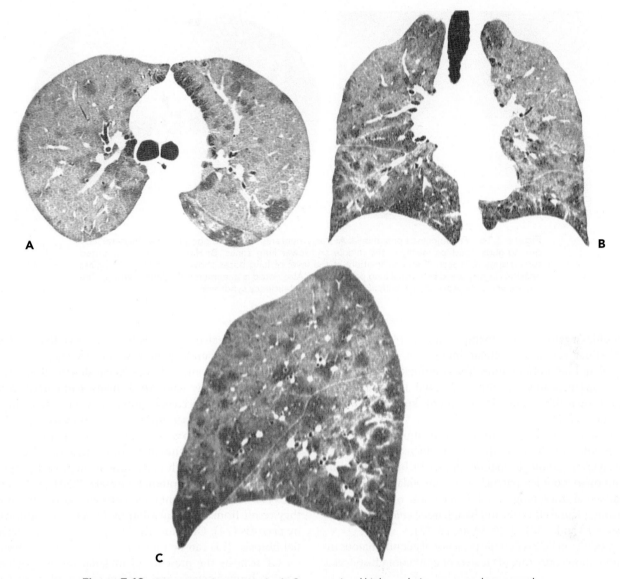

Figure 7.18 *Pneumocystis* pneumonia. **A:** Cross-sectional high-resolution computed tomography (CT) image (1-mm collimation) obtained on a multidetector CT scanner shows extensive bilateral ground-glass opacities. Coronal **(B)** and sagittal **(C)** images demonstrate the overall distribution of the findings. Note relative sparing of the lung apices and lung bases. The patient was a 36-year-old man with acquired immunodeficiency syndrome.

low CD4 counts, the introduction of HAART, and the increased use of corticosteroids as part of the treatment of PCP (82, 83).

Angioinvasive aspergillosis, airway invasive aspergillosis, pseudomembranous necrotizing tracheobronchial aspergillosis, obstructing bronchial aspergillosis, and chronic cavitary forms of aspergillosis have been described in AIDS (26, 75).

The most common radiographic and high-resolution CT scan finding of invasive aspergillosis in AIDS is the presence of thick-walled cavitary lesions (see Fig. 7.25) (84). The main histologic abnormalities include tissue invasion, abscess formation, and angioinvasion with or without infarction (74). Less common radiologic findings include single or multiple nodules, patchy areas of consolidation,

and pleural effusions (74). Nodules represent pulmonary infarction and may have a surrounding halo of ground-glass attenuation due to hemorrhage (see Fig. 7.26) (74, 85, 86).

Airway invasive aspergillosis occurs most commonly in the setting of severe neutropenia and in patients with AIDS (83, 87). Clinical manifestations include acute tracheobronchitis, bronchiolitis, and bronchopneumonia. Patients with acute tracheobronchitis usually have normal radiologic findings. *Aspergillus* bronchiolitis is characterized on high-resolution CT scan by the presence of centrilobular nodules and branching linear and nodular opacities ("tree-in-bud" pattern) (25, 34, 75, 83, 85, 86). *Aspergillus* bronchopneumonia results in predominantly peribronchial or lobular areas of consolidation (86). The

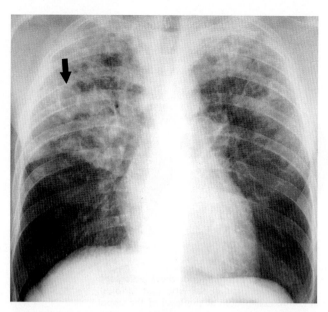

Figure 7.19 *Pneumocystis* pneumonia. Posteroanterior chest radiograph shows bilateral hazy ground-glass opacities small foci of consolidation and poorly defined nodules involving mainly the upper lobes. Also noted is a cyst (*arrow*) in the right upper lobe. The patient was a 28-year-old man with acquired immunodeficiency syndrome and *Pneumocystis* pneumonia.

radiographic and high-resolution CT scan manifestations of *Aspergillus* bronchiolitis and bronchopneumonia are indistinguishable from those caused by other organisms.

Obstructive bronchopulmonary aspergillosis (86, 88) is a descriptive term for the unusual pattern of a noninvasive form of aspergillosis characterized by the massive intraluminal overgrowth of *Aspergillus* sp, usually *A. fumigatus*, in patients with AIDS (34, 83, 85, 87). Patients may cough up fungal casts of their bronchi and present with severe hypoxemia. The CT scan findings mimic those

of allergic bronchopulmonary aspergillosis and consist of bilateral bronchiectasis and bronchiolectasis, mucoid impaction mainly in the lower lobes, and diffuse lower lobe consolidation due to postobstructive pneumonitis and atelectasis (see Fig. 7.27) (34, 85, 86).

Cryptococcus neoformans (Cryptococcosis)

Cryptococcus neoformans is an encapsulated nonmycelial, budding yeast found worldwide, particularly in the soil contaminated by bird droppings (89). *Cryptococcus* is a relatively common pulmonary fungal pathogen in the AIDS patients with a CD4 count <100 cells per mm^3 (57, 67, 90). Cryptococcosis in patients with AIDS usually manifests as disseminated disease, the main clinical manifestation being meningitis. The histologic response to cryptococcal infection depends on the immune status of the patient. In patients with normal or nearly normal immune response, the organisms result in nodular granulomas similar to other fungal pulmonary infections (89). In severely immunosuppressed patients there may be extensive tissue infiltration by organisms in a pneumonic fashion, with little tissue response. Although the central nervous system is the commonest affected organ, the lungs are also often involved. In a series of 31 HIV-infected patients with cryptococcal infection, 12 (39%) had cryptococcal pneumonia (68, 91). Presenting symptoms include fever, cough, dyspnea, sputum production, and pleuritic chest pain. Radiographic findings include a reticular or reticulonodular interstitial pattern (68, 92). Other less common manifestations are ground-glass opacities, airspace consolidation, and miliary nodules (see Fig. 7.28) (89, 93). The CT scan pattern in immunocompromised non-AIDS patients seems to differ from that of patients with AIDS by the presence of nodules and the

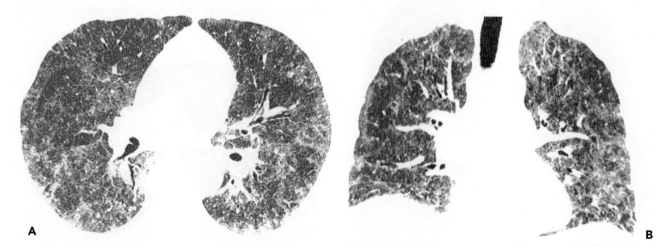

A   **B**

Figure 7.20 *Pneumocystis* pneumonia. **A:** Cross-sectional high-resolution computed tomography (CT) image (1-mm collimation) obtained on a multidetector CT scanner shows bilateral ground-glass opacities, mild reticulation, small foci of consolidation in the lower lobes, and numerous small nodules. **B:** Coronal image shows diffuse distribution of the abnormalities. The patient was a 51-year-old man with acquired immunodeficiency syndrome.

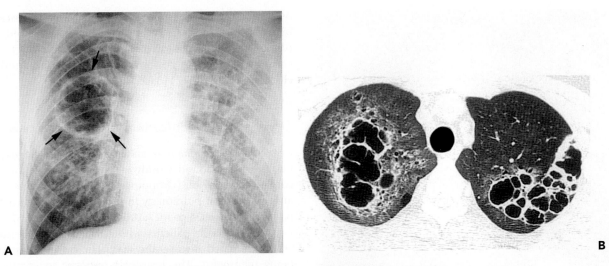

Figure 7.21 *Pneumocystis* pneumonia with cyst formation. **A:** Posteroanterior chest radiograph shows bilateral ground-glass opacities and a large thin-walled right upper lobe cyst (*arrows*). **B:** High-resolution computed tomography (CT) scan (2-mm collimation) at the level of the upper lobes demonstrates numerous bilateral thin-walled cystic lesions and adjacent ground-glass opacities. The patient was a 43-year-old man with acquired immunodeficiency syndrome.

absence of reticular or reticulonodular interstitial opacities (68, 93).

Histoplasma capsulatum (Histoplasmosis)

H. capsulatum is a dimorphic yeast found in temperate regions throughout the world. Histoplasmosis occurs mainly in endemic areas along the Mississippi and Ohio river valleys in the United States, the St. Lawrence river valley in Canada, and in South America (94). Histoplasmosis is seen in approximately 2% of patients with AIDS. Most cases of disseminated histoplasmosis in patients with AIDS are thought to be due to endogenous reactivation rather than primary infection. Approximately 40% of patients with pulmonary disseminated histoplasmosis have a normal chest radiograph (94). CT scan can be helpful in the assessment of patients who have symptoms of pulmonary disease and normal or nonspecific radiographic findings (95). The most common radiographic findings are diffuse nodular opacities 3 mm or less in diameter, nodules >3 mm in diameter, small linear opacities, and focal or patchy areas of consolidation (95). The high-resolution CT scan findings consist of a miliary pattern, or, less commonly, diffuse airspace consolidation (see Fig. 7.29) (95). The miliary lesions result from hematogenous dissemination and consist of small foci of acute inflammation with neutrophils and macrophages

Figure 7.22 *Pneumocystis* pneumonia with cyst formation. Coronal image from a high-resolution computed tomography (CT) scan (1-mm collimation) obtained on a multidetector scanner shows symmetric bilateral ground-glass opacities and thin-walled right upper lobe cyst (*arrow*). The patient was a 45-year-old man with acquired immunodeficiency syndrome.

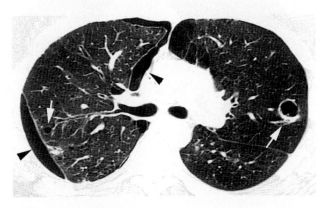

Figure 7.23 *Pneumocystis* pneumonia with cyst formation and pneumothorax. High-resolution computed tomography (CT) image (1-mm collimation) at the level of the main bronchi shows several thin-walled cystic lesions (*arrows*), mild emphysema, and a right pneumothorax (*arrowheads*).

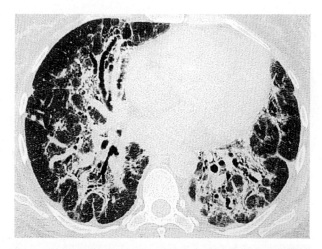

Figure 7.24 *Pneumocystis* pneumonia with fibrosis. High-resolution computed tomography (CT) scan (1-mm collimation) shows bilateral ground-glass opacities and reticulation involving mainly the central lung regions. Note associated distortion of the lung architecture and traction bronchiectasis consistent with fibrosis. The patient was a 49-year-old man with acquired immunodeficiency syndrome.

and granulomas. Diffuse airspace consolidation is typically associated with large numbers of organisms in the alveoli and an inflammatory response consisting of neutrophils with a mixture of fibrin, red blood cells, and macrophages.

Coccidioides immitis (Coccidioidomycosis)

Coccidioidomycosis is common in patients who have AIDS and live in endemic areas, particularly the southwestern United States and northern Mexico (96). The most common radiologic manifestations include focal or diffuse areas of consolidation. Other less common findings include nodules, cavitation, miliary pattern, hilar nodal enlargement, and pleural effusion. BAL or biopsy is required to confirm the diagnosis and exclude other coexisting diseases.

Blastomyces dermatitidis (North American Blastomycosis)

Blastomycosis is an endemic fungal infection seen most commonly in the central and southeastern United States (endemic areas include the Ohio, Mississippi, and Missouri river valleys) and southern Canada (mainly Quebec, Ontario, and Manitoba). Blastomycosis may occur more commonly in immunocompromised patients than in previously healthy patients (97–99). The most common sites of involvement are the skin, bones, prostate, and central nervous system (97). Pulmonary disease is rare and seen mainly in HIV-positive patients with CD4 lymphocyte counts <200 cells per mm^3 (100, 101). Clinical presentation is variable and includes flu-like illness, acute pneumonia, subacute or chronic respiratory illness, and fulminant acute respiratory distress syndrome (97, 98). The radiologic manifestation is usually that of bronchopneumonia. Less common findings include miliary dissemination, hilar and mediastinal lymph node enlargement, and pleural effusion.

MISCELLANEOUS INFECTIONS

Bartonella henselae (Bacillary angiomatosis)

Bacillary angiomatosis is an unusual bacterial infection encountered in patients with AIDS that is caused by *Bartonella henselae* (formerly *Rochalimaea henselae*) (102–104). Vascular skin nodules caused by this infection may mimic Kaposi sarcoma (105). Infection may spread to the lymph nodes, liver (peliosis), spleen, central nervous system, skeleton (osteolytic lesions), and lungs (106–109). In the chest, endobronchial lesions, lung nodules, endobronchial masses, interstitial lung disease, mediastinal lymphadenopathy, pleural disease, and chest wall masses have all been reported (102, 103, 106). Mass lesions may demonstrate marked contrast enhancement on CT scan. Diagnosis is

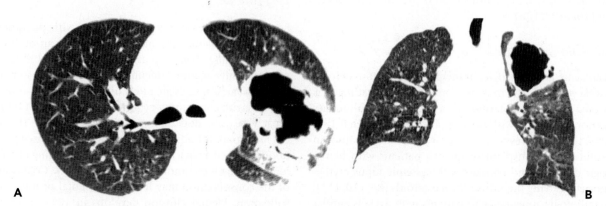

A

B

Figure 7.25 Invasive aspergillosis. **A:** Cross-sectional high-resolution computed tomography (CT) image (1-mm collimation) obtained on a multidetector scanner shows thick-walled left upper lobe cavity, mild adjacent consolidation, and ground-glass opacities. **B:** Coronal image demonstrates the location of the cavity in the cephalocaudal plane. The patient was a 38-year old with acquired immunodeficiency syndrome.

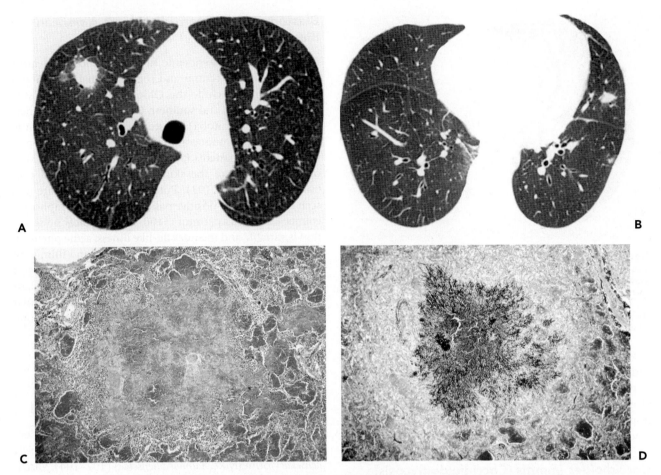

Figure 7.26 Angioinvasive pulmonary aspergillosis. High-resolution computed tomography (CT) images (2-mm collimation) at the level of the upper **(A)** and lower lung zones **(B)** show a nodule with surrounding halo of ground-glass opacity in the right upper lobe, and small nodules in the lingula and left lower lobe. **C:** Histologic section of one of the small nodules shows necrotic center surrounded by a leukocyte infiltrate and more peripherally by alveolar hemorrhage (hematoxylin and eosin ×40). **D:** Grocott stain demonstrates in black the hyphae of *Aspergillus* inside the nodule. The hyphae are in a radial distribution from the center to the periphery of the nodule (×40). The patient was a 62-year-old man with acquired immunodeficiency syndrome. (From Marchiori E, Müller NL, Soares Souza A Jr, et al. Pulmonary disease in patients with AIDS: High-resolution CT and pathologic findings. *Am J Roentgenol.* 2005;184:757–764., with permission.)

made by biopsy and identification of bacilli in the specimen (102, 103, 106).

Nocardia asteroides

Nocardia are gram-positive, branching, filamentous aerobic bacteria of which the most important human pathogen is *Nocardia asteroides*. Nocardiosis is a rare cause of pulmonary infection in patients with AIDS (prevalence between 0.19% to 2%) (110). However, it is a relatively common pathogen in solid organ transplant recipients, patients with hematologic diseases, and patients with systemic lupus erythematosus receiving high-dose corticosteroids (88, 110, 111). The radiologic appearance in patients with AIDS is similar to that seen in non-AIDS patients and consists of solitary or multiple nodules or masses and nonsegmental lobar or multifocal consolidation (bronchopneumonia) (112, 113). Pleural effusion is rare.

Legionella

Legionnaires disease is a febrile illness with pneumonia caused by *Legionella* sp. This illness presents in outbreaks or sporadically. *Legionella* is responsible for 1% to 5% of community-acquired pneumonias requiring hospitalization. *Legionella* species are rarely diagnosed in HIV-infected patients with community-acquired pneumonia (114, 115). Most cases are due to *Legionella pneumophila*. The initial radiographic findings include unilateral, nonsegmental poorly defined airspace consolidation. Worsening of radiologic findings is common during the first week. Coalescence of the consolidation may lead to segmental or lobar consolidation. Pleural effusion develops in 10% to 30% of patients during the first week of hospitalization (116). Cavitation is rare. Legionnaires disease has a more severe clinical presentation and increased morbidity in patients with HIV (115).

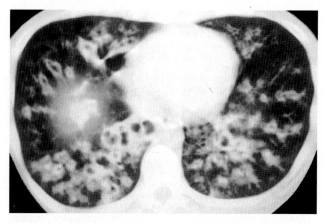

Figure 7.27 Obstructive bronchopulmonary aspergillosis. Computed tomography (CT) image (8-mm collimation) at the level of lower lung zones shows bilateral bifurcating tubular shadows caused by impacted mucous material within markedly dilated bronchi. Bronchoscopy revealed that the lumen of the bronchi was packed with inflammatory material. CT scan findings resemble those of allergic bronchopulmonary aspergillosis. The patient was a 24-year-old man with acquired immunodeficiency syndrome. (From Franquet T, Müller NL, Oikonomou A, et al. Aspergillus infection of the airways: Computed tomography and pathologic findings. *J Comput Assist Tomogr.* 2004;28:10–16., with permission.)

Toxoplasma gondii

Toxoplasma gondii is an obligate intracellular protozoan parasite, which invades subclinically (latent form) a large portion of the adult population (up to 70% in some areas) (117). Toxoplasmosis is the most frequent opportunistic brain infection in patients with AIDS (117). Pulmonary toxoplasmosis is rare (118, 119). The most common radiographic findings include a fine reticulonodular or ground-glass pattern similar to that seen in patients with PCP (120).

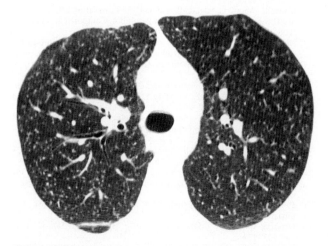

Figure 7.28 Cryptococcosis. High-resolution computed tomography (CT) scan (1-mm collimation) at the level of the upper lobes shows numerous small nodules in a random distribution characteristic of miliary disease. The patient was a 37-year-old man with acquired immunodeficiency syndrome.

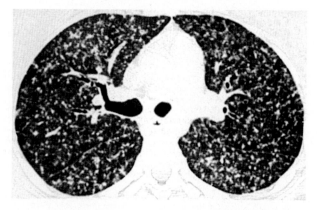

Figure 7.29 Histoplasmosis. High-resolution computed tomography (CT) scan (1-mm collimation) at the level of carina shows numerous small nodules in a random distribution characteristic of miliary disease. The patient was a 19-year-old man with acquired immunodeficiency syndrome. (From Marchiori E, Müller NL, Soares Souza A Jr, et al. Pulmonary disease in patients with AIDS: High-resolution CT and pathologic findings. *Am J Roentgenol.* 2005;184:757–764, with permission.)

REFERENCES

1. Maki DD. Pulmonary infections in HIV/AIDS. *Semin Roentgenol.* 2000; 35:124–139.
2. Meduri GU, Stein DS. Pulmonary manifestations of acquired immunodeficiency syndrome. *Clin Infect Dis.* 1992;14:98–113.
3. Afessa B, Green B. Clinical course, prognostic factors, and outcome prediction for HIV patients in the ICU. The PIP (Pulmonary Complications, ICU Support, and Prognostic Factors in Hospitalized Patients with HIV) Study. *Chest.* 2000;118:138–145.
4. Afessa B, Green B. Bacterial pneumonia in hospitalized patients with HIV infection: The Pulmonary Complications, ICU Support, and Prognostic Factors of Hospitalized Patients with HIV (PIP) Study. *Chest.* 2000;117:1017–1022.
5. Yabuuchi H, Murayama S, Murakami J, et al. Correlation of immunologic status with high-resolution CT and distributions of pulmonary tuberculosis. *Acta Radiol.* 2002;43:44–47.
6. Boiselle PM, Aviram G, Fishman JE. Update on lung disease in AIDS. *Semin Roentgenol.* 2002;37:54–71.
7. Castaner E, Gallardo X, Mata JM, et al. Radiologic approach to the diagnosis of infectious pulmonary diseases in patients infected with the human immunodeficiency virus. *Eur J Radiol.* 2004;51:114–129.
8. Barry SM, Lipman MC, Johnson MA, et al. Respiratory infections in immunocompromised patients. *Curr Opin Pulm Med.* 1999;5:168–173.
9. Boiselle PM, Crans CA Jr, Kaplan MA. The changing face of Pneumocystis carinii pneumonia in AIDS patients. *Am J Roentgenol.* 1999;172: 1301–1309.
10. Bankier AA, Stauffer F, Fleischmann D, et al. Radiographic findings in patients with acquired immunodeficiency syndrome, pulmonary infection, and microbiologic evidence of Mycobacterium xenopi. *J Thorac Imaging.* 1998;13:282–288.
11. Crans CA Jr, Boiselle PM. Imaging features of Pneumocystis carinii pneumonia. *Crit Rev Diagn Imaging.* 1999;40:251–284.
12. Boiselle PM, Tocino I, Hooley RJ, et al. Chest radiograph interpretation of Pneumocystis carinii pneumonia, bacterial pneumonia, and pulmonary tuberculosis in HIV-positive patients: Accuracy, distinguishing features, and mimics. *J Thorac Imaging.* 1997;12:47–53.
13. Busi Rizzi E, Schinina V, Palmieri F, et al. Radiological patterns in HIV-associated pulmonary tuberculosis: Comparison between HAART-treated and non-HAART-treated patients. *Clin Radiol.* 2003;58:469–473.
14. Worthy S, Kang EY, Müller NL. Acute lung disease in the immunocompromised host: Differential diagnosis at high-resolution CT. *Semin Ultrasound CT MR.* 1995;16:353–360.
15. Huang L, Stansell JD. AIDS and the lung. *Med Clin North Am.* 1996;80: 775–801.
16. Hiorns MP, Screaton NJ, Müller NL. Acute lung disease in the immunocompromised host. *Radiol Clin North Am.* 2001;39:1137–1151.
17. Hirschtick RE, Glassroth J, Jordan MC, et al. Pulmonary Complications of HIV Infection Study Group. Bacterial pneumonia in persons infected with the human immunodeficiency virus. *N Engl J Med.* 1995;333:845–851.
18. Mayaud C, Parrot A, Cadranel J. Pyogenic bacterial lower respiratory tract infection in human immunodeficiency virus-infected patients. *Eur Respir J Suppl.* 2002;36:28s–39s.

19. McGuinness G. Changing trends in the pulmonary manifestations of AIDS. *Radiol Clin North Am.* 1997;35:1029–1082.
20. Afessa B, Green W, Chiao J, et al. Pulmonary complications of HIV infection: Autopsy findings. *Chest.* 1998;113:1225–1229.
21. Levy H, Kallenbach JM, Feldman C, et al. Acute respiratory failure in active tuberculosis. *Crit Care Med.* 1987;15:221–225.
22. Janoff EN, Breiman RF, Daley CL, et al. Pneumococcal disease during HIV infection. Epidemiologic, clinical, and immunologic perspectives. *Ann Intern Med.* 1992;117:314–324.
23. Janoff EN, Rubins JB. Invasive pneumococcal disease in the immunocompromised host. *Microb Drug Resist.* 1997;3:215–232.
24. Aaron L, Saadoun D, Calatroni I, et al. Tuberculosis in HIV-infected patients: A comprehensive review. *Clin Microbiol Infect.* 2004;10:388–398.
25. Franquet T. Respiratory infection in the AIDS and immunocompromised patient. *Eur Radiol.* 2004;14(suppl 3):E21–E33.
26. Kuhlman JE. Imaging pulmonary disease in AIDS: State of the art. *Eur Radiol.* 1999;9:395–408.
27. Shah RM, Salazar AM. CT manifestations of human immunodeficiency virus (HIV)-related pulmonary infections. *Semin Ultrasound CT MR.* 1998; 19:167–174.
28. Aviram G, Fishman JE, Sagar M. Cavitary lung disease in AIDS: Etiologies and correlation with immune status. *AIDS Patient Care STDS.* 2001; 15:353–361.
29. Padley SP, King LJ. Computed tomography of the thorax in HIV disease. *Eur Radiol.* 1999;9:1556–1569.
30. Primack SL, Müller NL. High-resolution computed tomography in acute diffuse lung disease in the immunocompromised patient. *Radiol Clin North Am.* 1994;32:731–744.
31. McGuinness G, Naidich DP, Garay S, et al. AIDS associated bronchiectasis: CT features. *J Comput Assist Tomogr.* 1993;17:260–266.
32. McGuinness G, Gruden JF, Bhalla M, et al. AIDS-related airway disease. *Am J Roentgenol.* 1997;168:67–77.
33. Im JG, Itoh H, Shim YS, et al. Pulmonary tuberculosis: CT findings—early active disease and sequential change with antituberculous therapy. *Radiology.* 1993;186:653–660.
34. Aquino SL, Gamsu G, Webb WR, et al. Tree-in-bud pattern: Frequency and significance on thin section CT. *J Comput Assist Tomogr.* 1996;20:594–599.
35. Girardi E, Raviglione MC, Antonucci G, et al. Impact of the HIV epidemic on the spread of other diseases: The case of tuberculosis. *Aids.* 2000;14(suppl 3):S47–S56.
36. Barnes PF, Bloch AB, Davidson PT, et al. Tuberculosis in patients with human immunodeficiency virus infection. *N Engl J Med.* 1991;324: 1644–1650.
37. Laissy JP, Cadi M, Cinqualbre A, et al. Mycobacterium tuberculosis versus nontuberculous mycobacterial infection of the lung in AIDS patients: CT and HRCT patterns. *J Comput Assist Tomogr.* 1997;21:312–317.
38. Bock N, Reichman LB. Tuberculosis and HIV/AIDS: Epidemiological and clinical aspects (world perspective). *Semin Respir Crit Care Med.* 2004;25: 337–344.
39. Keiper MD, Beumont M, Elshami A, et al. CD4 T lymphocyte count and the radiographic presentation of pulmonary tuberculosis. A study of the relationship between these factors in patients with human immunodeficiency virus infection. *Chest.* 1995;107:74–80.
40. Leung AN. Pulmonary tuberculosis: The essentials. *Radiology.* 1999;210: 307–322.
41. Perlman DC, el-Sadr WM, Nelson ET, et al. Variation in chest radiographic patterns in pulmonary tuberculosis by degree of human immunodeficiency virus-related immunosuppression. The Terry Beirn Community Programs for Clinical Research on AIDS (CPCRA). The AIDS Clinical Trials Group (ACTG). *Clin Infect Dis.* 1997;25:242–246.
42. Pastores SM, Naidich DP, Aranda CP, et al. Intrathoracic adenopathy associated with pulmonary tuberculosis in patients with human immunodeficiency virus infection. *Chest.* 1993;103:1433–1437.
43. Im JG, Song KS, Kang HS, et al. Mediastinal tuberculous lymphadenitis: CT manifestations. *Radiology.* 1987;164:115–119.
44. Greenberg SD, Frager D, Suster B, et al. Active pulmonary tuberculosis in patients with AIDS: Spectrum of radiographic findings (including a normal appearance). *Radiology.* 1994;193:115–119.
45. Kramer F, Modilevsky T, Waliany AR, et al. Delayed diagnosis of tuberculosis in patients with human immunodeficiency virus infection. *Am J Med.* 1990;89:451–456.
46. Hartman TE, Primack SL, Müller NL, et al. Diagnosis of thoracic complications in AIDS: Accuracy of CT. *Am J Roentgenol.* 1994;162:547–553.
47. Leung AN, Brauner MW, Gamsu G, et al. Pulmonary tuberculosis: Comparison of CT findings in HIV-seropositive and HIV-seronegative patients. *Radiology.* 1996;198:687–691.
48. Haramati LB, Jenny-Avital ER, Alterman DD. Effect of HIV status on chest radiographic and CT findings in patients with tuberculosis. *Clin Radiol.* 1997;52:31–35.
49. Im JG, Itoh H, Lee KS, et al. CT-pathology correlation of pulmonary tuberculosis. *Crit Rev Diagn Imaging.* 1995;36:227–285.
50. Marinelli DL, Albelda SM, Williams TM, et al. Nontuberculous mycobacterial infection in AIDS: Clinical, pathologic, and radiographic features. *Radiology.* 1986;160:77–82.
51. Primack SL, Logan PM, Hartman TE, et al. Pulmonary tuberculosis and Mycobacterium avium-intracellulare: A comparison of CT findings. *Radiology.* 1995;194:413–417.
52. Monill JM, Franquet T, Sambeat MA, et al. Mycobacterium genavense infection in AIDS: Imaging findings in eight patients. *Eur Radiol.* 2001;11: 193–196.
53. Erasmus JJ, McAdams HP, Farrell MA, et al. Pulmonary nontuberculous mycobacterial infection: Radiologic manifestations. *Radiographics.* 1999;19: 1487–1505.
54. Moore EH. Atypical mycobacterial infection in the lung: CT appearance. *Radiology.* 1993;187:777–782.
55. Shelburne SA III, Hamill RJ. The immune reconstitution inflammatory syndrome. *AIDS Rev.* 2003;5:67–79.
56. Lawn SD, Bekker LG, Miller RF. Immune reconstitution disease associated with mycobacterial infections in HIV-infected individuals receiving antiretrovirals. *Lancet Infect Dis.* 2005;5:361–373.
57. Vilchez RA, Irish W, Lacomis J, et al. The clinical epidemiology of pulmonary cryptococcosis in non-AIDS patients at a tertiary care medical center. *Medicine (Baltimore).* 2001;80:308–312.
58. Breen RA, Smith CJ, Cropley I, et al. Does immune reconstitution syndrome promote active tuberculosis in patients receiving highly active antiretroviral therapy? *Aids.* 2005;19:1201–1206.
59. Buckingham SJ, Haddow LJ, Shaw PJ, et al. Immune reconstitution inflammatory syndrome in HIV-infected patients with mycobacterial infections starting highly active anti-retroviral therapy. *Clin Radiol.* 2004;59: 505–513.
60. McGuinness G, Scholes JV, Garay SM, et al. Cytomegalovirus pneumonitis: Spectrum of parenchymal CT findings with pathologic correlation in 21 AIDS patients. *Radiology.* 1994;192:451–459.
61. Waxman AB, Goldie SJ, Brett-Smith H, et al. Cytomegalovirus as a primary pulmonary pathogen in AIDS. *Chest.* 1997;111:128–134.
62. Olliff JF, Williams MP. Radiological appearances of cytomegalovirus infections. *Clin Radiol.* 1989;40:463–467.
63. Kang EY, Patz EF Jr, Müller NL. Cytomegalovirus pneumonia in transplant patients: CT findings. *J Comput Assist Tomogr.* 1996;20:295–299.
64. Tamm M, Traenkle P, Grilli B, et al. Pulmonary cytomegalovirus infection in immunocompromised patients. *Chest.* 2001;119:838–843.
65. Moon JH, Kim EA, Lee KS, et al. Cytomegalovirus pneumonia: High-resolution CT findings in ten non-AIDS immunocompromised patients. *Korean J Radiol.* 2000;1:73–78.
66. Davies SF, Sarosi GA. Fungal pulmonary complications. *Clin Chest Med.* 1996;17:725–744.
67. Stansell JD. Pulmonary fungal infections in HIV-infected persons. *Semin Respir Infect.* 1993;8:116–123.
68. Sider L, Westcott MA. Pulmonary manifestations of cryptococcosis in patients with AIDS: CT features. *J Thorac Imaging.* 1994;9:78–84.
69. Sarosi GA, Johnson PC. Progressive disseminated histoplasmosis in the acquired immunodeficiency syndrome: A model for disseminated disease. *Semin Respir Infect.* 1990;5:146–150.
70. Sarosi GA, Johnson PC. Disseminated histoplasmosis in patients infected with human immunodeficiency virus. *Clin Infect Dis.* 1992;14(suppl 1): S60–S67.
71. Gruden JF, Huang L, Turner J, et al. High-resolution CT in the evaluation of clinically suspected Pneumocystis carinii pneumonia in AIDS patients with normal, equivocal, or nonspecific radiographic findings. *Am J Roentgenol.* 1997;169:967–975.
72. Bianco R, Arborio G, Mariani P, et al. Pneumocystis carinii lung infections in AIDS patients: A study with High-Resolution Computed Tomography (HRCT). *Radiol Med (Torino).* 1996;91:370–376.
73. Hidalgo A, Falco V, Mauleon S, et al. Accuracy of high-resolution CT in distinguishing between Pneumocystis carinii pneumonia and non-Pneumocystis carinii pneumonia in AIDS patients. *Eur Radiol.* 2003;13: 1179–1184.
74. Marchiori E, Müller NL, Soares Souza A Jr, et al. Pulmonary disease in patients with AIDS: High-resolution CT and pathologic findings. *Am J Roentgenol.* 2005;184:757–764.
75. Franquet T, Gimenez A, Hidalgo A. Imaging of opportunistic fungal infections in immunocompromised patient. *Eur J Radiol.* 2004;51:130–138.
76. Logan PM, Finnegan MM. Pulmonary complications in AIDS: CT appearances. *Clin Radiol.* 1998;53:567–573.
77. Logan PM, Primack SL, Staples C, et al. Acute lung disease in the immunocompromised host. Diagnostic accuracy of the chest radiograph. *Chest.* 1995;108:1283–1287.
78. Denning DW. Invasive aspergillosis. *Clin Infect Dis.* 1998;26:781–803; quiz 804–785.
79. Denning DW. Early diagnosis of invasive aspergillosis. *Lancet.* 2000; 355:423–424.
80. Flores KM, White CS, Wisniewski P, et al. Invasive pulmonary aspergillosis: CT diagnosis of a peribronchial sinus track in an AIDS patient. *J Comput Assist Tomogr.* 1994;18:495–496.
81. Miller WT Jr, Sais GJ, Frank I, et al. Pulmonary aspergillosis in patients with AIDS. Clinical and radiographic correlations. *Chest.* 1994;105: 37–44.

82. Marr KA, Patterson T, Denning D. Aspergillosis. Pathogenesis, clinical manifestations, and therapy. *Infect Dis Clin North Am.* 2002;16:875–894, vi.

83. Franquet T, Müller NL, Oikonomou A, et al. Aspergillus infection of the airways: Computed tomography and pathologic findings. *J Comput Assist Tomogr.* 2004;28:10–16.

84. Staples CA, Kang EY, Wright JL, et al. Invasive pulmonary aspergillosis in AIDS: Radiographic, CT, and pathologic findings. *Radiology.* 1995;196:409–414.

85. Aquino SL, Kee ST, Warnock ML, et al. Pulmonary aspergillosis: Imaging findings with pathologic correlation. *Am J Roentgenol.* 1994;163:811–815.

86. Franquet T, Müller NL, Gimenez A, et al. Spectrum of pulmonary aspergillosis: Histologic, clinical, and radiologic findings. *Radiographics.* 2001; 21:825–837.

87. Franquet T, Serrano F, Gimenez A, et al. Necrotizing aspergillosis of large airways: CT findings in eight patients. *J Comput Assist Tomogr.* 2002; 26:342–345.

88. Mamelak AN, Obana WG, Flaherty JF, et al. Nocardial brain abscess: Treatment strategies and factors influencing outcome. *Neurosurgery.* 1994; 35:622–631.

89. Cameron ML, Bartlett JA, Gallis HA, et al. Manifestations of pulmonary cryptococcosis in patients with acquired immunodeficiency syndrome. *Rev Infect Dis.* 1991;13:64–67.

90. Stansell JD. Fungal disease in HIV-infected persons: Cryptococcosis, histoplasmosis, and coccidioidomycosis. *J Thorac Imaging.* 1991;6:28–35.

91. Minamoto G, Armstrong D. Fungal infections in AIDS. Histoplasmosis and coccidioidomycosis. *Infect Dis Clin North Am.* 1988;2:447–456.

92. Lacomis JM, Costello P, Vilchez R, et al. The radiology of pulmonary cryptococcosis in a tertiary medical center. *J Thorac Imaging.* 2001;16: 139–148.

93. Zinck SE, Leung AN, Frost M, et al. Pulmonary cryptococcosis: CT and pathologic findings. *J Comput Assist Tomogr.* 2002;26:330–334.

94. Conces DJ Jr, Stockberger SM, Tarver RD, et al. Disseminated histoplasmosis in AIDS: Findings on chest radiographs. *Am J Roentgenol.* 1993;160: 15–19.

95. McAdams HP, Rosado-de-Christenson ML, Lesar M, et al. Thoracic mycoses from endemic fungi: Radiologic-pathologic correlation. *Radiographics.* 1995;15:255–270.

96. Ampel NM, Ryan KJ, Carry PJ, et al. Fungemia due to Coccidioides immitis. An analysis of 16 episodes in 15 patients and a review of the literature. *Medicine (Baltimore).* 1986;65:312–321.

97. Sarosi GA, Davies SF. Blastomycosis. *Am Rev Respir Dis.* 1979;120:911–938.

98. Davies SF, Sarosi GA. Blastomycosis. *Eur J Clin Microbiol Infect Dis.* 1989; 8:474–479.

99. Pappas PG, Threlkeld MG, Bedsole GD, et al. Blastomycosis in immunocompromised patients. *Medicine (Baltimore).* 1993;72:311–325.

100. Recht LD, Davies SF, Eckman MR, et al. Blastomycosis in immunosuppressed patients. *Am Rev Respir Dis.* 1982;125:359–362.

101. Harding CV. Blastomycosis and opportunistic infections in patients with acquired immunodeficiency syndrome. An autopsy study. *Arch Pathol Lab Med.* 1991;115:1133–1136.

102. Foltzer MA, Guiney WB Jr, Wager GC, et al. Bronchopulmonary Bacillary angiomatosis. *Chest.* 1993;104:973–975.

103. Goodman P, Balachandran S. Bacillary angiomatosis in a patient with HIV infection. *Am J Roentgenol.* 1993;160:207–208.

104. Slater LN, Min KW. Polypoid endobronchial lesions. A manifestation of Bacillary angiomatosis. *Chest.* 1992;102:972–974.

105. Blanche P, Bachmeyer C, Salmon-Ceron D, et al. Muscular bacillary angiomatosis in AIDS. *J Infect.* 1998;37:193.

106. Gasquet S, Maurin M, Brouqui P, et al. Bacillary angiomatosis in immunocompromised patients. *Aids.* 1998;12:1793–1803.

107. Rosales CM, McLaughlin MD, Sata T, et al. AIDS presenting with cutaneous Kaposi's sarcoma and bacillary angiomatosis in the bone marrow mimicking Kaposi's sarcoma. *AIDS Patient Care STDS.* 2002;16:573–577.

108. Sandrasegaran K, Hawes DR, Matthew G. Hepatic peliosis (Bacillary angiomatosis) in AIDS: CT findings. *Abdom Imaging.* 2005;30:738–740.

109. Santos R, Cardoso O, Rodrigues P, et al. Bacillary angiomatosis by Bartonella quintana in an HIV-infected patient. *J Am Acad Dermatol.* 2000; 42:299–301.

110. Simpson GL, Stinson EB, Egger MJ, et al. Nocardial infections in the immunocompromised host: A detailed study in a defined population. *Rev Infect Dis.* 1981;3:492–507.

111. Choucino C, Goodman SA, Greer JP, et al. Nocardial infections in bone marrow transplant recipients. *Clin Infect Dis.* 1996;23:1012–1019.

112. Yoon HK, Im JG, Ahn JM, et al. Pulmonary nocardiosis: CT findings. *J Comput Assist Tomogr.* 1995;19:52–55.

113. Buckley JA, Padhani AR, Kuhlman JE. CT features of pulmonary nocardiosis. *J Comput Assist Tomogr.* 1995;19:726–732.

114. Rimland D, Navin TR, Lennox JL, et al. Prospective study of etiologic agents of community-acquired pneumonia in patients with HIV infection. *Aids.* 2002;16:85–95.

115. Pedro-Botet ML, Sabria M, Sopena N, et al. Legionnaires disease and HIV infection. *Chest.* 2003;124:543–547.

116. Tan MJ, Tan JS, Hamor RH, et al. The Ohio Community-Based Pneumonia Incidence Study Group. The radiologic manifestations of Legionnaire's disease. *Chest.* 2000;117:398–403.

117. Hofman P, Michiels JF, Saint-Paul MC, et al. Toxoplasmosis in AIDS patients. Pathoclinical study of 78 cases. *Ann Pathol.* 1993;13:233–240.

118. Schnapp LM, Geaghan SM, Campagna A, et al. Toxoplasma gondii pneumonitis in patients infected with the human immunodeficiency virus. *Arch Intern Med.* 1992;152:1073–1077.

119. Campagna AC. Pulmonary toxoplasmosis. *Semin Respir Infect.* 1997;12: 98–105.

120. Rottenberg GT, Miszkiel K, Shaw P, et al. Case report: Fulminant Toxoplasma gondii pneumonia in a patient with AIDS. *Clin Radiol.* 1997; 52:472–474.

Immunocompromised Host

8

INTRODUCTION

Infection is the main pulmonary complication and the commonest cause of radiographic abnormality in immuno-compromised non–acquired immunodeficiency syndrome (AIDS) patients (1–7). The number of these patients has increased considerably in the last two decades because of greater number of hematopoietic stem cell (bone marrow) and solid organ transplantations, advances in the treatment of cancer, and increased use of immunosuppressive ther-apy in a number of other conditions (8–16). A wide variety of pulmonary infections may occur in these patients and result in considerable morbidity and mortality (17–22).

Immunocompromised non–AIDS patients are at risk not only for developing infections that occur in immuno-competent patients but also for infections that do not affect patients with normal immunity (opportunistic infections).

Awareness of the type and severity of the immunologic defect can be helpful in predicting the most likely organisms responsible for the infection. For example, gram-negative bacteria, *Aspergillus* and *Candida*, should be the primary considerations in patients with severe neutropenia.

Imaging Approach

Chest radiography has been shown to be important in the diagnosis and management of immunocompromised patients with a suspected respiratory infection (1, 23–26). It remains the first and foremost imaging modality used in the evaluation of these patients and in most cases provides adequate imaging information. However, it has limited sensitivity for the detection of early infection being normal in up to 10% of patients with proved pulmonary disease (27,28). Serial chest radiographs are often requested to detect pulmonary disease, but faint opacities may be difficult to detect, especially in patients who are unable to take a full inspiration. Furthermore, neutrophil counts are often low, resulting in a poor inflammatory response, which may further decrease the sensitivity of the chest radiograph.

Computed tomography (CT) scan is more sensitive and specific than chest radiography in the detection of subtle pulmonary abnormalities. CT scan is particularly helpful in the assessment of patients with acute pulmonary disease and a high clinical suspicion for pneumonia but with normal or questionable radiographic findings. Heussel et al. (26) performed CT scan in neutropenic patients with unexplained fever and a normal chest radiograph. CT scan demonstrated findings consistent with pneumonia in 60% of cases 5 days before any abnormalities were evident on the chest radiograph.

The most common patterns seen on high-resolution CT scan in acute pulmonary infections are nodules,

TABLE 8.1

HIGH-RESOLUTION COMPUTED TOMOGRAPHY PATTERNS IN PULMONARY INFECTIONS: MOST COMMON CAUSES

Extensive bilateral ground-glass opacity: *Pneumocystis* and cytomegalovirus
Nodules:
  <1 cm diameter: Viral pneumonia
  >1 cm diameter: Invasive aspergillosis and septic embolism
  CT "halo sign": Invasive aspergillosis, candidiasis, cytomegalovirus pneumonia
  Cavitated nodules: Septic embolism, invasive aspergillosis
  "Tree-in-bud" pattern: Infectious bronchiolitis of any cause
Consolidation:
  Lobar: Pneumococcus, *Klebsiella*
  Rounded: Pneumococcus, *Legionella*
  Bronchopneumonia: Gram-negative bacteria, staphylococcus

CT, computed tomography.

centrilobular branching linear and nodular opacities ("tree-in-bud" pattern), ground-glass opacities, consolidation, or a combination of these (see Table 8.1) (1, 28). Ground-glass opacities are a common but nonspecific CT scan finding that may result from bacterial, fungal, or viral pneumonia (29–31) or from noninfectious conditions such as drug-induced lung disease, pulmonary edema, and pulmonary hemorrhage. However, in severely immunocompromised patients, particularly following hematopoietic stem cell or organ transplantation, extensive bilateral ground-glass opacities should raise the possibility of *Pneumocystis* or cytomegalovirus (CMV) pneumonia.

In the appropriate clinical setting, high-resolution CT scan findings may result in a change in clinical management or add confidence to the diagnosis. For example, focal airspace consolidation, with or without cavitation, has been shown to be most commonly caused by bacterial infection. Less commonly, it may result from invasive aspergillosis and mycobacterial infection. A predominantly nodular pattern is seen in a variety of infections. The presence of a halo of ground-glass attenuation, indicating hemorrhage surrounding the nodule, is characteristic of angioinvasive aspergillosis (32–34). Although the CT scan halo sign in patients with severe neutropenia is most suggestive of invasive aspergillosis, a similar pattern may also be seen in candida, CMV, varicella, and herpes simplex pneumonia (35–37).

Transplant Recipients

Pneumonia is a common complication following hematopoietic stem cell and solid organ transplantation (8, 14–16,

24, 38). The etiology of pneumonia includes bacteria and opportunistic organisms and can be established from sputum culture, bronchoalveolar lavage (BAL), blood culture, or fine needle aspiration (39–41).

Hematopoietic stem cell transplantation is currently the treatment of choice for various hematologic malignancies and severe congenital or acquired disorders of the hematopoietic or immune systems (19, 42). It is estimated that >50,000 stem cell transplantations are performed annually worldwide (19, 42). Infectious and noninfectious pulmonary complications can occur in 40% to 60% of hematopoietic stem cell transplant recipients, being most frequent in allogeneic transplant recipients (26, 43).

Complications following hematopoietic stem cell transplantation have been classified according to the time of presentation into early (pre-engraftment phase) and late (postengraftment phase) depending on whether they occur before or after 100 days following transplantation (see Table 8.2) (19, 42, 44, 45). During the initial post-transplantation period, patients are profoundly neutropenic (absolute neutrophil count <500 cells per μL) and most microbiologically documented pneumonias are caused by fungi or bacteria (46). If neutropenia is prolonged beyond 2 weeks, *Aspergillus* sp and other opportunistic fungi may cause life-threatening infections (47). While fungi are the most common cause of pulmonary infection in the early pre-engraftment phase (first 30 days post-transplantation), viruses most commonly occur in the postengraftment phase. Conversely, in the late postengraftment phase, from day 100 until the patient regains normal immunity, usually 1 to 2 years later, most infections are caused by bacteria (42, 45, 46).

Solid organ transplantation has become the treatment of choice for patients with end-stage diseases of the kidney, liver, heart, and lung. Renal transplantation accounts for more than half of all solid organ transplantations performed in the United States, and the liver is the second most commonly transplanted solid organ (25, 44).

The type of infection following solid organ transplantation is influenced by the type of transplantation and the

TABLE 8.2

PULMONARY INFECTIONS AFTER HEMATOPOIETIC STEM CELL TRANSPLANTATION

Type of infection is influenced by the time following transplantation
Early complications (<100 d post-transplantation)
  Pre-engraftment phase (0–30 d): Aspergillus, candida, bacteria
  Postengraftment phase (31–100 d): Cytomegalovirus, bacteria
Late complications (>100 d post-transplantation)
  Most infections caused by bacteria

time interval since transplantation (48–50). Infections are common following lung transplantation and relatively uncommon following kidney transplantation due to the less rigorous surgical procedure required to implant the allograft and the lower level of immunosuppression required to maintain it (43).

Post-transplantation complications have been classified according to the time following the surgical procedure. The post-transplantation period can be subdivided into postoperative (0 to 30 days), early (31 to 180 days post-transplantation) and late (>6 months post-transplantation) (43). Infections are more frequent and most varied during the first 6 months after transplantation (44). In the postoperative period, nosocomial transmission of respiratory viruses and common gram-positive and gram-negative organisms frequently occurs through contaminated hands of hospital personnel. After the first 6 months, the risk of infection correlates directly with the degree of immunosuppression needed to forestall graft rejection (43).

The differential diagnosis of pulmonary infiltrates in transplant recipients remains a difficult diagnostic challenge (1, 7, 42). The differential diagnosis is broad and includes both infectious and noninfectious causes such as hemorrhage, drug-induced lung disease, pulmonary edema, and pulmonary embolism (45). Unfortunately, the clinical data and radiographic findings often fail to lead to a definitive diagnosis of pneumonia because there is an extensive number of noninfectious processes associated with fever and pneumonitis that may mimic pulmonary infection, including drug-induced pulmonary disease, organizing pneumonia, and pulmonary vasculitis (1, 27, 45).

Aspirates obtained during fiberoptic bronchoscopy and BAL have the highest diagnostic yield and impact on therapeutic decisions (51). Diagnostic information may also be obtained by transbronchial biopsy or percutaneous needle aspiration (52, 53). The combined use of clinical information, knowledge of typical conditions associated with the host's immunodeficiency, and radiographic patterns offers a useful approach to the diagnosis of pulmonary disease in these patients.

FUNGI

Fungal infections are responsible for >10% of pulmonary infections in hematopoietic stem cell transplant recipients and approximately 5% of pulmonary infections in solid organ transplant recipients (34, 54, 55). Fungal infection can occur at any time but invasive disease occurs most commonly within the first 6 months of transplantation. The main risk factors for invasive aspergillosis are severe neutropenia and prolonged high-dose corticosteroid therapy (50).

Pneumocystis jiroveci (*carinii*), *Aspergillus fumigatus*, and *Candida albicans* are the most common fungi causing pulmonary infection in immunocompromised patients.

Other less common fungal pathogens are *Cryptococcus neoformans*, *Mucor*, and endemic fungi such as *Histoplasma capsulatum*, *Coccidioides immitis*, and *Blastomyces*.

Pneumocystis Jiroveci (Carinii)

Pneumocystises are unicellular organisms currently classified as fungi. They include several species that are host-specific. The *Pneumocystis* that infects humans does not infect animals and was recently renamed *P. jiroveci*. *Pneumocystis carinii* on the other hand infects only rats. *P. jiroveci* causes pneumonia only in immunocompromised patients, particularly patients with AIDS, lymphoproliferative disorders, and with organ or hematopoietic stem cell transplantation (see Table 8.3) (1, 12, 55–57). The organism probably resides normally on the alveolar surface, where it is maintained in low numbers by host defense mechanisms. The most common histologic pattern of pulmonary infection consists of finely vacuolated eosinophilic material within alveolar airspaces accompanied by a variably severe infiltrate of lymphocytes and plasma cells in the adjacent interstitium. The foamy material consists of solitary and encysted organisms, which can be detected with special stains as round or helmet-shaped structures admixed with host-derived material such as surfactant and fibrin. Other histologic reaction patterns include granulomatous inflammation and diffuse alveolar damage (58). Patients typically present with insidious symptoms of fever, nonproductive cough, and dyspnea. A definitive diagnosis of *Pneumocystis* pneumonia (PCP) requires the demonstration of organisms in sputum or BAL fluid.

The characteristic initial radiographic manifestation is that of bilateral symmetric ground-glass opacities. These tend to involve mainly the perihilar regions but may be diffuse or involve mainly the lower or upper lung zones (see Fig. 8.1). Unless the patient is treated, the ground-glass

TABLE 8.3
***PNEUMOCYSTIS* PNEUMONIA**

Risk factors: Lymphoproliferative disorders, transplantation, AIDS

Common radiographic findings:

    Bilateral symmetric ground-glass opacities or fine reticulonodular pattern

    Tends to involve mainly the perihilar regions

    May be diffuse or involve mainly the lower or upper lung zones

Common high-resolution CT scan findings:

    Bilateral symmetric ground-glass opacities

    May be patchy or diffuse

    May have superimposed fine linear pattern ("crazy paving" pattern)

AIDS, acquired immunodeficiency syndrome; CT, computed tomography.

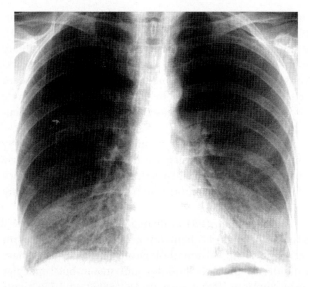

Figure 8.1 *Pneumocystis* pneumonia in lymphoma. Anteroposterior chest radiograph shows bilateral ground-glass opacities and small areas of consolidation involving mainly the lower lung zones. The patient was a 55-year-old woman undergoing chemotherapy for lymphoma.

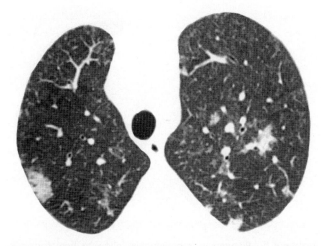

Figure 8.3 *Pneumocystis* pneumonia following allogeneic hematopoietic stem cell transplantation. High-resolution computed tomography (CT) (2-mm collimation) image at the level of upper lobes shows bilateral ground-glass opacities and several small foci of consolidation. Also noted are several poorly defined small nodules. The patient was a 41-year-old man.

opacities progress over 3 to 5 days to homogeneous diffuse airspace consolidation. The pattern may be mistaken for pulmonary edema, but the heart size is usually normal (59). Hilar lymphadenopathy and pleural effusion are distinctly unusual.

The characteristic high-resolution CT scan manifestations of PCP include extensive symmetric bilateral ground-glass opacities (see Fig. 8.2). Small nodules, foci of consolidation, and linear opacities may be seen in association with the ground-glass opacities (see Figs. 8.3 and 8.4). The presence of septal lines and smooth intralobular linear opacities superimposed on the ground-glass opacities results in a pattern known as *crazy paving* (60–63). Sharp demarcation between normal and

abnormal parenchyma results in a mosaic or geographic appearance (see Fig. 8.5).

Thin-walled cystic spaces superimposed on the ground-glass opacities are relatively uncommon in non–AIDS patients. The cystic lesions represent pneumatoceles and are associated with an increased prevalence of pneumothorax (64, 65). The cysts are usually multiple and tend to decrease in size or resolve after the acute stage of the infection (see Fig. 8.6). They are most common in the upper lobes.

Atypical manifestations of PCP include miliary nodules, nodular areas of consolidation (see Fig. 8.7), large nodules, and focal masses or mass-like areas of consolidation.

Candida Albicans

Candida albicans is a ubiquitous dimorphic fungus identified in tissue as both oval budding yeast and hyphae. Pulmonary candidiasis is seen mainly in patients with

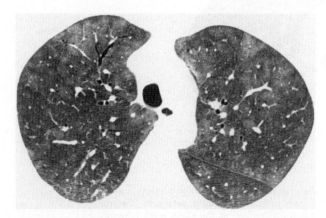

Figure 8.2 *Pneumocystis* pneumonia (PCP) in lymphoma. High-resolution computed tomography (CT) image (1-mm collimation) at the level of aortic arch shows extensive bilateral ground-glass opacities. The findings are a common and characteristic feature of PCP. The patient was a 55-year-old woman (same patient as in Figure 8.1).

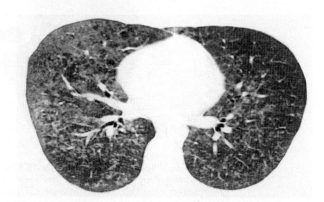

Figure 8.4 *Pneumocystis* pneumonia in acute myeloid leukemia. High-resolution computed tomography (CT) image (2-mm collimation) at the level of inferior pulmonary veins shows extensive bilateral ground-glass opacities and several poorly defined small nodules. The patient was a 28-year-old man.

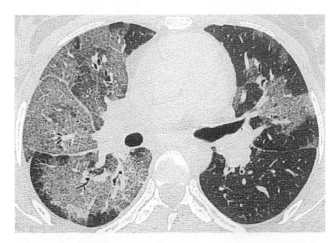

Figure 8.5 *Pneumocystis* pneumonia following hematopoietic stem cell transplantation. High-resolution computed tomography (CT) image (1-mm collimation) at the level of the bronchus intermedius shows asymmetric bilateral ground-glass opacities. Note sharp demarcation between the normal and abnormal lung resulting in a mosaic or geographic pattern. The patient was a 34-year-old man.

hematologic malignancies (acute leukemia and lymphoma) and in intravenous drug users (see Table 8.4) (49). It usually accompanies widespread infection of the urinary tract, gastrointestinal tract, liver, spleen, or central nervous system. Factors that predispose hematopoietic stem cell transplant recipients to candida infections include allogeneic transplant, increased age, and a prolonged neutropenia (49, 66).

The chest radiographic manifestations include patchy unilateral or bilateral airspace consolidation and poorly defined nodules (67,68). These findings reflect the presence of necrotizing bronchopneumonia. Occasionally, miliary disease is seen (68).

Franquet et al. (69) evaluated the high-resolution CT scan findings in 17 hematopoietic stem cell transplant recipients with histopathologically proved pulmonary candidiasis. Multiple nodules and tree-in-bud opacities were common, being seen in 15 (88%) of 17 patients and 7 (41%), respectively (see Fig. 8.8). The nodules were bilateral in 12 patients and unilateral in 3. Nodules were

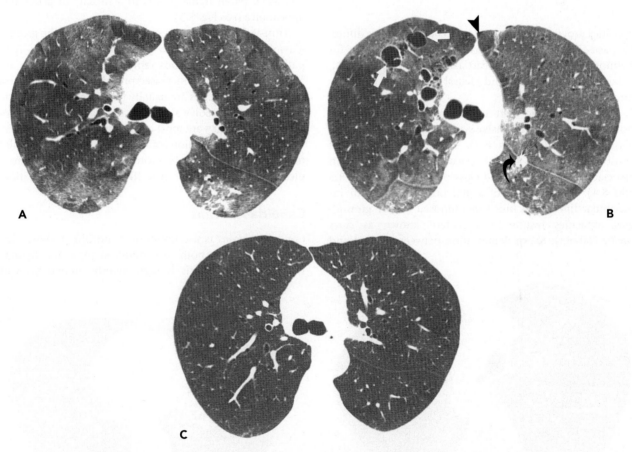

Figure 8.6 *Pneumocystis* pneumonia (PCP) with pneumatocele formation. High-resolution computed tomography (CT) image at the level of the main bronchi **(A)** shows extensive bilateral ground-glass opacities. High-resolution CT image (1-mm collimation) at the same level 1 month later **(B)** shows several pneumatoceles (straight *arrows*) in the right upper lobe. Also noted is a small left pneumothorax (*arrowhead*) and a left chest tube in the major fissure (*curved arrow*). The patient was a 55-year-old woman who developed PCP while undergoing treatment for non-Hodgkin lymphoma. The pneumonia resolved but no follow-up images immediately following resolution of the pneumonia were available. High-resolution CT image 3 years later **(C)** demonstrates resolution of the pneumatoceles.

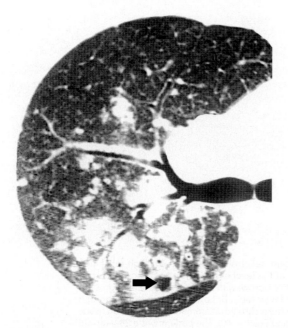

Figure 8.7 Atypical presentation of *Pneumocystis* pneumonia (PCP). View of the right upper lobe on high-resolution computed tomography (CT) scan (1-mm collimation) shows ground-glass opacities, multiple nodular opacities, and foci of consolidation. Also noted is a small cavity (*arrow*). The patient was a 28-year-old man hematopoietic stem cell recipient. Large nodules and nodular areas of consolidation are an uncommon presentation of PCP. Cavitation is rare.

an isolated CT scan finding in 5 patients. An associated halo of ground-glass opacity was present in five of 15 (33%) patients with nodules (see Fig. 8.9). Airspace consolidation was present in 11 (65%) patients and ground-glass opacities in 6 (35%) (see Figs. 8.9 and 8.10). They concluded that the most common high-resolution CT

TABLE 8.4
PULMONARY CANDIDIASIS

Main risk factors: Leukemia, allogeneic hematopoietic stem cell transplantation, intravenous drug abuse
Common radiographic findings:
    Unilateral or bilateral areas of consolidation
    Poorly defined nodules
Common high-resolution CT scan findings:
    Multiple bilateral nodules
    CT halo sign
    Patchy or confluent areas of consolidation

CT, computed tomography.

scan findings of pulmonary candidiasis in hematopoietic stem cell transplant recipients are multiple bilateral nodular opacities often associated with consolidation. Definitive diagnosis of pulmonary candidiasis requires demonstration of the organism in tissue (68, 69).

Aspergillus Fumigatus

Pulmonary aspergillosis is usually acquired by inhalation of the organisms normally present in the environment. It occurs almost exclusively in individuals who have structural lung abnormality (such as a cavity), atopy, or deficiency of the inflammatory or immunologic reactions. The pathologic and radiologic manifestations of the disease can be divided into three main forms: Aspergilloma, allergic bronchopulmonary aspergillosis (ABPA), and invasive aspergillosis. The last named in turn can be subdivided into

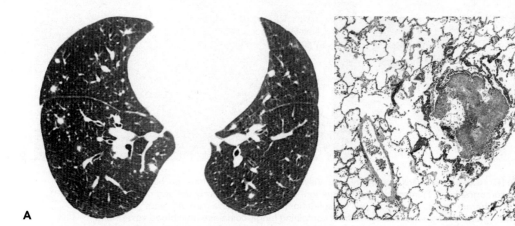

Figure 8.8 Candida pneumonia following hematopoietic stem cell transplantation. **A:** High-resolution computed tomography (CT) image (1-mm collimation) at the level of the inferior pulmonary veins shows multiple bilateral nodules with surrounding halo of ground-glass attenuation. **B:** Photomicrograph of lung specimen shows nodular inflammatory focus consisting of colonies of *Candida* centered on a blood vessel. Surrounding the nodule there is mild inflammatory interstitial thickening and engorgement of alveolar capillaries. (Hematoxylin and Eosin × 200). The patient was a 52-year-old man. (From Franquet T, Müller NL, Lee KS, et al. Pulmonary candidiasis after hematopoietic stem cell transplantation: Thin-section CT findings. *Radiology.* 2005;236:332–337, with permission.)

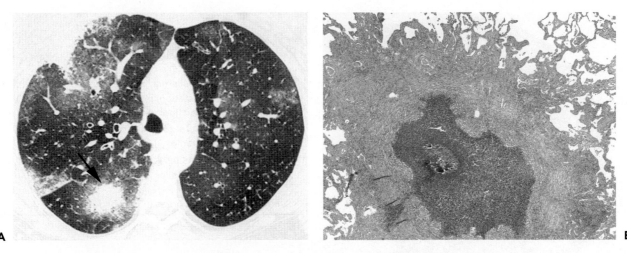

A
B

Figure 8.9 Candidiasis following hematopoietic stem cell transplantation. **A:** High-resolution computed tomography (CT) image (1-mm collimation) at the level of the aortic arch shows bilateral ground-glass opacities, foci of consolidation, and a nodule (*arrow*) with a surrounding halo of ground-glass attenuation in the superior segment of the right lower lobe. **B:** Low power photomicrograph of lung specimen shows intravascular candidiasis and diffuse chronic inflammatory granulation tissue response centered on pulmonary artery. (Hematoxylin and Eosin × 40). The patient was a 28-year-old man. (From Franquet T, Müller NL, Lee KS, et al. Pulmonary candidiasis after hematopoietic stem cell transplantation: Thin-section CT findings. *Radiology.* 2005;236:332–337, with permission.)

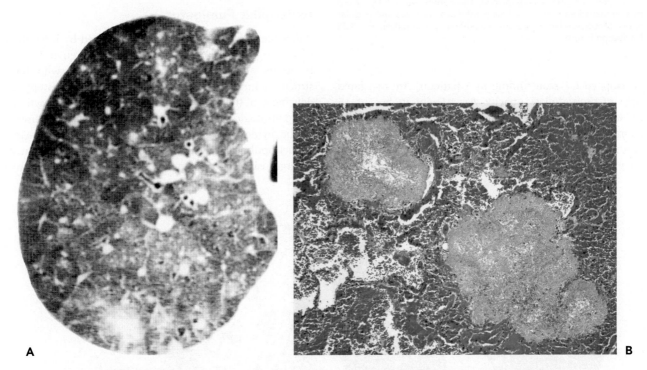

A
B

Figure 8.10 *Candida albicans* pneumonia. **A:** View of the right upper lobe on high-resolution computed tomography (CT) image (1-mm collimation) shows multiple poorly defined centrilobular nodules of different sizes, small foci of consolidation, and extensive ground-glass opacities. **B:** Photomicrograph shows a hemorrhagic infarct containing fungal colonies within blood vessels and the infarcted tissue. (Hematoxylin and Eosin × 400). The patient was a 25-year-old man with acute myeloid leukemia and hematopoietic stem cell transplant. (From Franquet T, Müller NL, Lee KS, et al. Pulmonary candidiasis after hematopoietic stem cell transplantation: Thin-section CT findings. *Radiology.* 2005;236:332–337, with permission.)

angioinvasive, bronchopneumonic (airway invasive), and chronic necrotizing (semi-invasive) forms (64, 65, 70–72).

Invasive Pulmonary Aspergillosis

Invasive pulmonary aspergillosis occurs only in immuno-compromised patients and it is the most common opportunistic pulmonary fungal infection. Risk factors for invasive aspergillosis include severe or prolonged neutropenia (absolute neutrophil count <500 per mm^3), prolonged corticosteroid therapy, graft-versus-host disease after hematopoietic stem cell transplantation, and late-stage AIDS (see Table 8.5) (32, 50). Infection begins when aerosolized spores are inhaled into the distal airways and airspaces. In the absence of an effective host immune response, the spores mature into hyphae that can invade the pulmonary arteries. This results in pulmonary arterial thrombosis, hemorrhage, lung necrosis, and systemic dissemination (50, 73, 74).

Affected patients present with fever, cough, and dyspnea. Symptoms suggestive of pulmonary embolism, such as pleuritic chest pain, may also occur. The diagnosis of invasive aspergillosis is difficult because the organism can normally colonize the upper airway. The diagnosis is based on clinical, radiologic, and mycological data. On the basis of the findings, the likelihood of *Aspergillus* infection can be classified into proved, likely, and possible (10). Specimens obtained from normally sterile but clinically abnormal sites (e.g., needle biopsy of the lung lesion or surgical lung biopsy) are the most reliable and considered necessary to prove the diagnosis. Mycologic evidence acquired by means of either direct examination or culture of specimens from sites that may be colonized (e.g., sputum, BAL fluid) are helpful in supporting the likely diagnosis but do not prove the diagnosis. Similarly, galactomannan and nucleic acid detection in serum or in BAL fluid are supportive of the diagnosis but do not prove it; definite diagnosis of invasive

aspergillosis requires the demonstration of the fungus in tissue specimens (75). Furthermore, the potential value of early diagnostic tests such as the galactomannan needs to be confirmed in prospective trials (76).

Thrombocytopenia in these patients may preclude invasive diagnostic procedures such as percutaneous or transbronchial biopsy. Cultures of BAL fluid are positive in 30% to 68% of infected patients.

Mortality rates from infection are high (50% to 70%). Patient outcomes are influenced by early institution of antifungal therapy, severity of the underlying disease, and rapidity of granulocyte recovery.

The radiographic manifestations of angioinvasive pulmonary aspergillosis usually include multiple, ill-defined 1- to 3-cm diameter nodular opacities (see Fig. 8.11). The nodular opacities gradually increase in size and may progress to subsegmental, segmental, or lobar consolidation.

The high-resolution CT scan findings include multiple nodules involving mainly the peripheral lung and the lower lobes. Another common finding is the presence of pleural-based wedge-shaped areas of consolidation. High-resolution CT scan frequently demonstrates a rim of ground-glass attenuation surrounding several of the nodules (CT halo sign) (see Fig. 8.12) (32). Although the CT halo sign has been described in several other entities (37), in the appropriate clinical setting of a patient with severe neutropenia and recent onset of fever, it is highly suggestive of invasive aspergillosis. Cavitation of the nodules occurs in 40% of affected patients and often has a

---

TABLE 8.5

ANGIOINVASIVE PULMONARY ASPERGILLOSIS

Main risk factor: Severe neutropenia (absolute neutrophil count <500/mm^3)

Common radiographic findings:

　Bilateral poorly defined nodules

　Single or multiple foci of consolidation

Common high-resolution CT scan findings:

　Multiple, 1 to 3 cm diameter nodules

　CT halo sign (nodule surrounded by rim of ground-glass opacity)

　Pleural-based wedge-shaped areas of consolidation

　Cavitation with or without air-crescent sign

CT, computed tomography.

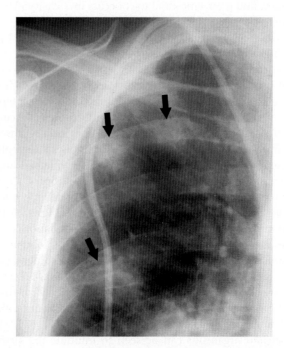

Figure 8.11 Angioinvasive aspergillosis following hematopoietic stem cell transplantation. View of the right upper lobe on a posteroanterior chest radiograph shows ill-defined nodular opacities (*arrows*). Also noted is a central venous line. The patient was a 54-year-old man.

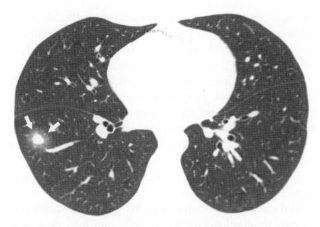

Figure 8.12 Computed tomography (CT) halo sign in angioinvasive aspergillosis. High-resolution CT image (1-mm collimation) shows right lower lobe nodule surrounded by rim of ground-glass attenuation (CT halo sign) (*arrows*). The patient was a 28-year-old woman with severe neutropenia due to acute myelogenous leukemia and chemotherapy.

distinctive radiologic appearance, the air-crescent sign (see Fig. 8.13) (32, 50, 77). The air-crescent sign results from an intracavitary mass composed of necrotic lung that has separated from the adjacent viable tissue and filling of the remaining space by air. It characteristically occurs 2 to 3 weeks after initiation of treatment and is concomitant with resolution of the neutropenia, and usually indicates a good prognosis (32, 50).

Pleural effusion is uncommon and lymphadenopathy is rare. Systemic dissemination to the central nervous system, kidney, and gastrointestinal tract occurs in 25% to 50% of patients.

Airway invasive aspergillosis accounts for about 15% to 30% of cases of invasive disease (54, 78, 79). The most common manifestations are *Aspergillus* bronchiolitis and bronchopneumonia. The histologic findings include liquefactive necrosis and a neutrophilic infiltrate centered on membranous and respiratory bronchioles. Vascular infiltration and coagulative necrosis are usually absent or minimal in extent. The most common radiographic presentation includes patchy unilateral or bilateral areas of consolidation (see Fig. 8.14). High-resolution CT scan demonstrates centrilobular nodular and branching linear opacities ("tree-in-bud" pattern) (see Figs. 8.14, 8.15, 8.16) and unilateral or bilateral areas of consolidation (77). The areas of consolidation often have a lobular or segmental distribution but may become confluent (see Fig. 8.17). Histologically, the high-resolution CT scan findings correspond to foci of necrotizing bronchitis and bronchiolitis, typically associated with a neutrophilic inflammatory reaction (Figs. 8.15 and 8.16) (73, 74). *Aspergillus* organisms can be seen to infiltrate the airway walls and the immediately adjacent parenchyma (79).

Another distinct form of airway invasive aspergillosis is chronic necrotizing bronchial aspergillosis. This is an infrequent but serious complication seen in approximately 5% of lung transplant recipients (79). The histologic findings include *Aspergillus* invasion of tracheal and bronchial mucosa without extension into the lung parenchyma. As with more invasive forms of fungal infection, the degree of immunosuppression is probably the most important factor leading to bronchial wall invasion (79). High-resolution CT scan demonstrates bronchial wall thickening, smooth or irregular bronchial narrowing, and multiple endobronchial nodules.

Mucormycosis (Zygomycosis)

Mucormycosis is an uncommon opportunistic infection caused by fungi of the class *Zygomycetes*, order *Mucorales* (80). The main risk factors are diabetes mellitus, hematologic malignancy, renal failure, organ transplantation, and metabolic acidosis (see Table 8.6) (80, 81). Pulmonary mucormycosis occurs almost exclusively in immunocompromised patients, particularly in those with hematologic malignancies. Pathologic examination demonstrates confluent pneumonia or pulmonary infarction and hemorrhage secondary to vascular thrombosis. Abscess formation may occur (36, 82).

Radiographs show areas of consolidation and solitary or multiple nodules or masses. The consolidation may be patchy or confluent, unilateral or bilateral (see Fig. 8.18). Cavitation is frequent. Pleural effusion is seen in up to 20% of patients and hilar or mediastinal lymphadenopathy in <10% of patients (36, 82, 83). CT scan findings include focal or diffuse areas of consolidation, single or multiple nodules or masses and, frequently, cavitation (Fig. 8.18). CT scan may demonstrate findings not apparent on chest radiography including bronchial occlusion due to endobronchial mucormycosis, CT halo sign, and pulmonary artery pseudoaneurysm formation (36).

TABLE 8.6
MUCORMYCOSIS
Uncommon opportunistic infection
Caused by fungi of the class *Zygomycetes*, order *Mucorales*
Risk factors: Hematologic malignancy, transplantation, diabetes mellitus
Common radiographic findings:
Unilateral or bilateral areas of consolidation
Single or multiple nodules
Cavitation is common
Common high-resolution CT scan findings:
Focal or diffuse areas of consolidation
Single or multiple nodules or masses
Cavitation is common

CT, computed tomography.

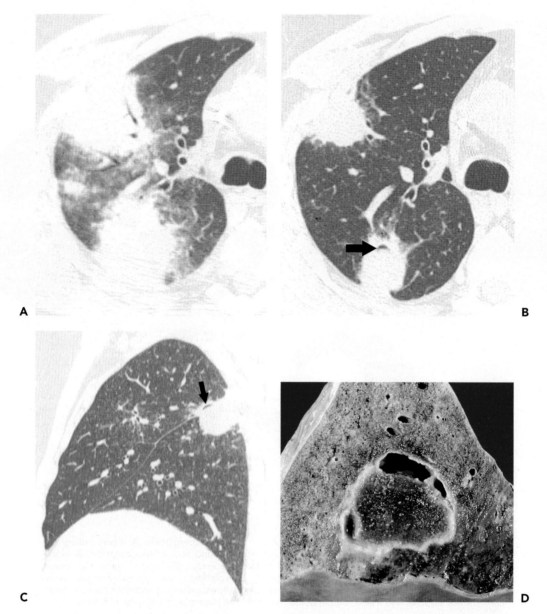

Figure 8.13 Air-crescent sign in angioinvasive aspergillosis. **A:** View of the right upper lobe on high-resolution computed tomography (CT) scan (1-mm collimation) obtained on a multidetector CT scanner shows pleural-based wedge-shaped areas of consolidation and small nodule with surrounding halo of ground-glass attenuation (CT halo sign). **B:** View of the right upper lobe on high-resolution CT scan (1-mm collimation) obtained 27 days later shows improvement. Note crescent shaped gas collection in the periphery of the nodule (*arrow*) (air-crescent sign). **C:** Sagittal image better demonstrates the air-crescent (*arrow*). The patient was a 33-year-old man with acute myelogenous leukemia. **D:** Photograph of pathologic specimen in a different patient shows a thick-walled cavity with corresponding air-crescent formation. The intracavitary mass represents necrotic lung that has separated from the adjacent viable tissue.

Although the presence of organisms in a culture from the respiratory tract is suggestive, definite diagnosis requires histologic demonstration of the organism in affected tissue. Overall mortality rate of pulmonary mucormycosis is 45% (80). Early recognition and aggressive management are required to maximize the chances for a cure. Patients treated with a combined medical–surgical approach have a better outcome than those who do not undergo surgery (80).

BACTERIA

Bacterial infections are common particularly in patients with neutropenia (46). The list of pathogens that can cause pneumonia in these patients is extensive, but a narrow spectrum accounts for most cases. The most common bacterial pathogen seen following hematopoietic stem cell transplantation is *Pseudomonas*; other common organisms include *Nocardia*, *Legionella*, *Haemophilus influenzae*, and

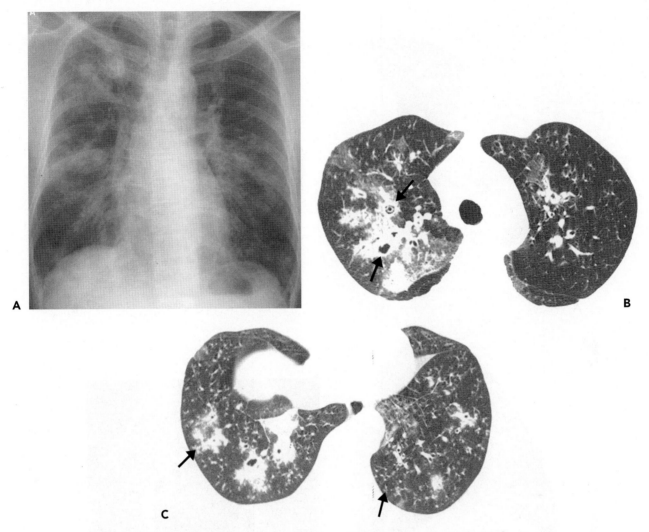

Figure 8.14 *Aspergillus* bronchopneumonia (airway invasive aspergillosis). **A:** Chest radiograph shows poorly defined multifocal bilateral nodular opacities and foci of consolidation. **B:** High-resolution computed tomography (CT) image (1-mm collimation) at the level of aortic arch shows cavitating nodular opacities (*arrows*), focal areas of consolidation, and ground-glass opacities. **C:** CT scan obtained at level of the right hemidiaphragm shows cavitating nodular opacities, small centrilobular nodules and tree-in-bud opacities (*arrows*). The patient was a 49-year-old man.

Enterobacter (1, 9, 10, 84, 85). Clinical symptoms of bacterial infection include fever, cough, and progressive dyspnea.

Bacterial pneumonias following solid organ transplantation do not differ appreciably from pneumonias seen in the normal host (20). Infections may be either nosocomial or community-acquired and may be caused by single or multiple pathogens, including *Staphylococcus aureus*, and gram-negative organisms, such as *Pseudomonas aeruginosa* or *Klebsiella pneumoniae* (20). *Nocardia* infections were common in the early era of organ transplantation but are now relatively uncommon (86, 87). Most bacterial infections occur during the immediate postoperative period and mainly affect patients receiving mechanical ventilation (8, 11). Other infectious complications are mediastinitis and empyema.

Streptococcus pneumoniae is the most common cause of pneumonia following heart–lung and lung transplantation.

It occurs in up to 50% of cases during the first 6 months after transplantation and accounts for up to 50% of early postoperative mortality (11). Community-acquired bacterial pneumonias occur later in the post-transplantation period. *H. influenzae, S. pneumoniae*, and *Legionella* species are among the commonly identified organisms (43, 88). Lung transplant recipients with cystic fibrosis show a particularly high incidence of pneumonia, presumably because of chronic colonization by *P. aeruginosa* or *Burkholderia cepacia complex* (14–16).

Gram-negative bacterial pneumonia is the most common infection during the first month after heart transplantation because of prolonged intubation, pulmonary edema, and effects of surgery on lung mechanics (11). Gram-negative bacteria (*Enterobacter* and *Pseudomonas*) are also a common cause of infection after kidney and liver transplantation (14–16).

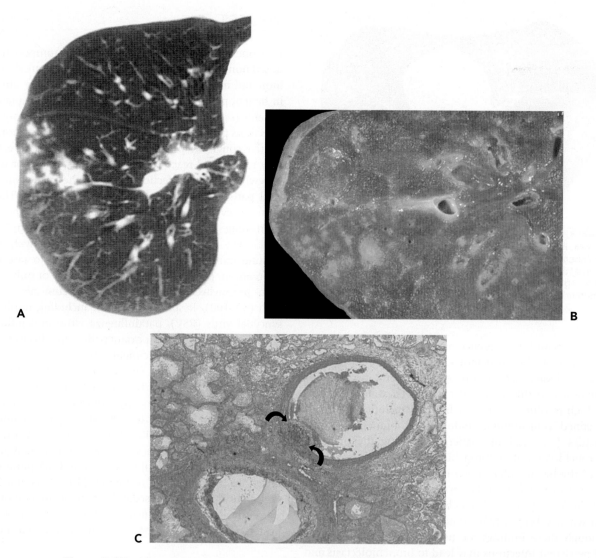

Figure 8.15 *Aspergillus* bronchiolitis. **A:** High-resolution computed tomography (CT) image (2-mm collimation) at the level of the carina shows focal small centrilobular nodules and branching linear opacities ("tree-in-bud" pattern). **B:** Magnified view of gross lung specimen shows multiple branching lesions suggesting a relation with small airways. **C:** Highly magnified view of bronchioles shows a small colony of *Aspergillus* invading the bronchiolar wall (*arrows*). Peribronchiolar areas of consolidation can also be seen. The patient was a 23-year-old man with acute myeloid leukemia and hematopoietic stem cell transplant.

The radiographic findings include single or multiple foci of consolidation, that may be patchy or have a segmental or lobar distribution (1, 8, 9, 11). Pseudomonas, *Escherichia coli* and *S. aureus* usually present with patchy unilateral or bilateral areas of consolidation typical of bronchopneumonia. *Enterobacter* may result in bronchopneumonia or confluent consolidation occupying a segment or lobe. *Legionella pneumophila* most commonly results in lobar or multilobar consolidation (see Fig. 8.19) or in round areas of consolidation (2, 3, 24). A rounded appearance (rounded pneumonia) is most commonly due to *S. pneumoniae* but a more typical presentation of pneumococcal pneumonia is the lobar consolidation (see Fig. 8.20).

The chest radiograph may be normal in up to 30% of patients with bacterial pneumonia (1, 2, 24, 89). A normal radiograph is particularly common in the early phases of pneumonia and in patients with severe neutropenia. High-resolution CT scan may demonstrate parenchymal abnormalities consistent with pneumonia in patients with normal radiographs. The high-resolution CT scan findings include unilateral or bilateral areas of airspace consolidation in a patchy or lobar distribution (see Fig. 8.21). Other findings may include ground-glass opacities, centrilobular nodules, and centrilobular branching structures ("tree-in-bud" pattern) (89).

Pyogenic airways disease, usually caused by *S. pneumoniae* and *Staphylococcus*, is common in hematopoietic stem cell transplant recipients. Pyogenic bronchiolitis is characterized histologically by an active cellular bronchitis and bronchiolitis with mononuclear cell inflammation of

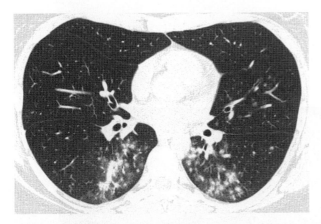

Figure 8.16 *Aspergillus* bronchiolitis in acute lymphoblastic leukemia. High-resolution computed tomography (CT) scan shows centrilobular nodular and branching opacities ("tree-in-bud" pattern) in both lower lobes. Also noted are a few centrilobular nodules in the lingula. The patient was a 38-year-old woman receiving chemotherapy for acute lymphoblastic leukemia.

the airways and the presence of an inflammatory exudate and mucus in the bronchiolar lumen (30, 90–92). Bronchogenic dissemination of pyogenic bacteria can result in dilatation and thickening of bronchiolar walls. The typical high-resolution CT scan findings include: (a) Small ill-defined centrilobular nodular and branching linear opacities ("tree-in-bud" pattern) reflecting the presence of bronchiolar and peribronchiolar inflammation and filling of the bronchiolar lumen inflammatory material and (b) focal areas of consolidation due to bronchopneumonia (see Fig. 8.22) (90, 93). Larger branching opacities are also seen when subsegmental bronchial impaction is present. Although these findings are usually reversible, recurrent and persistent infections may lead to bronchiolectasis and bronchiectasis (93).

VIRUSES

Viral pneumonias occur in up to 50% of immunocompromised non–AIDS patients (30, 94–96). Viruses are the common and important causes of serious respiratory illnesses in hematopoietic stem cell and solid organ transplant recipients (see Table 8.7) (17, 95–97). Most respiratory viral infections produce acute symptoms such as fever, nonproductive cough, dyspnea, and hypoxemia. These infections may result from reactivation of a latent process or reflect a newly acquired infection. CMV is the most common viral pathogen in transplant recipients (43, 98). The reported prevalence of CMV pneumonia in renal, heart or heart–lung, and liver transplantations ranges from 5% to 30%, 16% to 34%, and 2% to 32%, respectively (43). In lung transplant recipients CMV appears to target the graft, and in patients who have received no or only short-term prophylaxis the incidence of pneumonia is very high (99, 100). Respiratory viruses, including respiratory syncytial virus (RSV), parainfluenza virus, and influenza virus, have emerged as important pathogens affecting up to 20% of lung transplant recipients (101, 102).

In hematopoietic stem cell recipients, CMV pulmonary infection remains one of the major complications in the postengraftment phase, mostly within the first 4 months, being responsible for up to 50% of cases of pneumonia in some large series (24, 43, 88, 98). Community-acquired respiratory viral infections such as RSV, influenza A and B, and parainfluenza, account for most non–CMV pulmonary infections in transplant recipients (19, 84, 94, 95, 103). Pulmonary infections caused by human metapneumovirus, a recently identified ribonucleic acid (RNA) virus, have also been reported in hematopoietic stem cell recipients (104).

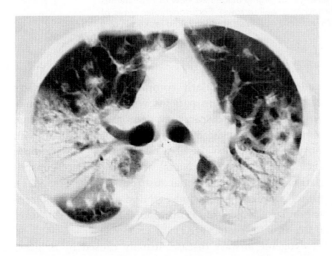

Figure 8.17 *Aspergillus* bronchopneumonia in a liver transplant recipient. Computed tomography (CT) scan (8-mm collimation) at the level of the main bronchi shows extensive bilateral airspace consolidation with air-bronchograms. The patient was a 52-year-old man.

TABLE 8.7
VIRAL PULMONARY INFECTIONS

Occur in up to 50% of immunocompromised non–AIDS patients

Main risk factor: Transplantation

Cytomegalovirus is the commonest viral pathogen in transplant recipients

Respiratory viruses occur in up to 20% of lung transplant recipients

Common radiographic findings:
    Bilateral reticulonodular pattern
    Patchy bilateral areas of consolidation

Common high-resolution CT scan findings:
    Multiple small centrilobular nodules
    Unilateral or bilateral
    Patchy areas of consolidation
    Ground-glass opacities

CT, computed tomography.

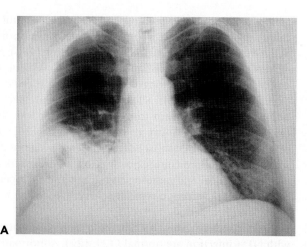
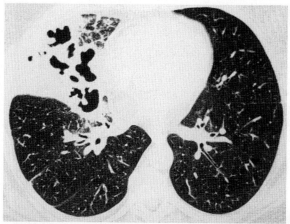

Figure 8.18   Mucormycosis. **A:** Posteroanterior chest radiograph demonstrates consolidation with cavitation in the right lower lung zone. **B:** High-resolution computed tomography (CT) image (1-mm collimation) shows cavitated consolidation in the middle lobe and several septal lines. The patient was a 58-year-old man with severe neutropenia.

The chest radiograph is frequently normal in patients with viral infection but may show bronchopneumonia or focal or diffuse reticulonodular opacities. Other radiographic manifestations include ground-glass opacities and small nodules (7, 88, 105).

High-resolution CT scan manifestations of CMV pneumonia include multiple small nodular opacities, areas of consolidation, and ground-glass opacities (see Figs. 8.23–8.25) (29, 31, 106). The abnormalities are usually bilateral and may be symmetric or asymmetric. The nodules tend to have a centrilobular distribution reflecting the presence of bronchiolitis. Small nodular opacities have also been reported in patients with adenovirus, influenza virus, herpes simplex virus, and herpes varicella-zoster virus pulmonary infections (107–109). The CT scan features of metapneumovirus infection in hematopoietic stem cell recipients are indistinguishable from those of other causes

of viral pneumonia. They most commonly consist of a mixture of patterns including small nodules, ground-glass opacities, and patchy areas of consolidation. The nodules are centrilobular in distribution and tend to be associated with branching opacities ("tree-in-bud" pattern) (see Fig. 8.26) (110). Nodule size has been shown to be helpful in the differential diagnosis of pulmonary infections in immunocompromised patients. Patients whose nodules are all <10 mm in diameter are most likely to have a viral infection (35).

MYCOBACTERIA

Although the risk of active tuberculosis in transplant recipients is 30 to 50 times higher than in the general

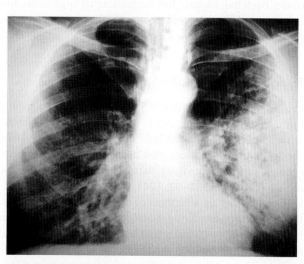

Figure 8.19   *Legionella* pneumonia in a renal transplant recipient. Posteroanterior chest radiograph shows extensive left upper lobe consolidation. The patient was a 56-year-old man.

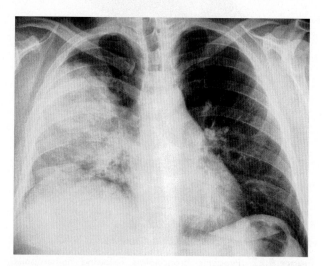

Figure 8.20   Pneumococcal pneumonia in a renal transplant recipient. Posteroanterior chest radiograph shows dense consolidation in the right lung involving mainly the right upper lobe. *Streptococcus pneumoniae* was isolated from the sputum. The patient was a 45-year-old man.

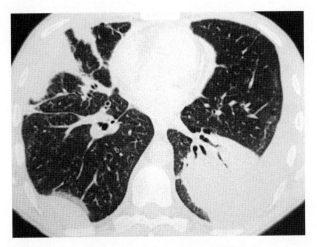

Figure 8.21 Pneumococcal pneumonia following liver transplantation. High-resolution computed tomography (CT) image (2-mm collimation) at the level of the lower lung zones shows multiple peripheral pleural-based areas of consolidation. Bilateral pleural effusions with some loculated collections are also demonstrated. The patient was a 48-year-old man.

population, infection with *M. tuberculosis* is an uncommon post-transplant infection in developed countries. Tuberculosis has been reported in about 0.5% to 2% of organ transplant recipients in the United States and Europe (111–116).

Major risk factors for development of tuberculosis include reactivation of latent infection acquired prior to transplantation or transmission through the donor

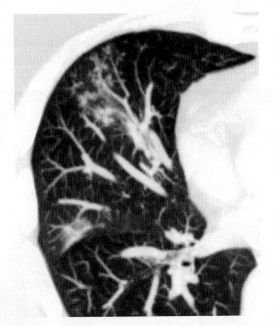

Figure 8.22 Pyogenic bronchiolitis following hematopoietic stem cell transplantation. A magnified maximum-intensity projection computed tomography (CT) image of the right lung shows multiple branching linear opacities and a few centrilobular nodules in the right middle lobe. The findings are characteristic of infectious bronchiolitis. The patient was a 51-year-old man.

organ (117). Among lung transplant recipients, nontuberculous mycobacteria (NTM) may be more common than *M. tuberculosis* as a cause of pulmonary infection (118). *Mycobacterium avium-intracellulare complex* (MAC), *M. kansasii*, *and M. abscessus* are among the most common causative organisms. Diagnosis of NTM is often difficult because isolation of the organism from the sputum or BAL fluid can merely denote airway colonization (119, 120). The diagnosis may be established by the combination of a sputum or BAL fluid culture positive for the organism, appropriate clinical and radiologic findings, and therapeutic response. NTM infection typically occurs late in the post-transplantation period (119, 120).

Approximately 20% of chest radiographs in patients with NTM infection are normal (121, 122). Abnormalities seen on chest radiographs and CT scan included multifocal patchy consolidation and ill-defined nodules that may cavitate (121, 122). While pleural effusions are more common in NTM infection than in tuberculosis, miliary disease is rare in NTM pulmonary disease (121, 123).

MILDLY IMMUNOCOMPROMISED PATIENTS

Mildly immunocompromised patients such as the elderly, heavy smokers and alcoholics, and patients with underlying lung disease such as bronchiectasis, chronic obstructive lung disease, or previous tuberculosis, are at increased risk of developing the pulmonary infections. Recent data suggest that these infections are increasing in frequency and may be fatal if untreated (1–4). Clinical symptoms are often insidious and include chronic cough, sputum production, fever, and constitutional symptoms (weight loss and weakness). The slow progression of clinical and radiographic findings (several months to years) may contribute to a delay in diagnosis (1–4). The etiology of infection includes bacterial, fungal, and mycobacterial organisms and is influenced by the predisposing clinical setting and the patient's immunologic status (4, 35, 92).

Pyogenic Airway Infection

Pyogenic airway infection is commonly seen in mildly immunocompromised hosts (30, 90–92, 124). It is characterized histologically by an inflammatory process involving the walls of the bronchi and bronchioles and the presence of an inflammatory exudate and mucus in the airway lumen (30, 90–92, 124). The most common presenting features are shortness of breath, cough, and fever. Bronchiolar abnormalities due to granulomas are also seen in patients with endobronchial spread of tuberculosis and nontuberculous mycobacterial infections (125–132). The high-resolution CT scan findings of infectious bronchiolitis and endobronchial spread of mycobacterial infection include small centrilobular, nodular, and branching linear

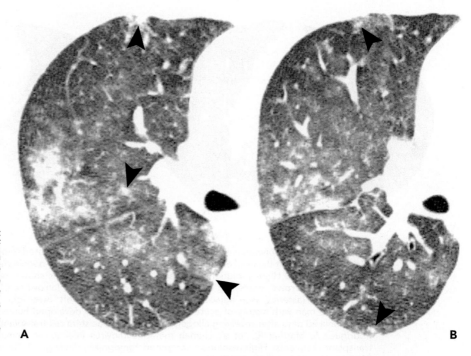

Figure 8.23 Cytomegalovirus pneumonia following hematopoietic stem cell transplantation. Views of the right lung on high-resolution computed tomography (CT) image (1-mm collimation) at the level of the bronchus intermedius **(A)**, slightly more caudally **(B)**, show ground-glass opacities, small foci of consolidation, and a few small nodules (*arrows*). The patient was a 23-year-old man.

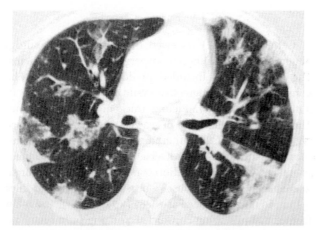

Figure 8.24 Cytomegalovirus pneumonia following liver transplantation. High-resolution computed tomography (CT) image (2-mm collimation) at the level of the bronchus intermedius shows multiple peripheral lobular and subsegmental areas of consolidation and ground-glass opacities in both lungs. The patient was a 52-year-old man. (From Franquet T, Lee KS, Müller NL. Thin-section CT findings in 32 immunocompromised patients with cytomegalovirus pneumonia who do not have AIDS. *Am J Roentgenol.* 2003;181:1059–1063, with permission.)

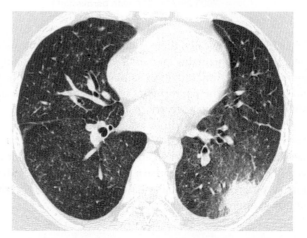

Figure 8.25 Cytomegalovirus pneumonia. High-resolution computed tomography (CT) image (2-mm collimation) at the level of inferior pulmonary veins shows focal area of consolidation in left lower lobe surrounded by halo of ground-glass attenuation. The patient was a 23-year-old man with acute myeloid leukemia and hematopoietic stem cell transplant. (From Franquet T, Lee KS, Müller NL. Thin-section CT findings in 32 immunocompromised patients with cytomegalovirus pneumonia who do not have AIDS. *Am J Roentgenol.* 2003;181:1059–1063, with permission.)

opacities ("tree-in-bud" pattern). The abnormalities tend to have a patchy unilateral or bilateral distribution (Fig. 8.22).

Semi-invasive Pulmonary Aspergillosis

Semi-invasive pulmonary aspergillosis is a chronic localized granulomatous form of aspergillosis, arising in the setting of mild immunologic compromise (see Table 8.8) (70, 133). It clinically resembles a number of other chronic pulmonary diseases including tuberculosis, actinomycosis, and histoplasmosis. The patients are usually middle-aged and have poor nutrition due to alcoholism, diabetes mellitus, chronic granulomatous disease, prolonged corticosteroid administration, chronic obstructive lung disease, or connective tissue disorders (70–72). These patients may have underlying pulmonary abnormalities that result in lowered defense mechanisms, such as scarring from previous mycobacterial infection, chronic obstructive lung disease, previous surgery, radiation therapy, pulmonary infarction or pneumoconiosis (134). Gross specimens show ill-defined consolidation and fibrosis with single or multiple thick-walled cavities; some of the latter represent ectatic

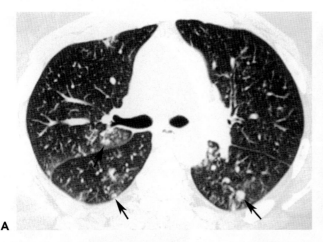 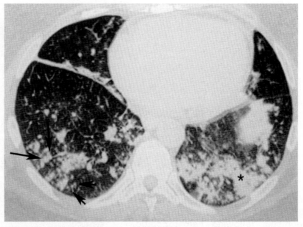

A   **B**

Figure 8.26 Metapneumovirus pneumonia. **A:** High-resolution computed tomography (CT) image (2-mm collimation) at the level of the main bronchi shows bilateral small nodules (*arrows*) and ground-glass opacities. **B:** High-resolution CT image at level of lung bases shows multiple centrilobular nodules (*solid arrows*), branching opacities ("tree-in-bud" pattern) (*arrowheads*), and focal areas of consolidation (*asterisk*) with adjacent ground-glass opacity in left lower lobe. The patient was a 58-year-old man with history of acute myeloid leukemia who developed human metapneumovirus pneumonia 80 days after receiving allogeneic hematopoietic stem cell transplant. (From Franquet T, Rodriguez S, Martino R, et al. Human metapneumovirus infection in hematopoietic stem cell transplant recipients: High-resolution computed tomography findings. *J Comput Assist Tomogr.* 2005;29:223–227, with permission.)

bronchi. Histologically, there is often a mixture of fibrosis and acute or organizing pneumonia. Foci of necrotizing granulomatous inflammation containing fungal hyphae may be seen in the parenchyma or in relation to large or small airways (bronchocentric granulomatosis).

Clinical symptoms include cough, sputum production, fever, and constitutional symptoms (weight loss and weakness), persisting over several months. This time course is different from that of invasive aspergillosis in which the rate of progression is usually days or weeks. Hemoptysis occurs in approximately 15% of patients.

TABLE 8.8
SEMI-INVASIVE PULMONARY ASPERGILLOSIS

Typically seen in mildly immunocompromised patients
Risk factors: COPD, heavy smoking, alcoholism
Symptoms: Chronic cough, sputum production, fever and
  constitutional symptoms over several months
Slow progression of radiographic findings (several months
  to years)
Diagnosis often delayed
Common high-resolution CT scan findings:
  Upper lobe consolidation
  Pleural thickening
  Cavitary consolidation with/without aspergilloma
  Solitary or multiple cavitated or spiculated nodules
    >1 cm

COPD, chronic obstructive pulmonary disease; CT, computed tomography.

Gefter et al. (71) reviewed the radiographic findings of semi-invasive pulmonary aspergillosis in five patients. The abnormalities included predominantly upper lobe consolidation or progressive cystic infiltrate resulting in a thick-walled cavity. Pleural thickening was common. The findings mimic those of reactivation tuberculosis (see Fig. 8.27) (71). CT scan findings of semi-invasive pulmonary aspergillosis are diverse including bronchopneumonia, cavitary consolidation containing an aspergilloma, and solitary or multiple smooth or spiculated nodules >1 cm in diameter (see Fig. 8.28) (70–72, 133). The main feature distinguishing chronic necrotizing pulmonary aspergillosis from aspergilloma developing in a previous cavity is the presence of tissue invasion and destruction (70–72).

Diagnosis is often difficult to make because *Aspergillus* organisms may be present in the sputum or BAL fluid in patients who have colonization of the airways without tissue invasion (135,136). In clinical practice, the diagnosis is usually based on the presence of multiple cultures that are positive for *Aspergillus*, abnormal chest radiograph, and bronchoscopy biopsy specimen consistent with tissue invasion (71). Pathologically, the findings of angioinvasion are lacking.

Nontuberculous Mycobacteria

NTM are a group of ubiquitous, low-grade pathogens that may cause chronic indolent pulmonary infection (120). They are responsible for 0.5% to 30% of all mycobacterial infections. Patients at increased risk for developing pulmonary NTM infection include immunocompromised patients and those with chronic obstructive

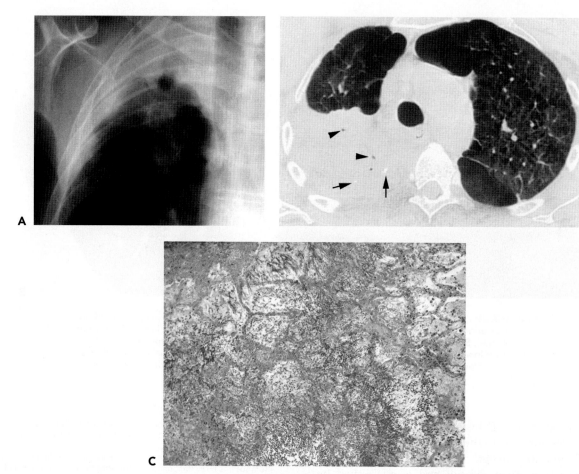

Figure 8.27 Semi-invasive pulmonary aspergillosis. **A:** Posteroanterior chest radiograph shows right apical pleural thickening and poorly defined right upper lobe nodular opacities and consolidation. **B:** Computed tomography (CT) image (8-mm collimation) at the level of the aortic arch shows consolidation in posterior segment of right upper lobe. Multiple small air bubbles (*arrowheads*) and punctate calcifications (*arrows*) are seen within the consolidation. Also noted are bilateral centrilobular and paraseptal emphysema. **C:** Photomicrograph of biopsy specimen obtained from right upper lobe reveals widespread intra-alveolar exudative eosinophil material mixed with acute inflammatory cells, macrophages, and fungal hyphae (Hematoxylin and Eosin × 400). The patient was a 72-year-old man with emphysema and 2-month history of cough and chest discomfort.

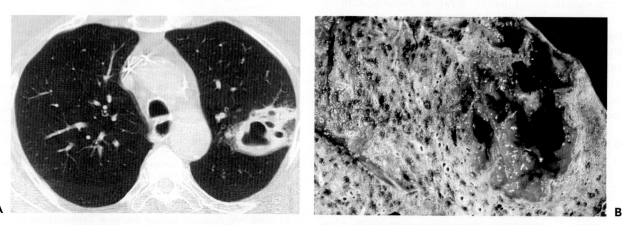

Figure 8.28 Semi-invasive aspergillosis. **A:** High-resolution computed tomography (CT) image (2-mm collimation) at the level of the tracheal carina shows cavitary consolidation in left upper lobe. **B:** Photograph of left upper lobe pathologic specimen from autopsy shows irregular cavitary lesion with regular margins and dark-brown appearance, consisting of necrotic material and *Aspergillus* organisms. The patient was a 68-year-old man with chronic bronchitis and recurrent episodes of mild hemoptysis.

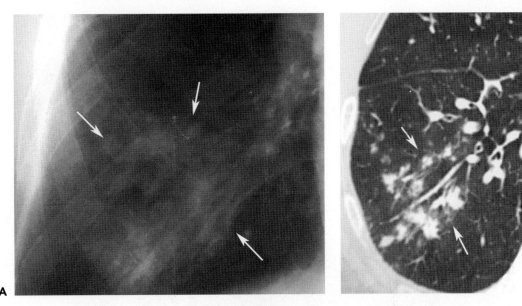

Figure 8.29 *Mycobacterium avium-intracellulare* complex infection. **A:** Close-up view of an anteroposterior chest radiograph shows ill-defined nodular and linear opacities in the right lower lobe (*arrows*). **B:** High-resolution computed tomography (CT) image (2-mm collimation) at the level of the right lower lobe shows multiple centrilobular ill-defined nodules with associated ground-glass opacities (*arrows*). The patient was a 56-year-old woman on long-term steroids for rheumatoid arthritis.

airway disease, smoking history, and alcoholism, and on corticosteroids (137). The most common pathogens are *MAC* and *M. kansasii*. The definite diagnosis of NTM infection is often difficult and is established by a combination of clinical manifestations, culture results positive for the organism, radiologic findings, and response to appropriate therapy (123, 138).

MAC pulmonary disease may manifest as two main patterns: Upper lobe cavitary form and nodular bronchiectatic form (see Chapter 4). The upper lobe cavitary form is the one typically seen in mildly immunocompromised patients. Chest radiographs show ill-defined nodular and linear opacities and patchy areas of consolidation involving mainly the upper lobes. Cavitation is common. High-resolution CT scan demonstrates nodules typically ranging from 0.5 to 2 cm in diameter; small centrilobular, nodular, and branching linear opacities ("tree-in-bud" pattern); focal areas of consolidation; and bronchiectasis (see Fig. 8.29) (120, 121, 138, 139). The findings radiologically resemble those of postprimary tuberculosis (125, 126).

REFERENCES

1. Brown MJ, Miller RR, Müller NL. Acute lung disease in the immuno-compromised host: CT and pathologic examination findings. *Radiology.* 1994;190:247–254.
2. Conces DJ Jr. Pulmonary infections in immunocompromised patients who do not have acquired immunodeficiency syndrome: A systematic approach. *J Thorac Imaging.* 1998;13:234–246.
3. Franquet T. High-resolution computed tomography (HRCT) of lung infections in non–AIDS immunocompromised patients. *Eur Radiol.* 2006; 16:707–718.
4. Gosselin MV. Diffuse lung disease in the immunocompromised non–HIV patient. *Semin Roentgenol.* 2002;37:37–53.
5. Janzen DL, Padley SP, Adler BD, et al. Acute pulmonary complications in immunocompromised non–AIDS patients: Comparison of diagnostic accuracy of CT and chest radiography. *Clin Radiol.* 1993;47:159–165.
6. Logan PM, Primack SL, Staples C, et al. Acute lung disease in the immunocompromised host. Diagnostic accuracy of the chest radiograph. *Chest.* 1995;108:1283–1287.
7. Oh YW, Effmann EL, Godwin JD. Pulmonary infections in immunocom-promised hosts: The importance of correlating the conventional radiologic appearance with the clinical setting. *Radiology.* 2000;217:647–656.
8. Afessa B, Gay PC, Plevak DJ, et al. Pulmonary complications of orthotopic liver transplantation. *Mayo Clin Proc.* 1993;68:427–434.
9. Aronchick JM. Pulmonary infections in cancer and bone marrow transplant patients. *Semin Roentgenol.* 2000;35:140–151.
10. Ascioglu S, Rex JH, de Pauw B, et al. Defining opportunistic invasive fungal infections in immunocompromised patients with cancer and hematopoietic stem cell transplants: An international consensus. *Clin Infect Dis.* 2002;34:7–14.
11. Austin JH, Schulman LL, Mastrobattista JD. Pulmonary infection after cardiac transplantation: Clinical and radiologic correlations. *Radiology.* 1989; 172:259–265.
12. Bag R. Fungal pneumonias in transplant recipients. *Curr Opin Pulm Med.* 2003;9:193–198.
13. Chan CK, Hyland RH, Hutcheon MA. Pulmonary complications following bone marrow transplantation. *Clin Chest Med.* 1990;11:323–332.
14. Ettinger NA, Trulock EP. Pulmonary considerations of organ transplantation. Part I. *Am Rev Respir Dis.* 1991;143:1386–1405.
15. Ettinger NA, Trulock EP. Pulmonary considerations of organ transplantation. Part 3. *Am Rev Respir Dis.* 1991;144:433–451.
16. Ettinger NA, Trulock EP. Pulmonary considerations of organ transplantation. Part 2. *Am Rev Respir Dis.* 1991;144:213–223.
17. Shreeniwas R, Schulman LL, Berkmen YM, et al. Opportunistic bronchopul-monary infections after lung transplantation: Clinical and radiographic findings. *Radiology.* 1996;200:349–356.
18. Singh N, Paterson DL. Aspergillus infections in transplant recipients. *Clin Microbiol Rev.* 2005;18:44–69.
19. Soubani AO, Miller KB, Hassoun PM. Pulmonary complications of bone marrow transplantation. *Chest.* 1996;109:1066–1077.
20. Torres A, Ewig S, Insausti J, et al. Etiology and microbial patterns of pulmonary infiltrates in patients with orthotopic liver transplantation. *Chest.* 2000;117:494–502.
21. Webb WR, Gamsu G, Rohlfing BM, et al. Pulmonary complications of renal transplantation: A survey of patients treated by low-dose immunosuppression. *Radiology.* 1978;126:1–8.
22. Winer-Muram HT, Gurney JW, Bozeman PM, et al. Pulmonary complications after bone marrow transplantation. *Radiol Clin North Am.* 1996; 34:97–117.
23. Choi YH, Leung AN. Radiologic findings: Pulmonary infections after bone marrow transplantation. *J Thorac Imaging.* 1999;14:201–206.

24. Collin BA, Ramphal R. Pneumonia in the compromised host including cancer patients and transplant patients. *Infect Dis Clin North Am.* 1998; 12:781–805.
25. Fishman JE, Rabkin JM. Thoracic radiology in kidney and liver transplantation. *J Thorac Imaging.* 2002;17:122–131.
26. Heussel CP, Kauczor HU, Heussel GE, et al. Pneumonia in febrile neutropenic patients and in bone marrow and blood stem-cell transplant recipients: Use of high-resolution computed tomography. *J Clin Oncol.* 1999;17:796–805.
27. Primack SL, Müller NL. High-resolution computed tomography in acute diffuse lung disease in the immunocompromised patient. *Radiol Clin North Am.* 1994;32:731–744.
28. Worthy S, Kang EY, Müller NL. Acute lung disease in the immunocompromised host: Differential diagnosis at high-resolution CT. *Semin Ultrasound CT MR.* 1995;16:353–360.
29. Kang EY, Patz EF Jr, Müller NL. Cytomegalovirus pneumonia in transplant patients: CT findings. *J Comput Assist Tomogr.* 1996;20:295–299.
30. Franquet T. Respiratory infection in the AIDS and immunocompromised patient. *Eur Radiol.* 2004;14(Suppl 3):E21–E33.
31. Franquet T, Lee KS, Müller NL. Thin-section CT findings in 32 immunocompromised patients with cytomegalovirus pneumonia who do not have AIDS. *Am J Roentgenol.* 2003;181:1059–1063.
32. Kuhlman JE, Fishman EK, Siegelman SS. Invasive pulmonary aspergillosis in acute leukemia: Characteristic findings on CT, the CT halo sign, and the role of CT in early diagnosis. *Radiology.* 1985;157:611–614.
33. Mehrad B, Paciocco G, Martinez FJ, et al. Spectrum of Aspergillus infection in lung transplant recipients: Case series and review of the literature. *Chest.* 2001;119:169–175.
34. Somboonwit C, Greene JN. Diagnostic methodologies for invasive fungal infections in hematopoietic stem-cell transplant recipients. *Semin Respir Infect.* 2002;17:151–157.
35. Franquet T, Müller NL, Gimenez A, et al. Infectious pulmonary nodules in immunocompromised patients: Usefulness of computed tomography in predicting their etiology. *J Comput Assist Tomogr.* 2003;27:461–468.
36. McAdams HP, Rosado de Christenson M, Strollo DC, et al. Pulmonary mucormycosis: Radiologic findings in 32 cases. *Am J Roentgenol.* 1997; 168:1541–1548.
37. Primack SL, Hartman TE, Lee KS, et al. Pulmonary nodules and the CT halo sign. *Radiology.* 1994;190:513–515.
38. Golfieri R, Giampalma E, Morselli Labate AM, et al. Pulmonary complications of liver transplantation: Radiological appearance and statistical evaluation of risk factors in 300 cases. *Eur Radiol.* 2000;10:1169–1183.
39. Wong PW, Stefanec T, Brown K, et al. Role of fine-needle aspirates of focal lung lesions in patients with hematologic malignancies. *Chest.* 2002; 121:527–532.
40. Young JA, Hopkin JM, Cuthbertson WP. Pulmonary infiltrates in immunocompromised patients: Diagnosis by cytological examination of bronchoalveolar lavage fluid. *J Clin Pathol.* 1984;37:390–397.
41. Zihlif M, Khanchandani G, Ahmed HP, et al. Surgical lung biopsy in patients with hematological malignancy or hematopoietic stem cell transplantation and unexplained pulmonary infiltrates: Improved outcome with specific diagnosis. *Am J Hematol.* 2005;78:94–99.
42. Leung AN, Gosselin MV, Napper CH, et al. Pulmonary infections after bone marrow transplantation: Clinical and radiographic findings. *Radiology.* 1999;210:699–710.
43. Kotloff RM, Ahya VN, Crawford SW. Pulmonary complications of solid organ and hematopoietic stem cell transplantation. *Am J Respir Crit Care Med.* 2004;170:22–48.
44. Fishman JA, Rubin RH. Infection in organ-transplant recipients. *N Engl J Med.* 1998;338:1741–1751.
45. Worthy SA, Flint JD, Müller NL. Pulmonary complications after bone marrow transplantation: High-resolution CT and pathologic findings. *Radiographics.* 1997;17:1359–1371.
46. Sable CA, Donowitz GR. Infections in bone marrow transplant recipients. *Clin Infect Dis.* 1994;18:273–281, quiz 282–274.
47. Leather HL, Wingard JR. Infections following hematopoietic stem cell transplantation. *Infect Dis Clin North Am.* 2001;15:483–520.
48. Curtis DJ, Smale A, Thien F, et al. Chronic airflow obstruction in long-term survivors of allogeneic bone marrow transplantation. *Bone Marrow Transplant.* 1995;16:169–173.
49. Dubois PJ, Myerowitz RL, Allen CM. Pathoradiologic correlation of pulmonary candidiasis in immunosuppressed patients. *Cancer.* 1977;40: 1026–1036.
50. Gefter WB, Albelda SM, Talbot GH, et al. Invasive pulmonary aspergillosis and acute leukemia. Limitations in the diagnostic utility of the air crescent sign. *Radiology.* 1985;157:605–610.
51. Ramila E, Sureda A, Martino R, et al. Bronchoscopy guided by high-resolution computed tomography for the diagnosis of pulmonary infections in patients with hematologic malignancies and normal plain chest X-ray. *Haematologica.* 2000;85:961–966.
52. Castellino RA, Blank N. Etiologic diagnosis of focal pulmonary infection in immunocompromised patients by fluoroscopically guided percutaneous needle aspiration. *Radiology.* 1979;132:563–567.
53. Hwang SS, Kim HH, Park SH, et al. The value of CT-guided percutaneous needle aspiration in immunocompromised patients with suspected pulmonary infection. *Am J Roentgenol.* 2000;175:235–238.
54. Franquet T, Gimenez A, Hidalgo A. Imaging of opportunistic fungal infections in immunocompromised patient. *Eur J Radiol.* 2004;51:130–138.
55. Connolly JE Jr, McAdams HP, Erasmus JJ, et al. Opportunistic fungal pneumonia. *J Thorac Imaging.* 1999;14:51–62.
56. Davies SF, Sarosi GA. Fungal pulmonary complications. *Clin Chest Med.* 1996;17:725–744.
57. Russian DA, Levine SJ. Pneumocystis carinii pneumonia in patients without HIV infection. *Am J Med Sci.* 2001;321:56–65.
58. Marchiori E, Müller NL, Soares Souza A Jr, et al. Pulmonary disease in patients with AIDS: High-resolution CT and pathologic findings. *Am J Roentgenol.* 2005;184:757–764.
59. Lyon R, Haque AK, Asmuth DM, et al. Changing patterns of infections in patients with AIDS: A study of 279 autopsies of prison inmates and nonincarcerated patients at a university hospital in eastern Texas, 1984–1993. *Clin Infect Dis.* 1996;23:241–247.
60. Boiselle PM, Aviram G, Fishman JE. Update on lung disease in AIDS. *Semin Roentgenol.* 2002;37:54–71.
61. Boiselle PM, Crans CA Jr, Kaplan MA. The changing face of Pneumocystis carinii pneumonia in AIDS patients. *Am J Roentgenol.* 1999;172: 1301–1309.
62. Boiselle PM, Tocino I, Hooley RJ, et al. Chest radiograph interpretation of Pneumocystis carinii pneumonia, bacterial pneumonia, and pulmonary tuberculosis in HIV-positive patients: Accuracy, distinguishing features, and mimics. *J Thorac Imaging.* 1997;12:47–53.
63. Crans CA Jr, Boiselle PM. Imaging features of Pneumocystis carinii pneumonia. *Crit Rev Diagn Imaging.* 1999;40:251–284.
64. Aviram G, Fishman JE, Sagar M. Cavitary lung disease in AIDS: Etiologies and correlation with immune status. *AIDS Patient Care STDS.* 2001; 15:353–361.
65. Evlogias NE, Leonidas JC, Rooney J, et al. Severe cystic pulmonary disease associated with chronic Pneumocystis carinii infection in a child with AIDS. *Pediatr Radiol.* 1994;24:606–608.
66. Verfaillie C, Weisdorf D, Haake R, et al. Candida infections in bone marrow transplant recipients. *Bone Marrow Transplant.* 1991;8:177–184.
67. Buff SJ, McLelland R, Gallis HA, et al. Candida albicans pneumonia: Radiographic appearance. *Am J Roentgenol.* 1982;138:645–648.
68. Kassner EG, Kauffman SL, Yoon JJ, et al. Pulmonary candidiasis in infants: Clinical, radiologic, and pathologic features. *Am J Roentgenol.* 1981;137: 707–716.
69. Franquet T, Müller NL, Lee KS, et al. Pulmonary candidiasis after hematopoietic stem cell transplantation: Thin-section CT findings. *Radiology.* 2005;236:332–337.
70. Franquet T, Müller NL, Gimenez A, et al. Semiinvasive pulmonary aspergillosis in chronic obstructive pulmonary disease: Radiologic and pathologic findings in nine patients. *Am J Roentgenol.* 2000;174:51–56.
71. Gefter WB, Weingrad TR, Epstein DM, et al. "Semi-invasive" pulmonary aspergillosis: A new look at the spectrum of aspergillus infections of the lung. *Radiology.* 1981;140:313–321.
72. Kim SY, Lee KS, Han J, et al. Semiinvasive pulmonary aspergillosis: CT and pathologic findings in six patients. *Am J Roentgenol.* 2000;174:795–798.
73. Aquino SL, Kee ST, Warnock ML, et al. Pulmonary aspergillosis: Imaging findings with pathologic correlation. *Am J Roentgenol.* 1994;163:811–815.
74. Franquet T, Müller NL, Gimenez A, et al. Spectrum of pulmonary aspergillosis: Histologic, clinical, and radiologic findings. *Radiographics.* 2001;21:825–837.
75. Maertens J, Verhaegen J, Lagrou K, et al. Screening for circulating galactomannan as a noninvasive diagnostic tool for invasive aspergillosis in prolonged neutropenic patients and stem cell transplantation recipients: A prospective validation. *Blood.* 2001;97:1604–1610.
76. Meersseman W, Vandecasteele SJ, Wilmer A, et al. Invasive aspergillosis in critically ill patients without malignancy. *Am J Respir Crit Care Med.* 2004; 170:621–625.
77. Logan PM, Primack SL, Miller RR, et al. Invasive aspergillosis of the airways: Radiographic, CT, and pathologic findings. *Radiology.* 1994;193: 383–388.
78. Franquet T, Müller NL, Oikonomou A, et al. Aspergillus infection of the airways: Computed tomography and pathologic findings. *J Comput Assist Tomogr.* 2004;28:10–16.
79. Franquet T, Serrano F, Gimenez A, et al. Necrotizing Aspergillosis of large airways: CT findings in eight patients. *J Comput Assist Tomogr.* 2002; 26:342–345.
80. Prabhu RM, Patel R. Mucormycosis and entomophthoramycosis: A review of the clinical manifestations, diagnosis and treatment. *Clin Microbiol Infect.* 2004;10(Suppl 1):31–47.
81. Gaziev D, Baronciani D, Galimberti M, et al. Mucormycosis after bone marrow transplantation: Report of four cases in thalassemia and review of the literature. *Bone Marrow Transplant.* 1996;17:409–414.
82. Morrison VA, McGlave PB. Mucormycosis in the BMT population. *Bone Marrow Transplant.* 1993;11:383–388.
83. Allan BT, Patton D, Ramsey NK, et al. Pulmonary fungal infections after bone marrow transplantation. *Pediatr Radiol.* 1988;18:118–122.
84. Buckner CD, Clift RA, Thomas ED, et al. Early infectious complications in allogeneic marrow transplant recipients with acute leukemia: Effects of prophylactic measures. *Infection.* 1983;11:243–250.

85. Busca A, Locatelli F, Barbui A, et al. Infectious complications following nonmyeloablative allogeneic hematopoietic stem cell transplantation. *Transpl Infect Dis.* 2003;5:132–139.

86. Shearer C, Chandrasekar PH. Pulmonary nocardiosis in a patient with a bone marrow transplant. Bone marrow transplantation team. *Bone Marrow Transplant.* 1995;15:479–481.

87. Simpson GL, Stinson EB, Egger MJ, et al. Nocardial infections in the immunocompromised host: A detailed study in a defined population. *Rev Infect Dis.* 1981;3:492–507.

88. Matar LD, McAdams HP, Palmer SM, et al. Respiratory viral infections in lung transplant recipients: Radiologic findings with clinical correlation. *Radiology.* 1999;213:735–742.

89. Franquet T. Imaging of pneumonia: Trends and algorithms. *Eur Respir J.* 2001;18:196–208.

90. Aquino SL, Gamsu G, Webb WR, et al. Tree-in-bud pattern: Frequency and significance on thin section CT. *J Comput Assist Tomogr.* 1996;20:594–599.

91. Franquet T, Müller NL. Disorders of the small airways: High-resolution computed tomographic features. *Semin Respir Crit Care Med.* 2003;24:437–444.

92. Hiorns MP, Screaton NJ, Müller NL. Acute lung disease in the immunocompromised host. *Radiol Clin North Am.* 2001;39:1137–1151.

93. Rossi SE, Franquet T, Volpacchio M, et al. Tree-in-bud pattern at thin-section CT of the lungs: Radiologic-pathologic overview. *Radiographics.* 2005;25:789–801.

94. Burgart LJ, Heller MJ, Reznicek MJ, et al. Cytomegalovirus detection in bone marrow transplant patients with idiopathic pneumonitis. A clinicopathologic study of the clinical utility of the polymerase chain reaction on open lung biopsy specimen tissue. *Am J Clin Pathol.* 1991;96:572–576.

95. Chen CS, Boeckh M, Seidel K, et al. Incidence, risk factors, and mortality from pneumonia developing late after hematopoietic stem cell transplantation. *Bone Marrow Transplant.* 2003;32:515–522.

96. Cunningham I. Pulmonary infections after bone marrow transplant. *Semin Respir Infect.* 1992;7:132–138.

97. Taplitz RA, Jordan MC. Pneumonia caused by herpesviruses in recipients of hematopoietic cell transplants. *Semin Respir Infect.* 2002;17:121–129.

98. Khushalani NI, Bakri FG, Wentling D, et al. Respiratory syncytial virus infection in the late bone marrow transplant period: Report of three cases and review. *Bone Marrow Transplant.* 2001;27:1071–1073.

99. Dauber JH, Paradis IL, Dummer JS. Infectious complications in pulmonary allograft recipients. *Clin Chest Med.* 1990;11:291–308.

100. Duncan AJ, Dummer JS, Paradis IL, et al. Cytomegalovirus infection and survival in lung transplant recipients. *J Heart Lung Transplant.* 1991;10:638–644, discussion 645-636.

101. Billings JL, Hertz MI, Savik K, et al. Respiratory viruses and chronic rejection in lung transplant recipients. *J Heart Lung Transplant.* 2002;21:559–566.

102. Billings JL, Hertz MI, Wendt CH. Community respiratory virus infections following lung transplantation. *Transpl Infect Dis.* 2001;3:138–148.

103. Tamm M, Traenkle P, Grilli B, et al. Pulmonary cytomegalovirus infection in immunocompromised patients. *Chest.* 2001;119:838–843.

104. Madhi SA, Ludewick H, Abed Y, et al. Human metapneumovirus-associated lower respiratory tract infections among hospitalized human immunodeficiency virus type 1 (HIV-1)-infected and HIV-1-uninfected African infants. *Clin Infect Dis.* 2003;37:1705–1710.

105. Maki DD. Pulmonary infections in HIV/AIDS. *Semin Roentgenol.* 2000;35:124–139.

106. Gasparetto EL, Ono SE, Escuissato D, et al. Cytomegalovirus pneumonia after bone marrow transplantation: High resolution CT findings. *Br J Radiol.* 2004;77:724–727.

107. Gasparetto EL, Escuissato DL, Inoue C, et al. Herpes simplex virus type 2 pneumonia after bone marrow transplantation: High-resolution CT findings in 3 patients. *J Thorac Imaging.* 2005;20:71–73.

108. Gasparetto EL, Escuissato DL, Marchiori E, et al. High-resolution CT findings of respiratory syncytial virus pneumonia after bone marrow transplantation. *Am J Roentgenol.* 2004;182:1133–1137.

109. Oikonomou A, Müller NL, Nantel S. Radiographic and high-resolution CT findings of influenza virus pneumonia in patients with hematologic malignancies. *Am J Roentgenol.* 2003;181:507–511.

110. Franquet T, Rodriguez S, Martino R, et al. Human metapneumovirus infection in hematopoietic stem cell transplant recipients: High-resolution computed tomography findings. *J Comput Assist Tomogr.* 2005;29:223–227.

111. Meyers JD, Atkinson K. Infection in bone marrow transplantation. *Clin Haematol.* 1983;12:791–811.

112. Mohite U, Das M, Saikia T, et al. Mycobacterial pulmonary infection post allogeneic bone marrow transplantation. *Leuk Lymphoma.* 2001;40:675–678.

113. Schulman LL, Htun T, Staniloae C, et al. Pulmonary nodules and masses after lung and heart-lung transplantation. *J Thorac Imaging.* 2000;15:173–179.

114. Singh N, Paterson DL. Mycobacterium tuberculosis infection in solid-organ transplant recipients: Impact and implications for management. *Clin Infect Dis.* 1998;27:1266–1277.

115. Martino R, Martinez C, Brunet S, et al. Tuberculosis in bone marrow transplant recipients: Report of two cases and review of the literature. *Bone Marrow Transplant.* 1996;18:809–812.

116. Gupta R, Espinal MA, Raviglione MC. Tuberculosis as a major global health problem in the 21st century: A WHO perspective. *Semin Respir Crit Care Med.* 2004;25:245–253.

117. Sinnott JT, Emmanuel PJ. Mycobacterial infections in the transplant patient. *Semin Respir Infect.* 1990;5:65–73.

118. Kesten S, Chaparro C. Mycobacterial infections in lung transplant recipients. *Chest.* 1999;115:741–745.

119. Afessa B. Mycobacterial and nonbacterial pulmonary complications in hospitalized patients with human immunodeficiency virus infection: A prospective, cohort study. *BMC Pulm Med.* 2001;1:1.

120. Doucette K, Fishman JA. Nontuberculous mycobacterial infection in hematopoietic stem cell and solid organ transplant recipients. *Clin Infect Dis.* 2004;38:1428–1439.

121. Erasmus JJ, McAdams HP, Farrell MA, et al. Pulmonary nontuberculous mycobacterial infection: Radiologic manifestations. *Radiographics.* 1999;19:1487–1505.

122. Leung AN. Pulmonary tuberculosis: The essentials. *Radiology.* 1999;210:307–322.

123. Koh DM, Bell JR, Burkill GJ, et al. Mycobacterial infections: Still a millennium bug—the imaging features of mycobacterial infections. *Clin Radiol.* 2001;56:535–544.

124. Hartman TE, Primack SL, Lee KS, et al. CT of bronchial and bronchiolar diseases. *Radiographics.* 1994;14:991–1003.

125. Im JG, Itoh H, Han MC. CT of pulmonary tuberculosis. *Semin Ultrasound CT MR.* 1995;16:420–434.

126. Im JG, Itoh H, Lee KS, et al. CT-pathology correlation of pulmonary tuberculosis. *Crit Rev Diagn Imaging.* 1995;36:227–285.

127. Im JG, Itoh H, Shim YS, et al. Pulmonary tuberculosis: CT findings—early active disease and sequential change with antituberculous therapy. *Radiology.* 1993;186:653–660.

128. Kim Y, Lee KS, Yoon JH, et al. Tuberculosis of the trachea and main bronchi: CT findings in 17 patients. *Am J Roentgenol.* 1997;168:1051–1056.

129. King MA, Neal DE, St John R, et al. Bronchial dilatation in patients with HIV infection: CT assessment and correlation with pulmonary function tests and findings at bronchoalveolar lavage. *Am J Roentgenol.* 1997;168:1535–1540.

130. Kuhlman JE, Deutsch JH, Fishman EK, et al. CT features of thoracic mycobacterial disease. *Radiographics.* 1990;10:413–431.

131. Lee JY, Lee KS, Jung KJ, et al. Pulmonary tuberculosis: CT and pathologic correlation. *J Comput Assist Tomogr.* 2000;24:691–698.

132. Lee KS, Hwang JW, Chung MP, et al. Utility of CT in the evaluation of pulmonary tuberculosis in patients without AIDS. *Chest.* 1996;110:977–984.

133. Marr KA, Patterson T, Denning D. Aspergillosis. Pathogenesis, clinical manifestations, and therapy. *Infect Dis Clin North Am.* 2002;16:875–894.

134. Kato T, Usami I, Morita H, et al. Chronic necrotizing pulmonary aspergillosis in pneumoconiosis: Clinical and radiologic findings in 10 patients. *Chest.* 2002;121:118–127.

135. Denning DW. Early diagnosis of invasive aspergillosis. *Lancet.* 2000;355:423–424.

136. Denning DW. Chronic forms of pulmonary aspergillosis. *Clin Microbiol Infect.* 2001;7(Suppl 2):25–31.

137. Moore EH. Atypical mycobacterial infection in the lung: CT appearance. *Radiology.* 1993;187:777–782.

138. Laissy JP, Cadi M, Cinqualbre A, et al. Mycobacterium tuberculosis versus nontuberculous mycobacterial infection of the lung in AIDS patients: CT and HRCT patterns. *J Comput Assist Tomogr.* 1997;21:312–317.

139. Marinelli DL, Albelda SM, Williams TM, et al. Nontuberculous mycobacterial infection in AIDS: Clinical, pathologic, and radiographic features. *Radiology.* 1986;160:77–82.

Index

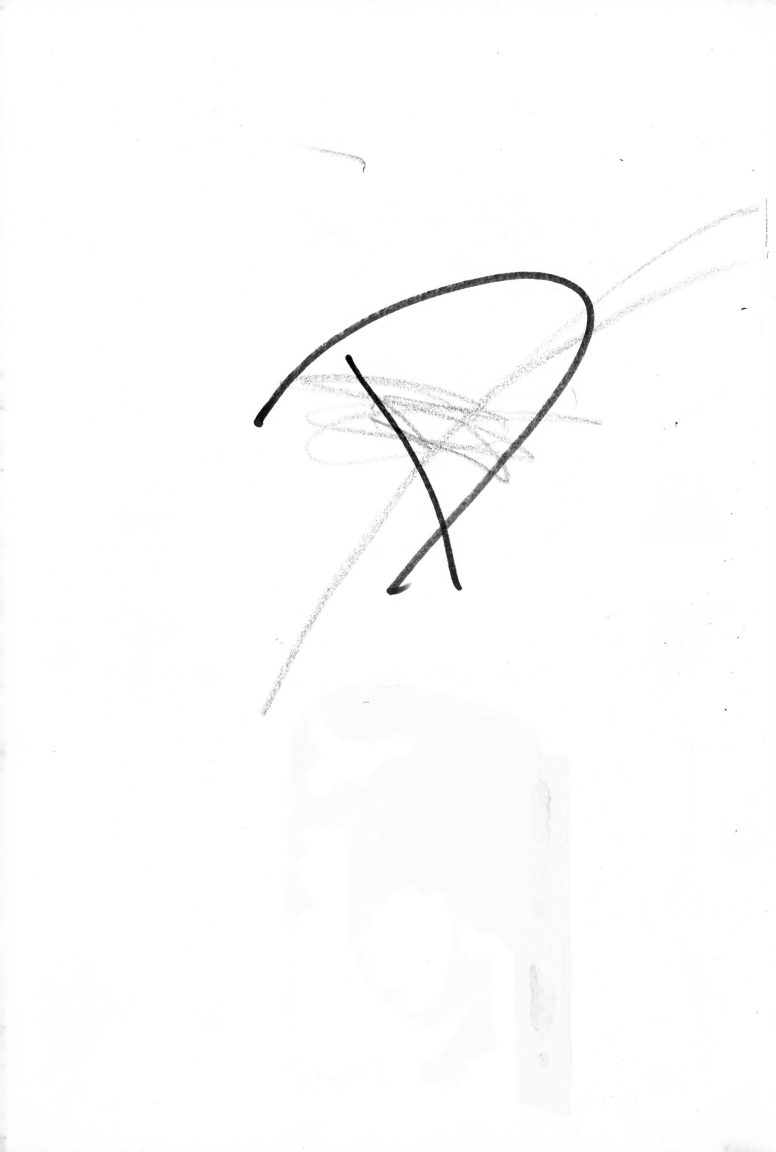

BY INGRI AND EDGAR PARIN D'AULAIRE

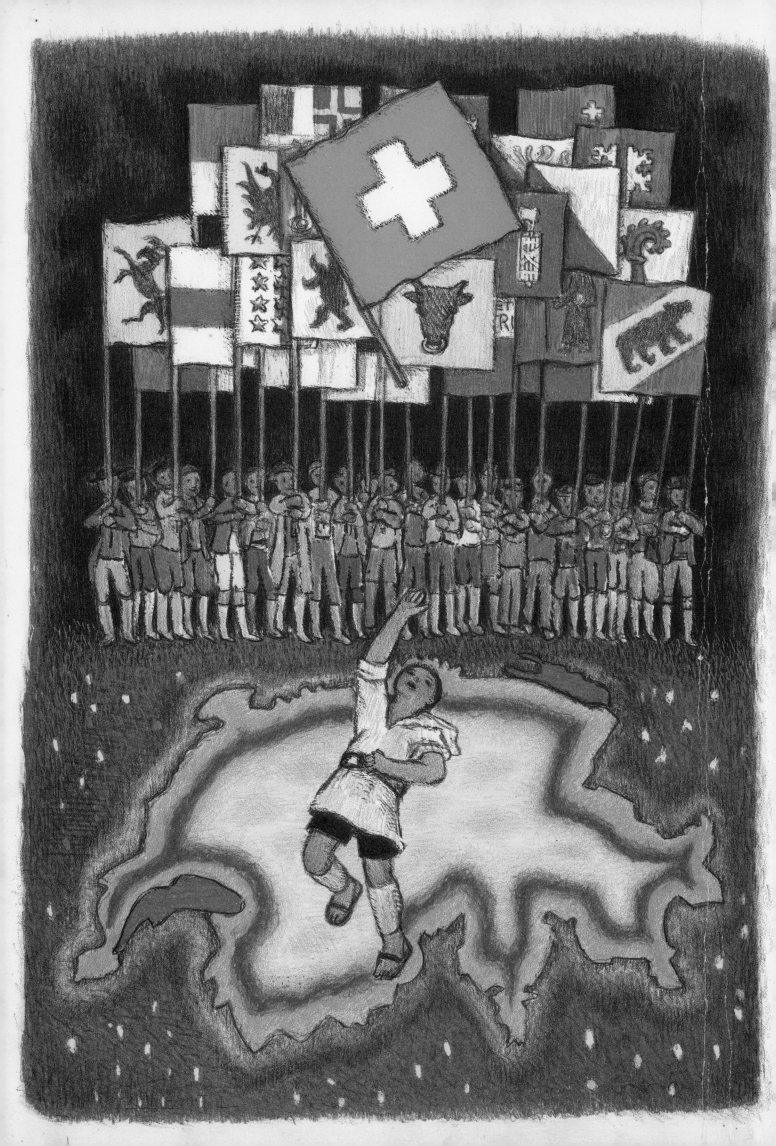

INGRI and EDGAR PARIN D'AULAIRE

THE
MAGIC
MEADOW

DOUBLEDAY & COMPANY, INC.
Garden City, New York

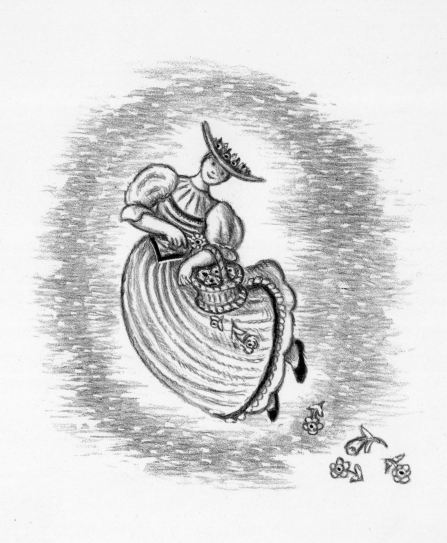

High up in the Alps, under the peaks of wild mountains, against the eternal ice and snow of a glacier, lies the loveliest flowering meadow. Nowhere is the sky so blue, the grass so dewy and green, the herbs and flowers so sparkling and gay.

Deep down below, a nest of black farmhouses clings to the steep mountain slope.

In the farm that lies highest up on the slope lived a little Swiss boy, whose name was Peterli, and his old grandfather. All summer long Peterli herded his grandfather's cows and goats to pasture up in the flowery meadow. It was his magic meadow. No other place in the world could be as lovely, Peterli thought.

Long ago, long before Grandfather's grandfather was born, a strong and fearless huntsman roamed these Alpine meadows, free as an eagle. He never missed his aim with his bow and arrow. His name was William Tell.

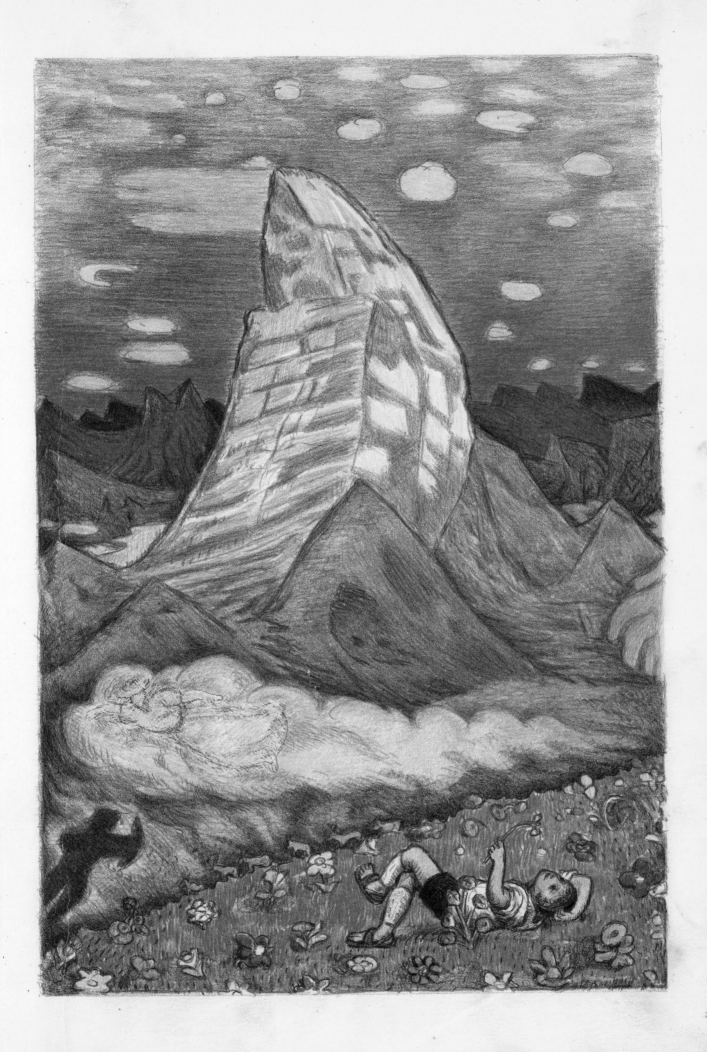

At that time there was no country called Switzerland. Free farmers and hunters like William Tell lived in small cantons, or states, on the high Alps and in the deep valleys. They were free men. They wanted no masters and had little to do with strangers. Even men of neighboring cantons did not mingle with each other.

But there were foreign lords and princes who thought they had a right to rule over the Alps and its freedom-loving people. They sent harsh overseers and soldiers to live there and collect taxes.

The harshest of these was a man called Gessler. To humble the free men of the mountains, he put his hat on a stake and ordered every passer-by to bow or lose his head.

"I shall never bow my head to an empty foreign hat," said William Tell. He walked straight by with his head high.

So Gessler's men seized him. But as they were about to chop off his head Gessler called, "Stop! I have heard that you are such a famous bowman! Now, shoot this apple off the head of your son, and I shall give you your life."

Gessler wanted to humiliate the proud William Tell before he killed him.

For who would dare to shoot an apple off his own son's head?

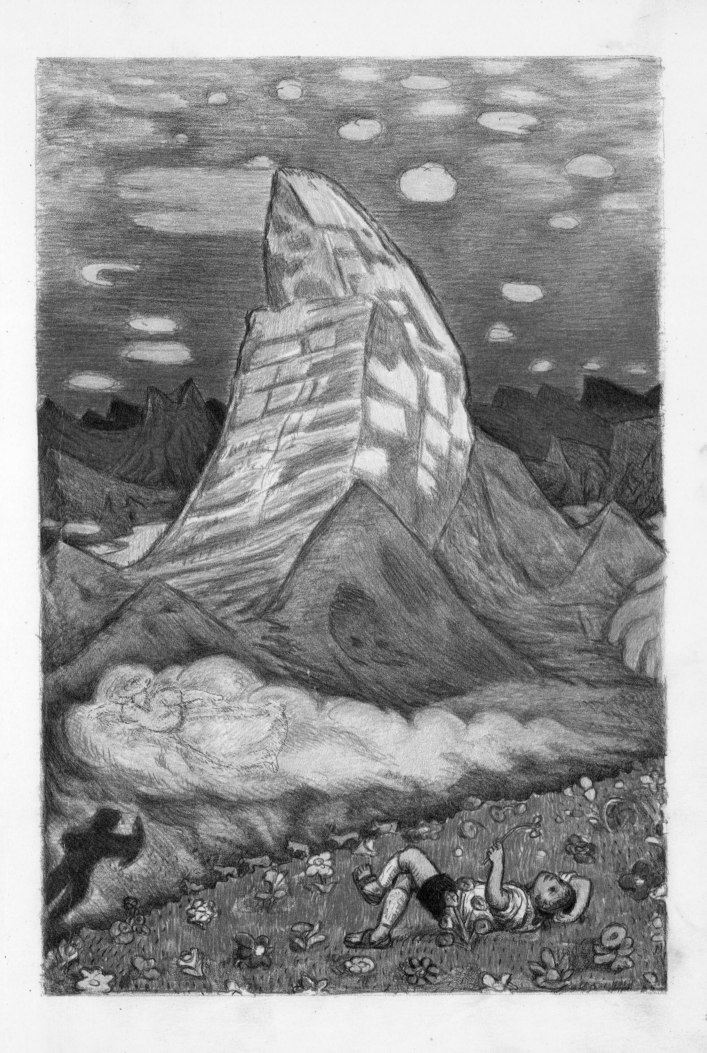

At that time there was no country called Switzerland. Free farmers and hunters like William Tell lived in small cantons, or states, on the high Alps and in the deep valleys. They were free men. They wanted no masters and had little to do with strangers. Even men of neighboring cantons did not mingle with each other.

But there were foreign lords and princes who thought they had a right to rule over the Alps and its freedom-loving people. They sent harsh overseers and soldiers to live there and collect taxes.

The harshest of these was a man called Gessler. To humble the free men of the mountains, he put his hat on a stake and ordered every passer-by to bow or lose his head.

"I shall never bow my head to an empty foreign hat," said William Tell. He walked straight by with his head high.

So Gessler's men seized him. But as they were about to chop off his head Gessler called, "Stop! I have heard that you are such a famous bowman! Now, shoot this apple off the head of your son, and I shall give you your life."

Gessler wanted to humiliate the proud William Tell before he killed him.

For who would dare to shoot an apple off his own son's head?

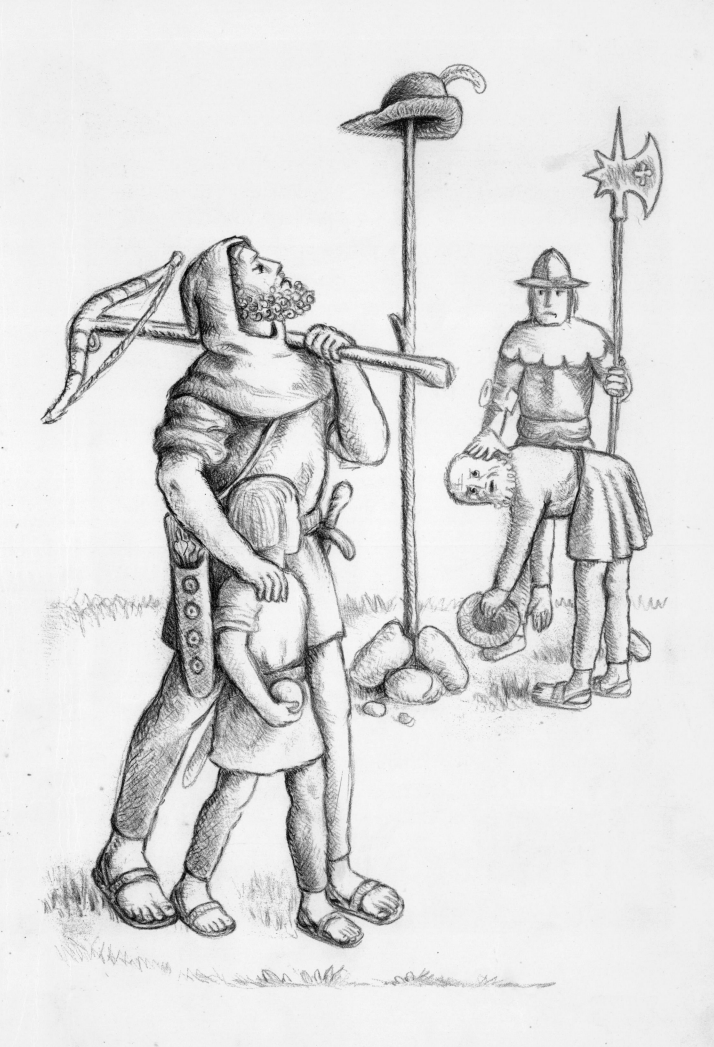

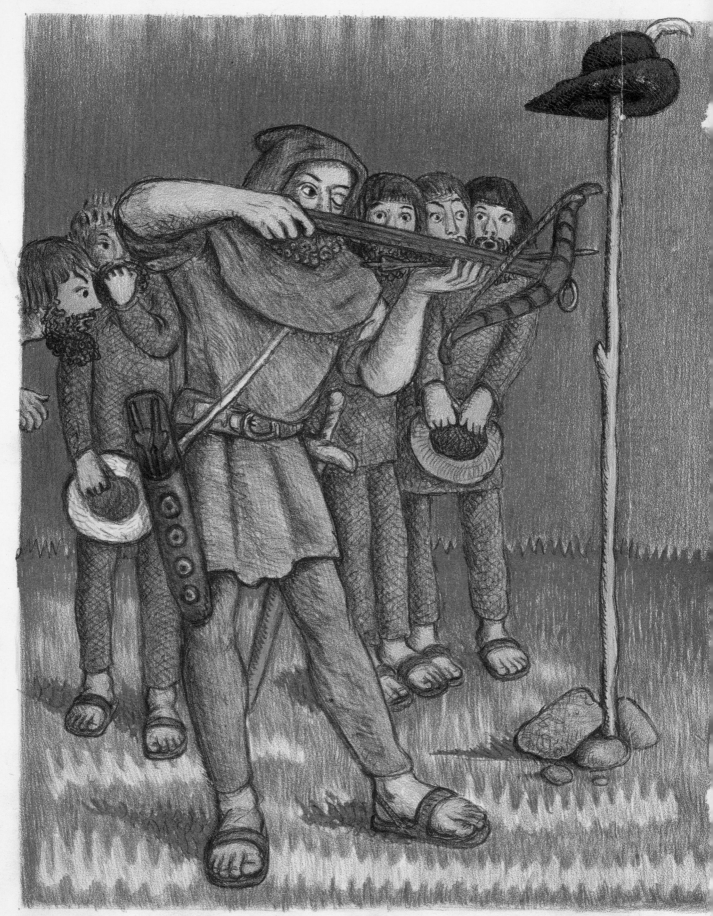

But with a steady hand William Tell took two arrows out of his quiver, put one in his bow, took careful aim, and shot. His son had

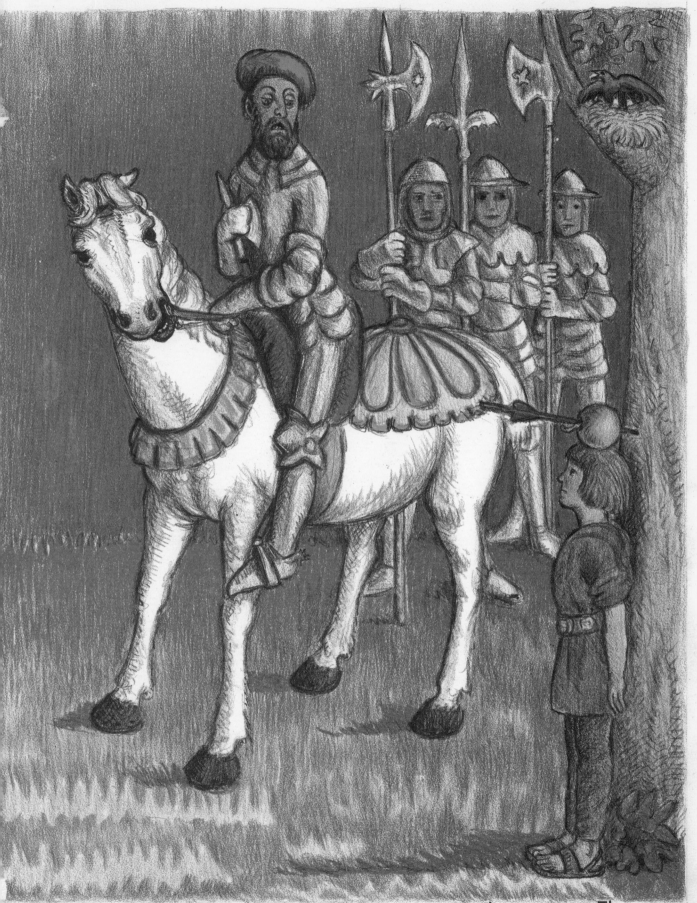

such faith in his father that he did not move or bat an eye. The arrow pierced the core of the apple.

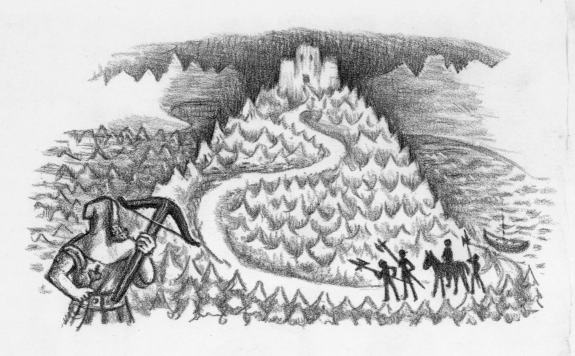

"You have won your life," said Gessler grudgingly, "but tell me, why did you take two arrows out of your quiver, marksman that you are?"

"The second arrow was meant for you if the first had killed my son," said William Tell.

"Into the deepest dungeon with him," shouted Gessler to his men. "There in damp and darkness he shall spend the life I have given him."

They tied him hand and foot and sailed off to take him to the dungeon in Gessler's castle on the far side of the long Vierwaldstaetter Lake. But suddenly a gust of wind came howling down from the mountains. The boat tossed wildly in the waves. "Only the steady hand of William Tell can keep us from capsizing," cried Gessler's men. "Free him from his chains." William Tell grasped the rudder. Daringly he steered the boat close to the rocky shore. There, with a mighty bound he jumped up on a rock, kicking the boat out into the lake again.

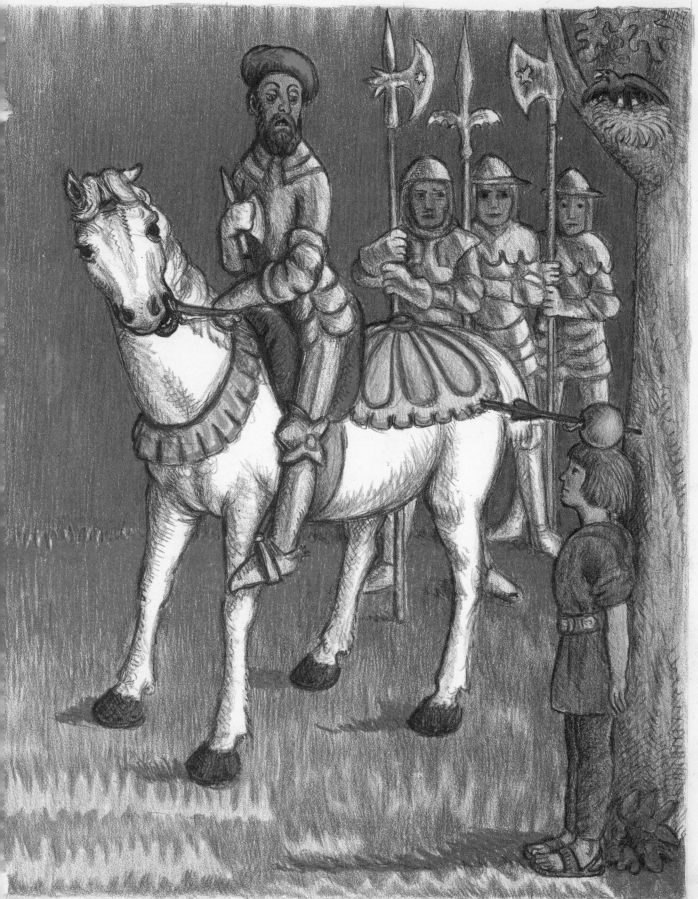

such faith in his father that he did not move or bat an eye. The arrow
pierced the core of the apple.

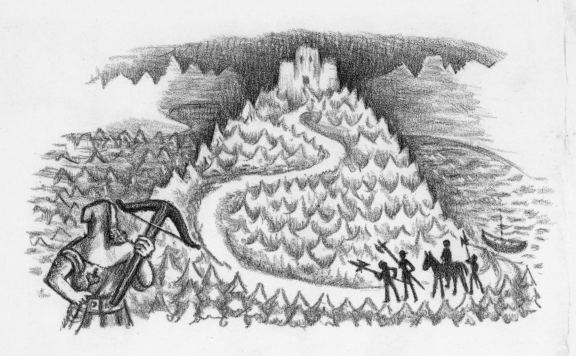

"You have won your life," said Gessler grudgingly, "but tell me, why did you take two arrows out of your quiver, marksman that you are?"

"The second arrow was meant for you if the first had killed my son," said William Tell.

"Into the deepest dungeon with him," shouted Gessler to his men. "There in damp and darkness he shall spend the life I have given him."

They tied him hand and foot and sailed off to take him to the dungeon in Gessler's castle on the far side of the long Vierwaldstaetter Lake. But suddenly a gust of wind came howling down from the mountains. The boat tossed wildly in the waves. "Only the steady hand of William Tell can keep us from capsizing," cried Gessler's men. "Free him from his chains." William Tell grasped the rudder. Daringly he steered the boat close to the rocky shore. There, with a mighty bound he jumped up on a rock, kicking the boat out into the lake again.

Strangely enough, the storm calmed down, so Gessler and his men did not drown. But the wicked overseer found his end anyway. For as he came riding up to his castle, William Tell lay in wait for him with his second arrow. He had run the long way through forests and ravines to free his mountains and himself of Gessler's evil rule. Gessler's men fled in terror and William Tell returned to his mountains, free as he came.

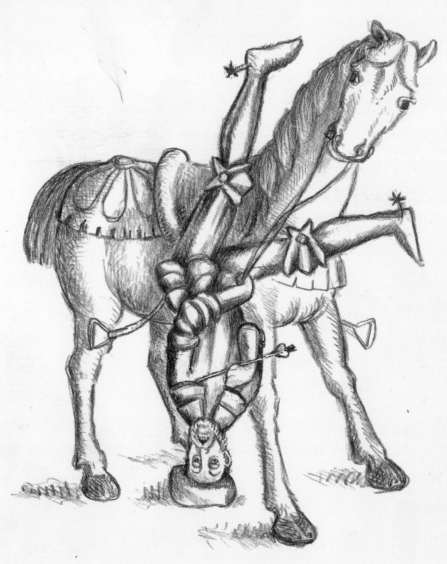

The tale of his brave deed spread through mountains and valleys. And soon other freedom-loving men from different cantons in the Alps came together at the meadow of Gruetli on the Vierwaldstaetter Lake. There they swore to unite and help each other defend their freedom.

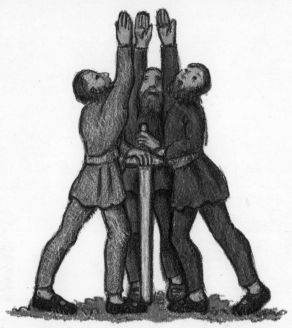

By and by all the people who lived in the Swiss Alps had united and the twenty-two cantons had become one country, Switzerland.

Still each canton kept the right to make its own laws. To this day, the men of each canton meet once a year to decide how they want their homeland run. In Peterli's canton, they still meet under the open sky, as they did at Gruetli in William Tell's day more than six hundred years ago.

And there was nothing his old grandfather loved so much as to go to the meeting in the valley.

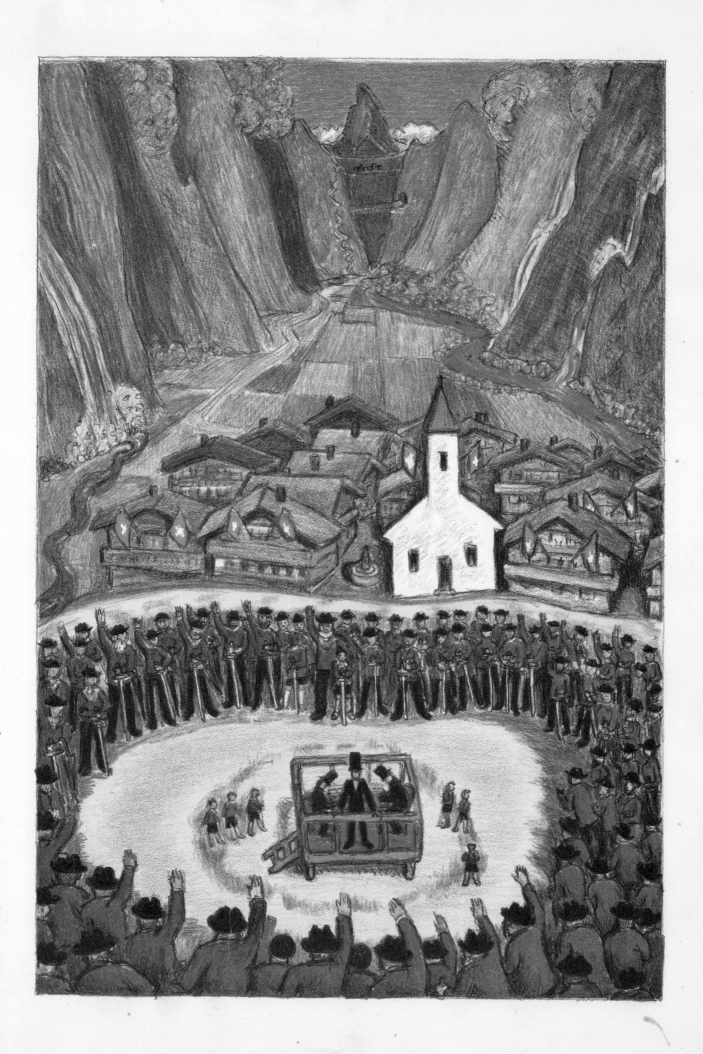

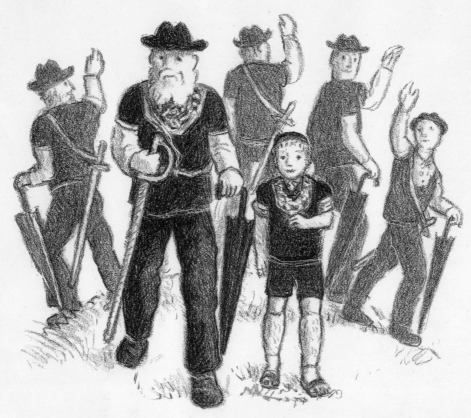

Like all the other men, Grandfather held a sword in one hand as a token that he was a freeman, ready to defend his country. In his other hand he carried an umbrella, for no one could tell what kinds of clouds lay in wait behind the mountains. Peterli and the other boys went to the meeting too, for one day they would be the ones who carried the swords. After the meeting, they all shook hands and set off— each one to his own village.

Nobody had as long and steep a road to walk as Peterli and his grandfather. The path up to their village was so crooked and steep that no car, not even a horse and cart, could make it.

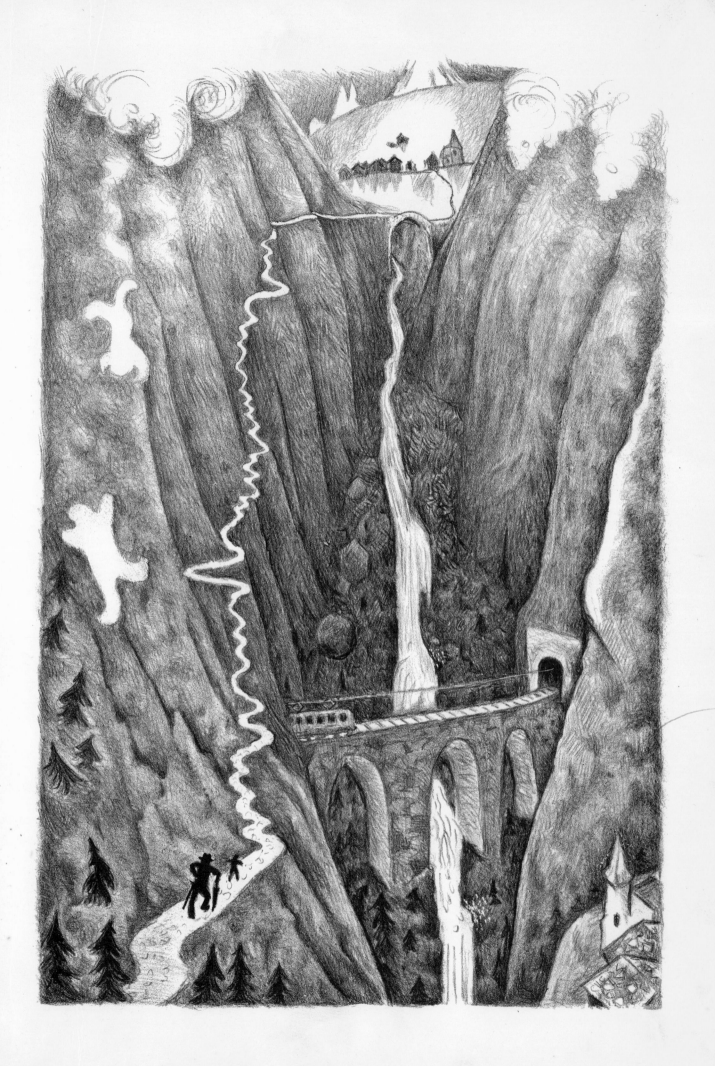

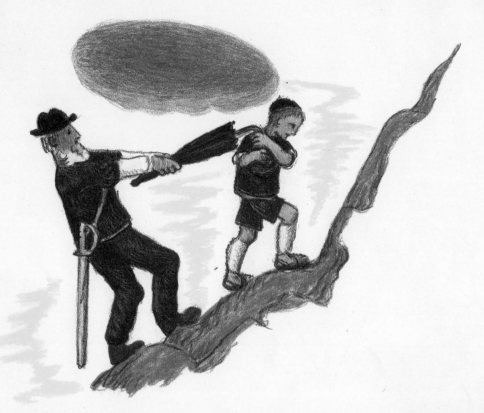

Peterli's legs were strong and sturdy. Grandfather's were old and stiff. Grandfather panted. Peterli pushed and pulled. At long last they came to their village, where the little white church seemed to be keeping an eye on the farmhouses. And there, too, a wooden figure of William Tell stood on watch over the village fountain. Doors and windows flew open and their neighbors welcomed them home.

"If it weren't for Peterli, I would not have made it," sighed Grandfather. "I am afraid it is the last time. My old legs can no longer carry me up these hills."

"One more little climb and we will be home," said Peterli, and looked up to their farm.

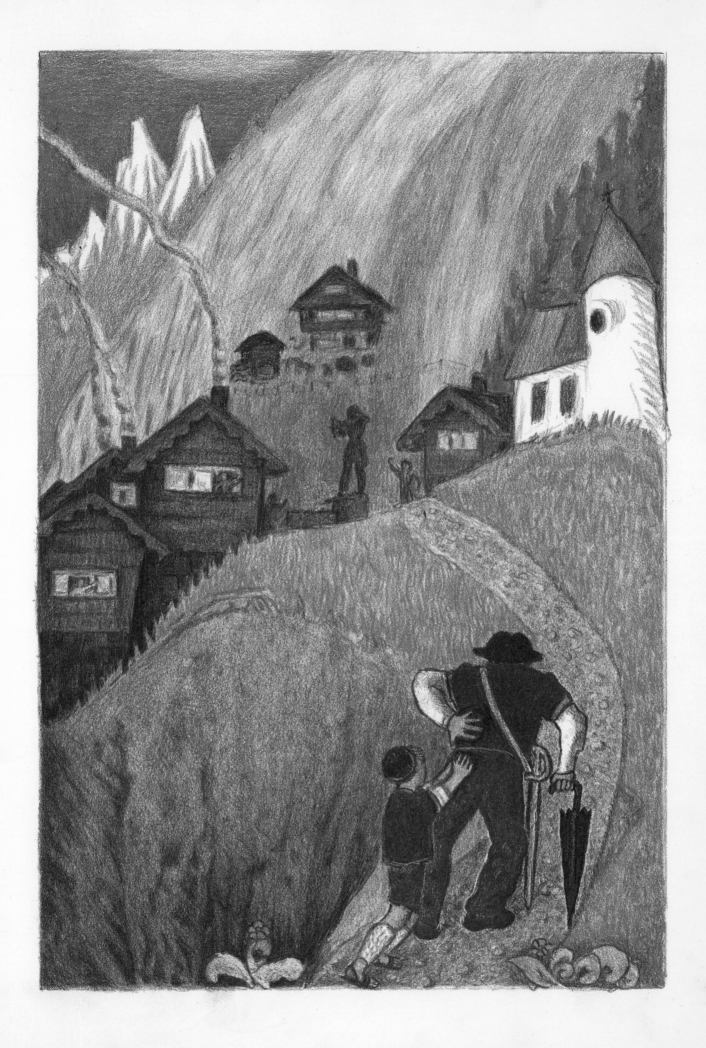

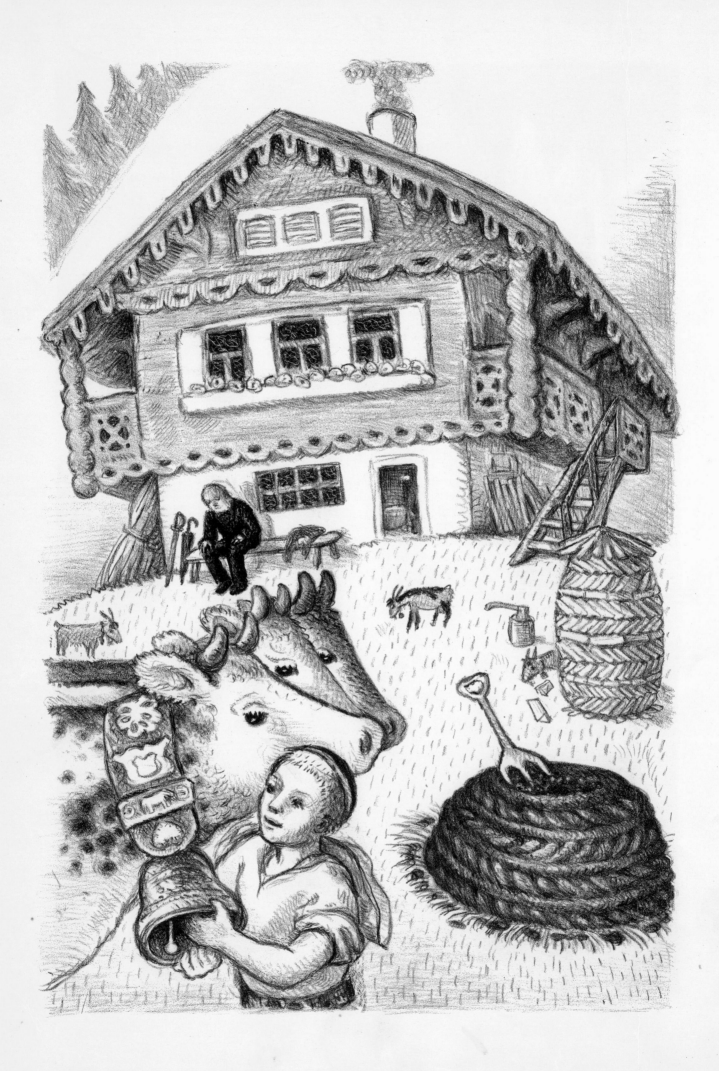

The old black farmhouse was trimmed with curlicues and fancy woodwork, and the farmyard was as tidy as a living room. It looked as if every blade of grass had been combed and counted. The firewood was neatly stacked and even the manure heap was piled in a pattern. The goats and the fat and glossy cows were waiting impatiently for Peterli to take them to the flowery meadow.

"Come Rosli, come Sternli, come Gretli, come all," sang Peterli as he buckled on their silver bells. Gaily he led them up the steep slope.

There lay the magic meadow, lovely and green. The sparkling flowers were bowing their heads in the fresh mountain wind. It looked as if they were bidding Peterli welcome.

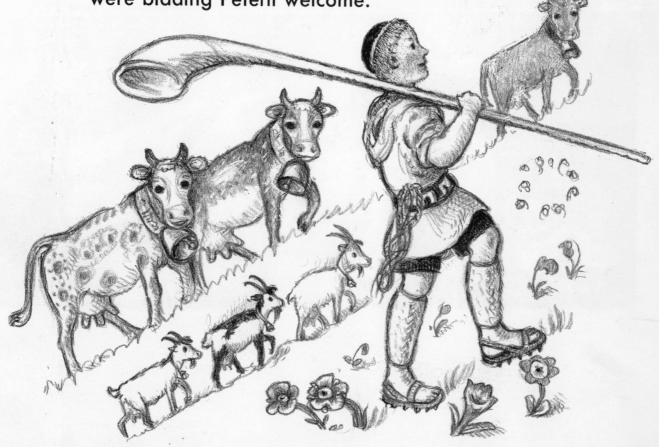

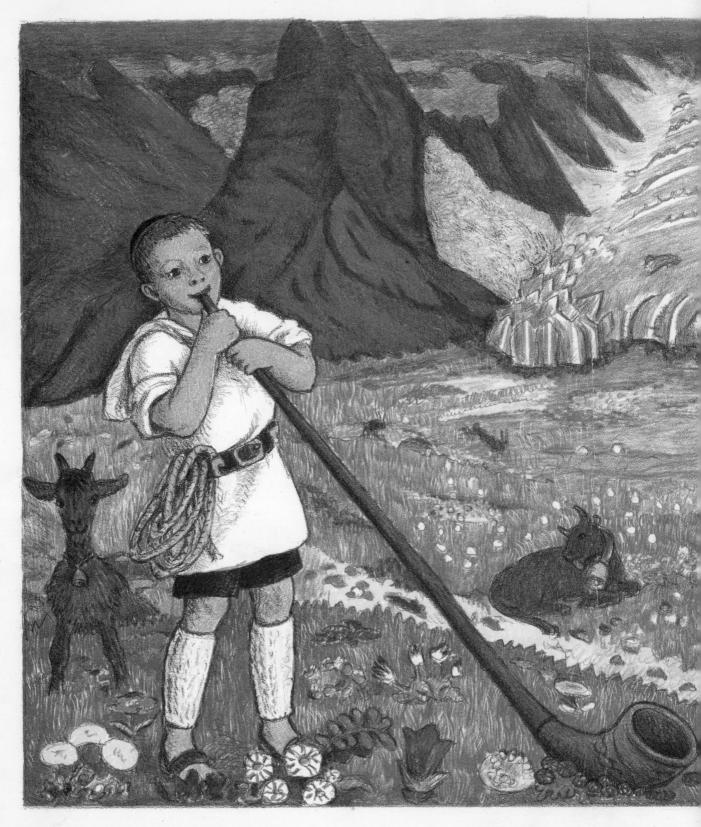

Joyfully Peterli yodeled and blew on his alpenhorn. The goats and cows nodded their heads. Their silver bells jingled and rang. Echoes answered from the mountains all around until the meadow was filled with melody.

Over the grass floated a light wisp of cloud. Or could it be the

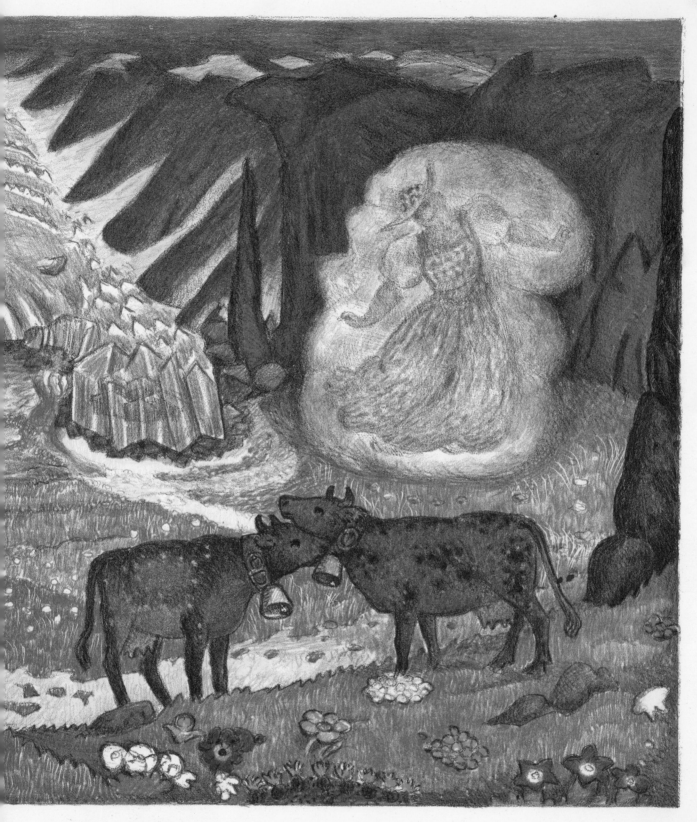

Princess of Spring who danced so lightly over her flowery carpet? Peterli did not dare to go closer, for the Princess of Spring must not mingle with people. Her heart might warm with love for them, and her heart must stay cool as the fresh spring breeze if the magic of spring flowering were to last all summer long.

Peterli knew well that it was her magic flowers and herbs that made the cows so glossy and fat; the cheeses made from their milk so rich and sweet and highly paid for. And how would he and Grandfather live without the good cheeses to sell?

Peterli loved the gentle Princess of Spring, but he feared her father, the fierce Ice King. He ruled over the glacier and the wild mountains, and his heart was made of ice. He huffed and coughed and blew raging storms. If people let their hearts grow cold as his, he had them in his power.

Peterli shivered as he looked down into the glacier. Was it a house he saw there, encased in the ice? Grandfather had told him that once, long ago, a rich man had his farm right by the glacier. His lands were wide, his cows were fat, and he lived in plenty. He even paved his floors with cheeses and filled the cracks with butter so they would be soft for his feet to tread upon. But his heart was hard and cold. One stormy night a freezing traveler knocked at his door and begged for shelter. The rich man turned him away and closed his door. "Ha, he is mine," laughed the Ice King. "His heart is cold as ice."

The glacier began to crack and thunder and creep toward the farm. From all sides the ice closed in and buried farmer and farm.

Was it still there? Peterli wondered. Maybe he could find some of the treasures the rich man had owned, so he could help Grandfather. But how?

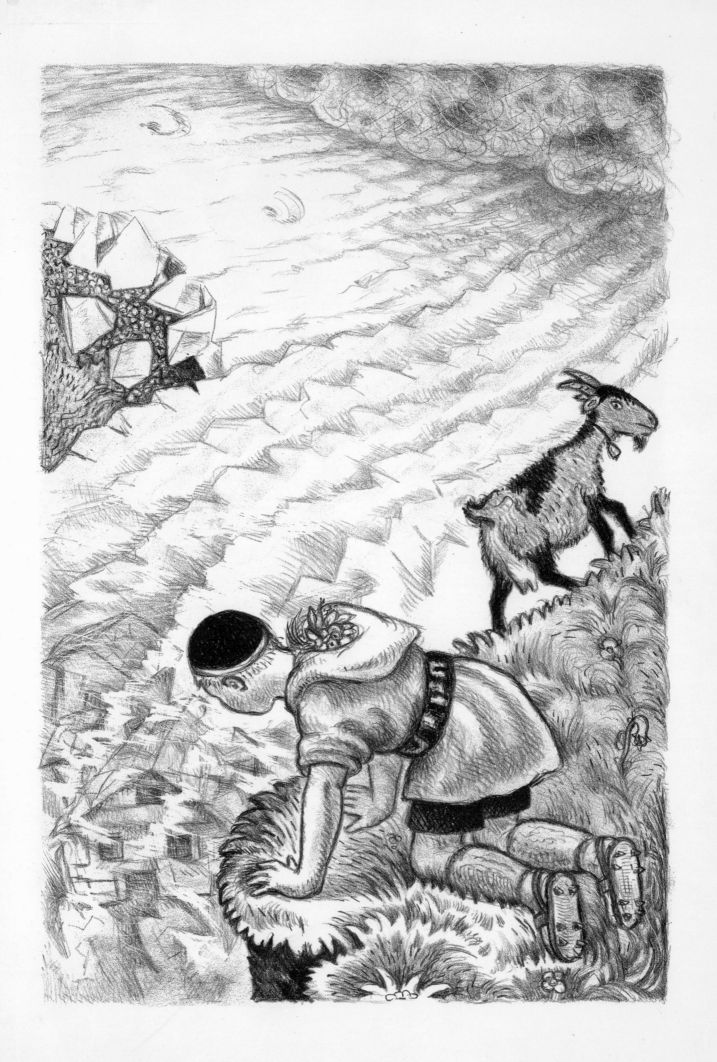

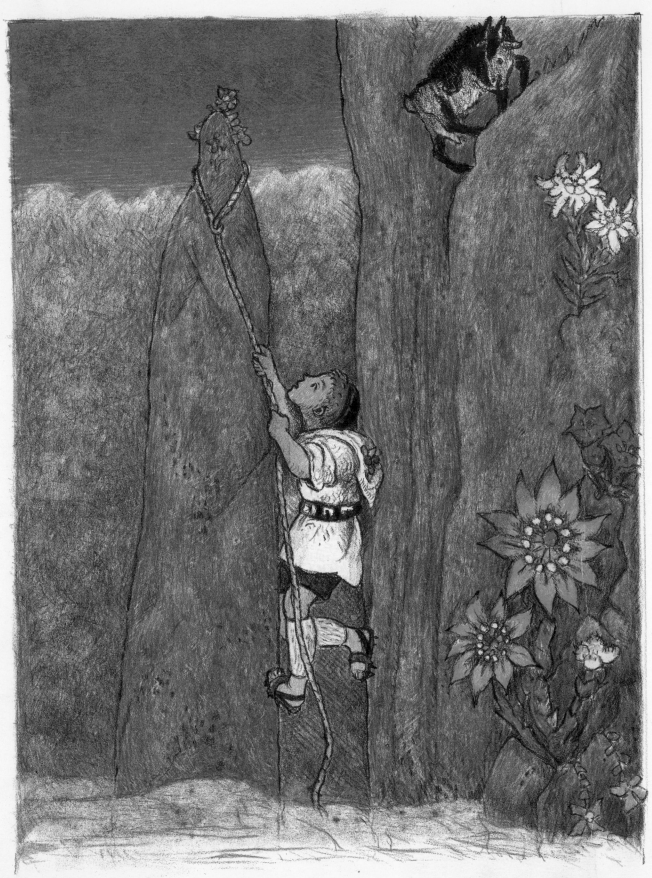

He found neither silver nor gold, but in the mountains above the glacier grew rare flowers and health-giving herbs. Peterli's goats climbed for them. So did Peterli.

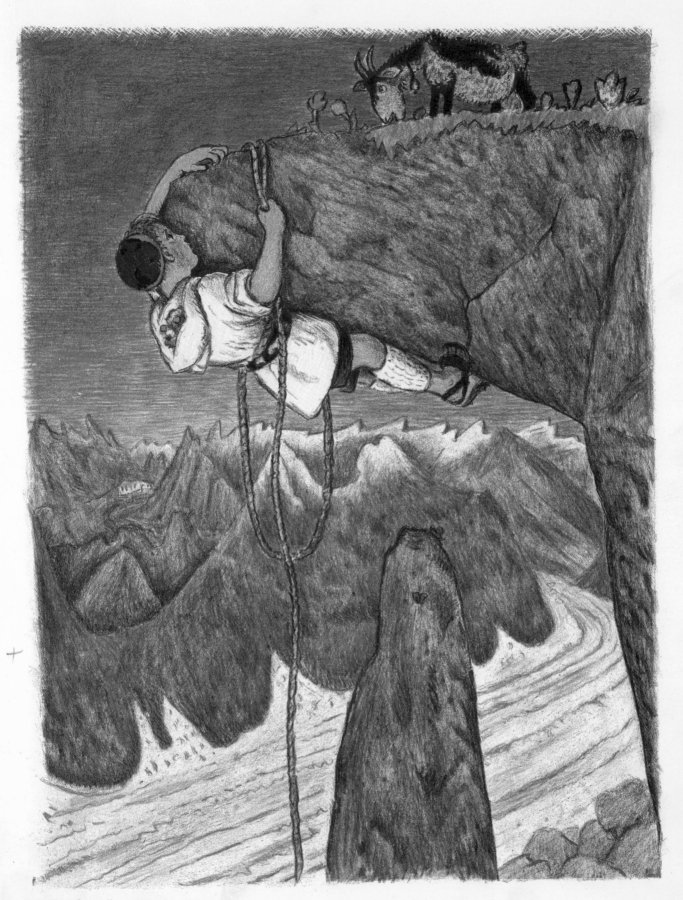

For the herbs brought a pretty penny in town!
Peterli climbed as well as any goat. He climbed all the way to the top of a crag. From there he could see far and wide.

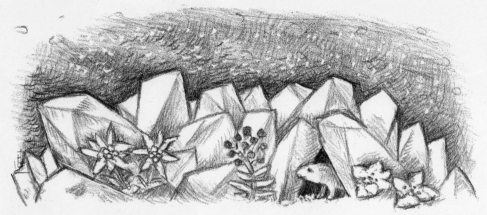

In the distance he saw a small monastery at a rugged mountain pass. A road wound its way through the pass. Before railroads were built and tunnels blasted under the mountains, people who wanted to go to the part of Switzerland that lay south of the Alps had to walk over the mountains. Often travelers were caught in snowstorms and avalanches. To help them, kindhearted monks had built the monastery and had trained huge St. Bernard dogs to sniff their way through the snowdrifts and rescue half-frozen travelers buried under the snow.

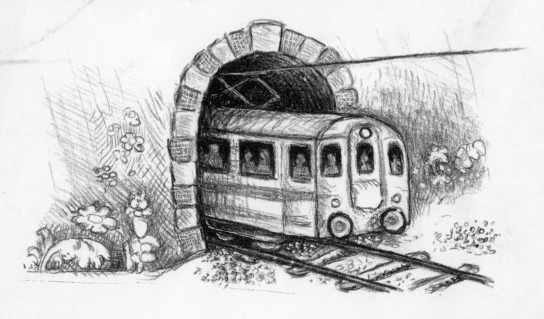

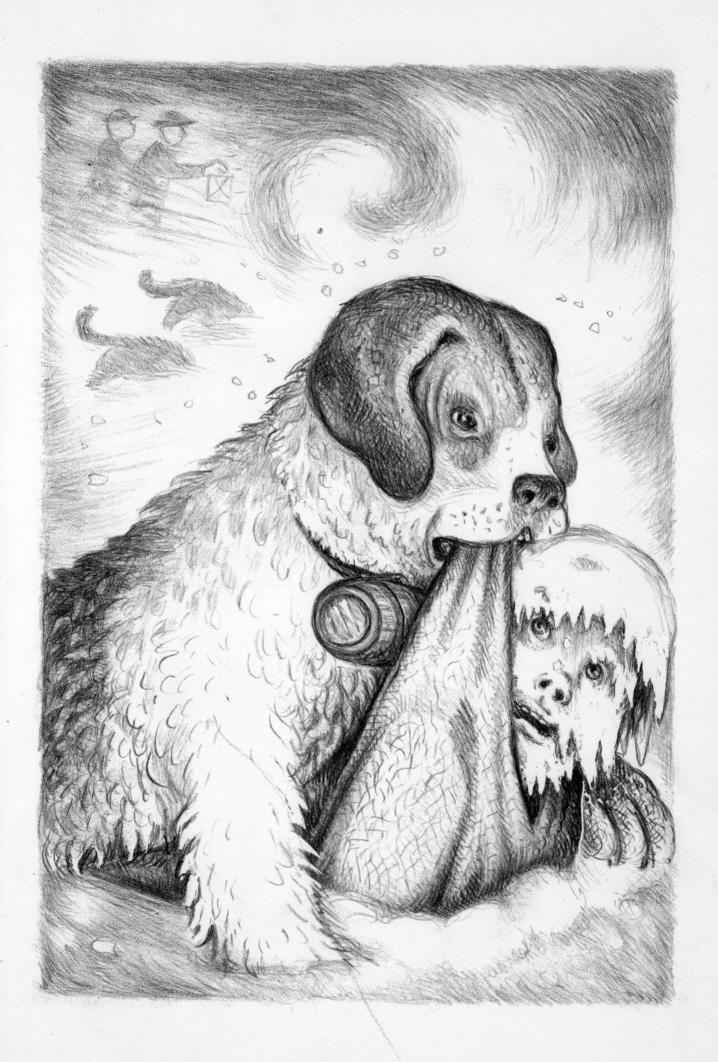

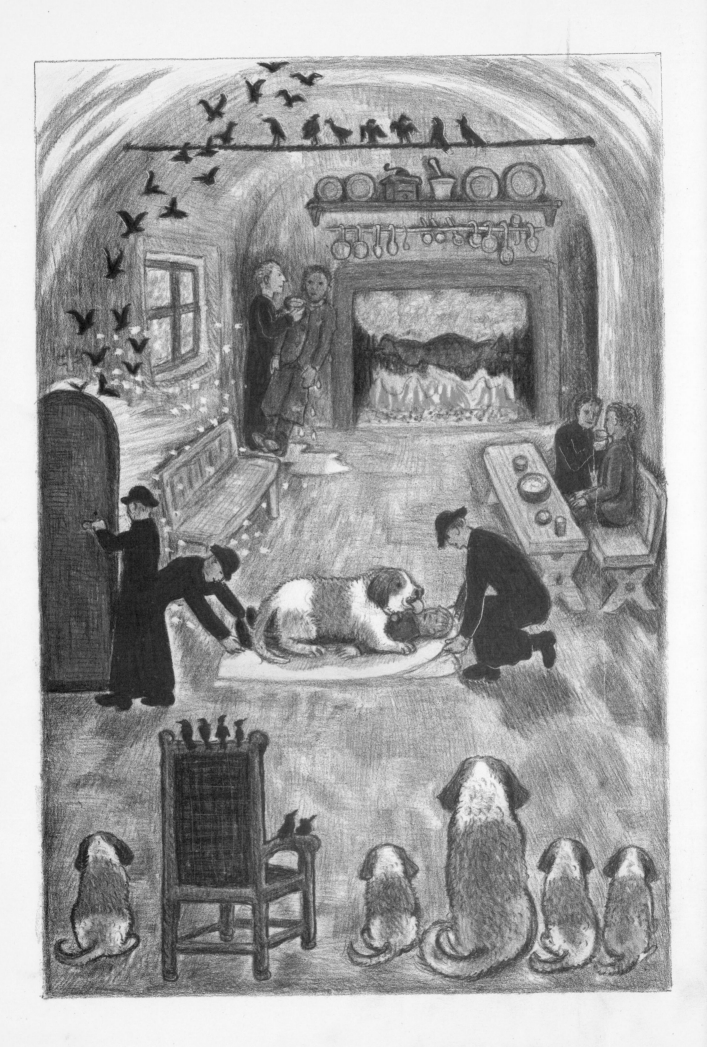

At the monastery, the monks thawed out their frozen clothes and cared for them. The monks did not close their doors to anyone. Even little birds came flying in when a snowstorm raged. They settled on benches and chairs and preened their feathers until the weather had cleared. Then birds and people traveled on south to the sunny slopes where chestnut trees and vineyards grow around blue lakes.

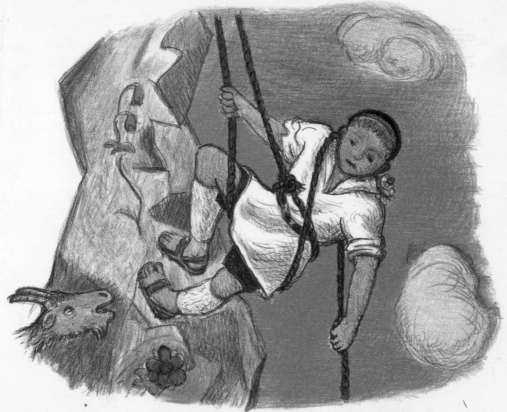

When Peterli had filled his hood with herbs and the goats had eaten their fill, they all had to climb down again. It is easier to climb up a steep mountain than down! Peterli had his rope and could slide straight down the precipice. But a goat often got stuck. Then Peterli had to go to its rescue.

Far down below he could see Grandfather getting ready to milk. He looked as if he had three legs, for he had his milking stool strapped on. Peterli and his cows and goats hurried home. Grandfather milked and Peterli helped him pour the milk into a huge copper kettle that hung over the fire. Grandfather poured in rennet to make the milk curdle. Then he stirred, first slowly, then fast, until the solids and the liquids in the milk had popped apart. Gently he herded all the little solid balls together until they made a big ball in the bottom of the kettle. That was the new cheese. Together he and Peterli lifted it out of the kettle and pressed it into a cheese mold.

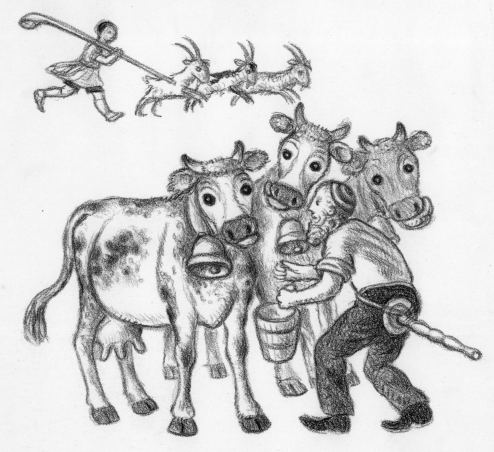

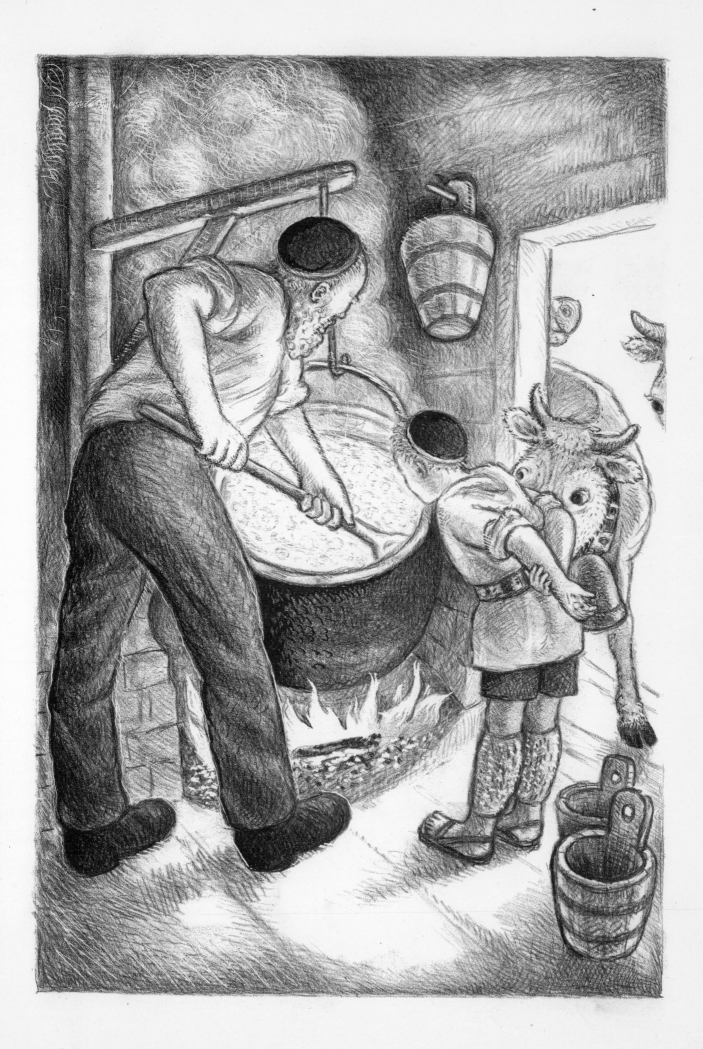

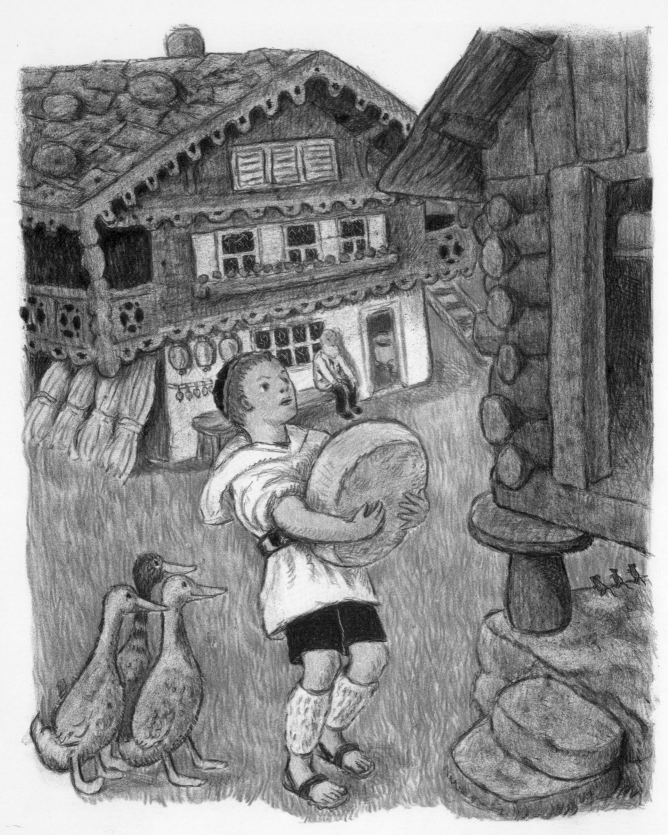

Peterli carried the newly made cheese to the cheese house and put it on a shelf to cure together with the other cheeses. There they sat, side by side, big cheeses and little cheeses, aging and fermenting. Tenderly Peterli rubbed them with salt and polished them with icy glacier water from the fountain.

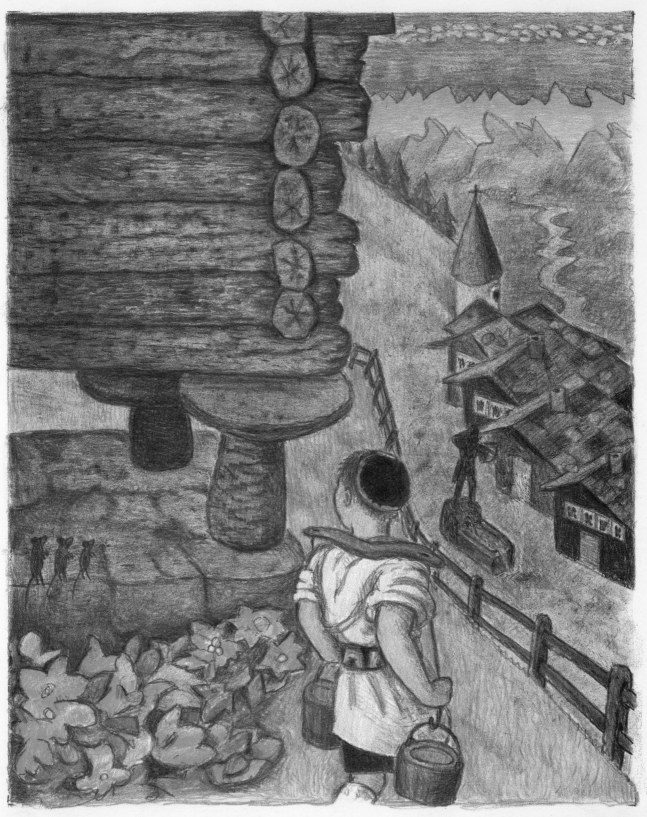

Outside the mice stood on their toes, sniffing the cheesy smell. Peterli laughed, for he knew they could not get in. The house stood on stilts! The sun was setting and the Alps were glowing, golden and red. Over the fountain the carved wooden figure of William Tell stood as if keeping watch.

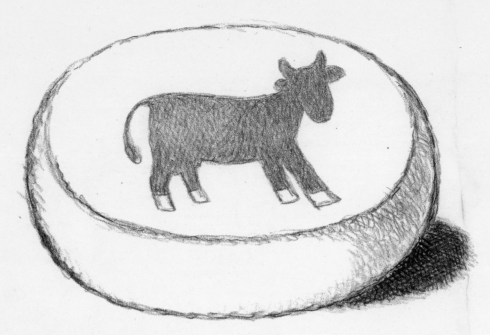

One day the shelf was full of fine ripe cheeses. They all had big holes and little holes in them as good Swiss cheese should have.

"You'll have to be my legs and take the cheeses to market in town," said Grandfather to Peterli.

Bravely Peterli set off down the path, with a big load of cheese on his back and a bunch of herbs in his hand.

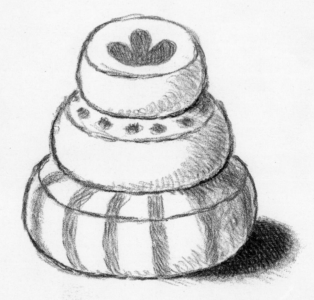

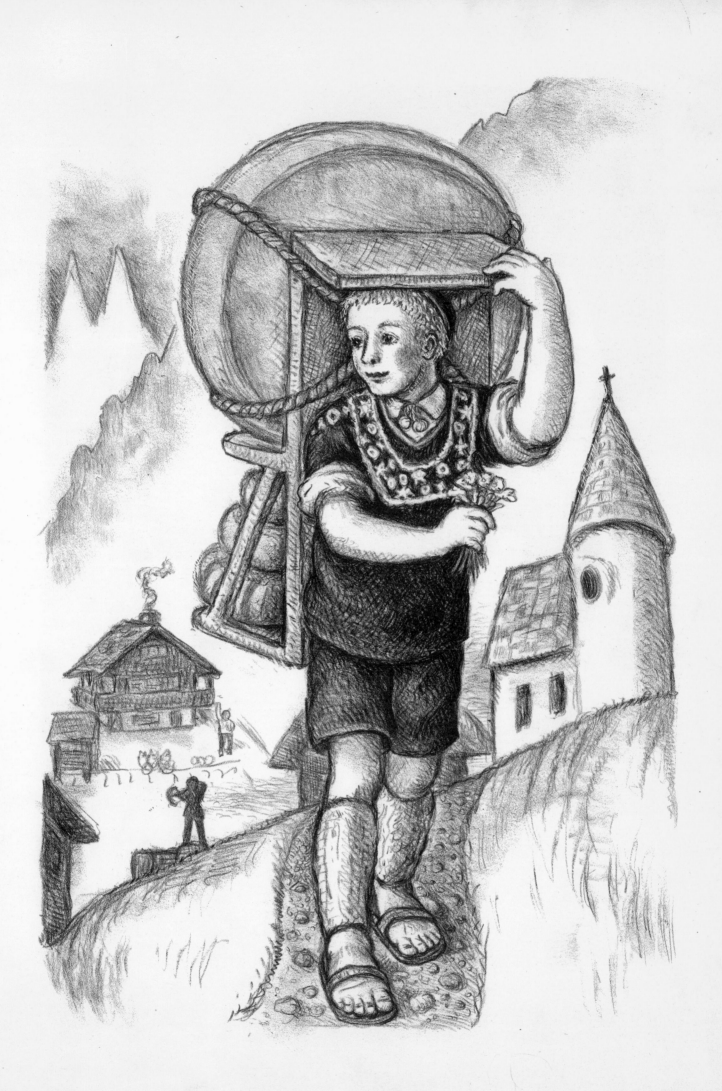

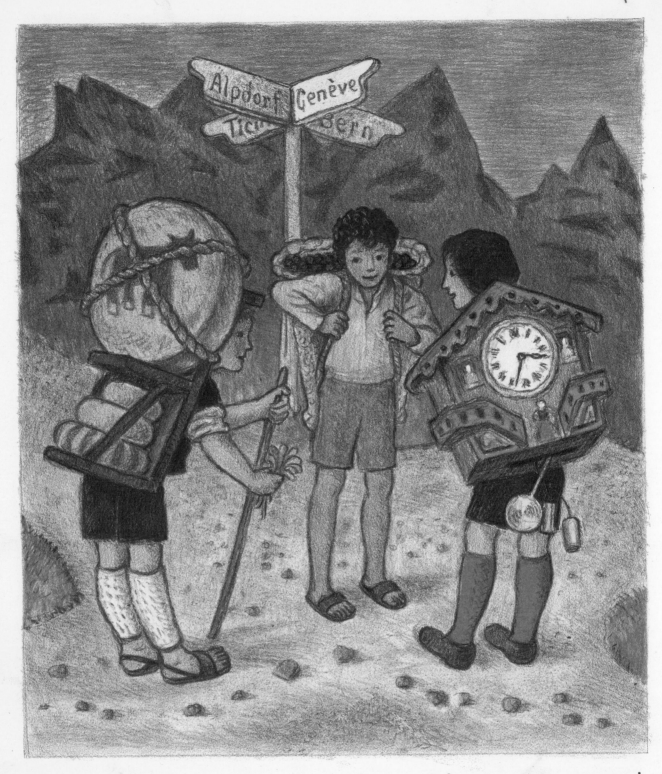

Down in the valley he came to a highway and soon to a crossroad. There he met two boys, one with a huge clock on his back, the other with a basket full of chestnuts.

"*Bonjour,*" said Pierre, the boy with the clock. He came from the west, where French is spoken.

"*Buon giorno,*" said Pietro, the boy with the chestnuts. He came from the south, where Italian is spoken.

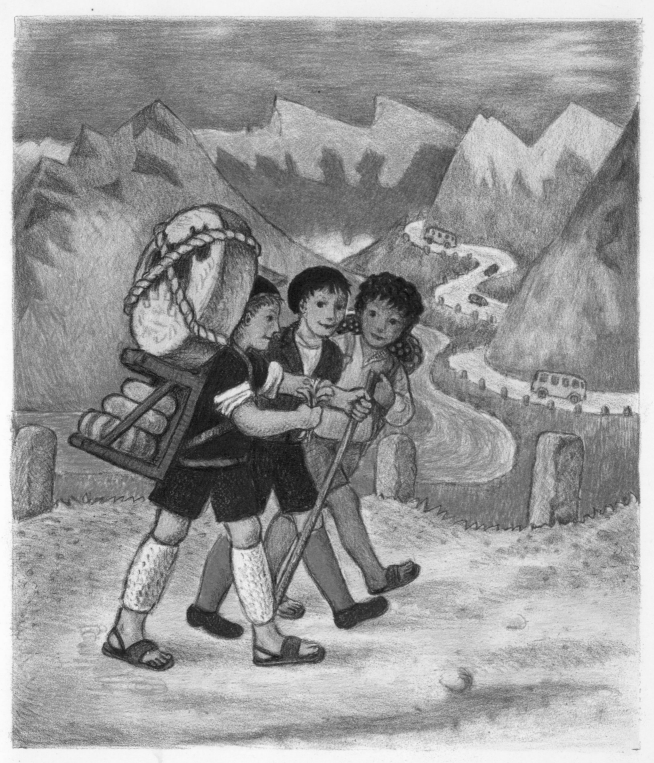

"*Gruessli,*" said Peterli in German Swiss, which was his language. Though their mother tongues were different, they were all three Swiss. They had the same fatherland and understood each other. Pierre and Pietro were going to the capital to sell their goods, and Peterli joined them.

They walked up and down, over mountains and valleys, until they came to the capital.

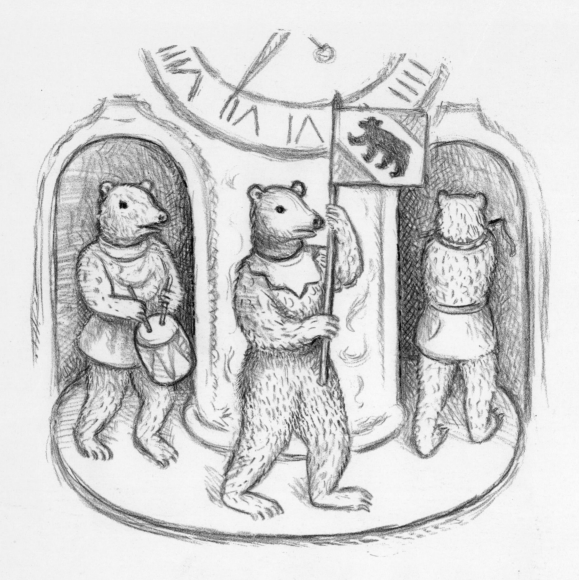

It was a beautiful city, circled by a river, with steep roofs and pointed towers.

Outside the city there was a pit with playful bears. There were bears on the flags, bears on the fountains, wooden bears dancing around the clock in the clock tower. The city was called Berne, which means bears. The streets were filled with people. Each spoke the language of his own canton. Some people even spoke a very old fourth language, which is called Romansch. A lovely smell came to Peterli's nose. Melted cheese!

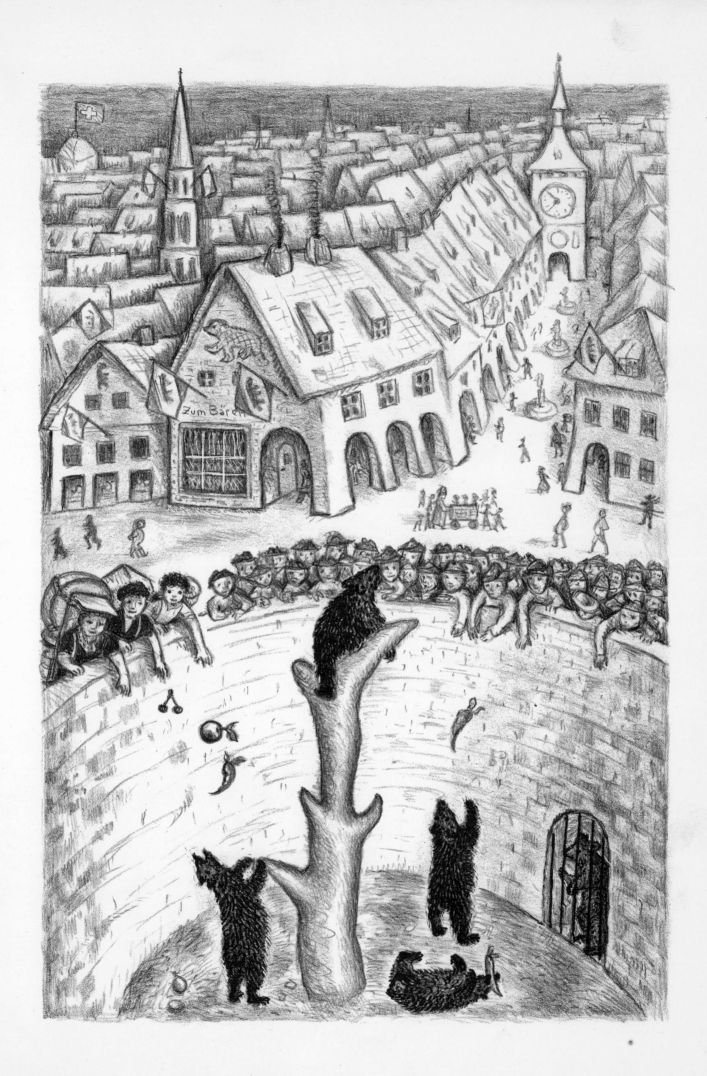

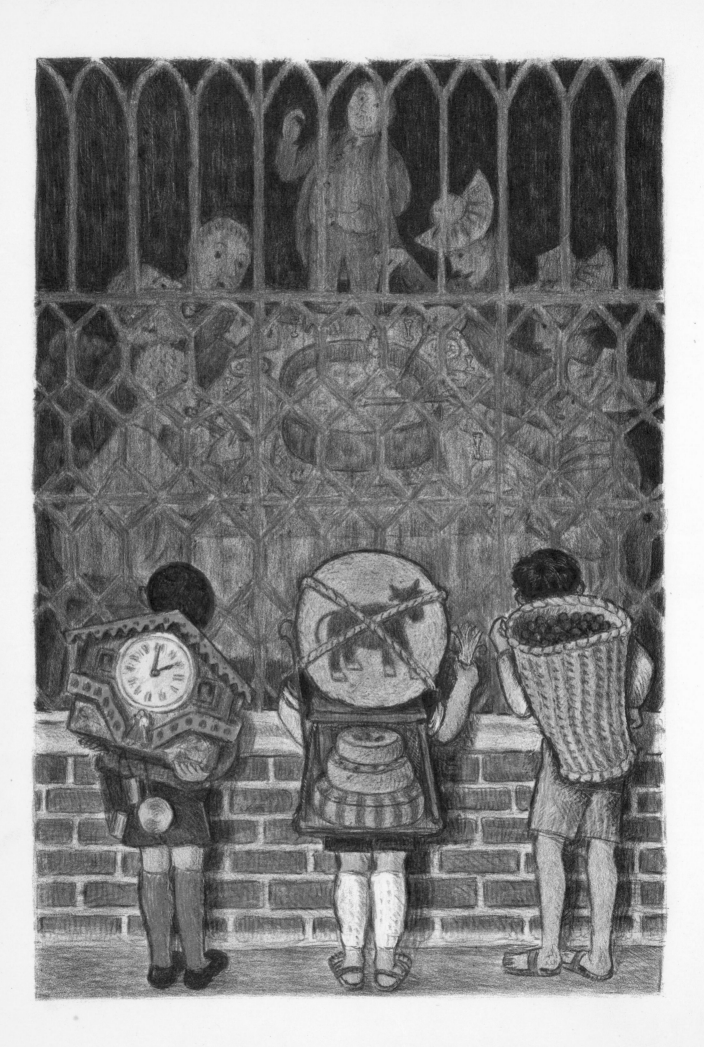

He followed his nose till he came to an inn where people were busy dipping small pieces of bread into melted cheese. It is a Swiss national dish called fondue. The landlord was standing by the window looking happy. His guests were getting fat and he was getting rich. When he saw the load of fine

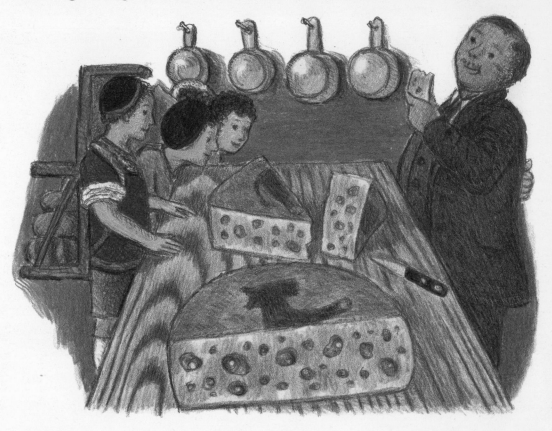

cheese on Peterli's back, he beckoned, and the three boys walked in the kitchen door. "I have never seen a finer cheese," he said when he had cut one to taste and saw the glistening dewdrops in every hole.

"Grandfather's cheese is fine," said Peterli proudly. "Our cattle graze in a magic meadow."

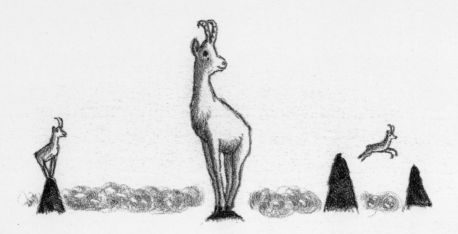

Then Peterli began to tell about the Princess of Spring who floated over her flowery meadow, about the glistening glacier and the mountains that rose like teeth and horns all around it.

As Peterli spoke, the landlord felt he was almost breathing the fresh mountain air. He looked very thoughtful.

"When the Lord created the world," he said, "he put treasures of precious metals into the mountains of every country. When he had finished and looked around, pleased with his work, he saw that there was one small land which he had quite forgotten.

" 'Done is done,' said the Lord, 'I can't start all over again and put treasures into the mountains, but I can make the mountains so steep and the valleys so lovely that they will make the poor people who live there happy.'

"That is why foreigners come to Switzerland from all over the world to be healthy and happy. They have become our treasure. I will build a hotel up in your magic meadow," said the landlord. "It sounds like a place where people would be very happy."

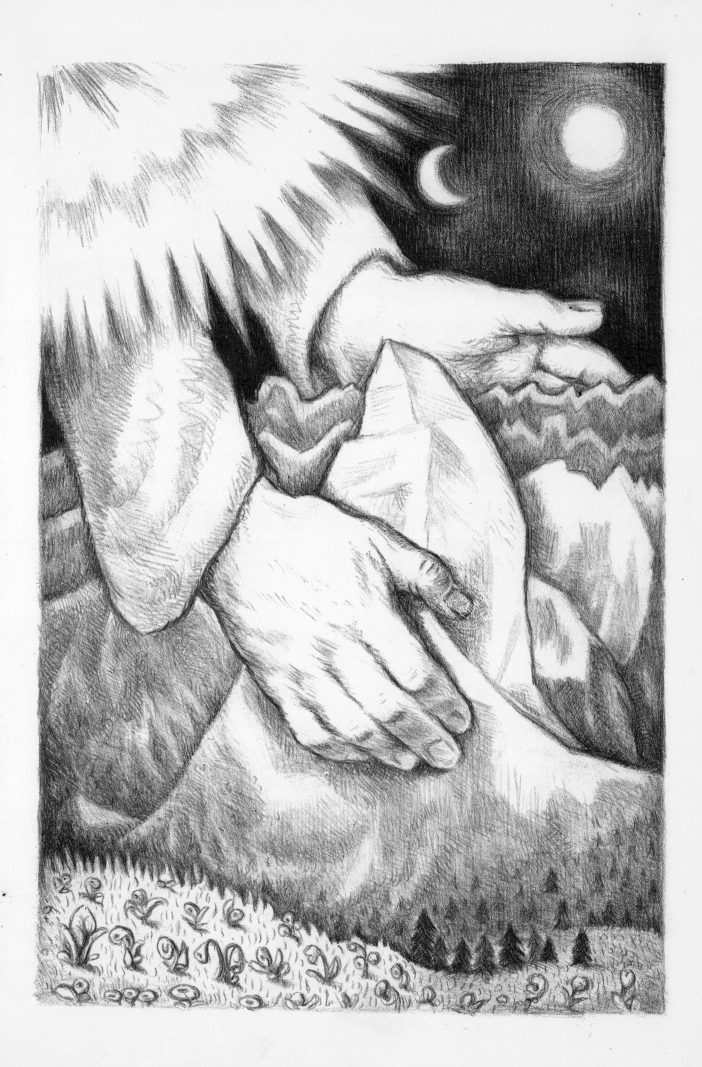

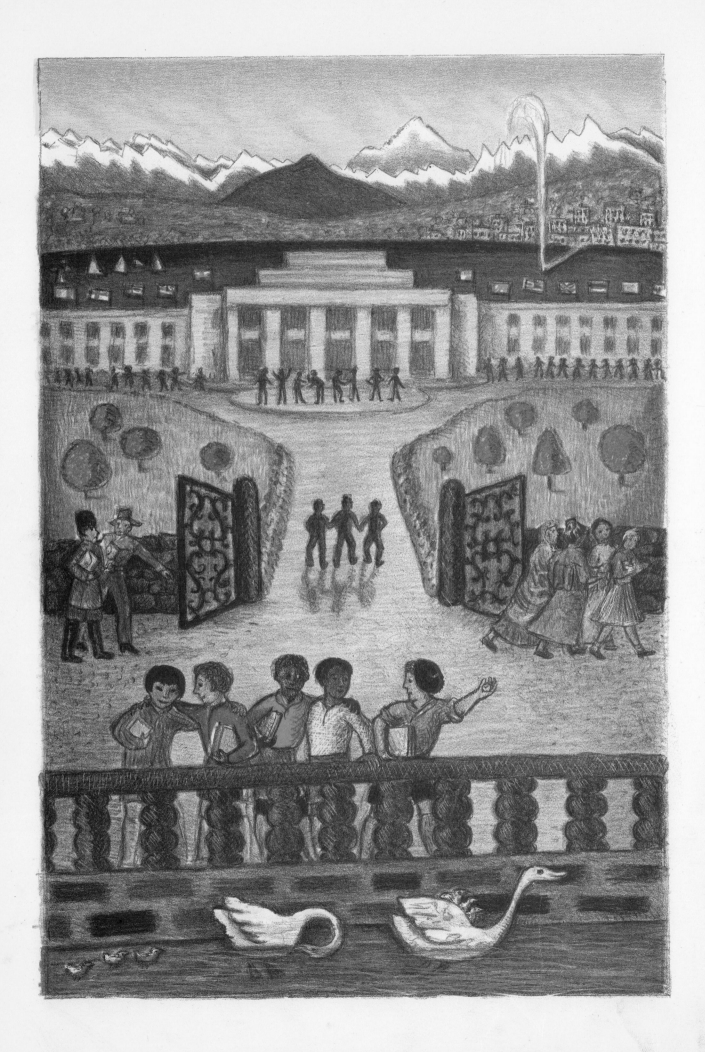

"Strangers in our mountains?" asked Peterli. "But it was to free us from strangers that William Tell killed the wicked Gessler."

"Gessler and his soldiers were strangers who wanted to rule over us," said Pierre. "My town, Geneva, is full of friendly strangers who have come to learn from us that different peoples can live in peace.

"They have even built a Peace Palace where men from many nations are trying to settle their quarrels with words instead of with wars. I go to school with children who are white, black and brown and yellow, and we are all friends."

"Even friendly strangers can never climb up to my meadow. Only the strongest Swiss legs can climb our mountainside," said Peterli.

"We'll build a cable car and lift them up," said the landlord.

"Then Grandfather will be able to go again to the meeting in the valley," said Peterli. "He likes his meeting as much as I love my meadow."

He thanked the landlord, who paid him handsomely for the cheeses and bought the herbs too.

He said "Gruessli" to his friends and wished them luck. Then he hurried homeward to tell Grandfather that he had not been to his last meeting in the valley. Soon he would be swooping up and down through the air like an eagle.

The landlord from Berne was as good as his word.
Cables were slung from the valley up to the
mountains. Peterli and Grandfather were
the first to ride in the cable car as it
soared between the earth and sky.
Down below in the village all the
windows and doors flew open
and their friends and neighbors waved up to them.
Later the cable car ran
up and down all day
long, with tourists
from all corners
of the earth.

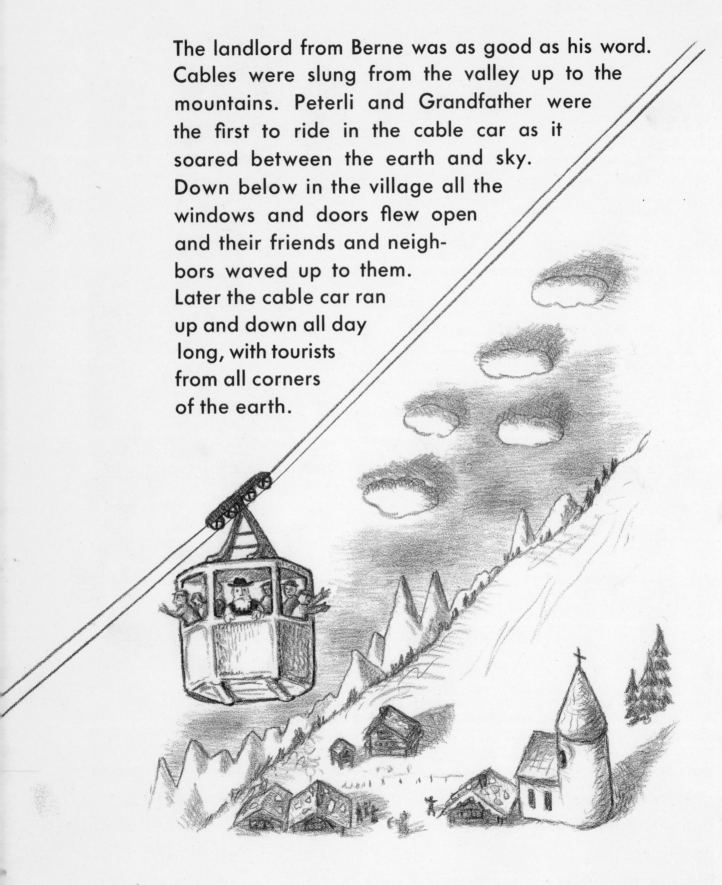

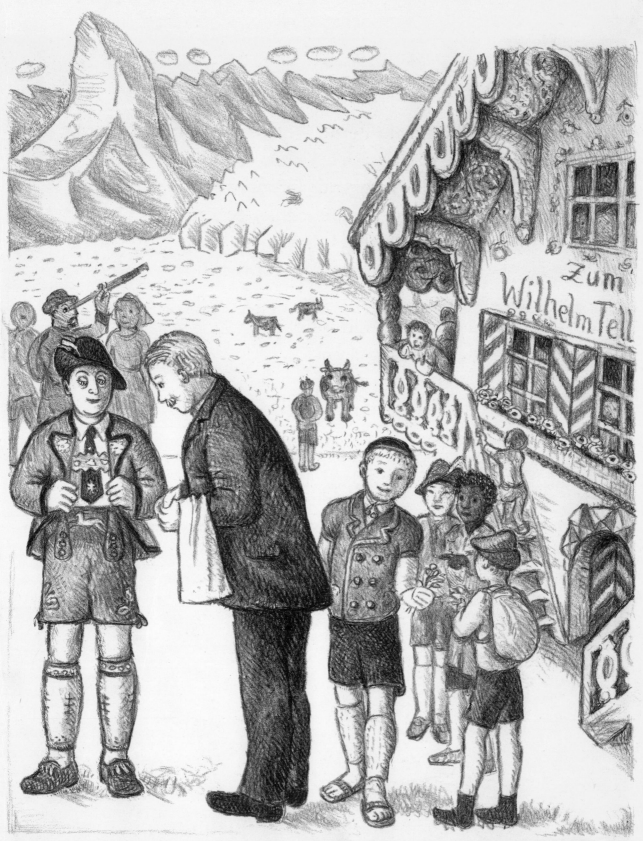

For up in the flowery meadow stood a fine big hotel, with curlicues and fancy woodwork. It looked like Grandfather's house, only it was much bigger. The landlord from Berne stood smiling in front of the hotel, waiting for his guests. At his side stood Peterli. The brass buttons on his new coat glittered and shone.

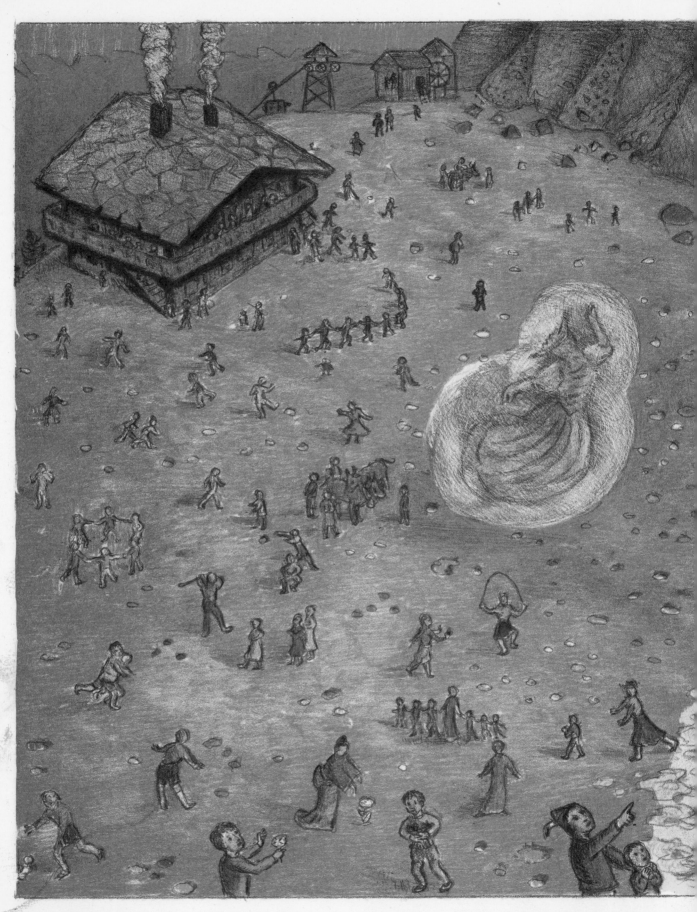

He had little time to herd his grandfather's cows and goats. He guided tourists instead. Their cheeks became rosy, their legs strong

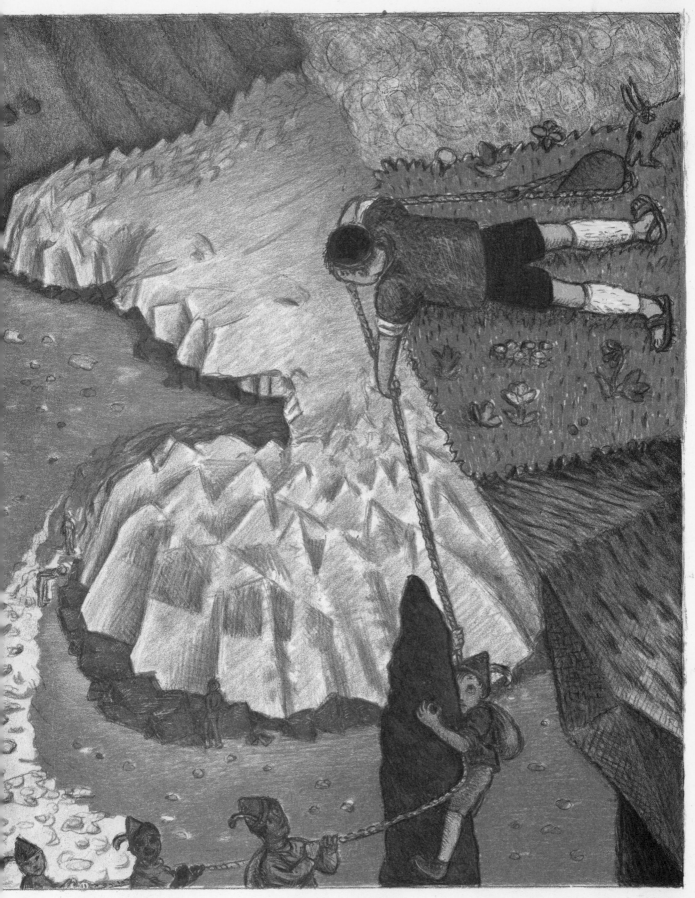

as his. They loved his magic meadow and Peterli too. And then
Peterli understood what the landlord had meant.

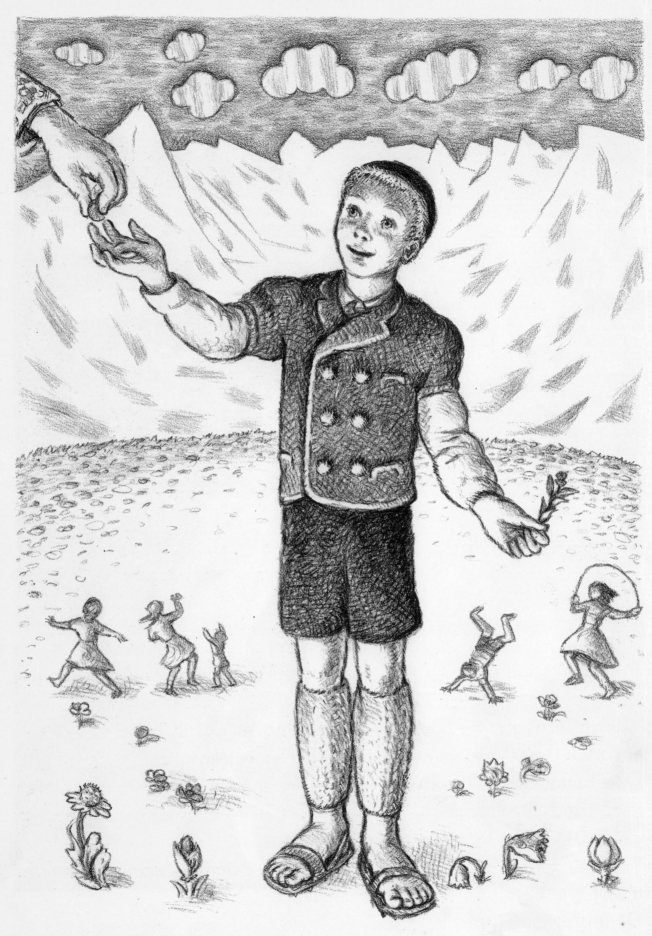

The treasure lay in the tourist's pocket!

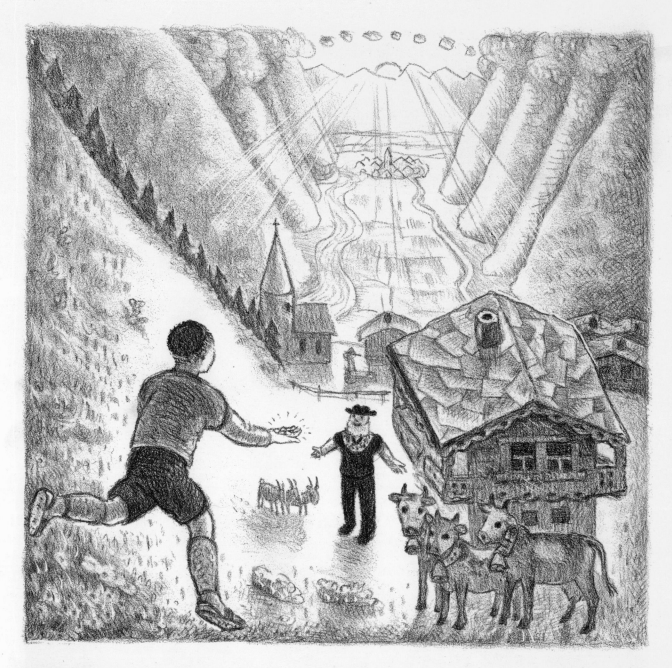

The setting sun gilded the coins in Peterli's hand as he came running
home in the evening.

"Grandfather," he called, "you will never again have to work so
hard. Our magic meadow has brought us a treasure."

"Our meadows and mountains won't change if strangers enjoy them
too," said Grandfather. "But don't forget, tourists come and tourists
go, but our old farm will always be here."

"I won't forget," said Peterli, "and when I am big enough, I will be
making cheese just the way you have taught me."

Grandfather patted Peterli's head, and the alpenglow painted his
old cheeks pink.

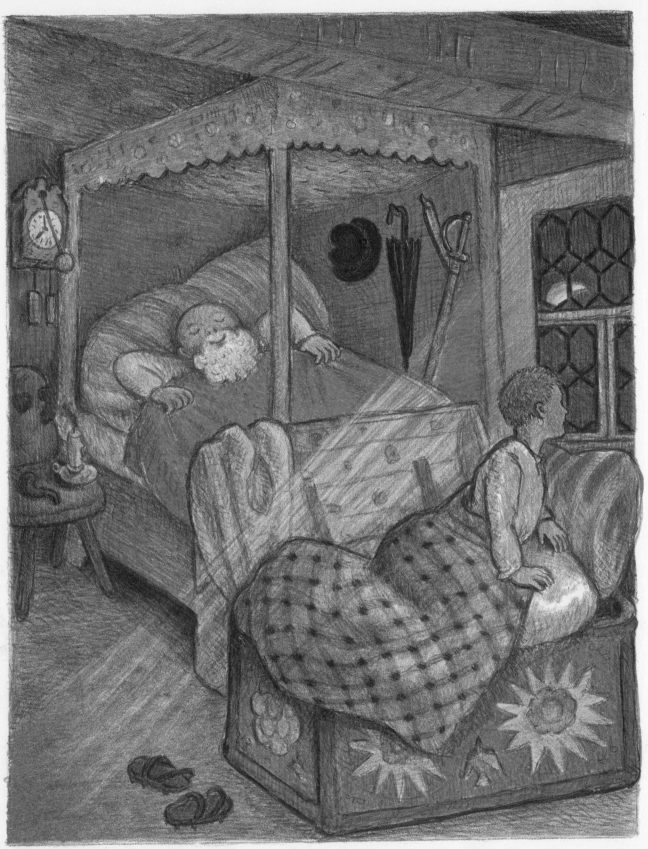

The sun set and Peterli and Grandfather went into the house and closed the door behind them. Grandfather went peacefully to sleep in his high bed. Peterli lay down on the sack of dry leaves at his feet as always before.

Outside in the moonlight, Peterli could see the fountain, where the sturdy figure of William Tell stood watching over his mountains. At his feet, the silvery water flowed as pure as ever. Over his head floated a light wisp of cloud. Or was it the Princess of Spring who was whispering into his ear: "Let the strangers play in the magic meadow. It is still yours and mine and Peterli's."

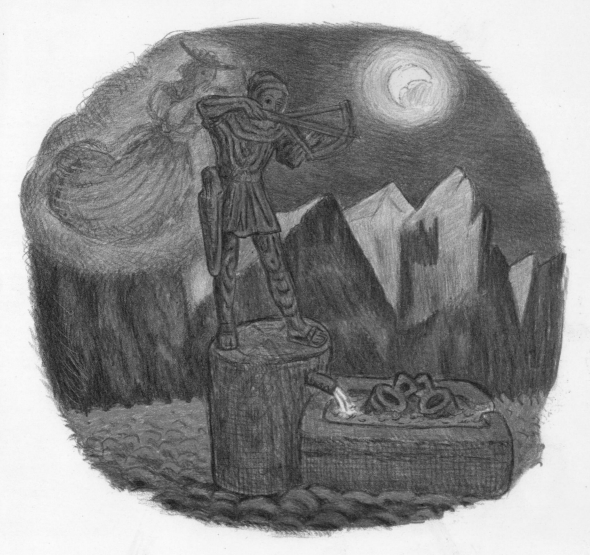

It looked as if William Tell winked in the moonlight.

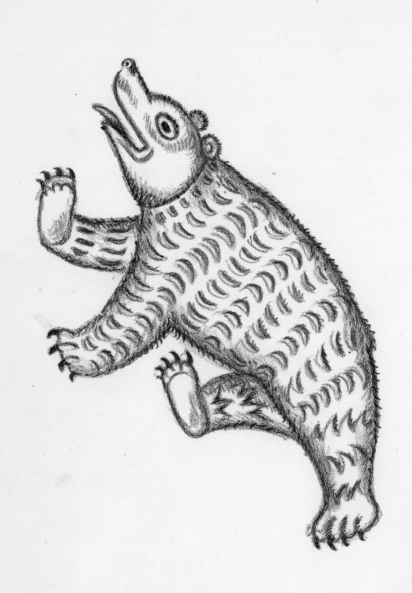